2019

ICD-10-PCS Code Book
Professional Edition

Anne B. Casto, RHIA, CCS
Consulting Editor

AHIMA
American Health Information
Management Association®

ISBN: 978-1-58426-670-9
AHIMA Product No.: AC222218

AHIMA Staff:
Chelsea Brotherton, MA, Assistant Editor
Megan Grennan, Managing Editor
Caitlin Wilson, Project Editor

Cover image: © knikola, Shutterstock

The Centers for Medicare and Medicaid Services (CMS) and the National Center for Health Statistics (NCHS), two departments within the US Federal Government's Department of Health and Human Services (HHS) provide the *International Classification of Diseases, Tenth Revision, Clinical Modification* (ICD-10-CM) for coding and reporting. ICD-10-CM is the US modification to the World Health Organization's (WHO) International Classification of Diseases, Tenth Revision (ICD-10).

Coding Clinic for ICD-10-CM and ICD-10-PCS is a publication of the American Hospital Association (AHA).

For more information about AHIMA Press publications, including updates, visit http://www.ahima.org/publications/updates.aspx.

American Health Information Management Association
233 North Michigan Avenue, 21st Floor
Chicago, Illinois 60601-5809
ahima.org

Contents

About the Consulting Editor iv
Acknowledgments iv

Introduction **v**
ICD-10-PCS Overview v
ICD-10-PCS Code Structure vii
ICD-10-PCS Organization and Official Conventions ix
AHA *Coding Clinic* for ICD-10-CM and ICD-10-PCS xi
ICD-10-PCS Official Guidelines for Coding and Reporting, 2019 xii

Index **1**

Medical and Surgical **88**
Central Nervous System and Cranial Nerves (001–00X) 98
Peripheral Nervous System (012–01X) 111
Heart and Great Vessels (021–02Y) 121
Upper Arteries (031–03W) 137
Lower Arteries (041–04W) 152
Upper Veins (051–05W) 168
Lower Veins (061–06W) 179
Lymphatic and Hemic System (072–07Y) 191
Eye (080–08X) 202
Ear, Nose, Sinus (090–09W) 215
Respiratory System (0B1–0BY) 230
Mouth and Throat (0C0–0CX) 245
Gastrointestinal System (0D1–0DY) 258
Hepatobiliary System and Pancreas (0F1–0FY) 281
Endocrine System (0G2–0GW) 291
Skin and Breast (0H0–0HX) 298
Subcutaneous Tissue and Fascia (0J0–0JX) 312
Muscles (0K2–0KX) 325
Tendons (0L2–0LX) 338
Bursae and Ligaments (0M2–0MX) 350
Head and Facial Bones (0N2–0NW) 363
Upper Bones (0P2–0PW) 374
Lower Bones (0Q2–0QW) 388
Upper Joints (0R2–0RW) 402
Lower Joints (0S2–0SW) 417
Urinary System (0T1–0TY) 437
Female Reproductive System (0U1–0UY) 451
Male Reproductive System (0V1–0VX) 465
Anatomical Regions, General (0W0–0WY) 477
Anatomical Regions, Upper Extremities (0X0–0XY) 488
Anatomical Regions, Lower Extremities (0Y0–0YW) 495

Obstetrics **502**

Placement **508**

Administration **517**

Measurement and Monitoring **535**

Extracorporeal or Systemic Assistance and Performance **541**

Extracorporeal or Systemic Therapies **544**

Osteopathic **547**

Other Procedures **549**

Chiropractic **552**

Imaging **554**

Nuclear Medicine **590**

Radiation Therapy **602**

Physical Rehabilitation and Diagnostic Audiology **618**

Mental Health **633**

Substance Abuse **637**

New Technology **640**

Appendix A: Root Operations Definitions **646**

Appendix B: Type and Qualifier Definitions **650**

Appendix C: Approach Definitions **658**

Appendix D: Medical and Surgical Body Parts **660**

Appendix E: Medical and Surgical Device Table (Device Key) and Device Aggregation Table **673**

Appendix F: Substance Qualifier Table (Key) **682**

Online Appendices:

Appendix G: New ICD-10-PCS Codes FY2019 **683**

Appendix H: Deleted ICD-10-PCS Codes FY2019 **684**

About the Consulting Editor

Anne B. Casto, RHIA, CCS, is the president of Casto Consulting, LLC. Casto Consulting, LLC is a consulting firm that provides services to hospitals and other healthcare stakeholders primarily in the areas of reimbursement and coding. Casto Consulting, LLC specializes in linking coding and billing practices to positive revenue cycle outcomes. Additionally, the firm provides guidance to consulting firms, healthcare organizations and healthcare insurers regarding reimbursement methodologies and Medicare regulations. Additionally, Ms. Casto serves as a lecturer in the HIMS Division at The Ohio State University. Her course topics include healthcare reimbursement, revenue cycle analysis, code set mapping, and RHIA preparation.

Prior to founding the firm, Ms. Casto was the program manager of the HIMS Division at The Ohio State University School of Allied Medical Professions. Ms. Casto taught healthcare reimbursement, ICD-9-CM coding, and CPT coding courses for several years. Additionally, Ms. Casto was responsible for curriculum revisions in the areas of chargemaster management, clinical data management, and healthcare reimbursement.

Additionally, Ms. Casto was the vice president of clinical information for Cleverley & Associates where she worked very closely with APC regulations and guidelines, preparing hospitals for the implementation of the Medicare OPPS. Ms. Casto was also the clinical information product manager for CHIPS/Ingenix. She joined CHIPS/Ingenix in 1998 and spent the majority of her time developing coding compliance products for the inpatient and outpatient settings.

Ms. Casto has been responsible for inpatient and outpatient coding activities in several large hospitals including Mt. Sinai Medical Center (NYC), Beth Israel Medical Center (NYC), and The Ohio State University. She worked extensively with CMI, quality measures, physician documentation, and coding accuracy efforts at these facilities.

Ms. Casto received her degree in Health Information Management at The Ohio State University in 1995. She received her Certified Coding Specialist credential in 1998 from the American Health Information Management Association. In 2009 Ms. Casto received her ICD-10-CM/PCS Trainer certificate from AHIMA. Ms. Casto is the author of an AHIMA-published textbook entitled *Principles of Healthcare Reimbursement*. Additionally, Ms. Casto was a contributing author to the published AHIMA books: *Severity DRGs and Reimbursement; A MS-DRG Primer* and *Effective Management of Coding Services.*

Ms. Casto received the AHIMA Legacy Award, part of the FORE Triumph Awards, in 2007 which honors a significant contribution to the knowledge base of the HIM field through an insightful publication. Additionally, Ms. Casto was honored with the Ohio Health Information Management Association's Distinguished Member Award in 2008 and the Ohio Health Information Management Association's Professional Achievement Award in 2011.

Acknowledgments

Many thanks to my family for their support during this project. Thanks to Dr. Susan White, The Ohio State University; your data manipulation skills are second to none. I thank the reviewers for their thoughtful comments and suggestions. Many thanks to Linda Hyde, RHIA, and Tina Cressman MALS, CCS, CCS-P, CPC, COC, CPC-P, CEMC, CPMA, CPEDC, CPC-I, MCS-P, MCS-I, CHEP, for their very thorough technical review of the book.

Introduction

ICD-10-PCS Overview

The *International Classification of Diseases, Tenth Revision, Procedure Coding System* (ICD-10-PCS) was created to accompany the World Health Organization's (WHO) ICD-10 diagnosis classification. This coding system was developed to replace ICD-9-CM procedure codes for reporting inpatient procedures. ICD-10-PCS was designed to enable each code to have a standard structure and be very descriptive, and yet flexible enough to accommodate future needs.

History of ICD-10-PCS

The WHO has maintained the International Classification of Diseases (ICD) for recording cause of death since 1893. It has updated the ICD periodically to reflect new discoveries in epidemiology and changes in medical understanding of disease. The International Classification of Diseases Tenth Revision (ICD-10), published in 1992, is the latest revision of the ICD. The WHO authorized the National Center for Health Statistics (NCHS) to develop a clinical modification of ICD-10 for use in the United States. This version of ICD-10 is called ICD-10-CM, and is intended to replace the previous US clinical modification, ICD-9-CM, that had been in use since 1979. ICD-9-CM contains a procedure classification; ICD-10-CM does not.

The Centers for Medicare and Medicaid Services (CMS), the agency responsible for maintaining the inpatient procedure code set in the United States, contracted with 3M Health Information Systems in 1993 to design and then develop a procedure classification system to replace Volume 3 of ICD-9-CM. ICD-10-PCS is the result. ICD-10-PCS was initially released in 1998. It has been updated annually since that time.

ICD-10-PCS Design

ICD-10-PCS is fundamentally different from previous procedure classification systems in its structure, organization, and capabilities. It was designed and developed to adhere to recommendations made by the National Committee on Vital and Health Statistics (NCVHS). It also incorporates input from a wide range of organizations, individual physicians, healthcare professionals, and researchers. Several structural attributes were recommended for a new procedure coding system. These attributes include a multiaxial structure, completeness, and expandability.

Multiaxial Structure

The key attribute that provides the framework for all other structural attributes is multiaxial code structure. *Multiaxial code structure* makes it possible for the ICD-10-PCS to be complete, expandable, and provide a high degree of flexibility and functionality.

ICD-10-PCS codes are composed of seven characters. Each character represents a category of information that can be specified about the procedure performed. A character defines both the category of information and its physical position in the code. A character's position can be understood as a semi-independent axis of classification that allows different specific values to be inserted into that space, and whose physical position remains stable. Within a defined code range, a character retains the general meaning that it confers on any value in that position.

Completeness

Completeness is considered a key structural attribute for a new procedure coding system. The specific recommendation for completeness included that a unique code be available for each significant procedure, that each code retain its unique definition, and that codes that have been deleted are not reused.

In ICD-10-PCS, a unique code is constructed for every significantly different procedure. Within each section, a character defines a consistent component of a code, and contains all applicable values for that character. The values define individual expressions (Open, Percutaneous) of the character's general meaning (approach) that are then used to construct unique procedure codes. Because all approaches by which a procedure is performed are assigned a separate approach value, every procedure which uses a different approach will have its own unique code. This is true of the other characters as well. The same procedure performed on a different body part has its own unique code; the same procedure performed using a different device has its own unique code, and so on.

Because ICD-10-PCS codes are constructed of individual values rather than lists of fixed codes and text descriptions, the unique, stable definition of a code in the system is retained. New values may be added to the system to represent a specific new approach or device or qualifier, but whole codes by design cannot be given new meanings and reused.

Expandability

Expandability was also recommended as a key structural attribute. The specific recommendation for expandability included that the system be capable of accommodating new procedures and technology and that these new codes could be added to the system without disrupting the existing structure.

ICD-10-PCS is designed to be easily updated as new codes are required for new procedures and new techniques. Changes to ICD-10-PCS can all be made within the existing structure because whole codes are not added. Instead, a new value for a character can be added to the system as needed. Likewise, an existing value for a character can be added to a table(s) in the system.

ICD-10-PCS Additional Characteristics

ICD-10-PCS possesses several additional characteristics in response to government and industry recommendations. These characteristics are

- Standardized terminology within the coding system
- Standardized level of specificity
- No diagnostic information
- No explicit "not otherwise specified" (NOS) code options
- Limited use of "not elsewhere classified" (NEC) code options

Standardized Terminology

Words commonly used in clinical vocabularies may have multiple meanings. This can cause confusion and result in inaccurate data. ICD-10-PCS is standardized and self-contained. Characters and values used in the system are defined in the system. For example, the word *excision* is used to describe a wide variety of surgical procedures. In ICD-10-PCS, the word *excision* describes a single, precise surgical objective, defined as "cutting out or off, without replacement, a portion of a body part."

No Eponyms or Common Procedure Names

The terminology used in ICD-10-PCS is standardized to provide precise and stable definitions of all procedures performed. This standardized terminology is used in all ICD-10-PCS code descriptions. As a result, ICD-10-PCS code descriptions do not include eponyms or common procedure names.

In ICD-10-PCS, physicians' names are not included in a code description, nor are procedures identified by common terms or acronyms such as appendectomy or CABG. Instead, such procedures are coded to the root operation that accurately identifies the objective of the procedure.

ICD-10-PCS assigns procedure codes according to the root operation that matches the objective of the procedure. By relying on the universal objectives defined in root operations rather than eponyms or specific procedure titles that change or become obsolete, ICD-10-PCS preserves the capacity to define past, present, and future procedures accurately using stable terminology in the form of characters and values.

No Combination Codes

With rare exceptions, ICD-10-PCS does not define multiple procedures with one code. This is to preserve standardized terminology and consistency across the system. A procedure that meets the reporting criteria for a separate procedure is coded separately in ICD-10-PCS. This allows the system to respond to changes in technology and medical practice with the maximum degree of stability and flexibility.

Standardized Level of Specificity

ICD-10-PCS provides a standardized level of specificity for each code, so each code represents a single procedure variation. In general, ICD-10-PCS code descriptions are much more specific than previous procedure classification systems but sometimes an ICD-10-PCS code description is actually less specific. ICD-10-PCS provides a standardized level of specificity that can be predicted across the system.

Diagnosis Information Excluded

Another key feature of ICD-10-PCS is that information pertaining to a diagnosis is excluded from the code descriptions. Adding diagnosis information limits the flexibility and functionality of a procedure coding system. It has the effect of placing a code "off limits" because the diagnosis in the medical record does not match the diagnosis in the procedure code description. The code cannot be used even though the procedural part of the code description precisely matches the procedure performed. Diagnosis information is not contained in any ICD-10-PCS code. The diagnosis codes, not the procedure codes, will specify the reason the procedure is performed.

Not Otherwise Specified (NOS) Code Options Restricted

The standardized level of specificity designed into ICD-10-PCS restricts the use of broadly applicable NOS or unspecified code options in the system. A minimal level of specificity is required to construct a valid code.

Limited Not Elsewhere Classified (NEC) Code Options

NEC options are provided in ICD-10-PCS, but only for specific, limited use. In the Medical and Surgical section, two significant NEC options are the root operation value Q, Repair, and the device value Y, Other Device. The root operation Repair is a true NEC value. It is used only when the procedure performed is not one of the other root operations in the Medical and Surgical section. Other Device, on the other hand, is intended to be used to temporarily define new devices that do not have a specific value assigned, until one can be added to the system. No categories of medical or surgical devices are permanently classified to Other Device.

ICD-10-PCS Code Structure

Undergirding ICD-10-PCS is a logical, consistent structure that informs the system as a whole, down to the level of a single code. This means the process of constructing codes in ICD-10-PCS is also logical and consistent: the spaces of the code, called *characters* are filled with individual letters and numbers, called *values*.

Characters

All codes in ICD-10-PCS are seven characters long. Each character in the seven-character code represents an aspect of the procedure. The following are two examples of the code structure: one from the Medical and Surgical section and one from the Ancillary section.

Medical and Surgical Code Structure

Character 1	Character 2	Character 3	Character 4	Character 5	Character 6	Character 7
Section	Body System	Operation	Body Part	Approach	Device	Qualifier

Imaging Section Code Structure

Character 1	Character 2	Character 3	Character 4	Character 5	Character 6	Character 7
Section	Body System	Type	Body Part	Contrast	Qualifier	Qualifier

An ICD-10-PCS code is best understood as the result of a process rather than as an isolated, fixed quantity. The process consists of assigning values from among the valid choices for that part of the system, according to the rules governing the construction of codes.

Values

One of 34 possible values can be assigned to each character in a code: the numbers 0 through 9 and the alphabet (except the letters I and O, because they are easily confused with the numbers 1 and 0). A finished code looks like this: 02103D4.

This code is derived by choosing a specific value for each of the seven characters. Based on details about the procedure performed, values for each character specifying the section, body system, root operation, body part, approach, device, and qualifier are assigned. Because the definition of each character is a function of its physical position in the code, the same value placed in a different position in the code means something different. The value 0 in the first character means something different than 0 in the second character, or 0 in the third character, and so on.

Code Structure Example

The following example defines each character using the code 0LB50ZZ, Excision of right lower arm and wrist tendon, Open approach. This example comes from the Medical and Surgical section of ICD-10-PCS.

Character 1: Section

The first character in the code determines the broad procedure category, or section, where the code is found. In this example, the section is Medical and Surgical. 0 is the value that represents Medical and Surgical in the first character.

Character 1	Character 2	Character 3	Character 4	Character 5	Character 6	Character 7
Section	Body System	Root Operation	Body Part	Approach	Device	Qualifier
0						

Character 2: Body System

The second character defines the body system—the general physiological system or anatomical region involved. Examples of body systems include Lower Arteries, Central Nervous System, and Respiratory System. In this example, the body system is Tendons, represented by the value L.

Character 1	Character 2	Character 3	Character 4	Character 5	Character 6	Character 7
Section	Body System	Root Operation	Body Part	Approach	Device	Qualifier
0	L					

Character 3: Root Operation

The third character defines the root operation, or the objective of the procedure. Some examples of root operations are Bypass, Drainage, and Reattachment. In this example code, the root operation is Excision. When used in the third character of the code, the value B represents Excision.

Character 1	Character 2	Character 3	Character 4	Character 5	Character 6	Character 7
Section	Body System	Root Operation	Body Part	Approach	Device	Qualifier
0	L	B				

Character 4: Body Part

The fourth character defines the body part or specific anatomical site where the procedure was performed. The body system (second character) provides only a general indication of the procedure site. The body part and body system values together provide a precise description of the procedure site. Examples of body parts are Kidney, Tonsils, and Thymus. In this example, the body part value is 5, Lower Arm and Wrist, Right. When the second character is L, the value 5 when used in the fourth character of the code represents the right lower arm and wrist tendon.

Character 1	Character 2	Character 3	Character 4	Character 5	Character 6	Character 7
Section	Body System	Root Operation	Body Part	Approach	Device	Qualifier
0	L	B	5			

Character 5: Approach

The fifth character defines the approach, or the technique used to reach the procedure site. Seven different approach values are used in the Medical and Surgical section to define the approach. Examples of approaches include Open and Percutaneous Endoscopic. In this example code, the approach is Open and is represented by the value 0.

Character 1	Character 2	Character 3	Character 4	Character 5	Character 6	Character 7
Section	Body System	Root Operation	Body Part	Approach	Device	Qualifier
0	L	B	5	0		

Character 6: Device

Depending on the procedure performed, there may be a device left in place at the end of the procedure. The sixth character defines the device. Device values fall into four basic categories:

- Grafts and Prostheses
- Implants
- Simple or Mechanical Appliances
- Electronic Appliances

In this example, there is no device used in the procedure. The value Z is used to represent No Device, as shown here:

Character 1	Character 2	Character 3	Character 4	Character 5	Character 6	Character 7
Section	Body System	Operation	Body Part	Approach	Device	Qualifier
0	L	B	5	0	Z	

Character 7: Qualifier

The seventh character defines a qualifier for the code. A qualifier specifies an additional attribute of the procedure, if applicable. Examples of qualifiers include Diagnostic and Stereotactic. Qualifier choices vary depending on the previous values selected. In this example, there is no specific qualifier applicable to this procedure, so the value is No Qualifier, represented by the letter Z.

Character 1	Character 2	Character 3	Character 4	Character 5	Character 6	Character 7
Section	Body System	Operation	Body Part	Approach	Device	Qualifier
0	L	B	5	0	Z	Z

0LB50ZZ is the complete specification of the procedure "Excision of right lower arm and wrist tendon, Open approach."

ICD-10-PCS Organization and Official Conventions

The *ICD-10-PCS Code Book, Professional Edition,* 2019 is based on the official *International Classification of Diseases, Tenth Revision, Procedure Coding System,* issued by the US Department of Health and Human Services (HHS) and CMS. This book is consistent with the content of the government's version of ICD-10-PCS and follows the official conventions.

Index

The Alphabetic Index is provided to assist the user with locating the appropriate table to construct procedure codes. Each table contains all the information required to construct valid procedure codes. Coders should not code from the PCS Index alone; the PCS code tables should always be consulted before assigning a PCS procedure code.

Main Terms

Main terms in the Alphabetic Index reflect the root operations, third character, of procedures. The Index includes not only root operation terms, but also other common procedural terms, anatomical sites, and device terms. The main terms are listed alphabetically. After the coder has located the correct main term and subterm in the Alphabetic Index, he or she is provided with the first three to four digits of the procedure code. The coder should then move to the Tables section of the code book and locate the appropriate table to complete the code construction. Even if the entire seven-digit code is provided in the Index, the coder should still reference the Tables to ensure the correct PCS code has been constructed.

See Reference

Common procedure terms are often listed with the *see* reference. The coder is instructed to follow the reference provided in order to locate the appropriate table to construct the code. For example, the *see* reference is present for the main term Colectomy. The Index excerpt is as follows:

Colectomy

see Excision, Gastrointestinal System 0DB

see Resection, Gastrointestinal System 0DT

In this example, the coder should review the definition of the root operations Excision and Resection to determine which is consistent with the medical record documentation. The coder should then proceed to the corresponding table as suggested by the *see* reference.

Use Reference

Anatomical site terms and device terms are often listed with the *use* reference. The coder is instructed to follow the reference provided in order to locate the appropriate main term for the procedure in question. For example, the *use* reference is present for the main term Inferior rectus muscle. The Index excerpt is as follows:

Inferior rectus muscle

use Muscle, Extraocular, Left

use Muscle, Extraocular, Right

In this example, the coder should identify the root operation for the procedure, and then look for the subterm that identifies the body part indicated in the *use* reference. For example, the procedure is excision of the inferior rectus muscle. The coder would locate the main term Excision. The Index excerpt is as follows:

Excision

Muscle

Extraocular

Left 08BM

Right 08BL

In this example, the coder knows that the Code Table 08B is the correct table because the previous review of the *use* reference identified that the inferior rectus muscle is an extraocular muscle. The coder can now proceed to the 08B Table to finish constructing the PCS code.

In addition to the *use* reference, the coder may also consult appendix D for Body Part Table or appendix E for the Device Table.

Code Tables

ICD-10-PCS contains 17 sections of Code Tables, represented by the numbers 0 through 9 and the letters B through D, F through H, and X. The Tables are organized by general type of procedure. The three main sections of tables include:

1. **Medical and Surgical section**
    - Medical and Surgical (first character 0)
2. **Medical and Surgical Related sections**
    - Obstetrics (first character 1)
    - Placement (first character 2)
    - Administration (first character 3)
    - Measurement and Monitoring (first character 4)
    - Extracorporeal Assistance and Performance (first character 5)
    - Extracorporeal Therapies (first character 6)
    - Osteopathic (first character 7)
    - Other Procedures (first character 8)
    - Chiropractic (first character 9)
3. **Ancillary sections**
    - Imaging (first character B)
    - Nuclear Medicine (first character C)
    - Radiation Therapy (first character D)
    - Physical Rehabilitation and Diagnostic Audiology (first character F)
    - Mental Health (first character G)
    - Substance Abuse (first character H)
    - New Technology (first character X)

Each code table is defined by the first three characters of the PCS code. Each of these characters is displayed above the table. The table consists of all the options for characters 4 through 7. The root operation or root type, character 3, is present along with its official definition. Table 097 is provided here as an example of the table structure.

0 Medical and Surgical

9 Ear, Nose, Sinus

7 Dilation, Expanding an orifice or the lumen of a tubular body part

Body Part Character 4	Approach Character 5	Device Character 6	Qualifier Character 7
F Eustachian Tube, Right **G** Eustachian Tube, Left	**0** Open **7** Via Natural or Artificial Opening **8** Via Natural or Artificial Opening Endoscopic	**D** Intraluminal Device **Z** No Device	**Z** No Qualifier
F Eustachian Tube, Right **G** Eustachian Tube, Left	**3** Percutaneous **4** Percutaneous Endoscopic	**Z** No Device	**Z** No Qualifier

There can be multiple rows within the table for the first three characters, so the coder must carefully review all the applicable rows. Additionally, a table may cover multiple pages. Therefore, the coder must continue to review the code table options until the end of the table is reached to ensure the correct PCS code has been constructed.

AHA *Coding Clinic* for ICD-10-CM and ICD-10-PCS

The American Hospital Association began publishing coding guidance for ICD-10-CM and ICD-10-PCS in the fourth quarter of 2012. In this code book we identify procedure codes that are discussed in the *Coding Clinic* guidance fourth quarter 2012 through second quarter 2018. In the Medical and Surgical section, after each body system table section, there is an AHA *Coding Clinic* section that lists the references. For all other sections of the code book, the AHA *Coding Clinic* section follows the Tables section. In the AHA *Coding Clinic* section, the PCS codes included in AHA *Coding Clinic* guidance are listed with a sky blue note that alerts the coder to review the AHA *Coding Clinic* prior to assignment of the code to ensure appropriate and accurate reporting. The quarter of publication, year and page number(s) are provided in the note.

AHA CC: 4Q; 2012; pg#-pg#

AHA Coding Clinic Crosswalk for Deleted Codes

Deleted Code	Coding Clinic Reference	Replacement Code
0B5S0ZZ	2Q, 2016, 17-18	See 0B5T0ZZ
0BQR0ZZ	2Q, 2016, 22-23	See 0BQT0ZZ
0BQR4ZZ	3Q, 2014, 28	See 0BQT4ZZ
0BQS0ZZ	2Q, 2016, 22-23	See 0BQT0ZZ
0BQS4ZZ	3Q, 2014, 28	See 0BQT4ZZ
0NQS0ZZ	3Q, 2016, 29-30	See 0NQR0ZZ
0NSS04Z	3Q, 2014, 23-24	See 0NSR04Z
0NSS0ZZ	1Q, 2017, 20-21	See 0NSR0ZZ
0NR80JZ	3Q, 2017, 17	See 0NR70JZ

ICD-10-PCS Coding Guidelines

The ICD-10-PCS Coding Guidelines are presented here in the introduction and throughout this manual. Within the manual, the Medical and Surgical Section Guidelines are presented after the Introduction of the Medical and Surgical section. The Obstetric Section Guidelines are presented after the Introduction of the Obstetrics section. Lastly, the New Technology Guidelines are presented after the Introduction of the New Technology section.

ICD-10-PCS Official Guidelines for Coding and Reporting, 2019

The Centers for Medicare and Medicaid Services (CMS) and the National Center for Health Statistics (NCHS), two departments within the US federal government's Department of Health and Human Services (HHS) provide the following guidelines for coding and reporting using the International Classification of Diseases, 10th Revision, Procedure Coding System (ICD-10-PCS). These guidelines should be used as a companion document to the official version of the ICD-10-PCS as published on the CMS website. The ICD-10-PCS is a procedure classification published by the United States for classifying procedures performed in hospital inpatient health care settings.

These guidelines have been approved by the four organizations that make up the Cooperating Parties for the ICD-10-PCS: the American Hospital Association (AHA), the American Health Information Management Association (AHIMA), CMS, and NCHS.

These guidelines are a set of rules that have been developed to accompany and complement the official conventions and instructions provided within the ICD-10-PCS itself. The instructions and conventions of the classification take precedence over guidelines. These guidelines are based on the coding and sequencing instructions in the Tables, Index, and Definitions of ICD-10-PCS, but provide additional instruction. Adherence to these guidelines when assigning ICD-10-PCS procedure codes is required under the Health Insurance Portability and Accountability Act (HIPAA). The procedure codes have been adopted under HIPAA for hospital inpatient healthcare settings. A joint effort between the healthcare provider and the coder is essential to achieve complete and accurate documentation, code assignment, and reporting of diagnoses and procedures. These guidelines have been developed to assist both the healthcare provider and the coder in identifying those procedures that are to be reported. The importance of consistent, complete documentation in the medical record cannot be overemphasized. Without such documentation, accurate coding cannot be achieved.

Conventions

A1. ICD-10-PCS codes are composed of seven characters. Each character is an axis of classification that specifies information about the procedure performed. Within a defined code range, a character specifies the same type of information in that axis of classification.

Example: The fifth axis of classification specifies the approach in sections 0 through 4 and 7 through 9 of the system.

A2. One of 34 possible values can be assigned to each axis of classification in the seven-character code: they are the numbers 0 through 9 and the alphabet (except the letters I and O because they are easily confused with the numbers 1 and 0). The number of unique values used in an axis of classification differs as needed.

Example: Where the fifth axis of classification specifies the approach, seven different approach values are currently used to specify the approach.

A3. The valid values for an axis of classification can be added to as needed.

Example: If a significantly distinct type of device is used in a new procedure, a new device value can be added to the system.

A4. As with words in their context, the meaning of any single value is a combination of its axis of classification and any preceding values on which it may be dependent.

Example: The meaning of a body part value in the Medical and Surgical section is always dependent on the body system value. The body part value 0 in the Central Nervous body system specifies Brain and the body part value 0 in the Peripheral Nervous body system specifies Cervical Plexus.

A5. As the system is expanded to become increasingly detailed, over time more values will depend on preceding values for their meaning.

Example: In the Lower Joints body system, the device value 3 in the root operation Insertion specifies Infusion Device and the device value 3 in the root operation Replacement specifies Ceramic Synthetic Substitute.

A6. The purpose of the Alphabetic Index is to locate the appropriate table that contains all information necessary to construct a procedure code. The PCS Tables should always be consulted to find the most appropriate valid code.

A7. It is not required to consult the Index first before proceeding to the tables to complete the code. A valid code may be chosen directly from the Tables.

A8. All seven characters must be specified to be a valid code. If the documentation is incomplete for coding purposes, the physician should be queried for the necessary information.

A9. Within a PCS Table, valid codes include all combinations of choices in characters 4 through 7 contained in the same row of the table. In the example below, 0JHT3VZ is a valid code, and 0JHW3VZ is *not* a valid code.

Section:	**0**	**Medical and Surgical**
Body System:	**J**	**Subcutaneous Tissue and Fascia**
Operation:	**H**	**Insertion:** Putting in a nonbiological appliance that monitors, assists, performs, or prevents a physiological function but does not physically take the place of a body part

Body Part (4th)	Approach (5th)	Device (6th)	Qualifier (7th)
S Subcutaneous Tissue and Fascia, Head and Neck **V** Subcutaneous Tissue and Fascia, Upper Extremity **W** Subcutaneous Tissue and Fascia, Lower Extremity	**0** Open **3** Percutaneous	**1** Radioactive Element **3** Infusion Device	**Z** No Qualifier
T Subcutaneous Tissue and Fascia, Trunk	**0** Open **3** Percutaneous	**1** Radioactive Element **3** Infusion Device **V** Infusion Pump	**Z** No Qualifier

A10. "And," when used in a code description, means "and/or," except when used to describe a combination of multiple body parts for which separate values exist for each body part (e.g., Skin and Subcutaneous Tissue used as a qualifier, where there are separate body part values for "Skin" and "Subcutaneous Tissue").

Example: Lower Arm and Wrist Muscle means lower arm and/or wrist muscle.

A11. Many of the terms used to construct PCS codes are defined within the system. It is the coder's responsibility to determine what the documentation in the medical record equates to in the PCS definitions. The physician is not expected to use the terms used in PCS code descriptions, nor is the coder required to query the physician when the correlation between the documentation and the defined PCS terms is clear.

Example: When the physician documents "partial resection" the coder can independently correlate "partial resection" to the root operation Excision without querying the physician for clarification.

Medical and Surgical Section Guidelines (section 0)

B2. Body System

General guidelines

B2.1a

The procedure codes in the general anatomical regions body systems can be used when the procedure is performed on an anatomical region rather than a specific body part (e.g., root operations Control and Detachment, Drainage of a body cavity) or on the rare occasion when no information is available to support assignment of a code to a specific body part.

Examples: Control of postoperative hemorrhage is coded to the root operation Control found in the general anatomical regions body systems. Chest tube drainage of the pleural cavity is coded to the root operation Drainage found in the general anatomical regions body systems. Suture repair of the abdominal wall is coded to the root operation Repair in the general anatomical regions body system.

B2.1b

Where the general body part values "upper" and "lower" are provided as an option in the Upper Arteries, Lower Arteries, Upper Veins, Lower Veins, Muscles and Tendons body systems, "upper" or "lower "specifies body parts located above or below the diaphragm respectively.

Example: Vein body parts above the diaphragm are found in the Upper Veins body system; vein body parts below the diaphragm are found in the Lower Veins body system.

B3. Root Operation

General guidelines

B3.1a

In order to determine the appropriate root operation, the full definition of the root operation as contained in the PCS Tables must be applied.

B3.1b

Components of a procedure specified in the root operation definition and explanation are not coded separately. Procedural steps necessary to reach the operative site and close the operative site, including anastomosis of a tubular body part, are also not coded separately.

Example: Resection of a joint as part of a joint replacement procedure is included in the root operation definition of Replacement and is not coded separately. Laparotomy performed to reach the site of an open liver biopsy is not coded separately. In a resection of sigmoid colon with anastomosis of descending colon to rectum, the anastomosis is not coded separately.

Multiple procedures
B3.2

During the same operative episode, multiple procedures are coded if:

a. The same root operation is performed on different body parts as defined by distinct values of the body part character.

   Examples: Diagnostic excision of liver and pancreas are coded separately. Excision of lesion in the ascending colon and excision of lesion in the transverse colon are coded separately.

b. The same root operation is repeated in multiple body parts, and those body parts are separate and distinct body parts classified to a single ICD-10-PCS body part value.

   Examples: Excision of the sartorius muscle and excision of the gracilis muscle are both included in the upper leg muscle body part value, and multiple procedures are coded. Extraction of multiple toenails are coded separately.

c. Multiple root operations with distinct objectives are performed on the same body part.

   Example: Destruction of sigmoid lesion and bypass of sigmoid colon are coded separately.

d. The intended root operation is attempted using one approach, but is converted to a different approach.

   Example: Laparoscopic cholecystectomy converted to an open cholecystectomy is coded as percutaneous endoscopic Inspection and open Resection.

Discontinued or incomplete procedures
B3.3

If the intended procedure is discontinued or otherwise not completed, code the procedure to the root operation performed. If a procedure is discontinued before any other root operation is performed, code the root operation Inspection of the body part or anatomical region inspected.

Example: A planned aortic valve replacement procedure is discontinued after the initial thoracotomy and before any incision is made in the heart muscle, when the patient becomes hemodynamically unstable. This procedure is coded as an open Inspection of the mediastinum.

Biopsy procedures
B3.4a

Biopsy procedures are coded using the root operations Excision, Extraction, or Drainage and the qualifier Diagnostic. *Examples:* Fine needle aspiration biopsy of fluid in the lung is coded to the root operation Drainage with the qualifier Diagnostic. Biopsy of bone marrow is coded to the root operation Extraction with the qualifier Diagnostic. Lymph node sampling for biopsy is coded to the root operation Excision with the qualifier Diagnostic.

Biopsy followed by more definitive treatment
B3.4b

If a diagnostic Excision, Extraction, or Drainage procedure (biopsy) is followed by a more definitive procedure, such as Destruction, Excision or Resection at the same procedure site, both the biopsy and the more definitive treatment are coded.

Example: Biopsy of breast followed by partial mastectomy at the same procedure site, both the biopsy and the partial mastectomy procedure are coded.

Overlapping body layers

B3.5

If the root operations Excision, Repair or Inspection are performed on overlapping layers of the musculoskeletal system, the body part specifying the deepest layer is coded.

Example: Excisional debridement that includes skin and subcutaneous tissue and muscle is coded to the muscle body part.

Bypass procedures

B3.6a

Bypass procedures are coded by identifying the body part bypassed "from" and the body part bypassed "to." The fourth character body part specifies the body part bypassed from, and the qualifier specifies the body part bypassed to.

Example: Bypass from stomach to jejunum, stomach is the body part and jejunum is the qualifier.

B3.6b

Coronary artery bypass procedures are coded differently than other bypass procedures as described in the previous guideline. Rather than identifying the body part bypassed from, the body part identifies the number of coronary artery sites bypassed to, and the qualifier specifies the vessel bypassed from.

Example: Aortocoronary artery bypass of the left anterior descending coronary artery and the obtuse marginal coronary artery is classified in the body part axis of classification as two coronary arteries and the qualifier specifies the aorta as the body part bypassed from.

B3.6c

If multiple coronary arteries are bypassed, a separate procedure is coded for each coronary artery that uses a different device and/or qualifier.

Example: Aortocoronary artery bypass and internal mammary coronary artery bypass are coded separately.

Control vs. more definitive root operations

B3.7

The root operation Control is defined as, "Stopping, or attempting to stop, postprocedural or other acute bleeding." If an attempt to stop postprocedural or other acute bleeding is initially unsuccessful, and to stop the bleeding requires performing a more definitive root operation, such as Bypass, Detachment, Excision, Extraction, Reposition, Replacement, or Resection, then the more definitive root operation is coded instead of Control.

Example: Resection of spleen to stop bleeding is coded to Resection instead of Control.

Excision vs. Resection

B3.8

PCS contains specific body parts for anatomical subdivisions of a body part, such as lobes of the lungs or liver and regions of the intestine. Resection of the specific body part is coded whenever all of the body part is cut out or off, rather than coding Excision of a less specific body part.

Example: Left upper lung lobectomy is coded to Resection of Upper Lung Lobe, Left rather than Excision of Lung, Left.

Excision for graft

B3.9

If an autograft is obtained from a different procedure site in order to complete the objective of the procedure, a separate procedure is coded.

Example: Coronary bypass with excision of saphenous vein graft, excision of saphenous vein is coded separately.

Fusion procedures of the spine

B3.10a

The body part coded for a spinal vertebral joint(s) rendered immobile by a spinal fusion procedure is classified by the level of the spine (e.g. thoracic). There are distinct body part values for a single vertebral joint and for multiple vertebral joints at each spinal level.

Example: Body part values specify Lumbar Vertebral Joint, Lumbar Vertebral Joints, 2 or More and Lumbosacral Vertebral Joint.

B3.10b

If multiple vertebral joints are fused, a separate procedure is coded for each vertebral joint that uses a different device and/or qualifier.

Example: Fusion of lumbar vertebral joint, posterior approach, anterior column and fusion of lumbar vertebral joint, posterior approach, posterior column are coded separately.

B3.10c

Combinations of devices and materials are often used on a vertebral joint to render the joint immobile. When combinations of devices are used on the same vertebral joint, the device value coded for the procedure is as follows:

- If an interbody fusion device is used to render the joint immobile (alone or containing other material like bone graft), the procedure is coded with the device value Interbody Fusion Device
- If bone graft is the *only* device used to render the joint immobile, the procedure is coded with the device value Nonautologous Tissue Substitute or Autologous Tissue Substitute
- If a mixture of autologous and nonautologous bone graft (with or without biological or synthetic extenders or binders) is used to render the joint immobile, code the procedure with the device value Autologous Tissue Substitute

Examples: Fusion of a vertebral joint using a cage style interbody fusion device containing morsellized bone graft is coded to the device Interbody Fusion Device. Fusion of a vertebral joint using a bone dowel interbody fusion device made of cadaver bone and packed with a mixture of local morsellized bone and demineralized bone matrix is coded to the device Interbody Fusion Device. Fusion of a vertebral joint using both autologous bone graft and bone bank bone graft is coded to the device Autologous Tissue Substitute.

Inspection procedures

B3.11a

Inspection of a body part(s) performed in order to achieve the objective of a procedure is not coded separately.

Example: Fiberoptic bronchoscopy performed for irrigation of bronchus, only the irrigation procedure is coded.

B3.11b

If multiple tubular body parts are inspected, the most distal body part (the body part furthest from the starting point of the inspection) is coded. If multiple non-tubular body parts in a region are inspected, the body part that specifies the entire area inspected is coded.

Examples: Cystoureteroscopy with inspection of bladder and ureters is coded to the ureter body part value. Exploratory laparotomy with general inspection of abdominal contents is coded to the peritoneal cavity body part value.

B3.11c

When both an Inspection procedure and another procedure are performed on the same body part during the same episode, if the Inspection procedure is performed using a different approach than the other procedure, the Inspection procedure is coded separately.

Example: Endoscopic Inspection of the duodenum is coded separately when open Excision of the duodenum is performed during the same procedural episode.

Occlusion vs. Restriction for vessel embolization procedures

B3.12

If the objective of an embolization procedure is to completely close a vessel, the root operation Occlusion is coded. If the objective of an embolization procedure is to narrow the lumen of a vessel, the root operation Restriction is coded.

Examples: Tumor embolization is coded to the root operation Occlusion, because the objective of the procedure is to cut off the blood supply to the vessel. Embolization of a cerebral aneurysm is coded to the root operation Restriction, because the objective of the procedure is not to close off the vessel entirely, but to narrow the lumen of the vessel at the site of the aneurysm where it is abnormally wide.

Release procedures

B3.13

In the root operation Release, the body part value coded is the body part being freed and not the tissue being manipulated or cut to free the body part.

Example: Lysis of intestinal adhesions is coded to the specific intestine body part value.

Release vs. Division

B3.14

If the sole objective of the procedure is freeing a body part without cutting the body part, the root operation is Release. If the sole objective of the procedure is separating or transecting a body part, the root operation is Division.

Examples: Freeing a nerve root from surrounding scar tissue to relieve pain is coded to the root operation Release. Severing a nerve root to relieve pain is coded to the root operation Division.

Reposition for fracture treatment

B3.15

Reduction of a displaced fracture is coded to the root operation Reposition and the application of a cast or splint in conjunction with the Reposition procedure is not coded separately. Treatment of a nondisplaced fracture is coded to the procedure performed.

Examples: Casting of a nondisplaced fracture is coded to the root operation Immobilization in the Placement section.

Putting a pin in a nondisplaced fracture is coded to the root operation Insertion.

Transplantation vs. Administration

B3.16

Putting in a mature and functioning living body part taken from another individual or animal is coded to the root operation Transplantation. Putting in autologous or nonautologous cells is coded to the Administration section.

Example: Putting in autologous or nonautologous bone marrow, pancreatic islet cells or stem cells is coded to the Administration section.

Transfer procedures using multiple tissue layers

B3.17

The root operation Transfer contains qualifiers that can be used to specify when a transfer flap is composed of more than one tissue layer, such as a musculocutaneous flap. For procedures involving transfer of multiple tissue layers including skin, subcutaneous tissue, fascia or muscle, the procedure is coded to the body part value that describes the deepest tissue layer in the flap, and the qualifier can be used to describe the other tissue layer(s) in the transfer flap.

Example: A musculocutaneous flap transfer is coded to the appropriate body part value in the body system Muscles, and the qualifier is used to describe the additional tissue layer(s) in the transfer flap.

B4. Body Part

General guidelines

B4.1a

If a procedure is performed on a portion of a body part that does not have a separate body part value, code the body part value corresponding to the whole body part.

Example: A procedure performed on the alveolar process of the mandible is coded to the mandible body part.

B4.1b

If the prefix "peri" is combined with a body part to identify the site of the procedure, and the site of the procedure is not further specified, then the procedure is coded to the body part named. This guideline applies only when a more specific body part value is not available.

Examples: A procedure site identified as perirenal is coded to the kidney body part when the site of the procedure is not further specified. A procedure site described in the documentation as peri-urethral, and the documentation also indicates that it is the vulvar tissue and not the urethral tissue that is the site of the procedure, then the procedure is coded to the vulva body part.

B4.1c

If a procedure is performed on a continuous section of a tubular body part, code the body part value corresponding to the furthest anatomical site from the point of entry.

Example: A procedure performed on a continuous section of artery from the femoral artery to the external iliac artery with the point of entry at the femoral artery is coded to the external iliac body part.

Branches of body parts

B4.2

Where a specific branch of a body part does not have its own body part value in PCS, the body part is typically coded to the closest proximal branch that has a specific body part value. In the cardiovascular body systems, if a general body part is available in the correct root operation table, and coding to a proximal branch would require assigning a code in a different body system, the procedure is coded using the general body part value.

Examples: A procedure performed on the mandibular branch of the trigeminal nerve is coded to the trigeminal nerve body part value. Occlusion of the bronchial artery is coded to the body part value Upper Artery in the body system Upper Arteries, and not to the body part value Thoracic Aorta, Descending in the body system Heart and Great Vessels.

Bilateral body part values

B4.3

Bilateral body part values are available for a limited number of body parts. If the identical procedure is performed on contralateral body parts, and a bilateral body part value exists for that body part, a single procedure is coded using the bilateral body part value. If no bilateral body part value exists, each procedure is coded separately using the appropriate body part value.

Example: The identical procedure performed on both fallopian tubes is coded once using the body part value Fallopian Tube, Bilateral. The identical procedure performed on both knee joints is coded twice using the body part values Knee Joint, Right and Knee Joint, Left.

Coronary arteries

B4.4

The coronary arteries are classified as a single body part that is further specified by number of arteries treated. One procedure code specifying multiple arteries is used when the same procedure is performed, including the same device and qualifier values.

Examples: Angioplasty of two distinct coronary arteries with placement of two stents is coded as Dilation of Coronary Artery, Two Arteries, with Two Intraluminal Devices. Angioplasty of two distinct coronary arteries, one with stent placed and one without, is coded separately as Dilation of Coronary Artery, One Artery with Intraluminal Device, and Dilation of Coronary Artery, One Artery with no device.

Tendons, ligaments, bursae and fascia near a joint

B4.5

Procedures performed on tendons, ligaments, bursae and fascia supporting a joint are coded to the body part in the respective body system that is the focus of the procedure. Procedures performed on joint structures themselves are coded to the body part in the joint body systems.

Example: Repair of the anterior cruciate ligament of the knee is coded to the knee bursa and ligament body part in the Bursae and Ligaments body system. Knee arthroscopy with shaving of articular cartilage is coded to the knee joint body part in the Lower Joints body system.

Skin, subcutaneous tissue and fascia overlying a joint

B4.6

If a procedure is performed on the skin, subcutaneous tissue or fascia overlying a joint, the procedure is coded to the following body part:

- Shoulder is coded to Upper Arm
- Elbow is coded to Lower Arm
- Wrist is coded to Lower Arm
- Hip is coded to Upper Leg
- Knee is coded to Lower Leg
- Ankle is coded to Foot

Fingers and toes

B4.7

If a body system does not contain a separate body part value for fingers, procedures performed on the fingers are coded to the body part value for the hand. If a body system does not contain a separate body part value for toes, procedures performed on the toes are coded to the body part value for the foot.

Example: Excision of finger muscle is coded to one of the hand muscle body part values in the Muscles body system.

Upper and lower intestinal tract

B4.8

In the Gastrointestinal body system, the general body part values Upper Intestinal Tract and Lower Intestinal Tract are provided as an option for the root operations Change, Inspection, Removal and Revision. Upper Intestinal Tract includes the portion of the gastrointestinal tract from the esophagus down to and including the duodenum, and Lower Intestinal Tract includes the portion of the gastrointestinal tract from the jejunum down to and including the rectum and anus.

Example: In the root operation Change table, change of a device in the jejunum is coded using the body part Lower Intestinal Tract.

B5. Approach

Open approach with percutaneous endoscopic assistance

B5.2

Procedures performed using the open approach with percutaneous endoscopic assistance are coded to the approach Open.

Example: Laparoscopic-assisted sigmoidectomy is coded to the approach Open.

External approach

B5.3a

Procedures performed within an orifice on structures that are visible without the aid of any instrumentation are coded to the approach External.

Example: Resection of tonsils is coded to the approach External.

B5.3b

Procedures performed indirectly by the application of external force through the intervening body layers are coded to the approach External.

Example: Closed reduction of fracture is coded to the approach External.

Percutaneous procedure via device

B5.4

Procedures performed percutaneously via a device placed for the procedure are coded to the approach Percutaneous.

Example: Fragmentation of kidney stone performed via percutaneous nephrostomy is coded to the approach Percutaneous.

B6. Device

General guidelines

B6.1a

A device is coded only if a device remains after the procedure is completed. If no device remains, the device value No Device is coded. In limited root operations, the classification provides the qualifier values Temporary and Intraoperative, for specific procedures involving clinically significant devices, where the purpose of the device is to be utilized for a brief duration during the procedure or current inpatient stay. If a device that is intended to remain after the procedure is completed requires removal before the end of the operative episode in which it was inserted (for example, the device size is inadequate or a complication occurs), both the insertion and removal of the device should be coded.

B6.1b

Materials such as sutures, ligatures, radiological markers and temporary post-operative wound drains are considered integral to the performance of a procedure and are not coded as devices.

B6.1c

Procedures performed on a device only and not on a body part are specified in the root operations Change, Irrigation, Removal and Revision, and are coded to the procedure performed.

Example: Irrigation of percutaneous nephrostomy tube is coded to the root operation Irrigation of indwelling device in the Administration section.

Drainage device

B6.2

A separate procedure to put in a drainage device is coded to the root operation Drainage with the device value Drainage Device.

Obstetric Section Guidelines (section 1)

C. Obstetrics Section

Products of conception

C1

Procedures performed on the products of conception are coded to the Obstetrics section. Procedures performed on the pregnant female other than the products of conception are coded to the appropriate root operation in the Medical and Surgical section.

Example: Amniocentesis is coded to the products of conception body part in the Obstetrics section. Repair of obstetric urethral laceration is coded to the urethra body part in the Medical and Surgical section.

Procedures following delivery or abortion

C2

Procedures performed following a delivery or abortion for curettage of the endometrium or evacuation of retained products of conception are all coded in the Obstetrics section, to the root operation Extraction and the body part Products of Conception, Retained. Diagnostic or therapeutic dilation and curettage performed during times other than the postpartum or post-abortion period are all coded in the Medical and Surgical section, to the root operation Extraction and the body part Endometrium.

New Technology Section Guidelines (section X)

D. New Technology Section

General guidelines

D1

Section X codes are standalone codes. They are not supplemental codes. Section X codes fully represent the specific procedure described in the code title, and do not require any additional codes from other sections of ICD-10-PCS. When section X contains a code title which describes a specific new technology procedure, only that X code is reported for the procedure. There is no need to report a broader, non-specific code in another section of ICD-10-PCS.

Example: XW04321 Introduction of Ceftazidime-Avibactam Anti-infective into Central Vein, Percutaneous Approach, New Technology Group 1, can be coded to indicate that Ceftazidime-Avibactam Anti-infective was administered via a central vein. A separate code from table 3E0 in the Administration section of ICD-10-PCS is not coded in addition to this code.

Selection of Principal Procedure

The following instructions should be applied in the selection of principal procedure and clarification on the importance of the relation to the principal diagnosis when more than one procedure is performed:

1. Procedure performed for definitive treatment of both principal diagnosis and secondary diagnosis
   a. Sequence procedure performed for definitive treatment most related to principal diagnosis as principal procedure.
2. Procedure performed for definitive treatment and diagnostic procedures performed for both principal diagnosis and secondary diagnosis
   a. Sequence procedure performed for definitive treatment most related to principal diagnosis as principal procedure
3. A diagnostic procedure was performed for the principal diagnosis and a procedure is performed for definitive treatment of a secondary diagnosis.
   a. Sequence diagnostic procedure as principal procedure, since the procedure most related to the principal diagnosis takes precedence.
4. No procedures performed that are related to principal diagnosis; procedures performed for definitive treatment and diagnostic procedures were performed for secondary diagnosis
   a. Sequence procedure performed for definitive treatment of secondary diagnosis as principal procedure, since there are no procedures (definitive or nondefinitive treatment) related to principal diagnosis.

3

3f (Aortic) Bioprosthesis valve
use Zooplastic Tissue in Heart and Great Vessels

A

Abdominal aortic plexus
use Nerve, Abdominal Sympathetic
Abdominal esophagus
use Esophagus, Lower
Abdominohysterectomy
see Resection, Uterus 0UT9
Abdominoplasty
see Alteration, Abdominal Wall 0W0F
see Repair, Abdominal Wall 0WQF
see Supplement, Abdominal Wall 0WUF
Abductor hallucis muscle
use Muscle, Foot, Left
use Muscle, Foot, Right
AbioCor® Total Replacement Heart
use Synthetic Substitute
Ablation
see Destruction
Abortion
Abortifacient 10A07ZX
Laminaria 10A07ZW
Products of Conception 10A0
Vacuum 10A07Z6
Abrasion
see Extraction
Absolute Pro Vascular (OTW) Self-Expanding Stent System
use Intraluminal Device
Accessory cephalic vein
use Vein, Cephalic, Left
use Vein, Cephalic, Right
Accessory obturator nerve
use Nerve, Lumbar Plexus
Accessory phrenic nerve
use Nerve, Phrenic
Accessory spleen
use Spleen
Acculink (RX) Carotid Stent System
use Intraluminal Device
Acellular Hydrated Dermis
use Nonautologous Tissue Substitute
Acetabular cup
use Liner in Lower Joints
Acetabulectomy
see Excision, Lower Bones 0QB
see Resection, Lower Bones 0QT
Acetabulofemoral joint
use Joint, Hip, Left
use Joint, Hip, Right
Acetabuloplasty
see Repair, Lower Bones 0QQ
see Replacement, Lower Bones 0QR
see Supplement, Lower Bones 0QU
Achilles tendon
use Tendon, Lower Leg, Left
use Tendon, Lower Leg, Right
Achillorrhaphy
see Repair, Tendons 0LQ
Achillotenotomy, achillotomy
see Division, Tendons 0L8
see Drainage, Tendons 0L9
Acromioclavicular ligament
use Bursa and Ligament, Shoulder, Left
use Bursa and Ligament, Shoulder, Right
Acromion (process)
use Scapula, Left
use Scapula, Right
Acromionectomy
see Excision, Upper Joints 0RB
see Resection, Upper Joints 0RT
Acromioplasty
see Repair, Upper Joints 0RQ
see Replacement, Upper Joints 0RR
see Supplement, Upper Joints 0RU
Activa PC neurostimulator
use Stimulator Generator, Multiple Array in 0JH
Activa RC neurostimulator
use Stimulator Generator, Multiple Array Rechargeable in 0JH
Activa SC neurostimulator
use Stimulator Generator, Single Array in 0JH
Activities of Daily Living Assessment F02
Activities of Daily Living Treatment F08
ACUITY™ Steerable Lead
use Cardiac Lead, Defibrillator in 02H
use Cardiac Lead, Pacemaker in 02H
Acupuncture
Breast
Anesthesia 8E0H300
No Qualifier 8E0H30Z
Integumentary System
Anesthesia 8E0H300
No Qualifier 8E0H30Z
Adductor brevis muscle
use Muscle, Upper Leg, Left
use Muscle, Upper Leg, Right
Adductor hallucis muscle
use Muscle, Foot, Left
use Muscle, Foot, Right
Adductor longus muscle
use Muscle, Upper Leg, Left
use Muscle, Upper Leg, Right
Adductor magnus muscle
use Muscle, Upper Leg, Left
use Muscle, Upper Leg, Right
Adenohypophysis
use Gland, Pituitary
Adenoidectomy
see Excision, Adenoids 0CBQ
see Resection, Adenoids 0CTQ
Adenoidotomy
see Drainage, Adenoids 0C9Q
Adhesiolysis
see Release
Administration
Blood products
see Transfusion
Other substance
see Introduction of substance in or on
Adrenalectomy
see Excision, Endocrine System 0GB
see Resection, Endocrine System 0GT
Adrenalorrhaphy
see Repair, Endocrine System 0GQ
Adrenalotomy
see Drainage, Endocrine System 0G9
Advancement
see Reposition
see Transfer
Advisa (MRI)
use Pacemaker, Dual Chamber in 0JH
AFX® Endovascular AAA System
use Intraluminal Device
AIGISRx Antibacterial Envelope
use Anti-Infective Envelope
Alar ligament of axis
use Bursa and Ligament, Head and Neck
Alimentation
see Introduction of substance in or on
Alfieri Stitch Valvuloplasty
see Restriction, Valve, Mitral 02VG
Alteration
Abdominal Wall 0W0F
Ankle Region
Left 0Y0L
Right 0Y0K
Arm
Lower
Left 0X0F
Right 0X0D
Upper
Left 0X09
Right 0X08
Axilla
Left 0X05
Right 0X04
Back
Lower 0W0L
Upper 0W0K
Breast
Bilateral 0H0V
Left 0H0U
Right 0H0T
Buttock
Left 0Y01
Right 0Y00
Chest Wall 0W08
Ear
Bilateral 0902
Left 0901
Right 0900
Elbow Region
Left 0X0C
Right 0X0B
Extremity
Lower
Left 0Y0B
Right 0Y09
Upper
Left 0X07
Right 0X06
Eyelid
Lower
Left 080R
Right 080Q
Upper
Left 080P
Right 080N
Face 0W02
Head 0W00
Jaw
Lower 0W05
Upper 0W04
Knee Region
Left 0Y0G
Right 0Y0F
Leg
Lower
Left 0Y0J
Right 0Y0H
Upper
Left 0Y0D
Right 0Y0C
Lip
Lower 0C01X
Upper 0C00X
Nasal Mucosa and Soft Tissue 090K
Neck 0W06
Alteration (continued)
Perineum
Female 0W0N
Male 0W0M
Shoulder Region
Left 0X03
Right 0X02
Subcutaneous Tissue and Fascia
Abdomen 0J08
Back 0J07
Buttock 0J09
Chest 0J06
Face 0J01
Lower Arm
Left 0J0H
Right 0J0G
Lower Leg
Left 0J0P
Right 0J0N
Neck
Left 0J05
Right 0J04
Upper Arm
Left 0J0F
Right 0J0D
Upper Leg
Left 0J0M
Right 0J0L
Wrist Region
Left 0X0H
Right 0X0G
Alveolar process of mandible
use Mandible
Alveolar process of maxilla
use Maxilla
Alveolectomy
see Excision, Head and Facial Bones 0NB
see Resection, Head and Facial Bones 0NT
Alveoloplasty
see Repair, Head and Facial Bones 0NQ
see Replacement, Head and Facial Bones 0NR
see Supplement, Head and Facial Bones 0NU
Alveolotomy
see Division, Head and Facial Bones 0N8
see Drainage, Head and Facial Bones 0N9
Ambulatory cardiac monitoring 4A12X45
Amniocentesis
see Drainage, Products of Conception 1090
Amnioinfusion
see Introduction of substance in or on, Products of Conception 3E0E
Amnioscopy 10J08ZZ
Amniotomy
see Drainage, Products of Conception 1090
AMPLATZER® Muscular VSD Occluder
use Synthetic Substitute
Amputation
see Detachment
AMS 800® Urinary Control System
use Artificial Sphincter in Urinary System
Anal orifice
use Anus

Analog radiography
see Plain Radiography
Anastomosis
see Bypass
Anatomical snuffbox
use Muscle, Lower Arm and Wrist, Left
use Muscle, Lower Arm and Wrist, Right
Andexanet Alfa, Factor Xa Inhibitor Reversal Agent XW0
AneuRx® AAA Advantage®
use Intraluminal Device
Angiectomy
see Excision, Heart and Great Vessels 02B
see Excision, Upper Arteries 03B
see Excision, Lower Arteries 04B
see Excision, Upper Veins 05B
see Excision, Lower Veins 06B
Angiocardiography
Combined right and left heart
see Fluoroscopy, Heart, Right and Left B216
Left Heart
see Fluoroscopy, Heart, Left B215
Right Heart
see Fluoroscopy, Heart, Right B214
SPY system intravascular fluorescence
see Monitoring, Physiological Systems 4A1
Angiography
see Plain Radiography, Heart B20
see Fluoroscopy, Heart B21
Angioplasty
see Dilation, Heart and Great Vessels 027
see Repair, Heart and Great Vessels 02Q
see Replacement, Heart and Great Vessels 02R
see Dilation, Upper Arteries 037
see Repair, Upper Arteries 03Q
see Replacement, Upper Arteries 03R
see Dilation, Lower Arteries 047
see Repair, Lower Arteries 04Q
see Replacement, Lower Arteries 04R
see Supplement, Heart and Great Vessels 02U
see Supplement, Upper Arteries 03U
see Supplement, Lower Arteries 04U
Angiorrhaphy
see Repair, Heart and Great Vessels 02Q
see Repair, Upper Arteries 03Q
see Repair, Lower Arteries 04Q
Angioscopy
02JY4ZZ
03JY4ZZ
04JY4ZZ
Angiotensin II
use Synthetic Human Angiotensin II
Angiotripsy
see Occlusion, Upper Arteries 03L
see Occlusion, Lower Arteries 04L
Angular artery
use Artery, Face
Angular vein
use Vein, Face, Left
use Vein, Face, Right
Annular ligament
use Bursa and Ligament, Elbow, Left
use Bursa and Ligament, Elbow, Right
Annuloplasty
see Repair, Heart and Great Vessels 02Q
see Supplement, Heart and Great Vessels 02U
Annuloplasty ring
use Synthetic Substitute
Anoplasty
see Repair, Anus 0DQQ
see Supplement, Anus 0DUQ
Anorectal junction
use Rectum
Anoscopy 0DJD8ZZ
Ansa cervicalis
use Nerve, Cervical Plexus
Antabuse therapy HZ93ZZZ
Antebrachial fascia
use Subcutaneous Tissue and Fascia, Lower Arm, Left
use Subcutaneous Tissue and Fascia, Lower Arm, Right
Anterior (pectoral) lymph node
use Lymphatic, Axillary, Left
use Lymphatic, Axillary, Right
Anterior cerebral artery
use Artery, Intracranial
Anterior cerebral vein
use Vein, Intracranial
Anterior choroidal artery
use Artery, Intracranial
Anterior circumflex humeral artery
use Artery, Axillary, Left
use Artery, Axillary, Right
Anterior communicating artery
use Artery, Intracranial
Anterior cruciate ligament (ACL)
use Bursa and Ligament, Knee, Left
use Bursa and Ligament, Knee, Right
Anterior crural nerve
use Nerve, Femoral
Anterior facial vein
use Vein, Face, Left
use Vein, Face, Right
Anterior intercostal artery
use Artery, Internal Mammary, Left
use Artery, Internal Mammary, Right
Anterior interosseous nerve
use Nerve, Median
Anterior lateral malleolar artery
use Artery, Anterior Tibial, Left
use Artery, Anterior Tibial, Right
Anterior lingual gland
use Gland, Minor Salivary
Anterior medial malleolar artery
use Artery, Anterior Tibial, Left
use Artery, Anterior Tibial, Right
Anterior spinal artery
use Artery, Vertebral, Left
use Artery, Vertebral, Right
Anterior tibial recurrent artery
use Artery, Anterior Tibial, Left
use Artery, Anterior Tibial, Right
Anterior ulnar recurrent artery
use Artery, Ulnar, Left
use Artery, Ulnar, Right
Anterior vagal trunk
use Nerve, Vagus
Anterior vertebral muscle
use Muscle, Neck, Left
use Muscle, Neck, Right
Antigen-free air conditioning
see Atmospheric Control, Physiological Systems 6A0
Antihelix
use Ear, External, Bilateral
use Ear, External, Left
use Ear, External, Right
Antimicrobial envelope
use Anti-Infective Envelope
Antitragus
use Ear, External, Bilateral
use Ear, External, Left
use Ear, External, Right
Antrostomy
see Drainage, Ear, Nose, Sinus 099
Antrotomy
see Drainage, Ear, Nose, Sinus 099
Antrum of Highmore
use Sinus, Maxillary, Left
use Sinus, Maxillary, Right
Aortic annulus
use Valve, Aortic
Aortic arch
use Thoracic Aorta, Ascending/Arch
Aortic intercostal artery
use Upper Artery
Aortography
see Plain Radiography, Upper Arteries B30
see Fluoroscopy, Upper Arteries B31
see Plain Radiography, Lower Arteries B40
see Fluoroscopy, Lower Arteries B41
Aortoplasty
see Repair, Aorta, Thoracic, Descending 02QW
see Repair, Aorta, Thoracic, Ascending/Arch 02QX
see Replacement, Aorta, Thoracic, Descending 02RW
see Replacement, Aorta, Thoracic, Ascending/Arch 02RX
see Supplement, Aorta, Thoracic, Descending 02UW
see Supplement, Aorta, Thoracic, Ascending/Arch 02UX
see Repair, Aorta, Abdominal 04Q0
see Replacement, Aorta, Abdominal 04R0
see Supplement, Aorta, Abdominal 04U0
Apical (subclavicular) lymph node
use Lymphatic, Axillary, Left
use Lymphatic, Axillary, Right
Apneustic center use Pons
Appendectomy
see Excision, Appendix 0DBJ
see Resection, Appendix 0DTJ
Appendicolysis
see Release, Appendix 0DNJ
Appendicotomy
see Drainage, Appendix 0D9J
Application
see Introduction of substance in or on
Aquablation therapy, prostate XV508A4
Aquapheresis 6A550Z3
Aqueduct of Sylvius
use Cerebral Ventricle
Aqueous humour
use Anterior Chamber, Left
use Anterior Chamber, Right
Arachnoid mater, intracranial
use Cerebral Meninges
Arachnoid mater, spinal
use Spinal Meninges
Arcuate artery
use Artery, Foot, Left
use Artery, Foot, Right
Areola
use Nipple, Left
use Nipple, Right
AROM (artificial rupture of membranes) 10907ZC
Arterial canal (duct)
use Artery, Pulmonary, Left
Arterial pulse tracing
see Measurement, Arterial 4A03
Arteriectomy
see Excision, Heart and Great Vessels 02B
see Excision, Upper Arteries 03B
see Excision, Lower Arteries 04B
Arteriography
see Plain Radiography, Heart B20
see Fluoroscopy, Heart B21
Arteriography *(continued)*
see Plain Radiography, Upper Arteries B30
see Fluoroscopy, Upper Arteries B3
see Plain Radiography, Lower Arteries B40
see Fluoroscopy, Lower Arteries B41
Arterioplasty
see Repair, Heart and Great Vessels 02Q
see Replacement, Heart and Great Vessels 02R
see Repair, Upper Arteries 03Q
see Replacement, Upper Arteries 03R
see Repair, Lower Arteries 04Q
see Replacement, Lower Arteries 04R
see Supplement, Upper Arteries 03U
see Supplement, Lower Arteries 04U
see Supplement, Heart and Great Vessels 02U
Arteriorrhaphy
see Repair, Heart and Great Vessels 02Q
see Repair, Upper Arteries 03Q
see Repair, Lower Arteries 04Q
Arterioscopy
see Inspection, Artery, Lower 04JY
see Inspection, Artery, Upper 03JY
see Inspection, Great Vessel 02JY
Arthrectomy
see Excision, Upper Joints 0RB
see Resection, Upper Joints 0RT
see Excision, Lower Joints 0SB
see Resection, Lower Joints 0ST
Arthrocentesis
see Drainage, Upper Joints 0R9
see Drainage, Lower Joints 0S9
Arthrodesis
see Fusion, Upper Joints 0RG
see Fusion, Lower Joints 0SG
Arthrography
see Plain Radiography, Skull and Facial Bones BN0
see Plain Radiography, Non-Axial Upper Bones BP0
see Plain Radiography, Non-Axial Lower Bones BQ0
Arthrolysis
see Release, Upper Joints 0RN
see Release, Lower Joints 0SN
Arthropexy
see Repair, Upper Joints 0RQ
see Reposition, Upper Joints 0RS
see Repair, Lower Joints 0SQ
see Reposition, Lower Joints 0SS
Arthroplasty
see Repair, Upper Joints 0RQ
see Replacement, Upper Joints 0R
see Repair, Lower Joints 0SQ
see Replacement, Lower Joints 0S
see Supplement, Lower Joints 0SU
see Supplement, Upper Joints 0RU
Arthroplasty, radial head
see Replacement, Radius, Left 0P
see Replacement, Radius, Right 0PRH
Arthroscopy
see Inspection, Upper Joints 0RJ
see Inspection, Lower Joints 0SJ
Arthrotomy
see Drainage, Upper Joints 0R9
see Drainage, Lower Joints 0S9
Articulating Spacer (Antibiotic)
use Articulating Spacer in Lower Joints
Artificial anal sphincter (AAS)
use Artificial Sphincter in Gastrointestinal System

Artificial bowel sphincter (neosphincter)
- *use* Artificial Sphincter in Gastrointestinal System

Artificial Sphincter
- Insertion of device in
  - Anus 0DHQ
  - Bladder 0THB
  - Bladder Neck 0THC
  - Urethra 0THD
- Removal of device from
  - Anus 0DPQ
  - Bladder 0TPB
  - Urethra 0TPD
- Revision of device in
  - Anus 0DWQ
  - Bladder 0TWB
  - Urethra 0TWD

Artificial urinary sphincter (AUS)
- *use* Artificial Sphincter in Urinary System

Aryepiglottic fold
- *use* Larynx

Arytenoid cartilage
- *use* Larynx

Arytenoid muscle
- *use* Muscle, Neck, Left
- *use* Muscle, Neck, Right

Arytenoidectomy
- *see* Excision, Larynx 0CBS

Arytenoidopexy
- *see* Repair, Larynx 0CQS

Ascenda Intrathecal Catheter
- *use* Infusion Device

Ascending aorta
- *use* Thoracic Aorta, Ascending/Arch

Ascending palatine artery
- *use* Artery, Face

Ascending pharyngeal artery
- *use* Artery, External Carotid, Left
- *use* Artery, External Carotid, Right

Aspiration, fine needle
- Fluid or gas
  - *see* Drainage
- Tissue biopsy
  - *see* Excision
  - *see* Extraction

Assessment
- Activities of daily living
  - *see* Activities of Daily Living Assessment, Rehabilitation F02
- Hearing
  - *see* Hearing Assessment, Diagnostic Audiology F13
- Hearing aid
  - *see* Hearing Aid Assessment, Diagnostic Audiology F14
- Intravascular perfusion, using indocyanine green (ICG) dye
  - *see* Monitoring, Physiological Systems 4A1
- Motor function
  - *see* Motor Function Assessment, Rehabilitation F01
- Nerve function
  - *see* Motor Function Assessment, Rehabilitation F01
- Speech
  - *see* Speech Assessment, Rehabilitation F00
- Vestibular
  - *see* Vestibular Assessment, Diagnostic Audiology F15
- Vocational
  - *see* Activities of Daily Living Treatment, Rehabilitation F08

Assistance
- Cardiac
  - Continuous

Assistance *(continued)*
- Cardiac *(continued)*
  - Continuous *(continued)*
    - Balloon Pump 5A02210
    - Impeller Pump 5A0221D
    - Other Pump 5A02216
    - Pulsatile Compression 5A02215
  - Intermittent
    - Balloon Pump 5A02110
    - Impeller Pump 5A0211D
    - Other Pump 5A02116
    - Pulsatile Compression 5A02115
- Circulatory
  - Continuous
    - Hyperbaric 5A05221
    - Supersaturated 5A0522C
  - Intermittent
    - Hyperbaric 5A05121
    - Supersaturated 5A0512C
- Respiratory
  - 24-96 Consecutive Hours
    - Continuous Negative Airway Pressure 5A09459
    - Continuous Positive Airway Pressure 5A09457
    - Intermittent Negative Airway Pressure 5A0945B
    - Intermittent Positive Airway Pressure 5A09458
    - No Qualifier 5A0945Z
  - Continuous, Filtration 5A0920Z
  - Greater than 96 Consecutive Hours
    - Continuous Negative Airway Pressure 5A09559
    - Continuous Positive Airway Pressure 5A09557
    - Intermittent Negative Airway Pressure 5A0955B
    - Intermittent Positive Airway Pressure 5A09558
    - No Qualifier 5A0955Z
  - Less than 24 Consecutive Hours
    - Continuous Negative Airway Pressure 5A09359
    - Continuous Positive Airway Pressure 5A09357
    - Intermittent Negative Airway Pressure 5A0935B
  - Intermittent Positive Airway Pressure 5A09358
    - No Qualifier 5A0935Z

Assurant (Cobalt) stent
- *use* Intraluminal Device

Atherectomy
- *see* Extirpation, Heart and Great Vessels 02C
- *see* Extirpation, Upper Arteries 03C
- *see* Extirpation, Lower Arteries 04C

Atlantoaxial joint
- *use* Joint, Cervical Vertebral

Atmospheric Control 6A0Z

AtriClip LAA Exclusion System
- *use* Extraluminal Device

Atrioseptoplasty
- *see* Repair, Heart and Great Vessels 02Q
- *see* Replacement, Heart and Great Vessels 02R
- *see* Supplement, Heart and Great Vessels 02U

Atrioventricular node
- *use* Conduction Mechanism

Atrium dextrum cordis
- *use* Atrium, Right

Atrium pulmonale
- *use* Atrium, Left

Attain Ability® lead
- *use* Cardiac Lead, Pacemaker in 02H
- *use* Cardiac Lead, Defibrillator in 02H

Attain StarFix® (OTW) lead
- *use* Cardiac Lead, Defibrillator in 02H
- *use* Cardiac Lead, Pacemaker in 02H

Audiology, diagnostic
- *see* Hearing Assessment, Diagnostic Audiology F13
- *see* Hearing Aid Assessment, Diagnostic Audiology F14
- *see* Vestibular Assessment, Diagnostic Audiology F15

Audiometry
- *see* Hearing Assessment, Diagnostic Audiology F13

Auditory tube
- *use* Eustachian Tube, Left
- *use* Eustachian Tube, Right

Auerbach's (myenteric) plexus
- *use* Nerve, Abdominal Sympathetic

Auricle
- *use* Ear, External, Bilateral
- *use* Ear, External, Left
- *use* Ear, External, Right

Auricularis muscle
- *use* Muscle, Head

Autograft
- *use* Autologous Tissue Substitute

Autologous artery graft
- *use* Autologous Arterial Tissue in Heart and Great Vessels
- *use* Autologous Arterial Tissue in Lower Arteries
- *use* Autologous Arterial Tissue in Lower Veins
- *use* Autologous Arterial Tissue in Upper Arteries
- *use* Autologous Arterial Tissue in Upper Veins

Autologous vein graft
- *use* Autologous Venous Tissue in Heart and Great Vessels
- *use* Autologous Venous Tissue in Lower Arteries
- *use* Autologous Venous Tissue in Lower Veins
- *use* Autologous Venous Tissue in Upper Arteries
- *use* Autologous Venous Tissue in Upper Veins

Autotransfusion
- *see* Transfusion

Autotransplant
- Adrenal tissue
  - *see* Reposition, Endocrine System 0GS
- Kidney
  - *see* Reposition, Urinary System 0TS
- Pancreatic tissue
  - *see* Reposition, Pancreas 0FSG
- Parathyroid tissue
  - *see* Reposition, Endocrine System 0GS
- Thyroid tissue
  - *see* Reposition, Endocrine System 0GS
- Tooth
  - *see* Reattachment, Mouth and Throat 0CM

Avulsion
- *see* Extraction

Axial Lumbar Interbody Fusion System
- *use* Interbody Fusion Device in Lower Joints

AxiaLIF® System
- *use* Interbody Fusion Device in Lower Joints

Axicabtagene Ciloeucel
- *use* Engineered Autologous Chimeric Antigen Receptor T-cell Immunotherapy

Axillary fascia
- *use* Subcutaneous Tissue and Fascia, Upper Arm, Left
- *use* Subcutaneous Tissue and Fascia, Upper Arm, Right

Axillary nerve
- *use* Nerve, Brachial Plexus

B

BAK/C® Interbody Cervical Fusion System
- *use* Interbody Fusion Device in Upper Joints

BAL (bronchial alveolar lavage), diagnostic
- *see* Drainage, Respiratory System 0B9

Balanoplasty
- *see* Repair, Penis 0VQS
- *see* Supplement, Penis 0VUS

Balloon atrial septostomy (BAS) 02163Z7

Balloon Pump
- Continuous, Output 5A02210
- Intermittent, Output 5A02110

Bandage, Elastic
- *see* Compression

Banding
- *see* Occlusion
- *see* Restriction

Banding, esophageal varices
- *see* Occlusion, Vein, Esophageal 06L3

Banding, laparoscopic (adjustable) gastric
- Initial procedure 0DV64CZ
- Surgical correction
  - *see* Revision of device in, Stomach 0DW6

Bard® Composix® (E/X)(LP) mesh
- *use* Synthetic Substitute

Bard® Composix® Kugel® patch
- *use* Synthetic Substitute

Bard® Dulex™ mesh
- *use* Synthetic Substitute

Bard® Ventralex™ hernia patch
- *use* Synthetic Substitute

Barium swallow
- *see* Fluoroscopy, Gastrointestinal System BD1

Baroreflex Activation Therapy® (BAT®)
- Stimulator Generator in Subcutaneous Tissue and Fascia
- *use* Stimulator Lead in Upper Arteries

Bartholin's (greater vestibular) gland
- *use* Gland, Vestibular

Basal (internal) cerebral vein
- *use* Vein, Intracranial

Basal metabolic rate (BMR)
- *see* Measurement, Physiological Systems 4A0Z

Basal nuclei
- *use* Basal Ganglia

Base of Tongue
- *use* Pharynx

Basilar artery
- *use* Artery, Intracranial

Basis pontis
- *use* Pons

Beam Radiation
- Abdomen DW03
  - Intraoperative DW033Z0
- Adrenal Gland DG02
  - Intraoperative DG023Z0

Beam Radiation *(continued)*
Bile Ducts DF02
Intraoperative DF023Z0
Bladder DT02
Intraoperative DT023Z0
Bone
Intraoperative DP0C3Z0
Other DP0C
Bone Marrow D700
Intraoperative D7003Z0
Brain D000
Intraoperative D0003Z0
Brain Stem D001
Intraoperative D0013Z0
Breast
Left DM00
Intraoperative DM003Z0
Right DM01
Intraoperative DM013Z0
Bronchus DB01
Intraoperative DB013Z0
Cervix DU01
Intraoperative DU013Z0
Chest DW02
Intraoperative DW023Z0
Chest Wall DB07
Intraoperative DB073Z0
Colon DD05
Intraoperative DD053Z0
Diaphragm DB08
Intraoperative DB083Z0
Duodenum DD02
Intraoperative DD023Z0
Ear D900
Intraoperative D9003Z0
Esophagus DD00
Intraoperative DD003Z0
Eye D800
Intraoperative D8003Z0
Femur DP09
Intraoperative DP093Z0
Fibula DP0B
Intraoperative DP0B3Z0
Gallbladder DF01
Intraoperative DF013Z0
Gland
Adrenal DG02
Intraoperative DG023Z0
Parathyroid DG04
Intraoperative DG043Z0
Pituitary DG00
Intraoperative DG003Z0
Thyroid DG05
Intraoperative DG053Z0
Glands
Intraoperative D9063Z0
Salivary D906
Head and Neck DW01
Intraoperative DW013Z0
Hemibody DW04
Intraoperative DW043Z0
Humerus DP06
Intraoperative DP063Z0
Hypopharynx D903
Intraoperative D9033Z0
Ileum DD04
Intraoperative DD043Z0
Jejunum DD03
Intraoperative DD033Z0
Kidney DT00
Intraoperative DT003Z0
Larynx D90B
Intraoperative D90B3Z0
Liver DF00
Intraoperative DF003Z0
Lung DB02
Intraoperative DB023Z0
Lymphatics
Abdomen D706
Intraoperative D7063Z0

Beam Radiation *(continued)*
Lymphatics *(continued)*
Axillary D704
Intraoperative D7043Z0
Inguinal D708
Intraoperative D7083Z0
Neck D703
Intraoperative D7033Z0
Pelvis D707
Intraoperative D7073Z0
Thorax D705
Intraoperative D7053Z0
Mandible DP03
Intraoperative DP033Z0
Maxilla DP02
Intraoperative DP023Z0
Mediastinum DB06
Intraoperative DB063Z0
Mouth D904
Intraoperative D9043Z0
Nasopharynx D90D
Intraoperative D90D3Z0
Neck and Head DW01
Intraoperative DW013Z0
Nerve
Intraoperative D0073Z0
Peripheral D007
Nose D901
Intraoperative D9013Z0
Oropharynx D90F
Intraoperative D90F3Z0
Ovary DU00
Intraoperative DU003Z0
Palate
Hard D908
Intraoperative D9083Z0
Soft D909
Intraoperative D9093Z0
Pancreas DF03
Intraoperative DF033Z0
Parathyroid Gland DG04
Intraoperative DG043Z0
Pelvic Bones DP08
Intraoperative DP083Z0
Pelvic Region DW06
Intraoperative DW063Z0
Pineal Body DG01
Intraoperative DG013Z0
Pituitary Gland DG00
Intraoperative DG003Z0
Pleura DB05
Intraoperative DB053Z0
Prostate DV00
Intraoperative DV003Z0
Radius DP07
Intraoperative DP073Z0
Rectum DD07
Intraoperative DD073Z0
Rib DP05
Intraoperative DP053Z0
Sinuses D907
Intraoperative D9073Z0
Skin
Abdomen DH08
Intraoperative DH083Z0
Arm DH04
Intraoperative DH043Z0
Back DH07
Intraoperative DH073Z0
Buttock DH09
Intraoperative DH093Z0
Chest DH06
Intraoperative DH063Z0
Face DH02
Intraoperative DH023Z0
Leg DH0B
Intraoperative DH0B3Z0
Neck DH03
Intraoperative DH033Z0
Skull DP00
Intraoperative DP003Z0

Beam Radiation *(continued)*
Spinal Cord D006
Intraoperative D0063Z0
Spleen D702
Intraoperative D7023Z0
Sternum DP04
Intraoperative DP043Z0
Stomach DD01
Intraoperative DD013Z0
Testis DV01
Intraoperative DV013Z0
Thymus D701
Intraoperative D7013Z0
Thyroid Gland DG05
Intraoperative DG053Z0
Tibia DP0B
Intraoperative DP0B3Z0
Tongue D905
Intraoperative D9053Z0
Trachea DB00
Intraoperative DB003Z0
Ulna DP07
Intraoperative DP073Z0
Ureter DT01
Intraoperative DT013Z0
Urethra DT03
Intraoperative DT033Z0
Uterus DU02
Intraoperative DU023Z0
Whole Body DW05
Intraoperative DW053Z0
Bedside swallow F00ZJWZ
Berlin Heart Ventricular Assist Device
use Implantable Heart Assist System in Heart and Great Vessels
Bezlotoxumab Monoclonal Antibody XW0
Biceps brachii muscle
use Muscle, Upper Arm, Left
use Muscle, Upper Arm, Right
Biceps femoris muscle
use Muscle, Upper Leg, Left
use Muscle, Upper Leg, Right
Bicipital aponeurosis
use Subcutaneous Tissue and Fascia, Lower Arm, Left
use Subcutaneous Tissue and Fascia, Lower Arm, Right
Bicuspid valve
use Valve, Mitral
Bili light therapy
see Phototherapy, Skin 6A60
Bioactive embolization coil(s)
use Intraluminal Device, Bioactive in Upper Arteries
Biofeedback GZC9ZZZ
Biopsy
see Drainage with qualifier Diagnostic
see Excision with qualifier Diagnostic
see Extraction with qualifier Diagnostic
BiPAP
see Assistance, Respiratory v5A09
Bisection
see Division
Biventricular external heart assist system
use Short-term External Heart Assist System in Heart and Great Vessels
Blepharectomy
see Excision, Eye 08B
see Resection, Eye 08T
Blepharoplasty
see Repair, Eye 08Q
see Replacement, Eye 08R
see Reposition, Eye 08S
see Supplement, Eye 08U
Blepharorrhaphy
see Repair, Eye 08Q
Blepharotomy
see Drainage, Eye 089

Blinatumomab Antineoplastic Immunotherapy XW0
Block, Nerve, anesthetic injection 3E0T3CZ
Blood glucose monitoring system
use Monitoring Device
Blood pressure
see Measurement, Arterial 4A03
BMR (basal metabolic rate)
see Measurement, Physiological Systems 4A0Z
Body of femur
use Femoral Shaft, Left
use Femoral Shaft, Right
Body of fibula
use Fibula, Left
use Fibula, Right
Bone anchored hearing device
use Hearing Device, Bone Conduction in 09H
use Hearing Device in Head and Facia Bones
Bone bank bone graft
use Nonautologous Tissue Substitu
Bone Growth Stimulator
Insertion of device in
Bone
Facial 0NHW
Lower 0QHY
Nasal 0NHB
Upper 0PHY
Skull 0NH0
Removal of device from
Bone
Facial 0NPW
Lower 0QPY
Nasal 0NPB
Upper 0PPY
Skull 0NP0
Revision of device in
Bone
Facial 0NWW
Lower 0QWY
Nasal 0NWB
Upper 0PWY
Skull 0NW0
Bone marrow transplant
see Transfusion, Circulatory 302
Bone morphogenetic protein 2 (BMP
use Recombinant Bone Morphogenetic Protein
Bone screw (interlocking)(lag) (pedicle)(recessed)
use Internal Fixation Device in He and Facial Bones
use Internal Fixation Device in Lower Bones
use Internal Fixation Device in Upp Bones
Bony labyrinth
use Ear, Inner, Left
use Ear, Inner, Right
Bony orbit
use Orbit, Left
use Orbit, Right
Bony vestibule
use Ear, Inner, Left
use Ear, Inner, Right
Botallo's duct
use Artery, Pulmonary, Left
Bovine pericardial valve
use Zooplastic Tissue in Heart and Great Vessels
Bovine pericardium graft
use Zooplastic Tissue in Heart and Great Vessels
BP (blood pressure)
see Measurement, Arterial 4A03
Brachial (lateral) lymph node
use Lymphatic, Axillary, Left
use Lymphatic, Axillary, Right

Brachialis muscle
use Muscle, Upper Arm, Left
use Muscle, Upper Arm, Right
Brachiocephalic artery
use Artery, Innominate
Brachiocephalic trunk
use Artery, Innominate
Brachiocephalic vein
use Vein, Innominate, Left
use Vein, Innominate, Right
Brachioradialis muscle
use Muscle, Lower Arm and Wrist, Left
use Muscle, Lower Arm and Wrist, Right
Brachytherapy
Abdomen DW13
Adrenal Gland DG12
Bile Ducts DF12
Bladder DT12
Bone Marrow D710
Brain D010
Brain Stem D011
Breast
Left DM10
Right DM11
Bronchus DB11
Cervix DU11
Chest DW12
Chest Wall DB17
Colon DD15
Diaphragm DB18
Duodenum DD12
Ear D910
Esophagus DD10
Eye D810
Gallbladder DF11
Gland
Adrenal DG12
Parathyroid DG14
Pituitary DG10
Thyroid DG15
Glands, Salivary D916
Head and Neck DW11
Hypopharynx D913
Ileum DD14
Jejunum DD13
Kidney DT10
Larynx D91B
Liver DF10
Lung DB12
Lymphatics
Abdomen D716
Axillary D714
Inguinal D718
Neck D713
Pelvis D717
Thorax D715
Mediastinum DB16
Mouth D914
Nasopharynx D91D
Neck and Head DW11
Nerve, Peripheral D017
Nose D911
Oropharynx D91F
Ovary DU10
Palate
Hard D918
Soft D919
Pancreas DF13
Parathyroid Gland DG14
Pelvic Region DW16
Pineal Body DG11
Pituitary Gland DG10
Pleura DB15
Prostate DV10
Rectum DD17
Sinuses D917
Spinal Cord D016
Spleen D712
Stomach DD11

Brachytherapy *(continued)*
Testis DV11
Thymus D711
Thyroid Gland DG15
Tongue D915
Trachea DB10
Ureter DT11
Urethra DT13
Uterus DU12
Brachytherapy seeds
use Radioactive Element
Broad ligament
use Uterine Supporting Structure
Bronchial artery
use Upper Artery
Bronchography
see Fluoroscopy, Respiratory System BB1
see Plain Radiography, Respiratory System BB0
Bronchoplasty
see Repair, Respiratory System 0BQ
see Supplement, Respiratory System 0BU
Bronchorrhaphy
see Repair, Respiratory System 0BQ
Bronchoscopy 0BJ08ZZ
Bronchotomy
see Drainage, Respiratory System 0B9
Bronchus Intermedius
use Main Bronchus, Right
BRYAN® Cervical Disc System
use Synthetic Substitute
Buccal gland
use Buccal Mucosa
Buccinator lymph node
use Lymphatic, Head
Buccinator muscle
use Muscle, Facial
Buckling, scleral with implant
see Supplement, Eye 08U
Bulbospongiosus muscle
use Muscle, Perineum
Bulbourethral (Cowper's) gland
use Urethra
Bundle of His
use Conduction Mechanism
Bundle of Kent
use Conduction Mechanism
Bunionectomy
see Excision, Lower Bones 0QB
Bursectomy
see Excision, Bursae and Ligaments 0MB
see Resection, Bursae and Ligaments 0MT
Bursocentesis
see Drainage, Bursae and Ligaments 0M9
Bursography
see Plain Radiography, Non-Axial Upper Bones BP0
see Plain Radiography, Non-Axial Lower Bones BQ0
Bursotomy
see Division, Bursae and Ligaments 0M8
see Drainage, Bursae and Ligaments 0M9
BVS 5000 Ventricular Assist Device
use Short-term External Heart Assist System in Heart and Great Vessels
Bypass
Anterior Chamber
Left 08133
Right 08123
Aorta
Abdominal 0410
Thoracic
Ascending/Arch 021X
Descending 021W

Bypass *(continued)*
Artery
Anterior Tibial
Left 041Q
Right 041P
Axillary
Left 03160
Right 03150
Brachial
Left 03180
Right 03170
Common Carotid
Left 031J0
Right 031H0
Common Iliac
Left 041D
Right 041C
Coronary
Four or More Arteries 0213
One Artery 0210
Three Arteries 0212
Two Arteries 0211
External Carotid
Left 031N0
Right 031M0
External Iliac
Left 041J
Right 041H
Femoral
Left 041L
Right 041K
Foot
Left 041W
Right 041V
Hepatic 0413
Innominate 03120
Internal Carotid
Left 031L0
Right 031K0
Internal Iliac
Left 041F
Right 041E
Intracranial 031G0
Peroneal
Left 041U
Right 041T
Popliteal
Left 041N
Right 041M
Posterior Tibial
Left 041S
Right 041R
Pulmonary
Left 021R
Right 021Q
Pulmonary Trunk 021P
Radial
Left 031C0
Right 031B0
Splenic 0414
Subclavian
Left 03140
Right 03130
Temporal
Left 031T0
Right 031S0
Ulnar
Left 031A0
Right 03190
Atrium
Left 0217
Right 0216
Bladder 0T1B
Cavity, Cranial 0W110J
Cecum 0D1H
Cerebral Ventricle 0016
Colon
Ascending 0D1K
Descending 0D1M
Sigmoid 0D1N
Transverse 0D1L

Bypass *(continued)*
Duct
Common Bile 0F19
Cystic 0F18
Hepatic
Common 0F17
Left 0F16
Right 0F15
Lacrimal
Left 081Y
Right 081X
Pancreatic 0F1D
Accessory 0F1F
Duodenum 0D19
Ear
Left 091E0
Right 091D0
Esophagus 0D15
Lower 0D13
Middle 0D12
Upper 0D11
Fallopian Tube
Left 0U16
Right 0U15
Gallbladder 0F14
Ileum 0D1B
Jejunum 0D1A
Kidney Pelvis
Left 0T14
Right 0T13
Pancreas 0F1G
Pelvic Cavity 0W1J
Peritoneal Cavity 0W1G
Pleural Cavity
Left 0W1B
Right 0W19
Spinal Canal 001U
Stomach 0D16
Trachea 0B11
Ureter
Left 0T17
Right 0T16
Ureters, Bilateral 0T18
Vas Deferens
Bilateral 0V1Q
Left 0V1P
Right 0V1N
Vein
Axillary
Left 0518
Right 0517
Azygos 0510
Basilic
Left 051C
Right 051B
Brachial
Left 051A
Right 0519
Cephalic
Left 051F
Right 051D
Colic 0617
Common Iliac
Left 061D
Right 061C
Esophageal 0613
External Iliac
Left 061G
Right 061F
External Jugular
Left 051Q
Right 051P
Face
Left 051V
Right 051T
Femoral
Left 061N
Right 061M
Foot
Left 061V
Right 061T

Bypass *(continued)*
Vein *(continued)*
Gastric 0612
Hand
Left 051H
Right 051G
Hemiazygos 0511
Hepatic 0614
Hypogastric
Left 061J
Right 061H
Inferior Mesenteric 0616
Innominate
Left 0514
Right 0513
Internal Jugular
Left 051N
Right 051M
Intracranial 051L
Portal 0618
Renal
Left 061B
Right 0619
Saphenous
Left 061Q
Right 061P
Splenic 0611
Subclavian
Left 0516
Right 0515
Superior Mesenteric 0615
Vertebral
Left 051S
Right 051R
Vena Cava
Inferior 0610
Superior 021V
Ventricle
Left 021L
Right 021K
Bypass, cardiopulmonary 5A1221Z

C

Caesarean section
see Extraction, Products of Conception 10D0
Calcaneocuboid joint
use Joint, Tarsal, Left
use Joint, Tarsal, Right
Calcaneocuboid ligament
use Bursa and Ligament, Foot, Left
use Bursa and Ligament, Foot, Right
Calcaneofibular ligament
use Bursa and Ligament, Ankle, Left
use Bursa and Ligament, Ankle, Right
Calcaneus
use Tarsal, Left
use Tarsal, Right
Cannulation
see Bypass
see Dilation
see Drainage
see Irrigation
Canthorrhaphy
see Repair, Eye 08Q
Canthotomy
see Release, Eye 08N
Capitate bone
use Carpal, Left
use Carpal, Right
Capsulectomy, lens
see Excision, Eye 08B
Capsulorrhaphy, joint
see Repair, Lower Joints 0SQ
see Repair, Upper Joints 0RQ
Cardia
use Esophagogastric Junction
Cardiac contractility modulation lead
use Cardiac Lead in Heart and Great Vessels
Cardiac event recorder
use Monitoring Device
Cardiac Lead
Defibrillator
Atrium
Left 02H7
Right 02H6
Pericardium 02HN
Vein, Coronary 02H4
Ventricle
Left 02HL
Right 02HK
Insertion of device in
Atrium
Left 02H7Z
Right 02H6
Pericardium 02HN
Vein, Coronary 02H4
Ventricle
Left 02HL
Right 02HK
Pacemaker
Atrium
Left 02H7
Right 02H6
Pericardium 02HN
Vein, Coronary 02H4
Ventricle
Left 02HL
Right 02HK
Removal of device from, Heart 02PA
Revision of device in, Heart 02WA
Cardiac plexus
use Nerve, Thoracic Sympathetic
Cardiac Resynchronization Defibrillator Pulse Generator
Abdomen 0JH8
Chest 0JH6
Cardiac Resynchronization Pacemaker Pulse Generator
Abdomen 0JH8
Chest 0JH6
Cardiac resynchronization therapy (CRT) lead
use Cardiac Lead, Defibrillator in 02H
use Cardiac Lead, Pacemaker in 02H
Cardiac Rhythm Related Device
Insertion of device in
Abdomen 0JH8
Chest 0JH6
Removal of device from, Subcutaneous Tissue and Fascia, Trunk 0JPT
Revision of device in, Subcutaneous Tissue and Fascia, Trunk 0JWT
Cardiocentesis
see Drainage, Pericardial Cavity 0W9D
Cardioesophageal junction
use Esophagogastric Junction
Cardiolysis
see Release, Heart and Great Vessels 02N
CardioMEMS® pressure sensor
use Monitoring Device, Pressure Sensor in 02H
Cardiomyotomy
see Division, Esophagogastric Junction 0D84
Cardioplegia
see Introduction of substance in or on, Heart 3E08
Cardiorrhaphy
see Repair, Heart and Great Vessels 02Q
Cardioversion 5A2204Z
Caregiver Training F0FZ
Caroticotympanic artery
use Artery, Internal Carotid, Left
use Artery, Internal Carotid, Right
Carotid (artery) sinus (baroreceptor) lead
use Stimulator Lead in Upper Arteries
Carotid glomus
use Carotid Bodies, Bilateral
use Carotid Body, Left
use Carotid Body, Right
Carotid sinus
use Artery, Internal Carotid, Left
use Artery, Internal Carotid, Right
Carotid sinus nerve
use Nerve, Glossopharyngeal
Carotid WALLSTENT® Monorail® Endoprosthesis
use Intraluminal Device
Carpectomy
see Excision, Upper Bones 0PB
see Resection, Upper Bones 0PT
Carpometacarpal ligament
use Bursa and Ligament, Hand, Left
use Bursa and Ligament, Hand, Right
Casting
see Immobilization
CAT scan
see Computerized Tomography (CT Scan)
Catheterization
see Dilation
see Drainage
Heart
see Measurement, Cardiac 4A02
see Irrigation
see Insertion of device in
Umbilical vein, for infusion 06H033T
Cauda equina
use Spinal Cord, Lumbar
Cauterization
see Destruction
see Repair
Cavernous plexus
use Nerve, Head and Neck Sympathetic
CBMA (Concentrated Bone Marrow Aspirate)
use Concentrated Bone Marrow Aspirate
CBMA (Concentrated Bone Marrow Aspirate) injection, intramuscular XK02303
Cecectomy
see Excision, Cecum 0DBH
see Resection, Cecum 0DTH
Cecocolostomy
see Bypass, Gastrointestinal System 0D1
see Drainage, Gastrointestinal System 0D9
Cecopexy
see Repair, Cecum 0DQH
see Reposition, Cecum 0DSH
Cecoplication
see Restriction, Cecum 0DVH
Cecorrhaphy
see Repair, Cecum 0DQH
Cecostomy
see Bypass, Cecum 0D1H
see Drainage, Cecum 0D9H
Cecotomy
see Drainage, Cecum 0D9H
Ceftazidime-Avibactam Anti-infective XW0
Celiac (solar) plexus
use Nerve, Abdominal Sympathetic
Celiac ganglion
use Nerve, Abdominal Sympathetic
Celiac lymph node
use Lymphatic, Aortic
Celiac trunk
use Artery, Celiac
Central axillary lymph node
use Lymphatic, Axillary, Left
use Lymphatic, Axillary, Right
Central venous pressure
see Measurement, Venous 4A04
Centrimag® Blood Pump
use Short-term External Heart As System in Heart and Great Vessels
Cephalogram BN00ZZZ
Ceramic on ceramic bearing surfa
use Synthetic Substitute, Cerami in 0SR
Cerclage
see Restriction
Cerebral aqueduct (Sylvius)
use Cerebral Ventricle
Cerebral Embolic Filtration, Dual Filter X2A5312
Cerebrum
use Brain
Cervical esophagus
use Esophagus, Upper
Cervical facet joint
use Joint, Cervical Vertebral
use Joint, Cervical Vertebral, 2 o more
Cervical ganglion
use Nerve, Head and Neck Sympathetic
Cervical interspinous ligament
use Bursa and Ligament, Head a Neck
Cervical intertransverse ligament
use Bursa and Ligament, Head a Neck
Cervical ligamentum flavum
use Bursa and Ligament, Head a Neck
Cervical lymph node
use Lymphatic, Neck, Left
use Lymphatic, Neck, Right
Cervicectomy
see Excision, Cervix 0UBC
see Resection, Cervix 0UTC
Cervicothoracic facet joint
use Joint, Cervicothoracic Vertebral
Cesarean section
see Extraction, Products of Conception 10D0
Cesium-131 Collagen Implant
use Radioactive Element, Cesium-131 Collagen Impla in 00H
Change device in
Abdominal Wall 0W2FX
Back
Lower 0W2LX
Upper 0W2KX
Bladder 0T2BX
Bone
Facial 0N2WX
Lower 0Q2YX
Nasal 0N2BX
Upper 0P2YX
Bone Marrow 072TX
Brain 0020X
Breast
Left 0H2UX
Right 0H2TX
Bursa and Ligament
Lower 0M2YX
Upper 0M2XX
Cavity, Cranial 0W21X
Chest Wall 0W28X

Change device in *(continued)*
Cisterna Chyli 072LX
Diaphragm 0B2TX
Duct
Hepatobiliary 0F2BX
Pancreatic 0F2DX
Ear
Left 092JX
Right 092HX
Epididymis and Spermatic Cord 0V2MX
Extremity
Lower
Left 0Y2BX
Right 0Y29X
Upper
Left 0X27X
Right 0X26X
Eye
Left 0821X
Right 0820X
Face 0W22X
Fallopian Tube 0U28X
Gallbladder 0F24X
Gland
Adrenal 0G25X
Endocrine 0G2SX
Pituitary 0G20X
Salivary 0C2AX
Head 0W20X
Intestinal Tract
Lower 0D2DXUZ
Upper 0D20XUZ
Jaw
Lower 0W25X
Upper 0W24X
Joint
Lower 0S2YX
Upper 0R2YX
Kidney 0T25X
Larynx 0C2SX
Liver 0F20X
Lung
Left 0B2LX
Right 0B2KX
Lymphatic 072NX
Thoracic Duct 072KX
Mediastinum 0W2CX
Mesentery 0D2VX
Mouth and Throat 0C2YX
Muscle
Lower 0K2YX
Upper 0K2XX
Nasal Mucosa and Soft Tissue 092KX
Neck 0W26X
Nerve
Cranial 002EX
Peripheral 012YX
Omentum 0D2UX
Ovary 0U23X
Pancreas 0F2GX
Parathyroid Gland 0G2RX
Pelvic Cavity 0W2JX
Penis 0V2SX
Pericardial Cavity 0W2DX
Perineum
Female 0W2NX
Male 0W2MX
Peritoneal Cavity 0W2GX
Peritoneum 0D2WX
Pineal Body 0G21X
Pleura 0B2QX
Pleural Cavity
Left 0W2BX
Right 0W29X
Products of Conception 10207
Prostate and Seminal Vesicles 0V24X
Retroperitoneum 0W2HX

Change device in *(continued)*
Scrotum and Tunica Vaginalis 0V28X
Sinus 092YX
Skin 0H2PX
Skull 0N20X
Spinal Canal 002UX
Spleen 072PX
Subcutaneous Tissue and Fascia
Head and Neck 0J2SX
Lower Extremity 0J2WX
Trunk 0J2TX
Upper Extremity 0J2VX
Tendon
Lower 0L2YX
Upper 0L2XX
Testis 0V2DX
Thymus 072MX
Thyroid Gland 0G2KX
Trachea 0B21
Tracheobronchial Tree 0B20X
Ureter 0T29X
Urethra 0T2DX
Uterus and Cervix 0U2DXHZ
Vagina and Cul-de-sac 0U2HXGZ
Vas Deferens 0V2RX
Vulva 0U2MX
Change device in or on
Abdominal Wall 2W03X
Anorectal 2Y03X5Z
Arm
Lower
Left 2W0DX
Right 2W0CX
Upper
Left 2W0BX
Right 2W0AX
Back 2W05X
Chest Wall 2W04X
Ear 2Y02X5Z
Extremity
Lower
Left 2W0MX
Right 2W0LX
Upper
Left 2W09X
Right 2W08X
Face 2W01X
Finger
Left 2W0KX
Right 2W0JX
Foot
Left 2W0TX
Right 2W0SX
Genital Tract, Female 2Y04X5Z
Hand
Left 2W0FX
Right 2W0EX
Head 2W00X
Inguinal Region
Left 2W07X
Right 2W06X
Leg
Lower
Left 2W0RX
Right 2W0QX
Upper
Left 2W0PX
Right 2W0NX
Mouth and Pharynx 2Y00X5Z
Nasal 2Y01X5Z
Neck 2W02X
Thumb
Left 2W0HX
Right 2W0GX
Toe
Left 2W0VX
Right 2W0UX
Urethra 2Y05X5Z

Chemoembolization
see Introduction of substance in or on
Chemosurgery, Skin 3E00XTZ
Chemothalamectomy
see Destruction, Thalamus 0059
Chemotherapy, Infusion for cancer
see Introduction of substance in or on
Chest x-ray
see Plain Radiography, Chest BW03
Chiropractic Manipulation
Abdomen 9WB9X
Cervical 9WB1X
Extremities
Lower 9WB6X
Upper 9WB7X
Head 9WB0X
Lumbar 9WB3X
Pelvis 9WB5X
Rib Cage 9WB8X
Sacrum 9WB4X
Thoracic 9WB2X
Choana
use Nasopharynx
Cholangiogram
see Plain Radiography, Hepatobiliary System and Pancreas BF0
see Fluoroscopy, Hepatobiliary System and Pancreas BF1
Cholecystectomy
see Excision, Gallbladder 0FB4
see Resection, Gallbladder 0FT4
Cholecystojejunostomy
see Bypass, Hepatobiliary System and Pancreas 0F1
see Drainage, Hepatobiliary System and Pancreas 0F9
Cholecystopexy
see Repair, Gallbladder 0FQ4
see Reposition, Gallbladder 0FS4
Cholecystoscopy 0FJ44ZZ
Cholecystostomy
see Drainage, Gallbladder 0F94
see Bypass, Gallbladder 0F14
Cholecystotomy
see Drainage, Gallbladder 0F94
Choledochectomy
see Excision, Hepatobiliary System and Pancreas 0FB
see Resection, Hepatobiliary System and Pancreas 0FT
Choledocholithotomy
see Extirpation, Duct, Common Bile 0FC9
Choledochoplasty
see Repair, Hepatobiliary System and Pancreas 0FQ
see Replacement, Hepatobiliary System and Pancreas 0FR
see Supplement, Hepatobiliary System and Pancreas 0FU
Choledochoscopy 0FJB8ZZ
Choledochotomy
see Drainage, Hepatobiliary System and Pancreas 0F9
Cholelithotomy
see Extirpation, Hepatobiliary System and Pancreas 0FC
Chondrectomy
see Excision, Lower Joints 0SB
see Excision, Upper Joints 0RB
Knee
see Excision, Lower Joints 0SB
Semilunar cartilage
see Excision, Lower Joints 0SB
Chondroglossus muscle
use Muscle, Tongue, Palate, Pharynx

Chorda tympani
use Nerve, Facial
Chordotomy
see Division, Central Nervous System and Cranial Nerves 008
Choroid plexus
use Cerebral Ventricle
Choroidectomy
see Excision, Eye 08B
see Resection, Eye 08T
Ciliary body
use Eye, Left
use Eye, Right
Ciliary ganglion
use Nerve, Head and Neck Sympathetic
Circle of Willis
use Artery, Intracranial
Circumcision 0VTTXZZ
Circumflex iliac artery
use Artery, Femoral, Left
use Artery, Femoral, Right
Clamp and rod internal fixation system (CRIF)
use Internal Fixation Device in Lower Bones
use Internal Fixation Device in Upper Bones
Clamping
see Occlusion
Claustrum
use Basal Ganglia
Claviculectomy
see Excision, Upper Bones 0PB
see Resection, Upper Bones 0PT
Claviculotomy
see Division, Upper Bones 0P8
see Drainage, Upper Bones 0P9
Clipping, aneurysm
see Occlusion using Extraluminal Device
see Restriction using Extraluminal Device
Clitorectomy, clitoridectomy
see Excision, Clitoris 0UBJ
see Resection, Clitoris 0UTJ
Clolar
use Clofarabine
Closure
see Occlusion
see Repair
Clysis
see Introduction of substance in or on
Coagulation
see Destruction
COALESCE® radiolucent interbody fusion device
use Interbody Fusion Device, Radiolucent Porous in New Technology
CoAxia NeuroFlo catheter
use Intraluminal Device
Cobalt/chromium head and polyethylene socket
use Synthetic Substitute, Metal on Polyethylene in 0SR
Cobalt/chromium head and socket
use Synthetic Substitute, Metal in 0SR
Coccygeal body
use Coccygeal Glomus
Coccygeus muscle
use Muscle, Trunk, Left
use Muscle, Trunk, Right
Cochlea
use Ear, Inner, Left
use Ear, Inner, Right

Cochlear implant (CI), multiple channel (electrode)
  use Hearing Device, Multiple Channel Cochlear Prosthesis in 09H
Cochlear implant (CI), single channel (electrode)
  use Hearing Device, Single Channel Cochlear Prosthesis in 09H
Cochlear Implant Treatment F0BZ0
Cochlear nerve
  use Nerve, Acoustic
COGNIS® CRT-D
  use Cardiac Resynchronization Defibrillator Pulse Generator in 0JH
COHERE® radiolucent interbody fusion device
  use Interbody Fusion Device, Radiolucent Porous in New Technology
Colectomy
  see Excision, Gastrointestinal System 0DB
  see Resection, Gastrointestinal System 0DT
Collapse
  see Occlusion
Collection from
  Breast, Breast Milk 8E0HX62
  Indwelling Device
    Circulatory System
      Blood 8C02X6K
      Other Fluid 8C02X6L
    Nervous System
      Cerebrospinal Fluid 8C01X6J
      Other Fluid 8C01X6L
  Integumentary System, Breast Milk 8E0HX62
  Reproductive System, Male, Sperm 8E0VX63
Colocentesis
  see Drainage, Gastrointestinal System 0D9
Colofixation
  see Repair, Gastrointestinal System 0DQ
  see Reposition, Gastrointestinal System 0DS
Cololysis
  see Release, Gastrointestinal System 0DN
Colonic Z-Stent®
  use Intraluminal Device
Colonoscopy 0DJD8ZZ
Colopexy
  see Repair, Gastrointestinal System 0DQ
  see Reposition, Gastrointestinal System 0DS
Coloplication
  see Restriction, Gastrointestinal System 0DV
Coloproctectomy
  see Excision, Gastrointestinal System 0DB
  see Resection, Gastrointestinal System 0DT
Coloproctostomy
  see Bypass, Gastrointestinal System 0D1
  see Drainage, Gastrointestinal System 0D9
Colopuncture
  see Drainage, Gastrointestinal System 0D9
Colorrhaphy
  see Repair, Gastrointestinal System 0DQ
Colostomy
  see Bypass, Gastrointestinal System 0D1
  see Drainage, Gastrointestinal System 0D9
Colpectomy
  see Excision, Vagina 0UBG
  see Resection, Vagina 0UTG
Colpocentesis
  see Drainage, Vagina 0U9G
Colpopexy
  see Repair, Vagina 0UQG
  see Reposition, Vagina 0USG
Colpoplasty
  see Repair, Vagina 0UQG
  see Supplement, Vagina 0UUG
Colporrhaphy
  see Repair, Vagina 0UQG
Colposcopy 0UJH8ZZ
Columella
  use Nasal Mucosa and Soft Tissue
Common digital vein
  use Vein, Foot, Left
  use Vein, Foot, Right
Common facial vein
  use Vein, Face, Left
  use Vein, Face, Right
Common fibular nerve
  use Nerve, Peroneal
Common hepatic artery
  use Artery, Hepatic
Common iliac (subaortic) lymph node
  use Lymphatic, Pelvis
Common interosseous artery
  use Artery, Ulnar, Left
  use Artery, Ulnar, Right
Common peroneal nerve
  use Nerve, Peroneal
Complete (SE) stent
  use Intraluminal Device
Compression
  see Restriction
  Abdominal Wall 2W13X
  Arm
    Lower
      Left 2W1DX
      Right 2W1CX
    Upper
      Left 2W1BX
      Right 2W1AX
  Back 2W15X
  Chest Wall 2W14X
  Extremity
    Lower
      Left 2W1MX
      Right 2W1LX
    Upper
      Left 2W19X
      Right 2W18X
  Face 2W11X
  Finger
    Left 2W1KX
    Right 2W1JX
  Foot
    Left 2W1TX
    Right 2W1SX
  Hand
    Left 2W1FX
    Right 2W1EX
  Head 2W10X
  Inguinal Region
    Left 2W17X
    Right 2W16X
  Leg
    Lower
      Left 2W1RX
      Right 2W1QX
Compression *(continued)*
  Leg *(continued)*
    Upper
      Left 2W1PX
      Right 2W1NX
  Neck 2W12X
  Thumb
    Left 2W1HX
    Right 2W1GX
  Toe
    Left 2W1VX
    Right 2W1UX
Computer Assisted Procedure
  Extremity
    Lower
      No Qualifier 8E0YXBZ
      With Computerized Tomography 8E0YXBG
      With Fluoroscopy 8E0YXBF
      With Magnetic Resonance Imaging 8E0YXBH
    Upper
      No Qualifier 8E0XXBZ
      With Computerized Tomography 8E0XXBG
      With Fluoroscopy 8E0XXBF
      With Magnetic Resonance Imaging 8E0XXBH
  Head and Neck Region
    No Qualifier 8E09XBZ
    With Computerized Tomography 8E09XBG
    With Fluoroscopy 8E09XBF
    With Magnetic Resonance Imaging 8E09XBH
  Trunk Region
    No Qualifier 8E0WXBZ
    With Computerized Tomography 8E0WXBG
    With Fluoroscopy 8E0WXBF
    With Magnetic Resonance Imaging 8E0WXBH
Computerized Tomography (CT Scan)
  Abdomen BW20
    Chest and Pelvis BW25
  Abdomen and Chest BW24
  Abdomen and Pelvis BW21
  Airway, Trachea BB2F
  Ankle
    Left BQ2H
    Right BQ2G
  Aorta
    Abdominal B420
      Intravascular Optical Coherence B420Z2Z
    Thoracic B320
      Intravascular Optical Coherence B320Z2Z
  Arm
    Left BP2F
    Right BP2E
  Artery
    Celiac B421
      Intravascular Optical Coherence B421Z2Z
    Common Carotid
      Bilateral B325
      Intravascular Optical Coherence B325Z2Z
    Coronary
      Bypass Graft
        Multiple B223
        Intravascular Optical Coherence B223Z2Z
      Multiple B221
        Intravascular Optical Coherence B221Z2Z
Computerized Tomography (CT Scan) *(continued)*
  Artery *(continued)*
    Internal Carotid
      Bilateral B328
        Intravascular Optical Coherence B328Z2Z
    Intracranial B32R
      Intravascular Optical Coherence B32RZ2Z
    Lower Extremity
      Bilateral B42H
        Intravascular Optical Coherence B42HZ2Z
      Left B42G
        Intravascular Optical Coherence B42GZ2Z
      Right B42F
        Intravascular Optical Coherence B42FZ2Z
    Pelvic B42C
      Intravascular Optical Coherence B42CZ2Z
    Pulmonary
      Left B32T
        Intravascular Optical Coherence B32TZ2Z
      Right B32S
        Intravascular Optical Coherence B32SZ2Z
    Renal
      Bilateral B428
        Intravascular Optical Coherence B428Z2Z
      Transplant B42M
        Intravascular Optical Coherence B42MZ2Z
    Superior Mesenteric B424
      Intravascular Optical Coherence B424Z2Z
    Vertebral
      Bilateral B32G
      Intravascular Optical Coherence B32GZ2Z
  Bladder BT20
  Bone
    Facial BN25
    Temporal BN2F
  Brain B020
  Calcaneus
    Left BQ2K
    Right BQ2J
  Cerebral Ventricle B028
  Chest, Abdomen and Pelvis BW25
  Chest and Abdomen BW24
  Cisterna B027
  Clavicle
    Left BP25
    Right BP24
  Coccyx BR2F
  Colon BD24
  Ear B920
  Elbow
    Left BP2H
    Right BP2G
  Extremity
    Lower
      Left BQ2S
      Right BQ2R
    Upper
      Bilateral BP2V
      Left BP2U
      Right BP2T
  Eye
    Bilateral B827
    Left B826
    Right B825

Computerized Tomography (CT Scan) *(continued)*
Femur
Left BQ24
Right BQ23
Fibula
Left BQ2C
Right BQ2B
Finger
Left BP2S
Right BP2R
Foot
Left BQ2M
Right BQ2L
Forearm
Left BP2K
Right BP2J
Gland
Adrenal, Bilateral BG22
Parathyroid BG23
Parotid, Bilateral B926
Salivary, Bilateral B92D
Submandibular, Bilateral B929
Thyroid BG24
Hand
Left BP2P
Right BP2N
Hands and Wrists, Bilateral BP2Q
Head BW28
Head and Neck BW29
Heart
Intravascular Optical Coherence B226Z2Z
Right and Left B226
Hepatobiliary System, All BF2C
Hip
Left BQ21
Right BQ20
Humerus
Left BP2B
Right BP2A
Intracranial Sinus B522
Intravascular Optical Coherence B522Z2Z
Joint
Acromioclavicular, Bilateral BP23
Finger
Left BP2DZZZ
Right BP2CZZZ
Foot
Left BQ2Y
Right BQ2X
Hand
Left BP2DZZZ
Right BP2CZZZ
Sacroiliac BR2D
Sternoclavicular
Bilateral BP22
Left BP21
Right BP20
Temporomandibular, Bilateral BN29
Toe
Left BQ2Y
Right BQ2X
Kidney
Bilateral BT23
Left BT22
Right BT21
Transplant BT29
Knee
Left BQ28
Right BQ27
Larynx B92J
Leg
Left BQ2F
Right BQ2D
Liver BF25

Computerized Tomography (CT Scan) *(continued)*
Liver and Spleen BF26
Lung, Bilateral BB24
Mandible BN26
Nasopharynx B92F
Neck BW2F
Neck and Head BW29
Orbit, Bilateral BN23
Oropharynx B92F
Pancreas BF27
Patella
Left BQ2W
Right BQ2V
Pelvic Region BW2G
Pelvis BR2C
Chest and Abdomen BW25
Pelvis and Abdomen BW21
Pituitary Gland B029
Prostate BV23
Ribs
Left BP2Y
Right BP2X
Sacrum BR2F
Scapula
Left BP27
Right BP26
Sella Turcica B029
Shoulder
Left BP29
Right BP28
Sinus
Intracranial B522
Intravascular Optical Coherence B522Z2Z
Paranasal B922
Skull BN20
Spinal Cord B02B
Spine
Cervical BR20
Lumbar BR29
Thoracic BR27
Spleen and Liver BF26
Thorax BP2W
Tibia
Left BQ2C
Right BQ2B
Toe
Left BQ2Q
Right BQ2P
Trachea BB2F
Tracheobronchial Tree
Bilateral BB29
Left BB28
Right BB27
Vein
Pelvic (Iliac)
Left B52G
Intravascular Optical Coherence B52GZ2Z
Right B52F
Intravascular Optical Coherence B52FZ2Z
Pelvic (Iliac) Bilateral B52H
Intravascular Optical Coherence B52HZ2Z
Portal B52T
Intravascular Optical Coherence B52TZ2Z
Pulmonary
Bilateral B52S
Intravascular Optical Coherence B52SZ2Z
Left B52R
Intravascular Optical Coherence B52RZ2Z

Computerized Tomography (CT Scan) *(continued)*
Vein *(continued)*
Pulmonary *(continued)*
Right B52Q
Intravascular Optical Coherence B52QZ2Z
Renal
Bilateral B52L
Intravascular Optical Coherence B52LZ2Z
Left B52K
Intravascular Optical Coherence B52KZ2Z
Right B52J
Intravascular Optical Coherence B52JZ2Z
Spanchnic B52T
Intravascular Optical Coherence B52TZ2Z
Vena Cava
Inferior B529
Intravascular Optical Coherence B529Z2Z
Superior B528
Intravascular Optical Coherence B528Z2Z
Ventricle, Cerebral B028
Wrist
Left BP2M
Right BP2L
Concentrated Bone Marrow Aspirate (CBMA) injection, intramuscular XK02303
Concerto II CRT-D
use Cardiac Resynchronization Defibrillator Pulse Generator in 0JH
Condylectomy
see Excision, Head and Facial Bones 0NB
see Excision, Lower Bones 0QB
see Excision, Upper Bones 0PB
Condyloid process
use Mandible, Left
use Mandible, Right
Condylotomy
see Division, Head and Facial Bones 0N8
see Division, Lower Bones 0Q8
see Division, Upper Bones 0P8
see Drainage, Head and Facial Bones 0N9
see Drainage, Lower Bones 0Q9
see Drainage, Upper Bones 0P9
Condylysis
see Release, Head and Facial Bones 0NN
see Release, Lower Bones 0QN
see Release, Upper Bones 0PN
Conization, cervix
see Excision, Cervix 0UBC
Conjunctivoplasty
see Repair, Eye 08Q
see Replacement, Eye 08R
CONSERVE® PLUS Total Resurfacing Hip System
use Resurfacing Device in Lower Joints
Construction
Auricle, ear
see Bypass, Urinary System 0T1
Ileal conduit
see Replacement, Ear, Nose, Sinus 09R

Consulta CRT-D
use Cardiac Resynchronization Defibrillator Pulse Generator in 0JH
Consulta CRT-P
use Cardiac Resynchronization Pacemaker Pulse Generator in 0JH
Contact Radiation
Abdomen DWY37ZZ
Adrenal Gland DGY27ZZ
Bile Ducts DFY27ZZ
Bladder DTY27ZZ
Bone, Other DPYC7ZZ
Brain D0Y07ZZ
Brain Stem D0Y17ZZ
Breast
Left DMY07ZZ
Right DMY17ZZ
Bronchus DBY17ZZ
Cervix DUY17ZZ
Chest DWY27ZZ
Chest Wall DBY77ZZ
Colon DDY57ZZ
Diaphragm DBY87ZZ
Duodenum DDY27ZZ
Ear D9Y07ZZ
Esophagus DDY07ZZ
Eye D8Y07ZZ
Femur DPY97ZZ
Fibula DPYB7ZZ
Gallbladder DFY17ZZ
Gland
Adrenal DGY27ZZ
Parathyroid DGY47ZZ
Pituitary DGY07ZZ
Thyroid DGY57ZZ
Glands, Salivary D9Y67ZZ
Head and Neck DWY17ZZ
Hemibody DWY47ZZ
Humerus DPY67ZZ
Hypopharynx D9Y37ZZ
Ileum DDY47ZZ
Jejunum DDY37ZZ
Kidney DTY07ZZ
Larynx D9YB7ZZ
Liver DFY07ZZ
Lung DBY27ZZ
Mandible DPY37ZZ
Maxilla DPY27ZZ
Mediastinum DBY67ZZ
Mouth D9Y47ZZ
Nasopharynx D9YD7ZZ
Neck and Head DWY17ZZ
Nerve, Peripheral D0Y77ZZ
Nose D9Y17ZZ
Oropharynx D9YF7ZZ
Ovary DUY07ZZ
Palate
Hard D9Y87ZZ
Soft D9Y97ZZ
Pancreas DFY37ZZ
Parathyroid Gland DGY47ZZ
Pelvic Bones DPY87ZZ
Pelvic Region DWY67ZZ
Pineal Body DGY17ZZ
Pituitary Gland DGY07ZZ
Pleura DBY57ZZ
Prostate DVY07ZZ
Radius DPY77ZZ
Rectum DDY77ZZ
Rib DPY57ZZ
Sinuses D9Y77ZZ
Skin
Abdomen DHY87ZZ
Arm DHY47ZZ
Back DHY77ZZ
Buttock DHY97ZZ
Chest DHY67ZZ
Face DHY27ZZ

Contact Radiation *(continued)*
Skin *(continued)*
Leg DHYB7ZZ
Neck DHY37ZZ
Skull DPY07ZZ
Spinal Cord D0Y67ZZ
Sternum DPY47ZZ
Stomach DDY17ZZ
Testis DVY17ZZ
Thyroid Gland DGY57ZZ
Tibia DPYB7ZZ
Tongue D9Y57ZZ
Trachea DBY07ZZ
Ulna DPY77ZZ
Ureter DTY17ZZ
Urethra DTY37ZZ
Uterus DUY27ZZ
Whole Body DWY57ZZ
CONTAK RENEWAL® 3 RF (HE) CRT-D
use Cardiac Resynchronization Defibrillator Pulse Generator in 0JH
Contegra Pulmonary Valved Conduit
use Zooplastic Tissue in Heart and Great Vessels
Continuous Glucose Monitoring (CGM) device
use Monitoring Device
Continuous Negative Airway Pressure
24-96 Consecutive Hours, Ventilation 5A09459
Greater than 96 Consecutive Hours, Ventilation 5A09559
Less than 24 Consecutive Hours, Ventilation 5A09359
Continuous Positive Airway Pressure
24-96 Consecutive Hours, Ventilation 5A09457
Greater than 96 Consecutive Hours, Ventilation 5A09557
Less than 24 Consecutive Hours, Ventilation 5A09357
Continuous renal replacement therapy (CRRT) 5A1D90Z
Contraceptive Device
Change device in, Uterus and Cervix 0U2DXHZ
Insertion of device in
Cervix 0UHC
Subcutaneous Tissue and Fascia
Abdomen 0JH8
Chest 0JH6
Lower Arm
Left 0JHH
Right 0JHG
Lower Leg
Left 0JHP
Right 0JHN
Upper Arm
Left 0JHF
Right 0JHD
Upper Leg
Left 0JHM
Right 0JHL
Uterus 0UH9
Removal of device from
Subcutaneous Tissue and Fascia
Lower Extremity 0JPW
Trunk 0JPT
Upper Extremity 0JPV
Uterus and Cervix 0UPD
Revision of device in
Subcutaneous Tissue and Fascia
Lower Extremity 0JWW
Trunk 0JWT
Upper Extremity 0JWV
Uterus and Cervix 0UWD
Contractility Modulation Device
Abdomen 0JH8
Chest 0JH6
Control, Epistaxis
see Control bleeding in, Nasal Mucosa and Soft Tissue 093K
Control bleeding in
Abdominal Wall 0W3F
Ankle Region
Left 0Y3L
Right 0Y3K
Arm
Lower
Left 0X3F
Right 0X3D
Upper
Left 0X39
Right 0X38
Axilla
Left 0X35
Right 0X34
Back
Lower 0W3L
Upper 0W3K
Buttock
Left 0Y31
Right 0Y30
Cavity, Cranial 0W31
Chest Wall 0W38
Elbow Region
Left 0X3C
Right 0X3B
Extremity
Lower
Left 0Y3B
Right 0Y39
Upper
Left 0X37
Right 0X36
Face 0W32
Femoral Region
Left 0Y38
Right 0Y37
Foot
Left 0Y3N
Right 0Y3M
Gastrointestinal Tract 0W3P
Genitourinary Tract 0W3R
Hand
Left 0X3K
Right 0X3J
Head 0W30
Inguinal Region
Left 0Y36
Right 0Y35
Jaw
Lower 0W35
Upper 0W34
Knee Region
Left 0Y3G
Right 0Y3F
Leg
Lower
Left 0Y3J
Right 0Y3H
Upper
Left 0Y3D
Right 0Y3C
Mediastinum 0W3C
Nasal Mucosa and Soft Tissue 093K
Neck 0W36
Oral Cavity and Throat 0W33
Pelvic Cavity 0W3J
Pericardial Cavity 0W3D
Perineum
Female 0W3N
Male 0W3M
Peritoneal Cavity 0W3G
Pleural Cavity
Left 0W3B
Right 0W39
Control bleeding in *(continued)*
Respiratory Tract 0W3Q
Retroperitoneum 0W3H
Shoulder Region
Left 0X33
Right 0X32
Wrist Region
Left 0X3H
Right 0X3G
Conus arteriosus
use Ventricle, Right
Conus medullaris
use Spinal Cord, Lumbar
Conversion
Cardiac rhythm 5A2204Z
Gastrostomy to jejunostomy feeding device
see Insertion of device in, Jejunum 0DHA
Cook Biodesign® Fistula Plug(s)
use Nonautologous Tissue Substitute
Cook Biodesign® Hernia Graft(s)
use Nonautologous Tissue Substitute
Cook Biodesign® Layered Graft(s)
use Nonautologous Tissue Substitute
Cook Zenapro™ Layered Graft(s)
use Nonautologous Tissue Substitute
Cook Zenith AAA Endovascular Graft
use Intraluminal Device
use Intraluminal Device, Branched or Fenestrated, One or Two Arteries in 04V
use Intraluminal Device, Branched or Fenestrated, Three or More Arteries in 04V
Coracoacromial ligament
use Bursa and Ligament, Shoulder, Left
use Bursa and Ligament, Shoulder, Right
Coracobrachialis muscle
use Muscle, Upper Arm, Left
use Muscle, Upper Arm, Right
Coracoclavicular ligament
use Bursa and Ligament, Shoulder, Left
use Bursa and Ligament, Shoulder, Right
Coracohumeral ligament
use Bursa and Ligament, Shoulder, Left
use Bursa and Ligament, Shoulder, Right
Coracoid process
use Scapula, Left
use Scapula, Right
Cordotomy
see Division, Central Nervous System and Cranial Nerves 008
Core needle biopsy
see Excision with qualifier Diagnostic
CoreValve transcatheter aortic valve
use Zooplastic Tissue in Heart and Great Vessels
Cormet Hip Resurfacing System
use Resurfacing Device in Lower Joints
Corniculate cartilage
use Larynx
CoRoent® XL
use Interbody Fusion Device in Lower Joints
Coronary arteriography
see Fluoroscopy, Heart B21
see Plain Radiography, Heart B20
Corox (OTW) Bipolar Lead
use Cardiac Lead, Defibrillator in 02H
use Cardiac Lead, Pacemaker in 02H
Corpus callosum
use Brain
Corpus cavernosum
use Penis
Corpus spongiosum
use Penis
Corpus striatum
use Basal Ganglia
Corrugator supercilii muscle
use Muscle, Facial
Cortical strip neurostimulator lead
use Neurostimulator Lead in Centr[al] Nervous System and Cranial Nerves
Costatectomy
see Excision, Upper Bones 0PB
see Resection, Upper Bones 0PT
Costectomy
see Excision, Upper Bones 0PB
see Resection, Upper Bones 0PT
Costocervical trunk
use Artery, Subclavian, Left
use Artery, Subclavian, Right
Costochondrectomy
see Excision, Upper Bones 0PB
see Resection, Upper Bones 0PT
Costoclavicular ligament
use Bursa and Ligament, Shoulder, Left
use Bursa and Ligament, Shoulder, Right
Costosternoplasty
see Repair, Upper Bones 0PQ
see Replacement, Upper Bones 0PR
see Supplement, Upper Bones 0PU
Costotomy
see Division, Upper Bones 0P8
see Drainage, Upper Bones 0P9
Costotransverse joint
use Joint, Thoracic Vertebral
Costotransverse ligament
use Rib(s) Bursa and Ligament
Costovertebral joint
use Joint, Thoracic Vertebral
Costoxiphoid ligament
use Sternum Bursa and Ligament
Counseling
Family, for substance abuse, Other Family Counseling HZ63ZZZ
Group
12-Step HZ43ZZZ
Behavioral HZ41ZZZ
Cognitive HZ40ZZZ
Cognitive-Behavioral HZ42ZZZ
Confrontational HZ48ZZZ
Continuing Care HZ49ZZZ
Infectious Disease
Post-Test HZ4CZZZ
Pre-Test HZ4CZZZ
Interpersonal HZ44ZZZ
Motivational Enhancement HZ47ZZZ
Psychoeducation HZ46ZZZ
Spiritual HZ4BZZZ
Vocational HZ45ZZZ
Individual
12-Step HZ33ZZZ
Behavioral HZ31ZZZ
Cognitive HZ30ZZZ
Cognitive-Behavioral HZ32ZZZ
Confrontational HZ38ZZZ
Continuing Care HZ39ZZZ
Infectious Disease
Post-Test HZ3CZZZ
Pre-Test HZ3CZZZ
Interpersonal HZ34ZZZ
Motivational Enhancement HZ37ZZZ
Psychoeducation HZ36ZZZ

Counseling *(continued)*
Individual *(continued)*
Spiritual HZ3BZZZ
Vocational HZ35ZZZ
Mental Health Services
Educational GZ60ZZZ
Other Counseling GZ63ZZZ
Vocational GZ61ZZZ
Countershock, cardiac 5A2204Z
Cowper's (bulbourethral) gland
use Urethra
CPAP (continuous positive airway pressure)
see Assistance, Respiratory 5A09
Craniectomy
see Excision, Head and Facial Bones 0NB
see Resection, Head and Facial Bones 0NT
Cranioplasty
see Repair, Head and Facial Bones 0NQ
see Replacement, Head and Facial Bones 0NR
see Supplement, Head and Facial Bones 0NU
Craniotomy
see Drainage, Central Nervous System and Cranial Nerves 009
see Division, Head and Facial Bones 0N8
see Drainage, Head and Facial Bones 0N9
reation
Perineum
Female 0W4N0
Male 0W4M0
Valve
Aortic 024F0
Mitral 024G0
Tricuspid 024J0
remaster muscle
use Muscle, Perineum
ribriform plate
use Bone, Ethmoid, Left
use Bone, Ethmoid, Right
ricoid cartilage
use Trachea
ricoidectomy
see Excision, Larynx 0CBS
ricothyroid artery
use Artery, Thyroid, Left
use Artery, Thyroid, Right
ricothyroid muscle
use Muscle, Neck, Left
use Muscle, Neck, Right
risis Intervention GZ2ZZZZ
RRT (Continuous renal replacement therapy) 5A1D90Z
rural fascia
use Subcutaneous Tissue and Fascia, Upper Leg, Left
use Subcutaneous Tissue and Fascia, Upper Leg, Right
rushing, nerve
Cranial
see Destruction, Central Nervous System and Cranial Nerves 005
Peripheral
see Destruction, Peripheral Nervous System 015
yoablation
see Destruction
yotherapy
see Destruction
yptorchidectomy
see Excision, Male Reproductive System 0VB
see Resection, Male Reproductive System 0VT
Cryptorchiectomy
see Excision, Male Reproductive System 0VB
see Resection, Male Reproductive System 0VT
Cryptotomy
see Division, Gastrointestinal System 0D8
see Drainage, Gastrointestinal System 0D9
CT scan
see Computerized Tomography (CT Scan)
CT sialogram
see Computerized Tomography (CT Scan), Ear, Nose, Mouth and Throat B92
Cubital lymph node
use Lymphatic, Upper Extremity, Left
use Lymphatic, Upper Extremity, Right
Cubital nerve
use Nerve, Ulnar
Cuboid bone
use Tarsal, Left
use Tarsal, Right
Cuboideonavicular joint
use Joint, Tarsal, Left
use Joint, Tarsal, Right
Culdocentesis
see Drainage, Cul-de-sac 0U9F
Culdoplasty
see Repair, Cul-de-sac 0UQF
see Supplement, Cul-de-sac 0UUF
Culdoscopy 0UJH8ZZ
Culdotomy
see Drainage, Cul-de-sac 0U9F
Culmen
use Cerebellum
Cultured epidermal cell autograft
use Autologous Tissue Substitute
Cuneiform cartilage
use Larynx
Cuneonavicular joint
use Joint, Tarsal, Left
use Joint, Tarsal, Right
Cuneonavicular ligament
use Bursa and Ligament, Foot, Left
use Bursa and Ligament, Foot, Right
Curettage
see Excision
see Extraction
Cutaneous (transverse) cervical nerve
use Nerve, Cervical Plexus
CVP (central venous pressure)
see Measurement, Venous 4A04
Cyclodiathermy
see Destruction, Eye 085
Cyclophotocoagulation
see Destruction, Eye 085
CYPHER® Stent
use Intraluminal Device, Drug-eluting in Heart and Great Vessels
Cystectomy
see Excision, Bladder 0TBB
see Resection, Bladder 0TTB
Cystocele repair
see Repair, Subcutaneous Tissue and Fascia, Pelvic Region 0JQC
Cystography
see Fluoroscopy, Urinary System BT1
see Plain Radiography, Urinary System BT0
Cystolithotomy
see Extirpation, Bladder 0TCB
Cystopexy
see Repair, Bladder 0TQB
see Reposition, Bladder 0TSB
Cystoplasty
see Repair, Bladder 0TQB
see Replacement, Bladder 0TRB
see Supplement, Bladder 0TUB
Cystorrhaphy
see Repair, Bladder 0TQB
Cystoscopy 0TJB8ZZ
Cystostomy
see Bypass, Bladder 0T1B
Cystostomy tube
use Drainage Device
Cystotomy
see Drainage, Bladder 0T9B
Cystourethrography
see Fluoroscopy, Urinary System BT1
see Plain Radiography, Urinary System BT0
Cystourethroplasty
see Repair, Urinary System 0TQ
see Replacement, Urinary System 0TR
see Supplement, Urinary System 0TU
Cytarabine and Daunorubicin Liposome Antineoplastic XW0

D

DBS lead
use Neurostimulator Lead in Central Nervous System and Cranial Nerves
DeBakey Left Ventricular Assist Device
use Implantable Heart Assist System in Heart and Great Vessels
Debridement
Excisional
see Excision
Non-excisional
see Extraction
Decompression, Circulatory 6A15
Decortication, lung
see Extirpation, Respiratory System 0BC
see Release, Respiratory System 0BN
Deep brain neurostimulator lead
use Neurostimulator Lead in Central Nervous System and Cranial Nerves
Deep cervical fascia
use Subcutaneous Tissue and Fascia, Neck, Left
use Subcutaneous Tissue and Fascia, Neck, Right
Deep cervical vein
use Vein, Vertebral, Left
use Vein, Vertebral, Right
Deep circumflex iliac artery
use Artery, External Iliac, Left
use Artery, External Iliac, Right
Deep facial vein
use Vein, Face, Left
use Vein, Face, Right
Deep femoral (profunda femoris) vein
use Vein, Femoral, Left
use Vein, Femoral, Right
Deep femoral artery
use Artery, Femoral, Left
use Artery, Femoral, Right
Deep Inferior Epigastric Artery Perforator Flap
Replacement
Bilateral 0HRV077
Left 0HRU077
Right 0HRT077
Transfer
Left 0KXG
Right 0KXF
Deep palmar arch
use Artery, Hand, Left
use Artery, Hand, Right
Deep transverse perineal muscle
use Muscle, Perineum
Deferential artery
use Artery, Internal Iliac, Left
use Artery, Internal Iliac, Right
Defibrillator Generator
Abdomen 0JH8
Chest 0JH6
Defibrotide Sodium Anticoagulant XW0
Defitelio
use Defibrotide Sodium Anticoagulant
Delivery
Cesarean
see Extraction, Products of Conception 10D0
Forceps
see Extraction, Products of Conception 10D0
Manually assisted 10E0XZZ
Products of Conception 10E0XZZ
Vacuum assisted
see Extraction, Products of Conception 10D0
Delta frame external fixator
use External Fixation Device, Hybrid in 0PH
use External Fixation Device, Hybrid in 0PS
use External Fixation Device, Hybrid in 0QH
use External Fixation Device, Hybrid in 0QS
Delta III Reverse shoulder prosthesis
use Synthetic Substitute, Reverse Ball and Socket in 0RR
Deltoid fascia
use Subcutaneous Tissue and Fascia, Upper Arm, Left
use Subcutaneous Tissue and Fascia, Upper Arm, Right
Deltoid ligament
use Bursa and Ligament, Ankle, Left
use Bursa and Ligament, Ankle, Right
Deltoid muscle
use Muscle, Shoulder, Left
use Muscle, Shoulder, Right
Deltopectoral (infraclavicular) lymph node
use Lymphatic, Upper Extremity, Left
use Lymphatic, Upper Extremity, Right
Denervation
Cranial nerve
see Destruction, Central Nervous System and Cranial Nerves 005
Peripheral nerve
see Destruction, Peripheral Nervous System 015
Dens
use Cervical Vertebra
Densitometry
Plain Radiography
Femur
Left BQ04ZZ1
Right BQ03ZZ1
Hip
Left BQ01ZZ1
Right BQ00ZZ1
Spine
Cervical BR00ZZ1
Lumbar BR09ZZ1

- **Densitometry** *(continued)*
  - Plain Radiography *(continued)*
    - Spine *(continued)*
      - Thoracic BR07ZZ1
      - Whole BR0GZZ1
  - Ultrasonography
    - Elbow
      - Left BP4HZZ1
      - Right BP4GZZ1
    - Hand
      - Left BP4PZZ1
      - Right BP4NZZ1
    - Shoulder
      - Left BP49ZZ1
      - Right BP48ZZ1
    - Wrist
      - Left BP4MZZ1
      - Right BP4LZZ1
- **Denticulate (dentate) ligament**
  - *use* Spinal Meninges
- **Depressor anguli oris muscle**
  - *use* Muscle, Facial
- **Depressor labii inferioris muscle**
  - *use* Muscle, Facial
- **Depressor septi nasi muscle**
  - *use* Muscle, Facial
- **Depressor supercilii muscle**
  - *use* Muscle, Facial
- **Dermabrasion**
  - *see* Extraction, Skin and Breast 0HD
- **Dermis**
  - *use* Skin
- **Descending genicular artery**
  - *use* Artery, Femoral, Left
  - *use* Artery, Femoral, Right
- **Destruction**
  - Acetabulum
    - Left 0Q55
    - Right 0Q54
  - Adenoids 0C5Q
  - Ampulla of Vater 0F5C
  - Anal Sphincter 0D5R
  - Anterior Chamber
    - Left 08533ZZ
    - Right 08523ZZ
  - Anus 0D5Q
  - Aorta
    - Abdominal 0450
    - Thoracic
      - Ascending/Arch 025X
      - Descending 025W
  - Aortic Body 0G5D
  - Appendix 0D5J
  - Artery
    - Anterior Tibial
      - Left 045Q
      - Right 045P
    - Axillary
      - Left 0356
      - Right 0355
    - Brachial
      - Left 0358
      - Right 0357
    - Celiac 0451
    - Colic
      - Left 0457
      - Middle 0458
      - Right 0456
    - Common Carotid
      - Left 035J
      - Right 035H
    - Common Iliac
      - Left 045D
      - Right 045C
    - External Carotid
      - Left 035N
      - Right 035M
    - External Iliac
      - Left 045J
      - Right 045H

- **Destruction** *(continued)*
  - Artery *(continued)*
    - Face 035R
    - Femoral
      - Left 045L
      - Right 045K
    - Foot
      - Left 045W
      - Right 045V
    - Gastric 0452
    - Hand
      - Left 035F
      - Right 035D
    - Hepatic 0453
    - Inferior Mesenteric 045B
    - Innominate 0352
    - Internal Carotid
      - Left 035L
      - Right 035K
    - Internal Iliac
      - Left 045F
      - Right 045E
    - Internal Mammary
      - Left 0351
      - Right 0350
    - Intracranial 035G
    - Lower 045Y
    - Peroneal
      - Left 045U
      - Right 045T
    - Popliteal
      - Left 045N
      - Right 045M
    - Posterior Tibial
      - Left 045S
      - Right 045R
    - Pulmonary
      - Left 025R
      - Right 025Q
    - Pulmonary Trunk 025P
    - Radial
      - Left 035C
      - Right 035B
    - Renal
      - Left 045A
      - Right 0459
    - Splenic 0454
    - Subclavian
      - Left 0354
      - Right 0353
    - Superior Mesenteric 0455
    - Temporal
      - Left 035T
      - Right 035S
    - Thyroid
      - Left 035V
      - Right 035U
    - Ulnar
      - Left 035A
      - Right 0359
    - Upper 035Y
    - Vertebral
      - Left 035Q
      - Right 035P
  - Atrium
    - Left 0257
    - Right 0256
  - Auditory Ossicle
    - Left 095A
    - Right 0959
  - Basal Ganglia 0058
  - Bladder 0T5B
  - Bladder Neck 0T5C
  - Bone
    - Ethmoid
      - Left 0N5G
      - Right 0N5F
    - Frontal 0N51
    - Hyoid 0N5X

- **Destruction** *(continued)*
  - Bone *(continued)*
    - Lacrimal
      - Left 0N5J
      - Right 0N5H
    - Nasal 0N5B
    - Occipital 0N57
    - Palatine
      - Left 0N5L
      - Right 0N5K
    - Parietal
      - Left 0N54
      - Right 0N53
    - Pelvic
      - Left 0Q53
      - Right 0Q52
    - Sphenoid 0N5C
    - Temporal
      - Left 0N56
      - Right 0N55
    - Zygomatic
      - Left 0N5N
      - Right 0N5M
  - Brain 0050
  - Breast
    - Bilateral 0H5V
    - Left 0H5U
    - Right 0H5T
  - Bronchus
    - Lingula 0B59
    - Lower Lobe
      - Left 0B5B
      - Right 0B56
    - Main
      - Left 0B57
      - Right 0B53
    - Middle Lobe, Right 0B55
    - Upper Lobe
      - Left 0B58
      - Right 0B54
  - Buccal Mucosa 0C54
  - Bursa and Ligament
    - Abdomen
      - Left 0M5J
      - Right 0M5H
    - Ankle
      - Left 0M5R
      - Right 0M5Q
    - Elbow
      - Left 0M54
      - Right 0M53
    - Foot
      - Left 0M5T
      - Right 0M5S
    - Hand
      - Left 0M58
      - Right 0M57
    - Head and Neck 0M50
    - Hip
      - Left 0M5M
      - Right 0M5L
    - Knee
      - Left 0M5P
      - Right 0M5N
    - Lower Extremity
      - Left 0M5W
      - Right 0M5V
    - Rib(s) 0M5G
    - Shoulder
      - Left 0M52
      - Right 0M51
    - Spine
      - Lower 0M5D
      - Upper 0M5C
    - Sternum 0M5F
    - Upper Extremity
      - Left 0M5B
      - Right 0M59
    - Wrist
      - Left 0M56
      - Right 0M55

- **Destruction** *(continued)*
  - Carina 0B52
  - Carotid Bodies, Bilateral 0G58
  - Carotid Body
    - Left 0G56
    - Right 0G57
  - Carpal
    - Left 0P5N
    - Right 0P5M
  - Cecum 0D5H
  - Cerebellum 005C
  - Cerebral Hemisphere 0057
  - Cerebral Meninges 0051
  - Cerebral Ventricle 0056
  - Cervix 0U5C
  - Chordae Tendineae 0259
  - Choroid
    - Left 085B
    - Right 085A
  - Cisterna Chyli 075L
  - Clavicle
    - Left 0P5B
    - Right 0P59
  - Clitoris 0U5J
  - Coccygeal Glomus 0G5B
  - Coccyx 0Q5S
  - Colon
    - Ascending 0D5K
    - Descending 0D5M
    - Sigmoid 0D5N
    - Transverse 0D5L
  - Conduction Mechanism 0258
  - Conjunctiva
    - Left 085TXZZ
    - Right 085SXZZ
  - Cord
    - Bilateral 0V5H
    - Left 0V5G
    - Right 0V5F
  - Cornea
    - Left 0859XZZ
    - Right 0858XZZ
  - Cul-de-sac 0U5F
  - Diaphragm 0B5T
  - Disc
    - Cervical Vertebral 0R53
    - Cervicothoracic Vertebral 0R55
    - Lumbar Vertebral 0S52
    - Lumbosacral 0S54
    - Thoracic Vertebral 0R59
    - Thoracolumbar Vertebral 0R5
  - Duct
    - Common Bile 0F59
    - Cystic 0F58
    - Hepatic
      - Common 0F57
      - Left 0F56
      - Right 0F55
    - Lacrimal
      - Left 085Y
      - Right 085X
    - Pancreatic 0F5D
      - Accessory 0F5F
    - Parotid
      - Left 0C5C
      - Right 0C5B
  - Duodenum 0D59
  - Dura Mater 0052
  - Ear
    - External
      - Left 0951
      - Right 0950
    - External Auditory Canal
      - Left 0954
      - Right 0953
    - Inner
      - Left 095E
      - Right 095D
    - Middle
      - Left 0956
      - Right 0955

Destruction *(continued)*
- Endometrium 0U5B
- Epididymis
  - Bilateral 0V5L
  - Left 0V5K
  - Right 0V5J
- Epiglottis 0C5R
- Esophagogastric Junction 0D54
- Esophagus 0D55
  - Lower 0D53
  - Middle 0D52
  - Upper 0D51
- Eustachian Tube
  - Left 095G
  - Right 095F
- Eye
  - Left 0851XZZ
  - Right 0850XZZ
- Eyelid
  - Lower
    - Left 085R
    - Right 085Q
  - Upper
    - Left 085P
    - Right 085N
- Fallopian Tube
  - Left 0U56
  - Right 0U55
- Fallopian Tubes, Bilateral 0U57
- Femoral Shaft
  - Left 0Q59
  - Right 0Q58
- Femur
  - Lower
    - Left 0Q5C
    - Right 0Q5B
  - Upper
    - Left 0Q57
    - Right 0Q56
- Fibula
  - Left 0Q5K
  - Right 0Q5J
- Finger Nail 0H5QXZZ
- Gallbladder 0F54
- Gingiva
  - Lower 0C56
  - Upper 0C55
- Gland
  - Adrenal
    - Bilateral 0G54
    - Left 0G52
    - Right 0G53
  - Lacrimal
    - Left 085W
    - Right 085V
  - Minor Salivary 0C5J
  - Parotid
    - Left 0C59
    - Right 0C58
  - Pituitary 0G50
  - Sublingual
    - Left 0C5F
    - Right 0C5D
  - Submaxillary
    - Left 0C5H
    - Right 0C5G
  - Vestibular 0U5L
- Glenoid Cavity
  - Left 0P58
  - Right 0P57
- Glomus Jugulare 0G5C
- Humeral Head
  - Left 0P5D
  - Right 0P5C
- Humeral Shaft
  - Left 0P5G
  - Right 0P5F
- Hymen 0U5K
- Hypothalamus 005A
- Ileocecal Valve 0D5C

Destruction *(continued)*
- Ileum 0D5B
- Intestine
  - Large 0D5E
    - Left 0D5G
    - Right 0D5F
  - Small 0D58
- Iris
  - Left 085D3ZZ
  - Right 085C3ZZ
- Jejunum 0D5A
- Joint
  - Acromioclavicular
    - Left 0R5H
    - Right 0R5G
  - Ankle
    - Left 0S5G
    - Right 0S5F
  - Carpal
    - Left 0R5R
    - Right 0R5Q
  - Carpometacarpal
    - Left 0R5T
    - Right 0R5S
  - Cervical Vertebral 0R51
  - Cervicothoracic Vertebral 0R54
  - Coccygeal 0S56
  - Elbow
    - Left 0R5M
    - Right 0R5L
  - Finger Phalangeal
    - Left 0R5X
    - Right 0R5W
  - Hip
    - Left 0S5B
    - Right 0S59
  - Knee
    - Left 0S5D
    - Right 0S5C
  - Lumbar Vertebral 0S50
  - Lumbosacral 0S53
  - Metacarpophalangeal
    - Left 0R5V
    - Right 0R5U
  - Metatarsal-Phalangeal
    - Left 0S5N
    - Right 0S5M
  - Occipital-cervical 0R50
  - Sacrococcygeal 0S55
  - Sacroiliac
    - Left 0S58
    - Right 0S57
  - Shoulder
    - Left 0R5K
    - Right 0R5J
  - Sternoclavicular
    - Left 0R5F
    - Right 0R5E
  - Tarsal
    - Left 0S5J
    - Right 0S5H
  - Tarsometatarsal
    - Left 0S5L
    - Right 0S5K
  - Temporomandibular
    - Left 0R5D
    - Right 0R5C
  - Thoracic Vertebral 0R56
  - Thoracolumbar Vertebral 0R5A
  - Toe Phalangeal
    - Left 0S5Q
    - Right 0S5P
  - Wrist
    - Left 0R5P
    - Right 0R5N
- Kidney
  - Left 0T51
  - Right 0T50

Destruction *(continued)*
- Kidney Pelvis
  - Left 0T54
  - Right 0T53
- Larynx 0C5S
- Lens
  - Left 085K3ZZ
  - Right 085J3ZZ
- Lip
  - Lower 0C51
  - Upper 0C50
- Liver 0F50
  - Left Lobe 0F52
  - Right Lobe 0F51
- Lung
  - Bilateral 0B5M
  - Left 0B5L
  - Lower Lobe
    - Left 0B5J
    - Right 0B5F
  - Middle Lobe, Right 0B5D
  - Right 0B5K
  - Upper Lobe
    - Left 0B5G
    - Right 0B5C
- Lung Lingula 0B5H
- Lymphatic
  - Aortic 075D
  - Axillary
    - Left 0756
    - Right 0755
  - Head 0750
  - Inguinal
    - Left 075J
    - Right 075H
  - Internal Mammary
    - Left 0759
    - Right 0758
  - Lower Extremity
    - Left 075G
    - Right 075F
  - Mesenteric 075B
  - Neck
    - Left 0752
    - Right 0751
  - Pelvis 075C
  - Thoracic Duct 075K
  - Thorax 0757
  - Upper Extremity
    - Left 0754
    - Right 0753
- Mandible
  - Left 0N5V
  - Right 0N5T
- Maxilla 0N5R
- Medulla Oblongata 005D
- Mesentery 0D5V
- Metacarpal
  - Left 0P5Q
  - Right 0P5P
- Metatarsal
  - Left 0Q5P
  - Right 0Q5N
- Muscle
  - Abdomen
    - Left 0K5L
    - Right 0K5K
  - Extraocular
    - Left 085M
    - Right 085L
  - Facial 0K51
  - Foot
    - Left 0K5W
    - Right 0K5V
  - Hand
    - Left 0K5D
    - Right 0K5C
  - Head 0K50

Destruction *(continued)*
- Muscle *(continued)*
  - Hip
    - Left 0K5P
    - Right 0K5N
  - Lower Arm and Wrist
    - Left 0K5B
    - Right 0K59
  - Lower Leg
    - Left 0K5T
    - Right 0K5S
  - Neck
    - Left 0K53
    - Right 0K52
  - Papillary 025D
  - Perineum 0K5M
  - Shoulder
    - Left 0K56
    - Right 0K55
  - Thorax
    - Left 0K5J
    - Right 0K5H
  - Nasal Mucosa and Soft Tissue 095K
  - Tongue, Palate, Pharynx 0K54
  - Trunk
    - Left 0K5G
    - Right 0K5F
  - Upper Arm
    - Left 0K58
    - Right 0K57
  - Upper Leg
    - Left 0K5R
    - Right 0K5Q
- Nasal Mucosa and Soft Tissue 095K
- Nasopharynx 095N
- Nerve
  - Abdominal Sympathetic 015M
  - Abducens 005L
  - Accessory 005R
  - Acoustic 005N
  - Brachial Plexus 0153
  - Cervical 0151
  - Cervical Plexus 0150
  - Facial 005M
  - Femoral 015D
  - Glossopharyngeal 005P
  - Head and Neck Sympathetic 015K
  - Hypoglossal 005S
  - Lumbar 015B
  - Lumbar Plexus 0159
  - Lumbar Sympathetic 015N
  - Lumbosacral Plexus 015A
  - Median 0155
  - Oculomotor 005H
  - Olfactory 005F
  - Optic 005G
  - Peroneal 015H
  - Phrenic 0152
  - Pudendal 015C
  - Radial 0156
  - Sacral 015R
  - Sacral Plexus 015Q
  - Sacral Sympathetic 015P
  - Sciatic 015F
  - Thoracic 0158
  - Thoracic Sympathetic 015L
  - Tibial 015G
  - Trigeminal 005K
  - Trochlear 005J
  - Ulnar 0154
  - Vagus 005Q
- Nipple
  - Left 0H5X
  - Right 0H5W
- Omentum 0D5U
- Orbit
  - Left 0N5Q
  - Right 0N5P

Destruction *(continued)*
- Ovary
  - Bilateral 0U52
  - Left 0U51
  - Right 0U50
- Palate
  - Hard 0C52
  - Soft 0C53
- Pancreas 0F5G
- Para-aortic Body 0G59
- Paraganglion Extremity 0G5F
- Parathyroid Gland 0G5R
  - Inferior
    - Left 0G5P
    - Right 0G5N
  - Multiple 0G5Q
  - Superior
    - Left 0G5M
    - Right 0G5L
- Patella
  - Left 0Q5F
  - Right 0Q5D
- Penis 0V5S
- Pericardium 025N
- Peritoneum 0D5W
- Phalanx
  - Finger
    - Left 0P5V
    - Right 0P5T
  - Thumb
    - Left 0P5S
    - Right 0P5R
  - Toe
    - Left 0Q5R
    - Right 0Q5Q
- Pharynx 0C5M
- Pineal Body 0G51
- Pleura
  - Left 0B5P
  - Right 0B5N
- Pons 005B
- Prepuce 0V5T
- Prostate 0V50
  - Robotic Waterjet Ablation XV508A4
- Radius
  - Left 0P5J
  - Right 0P5H
- Rectum 0D5P
- Retina
  - Left 085F3ZZ
  - Right 085E3ZZ
- Retinal Vessel
  - Left 085H3ZZ
  - Right 085G3ZZ
- Rib (s)
  - 1 to 2 0P51
  - 3 or More 0P52
- Sacrum 0Q51
- Scapula
  - Left 0P56
  - Right 0P55
- Sclera
  - Left 0857XZZ
  - Right 0856XZZ
- Scrotum 0V55
- Septum
  - Atrial 0255
  - Nasal 095M
  - Ventricular 025M
- Sinus
  - Accessory 095P
  - Ethmoid
    - Left 095V
    - Right 095U
  - Frontal
    - Left 095T
    - Right 095S
  - Mastoid
    - Left 095C
    - Right 095B

Destruction *(continued)*
- Sinus *(continued)*
  - Maxillary
    - Left 095R
  - Maxillary
    - Right 095Q
  - Sphenoid
    - Left 095X
    - Right 095W
- Skin
  - Abdomen 0H57XZ
  - Back 0H56XZ
  - Buttock 0H58XZ
  - Chest 0H55XZ
  - Ear
    - Left 0H53XZ
    - Right 0H52XZ
  - Face 0H51XZ
  - Foot
    - Left 0H5NXZ
    - Right 0H5MXZ
  - Hand
    - Left 0H5GXZ
    - Right 0H5FXZ
  - Inguinal 0H5AXZ
  - Lower Arm
    - Left 0H5EXZ
    - Right 0H5DXZ
  - Lower Leg
    - Left 0H5LXZ
    - Right 0H5KXZ
  - Neck 0H54XZ
  - Perineum 0H59XZ
  - Scalp 0H50XZ
  - Upper Arm
    - Left 0H5CXZ
    - Right 0H5BXZ
  - Upper Leg
    - Left 0H5JXZ
    - Right 0H5HXZ
- Skull 0N50
- Spinal Cord
  - Cervical 005W
  - Lumbar 005Y
  - Thoracic 005X
- Spinal Meninges 005T
- Spleen 075P
- Sternum 0P50
- Stomach 0D56
  - Pylorus 0D57
- Subcutaneous Tissue and Fascia
  - Abdomen 0J58
  - Back 0J57
  - Buttock 0J59
  - Chest 0J56
  - Face 0J51
  - Foot
    - Left 0J5R
    - Right 0J5Q
  - Hand
    - Left 0J5K
    - Right 0J5J
  - Lower Arm
    - Left 0J5H
    - Right 0J5G
  - Lower Leg
    - Left 0J5P
    - Right 0J5N
  - Neck
    - Left 0J55
    - Right 0J54
  - Pelvic Region 0J5C
  - Perineum 0J5B
  - Scalp 0J50
  - Upper Arm
    - Left 0J5F
    - Right 0J5D
  - Upper Leg
    - Left 0J5M
    - Right 0J5L

Destruction *(continued)*
- Tarsal
  - Left 0Q5M
  - Right 0Q5L
- Tendon
  - Abdomen
    - Left 0L5G
    - Right 0L5F
  - Ankle
    - Left 0L5T
    - Right 0L5S
  - Foot
    - Left 0L5W
    - Right 0L5V
  - Hand
    - Left 0L58
    - Right 0L57
  - Head and Neck 0L50
  - Hip
    - Left 0L5K
    - Right 0L5J
  - Knee
    - Left 0L5R
    - Right 0L5Q
  - Lower Arm and Wrist
    - Left 0L56
    - Right 0L55
  - Lower Leg
    - Left 0L5P
    - Right 0L5N
  - Perineum 0L5H
  - Shoulder
    - Left 0L52
    - Right 0L51
  - Thorax
    - Left 0L5D
    - Right 0L5C
  - Trunk
    - Left 0L5B
    - Right 0L59
  - Upper Arm
    - Left 0L54
    - Right 0L53
  - Upper Leg
    - Left 0L5M
    - Right 0L5L
- Testis
  - Bilateral 0V5C
  - Left 0V5B
  - Right 0V59
- Thalamus 0059
- Thymus 075M
- Thyroid Gland 0G5K
  - Left Lobe 0G5G
  - Right Lobe 0G5H
- Tibia
  - Left 0Q5H
  - Right 0Q5G
- Toe Nail 0H5RXZZ
- Tongue 0C57
- Tonsils 0C5P
- Tooth
  - Lower 0C5X
  - Upper 0C5W
- Trachea 0B51
- Tunica Vaginalis
  - Left 0V57
  - Right 0V56
- Turbinate, Nasal 095L
- Tympanic Membrane
  - Left 0958
  - Right 0957
- Ulna
  - Left 0P5L
  - Right 0P5K
- Ureter
  - Left 0T57
  - Right 0T56
- Urethra 0T5D
- Uterine Supporting Structure 0U54

Destruction *(continued)*
- Uterus 0U59
- Uvula 0C5N
- Vagina 0U5G
- Valve
  - Aortic 025F
  - Mitral 025G
  - Pulmonary 025H
  - Tricuspid 025J
- Vas Deferens
  - Bilateral 0V5Q
  - Left 0V5P
  - Right 0V5N
- Vein
  - Axillary
    - Left 0558
    - Right 0557
  - Azygos 0550
  - Basilic
    - Left 055C
    - Right 055B
  - Brachial
    - Left 055A
    - Right 0559
  - Cephalic
    - Left 055F
    - Right 055D
  - Colic 0657
  - Common Iliac
    - Left 065D
    - Right 065C
  - Coronary 0254
  - Esophageal 0653
  - External Iliac
    - Left 065G
    - Right 065F
  - External Jugular
    - Left 055Q
    - Right 055P
  - Face
    - Left 055V
    - Right 055T
  - Femoral
    - Left 065N
    - Right 065M
  - Foot
    - Left 065V
    - Right 065T
  - Gastric 0652
  - Hand
    - Left 055H
    - Right 055G
  - Hemiazygos 0551
  - Hepatic 0654
  - Hypogastric
    - Left 065J
    - Right 065H
  - Inferior Mesenteric 0656
  - Innominate
    - Left 0554
    - Right 0553
  - Internal Jugular
    - Left 055N
    - Right 055M
  - Intracranial 055L
  - Lower 065Y
  - Portal 0658
  - Pulmonary
    - Left 025T
    - Right 025S
  - Renal
    - Left 065B
    - Right 0659
  - Saphenous
    - Left 065Q
    - Right 065P
  - Splenic 0651
  - Subclavian
    - Left 0556
    - Right 0555
  - Superior Mesenteric 0655

Destruction *(continued)*
- Vein *(continued)*
  - Upper 055Y
  - Vertebral
    - Left 055S
    - Right 055R
- Vena Cava
  - Inferior 0650
  - Superior 025V
- Ventricle
  - Left 025L
  - Right 025K
- Vertebra
  - Cervical 0P53
  - Lumbar 0Q50
  - Thoracic 0P54
- Vesicle
  - Bilateral 0V53
  - Left 0V52
  - Right 0V51
- Vitreous
  - Left 08553ZZ
  - Right 08543ZZ
- Vocal Cord
  - Left 0C5V
  - Right 0C5T
- Vulva 0U5M

Detachment
- Arm
  - Lower
    - Left 0X6F0Z
    - Right 0X6D0Z
  - Upper
    - Left 0X690Z
    - Right 0X680Z
- Elbow Region
  - Left 0X6C0ZZ
  - Right 0X6B0ZZ
- Femoral Region
  - Left 0Y680ZZ
  - Right 0Y670ZZ
- Finger
  - Index
    - Left 0X6P0Z
    - Right 0X6N0Z
  - Little
    - Left 0X6W0Z
    - Right 0X6V0Z
  - Middle
    - Left 0X6R0Z
    - Right 0X6Q0Z
  - Ring
    - Left 0X6T0Z
    - Right 0X6S0Z
- Foot
  - Left 0Y6N0Z
  - Right 0Y6M0Z
- Forequarter
  - Left 0X610ZZ
  - Right 0X600ZZ
- Hand
  - Left 0X6K0Z
  - Right 0X6J0Z
- Hindquarter
  - Bilateral 0Y640ZZ
  - Left 0Y630ZZ
  - Right 0Y620ZZ
- Knee Region
  - Left 0Y6G0ZZ
  - Right 0Y6F0ZZ
- Leg
  - Lower
    - Left 0Y6J0Z
    - Right 0Y6H0Z
  - Upper
    - Left 0Y6D0Z
    - Right 0Y6C0Z
- Shoulder Region
  - Left 0X630ZZ
  - Right 0X620ZZ

Detachment *(continued)*
- Thumb
  - Left 0X6M0Z
  - Right 0X6L0Z
- Toe
  - 1st
    - Left 0Y6Q0Z
    - Right 0Y6P0Z
  - 2nd
    - Left 0Y6S0Z
    - Right 0Y6R0Z
  - 3rd
    - Left 0Y6U0Z
    - Right 0Y6T0Z
  - 4th
    - Left 0Y6W0Z
    - Right 0Y6V0Z
  - 5th
    - Left 0Y6Y0Z
    - Right 0Y6X0Z

Determination, Mental status GZ14ZZZ

Detorsion
- *see* Release
- *see* Reposition

Detoxification Services, for substance abuse HZ2ZZZZ

Device Fitting F0DZ

Diagnostic Audiology
- *see* Audiology, Diagnostic

Diagnostic imaging
- *see* Imaging, Diagnostic

Diagnostic radiology
- *see* Imaging, Diagnostic

Dialysis
- Hemodialysis *see* Performance, Urinary 5A1D
- Peritoneal 3E1M39Z

Diaphragma sellae
- *use* Dura Mater

Diaphragmatic pacemaker generator
- *use* Stimulator Generator in Subcutaneous Tissue and Fascia

Diaphragmatic Pacemaker Lead
- Insertion of device in, Diaphragm 0BHT
- Removal of device from, Diaphragm 0BPT
- Revision of device in, Diaphragm 0BWT

Digital radiography, plain
- *see* Plain Radiography

Dilation
- Ampulla of Vater 0F7C
- Anus 0D7Q
- Aorta
  - Abdominal 0470
  - Thoracic
    - Ascending/Arch 027X
    - Descending 027W
- Artery
  - Anterior Tibial
    - Left 047Q
    - Right 047P
  - Axillary
    - Left 0376
    - Right 0375
  - Brachial
    - Left 0378
    - Right 0377
  - Celiac 0471
  - Colic
    - Left 0477
    - Middle 0478
    - Right 0476
  - Common Carotid
    - Left 037J
    - Right 037H
  - Common Iliac
    - Left 047D

Dilation *(continued)*
- Artery *(continued)*
  - Common Iliac *(continued)*
    - Right 047C
  - Coronary
    - Four or More Arteries 0273
    - One Artery 0270
    - Three Arteries 0272
    - Two Arteries 0271
  - External Carotid
    - Left 037N
    - Right 037M
  - External Iliac
    - Left 047J
    - Right 047H
  - Face 037R
  - Femoral
    - Left 047L
    - Right 047K
  - Foot
    - Left 047W
    - Right 047V
  - Gastric 0472
  - Hand
    - Left 037F
    - Right 037D
  - Hepatic 0473
  - Inferior Mesenteric 047B
  - Innominate 0372
  - Internal Carotid
    - Left 037L
    - Right 037K
  - Internal Iliac
    - Left 047F
    - Right 047E
  - Internal Mammary
    - Left 0371
    - Right 0370
  - Intracranial 037G
  - Lower 047Y
  - Peroneal
    - Left 047U
    - Right 047T
  - Popliteal
    - Left 047N
    - Right 047M
  - Posterior Tibial
    - Left 047S
    - Right 047R
  - Pulmonary
    - Left 027R
    - Right 027Q
  - Pulmonary Trunk 027P
  - Radial
    - Left 037C
    - Right 037B
  - Renal
    - Left 047A
    - Right 0479
  - Splenic 0474
  - Subclavian
    - Left 0374
    - Right 0373
  - Superior Mesenteric 0475
  - Temporal
    - Left 037T
    - Right 037S
  - Thyroid
    - Left 037V
    - Right 037U
  - Ulnar
    - Left 037A
    - Right 0379
  - Upper 037Y
  - Vertebral
    - Left 037Q
    - Right 037P
- Bladder 0T7B
- Bladder Neck 0T7C

Dilation *(continued)*
- Bronchus
  - Lingula 0B79
  - Lower Lobe
    - Left 0B7B
    - Right 0B76
  - Main
    - Left 0B77
    - Right 0B73
  - Middle Lobe, Right 0B75
  - Upper Lobe
    - Left 0B78
    - Right 0B74
- Carina 0B72
- Cerebral Ventricle 0076
- Cecum 0D7H
- Cervix 0U7C
- Colon
  - Ascending 0D7K
  - Descending 0D7M
  - Sigmoid 0D7N
  - Transverse 0D7L
- Duct
  - Common Bile 0F79
  - Cystic 0F78
  - Hepatic
    - Common 0F77
    - Left 0F76
    - Right 0F75
  - Lacrimal
    - Left 087Y
    - Right 087X
  - Pancreatic 0F7D
    - Accessory 0F7F
  - Parotid
    - Left 0C7C
    - Right 0C7B
- Duodenum 0D79
- Esophagogastric Junction 0D74
- Esophagus 0D75
  - Lower 0D73
  - Middle 0D72
  - Upper 0D71
- Eustachian Tube
  - Left 097G
  - Right 097F
- Fallopian Tube
  - Left 0U76
  - Right 0U75
- Fallopian Tubes, Bilateral 0U77
- Hymen 0U7K
- Ileocecal Valve 0D7C
- Ileum 0D7B
- Intestine
  - Large 0D7E
    - Left 0D7G
    - Right 0D7F
  - Small 0D78
- Jejunum 0D7A
- Kidney Pelvis
  - Left 0T74
  - Right 0T73
- Larynx 0C7S
- Pharynx 0C7M
- Rectum 0D7P
- Stomach 0D76
  - Pylorus 0D77
- Trachea 0B71
- Ureter
  - Left 0T77
  - Right 0T76
- Ureters, Bilateral 0T78
- Urethra 0T7D
- Uterus 0U79
- Vagina 0U7G
- Valve
  - Aortic 027F
  - Mitral 027G
  - Pulmonary 027H
  - Tricuspid 027J

Dilation *(continued)*
- Vas Deferens
  - Bilateral 0V7Q
  - Left 0V7P
  - Right 0V7N
- Vein
  - Axillary
    - Left 0578
    - Right 0577
  - Azygos 0570
  - Basilic
    - Left 057C
    - Right 057B
  - Brachial
    - Left 057A
    - Right 0579
  - Cephalic
    - Left 057F
    - Right 057D
  - Colic 0677
  - Common Iliac
    - Left 067D
    - Right 067C
  - Esophageal 0673
  - External Iliac
    - Left 067G
    - Right 067F
  - External Jugular
    - Left 057Q
    - Right 057P
  - Face
    - Left 057V
    - Right 057T
  - Femoral
    - Left 067N
    - Right 067M
  - Foot
    - Left 067V
    - Right 067T
  - Gastric 0672
  - Hand
    - Left 057H
    - Right 057G
  - Hemiazygos 0571
  - Hepatic 0674
  - Hypogastric
    - Left 067J
    - Right 067H
  - Inferior Mesenteric 0676
  - Innominate
    - Left 0574
    - Right 0573
  - Internal Jugular
    - Left 057N
    - Right 057M
  - Intracranial 057L
  - Lower 067Y
  - Portal 0678
  - Pulmonary
    - Left 027T
    - Right 027S
  - Renal
    - Left 067B
    - Right 0679
  - Saphenous
    - Left 067Q
    - Right 067P
  - Splenic 0671
  - Subclavian
    - Left 0576
    - Right 0575
  - Superior Mesenteric 0675
  - Upper 057Y
  - Vertebral
    - Left 057S
    - Right 057R
- Vena Cava
  - Inferior 0670
  - Superior 027V
- Ventricle
  - Left 027L

Dilation *(continued)*
- Ventricle *(continued)*
  - Right 027K

Direct Lateral Interbody Fusion (DLIF) device
- *use* Interbody Fusion Device in Lower Joints

Disarticulation
- *see* Detachment

Discectomy, diskectomy
- *see* Excision, Lower Joints 0SB
- *see* Excision, Upper Joints 0RB
- *see* Resection, Lower Joints 0ST
- *see* Resection, Upper Joints 0RT

Discography
- *see* Fluoroscopy, Axial Skeleton, Except Skull and Facial Bones BR1
- *see* Plain Radiography, Axial Skeleton, Except Skull and Facial Bones BR0

Distal humerus
- *use* Humeral Shaft, Left
- *use* Humeral Shaft, Right

Distal humerus, involving joint
- *use* Joint, Elbow, Left
- *use* Joint, Elbow, Right

Distal radioulnar joint
- *use* Joint, Wrist, Left
- *use* Joint, Wrist, Right

Diversion
- *see* Bypass

Diverticulectomy
- *see* Excision, Gastrointestinal System 0DB

Division
- Acetabulum
  - Left 0Q85
  - Right 0Q84
- Anal Sphincter 0D8R
- Basal Ganglia 0088
- Bladder Neck 0T8C
- Bone
  - Ethmoid
    - Left 0N8G
    - Right 0N8F
  - Frontal 0N81
  - Hyoid 0N8X
  - Lacrimal
    - Left 0N8J
    - Right 0N8H
  - Nasal 0N8B
  - Occipital 0N87
  - Palatine
    - Left 0N8L
    - Right 0N8K
  - Parietal
    - Left 0N84
    - Right 0N83
  - Pelvic
    - Left 0Q83
    - Right 0Q82
  - Sphenoid 0N8C
  - Temporal
    - Left 0N86
    - Right 0N85
  - Zygomatic
    - Left 0N8N
    - Right 0N8M
- Brain 0080
- Bursa and Ligament
  - Abdomen
    - Left 0M8J
    - Right 0M8H
  - Ankle
    - Left 0M8R
    - Right 0M8Q
  - Elbow
    - Left 0M84
    - Right 0M83

Division *(continued)*
- Bursa and Ligament *(continued)*
  - Foot
    - Left 0M8T
    - Right 0M8S
  - Hand
    - Left 0M88
    - Right 0M87
  - Head and Neck 0M80
  - Hip
    - Left 0M8M
    - Right 0M8L
  - Knee
    - Left 0M8P
    - Right 0M8N
  - Lower Extremity
    - Left 0M8W
    - Right 0M8V
  - Perineum 0M8K
  - Rib(s) 0M8G
  - Shoulder
    - Left 0M82
    - Right 0M81
  - Spine
    - Lower 0M8D
    - Upper 0M8C
  - Sternum 0M8F
  - Upper Extremity
    - Left 0M8B
    - Right 0M89
  - Wrist
    - Left 0M86
    - Right 0M85
- Carpal
  - Left 0P8N
  - Right 0P8M
- Cerebral Hemisphere 0087
- Chordae Tendineae 0289
- Clavicle
  - Left 0P8B
  - Right 0P89
- Coccyx 0Q8S
- Conduction Mechanism 0288
- Esophagogastric Junction 0D84
- Femoral Shaft
  - Left 0Q89
  - Right 0Q88
- Femur
  - Lower
    - Left 0Q8C
    - Right 0Q8B
  - Upper
    - Left 0Q87
    - Right 0Q86
- Fibula
  - Left 0Q8K
  - Right 0Q8J
- Gland, Pituitary 0G80
- Glenoid Cavity
  - Left 0P88
  - Right 0P87
- Humeral Head
  - Left 0P8D
  - Right 0P8C
- Humeral Shaft
  - Left 0P8G
  - Right 0P8F
- Hymen 0U8K
- Kidneys, Bilateral 0T82
- Mandible
  - Left 0N8V
  - Right 0N8T
- Maxilla 0N8R
- Metacarpal
  - Left 0P8Q
  - Right 0P8P
- Metatarsal
  - Left 0Q8P
  - Right 0Q8N

Division *(continued)*
- Muscle
  - Abdomen
    - Left 0K8L
    - Right 0K8K
  - Facial 0K81
  - Foot
    - Left 0K8W
    - Right 0K8V
  - Hand
    - Left 0K8D
    - Right 0K8C
  - Head 0K80
  - Hip
    - Left 0K8P
    - Right 0K8N
  - Lower Arm and Wrist
    - Left 0K8B
    - Right 0K89
  - Lower Leg
    - Left 0K8T
    - Right 0K8S
  - Neck
    - Left 0K83
    - Right 0K82
  - Papillary 028D
  - Perineum 0K8M
  - Shoulder
    - Left 0K86
    - Right 0K85
  - Thorax
    - Left 0K8J
    - Right 0K8H
  - Tongue, Palate, Pharynx 0K84
  - Trunk
    - Left 0K8G
    - Right 0K8F
  - Upper Arm
    - Left 0K88
    - Right 0K87
  - Upper Leg
    - Left 0K8R
    - Right 0K8Q
- Nerve
  - Abdominal Sympathetic 018M
  - Abducens 008L
  - Accessory 008R
  - Acoustic 008N
  - Brachial Plexus 0183
  - Cervical 0181
  - Cervical Plexus 0180
  - Facial 008M
  - Femoral 018D
  - Glossopharyngeal 008P
  - Head and Neck Sympathetic 018K
  - Hypoglossal 008S
  - Lumbar 018B
  - Lumbar Plexus 0189
  - Lumbar Sympathetic 018N
  - Lumbosacral Plexus 018A
  - Median 0185
  - Oculomotor 008H
  - Olfactory 008F
  - Optic 008G
  - Peroneal 018H
  - Phrenic 0182
  - Pudendal 018C
  - Radial 0186
  - Sacral 018R
  - Sacral Plexus 018Q
  - Sacral Sympathetic 018P
  - Sciatic 018F
  - Thoracic 0188
  - Thoracic Sympathetic 018L
  - Tibial 018G
  - Trigeminal 008K
  - Trochlear 008J
  - Ulnar 0184
  - Vagus 008Q

Division *(continued)*
- Orbit
  - Left 0N8Q
  - Right 0N8P
- Ovary
  - Bilateral 0U82
  - Left 0U81
  - Right 0U80
- Pancreas 0F8G
- Patella
  - Left 0Q8F
  - Right 0Q8D
- Perineum, Female 0W8NXZZ
- Phalanx
  - Finger
    - Left 0P8V
    - Right 0P8T
  - Thumb
    - Left 0P8S
    - Right 0P8R
  - Toe
    - Left 0Q8R
    - Right 0Q8Q
- Radius
  - Left 0P8J
  - Right 0P8H
- Ribs
  - 1 to 2 0P81
  - 3 or More 0P82
- Sacrum 0Q81
- Scapula
  - Left 0P86
  - Right 0P85
- Skin
  - Abdomen 0H87XZZ
  - Back 0H86XZZ
  - Buttock 0H88XZZ
  - Chest 0H85XZZ
  - Ear
    - Left 0H83XZZ
    - Right 0H82XZZ
  - Face 0H81XZZ
  - Foot
    - Left 0H8NXZZ
    - Right 0H8MXZZ
  - Hand
    - Left 0H8GXZZ
    - Right 0H8FXZZ
  - Inguinal 0H8AXZZ
  - Lower Arm
    - Left 0H8EXZZ
    - Right 0H8DXZZ
  - Lower Leg
    - Left 0H8LXZZ
    - Right 0H8KXZZ
  - Neck 0H84XZZ
  - Perineum 0H89XZZ
  - Scalp 0H80XZZ
  - Upper Arm
    - Left 0H8CXZZ
    - Right 0H8BXZZ
  - Upper Leg
    - Left 0H8JXZZ
    - Right 0H8HXZZ
- Skull 0N80
- Spinal Cord
  - Cervical 008W
  - Lumbar 008Y
  - Thoracic 008X
- Sternum 0P80
- Stomach, Pylorus 0D87
- Subcutaneous Tissue and Fascia
  - Abdomen 0J88
  - Back 0J87
  - Buttock 0J89
  - Chest 0J86
  - Face 0J81
  - Foot
    - Left 0J8R
    - Right 0J8Q

Division *(continued)*
- Subcutaneous Tissue and Fascia *(continued)*
  - Hand
    - Left 0J8K
    - Right 0J8J
  - Head and Neck 0J8S
  - Lower Arm
    - Left 0J8H
    - Right 0J8G
  - Lower Extremity 0J8W
  - Lower Leg
    - Left 0J8P
    - Right 0J8N
  - Neck
    - Left 0J85
    - Right 0J84
  - Pelvic Region 0J8C
  - Perineum 0J8B
  - Scalp 0J80
  - Trunk 0J8T
  - Upper Arm
    - Left 0J8F
    - Right 0J8D
  - Upper Extremity 0J8V
  - Upper Leg
    - Left 0J8M
    - Right 0J8L
- Tarsal
  - Left 0Q8M
  - Right 0Q8L
- Tendon
  - Abdomen
    - Left 0L8G
    - Right 0L8F
  - Ankle
    - Left 0L8T
    - Right 0L8S
  - Foot
    - Left 0L8W
    - Right 0L8V
  - Hand
    - Left 0L88
    - Right 0L87
  - Head and Neck 0L80
  - Hip
    - Left 0L8K
    - Right 0L8J
  - Knee
    - Left 0L8R
    - Right 0L8Q
  - Lower Arm and Wrist
    - Left 0L86
    - Right 0L85
  - Lower Leg
    - Left 0L8P
    - Right 0L8N
  - Perineum 0L8H
  - Shoulder
    - Left 0L82
    - Right 0L81
  - Thorax
    - Left 0L8D
    - Right 0L8C
  - Trunk
    - Left 0L8B
    - Right 0L89
  - Upper Arm
    - Left 0L84
    - Right 0L83
  - Upper Leg
    - Left 0L8M
    - Right 0L8L
- Thyroid Gland Isthmus 0G8J
- Tibia
  - Left 0Q8H
  - Right 0Q8G
- Turbinate, Nasal 098L
- Ulna
  - Left 0P8L

Division *(continued)*
- Ulna *(continued)*
  - Right 0P8K
- Uterine Supporting Structure 0U84
- Vertebra
  - Cervical 0P83
  - Lumbar 0Q80
  - Thoracic 0P84

Doppler study
- *see* Ultrasonography

Dorsal digital nerve
- *use* Nerve, Radial

Dorsal metacarpal vein
- *use* Vein, Hand, Left
- *use* Vein, Hand, Right

Dorsal metatarsal artery
- *use* Artery, Foot, Left
- *use* Artery, Foot, Right

Dorsal metatarsal vein
- *use* Vein, Foot, Left
- *use* Vein, Foot, Right

Dorsal scapular artery
- *use* Artery, Subclavian, Left
- *use* Artery, Subclavian, Right

Dorsal scapular nerve
- *use* Nerve, Brachial Plexus

Dorsal venous arch
- *use* Vein, Foot, Left
- *use* Vein, Foot, Right

Dorsalis pedis artery
- *use* Artery, Anterior Tibial, Left
- *use* Artery, Anterior Tibial, Right

DownStream® System
- 5A0512C
- 5A0522C

Drainage
- Abdominal Wall 0W9F
- Acetabulum
  - Left 0Q95
  - Right 0Q94
- Adenoids 0C9Q
- Ampulla of Vater 0F9C
- Anal Sphincter 0D9R
- Ankle Region
  - Left 0Y9L
  - Right 0Y9K
- Anterior Chamber
  - Left 0893
  - Right 0892
- Anus 0D9Q
- Aorta, Abdominal 0490
- Aortic Body 0G9D
- Appendix 0D9J
- Arm
  - Lower
    - Left 0X9F
    - Right 0X9D
  - Upper
    - Left 0X99
    - Right 0X98
- Artery
  - Anterior Tibial
    - Left 049Q
    - Right 049P
  - Axillary
    - Left 0396
    - Right 0395
  - Brachial
    - Left 0398
    - Right 0397
  - Celiac 0491
  - Colic
    - Left 0497
    - Middle 0498
    - Right 0496
  - Common Carotid
    - Left 039J
    - Right 039H
  - Common Iliac
    - Left 049D
    - Right 049C

Drainage *(continued)*
- Artery *(continued)*
  - External Carotid
    - Left 039N
    - Right 039M
  - External Iliac
    - Left 049J
    - Right 049H
  - Face 039R
  - Femoral
    - Left 049L
    - Right 049K
  - Foot
    - Left 049W
    - Right 049V
  - Gastric 0492
  - Hand
    - Left 039F
    - Right 039D
  - Hepatic 0493
  - Inferior Mesenteric 049B
  - Innominate 0392
  - Internal Carotid
    - Left 039L
    - Right 039K
  - Internal Iliac
    - Left 049F
    - Right 049E
  - Internal Mammary
    - Left 0391
    - Right 0390
  - Intracranial 039G
  - Lower 049Y
  - Peroneal
    - Left 049U
    - Right 049T
  - Popliteal
    - Left 049N
    - Right 049M
  - Posterior Tibial
    - Left 049S
    - Right 049R
  - Radial
    - Left 039C
    - Right 039B
  - Renal
    - Left 049A
    - Right 0499
  - Splenic 0494
  - Subclavian
    - Left 0394
    - Right 0393
  - Superior Mesenteric 0495
  - Temporal
    - Left 039T
    - Right 039S
  - Thyroid
    - Left 039V
    - Right 039U
  - Ulnar
    - Left 039A
    - Right 0399
  - Upper 039Y
  - Vertebral
    - Left 039Q
    - Right 039P
- Auditory Ossicle
  - Left 099A
  - Right 0999
- Axilla
  - Left 0X95
  - Right 0X94
- Back
  - Lower 0W9L
  - Upper 0W9K
- Basal Ganglia 0098
- Bladder 0T9B

Drainage *(continued)*
- Bladder Neck 0T9C
- Bone
  - Ethmoid
    - Left 0N9G
    - Right 0N9F
  - Frontal 0N91
  - Hyoid 0N9X
  - Lacrimal
    - Left 0N9J
    - Right 0N9H
  - Nasal 0N9B
  - Occipital 0N97
  - Palatine
    - Left 0N9L
    - Right 0N9K
  - Parietal
    - Left 0N94
    - Right 0N93
  - Pelvic
    - Left 0Q93
    - Right 0Q92
  - Sphenoid 0N9C
  - Temporal
    - Left 0N96
    - Right 0N95
  - Zygomatic
    - Left 0N9N
    - Right 0N9M
- Bone Marrow 079T
- Brain 0090
- Breast
  - Bilateral 0H9V
  - Left 0H9U
  - Right 0H9T
- Bronchus
  - Lingula 0B99
  - Lower Lobe
    - Left 0B9B
    - Right 0B96
  - Main
    - Left 0B97
    - Right 0B93
  - Middle Lobe, Right 0B95
  - Upper Lobe
    - Left 0B98
    - Right 0B94
- Buccal Mucosa 0C94
- Bursa and Ligament
  - Abdomen
    - Left 0M9J
    - Right 0M9H
  - Ankle
    - Left 0M9R
    - Right 0M9Q
  - Elbow
    - Left 0M94
    - Right 0M93
  - Foot
    - Left 0M9T
    - Right 0M9S
  - Hand
    - Left 0M98
    - Right 0M97
  - Head and Neck 200M90
  - Hip
    - Left 0M9M
    - Right 0M9L
  - Knee
    - Left 0M9P
    - Right 0M9N
  - Lower Extremity
    - Left 0M9W
    - Right 0M9V
  - Perineum 0M9K
  - Rib(s) 0M9G
  - Shoulder
    - Left 0M92
    - Right 0M91

Drainage *(continued)*
- Bursa and Ligament *(continued)*
  - Spine
    - Lower 0M9D
    - Upper 0M9C
  - Sternum 0M9F
  - Upper Extremity
    - Left 0M9B
    - Right 0M99
  - Wrist
    - Left 0M96
    - Right 0M95
- Buttock
  - Left 0Y91
  - Right 0Y90
- Carina 0B92
- Carotid Bodies, Bilateral 0G98
- Carotid Body
  - Left 0G96
  - Right 0G97
- Carpal
  - Left 0P9N
  - Right 0P9M
- Cavity, Cranial 0W91
- Cecum 0D9H
- Cerebellum 009C
- Cerebral Hemisphere 0097
- Cerebral Meninges 0091
- Cerebral Ventricle 0096
- Cervix 0U9C
- Chest Wall 0W98
- Choroid
  - Left 089B
  - Right 089A
- Cisterna Chyli 079L
- Clavicle
  - Left 0P9B
  - Right 0P99
- Clitoris 0U9J
- Coccygeal Glomus 0G9B
- Coccyx 0Q9S
- Colon
  - Ascending 0D9K
  - Descending 0D9M
  - Sigmoid 0D9N
  - Transverse 0D9L
- Conjunctiva
  - Left 089T
  - Right 089S
- Cord
  - Bilateral 0V9H
  - Left 0V9G
  - Right 0V9F
- Cornea
  - Left 0899
  - Right 0898
- Cul-de-sac 0U9F
- Diaphragm 0B9T
- Disc
  - Cervical Vertebral 0R93
  - Cervicothoracic Vertebral 0R95
  - Lumbar Vertebral 0S92
  - Lumbosacral 0S94
  - Thoracic Vertebral 0R99
  - Thoracolumbar Vertebral 0R9B
- Duct
  - Common Bile 0F99
  - Cystic 0F98
  - Hepatic
    - Common 0F97
    - Left 0F96
    - Right 0F95
  - Lacrimal
    - Left 089Y
    - Right 089X
  - Pancreatic 0F9D
    - Accessory 0F9F
  - Parotid
    - Left 0C9C
    - Right 0C9B

Drainage *(continued)*
- Duodenum 0D99
- Dura Mater 0092
- Ear
  - External
    - Left 0991
    - Right 0990
  - External Auditory Canal
    - Left 0994
    - Right 0993
  - Inner
    - Left 099E
    - Right 099D
  - Middle
    - Left 0996
    - Right 0995
- Elbow Region
  - Left 0X9C
  - Right 0X9B
- Epididymis
  - Bilateral 0V9L
  - Left 0V9K
  - Right 0V9J
- Epidural Space, Intracranial 0093
- Epiglottis 0C9R
- Esophagogastric Junction 0D94
- Esophagus 0D95
  - Lower 0D93
  - Middle 0D92
  - Upper 0D91
- Eustachian Tube
  - Left 099G
  - Right 099F
- Extremity
  - Lower
    - Left 0Y9B
    - Right 0Y99
  - Upper
    - Left 0X97
    - Right 0X96
- Eye
  - Left 0891
  - Right 0890
- Eyelid
  - Lower
    - Left 089R
    - Right 089Q
  - Upper
    - Left 089P
    - Right 089N
- Face 0W92
- Fallopian Tube
  - Left 0U96
  - Right 0U95
- Fallopian Tubes, Bilateral 0U97
- Femoral Region
  - Left 0Y98
  - Right 0Y97
- Femoral Shaft
  - Left 0Q99
  - Right 0Q98
- Femur
  - Lower
    - Left 0Q9C
    - Right 0Q9B
  - Upper
    - Left 0Q97
    - Right 0Q96
- Fibula
  - Left 0Q9K
  - Right 0Q9J
- Finger Nail 0H9Q
- Foot
  - Left 0Y9N
  - Right 0Y9M
- Gallbladder 0F94
- Gingiva
  - Lower 0C96
  - Upper 0C95

Drainage *(continued)*
- Gland
  - Adrenal
    - Bilateral 0G94
    - Left 0G92
    - Right 0G93
  - Lacrimal
    - Left 089W
    - Right 089V
  - Minor Salivary 0C9J
  - Parotid
    - Left 0C99
    - Right 0C98
  - Pituitary 0G90
  - Sublingual
    - Left 0C9F
    - Right 0C9D
  - Submaxillary
    - Left 0C9H
    - Right 0C9G
  - Vestibular 0U9L
- Glenoid Cavity
  - Left 0P98
  - Right 0P97
- Glomus Jugulare 0G9C
- Hand
  - Left 0X9K
  - Right 0X9J
- Head 0W90
- Humeral Head
  - Left 0P9D
  - Right 0P9C
- Humeral Shaft
  - Left 0P9G
  - Right 0P9F
- Hymen 0U9K
- Hypothalamus 009A
- Ileocecal Valve 0D9C
- Ileum 0D9B
- Inguinal Region
  - Left 0Y96
  - Right 0Y95
- Intestine
  - Large 0D9E
    - Left 0D9G
    - Right 0D9F
  - Small 0D98
- Iris
  - Left 089D
  - Right 089C
- Jaw
  - Lower 0W95
  - Upper 0W94
- Jejunum 0D9A
- Joint
  - Acromioclavicular
    - Left 0R9H
    - Right 0R9G
  - Ankle
    - Left 0S9G
    - Right 0S9F
  - Carpal
    - Left 0R9R
    - Right 0R9Q
  - Carpometacarpal
    - Left 0R9T
    - Right 0R9S
  - Cervical Vertebral 0R91
  - Cervicothoracic Vertebral 0R94
  - Coccygeal 0S96
  - Elbow
    - Left 0R9M
    - Right 0R9L
  - Finger Phalangeal
    - Left 0R9X
    - Right 0R9W
  - Hip
    - Left 0S9B
    - Right 0S99

Drainage *(continued)*
Joint *(continued)*
Knee
Left 0S9D
Right 0S9C
Lumbar Vertebral 0S90
Lumbosacral 0S93
Metacarpophalangeal
Left 0R9V
Right 0R9U
Metatarsal-Phalangeal
Left 0S9N
Right 0S9M
Occipital-cervical 0R90
Sacrococcygeal 0S95
Sacroiliac
Left 0S98
Right 0S97
Shoulder
Left 0R9K
Right 0R9J
Sternoclavicular
Left 0R9F
Right 0R9E
Tarsal
Left 0S9J
Right 0S9H
Tarsometatarsal
Left 0S9L
Right 0S9K
Temporomandibular
Left 0R9D
Right 0R9C
Thoracic Vertebral 0R96
Thoracolumbar Vertebral 0R9A
Toe Phalangeal
Left 0S9Q
Right 0S9P
Wrist
Left 0R9P
Right 0R9N
Kidney
Left 0T91
Right 0T90
Kidney Pelvis
Left 0T94
Right 0T93
Knee Region
Left 0Y9G
Right 0Y9F
Larynx 0C9S
Leg
Lower
Left 0Y9J
Right 0Y9H
Upper
Left 0Y9D
Right 0Y9C
Lens
Left 089K
Right 089J
Lip
Lower 0C91
Upper 0C90
Liver 0F90
Left Lobe 0F92
Right Lobe 0F91
Lung
Bilateral 0B9M
Left 0B9L
Lower Lobe
Left 0B9J
Right 0B9F
Middle Lobe, Right 0B9D
Right 0B9K
Upper Lobe
Left 0B9G
Right 0B9C
Lung Lingula 0B9H

Drainage *(continued)*
Lymphatic
Aortic 079D
Axillary
Left 0796
Right 0795
Head 0790
Inguinal
Left 079J
Right 079H
Internal Mammary
Left 0799
Right 0798
Lower Extremity
Left 079G
Right 079F
Mesenteric 079B
Neck
Left 0792
Right 0791
Pelvis 079C
Thoracic Duct 079K
Thorax 0797
Upper Extremity
Left 0794
Right 0793
Mandible
Left 0N9V
Right 0N9T
Maxilla 0N9R
Mediastinum 0W9C
Medulla Oblongata 009D
Mesentery 0D9V
Metacarpal
Left 0P9Q
Right 0P9P
Metatarsal
Left 0Q9P
Right 0Q9N
Muscle
Abdomen
Left 0K9L
Right 0K9K
Extraocular
Left 089M
Right 089L
Facial 0K91
Foot
Left 0K9W
Right 0K9V
Hand
Left 0K9D
Right 0K9C
Head 0K90
Hip
Left 0K9P
Right 0K9N
Lower Arm and Wrist
Left 0K9B
Right 0K99
Lower Leg
Left 0K9T
Right 0K9S
Neck
Left 0K93
Right 0K92
Perineum 0K9M
Shoulder
Left 0K96
Right 0K95
Thorax
Left 0K9J
Right 0K9H
Tongue, Palate, Pharynx 0K94
Trunk
Left 0K9G
Right 0K9F
Upper Arm
Left 0K98
Right 0K97

Drainage *(continued)*
Muscle *(continued)*
Upper Leg
Left 0K9R
Right 0K9Q
Nasal Mucosa and Soft Tissue 099K
Nasopharynx 099N
Neck 0W96
Nerve
Abdominal Sympathetic 019M
Abducens 009L
Accessory 009R
Acoustic 009N
Brachial Plexus 0193
Cervical 0191
Cervical Plexus 0190
Facial 009M
Femoral 019D
Glossopharyngeal 009P
Head and Neck Sympathetic 019K
Hypoglossal 009S
Lumbar 019B
Lumbar Plexus 0199
Lumbar Sympathetic 019N
Lumbosacral Plexus 019A
Median 0195
Oculomotor 009H
Olfactory 009F
Optic 009G
Peroneal 019H
Phrenic 0192
Pudendal 019C
Radial 0196
Sacral 019R
Sacral Plexus 019Q
Sacral Sympathetic 019P
Sciatic 019F
Thoracic 0198
Thoracic Sympathetic 019L
Tibial 019G
Trigeminal 009K
Trochlear 009J
Ulnar 0194
Vagus 009Q
Nipple
Left 0H9X
Right 0H9W
Omentum 0D9U
Oral Cavity and Throat 0W93
Orbit
Left 0N9Q
Right 0N9P
Ovary
Bilateral 0U92
Left 0U91
Right 0U90
Palate
Hard 0C92
Soft 0C93
Pancreas 0F9G
Para-aortic Body 0G99
Paraganglion Extremity 0G9F
Parathyroid Gland 0G9R
Inferior
Left 0G9P
Right 0G9N
Multiple 0G9Q
Superior
Left 0G9M
Right 0G9L
Patella
Left 0Q9F
Right 0Q9D
Pelvic Cavity 0W9J
Penis 0V9S
Pericardial Cavity 0W9D
Perineum
Female 0W9N
Male 0W9M

Drainage *(continued)*
Peritoneal Cavity 0W9G
Peritoneum 0D9W
Phalanx
Finger
Left 0P9V
Right 0P9T
Thumb
Left 0P9S
Right 0P9R
Toe
Left 0Q9R
Right 0Q9Q
Pharynx 0C9M
Pineal Body 0G91
Pleura
Left 0B9P
Right 0B9N
Pleural Cavity
Left 0W9B
Right 0W99
Pons 009B
Prepuce 0V9T
Products of Conception
Amniotic Fluid
Diagnostic 1090
Therapeutic 1090
Fetal Blood 1090
Fetal Cerebrospinal Fluid 1090
Fetal Fluid, Other 1090
Fluid, Other 1090
Prostate 0V90
Radius
Left 0P9J
Right 0P9H
Rectum 0D9P
Retina
Left 089F
Right 089E
Retinal Vessel
Left 089H
Right 089G
Retroperitoneum 0W9H
Ribs
1 to 2 0P91
3 or More 0P92
Sacrum 0Q91
Scapula
Left 0P96
Right 0P95
Sclera
Left 0897
Right 0896
Scrotum 0V95
Septum, Nasal 099M
Shoulder Region
Left 0X93
Right 0X92
Sinus
Accessory 099P
Ethmoid
Left 099V
Right 099U
Frontal
Left 099T
Right 099S
Mastoid
Left 099C
Right 099B
Maxillary
Left 099R
Right 099Q
Sphenoid
Left 099X
Right 099W
Skin
Abdomen 0H97
Back 0H96
Buttock 0H98
Chest 0H95

Drainage *(continued)*
Skin *(continued)*
Ear
Left 0H93
Right 0H92
Face 0H91
Foot
Left 0H9N
Right 0H9M
Hand
Left 0H9G
Right 0H9F
Inguinal 0H9A
Lower Arm
Left 0H9E
Right 0H9D
Lower Leg
Left 0H9L
Right 0H9K
Neck 0H94
Perineum 0H99
Scalp 0H90
Upper Arm
Left 0H9C
Right 0H9B
Upper Leg
Left 0H9J
Right 0H9H
Skull 0N90
Spinal Canal 009U
Spinal Cord
Cervical 009W
Lumbar 009Y
Thoracic 009X
Spinal Meninges 009T
Spleen 079P
Sternum 0P90
Stomach 0D96
Pylorus 0D97
Subarachnoid Space, Intracranial 0095
Subcutaneous Tissue and Fascia
Abdomen 0J98
Back 0J97
Buttock 0J99
Chest 0J96
Face 0J91
Foot
Left 0J9R
Right 0J9Q
Hand
Left 0J9K
Right 0J9J
Lower Arm
Left 0J9H
Right 0J9G
Lower Leg
Left 0J9P
Right 0J9N
Neck
Left 0J95
Right 0J94
Pelvic Region 0J9C
Perineum 0J9B
Scalp 0J90
Upper Arm
Left 0J9F
Right 0J9D
Upper Leg
Left 0J9M
Right 0J9L
Subdural Space, Intracranial 0094
Tarsal
Left 0Q9M
Right 0Q9L
Tendon
Abdomen
Left 0L9G
Right 0L9F

Drainage *(continued)*
Tendon *(continued)*
Ankle
Left 0L9T
Right 0L9S
Foot
Left 0L9W
Right 0L9V
Hand
Left 0L98
Right 0L97
Head and Neck 0L90
Hip
Left 0L9K
Right 0L9J
Knee
Left 0L9R
Right 0L9Q
Lower Arm and Wrist
Left 0L96
Right 0L95
Lower Leg
Left 0L9P
Right 0L9N
Perineum 0L9H
Shoulder
Left 0L92
Right 0L91
Thorax
Left 0L9D
Right 0L9C
Electrocautery
Right 0L99
Upper Arm
Left 0L94
Right 0L93
Upper Leg
Left 0L9M
Right 0L9L
Testis
Bilateral 0V9C
Left 0V9B
Right 0V99
Thalamus 0099
Thymus 079M
Thyroid Gland 0G9K
Left Lobe 0G9G
Right Lobe 0G9H
Tibia
Left 0Q9H
Right 0Q9G
Toe Nail 0H9R
Tongue 0C97
Tonsils 0C9P
Tooth
Lower 0C9X
Upper 0C9W
Trachea 0B91
Tunica Vaginalis
Left 0V97
Right 0V96
Turbinate, Nasal 099L
Tympanic Membrane
Left 0998
Right 0997
Ulna
Left 0P9L
Right 0P9K
Ureter
Left 0T97
Right 0T96
Ureters, Bilateral 0T98
Urethra 0T9D
Uterine Supporting Structure 0U94
Uterus 0U99
Uvula 0C9N
Vagina 0U9G
Vas Deferens
Bilateral 0V9Q

Drainage *(continued)*
Vas Deferens *(continued)*
Left 0V9P
Right 0V9N
Vein
Axillary
Left 0598
Right 0597
Azygos 0590
Basilic
Left 059C
Right 059B
Brachial
Left 059A
Right 0599
Cephalic
Left 059F
Right 059D
Colic 0697
Common Iliac
Left 069D
Right 069C
Esophageal 0693
External Iliac
Left 069G
Right 069F
External Jugular
Left 059Q
Right 059P
Face
Left 059V
Right 059T
Femoral
Left 069N
Right 069M
Foot
Left 069V
Right 069T
Gastric 0692
Hand
Left 059H
Right 059G
Hemiazygos 0591
Hepatic 0694
Hypogastric
Left 069J
Right 069H
Inferior Mesenteric 0696
Innominate
Left 0594
Right 0593
Internal Jugular
Left 059N
Right 059M
Intracranial 059L
Lower 069Y
Portal 0698
Renal
Left 069B
Right 0699
Saphenous
Left 069Q
Right 069P
Splenic 0691
Subclavian
Left 0596
Right 0595
Superior Mesenteric 0695
Upper 059Y
Vertebral
Left 059S
Right 059R
Vena Cava, Inferior 0690
Vertebra
Cervical 0P93
Lumbar 0Q90
Thoracic 0P94

Drainage *(continued)*
Vesicle
Bilateral 0V93
Left 0V92
Right 0V91
Vitreous
Left 0895
Right 0894
Vocal Cord
Left 0C9V
Right 0C9T
Vulva 0U9M
Wrist Region
Left 0X9H
Right 0X9G
Dressing
Abdominal Wall 2W23X4Z
Arm
Lower
Left 2W2DX4Z
Right 2W2CX4Z
Upper
Left 2W2BX4Z
Right 2W2AX4Z
Back 2W25X4Z
Chest Wall 2W24X4Z
Extremity
Lower
Left 2W2MX4Z
Right 2W2LX4Z
Upper
Left 2W29X4Z
Right 2W28X4Z
Face 2W21X4Z
Finger
Left 2W2KX4Z
Right 2W2JX4Z
Foot
Left 2W2TX4Z
Right 2W2SX4Z
Hand
Left 2W2FX4Z
Right 2W2EX4Z
Head 2W20X4Z
Inguinal Region
Left 2W27X4Z
Right 2W26X4Z
Leg
Lower
Left 2W2RX4Z
Right 2W2QX4Z
Upper
Left 2W2PX4Z
Right 2W2NX4Z
Neck 2W22X4Z
Thumb
Left 2W2HX4Z
Right 2W2GX4Z
Toe
Left 2W2VX4Z
Right 2W2UX4Z
Driver stent (RX) (OTW)
use Intraluminal Device
Drotrecogin alfa, infusion
see Introduction of Recombinant Human-activated Protein C
Duct of Santorini
use Duct, Pancreatic, Accessory
Duct of Wirsung
use Duct, Pancreatic
Ductogram, mammary
see Plain Radiography, Skin, Subcutaneous Tissue and Brea BH0
Ductography, mammary
see Plain Radiography, Skin, Subcutaneous Tissue and Brea BH0
Ductus deferens
use Vas Deferens

Ductus deferens *(continued)*
use Vas Deferens, Bilateral
use Vas Deferens, Left
use Vas Deferens, Right
Duodenal ampulla
use Ampulla of Vater
Duodenectomy
see Excision, Duodenum 0DB9
see Resection, Duodenum 0DT9
Duodenocholedochotomy
see Drainage, Gallbladder 0F94
Duodenocystostomy
see Bypass, Gallbladder 0F14
see Drainage, Gallbladder 0F94
Duodenoenterostomy
see Bypass, Gastrointestinal System 0D1
see Drainage, Gastrointestinal System 0D9
Duodenojejunal flexure
use Jejunum
Duodenolysis
see Release, Duodenum 0DN9
Duodenorrhaphy
see Repair, Duodenum 0DQ9
Duodenostomy
see Bypass, Duodenum 0D19
see Drainage, Duodenum 0D99
Duodenotomy
see Drainage, Duodenum 0D99
DuraGraft® Endothelial Damage Inhibitor
use Endothelial Damage Inhibitor
DuraHeart Left Ventricular Assist System
use Implantable Heart Assist System in Heart and Great Vessels
Dural venous sinus
use Vein, Intracranial
Dura mater, intracranial
use Dura Mater
Dura mater, spinal
use Spinal Meninges
Durata® Defibrillation Lead
use Cardiac Lead, Defibrillator in 02H
Dynesys® Dynamic Stabilization System
use Spinal Stabilization Device, Pedicle-Based in 0RH
use Spinal Stabilization Device, Pedicle-Based in 0SH

E

E-Luminexx™ (Biliary)(Vascular) Stent
use Intraluminal Device
Earlobe
use Ear, External, Bilateral
use Ear, External, Left
use Ear, External, Right
ECCO2R (Extracorporeal Carbon Dioxide Removal) 5A0920Z
Echocardiogram
see Ultrasonography, Heart B24
Echography
see Ultrasonography
ECMO
see Performance, Circulatory 5A15
EDWARDS INTUITY Elite valve system
use Zooplastic Tissue, Rapid Deployment in New Technology
EEG (electroencephalogram)
see Measurement, Central Nervous 4A00
EGD (esophagogastroduodenoscopy) 0DJ08ZZ
Eighth cranial nerve
use Nerve, Acoustic
Ejaculatory duct
use Vas Deferens
use Vas Deferens, Bilateral
use Vas Deferens, Left
use Vas Deferens, Right
EKG (electrocardiogram)
see Measurement, Cardiac 4A02
Electrical bone growth stimulator (EBGS)
use Bone Growth Stimulator in Head and Facial Bones
use Bone Growth Stimulator in Lower Bones
use Bone Growth Stimulator in Upper Bones
Electrical muscle stimulation (EMS) lead
use Stimulator Lead in Muscles
Electrocautery
Destruction
see Destruction
Repair
see Repair
Electroconvulsive Therapy
Bilateral-Multiple Seizure GZB3ZZZ
Bilateral-Single Seizure GZB2ZZZ
Electroconvulsive Therapy, Other GZB4ZZZ
Unilateral-Multiple Seizure GZB1ZZZ
Unilateral-Single Seizure GZB0ZZZ
Electroencephalogram (EEG)
see Measurement, Central Nervous 4A00
Electromagnetic Therapy
Central Nervous 6A22
Urinary 6A21
Electronic muscle stimulator lead
use Stimulator Lead in Muscles
Electrophysiologic stimulation (EPS)
see Measurement, Cardiac 4A02
Electroshock therapy
see Electroconvulsive Therapy
Elevation, bone fragments, skull
see Reposition, Head and Facial Bones 0NS
Eleventh cranial nerve
use Nerve, Accessory
Embolectomy
see Extirpation
Embolization
see Occlusion
see Restriction
Embolization coil(s)
use Intraluminal Device
EMG (electromyogram)
see Measurement, Musculoskeletal 4A0F
Encephalon
use Brain
Endarterectomy
see Extirpation, Lower Arteries 04C
see Extirpation, Upper Arteries 03C
Endeavor® (III)(IV) (Sprint) Zotarolimus-eluting Coronary Stent System
use Intraluminal Device, Drug-eluting in Heart and Great Vessels
Endologix AFX® Endovascular AAA System
use Intraluminal Device
EndoSure® sensor
use Monitoring Device, Pressure Sensor in 02H
ENDOTAK RELIANCE® (G) Defibrillation Lead
use Cardiac Lead, Defibrillator in 02H
Endothelial damage inhibitor, applied to vein graft XY0VX83
Endotracheal tube (cuffed)(double-lumen)
use Intraluminal Device, Endotracheal Airway in Respiratory System
Endurant® II AAA stent graft system
use Intraluminal Device
Endurant® Endovascular Stent Graft
use Intraluminal Device
Engineered Autologous Chimeric Antigen Receptor T-cell Immunotherapy XW0
Enlargement
see Dilation
see Repair
EnRhythm
use Pacemaker, Dual Chamber in 0JH
Enterorrhaphy
see Repair, Gastrointestinal System 0DQ
Enterra gastric neurostimulator
use Stimulator Generator, Multiple Array in 0JH
Enucleation
Eyeball
see Resection, Eye 08T
Eyeball with prosthetic implant
see Replacement, Eye 08R
Ependyma
use Cerebral Ventricle
Epicel® cultured epidermal autograft
use Autologous Tissue Substitute
Epic™ Stented Tissue Valve (aortic)
use Zooplastic Tissue in Heart and Great Vessels
Epidermis
use Skin
Epididymectomy
see Excision, Male Reproductive System 0VB
see Resection, Male Reproductive System 0VT
Epididymoplasty
see Repair, Male Reproductive System 0VQ
see Supplement, Male Reproductive System 0VU
Epididymorrhaphy
see Repair, Male Reproductive System 0VQ
Epididymotomy
see Drainage, Male Reproductive System 0V9
Epidural space, spinal
use Spinal Canal
Epiphysiodesis
see Insertion of device in Lower Bones 0QH
see Insertion of device in Upper Bones 0PH
see Repair, Lower Bones 0QQ
see Repair, Upper Bones 0PQ
Epiploic foramen
use Peritoneum
Epiretinal Visual Prosthesis
Left 08H105Z
Right 08H005Z
Episiorrhaphy
see Repair, Perineum, Female 0WQN
Episiotomy
see Division, Perineum, Female 0W8N
Epithalamus
use Thalamus
Epitrochlear lymph node
use Lymphatic, Upper Extremity, Left
use Lymphatic, Upper Extremity, Right
EPS (electrophysiologic stimulation)
see Measurement, Cardiac 4A02
Eptifibatide, infusion
see Introduction of Platelet Inhibitor
ERCP (endoscopic retrograde cholangiopancreatography)
see Fluoroscopy, Hepatobiliary System and Pancreas BF1
Erector spinae muscle
use Muscle, Trunk, Left
use Muscle, Trunk, Right
Esophageal artery
use Upper Artery
Esophageal obturator airway (EOA)
use Intraluminal Device, Airway in Gastrointestinal System
Esophageal plexus
use Nerve, Thoracic Sympathetic
Esophagectomy
see Excision, Gastrointestinal System 0DB
see Resection, Gastrointestinal System 0DT
Esophagocoloplasty
see Repair, Gastrointestinal System 0DQ
see Supplement, Gastrointestinal System 0DU
Esophagoenterostomy
see Bypass, Gastrointestinal System 0D1
see Drainage, Gastrointestinal System 0D9
Esophagoesophagostomy
see Bypass, Gastrointestinal System 0D1
see Drainage, Gastrointestinal System 0D9
Esophagogastrectomy
see Excision, Gastrointestinal System 0DB
see Resection, Gastrointestinal System 0DT
Esophagogastroduodenoscopy (EGD) 0DJ08ZZ
Esophagogastroplasty
see Repair, Gastrointestinal System 0DQ
see Supplement, Gastrointestinal System 0DU
Esophagogastroscopy 0DJ68ZZ
Esophagogastrostomy
see Bypass, Gastrointestinal System 0D1
see Drainage, Gastrointestinal System 0D9
Esophagojejunoplasty
see Supplement, Gastrointestinal System 0DU
Esophagojejunostomy
see Bypass, Gastrointestinal System 0D1
see Drainage, Gastrointestinal System 0D9
Esophagomyotomy
see Division, Esophagogastric Junction 0D84
Esophagoplasty
see Repair, Gastrointestinal System 0DQ
see Replacement, Esophagus 0DR5
see Supplement, Gastrointestinal System 0DU

Esophagoplication
- *see* Restriction, Gastrointestinal System 0DV

Esophagorrhaphy
- *see* Repair, Gastrointestinal System 0DQ

Esophagoscopy 0DJ08ZZ

Esophagotomy
- *see* Drainage, Gastrointestinal System 0D9

Esteem® implantable hearing system
- *use* Hearing Device in Ear, Nose, Sinus

ESWL (extracorporeal shock wave lithotripsy)
- *see* Fragmentation

Ethmoidal air cell
- *use* Sinus, Ethmoid, Left
- *use* Sinus, Ethmoid, Right

Ethmoidectomy
- *see* Excision, Ear, Nose, Sinus 09B
- *see* Excision, Head and Facial Bones 0NB
- *see* Resection, Ear, Nose, Sinus 09T
- *see* Resection, Head and Facial Bones 0NT

Ethmoidotomy
- *see* Drainage, Ear, Nose, Sinus 099

Evacuation
- Hematoma
  - *see* Extirpation
- Other Fluid
  - *see* Drainage

Evera (XT)(S)(DR/VR)
- *use* Defibrillator Generator in 0JH

Everolimus-eluting coronary stent
- *use* Intraluminal Device, Drug-eluting in Heart and Great Vessels

Evisceration
- Eyeball
  - *see* Resection, Eye 08T
- Eyeball with prosthetic implant
  - *see* Replacement, Eye 08R

Ex-PRESS™ mini glaucoma shunt
- *use* Synthetic Substitute

Examination
- *see* Inspection

Exchange
- *see* Change device in

Excision
- Abdominal Wall 0WBF
- Acetabulum
  - Left 0QB5
  - Right 0QB4
- Adenoids 0CBQ
- Ampulla of Vater 0FBC
- Anal Sphincter 0DBR
- Ankle Region
  - Left 0YBL
  - Right 0YBK
- Anus 0DBQ
- Aorta
  - Abdominal 04B0
  - Thoracic
    - Ascending/Arch 02BX
    - Descending 02BW
- Aortic Body 0GBD
- Appendix 0DBJ
- Arm
  - Lower
    - Left 0XBF
    - Right 0XBD
  - Upper
    - Left 0XB9
    - Right 0XB8
- Artery
  - Anterior Tibial
    - Left 04BQ
    - Right 04BP
  - Axillary
    - Left 03B6
    - Right 03B5
  - Brachial
    - Left 03B8
    - Right 03B7
  - Celiac 04B1
  - Colic
    - Left 04B7
    - Middle 04B8
    - Right 04B6
  - Common Carotid
    - Left 03BJ
    - Right 03BH
  - Common Iliac
    - Left 04BD
    - Right 04BC
  - External Carotid
    - Left 03BN
    - Right 03BM
  - External Iliac
    - Left 04BJ
    - Right 04BH
  - Face 03BR
  - Femoral
    - Left 04BL
    - Right 04BK
  - Foot
    - Left 04BW
    - Right 04BV
  - Gastric 04B2
  - Hand
    - Left 03BF
    - Right 03BD
  - Hepatic 04B3
  - Inferior Mesenteric 04BB
  - Innominate 03B2
  - Internal Carotid
    - Left 03BL
    - Right 03BK
  - Internal Iliac
    - Left 04BF
    - Right 04BE
  - Internal Mammary
    - Left 03B1
    - Right 03B0
  - Intracranial 03BG
  - Lower 04BY
  - Peroneal
    - Left 04BU
    - Right 04BT
  - Popliteal
    - Left 04BN
    - Right 04BM
  - Posterior Tibial
    - Left 04BS
    - Right 04BR
  - Pulmonary
    - Left 02BR
    - Right 02BQ
  - Pulmonary Trunk 02BP
  - Radial
    - Left 03BC
    - Right 03BB
  - Renal
    - Left 04BA
    - Right 04B9
  - Splenic 04B4
  - Subclavian
    - Left 03B4
    - Right 03B3
  - Superior Mesenteric 04B5
  - Temporal
    - Left 03BT
    - Right 03BS
  - Thyroid
    - Left 03BV
    - Right 03BU
  - Ulnar
    - Left 03BA
    - Right 03B9
  - Upper 03BY
  - Vertebral
    - Left 03BQ
    - Right 03BP
- Atrium
  - Left 02B7
  - Right 02B6
- Auditory Ossicle
  - Left 09BA
  - Right 09B9
- Axilla
  - Left 0XB5
  - Right 0XB4
- Back
  - Lower 0WBL
  - Upper 0WBK
- Basal Ganglia 00B8
- Bladder 0TBB
- Bladder Neck 0TBC
- Bone
  - Ethmoid
    - Left 0NBG
    - Right 0NBF
  - Frontal 0NB1
  - Hyoid 0NBX
  - Lacrimal
    - Left 0NBJ
    - Right 0NBH
  - Nasal 0NBB
  - Occipital 0NB7
  - Palatine
    - Left 0NBL
    - Right 0NBK
  - Parietal
    - Left 0NB4
    - Right 0NB3
  - Pelvic
    - Left 0QB3
    - Right 0QB2
  - Sphenoid 0NBC
  - Temporal
    - Left 0NB6
    - Right 0NB5
  - Zygomatic
    - Left 0NBN
    - Right 0NBM
- Brain 00B0
- Breast
  - Bilateral 0HBV
  - Left 0HBU
  - Right 0HBT
  - Supernumerary 0HBY
- Bronchus
  - Lingula 0BB9
  - Lower Lobe
    - Left 0BBB
    - Right 0BB6
  - Main
    - Left 0BB7
    - Right 0BB3
  - Middle Lobe, Right 0BB5
  - Upper Lobe
    - Left 0BB8
    - Right 0BB4
- Buccal Mucosa 0CB4
- Bursa and Ligament
  - Abdomen
    - Left 0MBJ
    - Right 0MBH
  - Ankle
    - Left 0MBR
    - Right 0MBQ
  - Elbow
    - Left 0MB4
    - Right 0MB3
  - Foot
    - Left 0MBT
    - Right 0MBS
  - Hand
    - Left 0MB8
    - Right 0MB7
  - Head and Neck 0MB0
  - Hip
    - Left 0MBM
    - Right 0MBL
  - Knee
    - Left 0MBP
    - Right 0MBN
  - Lower Extremity
    - Left 0MBW
    - Right 0MBV
  - Rib(s) 0MBG
  - Perineum 0MBK
  - Shoulder
    - Left 0MB2
    - Right 0MB1
  - Spine
    - Lower 0MBD
    - Upper 0MBC
  - Sternum 0MBF
  - Upper Extremity
    - Left 0MBB
    - Right 0MB9
  - Wrist
    - Left 0MB6
    - Right 0MB5
- Buttock
  - Left 0YB1
  - Right 0YB0
- Carina 0BB2
- Carotid Bodies, Bilateral 0GB8
- Carotid Body
  - Left 0GB6
  - Right 0GB7
- Carpal
  - Left 0PBN
  - Right 0PBM
- Cecum 0DBH
- Cerebellum 00BC
- Cerebral Hemisphere 00B7
- Cerebral Meninges 00B1
- Cerebral Ventricle 00B6
- Cervix 0UBC
- Chest Wall 0WB8
- Chordae Tendineae 02B9
- Choroid
  - Left 08BB
  - Right 08BA
- Cisterna Chyli 07BL
- Clavicle
  - Left 0PBB
  - Right 0PB9
- Clitoris 0UBJ
- Coccygeal Glomus 0GBB
- Coccyx 0QBS
- Colon
  - Ascending 0DBK
  - Descending 0DBM
  - Sigmoid 0DBN
  - Transverse 0DBL
- Conduction Mechanism 02B8
- Conjunctiva
  - Left 08BTXZ
  - Right 08BSXZ
- Cord
  - Bilateral 0VBH
  - Left 0VBG
  - Right 0VBF
- Cornea
  - Left 08B9XZ
  - Right 08B8XZ
- Cul-de-sac 0UBF

Excision *(continued)*
- Diaphragm 0BBT
- Disc
  - Cervical Vertebral 0RB3
  - Cervicothoracic Vertebral 0RB5
  - Lumbar Vertebral 0SB2
  - Lumbosacral 0SB4
  - Thoracic Vertebral 0RB9
  - Thoracolumbar Vertebral 0RBB
- Duct
  - Common Bile 0FB9
  - Cystic 0FB8
  - Hepatic
    - Common 0FB7
    - Left 0FB6
    - Right 0FB5
  - Lacrimal
    - Left 08BY
    - Right 08BX
  - Pancreatic 0FBD
    - Accessory 0FBF
  - Parotid
    - Left 0CBC
    - Right 0CBB
- Duodenum 0DB9
- Dura Mater 00B2
- Ear
  - External
    - Left 09B1
    - Right 09B0
  - External Auditory Canal
    - Left 09B4
    - Right 09B3
  - Inner
    - Left 09BE
    - Right 09BD
  - Middle
    - Left 09B6
    - Right 09B5
- Elbow Region
  - Left 0XBC
  - Right 0XBB
- Epididymis
  - Bilateral 0VBL
  - Left 0VBK
  - Right 0VBJ
- Epiglottis 0CBR
- Esophagogastric Junction 0DB4
- Esophagus 0DB5
  - Lower 0DB3
  - Middle 0DB2
  - Upper 0DB1
- Eustachian Tube
  - Left 09BG
  - Right 09BF
- Extremity
  - Lower
    - Left 0YBB
    - Right 0YB9
  - Upper
    - Left 0XB7
    - Right 0XB6
- Eye
  - Left 08B1
  - Right 08B0
- Eyelid
  - Lower
    - Left 08BR
    - Right 08BQ
  - Upper
    - Left 08BP
    - Right 08BN
- Face 0WB2
- Fallopian Tube
  - Left 0UB6
  - Right 0UB5
- Fallopian Tubes, Bilateral 0UB7

Excision *(continued)*
- Femoral Region
  - Left 0YB8
  - Right 0YB7
- Femoral Shaft
  - Left 0QB9
  - Right 0QB8
- Femur
  - Lower
    - Left 0QBC
    - Right 0QBB
  - Upper
    - Left 0QB7
    - Right 0QB6
- Fibula
  - Left 0QBK
  - Right 0QBJ
- Finger Nail 0HBQXZ
- Floor of mouth
  - *see* Excision, Oral Cavity and Throat 0WB3
- Foot
  - Left 0YBN
  - Right 0YBM
- Gallbladder 0FB4
- Gingiva
  - Lower 0CB6
  - Upper 0CB5
- Gland
  - Adrenal
    - Bilateral 0GB4
    - Left 0GB2
    - Right 0GB3
  - Lacrimal
    - Left 08BW
    - Right 08BV
  - Minor Salivary 0CBJ
  - Parotid
    - Left 0CB9
    - Right 0CB8
  - Pituitary 0GB0
  - Sublingual
    - Left 0CBF
    - Right 0CBD
  - Submaxillary
    - Left 0CBH
    - Right 0CBG
  - Vestibular 0UBL
- Glenoid Cavity
  - Left 0PB8
  - Right 0PB7
- Glomus Jugulare 0GBC
- Hand
  - Left 0XBK
  - Right 0XBJ
- Head 0WB0
- Humeral Head
  - Left 0PBD
  - Right 0PBC
- Humeral Shaft
  - Left 0PBG
  - Right 0PBF
- Hymen 0UBK
- Hypothalamus 00BA
- Ileocecal Valve 0DBC
- Ileum 0DBB
- Inguinal Region
  - Left 0YB6
  - Right 0YB5
- Intestine
  - Large 0DBE
    - Left 0DBG
    - Right 0DBF
  - Small 0DB8
- Iris
  - Left 08BD3Z
  - Right 08BC3Z
- Jaw
  - Lower 0WB5
  - Upper 0WB4

Excision *(continued)*
- Jejunum 0DBA
- Joint
  - Acromioclavicular
    - Left 0RBH
    - Right 0RBG
  - Ankle
    - Left 0SBG
    - Right 0SBF
  - Carpal
    - Left 0RBR
    - Right 0RBQ
  - Carpometacarpal
    - Left 0RBT
    - Right 0RBS
  - Cervical Vertebral 0RB1
  - Cervicothoracic Vertebral 0RB4
  - Coccygeal 0SB6
  - Elbow
    - Left 0RBM
    - Right 0RBL
  - Finger Phalangeal
    - Left 0RBX
    - Right 0RBW
  - Hip
    - Left 0SBB
    - Right 0SB9
  - Knee
    - Left 0SBD
    - Right 0SBC
  - Lumbar Vertebral 0SB0
  - Lumbosacral 0SB3
  - Metacarpophalangeal
    - Left 0RBV
    - Right 0RBU
  - Metatarsal-Phalangeal
    - Left 0SBN
    - Right 0SBM
  - Occipital-cervical 0RB0
  - Sacrococcygeal 0SB5
  - Sacroiliac
    - Left 0SB8
    - Right 0SB7
  - Shoulder
    - Left 0RBK
    - Right 0RBJ
  - Sternoclavicular
    - Left 0RBF
    - Right 0RBE
  - Tarsal
    - Left 0SBJ
    - Right 0SBH
  - Tarsometatarsal
    - Left 0SBL
    - Right 0SBK
  - Temporomandibular
    - Left 0RBD
    - Right 0RBC
  - Thoracic Vertebral 0RB6
  - Thoracolumbar Vertebral 0RBA
  - Toe Phalangeal
    - Left 0SBQ
    - Right 0SBP
  - Wrist
    - Left 0RBP
    - Right 0RBN
- Kidney
  - Left 0TB1
  - Right 0TB0
- Kidney Pelvis
  - Left 0TB4
  - Right 0TB3
- Knee Region
  - Left 0YBG
  - Right 0YBF
- Larynx 0CBS

Excision *(continued)*
- Leg
  - Lower
    - Left 0YBJ
    - Right 0YBH
  - Upper
    - Left 0YBD
    - Right 0YBC
- Lens
  - Left 08BK3Z
  - Right 08BJ3Z
- Lip
  - Lower 0CB1
  - Upper 0CB0
- Liver 0FB0
  - Left Lobe 0FB2
  - Right Lobe 0FB1
- Lung
  - Bilateral 0BBM
  - Left 0BBL
  - Lower Lobe
    - Left 0BBJ
    - Right 0BBF
  - Middle Lobe, Right 0BBD
  - Right 0BBK
  - Upper Lobe
    - Left 0BBG
    - Right 0BBC
- Lung Lingula 0BBH
- Lymphatic
  - Aortic 07BD
  - Axillary
    - Left 07B6
    - Right 07B5
  - Head 07B0
  - Inguinal
    - Left 07BJ
    - Right 07BH
  - Internal Mammary
    - Left 07B9
    - Right 07B8
  - Lower Extremity
    - Left 07BG
    - Right 07BF
  - Mesenteric 07BB
  - Neck
    - Left 07B2
    - Right 07B1
  - Pelvis 07BC
  - Thoracic Duct 07BK
  - Thorax 07B7
  - Upper Extremity
    - Left 07B4
    - Right 07B3
- Mandible
  - Left 0NBV
  - Right 0NBT
- Maxilla 0NBR
- Mediastinum 0WBC
- Medulla Oblongata 00BD
- Mesentery 0DBV
- Metacarpal
  - Left 0PBQ
  - Right 0PBP
- Metatarsal
  - Left 0QBP
  - Right 0QBN
- Muscle
  - Abdomen
    - Left 0KBL
    - Right 0KBK
  - Extraocular
    - Left 08BM
    - Right 08BL
  - Facial 0KB1
  - Foot
    - Left 0KBW
    - Right 0KBV
  - Hand
    - Left 0KBD

Excision *(continued)*
- Muscle *(continued)*
  - Hand *(continued)*
    - Right 0KBC
  - Head 0KB0
  - Hip
    - Left 0KBP
    - Right 0KBN
  - Lower Arm and Wrist
    - Left 0KBB
    - Right 0KB9
  - Lower Leg
    - Left 0KBT
    - Right 0KBS
  - Neck
    - Left 0KB3
    - Right 0KB2
  - Papillary 02BD
  - Perineum 0KBM
  - Shoulder
    - Left 0KB6
    - Right 0KB5
  - Thorax
    - Left 0KBJ
    - Right 0KBH
  - Tongue, Palate, Pharynx 0KB4
  - Trunk
    - Left 0KBG
    - Right 0KBF
  - Upper Arm
    - Left 0KB8
    - Right 0KB7
  - Upper Leg
    - Left 0KBR
    - Right 0KBQ
- Nasal Mucosa and Soft Tissue 09BK
- Nasopharynx 09BN
- Neck 0WB6
- Nerve
  - Abdominal Sympathetic 01BM
  - Abducens 00BL
  - Accessory 00BR
  - Acoustic 00BN
  - Brachial Plexus 01B3
  - Cervical 01B1
  - Cervical Plexus 01B0
  - Facial 00BM
  - Femoral 01BD
  - Glossopharyngeal 00BP
  - Head and Neck Sympathetic 01BK
  - Hypoglossal 00BS
  - Lumbar 01BB
  - Lumbar Plexus 01B9
  - Lumbar Sympathetic 01BN
  - Lumbosacral Plexus 01BA
  - Median 01B5
  - Oculomotor 00BH
  - Olfactory 00BF
  - Optic 00BG
  - Peroneal 01BH
  - Phrenic 01B2
  - Pudendal 01BC
  - Radial 01B6
  - Sacral 01BR
  - Sacral Plexus 01BQ
  - Sacral Sympathetic 01BP
  - Sciatic 01BF
  - Thoracic 01B8
  - Thoracic Sympathetic 01BL
  - Tibial 01BG
  - Trigeminal 00BK
  - Trochlear 00BJ
  - Ulnar 01B4
  - Vagus 00BQ
- Nipple
  - Left 0HBX
  - Right 0HBW

Excision *(continued)*
- Omentum 0DBU
- Oral Cavity and Throat 0WB3
- Orbit
  - Left 0NBQ
  - Right 0NBP
- Ovary
  - Bilateral 0UB2
  - Left 0UB1
  - Right 0UB0
- Palate
  - Hard 0CB2
  - Soft 0CB3
- Pancreas 0FBG
- Para-aortic Body 0GB9
- Paraganglion Extremity 0GBF
- Parathyroid Gland 0GBR
  - Inferior
    - Left 0GBP
    - Right 0GBN
  - Multiple 0GBQ
  - Superior
    - Left 0GBM
    - Right 0GBL
- Patella
  - Left 0QBF
  - Right 0QBD
- Penis 0VBS
- Pericardium 02BN
- Perineum
  - Female 0WBN
  - Male 0WBM
- Peritoneum 0DBW
- Phalanx
  - Finger
    - Left 0PBV
    - Right 0PBT
  - Thumb
    - Left 0PBS
    - Right 0PBR
  - Toe
    - Left 0QBR
    - Right 0QBQ
- Pharynx 0CBM
- Pineal Body 0GB1
- Pleura
  - Left 0BBP
  - Right 0BBN
- Pons 00BB
- Prepuce 0VBT
- Prostate 0VB0
- Radius
  - Left 0PBJ
  - Right 0PBH
- Rectum 0DBP
- Retina
  - Left 08BF3Z
  - Right 08BE3Z
- Retroperitoneum 0WBH
- Ribs
  - 1 to 2 0PB1
  - 3 or More 0PB2
- Sacrum 0QB1
- Scapula
  - Left 0PB6
  - Right 0PB5
- Sclera
  - Left 08B7XZ
  - Right 08B6XZ
- Scrotum 0VB5
- Septum
  - Atrial 02B5
  - Nasal 09BM
  - Ventricular 02BM
- Shoulder Region
  - Left 0XB3
  - Right 0XB2
- Sinus
  - Accessory 09BP

Excision *(continued)*
- Sinus *(continued)*
  - Ethmoid
    - Left 09BV
    - Right 09BU
  - Frontal
    - Left 09BT
    - Right 09BS
  - Mastoid
    - Left 09BC
    - Right 09BB
  - Maxillary
    - Left 09BR
    - Right 09BQ
  - Sphenoid
    - Left 09BX
    - Right 09BW
- Skin
  - Abdomen 0HB7XZ
  - Back 0HB6XZ
  - Buttock 0HB8XZ
  - Chest 0HB5XZ
  - Ear
    - Left 0HB3XZ
    - Right 0HB2XZ
  - Face 0HB1XZ
  - Foot
    - Left 0HBNXZ
    - Right 0HBMXZ
  - Hand
    - Left 0HBGXZ
    - Right 0HBFXZ
  - Inguinal 0HBAXZ
  - Lower Arm
    - Left 0HBEXZ
    - Right 0HBDXZ
  - Lower Leg
    - Left 0HBLXZ
    - Right 0HBKXZ
  - Neck 0HB4XZ
  - Perineum 0HB9XZ
  - Scalp 0HB0XZ
  - Upper Arm
    - Left 0HBCXZ
    - Right 0HBBXZ
  - Upper Leg
    - Left 0HBJXZ
    - Right 0HBHXZ
- Skull 0NB0
- Spinal Cord
  - Cervical 00BW
  - Lumbar 00BY
  - Thoracic 00BX
- Spinal Meninges 00BT
- Spleen 07BP
- Sternum 0PB0
- Stomach 0DB6
  - Pylorus 0DB7
- Subcutaneous Tissue and Fascia
  - Abdomen 0JB8
  - Back 0JB7
  - Buttock 0JB9
  - Chest 0JB6
  - Face 0JB1
  - Foot
    - Left 0JBR
    - Right 0JBQ
  - Hand
    - Left 0JBK
    - Right 0JBJ
  - Lower Arm
    - Left 0JBH
    - Right 0JBG
  - Lower Leg
    - Left 0JBP
    - Right 0JBN
  - Neck
    - Left 0JB5
    - Right 0JB4
  - Pelvic Region 0JBC

Excision *(continued)*
- Subcutaneous Tissue and Fascia *(continued)*
  - Perineum 0JBB
  - Scalp 0JB0
  - Upper Arm
    - Left 0JBF
    - Right 0JBD
  - Upper Leg
    - Left 0JBM
    - Right 0JBL
- Tarsal
  - Left 0QBM
  - Right 0QBL
- Tendon
  - Abdomen
    - Left 0LBG
    - Right 0LBF
  - Ankle
    - Left 0LBT
    - Right 0LBS
  - Foot
    - Left 0LBW
    - Right 0LBV
  - Hand
    - Left 0LB8
    - Right 0LB7
  - Head and Neck 0LB0
  - Hip
    - Left 0LBK
    - Right 0LBJ
  - Knee
    - Left 0LBR
    - Right 0LBQ
  - Lower Arm and Wrist
    - Left 0LB6
    - Right 0LB5
  - Lower Leg
    - Left 0LBP
    - Right 0LBN
  - Perineum 0LBH
  - Shoulder
    - Left 0LB2
    - Right 0LB1
  - Thorax
    - Left 0LBD
    - Right 0LBC
  - Trunk
    - Left 0LBB
    - Right 0LB9
  - Upper Arm
    - Left 0LB4
    - Right 0LB3
  - Upper Leg
    - Left 0LBM
    - Right 0LBL
- Testis
  - Bilateral 0VBC
  - Left 0VBB
  - Right 0VB9
- Thalamus 00B9
- Thymus 07BM
- Thyroid Gland
  - Left Lobe 0GBG
  - Right Lobe 0GBH
- Thyroid Gland Isthmus 0GBJ
- Tibia
  - Left 0QBH
  - Right 0QBG
- Toe Nail 0HBRXZ
- Tongue 0CB7
- Tonsils 0CBP
- Tooth
  - Lower 0CBX
  - Upper 0CBW
- Trachea 0BB1
- Tunica Vaginalis
  - Left 0VB7
  - Right 0VB6

Excision *(continued)*
Turbinate, Nasal 09BL
Tympanic Membrane
Left 09B8
Right 09B7
Ulna
Left 0PBL
Right 0PBK
Ureter
Left 0TB7
Right 0TB6
Urethra 0TBD
Uterine Supporting Structure 0UB4
Uterus 0UB9
Uvula 0CBN
Vagina 0UBG
Valve
Aortic 02BF
Mitral 02BG
Pulmonary 02BH
Tricuspid 02BJ
Vas Deferens
Bilateral 0VBQ
Left 0VBP
Right 0VBN
Vein
Axillary
Left 05B8
Right 05B7
Azygos 05B0
Basilic
Left 05BC
Right 05BB
Brachial
Left 05BA
Right 05B9
Cephalic
Left 05BF
Right 05BD
Colic 06B7
Common Iliac
Left 06BD
Right 06BC
Coronary 02B4
Esophageal 06B3
External Iliac
Left 06BG
Right 06BF
External Jugular
Left 05BQ
Right 05BP
Face
Left 05BV
Right 05BT
Femoral
Left 06BN
Right 06BM
Foot
Left 06BV
Right 06BT
Gastric 06B2
Hand
Left 05BH
Right 05BG
Hemiazygos 05B1
Hepatic 06B4
Hypogastric
Left 06BJ
Right 06BH
Inferior Mesenteric 06B6
Innominate
Left 05B4
Right 05B3
Internal Jugular
Left 05BN
Right 05BM
Intracranial 05BL
Lower 06BY
Portal 06B8

Excision *(continued)*
Vein *(continued)*
Pulmonary
Left 02BT
Right 02BS
Renal
Left 06BB
Right 06B9
Saphenous
Left 06BQ
Right 06BP
Splenic 06B1
Subclavian
Left 05B6
Right 05B5
Superior Mesenteric 06B5
Upper 05BY
Vertebral
Left 05BS
Right 05BR
Vena Cava
Inferior 06B0
Superior 02BV
Ventricle
Left 02BL
Right 02BK
Vertebra
Cervical 0PB3
Lumbar 0QB0
Thoracic 0PB4
Vesicle
Bilateral 0VB3
Left 0VB2
Right 0VB1
Vitreous
Left 08B53Z
Right 08B43Z
Vocal Cord
Left 0CBV
Right 0CBT
Vulva 0UBM
Wrist Region
Left 0XBH
Right 0XBG
EXCLUDER® AAA Endoprosthesis
use Intraluminal Device
use Intraluminal Device, Branched or Fenestrated, One or Two Arteries in 04V
use Intraluminal Device, Branched or Fenestrated, Three or More Arteries in 04V
EXCLUDER® IBE Endoprosthesis
use Intraluminal Device, Branched or Fenestrated, One or Two Arteries in 04V
Exclusion, Left atrial appendage (LAA)
see Occlusion, Atrium, Left 02L7
Exercise, rehabilitation
see Motor Treatment, Rehabilitation F07
Exploration
see Inspection
Express® (LD) Premounted Stent System
use Intraluminal Device
Express® Biliary SD Monorail® Premounted Stent System
use Intraluminal Device
Express® SD Renal Monorail® Premounted Stent System
use Intraluminal Device
Extensor carpi radialis muscle
use Muscle, Lower Arm and Wrist, Left
Extensor carpi radialis muscle
use Muscle, Lower Arm and Wrist, Right

Extensor carpi ulnaris muscle
use Muscle, Lower Arm and Wrist, Left
use Muscle, Lower Arm and Wrist, Right
Extensor digitorum brevis muscle
use Muscle, Foot, Left
use Muscle, Foot, Right
Extensor digitorum longus muscle
use Muscle, Lower Leg, Left
use Muscle, Lower Leg, Right
Extensor hallucis brevis muscle
use Muscle, Foot, Left
use Muscle, Foot, Right
Extensor hallucis longus muscle
use Muscle, Lower Leg, Left
use Muscle, Lower Leg, Right
External anal sphincter
use Anal Sphincter
External auditory meatus
use Ear, External Auditory Canal, Left
use Ear, External Auditory Canal, Right
External fixator
use External Fixation Device in Head and Facial Bones
use External Fixation Device in Lower Bones
use External Fixation Device in Lower Joints
use External Fixation Device in Upper Bones
use External Fixation Device in Upper Joints
External maxillary artery
use Artery, Face
External naris
use Nasal Mucosa and Soft Tissue
External oblique aponeurosis
use Subcutaneous Tissue and Fascia, Trunk
External oblique muscle
use Muscle, Abdomen, Left
use Muscle, Abdomen, Right
External popliteal nerve
use Nerve, Peroneal
External pudendal artery
use Artery, Femoral, Left
use Artery, Femoral, Right
External pudendal vein
use Vein, Saphenous, Left
use Vein, Saphenous, Right
External urethral sphincter
use Urethra
Extirpation
Acetabulum
Left 0QC5
Right 0QC4
Adenoids 0CCQ
Ampulla of Vater 0FCC
Anal Sphincter 0DCR
Anterior Chamber
Left 08C3
Right 08C2
Anus 0DCQ
Aorta
Abdominal 04C0
Thoracic
Ascending/Arch 02CX
Descending 02CW
Aortic Body 0GCD
Appendix 0DCJ
Artery
Anterior Tibial
Left 04CQ
Right 04CP
Axillary
Left 03C6
Right 03C5

Extirpation *(continued)*
Artery *(continued)*
Brachial
Left 03C8
Right 03C7
Celiac 04C1
Colic
Left 04C7
Middle 04C8
Right 04C6
Common Carotid
Left 03CJ
Right 03CH
Common Iliac
Left 04CD
Right 04CC
Coronary
Four or More Arteries 02C3
One Artery 02C0
Three Arteries 02C2
Two Arteries 02C1
External Carotid
Left 03CN
Right 03CM
External Iliac
Left 04CJ
Right 04CH
Face 03CR
Femoral
Left 04CL
Right 04CK
Foot
Left 04CW
Right 04CV
Gastric 04C2
Hand
Left 03CF
Right 03CD
Hepatic 04C3
Inferior Mesenteric 04CB
Innominate 03C2
Internal Carotid
Left 03CL
Right 03CK
Internal Iliac
Left 04CF
Right 04CE
Internal Mammary
Left 03C1
Right 03C0
Intracranial 03CG
Lower 04CY
Peroneal
Left 04CU
Right 04CT
Popliteal
Left 04CN
Right 04CM
Posterior Tibial
Left 04CS
Right 04CR
Pulmonary
Left 02CR
Right 02CQ
Pulmonary Trunk 02CP
Radial
Left 03CC
Right 03CB
Renal
Left 04CA
Right 04C9
Splenic 04C4
Subclavian
Left 03C4
Right 03C3
Superior Mesenteric 04C5
Temporal
Left 03CT
Right 03CS

Extirpation *(continued)*
- Artery *(continued)*
  - Thyroid
    - Left 03CV
    - Right 03CU
  - Ulnar
    - Left 03CA
    - Right 03C9
  - Upper 03CY
  - Vertebral
    - Left 03CQ
    - Right 03CP
- Atrium
  - Left 02C7
  - Right 02C6
- Auditory Ossicle
  - Left 09CA
  - Right 09C9
- Basal Ganglia 00C8
- Bladder 0TCB
- Bladder Neck 0TCC
- Bone
  - Ethmoid
    - Left 0NCG
    - Right 0NCF
  - Frontal 0NC1
  - Hyoid 0NCX
  - Lacrimal
    - Left 0NCJ
    - Right 0NCH
  - Nasal 0NCB
  - Occipital 0NC7
  - Palatine
    - Left 0NCL
    - Right 0NCK
  - Parietal
    - Left 0NC4
    - Right 0NC3
  - Pelvic
    - Left 0QC3
    - Right 0QC2
  - Sphenoid 0NCC
  - Temporal
    - Left 0NC6
    - Right 0NC5
  - Zygomatic
    - Left 0NCN
    - Right 0NCM
- Brain 00C0
- Breast
  - Bilateral 0HCV
  - Left 0HCU
  - Right 0HCT
- Bronchus
  - Lingula 0BC9
  - Lower Lobe
    - Left 0BCB
    - Right 0BC6
  - Main
    - Left 0BC7
    - Right 0BC3
  - Middle Lobe, Right 0BC5
  - Upper Lobe
    - Left 0BC8
    - Right 0BC4
- Buccal Mucosa 0CC4
- Bursa and Ligament
  - Abdomen
    - Left 0MCJ
    - Right 0MCH
  - Ankle
    - Left 0MCR
    - Right 0MCQ
  - Elbow
    - Left 0MC4
    - Right 0MC3
  - Foot
    - Left 0MCT
    - Right 0MCS

Extirpation *(continued)*
- Bursa and Ligament *(continued)*
  - Hand
    - Left 0MC8
    - Right 0MC7
  - Head and Neck 0MC0
  - Hip
    - Left 0MCM
    - Right 0MCL
  - Knee
    - Left 0MCP
    - Right 0MCN
  - Lower Extremity
    - Left 0MCW
    - Right 0MCV
  - Perineum 0MCK
  - Rib(s) 0MCG
  - Shoulder
    - Left 0MC2
    - Right 0MC1
  - Spine
    - Lower 0MCD
    - Upper 0MCC
  - Sternum 0MCF
  - Upper Extremity
    - Left 0MCB
    - Right 0MC9
  - Wrist
    - Left 0MC6
    - Right 0MC5
- Carina 0BC2
- Carotid Bodies, Bilateral 0GC8
- Carotid Body
  - Left 0GC6
  - Right 0GC7
- Carpal
  - Left 0PCN
  - Right 0PCM
- Cavity, Cranial 0WC1
- Cecum 0DCH
- Cerebellum 00CC
- Cerebral Hemisphere 00C7
- Cerebral Meninges 00C1
- Cerebral Ventricle 00C6
- Cervix 0UCC
- Chordae Tendineae 02C9
- Choroid
  - Left 08CB
  - Right 08CA
- Cisterna Chyli 07CL
- Clavicle
  - Left 0PCB
  - Right 0PC9
- Clitoris 0UCJ
- Coccygeal Glomus 0GCB
- Coccyx 0QCS
- Colon
  - Ascending 0DCK
  - Descending 0DCM
  - Sigmoid 0DCN
  - Transverse 0DCL
- Conduction Mechanism 02C8
- Conjunctiva
  - Left 08CTXZZ
  - Right 08CSXZZ
- Cord
  - Bilateral 0VCH
  - Left 0VCG
  - Right 0VCF
- Cornea
  - Left 08C9XZZ
  - Right 08C8XZZ
- Cul-de-sac 0UCF
- Diaphragm 0BCT
- Disc
  - Cervical Vertebral 0RC3
  - Cervicothoracic Vertebral 0RC5
  - Lumbar Vertebral 0SC2
  - Lumbosacral 0SC4
  - Thoracic Vertebral 0RC9

Extirpation *(continued)*
- Disc *(continued)*
  - Thoracolumbar Vertebral 0RCB
- Duct
  - Common Bile 0FC9
  - Cystic 0FC8
  - Hepatic
    - Common 0FC7
    - Left 0FC6
    - Right 0FC5
  - Lacrimal
    - Left 08CY
    - Right 08CX
  - Pancreatic 0FCD
    - Accessory 0FCF
  - Parotid
    - Left 0CCC
    - Right 0CCB
- Duodenum 0DC9
- Dura Mater 00C2
- Ear
  - External
    - Left 09C1
    - Right 09C0
  - External Auditory Canal
    - Left 09C4
    - Right 09C3
  - Inner
    - Left 09CE
    - Right 09CD
  - Middle
    - Left 09C6
    - Right 09C5
- Endometrium 0UCB
- Epididymis
  - Bilateral 0VCL
  - Left 0VCK
  - Right 0VCJ
- Epidural Space, Intracranial 00C3
- Epiglottis 0CCR
- Esophagogastric Junction 0DC4
- Esophagus 0DC5
  - Lower 0DC3
  - Middle 0DC2
  - Upper 0DC1
- Eustachian Tube
  - Left 09CG
  - Right 09CF
- Eye
  - Left 08C1XZZ
  - Right 08C0XZZ
- Eyelid
  - Lower
    - Left 08CR
    - Right 08CQ
  - Upper
    - Left 08CP
    - Right 08CN
- Fallopian Tube
  - Left 0UC6
  - Right 0UC5
- Fallopian Tubes, Bilateral 0UC7
- Femoral Shaft
  - Left 0QC9
  - Right 0QC8
- Femur
  - Lower
    - Left 0QCC
    - Right 0QCB
  - Upper
    - Left 0QC7
    - Right 0QC6
- Fibula
  - Left 0QCK
  - Right 0QCJ
- Finger Nail 0HCQXZZ
- Gallbladder 0FC4
- Gastrointestinal Tract 0WCP
- Genitourinary Tract 0WCR

Extirpation *(continued)*
- Gingiva
  - Lower 0CC6
  - Upper 0CC5
- Gland
  - Adrenal
    - Bilateral 0GC4
    - Left 0GC2
    - Right 0GC3
  - Lacrimal
    - Left 08CW
    - Right 08CV
  - Minor Salivary 0CCJ
  - Parotid
    - Left 0CC9
    - Right 0CC8
  - Pituitary 0GC0
  - Sublingual
    - Left 0CCF
    - Right 0CCD
  - Submaxillary
    - Left 0CCH
    - Right 0CCG
  - Vestibular 0UCL
- Glenoid Cavity
  - Left 0PC8
  - Right 0PC7
- Glomus Jugulare 0GCC
- Humeral Head
  - Left 0PCD
  - Right 0PCC
- Humeral Shaft
  - Left 0PCG
  - Right 0PCF
- Hymen 0UCK
- Hypothalamus 00CA
- Ileocecal Valve 0DCC
- Ileum 0DCB
- Intestine
  - Large 0DCE
    - Left 0DCG
    - Right 0DCF
  - Small 0DC8
- Iris
  - Left 08CD
  - Right 08CC
- Jejunum 0DCA
- Joint
  - Acromioclavicular
    - Left 0RCH
    - Right 0RCG
  - Ankle
    - Left 0SCG
    - Right 0SCF
  - Carpal
    - Left 0RCR
    - Right 0RCQ
  - Carpometacarpal
    - Left 0RCT
    - Right 0RCS
  - Cervical Vertebral 0RC1
  - Cervicothoracic Vertebral 0RC4
  - Coccygeal 0SC6
  - Elbow
    - Left 0RCM
    - Right 0RCL
  - Finger Phalangeal
    - Left 0RCX
    - Right 0RCW
  - Hip
    - Left 0SCB
    - Right 0SC9
  - Knee
    - Left 0SCD
    - Right 0SCC
  - Lumbar Vertebral 0SC0
  - Lumbosacral 0SC3
  - Metacarpophalangeal
    - Left 0RCV
    - Right 0RCU

Extirpation *(continued)*
- Joint *(continued)*
  - Metatarsal-Phalangeal
    - Left 0SCN
    - Right 0SCM
  - Occipital-cervical 0RC0
  - Sacrococcygeal 0SC5
  - Sacroiliac
    - Left 0SC8
    - Right 0SC7
  - Shoulder
    - Left 0RCK
    - Right 0RCJ
  - Sternoclavicular
    - Left 0RCF
    - Right 0RCE
  - Tarsal
    - Left 0SCJ
    - Right 0SCH
  - Tarsometatarsal
    - Left 0SCL
    - Right 0SCK
  - Temporomandibular
    - Left 0RCD
    - Right 0RCC
  - Thoracic Vertebral 0RC6
  - Thoracolumbar Vertebral 0RCA
  - Toe Phalangeal
    - Left 0SCQ
    - Right 0SCP
  - Wrist
    - Left 0RCP
    - Right 0RCN
- Kidney
  - Left 0TC1
  - Right 0TC0
- Kidney Pelvis
  - Left 0TC4
  - Right 0TC3
- Larynx 0CCS
- Lens
  - Left 08CK
  - Right 08CJ
- Lip
  - Lower 0CC1
  - Upper 0CC0
- Liver 0FC0
  - Left Lobe 0FC2
  - Right Lobe 0FC1
- Lung
  - Bilateral 0BCM
  - Left 0BCL
  - Lower Lobe
    - Left 0BCJ
    - Right 0BCF
  - Middle Lobe, Right 0BCD
  - Right 0BCK
  - Upper Lobe
    - Left 0BCG
    - Right 0BCC
- Lung Lingula 0BCH
- Lymphatic
  - Aortic 07CD
  - Axillary
    - Left 07C6
    - Right 07C5
  - Head 07C0
  - Inguinal
    - Left 07CJ
    - Right 07CH
  - Internal Mammary
    - Left 07C9
    - Right 07C8
  - Lower Extremity
    - Left 07CG
    - Right 07CF
  - Mesenteric 07CB
  - Neck
    - Left 07C2
    - Right 07C1

Extirpation *(continued)*
- Lymphatic *(continued)*
  - Pelvis 07CC
  - Thoracic Duct 07CK
  - Thorax 07C7
  - Upper Extremity
    - Left 07C4
    - Right 07C3
- Mandible
  - Left 0NCV
  - Right 0NCT
- Maxilla 0NCR
- Mediastinum 0WCC
- Medulla Oblongata 00CD
- Mesentery 0DCV
- Metacarpal
  - Left 0PCQ
  - Right 0PCP
- Metatarsal
  - Left 0QCP
  - Right 0QCN
- Muscle
  - Abdomen
    - Left 0KCL
    - Right 0KCK
  - Extraocular
    - Left 08CM
    - Right 08CL
  - Facial 0KC1
  - Foot
    - Left 0KCW
    - Right 0KCV
  - Hand
    - Left 0KCD
    - Right 0KCC
  - Head 0KC0
  - Hip
    - Left 0KCP
    - Right 0KCN
  - Lower Arm and Wrist
    - Left 0KCB
    - Right 0KC9
  - Lower Leg
    - Left 0KCT
    - Right 0KCS
  - Neck
    - Left 0KC3
    - Right 0KC2
  - Papillary 02CD
  - Perineum 0KCM
  - Shoulder
    - Left 0KC6
    - Right 0KC5
  - Thorax
    - Left 0KCJ
    - Right 0KCH
  - Tongue, Palate, Pharynx 0KC4
  - Trunk
    - Left 0KCG
    - Right 0KCF
  - Upper Arm
    - Left 0KC8
    - Right 0KC7
  - Upper Leg
    - Left 0KCR
    - Right 0KCQ
- Nasal Mucosa and Soft Tissue 09CK
- Nasopharynx 09CN
- Nerve
  - Abdominal Sympathetic 01CM
  - Abducens 00CL
  - Accessory 00CR
  - Acoustic 00CN
  - Brachial Plexus 01C3
  - Cervical 01C1
  - Cervical Plexus 01C0
  - Facial 00CM
  - Femoral 01CD
  - Glossopharyngeal 00CP

Extirpation *(continued)*
- Nerve *(continued)*
  - Head and Neck Sympathetic 01CK
  - Hypoglossal 00CS
  - Lumbar 01CB
  - Lumbar Plexus 01C9
  - Lumbar Sympathetic 01CN
  - Lumbosacral Plexus 01CA
  - Median 01C5
  - Oculomotor 00CH
  - Olfactory 00CF
  - Optic 00CG
  - Peroneal 01CH
  - Phrenic 01C2
  - Pudendal 01CC
  - Radial 01C6
  - Sacral 01CR
  - Sacral Plexus 01CQ
  - Sacral Sympathetic 01CP
  - Sciatic 01CF
  - Thoracic 01C8
  - Thoracic Sympathetic 01CL
  - Tibial 01CG
  - Trigeminal 00CK
  - Trochlear 00CJ
  - Ulnar 01C4
  - Vagus 00CQ
- Nipple
  - Left 0HCX
  - Right 0HCW
- Omentum 0DCU
- Oral Cavity and Throat 0WC3
- Orbit
  - Left 0NCQ
  - Right 0NCP
- Orbital Atherectomy Technology X2C
- Ovary
  - Bilateral 0UC2
  - Left 0UC1
  - Right 0UC0
- Palate
  - Hard 0CC2
  - Soft 0CC3
- Pancreas 0FCG
- Para-aortic Body 0GC9
- Paraganglion Extremity 0GCF
- Parathyroid Gland 0GCR
  - Inferior
    - Left 0GCP
    - Right 0GCN
  - Multiple 0GCQ
  - Superior
    - Left 0GCM
    - Right 0GCL
- Patella
  - Left 0QCF
  - Right 0QCD
- Pelvic Cavity 0WCJ
- Penis 0VCS
- Pericardial Cavity 0WCD
- Pericardium 02CN
- Peritoneal Cavity 0WCG
- Peritoneum 0DCW
- Phalanx
  - Finger
    - Left 0PCV
    - Right 0PCT
  - Thumb
    - Left 0PCS
    - Right 0PCR
  - Toe
    - Left 0QCR
    - Right 0QCQ
- Pharynx 0CCM
- Pineal Body 0GC1
- Pleura
  - Left 0BCP

Extirpation *(continued)*
- Pleura *(continued)*
  - Right 0BCN
- Pleural Cavity
  - Left 0WCB
  - Right 0WC9
- Pons 00CB
- Prepuce 0VCT
- Prostate 0VC0
- Radius
  - Left 0PCJ
  - Right 0PCH
- Rectum 0DCP
- Respiratory Tract 0WCQ
- Retina
  - Left 08CF
  - Right 08CE
- Retinal Vessel
  - Left 08CH
  - Right 08CG
- Retroperitoneum 0WCH
- Ribs
  - 1 to 2 0PC1
  - 3 or More 0PC2
- Sacrum 0QC1
- Scapula
  - Left 0PC6
  - Right 0PC5
- Sclera
  - Left 08C7XZZ
  - Right 08C6XZZ
- Scrotum 0VC5
- Septum
  - Atrial 02C5
  - Nasal 09CM
  - Ventricular 02CM
- Sinus
  - Accessory 09CP
  - Ethmoid
    - Left 09CV
    - Right 09CU
  - Frontal
    - Left 09CT
    - Right 09CS
  - Mastoid
    - Left 09CC
    - Right 09CB
  - Maxillary
    - Left 09CR
    - Right 09CQ
  - Sphenoid
    - Left 09CX
    - Right 09CW
- Skin
  - Abdomen 0HC7XZZ
  - Back 0HC6XZZ
  - Buttock 0HC8XZZ
  - Chest 0HC5XZZ
  - Ear
    - Left 0HC3XZZ
    - Right 0HC2XZZ
  - Face 0HC1XZZ
  - Foot
    - Left 0HCNXZZ
    - Right 0HCMXZZ
  - Hand
    - Left 0HCGXZZ
    - Right 0HCFXZZ
  - Inguinal 0HCAXZZ
  - Lower Arm
    - Left 0HCEXZZ
    - Right 0HCDXZZ
  - Lower Leg
    - Left 0HCLXZZ
    - Right 0HCKXZZ
  - Neck 0HC4XZZ
  - Perineum 0HC9XZZ
  - Scalp 0HC0XZZ
  - Upper Arm
    - Left 0HCCXZZ

Extirpation *(continued)*
Skin *(continued)*
Upper Arm *(continued)*
Right 0HCBXZZ
Upper Leg
Left 0HCJXZZ
Right 0HCHXZZ
Spinal Canal 00CU
Spinal Cord
Cervical 00CW
Lumbar 00CY
Thoracic 00CX
Spinal Meninges 00CT
Spleen 07CP
Sternum 0PC0
Stomach 0DC6
Pylorus 0DC7
Subarachnoid Space, Intracranial 00C5
Subcutaneous Tissue and Fascia
Abdomen 0JC8
Back 0JC7
Buttock 0JC9
Chest 0JC6
Face 0JC1
Foot
Left 0JCR
Right 0JCQ
Hand
Left 0JCK
Right 0JCJ
Lower Arm
Left 0JCH
Right 0JCG
Lower Leg
Left 0JCP
Right 0JCN
Neck
Left 0JC5
Right 0JC4
Pelvic Region 0JCC
Perineum 0JCB
Scalp 0JC0
Upper Arm
Left 0JCF
Right 0JCD
Upper Leg
Left 0JCM
Right 0JCL
Subdural Space, Intracranial 00C4
Tarsal
Left 0QCM
Right 0QCL
Tendon
Abdomen
Left 0LCG
Right 0LCF
Ankle
Left 0LCT
Right 0LCS
Foot
Left 0LCW
Right 0LCV
Hand
Left 0LC8
Right 0LC7
Head and Neck 0LC0
Hip
Left 0LCK
Right 0LCJ
Knee
Left 0LCR
Right 0LCQ
Lower Arm and Wrist
Left 0LC6
Right 0LC5
Lower Leg
Left 0LCP
Right 0LCN
Perineum 0LCH

Extirpation *(continued)*
Tendon *(continued)*
Shoulder
Left 0LC2
Right 0LC1
Thorax
Left 0LCD
Right 0LCC
Trunk
Left 0LCB
Right 0LC9
Upper Arm
Left 0LC4
Right 0LC3
Upper Leg
Left 0LCM
Right 0LCL
Testis
Bilateral 0VCC
Left 0VCB
Right 0VC9
Thalamus 00C9
Thymus 07CM
Thyroid Gland 0GCK
Left Lobe 0GCG
Right Lobe 0GCH
Tibia
Left 0QCH
Right 0QCG
Toe Nail 0HCRXZZ
Tongue 0CC7
Tonsils 0CCP
Tooth
Lower 0CCX
Upper 0CCW
Trachea 0BC1
Tunica Vaginalis
Left 0VC7
Right 0VC6
Turbinate, Nasal 09CL
Tympanic Membrane
Left 09C8
Right 09C7
Ulna
Left 0PCL
Right 0PCK
Ureter
Left 0TC7
Right 0TC6
Urethra 0TCD
Uterine Supporting Structure 0UC4
Uterus 0UC9
Uvula 0CCN
Vagina 0UCG
Valve
Aortic 02CF
Mitral 02CG
Pulmonary 02CH
Tricuspid 02CJ
Vas Deferens
Bilateral 0VCQ
Left 0VCP
Right 0VCN
Vein
Axillary
Left 05C8
Right 05C7
Azygos 05C0
Basilic
Left 05CC
Right 05CB
Brachial
Left 05CA
Right 05C9
Cephalic
Left 05CF
Right 05CD
Colic 06C7
Common Iliac
Left 06CD
Right 06CC

Extirpation *(continued)*
Vein *(continued)*
Coronary 02C4
Esophageal 06C3
External Iliac
Left 06CG
Right 06CF
External Jugular
Left 05CQ
Right 05CP
Face
Left 05CV
Right 05CT
Femoral
Left 06CN
Right 06CM
Foot
Left 06CV
Right 06CT
Gastric 06C2
Hand
Left 05CH
Right 05CG
Hemiazygos 05C1
Hepatic 06C4
Hypogastric
Left 06CJ
Right 06CH
Inferior Mesenteric 06C6
Innominate
Left 05C4
Right 05C3
Internal Jugular
Left 05CN
Right 05CM
Intracranial 05CL
Lower 06CY
Portal 06C8
Pulmonary
Left 02CT
Right 02CS
Renal
Left 06CB
Right 06C9
Saphenous
Left 06CQ
Right 06CP
Splenic 06C1
Subclavian
Left 05C6
Right 05C5
Superior Mesenteric 06C5
Upper 05CY
Vertebral
Left 05CS
Right 05CR
Vena Cava
Inferior 06C0
Superior 02CV
Ventricle
Left 02CL
Right 02CK
Vertebra
Cervical 0PC3
Lumbar 0QC0
Thoracic 0PC4
Vesicle
Bilateral 0VC3
Left 0VC2
Right 0VC1
Vitreous
Left 08C5
Right 08C4
Vocal Cord
Left 0CCV
Right 0CCT
Vulva 0UCM
Extracorporeal shock wave lithotripsy
see Fragmentation

Extracranial-intracranial bypass (EC-IC)
see Bypass, Upper Arteries 031
Extracorporeal Carbon Dioxide Removal (ECCO2R) 5A0920Z
Extraction
Acetabulum
Left 0QD50ZZ
Right 0QD40ZZ
Ampulla of Vater 0FDC
Anus 0DDQ
Appendix 0DDJ
Auditory Ossicle
Left 09DA0ZZ
Right 09D90ZZ
Bone
Ethmoid
Left 0NDG0ZZ
Right 0NDF0ZZ
Frontal 0ND10ZZ
Hyoid 0NDX0ZZ
Lacrimal
Left 0NDJ0ZZ
Right 0NDH0ZZ
Nasal 0NDB0ZZ
Occipital 0ND70ZZ
Palatine
Left 0NDL0ZZ
Right 0NDK0ZZ
Parietal
Left 0ND40ZZ
Right 0ND30ZZ
Pelvic
Left 0QD30ZZ
Right 0QD20ZZ
Sphenoid 0NDC0ZZ
Temporal
Left 0ND60ZZ
Right 0ND50ZZ
Zygomatic
Left 0NDN0ZZ
Right 0NDM0ZZ
Bone Marrow
Iliac 07DR
Sternum 07DQ
Vertebral 07DS
Bronchus
Lingula 0BD9
Lower Lobe
Left 0BDB
Right 0BD6
Main
Left 0BD7
Right 0BD3
Middle Lobe, Right 0BD5
Upper Lobe
Left 0BD8
Right 0BD4
Bursa and Ligament
Abdomen
Left 0MDJ
Right 0MDH
Ankle
Left 0MDR
Right 0MDQ
Elbow
Left 0MD4
Right 0MD3
Foot
Left 0MDT
Right 0MDS
Hand
Left 0MD8
Right 0MD7
Head and Neck 0MD0
Hip
Left 0MDM
Right 0MDL
Knee
Left 0MDP
Right 0MDN

- xtraction *(continued)*
  - Bursa and Ligament *(continued)*
    - Lower Extremity
      - Left 0MDW
      - Right 0MDV
    - Perineum 0MDK
    - Rib(s) 0MDG
    - Shoulder
      - Left 0MD2
      - Right 0MD1
    - Spine
      - Lower 0MDD
      - Upper 0MDC
    - Sternum 0MDF
    - Upper Extremity
      - Left 0MDB
      - Right 0MD9
    - Wrist
      - Left 0MD6
      - Right 0MD5
  - Carina 0BD2
  - Carpal
    - Left 0PDN0ZZ
    - Right 0PDM0ZZ
  - Cecum 0DDH
  - Cerebral Meninges 00D1
  - Cisterna Chyli 07DL
  - Clavicle
    - Left 0PDB0ZZ
    - Right 0PD90ZZ
  - Coccyx 0QDS0ZZ
  - Colon
    - Ascending 0DDK
    - Descending 0DDM
    - Sigmoid 0DDN
    - Transverse 0DDL
  - Cornea
    - Left 08D9XZ
    - Right 08D8XZ
  - Duct
    - Common Bile 0FD9
    - Cystic 0FD8
    - Hepatic
      - Common 0FD7
      - Left 0FD6
      - Right 0FD5
    - Pancreatic 0FDD
      - Accessory 0FDF
  - Duodenum 0DD9
  - Dura Mater 00D2
  - Endometrium 0UDB
  - Esophagogastric Junction 0DD4
  - Esophagus 0DD5
    - Lower 0DD3
    - Middle 0DD2
    - Upper 0DD1
  - Femoral Shaft
    - Left 0QD90ZZ
    - Right 0QD80ZZ
  - Femur
    - Lower
      - Left 0QDC0ZZ
      - Right 0QDB0ZZ
    - Upper
      - Left 0QD70ZZ
      - Right 0QD60ZZ
  - Fibula
    - Left 0QDK0ZZ
    - Right 0QDJ0ZZ
  - Finger Nail 0HDQXZZ
  - Gallbladder 0FD4
  - Glenoid Cavity
    - Left 0PD80ZZ
    - Right 0PD70ZZ
  - Hair 0HDSXZZ
  - Humeral Head
    - Left 0PDD0ZZ
    - Right 0PDC0ZZ
  - Humeral Shaft
    - Left 0PDG0ZZ
    - Right 0PDF0ZZ

- **Extraction** *(continued)*
  - Ileocecal Valve 0DDC
  - Ileum 0DDB
  - Intestine
    - Large 0DDE
      - Left 0DDG
      - Right 0DDF
    - Small 0DD8
  - Jejunum 0DDA
  - Kidney
    - Left 0TD1
    - Right 0TD0
  - Lens
    - Left 08DK3ZZ
    - Right 08DJ3ZZ
  - Liver 0FD0
    - Left Lobe 0FD2
    - Right Lobe 0FD1
  - Lung
    - Bilateral 0BDM
    - Left 0BDL
    - Lower Lobe
      - Left 0BDJ
      - Right 0BDF
    - Middle Lobe, Right 0BDD
    - Right 0BDK
    - Upper Lobe
      - Left 0BDG
      - Right 0BDC
  - Lung Lingula 0BDH
  - Lymphatic
    - Aortic 07DD
    - Axillary
      - Left 07D6
      - Right 07D5
    - Head 07D0
    - Inguinal
      - Left 07DJ
      - Right 07DH
    - Internal Mammary
      - Left 07D9
      - Right 07D8
    - Lower Extremity
      - Left 07DG
      - Right 07DF
    - Mesenteric 07DB
    - Neck
      - Left 07D2
      - Right 07D1
    - Pelvis 07DC
    - Thoracic Duct 07DK
    - Thorax 07D7
    - Upper Extermity
      - Left 07D4
      - Right 07D3
  - Mandible
    - Left 0NDV0ZZ
    - Right 0NDT0ZZ
  - Maxilla 0NDR0ZZ
  - Metacarpal
    - Left 0PDQ0ZZ
    - Right 0PDP0ZZ
  - Metatarsal
    - Left 0QDP0ZZ
    - Right 0QDN0ZZ
  - Muscle
    - Abdomen
      - Left 0KDL0ZZ
      - Right 0KDK0ZZ
    - Facial 0KD10ZZ
    - Foot
      - Left 0KDW0ZZ
      - Right 0KDV0ZZ
    - Hand
      - Left 0KDD0ZZ
      - Right 0KDC0ZZ
    - Head 0KD00ZZ
    - Hip
      - Left 0KDP0ZZ
      - Right 0KD90ZZ

- **Extraction** *(continued)*
  - Muscle *(continued)*
    - Lower Arm and Wrist
      - Left 0KDB0ZZ
      - Right 0KD90ZZ
    - Lower Leg
      - Left 0KDT0ZZ
      - Right 0KDS0ZZ
    - Neck
      - Left 0KD30ZZ
      - Right 0KD20ZZ
    - Perineum 0KDM0ZZ
    - Shoulder
      - Left 0KD60ZZ
      - Right 0KD50ZZ
    - Thorax
      - Left 0KDJ0ZZ
      - Right 0KDH0ZZ
    - Tongue, Palate, Pharynx 0KD40ZZ
    - Trunk
      - Left 0KDG0ZZ
      - Right 0KDF0ZZ
    - Upper Arm
      - Left 0KD80ZZ
      - Right 0KD70ZZ
    - Upper Leg
      - Left 0KDR0ZZ
      - Right 0KDQ0ZZ
  - Nerve
    - Abdominal Sympathetic 01DM
    - Abducens 00DL
    - Accessory 00DR
    - Acoustic 00DN
    - Brachial Plexus 01D3
    - Cervical 01D1
    - Cervical Plexus 01D0
    - Facial 00DM
    - Femoral 01DD
    - Glossopharyngeal 00DP
    - Head and Neck Sympathetic 01DK
    - Hypoglossal 00DS
    - Lumbar 01DB
    - Lumbar Plexus 01D9
    - Lumbar Sympathetic 01DN
    - Lumbosacral Plexus 01DA
    - Median 01D5
    - Oculomotor 00DH
    - Olfactory 00DF
    - Optic 00DG
    - Peroneal 01DH
    - Phrenic 01D2
    - Pudendal 01DC
    - Radial 01D6
    - Sacral 01DR
    - Sacral Plexus 01DQ
    - Sacral Sympathetic 01DP
    - Sciatic 01DF
    - Thoracic 01D8
    - Thoracic Sympathetic 01DL
    - Tibial 01DG
    - Trigeminal 00DK
    - Trochlear 00DJ
    - Ulnar 01D4
    - Vagus 00DQ
  - Orbit
    - Left 0NDQ0ZZ
    - Right 0NDP0ZZ
  - Ova 0UDN
  - Pancreas 0FDG
  - Patella
    - Left 0QDF0ZZ
    - Right 0QDD0ZZ
  - Phalanx
    - Finger
      - Left 0PDV0ZZ
      - Right 0PDT0ZZ
    - Thumb
      - Left 0PDS0ZZ
      - Right 0PDR0ZZ

- **Extraction** *(continued)*
  - Phalanx *(continued)*
    - Toe
      - Left 0QDR0ZZ
      - Right 0QDQ0ZZ
  - Pleura
    - Left 0BDP
    - Right 0BDN
  - Products of Conception
    - Ectopic 10D2
    - Extraperitoneal 10D00Z2
    - High 10D00Z0
    - High Forceps 10D07Z5
    - Internal Version 10D07Z7
    - Low 10D00Z1
    - Low Forceps 10D07Z3
    - Mid Forceps 10D07Z4
    - Other 10D07Z8
    - Retained 10D1
    - Vacuum 10D07Z6
  - Radius
    - Left 0PDJ0ZZ
    - Right 0PDH0ZZ
  - Rectum 0DDP
  - Ribs
    - 1 to 2 0PD10ZZ
    - 3 or More 0PD20ZZ
  - Sacrum 0QD10ZZ
  - Scapula
    - Left 0PD60ZZ
    - Right 0PD50ZZ
  - Septum, Nasal 09DM
  - Sinus
    - Accessory 09DP
    - Ethmoid
      - Left 09DV
      - Right 09DU
    - Frontal
      - Left 09DT
      - Right 09DS
    - Mastoid
      - Left 09DC
      - Right 09DB
    - Maxillary
      - Left 09DR
      - Right 09DQ
    - Sphenoid
      - Left 09DX
      - Right 09DW
  - Skin
    - Abdomen 0HD7XZZ
    - Back 0HD6XZZ
    - Buttock 0HD8XZZ
    - Chest 0HD5XZZ
    - Ear
      - Left 0HD3XZZ
      - Right 0HD2XZZ
    - Face 0HD1XZZ
    - Foot
      - Left 0HDNXZZ
      - Right 0HDMXZZ
    - Hand
      - Left 0HDGXZZ
      - Right 0HDFXZZ
    - Inguinal 0HDAXZZ
    - Lower Arm
      - Left 0HDEXZZ
      - Right 0HDDXZZ
    - Lower Leg
      - Left 0HDLXZZ
      - Right 0HDKXZZ
    - Neck 0HD4XZZ
    - Perineum 0HD9XZZ
    - Scalp 0HD0XZZ
    - Upper Arm
      - Left 0HDCXZZ
      - Right 0HDBXZZ
    - Upper Leg
      - Left 0HDJXZZ
      - Right 0HDHXZZ

- **Extraction** *(continued)*
  - Skull 0ND00ZZ
  - Spinal Meninges 00DT
  - Spleen 07DP
  - Sternum 0PD00ZZ
  - Stomach 0DD6
    - Pylorus 0DD7
  - Subcutaneous Tissue and Fascia
    - Abdomen 0JD8
    - Back 0JD7
    - Buttock 0JD9
    - Chest 0JD6
    - Face 0JD1
    - Foot
      - Left 0JDR
      - Right 0JDQ
    - Hand
      - Left 0JDK
      - Right 0JDJ
    - Lower Arm
      - Left 0JDH
      - Right 0JDG
    - Lower Leg
      - Left 0JDP
      - Right 0JDN
    - Neck
      - Left 0JD5
      - Right 0JD4
    - Pelvic Region 0JDC
    - Perineum 0JDB
    - Scalp 0JD0
    - Upper Arm
      - Left 0JDF
      - Right 0JDD
    - Upper Leg
      - Left 0JDM
      - Right 0JDL
  - Tarsal
    - Left 0QDM0ZZ
    - Right 0QDL0ZZ
  - Tendon
    - Abdomen
      - Left 0LDG0ZZ
      - Right 0LDF0ZZ
    - Ankle
      - Left 0LDT0ZZ
      - Right 0LDS0ZZ
    - Foot
      - Left 0LDW0ZZ
      - Right 0LDV0ZZ
    - Hand
      - Left 0LD80ZZ
      - Right 0LD70ZZ
    - Head and Neck 0LD00ZZ
    - Hip
      - Left 0LDK0ZZ
      - Right 0LDJ0ZZ
    - Knee
      - Left 0LDR0ZZ
      - Right 0LDQ0ZZ
    - Lower Arm and Wrist
      - Left 0LD60ZZ
      - Right 0LD50ZZ
    - Lower Leg
      - Left 0LDP0ZZ
      - Right 0LDN0ZZ
    - Perineum 0LDH0ZZ
    - Shoulder
      - Left 0LD20ZZ
      - Right 0LD10ZZ
    - Thorax
      - Left 0LDD0ZZ
      - Right 0LDC0ZZ
    - Trunk
      - Left 0LDB0ZZ
      - Right 0LD90ZZ
    - Upper Arm
      - Left 0LD40ZZ
      - Right 0LD30ZZ

- **Extraction** *(continued)*
  - Tendon *(continued)*
    - Upper Leg
      - Left 0LDM0ZZ
      - Right 0LDL0ZZ
  - Thymus 07DM
  - Tibia
    - Left 0QDH0ZZ
    - Right 0QDG0ZZ
  - Toe Nail 0HDRXZZ
  - Tooth
    - Lower 0CDXXZ
    - Upper 0CDWXZ
  - Trachea 0BD1
  - Turbinate, Nasal 09DL
  - Tympanic Membrane
    - Left 09D8
    - Right 09D7
  - Ulna
    - Left 0PDL0ZZ
    - Right 0PDK0ZZ
  - Vein
    - Basilic
      - Left 05DC
      - Right 05DB
    - Brachial
      - Left 05DA
      - Right 05D9
    - Cephalic
      - Left 05DF
      - Right 05DD
    - Femoral
      - Left 06DN
      - Right 06DM
    - Foot
      - Left 06DV
      - Right 06DT
    - Hand
      - Left 05DH
      - Right 05DG
    - Lower 06DY
    - Saphenous
      - Left 06DQ
      - Right 06DP
    - Upper 05DY
  - Vertebra
    - Cervical 0PD30ZZ
    - Lumbar 0QD00ZZ
    - Thoracic 0PD40ZZ
  - Vocal Cord
    - Left 0CDV
    - Right 0CDT
- **Extradural space, intracranial**
  - *use* Epidural Space, Intracranial
- **Extradural space, spinal**
  - *use* Spinal Canal
- **EXtreme Lateral Interbody Fusion (XLIF) device**
  - *use* Interbody Fusion Device in Lower Joints

F

- **Face lift**
  - *see* Alteration, Face 0W02
- **Facet replacement spinal stabilization device**
  - *use* Spinal Stabilization Device, Facet Replacement in 0RH
  - *use* Spinal Stabilization Device, Facet Replacement in 0SH
- **Facial artery**
  - *use* Artery, Face
- **Factor Xa Inhibitor Reversal Agent, Andexanet Alfa**
  - *use* Andexanet Alfa, Factor Xa Inhibitor Reversal Agent
- **False vocal cord**
  - *use* Larynx
- **Falx cerebri**
  - *use* Dura Mater
- **Fascia lata**
  - *use* Subcutaneous Tissue and Fascia, Upper Leg, Left
  - *use* Subcutaneous Tissue and Fascia, Upper Leg, Right
- **Fasciaplasty, fascioplasty**
  - *see* Repair, Subcutaneous Tissue and Fascia 0JQ
  - *see* Replacement, Subcutaneous Tissue and Fascia 0JR
- **Fasciectomy**
  - *see* Excision, Subcutaneous Tissue and Fascia 0JB
  - *see* Release
- **Fasciorrhaphy**
  - *see* Repair, Subcutaneous Tissue and Fascia 0JQ
- **Fasciotomy**
  - *see* Division, Subcutaneous Tissue and Fascia 0J8
  - *see* Drainage, Subcutaneous Tissue and Fascia 0J9
  - *see* Release
- **Feeding Device**
  - Change device in
    - Lower 0D2DXUZ
    - Upper 0D20XUZ
  - Insertion of device in
    - Duodenum 0DH9
    - Esophagus 0DH5
    - Ileum 0DHB
    - Intestine, Small 0DH8
    - Jejunum 0DHA
    - Stomach 0DH6
  - Removal of device from
    - Esophagus 0DP5
    - Intestinal Tract
      - Lower 0DPD
      - Upper 0DP0
    - Stomach 0DP6
  - Revision of device in
    - Intestinal Tract
      - Lower 0DWD
      - Upper 0DW0
    - Stomach 0DW6
- **Femoral head**
  - *use* Femur, Upper, Left
  - *use* Femur, Upper, Right
- **Femoral lymph node**
  - *use* Lymphatic, Lower Extremity, Left
  - *use* Lymphatic, Lower Extremity, Right
- **Femoropatellar joint**
  - *use* Joint, Knee, Left
  - *use* Joint, Knee, Left, Femoral Surface
  - *use* Joint, Knee, Right
  - *use* Joint, Knee, Right, Femoral Surface
- **Femorotibial joint**
  - *use* Joint, Knee, Left
  - *use* Joint, Knee, Left, Tibial Surface
  - *use* Joint, Knee, Right
  - *use* Joint, Knee, Right, Tibial Surface
- **Fibular artery**
  - *use* Artery, Peroneal, Left
  - *use* Artery, Peroneal, Right
- **Fibularis brevis muscle**
  - *use* Muscle, Lower Leg, Left
  - *use* Muscle, Lower Leg, Right
- **Fibularis longus muscle**
  - *use* Muscle, Lower Leg, Left
  - *use* Muscle, Lower Leg, Right
- **Fifth cranial nerve**
  - *use* Nerve, Trigeminal
- **Filum terminale**
  - *use* Spinal Meninges
- **Fimbriectomy**
  - *see* Excision, Female Reproductive System 0UB
  - *see* Resection, Female Reproductive System 0UT
- **Fine needle aspiration**
  - Fluid or gas
    - *see* Drainage
  - Tissue biopsy
    - *see* Excision
    - *see* Extraction
- **First cranial nerve**
  - *use* Nerve, Olfactory
- **First intercostal nerve**
  - *use* Nerve, Brachial Plexus
- **Fistulization**
  - *see* Bypass
  - *see* Drainage
  - *see* Repair
- **Fitting**
  - Arch bars, for fracture reduction
    - *see* Reposition, Mouth and Throat 0CS
  - Arch bars, for immobilization
    - *see* Immobilization, Face 2W31
  - Artificial limb
    - *see* Device Fitting, Rehabilitation F0D
  - Hearing aid
    - *see* Device Fitting, Rehabilitation F0D
  - Ocular prosthesis F0DZ8UZ
  - Prosthesis, limb
    - *see* Device Fitting, Rehabilitation F0D
  - Prosthesis, ocular F0DZ8UZ
- **Fixation, bone**
  - External, with fracture reduction
    - *see* Reposition
  - External, without fracture reductic
    - *see* Insertion
  - Internal, with fracture reduction
    - *see* Reposition
  - Internal, without fracture reductio
    - *see* Insertion
- **FLAIR® Endovascular Stent Graft**
  - *use* Intraluminal Device
- **Flexible Composite Mesh**
  - *use* Synthetic Substitute
- **Flexor carpi radialis muscle**
  - *use* Muscle, Lower Arm and Wris Left
  - *use* Muscle, Lower Arm and Wris Right
- **Flexor carpi ulnaris muscle**
  - *use* Muscle, Lower Arm and Wris Left
  - *use* Muscle, Lower Arm and Wris Right
- **Flexor digitorum brevis muscle**
  - *use* Muscle, Foot, Left
  - *use* Muscle, Foot, Right
- **Flexor digitorum longus muscle**
  - *use* Muscle, Lower Leg, Left
  - *use* Muscle, Lower Leg, Right
- **Flexor hallucis brevis muscle**
  - *use* Muscle, Foot, Left
  - *use* Muscle, Foot, Right
- **Flexor hallucis longus muscle**
  - *use* Muscle, Lower Leg, Left
  - *use* Muscle, Lower Leg, Right
- **Flexor pollicis longus muscle**
  - *use* Muscle, Lower Arm and Wris Left
  - *use* Muscle, Lower Arm and Wris Right
- **Fluoroscopy**
  - Abdomen and Pelvis BW11
  - Airway, Upper BB1DZZZ
  - Ankle
    - Left BQ1
    - Right BQ1G
  - Aorta
    - Abdominal B410
      - Laser, Intraoperative B41

Fluoroscopy *(continued)*
- Aorta *(continued)*
  - Thoracic B310
    - Laser, Intraoperative B310
  - Thoraco-Abdominal B31P
    - Laser, Intraoperative B31P
- Aorta and Bilateral Lower Extremity
  - Arteries B41D
  - Laser, Intraoperative B41D
- Arm
  - Left BP1FZZZ
  - Right BP1EZZZ
- Artery
  - Brachiocephalic-Subclavian
    - Right B311
    - Laser, Intraoperative B311
  - Bronchial B31L
    - Laser, Intraoperative B31L
  - Bypass Graft, Other B21F
  - Cervico-Cerebral Arch B31Q
    - Laser, Intraoperative B31Q
  - Common Carotid
    - Bilateral B315
      - Laser, Intraoperative B315
    - Left B314
      - Laser, Intraoperative B314
    - Right B313
      - Laser, Intraoperative B313
  - Coronary
    - Bypass Graft
      - Multiple B213
        - Laser, Intraoperative B213
      - Single B212
        - Laser, Intraoperative B212
    - Multiple B211
      - Laser, Intraoperative B211
    - Single B210
      - Laser, Intraoperative B210
  - External Carotid
    - Bilateral B31C
      - Laser, Intraoperative B31C
    - Left B31B
      - Laser, Intraoperative B31B
    - Right B319
      - Laser, Intraoperative B319
  - Hepatic B412
    - Laser, Intraoperative B412
  - Inferior Mesenteric B415
    - Laser, Intraoperative B415
  - Intercostal B31L
    - Laser, Intraoperative B31L
  - Internal Carotid
    - Bilateral B318
      - Laser, Intraoperative B318
    - Left B317
      - Laser, Intraoperative B317
    - Right B316
      - Laser, Intraoperative B316
  - Internal Mammary Bypass Graft
    - Left B218
    - Right B217
  - Intra-Abdominal
    - Laser, Intraoperative B41B
    - Other B41B
  - Intracranial B31R
    - Laser, Intraoperative B31R

Fluoroscopy *(continued)*
- Artery *(continued)*
  - Lower
    - Laser, Intraoperative B41J
    - Other B41J
  - Lower Extremity
    - Bilateral and Aorta B41D
      - Laser, Intraoperative B41D
    - Left B41G
      - Laser, Intraoperative B41G
    - Right B41F
      - Laser, Intraoperative B41F
  - Lumbar B419
    - Laser, Intraoperative B419
  - Pelvic B41C
    - Laser, Intraoperative B41C
  - Pulmonary
    - Left B31T
      - Laser, Intraoperative B31T
    - Right B31S
      - Laser, Intraoperative B31S
  - Pulmonary Trunk B31U
    - Laser, Intraoperative B31U
  - Renal
    - Bilateral B418
      - Laser, Intraoperative B418
    - Left B417
      - Laser, Intraoperative B417
    - Right B416
      - Laser, Intraoperative B416
  - Spinal B31M
    - Laser, Intraoperative B31M
  - Splenic B413
    - Laser, Intraoperative B413
  - Subclavian
    - Laser, Intraoperative B312
    - Left B312
  - Superior Mesenteric B414
    - Laser, Intraoperative B414
  - Upper
    - Laser, Intraoperative B31N
    - Other B31N
  - Upper Extremity
    - Bilateral B31K
      - Laser, Intraoperative B31K
    - Left B31J
      - Laser, Intraoperative B31J
    - Right B31H
      - Laser, Intraoperative B31H
  - Vertebral
    - Bilateral B31G
      - Laser, Intraoperative B31G
    - Left B31F
      - Laser, Intraoperative B31F
    - Right B31D
      - Laser, Intraoperative B31D
- Bile Duct BF10
  - Pancreatic Duct and Gallbladder BF14
- Bile Duct and Gallbladder BF13
- Biliary Duct BF11

Fluoroscopy *(continued)*
- Bladder BT10
  - Kidney and Ureter BT14
    - Left BT1F
    - Right BT1D
- Bladder and Urethra BT1B
- Bowel, Small BD1
- Calcaneus
  - Left BQ1KZZZ
  - Right BQ1JZZZ
- Clavicle
  - Left BP15ZZZ
  - Right BP14ZZZ
- Coccyx BR1F
- Colon BD14
- Corpora Cavernosa BV10
- Dialysis Fistula B51W
- Dialysis Shunt B51W
- Diaphragm BB16ZZZ
- Disc
  - Cervical BR11
  - Lumbar BR13
  - Thoracic BR12
- Duodenum BD19
- Elbow
  - Left BP1H
  - Right BP1G
- Epiglottis B91G
- Esophagus BD11
- Extremity
  - Lower BW1C
  - Upper BW1J
- Facet Joint
  - Cervical BR14
  - Lumbar BR16
  - Thoracic BR15
- Fallopian Tube
  - Bilateral BU12
  - Left BU11
  - Right BU10
- Fallopian Tube and Uterus BU18
- Femur
  - Left BQ14ZZZ
  - Right BQ13ZZZ
- Finger
  - Left BP1SZZZ
  - Right BP1RZZZ
- Foot
  - Left BQ1MZZZ
  - Right BQ1LZZZ
- Forearm
  - Left BP1KZZZ
  - Right BP1JZZZ
- Gallbladder BF12
  - Bile Duct and Pancreatic Duct BF14
- Gallbladder and Bile Duct BF13
- Gastrointestinal, Upper BD1
- Hand
  - Left BP1PZZZ
  - Right BP1NZZZ
- Head and Neck BW19
- Heart
  - Left B215
  - Right B214
  - Right and Left B216
- Hip
  - Left BQ11
  - Right BQ10
- Humerus
  - Left BP1BZZZ
  - Right BP1AZZZ
- Ileal Diversion Loop BT1C
- Ileal Loop, Ureters and Kidney BT1G
- Intracranial Sinus B512
- Joint
  - Acromioclavicular, Bilateral BP13ZZZ

Fluoroscopy *(continued)*
- Joint *(continued)*
  - Finger
    - Left BP1D
    - Right BP1C
  - Foot
    - Left BQ1Y
    - Right BQ1X
  - Hand
    - Left BP1D
    - Right BP1C
  - Lumbosacral BR1B
  - Sacroiliac BR1D
  - Sternoclavicular
    - Bilateral BP12ZZZ
    - Left BP11ZZZ
    - Right BP10ZZZ
  - Temporomandibular
    - Bilateral BN19
    - Left BN18
    - Right BN17
  - Thoracolumbar BR18
  - Toe
    - Left BQ1Y
    - Right BQ1X
- Kidney
  - Bilateral BT13
  - Ileal Loop and Ureter BT1G
  - Left BT12
  - Right BT11
  - Ureter and Bladder BT14
    - Left BT1F
    - Right BT1D
- Knee
  - Left BQ18
  - Right BQ17
- Larynx B91J
- Leg
  - Left BQ1FZZZ
  - Right BQ1DZZZ
- Lung
  - Bilateral BB14ZZZ
  - Left BB13ZZZ
  - Right BB12ZZZ
- Mediastinum BB1CZZZ
- Mouth BD1B
- Neck and Head BW19
- Oropharynx BD1B
- Pancreatic Duct BF1
  - Gallbladder and Bile Buct BF14
- Patella
  - Left BQ1WZZZ
  - Right BQ1VZZZ
- Pelvis BR1C
- Pelvis and Abdomen BW11
- Pharynix B91G
- Ribs
  - Left BP1YZZZ
  - Right BP1XZZZ
- Sacrum BR1F
- Scapula
  - Left BP17ZZZ
  - Right BP16ZZZ
- Shoulder
  - Left BP19
  - Right BP18
- Sinus, Intracranial B512
- Spinal Cord B01B
- Spine
  - Cervical BR10
  - Lumbar BR19
  - Thoracic BR17
  - Whole BR1G
- Sternum BR1H
- Stomach BD12
- Toe
  - Left BQ1QZZZ
  - Right BQ1PZZZ

Fluoroscopy *(continued)*
Tracheobronchial Tree
Bilateral BB19YZZ
Left BB18YZZ
Right BB17YZZ
Ureter
Ileal Loop and Kidney BT1G
Kidney and Bladder BT14
Left BT1F
Right BT1D
Left BT17
Right BT16
Urethra BT15
Urethra and Bladder BT1B
Uterus BU16
Uterus and Fallopian Tube BU18
Vagina BU19
Vasa Vasorum BV18
Vein
Cerebellar B511
Cerebral B511
Epidural B510
Jugular
Bilateral B515
Left B514
Right B513
Lower Extremity
Bilateral B51D
Left B51C
Right B51B
Other B51V
Pelvic (Iliac)
Left B51G
Right B51F
Pelvic (Iliac) Bilateral B51H
Portal B51T
Pulmonary
Bilateral B51S
Left B51R
Right B51Q
Renal
Bilateral B51L
Left B51K
Right B51J
Spanchnic B51T
Subclavian
Left B517
Right B516
Upper Extremity
Bilateral B51P
Left B51N
Right B51M
Vena Cava
Inferior B519
Superior B518
Wrist
Left BP1M
Right BP1L
Fluoroscopy, laser intraoperative
Fluoroscopy, Heart B21
Fluoroscopy, Lower Arteries B41
Fluoroscopy, Upper Arteries B31
Flushing
see Irrigation
Foley catheter
use Drainage Device
Fontan completion procedure Stage II
see Bypass, Vena Cava, Inferior 0610
Foramen magnum
use Occipital Bone
Foramen of Monro (intraventricular)
use Cerebral Ventricle
Foreskin
use Prepuce
Formula™ Balloon-Expandable Renal Stent System
use Intraluminal Device
Fossa of Rosenmuller
use Nasopharynx
Fourth cranial nerve
use Nerve, Trochlear
Fourth ventricle
use Cerebral Ventricle
Fovea
use Retina, Left
use Retina, Right
Fragmentation
Ampulla of Vater 0FFC
Anus 0DFQ
Appendix 0DFJ
Bladder 0TFB
Bladder Neck 0TFC
Bronchus
Lingula 0BF9
Lower Lobe
Left 0BFB
Right 0BF6
Main
Left 0BF7
Right 0BF3
Middle Lobe, Right 0BF5
Upper Lobe
Left 0BF8
Right 0BF4
Carina 0BF2
Cavity, Cranial 0WF1
Cecum 0DFH
Cerebral Ventricle 00F6
Colon
Ascending 0DFK
Descending 0DFM
Sigmoid 0DFN
Transverse 0DFL
Duct
Common Bile 0FF9
Cystic 0FF8
Hepatic
Common 0FF7
Left 0FF6
Right 0FF5
Pancreatic 0FFD
Accessory 0FFF
Parotid
Left 0CFC
Right 0CFB
Duodenum 0DF9
Epidural Space, Intracranial 00F3
Esophagus 0DF5
Fallopian Tube
Left 0UF6
Right 0UF5
Fallopian Tubes, Bilateral 0UF7
Gallbladder 0FF4
Gastrointestinal Tract 0WFP
Genitourinary Tract 0WFR
Ileum 0DFB
Intestine
Large 0DFE
Left 0DFG
Right 0DFF
Small 0DF8
Jejunum 0DFA
Kidney Pelvis
Left 0TF4
Right 0TF3
Mediastinum 0WFC
Oral Cavity and Throat 0WF3
Pelvic Cavity 0WFJ
Pericardial Cavity 0WFD
Pericardium 02FN
Peritoneal Cavity 0WFG
Pleural Cavity
Left 0WFB
Right 0WF9
Rectum 0DFP
Respiratory Tract 0WFQ
Fragmentation *(continued)*
Spinal Canal 00FU
Stomach 0DF6
Subarachnoid Space, Intracranial 00F5
Subdural Space, Intracranial 00F4
Trachea 0BF1
Ureter
Left 0TF7
Right 0TF6
Urethra 0TFD
Uterus 0UF9
Vitreous
Left 08F5
Right 08F4
Freestyle (Stentless) Aortic Root Bioprosthesis
use Zooplastic Tissue in Heart and Great Vessels
Frenectomy
see Excision, Mouth and Throat 0CB
see Resection, Mouth and Throat 0CT
Frenoplasty, frenuloplasty
see Repair, Mouth and Throat 0CQ
see Replacement, Mouth and Throat 0CR
see Supplement, Mouth and Throat 0CU
Frenotomy
see Drainage, Mouth and Throat 0C9
see Release, Mouth and Throat 0CN
Frenulotomy
see Drainage, Mouth and Throat 0C9
see Release, Mouth and Throat 0CN
Frenulum labii inferioris
use Lip, Lower
Frenulum labii superioris
use Lip, Upper
Frenulum linguae
use Tongue
Frenulumectomy
see Excision, Mouth and Throat 0CB
see Resection, Mouth and Throat 0CT
Frontal lobe
use Cerebral Hemisphere
Frontal vein
use Vein, Face, Left
use Vein, Face, Right
Fulguration
see Destruction
Fundoplication, gastroesophageal
see Restriction, Esophagogastric Junction 0DV4
Fundus uteri
use Uterus
Fusion
Acromioclavicular
Left 0RGH
Right 0RGG
Ankle
Left 0SGG
Right 0SGF
Carpal
Left 0RGR
Right 0RGQ
Carpometacarpal
Left 0RGT
Right 0RGS
Cervical Vertebral 0RG1
2 or more 0RG2
Interbody Fusion Device
Nanotextured Surface XRG2092
Radiolucent Porous XRG20F3
Fusion *(continued)*
Cervical Vertebral *(continued)*
Interbody Fusion Device,
Nanotextured Surface XRG1092
Radiolucent Porous XRG10F3
Cervicothoracic Vertebral 0RG4
Interbody Fusion Device
Nanotextured Surface XRG4092
Radiolucent Porous XRG40F3
Coccygeal 0SG6
Elbow
Left 0RGM
Right 0RGL
Finger Phalangeal
Left 0RGX
Right 0RGW
Hip
Left 0SGB
Right 0SG9
Knee
Left 0SGD
Right 0SGC
Lumbar Vertebral 0SG0
2 or more 0SG1
Interbody Fusion Device
Nanotextured Surfac
XRGC092
Radiolucent Porous XRGC0F3
Interbody Fusion Device
Nanotextured Surface XRGB092
Radiolucent Porous XRGB0F3
Lumbosacral 0SG3
Interbody Fusion Device
Nanotextured Surface XRGD092
Radiolucent Porous XRGD0F3
Metacarpophalangeal
Left 0RGV
Right 0RGU
Metatarsal-Phalangeal
Left 0SGN
Right 0SGM
Occipital-cervical 0RG0
Interbody Fusion Device
Nanotextured Surface XRG0092
Radiolucent Porous XRG00F3
Sacrococcygeal 0SG5
Sacroiliac
Left 0SG8
Right 0SG7
Shoulder
Left 0RGK
Right 0RGJ
Sternoclavicular
Left 0RGF
Right 0RGE
Tarsal
Left 0SGJ
Right 0SGH
Tarsometatarsal
Left 0SGL
Right 0SGK
Temporomandibular
Left 0RGD
Right 0RGC

usion *(continued)*
Thoracic Vertebral 0RG6
2 to 7 0RG7
Interbody Fusion Device
Nanotextured Surface XRG7092
Radiolucent Porous XRG70F3
8 or more 0RG8
Interbody Fusion Device
Nanotextured Surface XRG8092
Radiolucent Porous XRG80F3
Interbody Fusion Device
Nanotextured Surface XRG6092
Radiolucent Porous XRG60F3
Thoracolumbar Vertebral 0RGA
Interbody Fusion Device
Nanotextured Surface XRGA092
Radiolucent Porous XRGA0F3
Toe Phalangeal
Left 0SGQ
Right 0SGP
Wrist
Left 0RGP
Right 0RGN
usion screw (compression)(lag) (locking)
use Internal Fixation Device in Lower Joints
use Internal Fixation Device in Upper Joints

G

ait training
see Motor Treatment, Rehabilitation F07
alea aponeurotica
use Subcutaneous Tissue and Fascia, Scalp
ammaTile™
use Radioactive Element, Cesium-131 Collagen Implant in 00H
anglion impar (ganglion of Walther)
use Nerve, Sacral Sympathetic
anglionectomy
Destruction of lesion
see Destruction
Excision of lesion
see Excision
asserian ganglion
use Nerve, Trigeminal
astrectomy
Partial
see Excision, Stomach 0DB6
Total
see Resection, Stomach 0DT6
Vertical (sleeve)
see Excision, Stomach 0DB6
astric electrical stimulation (GES) lead
use Stimulator Lead in Gastrointestinal System
astric lymph node
use Lymphatic, Aortic
astric pacemaker lead
use Stimulator Lead in Gastrointestinal System
astric plexus
use Nerve, Abdominal Sympathetic
astrocnemius muscle
use Muscle, Lower Leg, Left
use Muscle, Lower Leg, Right
Gastrocolic ligament
use Omentum
Gastrocolic omentum
use Omentum
Gastrocolostomy
see Bypass, Gastrointestinal System 0D1
see Drainage, Gastrointestinal System 0D9
Gastroduodenal artery
use Artery, Hepatic
Gastroduodenectomy
see Excision, Gastrointestinal System 0DB
see Resection, Gastrointestinal System 0DT
Gastroduodenoscopy 0DJ08ZZ
Gastroenteroplasty
see Repair, Gastrointestinal System 0DQ
see Supplement, Gastrointestinal System 0DU
Gastroenterostomy
see Bypass, Gastrointestinal System 0D1
see Drainage, Gastrointestinal System 0D9
Gastroesophageal (GE) junction
use Esophagogastric Junction
Gastrogastrostomy
see Bypass, Stomach 0D16
see Drainage, Stomach 0D96
Gastrohepatic omentum
use Omentum
Gastrojejunostomy
see Bypass, Stomach 0D16
see Drainage, Stomach 0D96
Gastrolysis
see Release, Stomach 0DN6
Gastropexy
see Repair, Stomach 0DQ6
see Reposition, Stomach 0DS6
Gastrophrenic ligament
use Omentum
Gastroplasty
see Repair, Stomach 0DQ6
see Supplement, Stomach 0DU6
Gastroplication
see Restriction, Stomach 0DV6
Gastropylorectomy
see Excision, Gastrointestinal System 0DB
Gastrorrhaphy
see Repair, Stomach 0DQ6
Gastroscopy 0DJ68ZZ
Gastrosplenic ligament
use Omentum
Gastrostomy
see Bypass, Stomach 0D16
see Drainage, Stomach 0D96
Gastrotomy
see Drainage, Stomach 0D96
Gemellus muscle
use Muscle, Hip, Left
use Muscle, Hip, Right
Geniculate ganglion
use Nerve, Facial
Geniculate nucleus
use Thalamus
Genioglossus muscle
use Muscle, Tongue, Palate, Pharynx
Genioplasty
see Alteration, Jaw, Lower 0W05
Genitofemoral nerve
use Nerve, Lumbar Plexus
GIAPREZA(™)
use Synthetic Human Angiotensin II
Gingivectomy
see Excision, Mouth and Throat 0CB
Gingivoplasty
see Repair, Mouth and Throat 0CQ
see Replacement, Mouth and Throat 0CR
see Supplement, Mouth and Throat 0CU
Glans penis
use Prepuce
Glenohumeral joint
use Joint, Shoulder, Left
use Joint, Shoulder, Right
Glenohumeral ligament
use Bursa and Ligament, Shoulder, Left
use Bursa and Ligament, Shoulder, Right
Glenoid fossa (of scapula)
use Glenoid Cavity, Left
use Glenoid Cavity, Right
Glenoid ligament (labrum)
use Shoulder Joint, Left
use Shoulder Joint, Right
Globus pallidus
use Basal Ganglia
Glomectomy
see Excision, Endocrine System 0GB
see Resection, Endocrine System 0GT
Glossectomy
see Excision, Tongue 0CB7
see Resection, Tongue 0CT7
Glossoepiglottic fold
use Epiglottis
Glossopexy
see Repair, Tongue 0CQ7
see Reposition, Tongue 0CS7
Glossoplasty
see Repair, Tongue 0CQ7
see Replacement, Tongue 0CR7
see Supplement, Tongue 0CU7
Glossorrhaphy
see Repair, Tongue 0CQ7
Glossotomy
see Drainage, Tongue 0C97
Glottis
use Larynx
Gluteal Artery Perforator Flap
Replacement
Bilateral 0HRV079
Left 0HRU079
Right 0HRT079
Transfer
Left 0KXG
Right 0KXF
Gluteal lymph node
use Lymphatic, Pelvis
Gluteal vein
use Vein, Hypogastric, Left
use Vein, Hypogastric, Right
Gluteus maximus muscle
use Muscle, Hip, Left
use Muscle, Hip, Right
Gluteus medius muscle
use Muscle, Hip, Left
use Muscle, Hip, Right
Gluteus minimus muscle
use Muscle, Hip, Left
use Muscle, Hip, Right
GORE® DUALMESH®
use Synthetic Substitute
GORE EXCLUDER® AAA Endoprosthesis
use Intraluminal Device
use Intraluminal Device, Branched or Fenestrated, One or Two Arteries in 04V
GORE EXCLUDER® AAA Endoprosthesis *(continued)*
use Intraluminal Device, Branched or Fenestrated, Three or More Arteries in 04V
GORE EXCLUDER® IBE Endoprosthesis
use Intraluminal Device, Branched or Fenestrated, One or Two Arteries in 04V
GORE TAG® Thoracic Endoprosthesis
use Intraluminal Device
Gracilis muscle
use Muscle, Upper Leg, Left
use Muscle, Upper Leg, Right
Graft
see Replacement
see Supplement
Great auricular nerve
use Nerve, Cervical Plexus
Great cerebral vein
use Vein, Intracranial
Great(er) saphenous vein
use Vein, Saphenous, Left
use Vein, Saphenous, Right
Greater alar cartilage
use Nasal Mucosa and Soft Tissue
Greater occipital nerve
use Nerve, Cervical
Greater Omentum
use Omentum
Greater splanchnic nerve
use Nerve, Thoracic Sympathetic
Greater superficial petrosal nerve
use Nerve, Facial
Greater trochanter
use Femur, Upper, Left
use Femur, Upper, Right
Greater tuberosity
use Humeral Head, Left
use Humeral Head, Right
Greater vestibular (Bartholin's) gland
use Gland, Vestibular
Greater wing
use Bone, Sphenoid
Guedel airway
use Intraluminal Device, Airway in Mouth and Throat
Guidance, catheter placement
EKG
see Measurement, Physiological Systems 4A0
Fluoroscopy
see Fluoroscopy, Veins B51
Ultrasound
see Ultrasonography, Veins B54

H

Hallux
use Toe, 1st, Left
use Toe, 1st, Right
Hamate bone
use Carpal, Left
use Carpal, Right
Hancock Bioprosthesis (aortic) (mitral) valve
use Zooplastic Tissue in Heart and Great Vessels
Hancock Bioprosthetic Valved Conduit
use Zooplastic Tissue in Heart and Great Vessels
Harvesting, stem cells
see Pheresis, Circulatory 6A55
Head of fibula
use Fibula, Left
use Fibula, Right
Hearing Aid Assessment F14Z
Hearing Assessment F13Z

- **Hearing Device**
  - Bone Conduction
    - Left 09HE
    - Right 09HD
  - Insertion of device in
    - Left 0NH6
    - Right 0NH5
  - Multiple Channel Cochlear Prosthesis
    - Left 09HE
    - Right 09HD
  - Removal of device from, Skull 0NP0
  - Revision of device in, Skull 0NW0
  - Single Channel Cochlear Prosthesis
    - Left 09HE
    - Right 09HD
- **Hearing Treatment** F09Z
- **Heart Assist System**
  - Implantable
    - Insertion of device in, Heart 02HA
    - Removal of device from, Heart 02PA
    - Revision of device in, Heart 02WA
  - Short-term External
    - Insertion of device in, Heart 02HA
    - Removal of device from, Heart 02PA
    - Revision of device in, Heart 02WA
- **HeartMate II® Left Ventricular Assist Device (LVAD)**
  - *use* Implantable Heart Assist System in Heart and Great Vessels
- **HeartMate 3™ LVAS**
  - *use* Implantable Heart Assist System in Heart and Great Vessels
- **HeartMate XVE® Left Ventricular Assist Device (LVAD)**
  - *use* Implantable Heart Assist System in Heart and Great Vessels
- **HeartMate® implantable heart assist system**
  - *see* Insertion of device in, Heart 02HA
- **Helix**
  - *use* Ear, External, Bilateral
  - *use* Ear, External, Left
  - *use* Ear, External, Right
- **Hematopoietic cell transplant (HCT)**
  - *see* Transfusion, Circulatory 302
- **Hemicolectomy**
  - *see* Resection, Gastrointestinal System 0DT
- **Hemicystectomy**
  - *see* Excision, Urinary System 0TB
- **Hemigastrectomy**
  - *see* Excision, Gastrointestinal System 0DB
- **Hemiglossectomy**
  - *see* Excision, Mouth and Throat 0CB
- **Hemilaminectomy**
  - *see* Excision, Lower Bones 0QB
  - *see* Excision, Upper Bones 0PB
- **Hemilaminotomy**
  - *see* Drainage, Lower Bones 0Q9
  - *see* Drainage, Upper Bones 0P9
  - *see* Excision, Lower Bones 0QB
  - *see* Excision, Upper Bones 0PB
  - *see* Release, Central Nervous System and Cranial Nerves 00N
  - *see* Release, Lower Bones 0QN
  - *see* Release, Peripheral Nervous System 01N
  - *see* Release, Upper Bones 0PN
- **Hemilaryngectomy**
  - *see* Excision, Larynx 0CBS
- **Hemimandibulectomy**
  - *see* Excision, Head and Facial Bones 0NB
- **Hemimaxillectomy**
  - *see* Excision, Head and Facial Bones 0NB
- **Hemipylorectomy**
  - *see* Excision, Gastrointestinal System 0DB
- **Hemispherectomy**
  - *see* Excision, Central Nervous System and Cranial Nerves 00B
  - *see* Resection, Central Nervous System and Cranial Nerves 00T
- **Hemithyroidectomy**
  - *see* Resection, Endocrine System 0GT
  - *see* Excision, Endocrine System 0GB
- **Hemodialysis**
  - *see* Performance, Urinary 5A1D
- **Hemolung® Respiratory Assist System (RAS)** 5A0920Z
- **Hepatectomy**
  - *see* Excision, Hepatobiliary System and Pancreas 0FB
  - *see* Resection, Hepatobiliary System and Pancreas 0FT
- **Hepatic artery proper**
  - *use* Artery, Hepatic
- **Hepatic flexure**
  - *use* Colon, Transverse
- **Hepatic lymph node**
  - *use* Lymphatic, Aortic
- **Hepatic plexus**
  - *use* Nerve, Abdominal Sympathetic
- **Hepatic portal vein**
  - *use* Vein, Portal
- **Hepaticoduodenostomy**
  - *see* Bypass, Hepatobiliary System and Pancreas 0F1
  - *see* Drainage, Hepatobiliary System and Pancreas 0F9
- **Hepaticotomy**
  - *see* Drainage, Hepatobiliary System and Pancreas 0F9
- **Hepatocholedochostomy**
  - *see* Drainage, Duct, Common Bile 0F99
- **Hepatogastric ligament**
  - *use* Omentum
- **Hepatopancreatic ampulla**
  - *use* Ampulla of Vater
- **Hepatopexy**
  - *see* Repair, Hepatobiliary System and Pancreas 0FQ
  - *see* Reposition, Hepatobiliary System and Pancreas 0FS
- **Hepatorrhaphy**
  - *see* Repair, Hepatobiliary System and Pancreas 0FQ
- **Hepatotomy**
  - *see* Drainage, Hepatobiliary System and Pancreas 0F9
- **Herculink (RX) Elite Renal Stent System**
  - *use* Intraluminal Device
- **Herniorrhaphy**
  - *see* Repair, Anatomical Regions, General 0WQ
  - *see* Repair, Anatomical Regions, Lower Extremities 0YQ
  - With synthetic substitute
    - *see* Supplement, Anatomical Regions, General 0WU
    - *see* Supplement, Anatomical Regions, Lower Extremities 0YU
- **Hip (joint) liner**
  - *use* Liner in Lower Joints
- **Holter monitoring** 4A12X45
- **Holter valve ventricular shunt**
  - *use* Synthetic Substitute
- **Human angiotensin II, synthetic**
  - *use* Synthetic Human Angiotensin II
- **Humeroradial joint**
  - *use* Joint, Elbow, Left
  - *use* Joint, Elbow, Right
- **Humeroulnar joint**
  - *use* Joint, Elbow, Left
  - *use* Joint, Elbow, Right
- **Humerus, distal**
  - *use* Humeral Shaft, Left
  - *use* Humeral Shaft, Right
- **Hydrocelectomy**
  - *see* Excision, Male Reproductive System 0VB
- **Hydrotherapy**
  - Assisted exercise in pool
    - *see* Motor Treatment, Rehabilitation F07
  - Whirlpool
    - *see* Activities of Daily Living Treatment, Rehabilitation F08
- **Hymenectomy**
  - *see* Excision, Hymen 0UBK
  - *see* Resection, Hymen 0UTK
- **Hymenoplasty**
  - *see* Repair, Hymen 0UQK
  - *see* Supplement, Hymen 0UUK
- **Hymenorrhaphy**
  - *see* Repair, Hymen 0UQK
- **Hymenotomy**
  - *see* Division, Hymen 0U8K
  - *see* Drainage, Hymen 0U9K
- **Hyoglossus muscle**
  - *use* Muscle, Tongue, Palate, Pharynx
- **Hyoid artery**
  - *use* Artery, Thyroid, Left
  - *use* Artery, Thyroid, Right
- **Hyperalimentation**
  - *see* Introduction of substance in or on
- **Hyperbaric oxygenation**
  - Decompression sickness treatment
    - *see* Decompression, Circulatory 6A15
  - Wound treatment
    - *see* Assistance, Circulatory 5A05
- **Hyperthermia**
  - Radiation Therapy
    - Abdomen DWY38ZZ
    - Adrenal Gland DGY28ZZ
    - Bile Ducts DFY28ZZ
    - Bladder DTY28ZZ
    - Bone, Other DPYC8ZZ
    - Bone Marrow D7Y08ZZ
    - Brain D0Y08ZZ
    - Brain Stem D0Y18ZZ
    - Breast
      - Left DMY08ZZ
      - Right DMY18ZZ
    - Bronchus DBY18ZZ
    - Cervix DUY18ZZ
    - Chest DWY28ZZ
    - Chest Wall DBY78ZZ
    - Colon DDY58ZZ
    - Diaphragm DBY88ZZ
    - Duodenum DDY28ZZ
    - Ear D9Y08ZZ
    - Esophagus DDY08ZZ
    - Eye D8Y08ZZ
    - Femur DPY98ZZ
    - Fibula DPYB8ZZ
    - Gallbladder DFY18ZZ
    - Gland
      - Adrenal DGY28ZZ
      - Parathyroid DGY48ZZ

Hyperthermia *(continued)*
  - Radiation Therapy *(continued)*
    - Gland *(continued)*
      - Pituitary DGY08ZZ
      - Thyroid DGY58ZZ
    - Glands, Salivary D9Y68ZZ
    - Head and Neck DWY18ZZ
    - Hemibody DWY48ZZ
    - Humerus DPY68ZZ
    - Hypopharynx D9Y38ZZ
    - Ileum DDY48ZZ
    - Jejunum DDY38ZZ
    - Kidney DTY08ZZ
    - Larynx D9YB8ZZ
    - Liver DFY08ZZ
    - Lung DBY28ZZ
    - Lymphatics
      - Abdomen D7Y68ZZ
      - Axillary D7Y48ZZ
      - Inguinal D7Y88ZZ
      - Neck D7Y38ZZ
      - Pelvis D7Y78ZZ
      - Thorax D7Y58ZZ
    - Mandible DPY38ZZ
    - Maxilla DPY28ZZ
    - Mediastinum DBY68ZZ
    - Mouth D9Y48ZZ
    - Nasopharynx D9YD8ZZ
    - Neck and Head DWY18ZZ
    - Nerve, Peripheral D0Y78ZZ
    - Nose D9Y18ZZ
    - Oropharynx D9YF8ZZ
    - Ovary DUY08ZZ
    - Palate
      - Hard D9Y88ZZ
      - Soft D9Y98ZZ
    - Pancreas DFY38ZZ
    - Parathyroid Gland DGY48ZZ
    - Pelvic Bones DPY88ZZ
    - Pelvic Region DWY68ZZ
    - Pineal Body DGY18ZZ
    - Pituitary Gland DGY08ZZ
    - Pleura DBY58ZZ
    - Prostate DVY08ZZ
    - Radius DPY78ZZ
    - Rectum DDY78ZZ
    - Rib DPY58ZZ
    - Sinuses D9Y78ZZ
    - Skin
      - Abdomen DHY88ZZ
      - Arm DHY48ZZ
      - Back DHY78ZZ
      - Buttock DHY98ZZ
      - Chest DHY68ZZ
      - Face DHY28ZZ
      - Leg DHYB8ZZ
      - Neck DHY38ZZ
    - Skull DPY08ZZ
    - Spinal Cord D0Y68ZZ
    - Spleen D7Y28ZZ
    - Sternum DPY48ZZ
    - Stomach DDY18ZZ
    - Testis DVY18ZZ
    - Thymus D7Y18ZZ
    - Thyroid Gland DGY58ZZ
    - Tibia DPYB8ZZ
    - Tongue D9Y58ZZ
    - Trachea DBY08ZZ
    - Ulna DPY78ZZ
    - Ureter DTY18ZZ
    - Urethra DTY38ZZ
    - Uterus DUY28ZZ
    - Whole Body DWY58ZZ
  - Whole Body 6A3Z
- **Hypnosis** GZFZZZZ
- **Hypogastric artery**
  - *use* Artery, Internal Iliac, Left
  - *use* Artery, Internal Iliac, Right
- **Hypopharynx**
  - *use* Pharynx

Hypophysectomy
see Excision, Gland, Pituitary 0GB0
see Resection, Gland, Pituitary 0GT0
Hypophysis
use Gland, Pituitary
Hypothalamotomy
see Destruction, Thalamus 0059
Hypothenar muscle
use Muscle, Hand, Left
use Muscle, Hand, Right
Hypothermia, Whole Body 6A4Z
Hysterectomy
Supracervical
see Resection, Uterus 0UT9
Total
see Resection, Uterus 0UT9
Hysterolysis
see Release, Uterus 0UN9
Hysteropexy
see Repair, Uterus 0UQ9
see Reposition, Uterus 0US9
Hysteroplasty
see Repair, Uterus 0UQ9
Hysterorrhaphy
see Repair, Uterus 0UQ9
Hysteroscopy 0UJD8ZZ
Hysterotomy
see Drainage, Uterus 0U99
Hysterotrachelectomy
see Resection, Cervix 0UTC
see Resection, Uterus 0UT9
Hysterotracheloplasty
see Repair, Uterus 0UQ9
Hysterotrachelorrhaphy
see Repair, Uterus 0UQ9

I

IABP (Intra-aortic balloon pump)
see Assistance, Cardiac 5A02
IAEMT (Intraoperative anesthetic effect monitoring and titration)
see Monitoring, Central Nervous 4A10
Idarucizumab, Dabigatran Reversal Agent XW0
IHD (Intermittent hemodialysis) 5A1D70Z
Ileal artery
use Artery, Superior Mesenteric
Ileectomy
see Excision, Ileum 0DBB
see Resection, Ileum 0DTB
Ileocolic artery
use Artery, Superior Mesenteric
Ileocolic vein
use Vein, Colic
Ileopexy
see Repair, Ileum 0DQB
see Reposition, Ileum 0DSB
Ileorrhaphy
see Repair, Ileum 0DQB
Ileoscopy 0DJD8ZZ
Ileostomy
see Bypass, Ileum 0D1B
see Drainage, Ileum 0D9B
Ileotomy
see Drainage, Ileum 0D9B
Ileoureterostomy
see Bypass, Urinary System 0T1
Iliac crest
use Bone, Pelvic, Left
use Bone, Pelvic, Right
Iliac fascia
use Subcutaneous Tissue and Fascia, Upper Leg, Left
use Subcutaneous Tissue and Fascia, Upper Leg, Right
Iliac lymph node
use Lymphatic, Pelvis
Iliacus muscle
use Muscle, Hip, Left
use Muscle, Hip, Right
Iliofemoral ligament
use Bursa and Ligament, Hip, Left
use Bursa and Ligament, Hip, Right
Iliohypogastric nerve
use Nerve, Lumbar Plexus
Ilioinguinal nerve
use Nerve, Lumbar Plexus
Iliolumbar artery
use Artery, Internal Iliac, Left
use Artery, Internal Iliac, Right
Iliolumbar ligament
use Bursa and Ligament, Lower Spine
Iliotibial tract (band)
use Subcutaneous Tissue and Fascia, Upper Leg, Left
use Subcutaneous Tissue and Fascia, Upper Leg, Right
Ilium
use Bone, Pelvic, Left
use Bone, Pelvic, Right
Ilizarov external fixator
use External Fixation Device, Ring in 0PH
use External Fixation Device, Ring in 0PS
use External Fixation Device, Ring in 0QH
use External Fixation Device, Ring in 0QS
Ilizarov-Vecklich device
use External Fixation Device, Limb Lengthening in 0QH
use External Fixation Device, Limb Lengthening in 0PH
Imaging, diagnostic
see Computerized Tomography (CT Scan)
see Fluoroscopy
see Magnetic Resonance Imaging (MRI)
see Plain Radiography
see Ultrasonography
Immobilization
Abdominal Wall 2W33X
Arm
Lower
Left 2W3DX
Right 2W3CX
Upper
Left 2W3BX
Right 2W3AX
Back 2W35X
Chest Wall 2W34X
Extremity
Lower
Left 2W3MX
Right 2W3LX
Upper
Left 2W39X
Right 2W38X
Face 2W31X
Finger
Left 2W3KX
Right 2W3JX
Foot
Left 2W3TX
Right 2W3SX
Hand
Left 2W3FX
Right 2W3EX
Head 2W30X
Inguinal Region
Left 2W37X
Right 2W36X
Immobilization *(continued)*
Leg
Lower
Left 2W3RX
Right 2W3QX
Upper
Left 2W3PX
Right 2W3NX
Neck 2W32X
Thumb
Left 2W3H
Right 2W3GX
Toe
Left 2W3VX
Right 2W3UX
Immunization
see Introduction of Serum, Toxoid, and Vaccine
Immunotherapy
see Introduction of Immunotherapeutic Substance
Immunotherapy, antineoplastic
Interferon
see Introduction of Low-dose Interleukin-2
Interleukin-2, high-dose
see Introduction of High-dose Interleukin-2
Interleukin-2, low-dose
see Introduction of Low-dose Interleukin-2
Monoclonal antibody
see Introduction of Monoclonal Antibody
Proleukin, high-dose
see Introduction of High-dose Interleukin-2
Proleukin, low-dose
see Introduction of Low-dose Interleukin-2
Impella® heart pump
use Short-term External Heart Assist System in Heart and Great Vessels
Impeller Pump
Continuous, Output 5A0221D
Intermittent, Output 5A0211D
Implantable cardioverter-defibrillator (ICD)
use Defibrillator Generator in 0JH
Implantable drug infusion pump (anti-spasmodic) (chemotherapy)(pain)
use Infusion Device, Pump in Subcutaneous Tissue and Fascia
Implantable glucose monitoring device
use Monitoring Device
Implantable hemodynamic monitor (IHM)
use Monitoring Device, Hemodynamic in 0JH
Implantable hemodynamic monitoring system (IHMS)
use Monitoring Device, Hemodynamic in 0JH
Implantable Miniature Telescope™ (IMT)
use Synthetic Substitute, Intraocular Telescope in 08R
Implantation
see Insertion
see Replacement
Implanted (venous)(access) port
use Vascular Access Device, Totally Implantable in Subcutaneous Tissue and Fascia
IMV (intermittent mandatory ventilation)
see Assistance, Respiratory 5A09
In Vitro Fertilization 8E0ZXY1
Incision, abscess
see Drainage
Incudectomy
see Excision, Ear, Nose, Sinus 09B
see Resection, Ear, Nose, Sinus 09T
Incudopexy
see Reposition, Ear, Nose, Sinus 09S
see Repair, Ear, Nose, Sinus 09Q
Incus
use Auditory Ossicle, Left
use Auditory Ossicle, Right
Induction of labor
Artificial rupture of membranes
see Drainage, Pregnancy 109
Oxytocin
see Introduction of Hormone
InDura, intrathecal catheter (1P) (spinal)
use Infusion Device
Inferior cardiac nerve
use Nerve, Thoracic Sympathetic
Inferior cerebellar vein
use Vein, Intracranial
Inferior cerebral vein
use Vein, Intracranial
Inferior epigastric artery
use Artery, External Iliac, Left
use Artery, External Iliac, Right
Inferior epigastric lymph node
use Lymphatic, Pelvis
Inferior genicular artery
use Artery, Popliteal, Left
use Artery, Popliteal, Right
Inferior gluteal artery
use Artery, Internal Iliac, Left
use Artery, Internal Iliac, Right
Inferior gluteal nerve
use Nerve, Sacral Plexus
Inferior hypogastric plexus
use Nerve, Abdominal Sympathetic
Inferior labial artery
use Artery, Face
Inferior longitudinal muscle
use Muscle, Tongue, Palate, Pharynx
Inferior mesenteric ganglion
use Nerve, Abdominal Sympathetic
Inferior mesenteric lymph node
use Lymphatic, Mesenteric
Inferior mesenteric plexus
use Nerve, Abdominal Sympathetic
Inferior oblique muscle
use Muscle, Extraocular, Left
use Muscle, Extraocular, Right
Inferior pancreaticoduodenal artery
use Artery, Superior Mesenteric
Inferior phrenic artery
use Aorta, Abdominal
Inferior rectus muscle
use Muscle, Extraocular, Left
use Muscle, Extraocular, Right
Inferior suprarenal artery
use Artery, Renal, Left
use Artery, Renal, Right
Inferior tarsal plate
use Eyelid, Lower, Left
use Eyelid, Lower, Right
Inferior thyroid vein
use Vein, Innominate, Left
use Vein, Innominate, Right
Inferior tibiofibular joint
use Joint, Ankle, Left
use Joint, Ankle, Right
Inferior turbinate
use Turbinate, Nasal
Inferior ulnar collateral artery
use Artery, Brachial, Left
use Artery, Brachial, Right

Inferior vesical artery
  use Artery, Internal Iliac, Left
  use Artery, Internal Iliac, Right
Infraauricular lymph node
  use Lymphatic, Head
Infraclavicular (deltopectoral) lymph node
  use Lymphatic, Upper Extremity, Left
  use Lymphatic, Upper Extremity, Right
Infrahyoid muscle
  use Muscle, Neck, Left
  use Muscle, Neck, Right
Infraparotid lymph node
  use Lymphatic, Head
Infraspinatus fascia
  use Subcutaneous Tissue and Fascia, Upper Arm, Left
  use Subcutaneous Tissue and Fascia, Upper Arm, Right
Infraspinatus muscle
  use Muscle, Shoulder, Left
  use Muscle, Shoulder, Right
Infundibulopelvic ligament
  use Uterine Supporting Structure
Infusion
  see Introduction of substance in or on
Infusion Device, Pump
  Insertion of device in
    Abdomen 0JH8
    Back 0JH7
    Chest 0JH6
    Lower Arm
      Left 0JHH
      Right 0JHG
    Lower Leg
      Left 0JHP
      Right 0JHN
    Trunk 0JHT
    Upper Arm
      Left 0JHF
      Right 0JHD
    Upper Leg
      Left 0JHM
      Right 0JHL
  Removal of device from
    Lower Extremity 0JPW
    Trunk 0JPT
    Upper Extremity 0JPV
  Revision of device in
    Lower Extremity 0JWW
    Trunk 0JWT
    Upper Extremity 0JWV
Infusion, glucarpidase
  Central vein 3E043GQ
  Peripheral vein 3E033GQ
Inguinal canal
  use Inguinal Region, Bilateral
  use Inguinal Region, Left
  use Inguinal Region, Right
Inguinal triangle
  use Inguinal Region, Bilateral
  use Inguinal Region, Left
  use Inguinal Region, Right
Injection
  see Introduction of substance in or on
Injection, Concentrated Bone Marrow Aspirate (CBMA), intramuscular XK02303
Injection reservoir, port
  use Vascular Access Device, Totally Implantable in Subcutaneous Tissue and Fascia
Injection reservoir, pump
  use Infusion Device, Pump in Subcutaneous Tissue and Fascia
Insemination, artificial 3E0P7LZ
Insertion
  Antimicrobial envelope
    see Introduction of Anti-infective
  Aqueous drainage shunt
    see Bypass, Eye 081
    see Drainage, Eye 089
  Products of Conception 10H0
  Spinal Stabilization Device
    see Insertion of device in, Upper Joints 0RH
    see Insertion of device in, Lower Joints 0SH
Insertion of device in
  Abdominal Wall 0WHF
  Acetabulum
    Left 0QH5
    Right 0QH4
  Anal Sphincter 0DHR
  Ankle Region
    Left 0YHL
    Right 0YHK
  Anus 0DHQ
  Aorta
    Abdominal 04H0
    Thoracic
      Ascending/Arch 02HX
      Descending 02HW
  Arm
    Lower
      Left 0XHF
      Right 0XHD
    Upper
      Left 0XH9
      Right 0XH8
  Artery
    Anterior Tibial
      Left 04HQ
      Right 04HP
    Axillary
      Left 03H6
      Right 03H5
    Brachial
      Left 03H8
      Right 03H7
    Celiac 04H1
    Colic
      Left 04H7
      Middle 04H8
      Right 04H6
    Common Carotid
      Left 03HJ
      Right 03HH
    Common Iliac
      Left 04HD
      Right 04HC
    External Carotid
      Left 03HN
      Right 03HM
    External Iliac
      Left 04HJ
      Right 04HH
    Face 03HR
    Femoral
      Left 04HL
      Right 04HK
    Foot
      Left 04HW
      Right 04HV
    Gastric 04H2
    Hand
      Left 03HF
      Right 03HD
    Hepatic 04H3
    Inferior Mesenteric 04HB
    Innominate 03H2
    Internal Carotid
      Left 03HL
      Right 03HK

Insertion of device in *(continued)*
  Artery *(continued)*
    Internal Iliac
      Left 04HF
      Right 04HE
    Internal Mammary
      Left 03H1
      Right 03H0
    Intracranial 03HG
    Lower 04HY
    Peroneal
      Left 04HU
      Right 04HT
    Popliteal
      Left 04HN
      Right 04HM
    Posterior Tibial
      Left 04HS
      Right 04HR
    Pulmonary
      Left 02HR
      Right 02HQ
    Pulmonary Trunk 02HP
    Radial
      Left 03HC
      Right 03HB
    Renal
      Left 04HA
      Right 04H9
    Splenic 04H4
    Subclavian
      Left 03H4
      Right 03H3
    Superior Mesenteric 04H5
    Temporal
      Left 03HT
      Right 03HS
    Thyroid
      Left 03HV
      Right 03HU
    Ulnar
      Left 03HA
      Right 03H9
    Upper 03HY
    Vertebral
      Left 03HQ
      Right 03HP
  Atrium
    Left 02H7
    Right 02H6
  Axilla
    Left 0XH5
    Right 0XH4
  Back
    Lower 0WHL
    Upper 0WHK
  Bladder 0THB
  Bladder Neck 0THC
  Bone
    Ethmoid
      Left 0NHG
      Right 0NHF
    Facial 0NHW
    Frontal 0NH1
    Hyoid 0NHX
    Lacrimal
      Left 0NHJ
      Right 0NHH
    Lower 0QHY
    Nasal 0NHB
    Occipital 0NH7
    Palatine
      Left 0NHL
      Right 0NHK
    Parietal
      Left 0NH4
      Right 0NH3
    Pelvic
      Left 0QH3
      Right 0QH2
    Sphenoid 0NHC

Insertion of device in *(continued)*
  Bone *(continued)*
    Temporal
      Left 0NH6
      Right 0NH5
    Upper 0PHY
    Zygomatic
      Left 0NHN
      Right 0NHM
  Brain 00H0
  Breast
    Bilateral 0HHV
    Left 0HHU
    Right 0HHT
  Bronchus
    Lingula 0BH9
    Lower Lobe
      Left 0BHB
      Right 0BH6
    Main
      Left 0BH7
      Right 0BH3
    Middle Lobe, Right 0BH5
    Upper Lobe
      Left 0BH8
      Right 0BH4
  Bursa and Ligament
    Lower 0MHY
    Upper 0MHX
  Buttock
    Left 0YH1
    Right 0YH0
  Carpal
    Left 0PHN
    Right 0PHM
  Cavity, Cranial 0WH1
  Cerebral Ventricle 00H6
  Cervix 0UHC
  Chest Wall 0WH8
  Cisterna Chyli 07HL
  Clavicle
    Left 0PHB
    Right 0PH9
  Coccyx 0QHS
  Cul-de-sac 0UHF
  Diaphragm 0BHT
  Disc
    Cervical Vertebral 0RH3
    Cervicothoracic Vertebral 0RH
    Lumbar Vertebral 0SH2
    Lumbosacral 0SH4
    Thoracic Vertebral 0RH9
    Thoracolumbar Vertebral 0RH
  Duct
    Hepatobiliary 0FHB
    Pancreatic 0FHD
  Duodenum 0DH9
  Ear
    Inner
      Left 09HE
      Right 09HD
    Left 09HJ
    Right 09HH
  Elbow Region
    Left 0XHC
    Right 0XHB
  Epididymis and Spermatic Cord 0VHM
  Esophagus 0DH5
  Extremity
    Lower
      Left 0YHB
      Right 0YH9
    Upper
      Left 0XH7
      Right 0XH6
  Eye
    Left 08H1
    Right 08H0
  Face 0WH2

Insertion of device in *(continued)*
- Fallopian Tube 0UH8
- Femoral Region
  - Left 0YH8
  - Right 0YH7
- Femoral Shaft
  - Left 0QH9
  - Right 0QH8
- Femur
  - Lower
    - Left 0QHC
    - Right 0QHB
  - Upper
    - Left 0QH7
    - Right 0QH6
- Fibula
  - Left 0QHK
  - Right 0QHJ
- Foot
  - Left 0YHN
  - Right 0YHM
- Gallbladder 0FH4
- Gastrointestinal Tract 0WHP
- Genitourinary Tract 0WHR
- Gland
  - Endocrine 0GHS
  - Salivary 0CHA
- Glenoid Cavity
  - Left 0PH8
  - Right 0PH7
- Hand
  - Left 0XHK
  - Right 0XHJ
- Head 0WH0
- Heart 02HA
- Humeral Head
  - Left 0PHD
  - Right 0PHC
- Humeral Shaft
  - Left 0PHG
  - Right 0PHF
- Ileum 0DHB
- Inguinal Region
  - Left 0YH6
  - Right 0YH5
- Intestinal Tract
  - Lower 0DHD
  - Upper 0DH0
- Intestine
  - Large 0DHE
  - Small 0DH8
- Jaw
  - Lower 0WH5
  - Upper 0WH4
- Jejunum 0DHA
- Joint
  - Acromioclavicular
    - Left 0RHH
    - Right 0RHG
  - Ankle
    - Left 0SHG
    - Right 0SHF
  - Carpal
    - Left 0RHR
    - Right 0RHQ
  - Carpometacarpal
    - Left 0RHT
    - Right 0RHS
  - Cervical Vertebral 0RH1
  - Cervicothoracic Vertebral 0RH4
  - Coccygeal 0SH6
  - Elbow
    - Left 0RHM
    - Right 0RHL
  - Finger Phalangeal
    - Left 0RHX
    - Right 0RHW
  - Hip
    - Left 0SHB
    - Right 0SH9

Insertion of device in *(continued)*
- Joint *(continued)*
  - Knee
    - Left 0SHD
    - Right 0SHC
  - Lumbar Vertebral 0SH0
  - Lumbosacral 0SH3
  - Metacarpophalangeal
    - Left 0RHV
    - Right 0RHU
  - Metatarsal-Phalangeal
    - Left 0SHN
    - Right 0SHM
  - Occipital-cervical 0RH0
  - Sacrococcygeal 0SH5
  - Sacroiliac
    - Left 0SH8
    - Right 0SH7
  - Shoulder
    - Left 0RHK
    - Right 0RHJ
  - Sternoclavicular
    - Left 0RHF
    - Right 0RHE
  - Tarsal
    - Left 0SHJ
    - Right 0SHH
  - Tarsometatarsal
    - Left 0SHL
    - Right 0SHK
  - Temporomandibular
    - Left 0RHD
    - Right 0RHC
  - Thoracic Vertebral 0RH6
  - Thoracolumbar Vertebral
  - Toe Phalangeal
    - Left 0SHQ
    - Right 0SHP
  - Wrist
    - Left 0RHP
    - Right 0RHN
- Kidney 0TH5
- Knee Region
  - Left 0YHG
  - Right 0YHF
- Larynx 0CHS
- Leg
  - Lower
    - Left 0YHJ
    - Right 0YHH
  - Upper
    - Left 0YHD
    - Right 0YHC
- Liver 0FH0
  - Left Lobe 0FH2
  - Right Lobe 0FH1
- Lung
  - Left 0BHL
  - Right 0BHK
- Lymphatic 07HN3
  - Thoracic Duct 07HK
- Mandible
  - Left 0NHV
  - Right 0NHT
- Maxilla 0NHR
- Mediastinum 0WHC
- Metacarpal
  - Left 0PHQ
  - Right 0PHP
- Metatarsal
  - Left 0QHP
  - Right 0QHN
- Mouth and Throat 0CHY
- Muscle
  - Lower 0KHY
  - Upper 0KHX
- Nasal Mucosa and Soft Tissue 09HK
- Nasopharynx 09HN
- Neck 0WH6

Insertion of device in *(continued)*
- Nerve
  - Cranial 00HE
  - Peripheral 01HY
- Nipple
  - Left 0HHX
  - Right 0HHW
- Oral Cavity and Throat 0WH3
- Orbit
  - Left 0NHQ
  - Right 0NHP
- Ovary 0UH3
- Pancreas 0FHG
- Patella
  - Left 0QHF
  - Right 0QHD
- Pelvic Cavity 0WHJ
- Penis 0VHS
- Pericardial Cavity 0WHD
- Pericardium 02HN
- Perineum
  - Female 0WHN
  - Male 0WHM
- Peritoneal Cavity 0WHG
- Phalanx
  - Finger
    - Left 0PHV
    - Right 0PHT
  - Thumb
    - Left 0PHS
    - Right 0PHR
  - Toe
    - Left 0QHR
    - Right 0QHQ
- Pleura 0BHQ
- Pleural Cavity
  - Left 0WHB
  - Right 0WH9
- Prostate 0VH0
- Prostate and Seminal Vesicles 0VH4
- Radius
  - Left 0PHJ
  - Right 0PHH
- Rectum 0DHP
- Respiratory Tract 0WHQ
- Retroperitoneum 0WHH
- Ribs
  - 1 to 2 0PH1
  - 3 or More 0PH2
- Sacrum 0QH1
- Scapula
  - Left 0PH6
  - Right 0PH5
- Scrotum and Tunica Vaginalis 0VH8
- Shoulder Region
  - Left 0XH3
  - Right 0XH2
- Sinus 09HY
- Skin 0HHPXYZ
- Skull 0NH0
- Spinal Canal 00HU
- Spinal Cord 00HV
- Spleen 07HP
- Sternum 0PH0
- Stomach 0DH6
- Subcutaneous Tissue and Fascia
  - Abdomen 0JH8
  - Back 0JH7
  - Buttock 0JH9
  - Chest 0JH6
  - Face 0JH1
  - Foot
    - Left 0JHR
    - Right 0JHQ
  - Hand
    - Left 0JHK
    - Right 0JHJ
  - Head and Neck 0JHS
  - Lower Arm
    - Left 0JHH

Insertion of device in *(continued)*
- Subcutaneous Tissue and Fascia *(continued)*
  - Lower Arm *(continued)*
    - Right 0JHG
  - Lower Extremity 0JHW
  - Lower Leg
    - Left 0JHP
    - Right 0JHN
  - Neck
    - Left 0JH5
    - Right 0JH4
  - Pelvic Region 0JHC
  - Perineum 0JHB
  - Scalp 0JH0
  - Trunk 0JHT
  - Upper Arm
    - Left 0JHF
    - Right 0JHD
  - Upper Extremity 0JHV
  - Upper Leg
    - Left 0JHM
    - Right 0JHL
- Tarsal
  - Left 0QHM
  - Right 0QHL
- Tendon
  - Lower 0LHY
  - Upper 0LHX
- Testis 0VHD
- Thymus 07HM
- Tibia
  - Left 0QHH
  - Right 0QHG
- Tongue 0CH7
- Trachea 0BH1
- Tracheobronchial Tree 0BH0
- Ulna
  - Left 0PHL
  - Right 0PHK
- Ureter 0TH9
- Urethra 0THD
- Uterus 0UH9
- Uterus and Cervix 0UHD
- Vagina 0UHG
- Vagina and Cul-de-sac 0UHH
- Vas Deferens 0VHR
- Vein
  - Axillary
    - Left 05H8
    - Right 05H7
  - Azygos 05H0
  - Basilic
    - Left 05HC
    - Right 05HB
  - Brachial
    - Left 05HA
    - Right 05H9
  - Cephalic
    - Left 05HF
    - Right 05HD
  - Colic 06H7
  - Common Iliac
    - Left 06HD
    - Right 06HC
  - Coronary 02H4
  - Esophageal 06H3
  - External Iliac
    - Left 06HG
    - Right 06HF
  - External Jugular
    - Left 05HQ
    - Right 05HP
  - Face
    - Left 05HV
    - Right 05HT
  - Femoral
    - Left 06HN
    - Right 06HM

- **Insertion of device in** *(continued)*
  - Vein *(continued)*
    - Foot
      - Left 06HV
      - Right 06HT
    - Gastric 06H2
    - Hand
      - Left 05HH
      - Right 05HG
    - Hemiazygos 05H1
    - Hepatic 06H4
    - Hypogastric
      - Left 06HJ
      - Right 06HH
    - Inferior Mesenteric 06H6
    - Innominate
      - Left 05H4
      - Right 05H3
    - Internal Jugular
      - Left 05HN
      - Right 05HM
    - Intracranial 05HL
    - Lower 06HY
    - Portal 06H8
    - Pulmonary
      - Left 02HT
      - Right 02HS
    - Renal
      - Left 06HB
      - Right 06H9
    - Saphenous
      - Left 06HQ
      - Right 06HP
    - Splenic 06H1
    - Subclavian
      - Left 05H6
      - Right 05H5
    - Superior Mesenteric 06H5
    - Upper 05HY
    - Vertebral
      - Left 05HS
      - Right 05HR
  - Vena Cava
    - Inferior 06H0
    - Superior 02HV
  - Ventricle
    - Left 02HL
    - Right 02HK
  - Vertebra
    - Cervical 0PH3
    - Lumbar 0QH0
    - Thoracic 0PH4
  - Wrist Region
    - Left 0XHH
    - Right 0XHG
- **Inspection**
  - Abdominal Wall 0WJF
  - Ankle Region
    - Left 0YJL
    - Right 0YJK
  - Arm
    - Lower
      - Left 0XJF
      - Right 0XJD
    - Upper
      - Left 0XJ9
      - Right 0XJ8
  - Artery
    - Lower 04JY
    - Upper 03JY
  - Axilla
    - Left 0XJ5
    - Right 0XJ4
  - Back
    - Lower 0WJL
    - Upper 0WJK
  - Bladder 0TJB
  - Bone
    - Facial 0NJW
    - Lower 0QJY
- **Inspection** *(continued)*
  - Bone *(continued)*
    - Nasal 0NJB
    - Upper 0PJY
  - Bone Marrow 07JT
  - Brain 00J0
  - Breast
    - Left 0HJU
    - Right 0HJT
  - Bursa and Ligament
    - Lower 0MJY
    - Upper 0MJX
  - Buttock
    - Left 0YJ1
    - Right 0YJ0
  - Cavity, Cranial 0WJ1
  - Chest Wall 0WJ8
  - Cisterna Chyli 07JL
  - Diaphragm 0BJT
  - Disc
    - Cervical Vertebral 0RJ3
    - Cervicothoracic Vertebral 0RJ5
    - Lumbar Vertebral 0SJ2
    - Lumbosacral 0SJ4
    - Thoracic Vertebral 0RJ9
    - Thoracolumbar Vertebral 0RJB
  - Duct
    - Hepatobiliary 0FJB
    - Pancreatic 0FJD
  - Ear
    - Inner
      - Left 09JE
      - Right 09JD
    - Left 09JJ
    - Right 09JH
  - Elbow Region
    - Left 0XJC
    - Right 0XJB
  - Epididymis and Spermatic Cord 0VJM
  - Extremity
    - Lower
      - Left 0YJB
      - Right 0YJ9
    - Upper
      - Left 0XJ7
      - Right 0XJ6
  - Eye
    - Left 08J1XZZ
    - Right 08J0XZZ
  - Face 0WJ2
  - Fallopian Tube 0UJ8
  - Femoral Region
    - Bilateral 0YJE
    - Left 0YJ8
    - Right 0YJ7
  - Finger Nail 0HJQXZZ
  - Foot
    - Left 0YJN
    - Right 0YJM
  - Gallbladder 0FJ4
  - Gastrointestinal Tract 0WJP
  - Genitourinary Tract 0WJR
  - Gland
    - Adrenal 0GJ5
    - Endocrine 0GJS
    - Pituitary 0GJ0
    - Salivary 0CJA
  - Great Vessel 02JY
  - Hand
    - Left 0XJK
    - Right 0XJJ
  - Head 0WJ0
  - Heart 02JA
  - Inguinal Region
    - Bilateral 0YJA
    - Left 0YJ6
    - Right 0YJ5
- **Inspection** *(continued)*
  - Intestinal Tract
    - Lower 0DJD
    - Upper 0DJ0
  - Jaw
    - Lower 0WJ5
    - Upper 0WJ4
  - Joint
    - Acromioclavicular
      - Left 0RJH
      - Right 0RJG
    - Ankle
      - Left 0SJG
      - Right 0SJF
    - Carpal
      - Left 0RJR
      - Right 0RJQ
    - Carpometacarpal
      - Left 0RJT
      - Right 0RJS
    - Cervical Vertebral 0RJ1
    - Cervicothoracic Vertebral 0RJ4
    - Coccygeal 0SJ6
    - Elbow
      - Left 0RJM
      - Right 0RJL
    - Finger Phalangeal
      - Left 0RJX
      - Right 0RJW
    - Hip
      - Left 0SJB
      - Right 0SJ9
    - Knee
      - Left 0SJD
      - Right 0SJC
    - Lumbar Vertebral 0SJ0
    - Lumbosacral 0SJ3
    - Metacarpophalangeal
      - Left 0RJV
      - Right 0RJU
    - Metatarsal-Phalangeal
      - Left 0SJN
      - Right 0SJM
    - Occipital-cervical 0RJ0
    - Sacrococcygeal 0SJ5
    - Sacroiliac
      - Left 0SJ8
      - Right 0SJ7
    - Shoulder
      - Left 0RJK
      - Right 0RJJ
    - Sternoclavicular
      - Left 0RJF
      - Right 0RJE
    - Tarsal
      - Left 0SJJ
      - Right 0SJH
    - Tarsometatarsal
      - Left 0SJL
      - Right 0SJK
    - Temporomandibular
      - Left 0RJD
      - Right 0RJC
    - Thoracic Vertebral 0RJ6
    - Thoracolumbar Vertebral 0RJA
    - Toe Phalangeal
      - Left 0SJQ
      - Right 0SJP
    - Wrist
      - Left 0RJP
      - Right 0RJN
  - Kidney 0TJ5
  - Knee Region
    - Left 0YJG
    - Right 0YJF
  - Larynx 0CJS
  - Leg
    - Lower
      - Left 0YJJ
      - Right 0YJH
- **Inspection** *(continued)*
  - Leg *(continued)*
    - Upper
      - Left 0YJD
      - Right 0YJC
  - Lens
    - Left 08JKXZZ
    - Right 08JJXZZ
  - Liver 0FJ0
  - Lung
    - Left 0BJL
    - Right 0BJK
  - Lymphatic 07JN
    - Thoracic Duct 07JK
  - Mediastinum 0WJC
  - Mesentery 0DJV
  - Mouth and Throat 0CJY
  - Muscle
    - Extraocular
      - Left 08JM
      - Right 08JL
    - Lower 0KJY
    - Upper 0KJX
  - Nasal Mucosa and Soft Tissue 09J
  - Neck 0WJ6
  - Nerve
    - Cranial 00JE
    - Peripheral 01JY
  - Omentum 0DJU
  - Oral Cavity and Throat 0WJ3
  - Ovary 0UJ3
  - Pancreas 0FJG
  - Parathyroid Gland 0GJR
  - Pelvic Cavity 0WJJ
  - Penis 0VJS
  - Pericardial Cavity 0WJD
  - Perineum
    - Female 0WJN
    - Male 0WJM
  - Peritoneal Cavity 0WJG
  - Peritoneum 0DJW
  - Pineal Body 0GJ1
  - Pleura 0BJQ
  - Pleural Cavity
    - Left 0WJB
    - Right 0WJ9
  - Products of Conception 10J0
    - Ectopic 10J2
    - Retained 10J1
  - Prostate and Seminal Vesicles 0VJ
  - Respiratory Tract 0WJQ
  - Retroperitoneum 0WJH
  - Scrotum and Tunica Vaginalis 0V
  - Shoulder Region
    - Left 0XJ3
    - Right 0XJ2
  - Sinus 09JY
  - Skin 0HJPXZZ
  - Skull 0NJ0
  - Spinal Canal 00JU
  - Spinal Cord 00JV
  - Spleen 07JP
  - Stomach 0DJ6
  - Subcutaneous Tissue and Fascia
    - Head and Neck 0JJS
    - Lower Extremity 0JJW
    - Trunk 0JJT
    - Upper Extremity 0JJV
  - Tendon
    - Lower 0LJY
    - Upper 0LJX
  - Testis 0VJD
  - Thymus 07JM
  - Thyroid Gland 0GJK
  - Toe Nail 0HJRX
  - Trachea 0BJ1
  - Tracheobronchial Tree 0BJ0
  - Tympanic Membrane
    - Left 09J8
    - Right 09J7

Inspection *(continued)*
- Ureter 0TJ9
- Urethra 0TJD
- Uterus and Cervix 0UJD
- Vagina and Cul-de-sac 0UJH
- Vas Deferens 0VJR
- Vein
  - Lower 06JY
  - Upper 05JY
- Vulva 0UJM
- Wrist Region
  - Left 0XJH
  - Right 0XJG

Instillation
- *see* Introduction of substance in or on

Insufflation
- *see* Introduction of substance in or on

Interatrial septum
- *use* Septum, Atrial

Interbody fusion (spine) cage
- *use* Interbody Fusion Device in Lower Joints
- *use* Interbody Fusion Device in Upper Joints

Interbody Fusion Device
- Nanotextured Surface
  - Cervical Vertebral XRG1092
    - 2 or more XRG2092
  - Cervicothoracic Vertebral XRG4092
  - Lumbar Vertebral XRGB092
    - 2 or more XRGC092
  - Lumbosacral XRGD092
  - Occipital-cervical XRG0092
  - Thoracic Vertebral XRG6092
    - 2 to 7 XRG7092
    - 8 or more XRG8092
  - Thoracolumbar Vertebral XRGA092
- Radiolucent Porous
  - Cervical Vertebral XRG10F3
    - 2 or more XRG20F3
  - Cervicothoracic Vertebral XRG40F3
  - Lumbar Vertebral XRGB0F3
    - 2 or more XRGC0F3
  - Lumbosacral XRGD0F3
  - Occipital-cervical XRG00F3
  - Thoracic Vertebral XRG60F3
    - 2 to 7 XRG70F3
    - 8 or more XRG80F3
  - Thoracolumbar Vertebral XRGA0F3

Intercarpal joint
- *use* Joint, Carpal, Left
- *use* Joint, Carpal, Right

Intercarpal ligament
- *use* Bursa and Ligament, Hand, Left
- *use* Bursa and Ligament, Hand, Right

Interclavicular ligament
- *use* Bursa and Ligament, Shoulder, Left
- *use* Bursa and Ligament, Shoulder, Right

Intercostal lymph node
- *use* Lymphatic, Thorax

Intercostal muscle
- *use* Muscle, Thorax, Left
- *use* Muscle, Thorax, Right

Intercostal nerve
- *use* Nerve, Thoracic

Intercostobrachial nerve
- *use* Nerve, Thoracic

Intercuneiform joint
- *use* Joint, Tarsal, Left
- *use* Joint, Tarsal, Right

Intercuneiform ligament
- *use* Bursa and Ligament, Foot, Left
- *use* Bursa and Ligament, Foot, Right

Intermediate bronchus
- *use* Main Bronchus, Right

Intermediate cuneiform bone
- *use* Tarsal, Left
- *use* Tarsal, Right

Intermittent hemodialysis (IHD) 5A1D70Z

Intermittent mandatory ventilation
- *see* Assistance, Respiratory 5A09

Intermittent Negative Airway Pressure
- 24-96 Consecutive Hours, Ventilation 5A0945B
- Greater than 96 Consecutive Hours, Ventilation 5A0955B
- Less than 24 Consecutive Hours, Ventilation 5A0935B

Intermittent Positive Airway Pressure
- 24-96 Consecutive Hours, Ventilation 5A09458
- Greater than 96 Consecutive Hours, Ventilation 5A09558
- Less than 24 Consecutive Hours, Ventilation 5A09358

Intermittent positive pressure breathing
- *see* Assistance, Respiratory 5A09

Internal anal sphincter
- *use* Anal Sphincter

Internal (basal) cerebral vein
- *use* Vein, Intracranial

Internal carotid artery, intracranial portion
- *use* Intracranial Artery

Internal carotid plexus
- *use* Nerve, Head and Neck Sympathetic

Internal iliac vein
- *use* Vein, Hypogastric, Left
- *use* Vein, Hypogastric, Right

Internal maxillary artery
- *use* Artery, External Carotid, Left
- *use* Artery, External Carotid, Right

Internal naris
- *use* Nasal Mucosa and Soft Tissue

Internal oblique muscle
- *use* Muscle, Abdomen, Left
- *use* Muscle, Abdomen, Right

Internal pudendal artery
- *use* Artery, Internal Iliac, Left
- *use* Artery, Internal Iliac, Right

Internal pudendal vein
- *use* Vein, Hypogastric, Left
- *use* Vein, Hypogastric, Right

Internal thoracic artery
- *use* Artery, Internal Mammary, Left
- *use* Artery, Internal Mammary, Right
- *use* Artery, Subclavian, Left
- *use* Artery, Subclavian, Right

Internal urethral sphincter
- *use* Urethra

Interphalangeal (IP) joint
- *use* Joint, Finger Phalangeal, Left
- *use* Joint, Finger Phalangeal, Right
- *use* Joint, Toe Phalangeal, Left
- *use* Joint, Toe Phalangeal, Right

Interphalangeal ligament
- *use* Bursa and Ligament, Foot, Left
- *use* Bursa and Ligament, Foot, Right
- *use* Bursa and Ligament, Hand, Left
- *use* Bursa and Ligament, Hand, Right

Interrogation, cardiac rhythm related device
- Interrogation only
  - *see* Measurement, Cardiac 4B02
- With cardiac function testing
  - *see* Measurement, Cardiac 4A02

Interruption
- *see* Occlusion

Interspinalis muscle
- *use* Muscle, Trunk, Left
- *use* Muscle, Trunk, Right

Interspinous ligament, cervical
- *use* Head and Neck Bursa and Ligament

Interspinous ligament, lumbar
- *use* Lower Spine Bursa and Ligament

Interspinous ligament, thoracic
- *use* Upper Spine Bursa and Ligament

Interspinous process spinal stabilization device
- *use* Spinal Stabilization Device, Interspinous Process in 0RH
- *use* Spinal Stabilization Device, Interspinous Process in 0SH

InterStim® Therapy lead
- *use* Neurostimulator Lead in Peripheral Nervous System

InterStim® Therapy neurostimulator
- *use* Stimulator Generator, Single Array in 0JH

Intertransversarius muscle
- *use* Muscle, Trunk, Left
- *use* Muscle, Trunk, Right

Intertransverse ligament, cervical
- *use* Head and Neck Bursa and Ligament

Intertransverse ligament, lumbar
- *use* Lower Spine Bursa and Ligament

Intertransverse ligament, thoracic
- *use* Upper Spine Bursa and Ligament

Interventricular foramen (Monro)
- *use* Cerebral Ventricle

Interventricular septum
- *use* Septum, Ventricular

Intestinal lymphatic trunk
- *use* Cisterna Chyli

Intraluminal Device
- Airway
  - Esophagus 0DH5
  - Mouth and Throat 0CHY
  - Nasopharynx 09HN
- Bioactive
  - Occlusion
    - Common Carotid
      - Left 03LJ
      - Right 03LH
    - External Carotid
      - Left 03LN
      - Right 03LM
    - Internal Carotid
      - Left 03LL
      - Right 03LK
    - Intracranial 03LG
    - Vertebral
      - Left 03LQ
      - Right 03LP
  - Restriction
    - Common Carotid
      - Left 03VJ
      - Right 03VH
    - External Carotid
      - Left 03VN
      - Right 03VM
    - Internal Carotid
      - Left 03VL
      - Right 03VK
    - Intracranial 03VG
    - Vertebral
      - Left 03VQ
      - Right 03VP

Intraluminal Device *(continued)*
- Endobronchial Valve
  - Lingula 0BH9
  - Lower Lobe
    - Left 0BHB
    - Right 0BH6
  - Main
    - Left 0BH7
    - Right 0BH3
  - Middle Lobe, Right 0BH5
  - Upper Lobe
    - Left 0BH8
    - Right 0BH4
- Endotracheal Airway
  - Change device in, Trachea 0B21XEZ
  - Insertion of device in, Trachea 0BH1
- Pessary
  - Change device in, Vagina and Cul-de-sac 0U2HXGZ
  - Insertion of device in
    - Cul-de-sac 0UHF
    - Vagina 0UHG

Intramedullary (IM) rod (nail)
- *use* Internal Fixation Device, Intramedullary in Lower Bones
- *use* Internal Fixation Device, Intramedullary in Upper Bones

Intramedullary skeletal kinetic distractor (ISKD)
- *use* Internal Fixation Device, Intramedullary in Lower Bones
- *use* Internal Fixation Device, Intramedullary in Upper Bones

Intraocular Telescope
- Left 08RK30Z
- Right 08RJ30Z

Intraoperative Knee Replacement Sensor XR2

Intraoperative Radiation Therapy (IORT)
- Anus DDY8CZZ
- Bile Ducts DFY2CZZ
- Bladder DTY2CZZ
- Cervix DUY1CZZ
- Colon DDY5CZZ
- Duodenum DDY2CZZ
- Gallbladder DFY1CZZ
- Ileum DDY4CZZ
- Jejunum DDY3CZZ
- Kidney DTY0CZZ
- Larynx D9YBCZZ
- Liver DFY0CZZ
- Mouth D9Y4CZZ
- Nasopharynx D9YDCZZ
- Ovary DUY0CZZ
- Pancreas DFY3CZZ
- Pharynx D9YCCZZ
- Prostate DVY0CZZ
- Rectum DDY7CZZ
- Stomach DDY1CZZ
- Ureter DTY1CZZ
- Urethra DTY3CZZ
- Uterus DUY2CZZ

Intrauterine device (IUD)
- *use* Contraceptive Device in Female Reproductive System

Intravascular fluorescence angiography (IFA)
- *see* Monitoring, Physiological Systems 4A1

Introduction of substance in or on
- Artery
  - Central 3E06
    - Analgesics 3E06
    - Anesthetic, Intracirculatory 3E06
    - Anti-infective 3E06
    - Anti-inflammatory 3E06

Introduction of substance in or on *(continued)*
Artery *(continued)*
Central *(continued)*
Antiarrhythmic 3E06
Antineoplastic 3E06
Destructive Agent 3E06
Diagnostic Substance, Other 3E06
Electrolytic Substance 3E06
Hormone 3E06
Hypnotics 3E06
Immunotherapeutic 3E06
Nutritional Substance 3E06
Platelet Inhibitor 3E06
Radioactive Substance 3E06
Sedatives 3E06
Serum 3E06
Thrombolytic 3E06
Toxoid 3E06
Vaccine 3E06
Vasopressor 3E06
Water Balance Substance 3E06
Coronary 3E07
Diagnostic Substance, Other 3E07
Platelet Inhibitor 3E07
Thrombolytic 3E07
Peripheral 3E05
Analgesics 3E05
Anesthetic, Intracirculatory 3E05
Anti-infective 3E052
Anti-inflammatory 3E05
Antiarrhythmic 3E05
Antineoplastic 3E05
Destructive Agent 3E05
Diagnostic Substance, Other 3E05
Electrolytic Substance 3E05
Hormone 3E05
Hypnotics 3E05
Immunotherapeutic 3E05
Nutritional Substance 3E05
Platelet Inhibitor 3E05
Radioactive Substance 3E05
Sedatives 3E05
Serum 3E05
Thrombolytic 3E05
Toxoid 3E05
Vaccine 3E05
Vasopressor 3E05
Water Balance Substance 3E05
Biliary Tract 3E0J
Analgesics 3E0J
Anesthetic, Agent 3E0J
Anti-infective 3E0J
Anti-inflammatory 3E0J
Antineoplastic 3E0J
Destructive Agent 3E0J
Diagnostic Substance, Other 3E0J
Electrolytic Substance 3E0J
Gas 3E0J
Hypnotics 3E0J
Islet Cells, Pancreatic 3E0J
Nutritional Substance 3E0J
Radioactive Substance 3E0J
Sedatives 3E0J
Water Balance Substance 3E0J
Bone 3E0V
Analgesics 3E0V3NZ
Anesthetic, Agent 3E0V3BZ
Anti-infective 3E0V32
Anti-inflammatory 3E0V33Z
Antineoplastic 3E0V30
Destructive Agent 3E0V3TZ

Introduction of substance in or on *(continued)*
Bone *(continued)*
Diagnostic Substance, Other 3E0V3KZ
Electrolytic Substance 3E0V37Z
Hypnotics 3E0V3NZ
Nutritional Substance 3E0V36Z
Radioactive Substance 3E0V3HZ
Sedatives 3E0V3NZ
Water Balance Substance 3E0V37Z
Bone Marrow 3E0A3GC
Antineoplastic 3E0A30
Brain 3E0Q
Analgesics 3E0Q
Anesthetic, Agent 3E0Q
Anti-infective 3E0Q
Anti-inflammatory 3E0Q
Antineoplastic 3E0Q
Destructive Agent 3E0Q
Diagnostic Substance, Other 3E0Q
Electrolytic Substance 3E0Q
Gas 3E0Q
Hypnotics 3E0Q
Nutritional Substance 3E0Q
Radioactive Substance 3E0Q
Sedatives 3E0Q
Stem Cells
Embryonic 3E0Q
Somatic 3E0Q
Water Balance Substance 3E0Q
Cranial Cavity 3E0Q
Analgesics 3E0Q
Anesthetic Agent 3E0Q
Anti-infective 3E0Q
Anti-inflammatory 3E0Q
Antineoplastic 3E0Q
Destructive Agent 3E0Q
Diagnostic Substance, Other 3E0Q
Electrolytic Substance 3E0Q
Gas 3E0Q
Hypnotics 3E0Q
Nutritional Substance 3E0Q
Radioactive Substance 3E0Q
Sedatives 3E0Q
Stem Cells
Embryonic 3E0Q
Somatic 3E0Q
Water Balance Substance 3E0Q
Ear 3E0B
Analgesics 3E0B
Anesthetic Agentl 3E0B
Anti-infective 3E0B
Anti-inflammatory 3E0B
Antineoplastic 3E0B
Destructive Agent 3E0B
Diagnostic Substance, Other 3E0B
Hypnotics 3E0B
Radioactive Substance 3E0B
Sedatives 3E0B
Epidural Space 3E0S3GC
Analgesics 3E0S3NZ
Anesthetic Agent 3E0S3BZ
Anti-infective 3E0S32
Anti-inflammatory 3E0S33Z
Antineoplastic 3E0S30
Destructive Agent 3E0S3TZ
Diagnostic Substance, Other 3E0S3KZ
Electrolytic Substance 3E0S37Z
Gas 3E0S

Introduction of substance in or on *(continued)*
Epidural Space *(continued)*
Hypnotics 3E0S3NZ
Nutritional Substance 3E0S36Z
Radioactive Substance 3E0S3HZ
Sedatives 3E0S3NZ
Water Balance Substance 3E0S37Z
Eye 3E0C
Analgesics 3E0C
Anesthetic Agent 3E0C
Anti-infective 3E0C
Anti-inflammatory 3E0C
Antineoplastic 3E0C
Destructive Agent 3E0C
Diagnostic Substance, Other 3E0C
Gas 3E0C
Hypnotics 3E0C
Pigment 3E0C
Radioactive Substance 3E0C
Sedatives 3E0C
Gastrointestinal Tract
Lower 3E0H
Analgesics 3E0H
Anesthetic Agent 3E0H
Anti-infective 3E0H
Anti-inflammatory 3E0H
Antineoplastic 3E0H
Destructive Agent 3E0H
Diagnostic Substance, Other 3E0H
Electrolytic Substance 3E0H
Gas 3E0H
Hypnotics 3E0H
Nutritional Substance 3E0H
Radioactive Substance 3E0H
Sedatives 3E0H
Water Balance Substance 3E0H
Upper 3E0G
Analgesics 3E0G
Anesthetic Agent 3E0G
Anti-infective 3E0G
Anti-inflammatory 3E0G
Antineoplastic 3E0G
Destructive Agent 3E0G
Diagnostic Substance, Other 3E0G
Electrolytic Substance 3E0G
Gas 3E0G
Hypnotics 3E0G
Nutritional Substance 3E0G
Radioactive Substance 3E0G
Sedatives 3E0G
Water Balance Substance 3E0G
Genitourinary Tract 3E0K
Analgesics 3E0K
Anesthetic Agent 3E0K
Anti-infective 3E0K
Anti-inflammatory 3E0K
Antineoplastic 3E0K
Destructive Agent 3E0K
Diagnostic Substance, Other 3E0K
Electrolytic Substance 3E0K
Gas 3E0K
Hypnotics 3E0K
Nutritional Substance 3E0K
Radioactive Substance 3E0K
Sedatives 3E0K
Water Balance Substance 3E0K
Heart 3E08
Diagnostic Substance, Other 3E08
Platelet Inhibitor 3E08
Thrombolytic 3E08

Introduction of substance in or on *(continued)*
Joint 3E0U
Analgesics 3E0U3NZ
Anesthetic Agent 3E0U3BZ
Anti-infective 3E0U
Anti-inflammatory 3E0U33Z
Antineoplastic 3E0U30
Destructive Agent 3E0U3TZ
Diagnostic Substance, Other 3E0U3KZ
Electrolytic Substance 3E0U37Z
Gas 3E0U3SF
Hypnotics 3E0U3NZ
Nutritional Substance 3E0U36Z
Radioactive Substance 3E0U3HZ
Sedatives 3E0U3NZ
Water Balance Substance 3E0U37Z
Lymphatic 3E0W3GC
Analgesics 3E0W3NZ
Anesthetic Agent 3E0W3BZ
Anti-infective 3E0W32
Anti-inflammatory 3E0W33Z
Antineoplastic 3E0W30
Destructive Agent 3E0W3TZ
Diagnostic Substance, Other 3E0W3KZ
Electrolytic Substance 3E0W37Z
Hypnotics 3E0W3NZ
Nutritional Substance 3E0W36
Radioactive Substance 3E0W3HZ
Sedatives 3E0W3NZ
Water Balance Substance 3E0W37Z
Mouth 3E0D
Analgesics 3E0D
Anesthetic Agent 3E0D
Anti-infective 3E0D
Anti-inflammatory 3E0D
Antiarrhythmic 3E0D
Antineoplastic 3E0D
Destructive Agent 3E0D
Diagnostic Substance, Other 3E0D
Electrolytic Substance 3E0D
Hypnotics 3E0D
Nutritional Substance 3E0D
Radioactive Substance 3E0D
Sedatives 3E0D
Serum 3E0D
Toxoid 3E0D
Vaccine 3E0D
Water Balance Substance 3E0D
Mucous Membrane 3E00XGC
Analgesics 3E00XNZ
Anesthetic Agent 3E00XBZ
Anti-infective 3E00X2
Anti-inflammatory 3E00X3Z
Antineoplastic 3E00X0
Destructive Agent 3E00XTZ
Diagnostic Substance, Other 3E00XKZ
Hypnotics 3E00XNZ
Pigment 3E00XMZ
Sedatives 3E00XNZ
Serum 3E00X4Z
Toxoid 3E00X4Z
Vaccine 3E00X4Z
Muscle 3E023GC
Analgesics 3E023NZ
Anesthetic Agent 3E023BZ
Anti-infective 3E0232
Anti-inflammatory 3E0233Z
Antineoplastic 3E0230
Destructive Agent 3E023TZ

Introduction of substance in or on (continued)
Muscle (continued)
Diagnostic Substance, Other 3E023KZ
Electrolytic Substance 3E0237Z
Hypnotics 3E023NZ
Nutritional Substance 3E0236Z
Radioactive Substance 3E023HZ
Sedatives 3E023NZ
Serum 3E0234Z
Toxoid 3E0234Z
Vaccine 3E0234Z
Water Balance Substance 3E0237Z
Nerve
Cranial 3E0X3GC
Anesthetic Agent 3E0X3BZ
Anti-inflammatory 3E0X33Z
Destructive Agent 3E0X3TZ
Peripheral 3E0T3GC
Anesthetic Agent 3E0T3BZ
Anti-inflammatory 3E0T33Z
Destructive Agent 3E0T3TZ
Plexus 3E0T3GC
Agent 3E0T3BZ
Anti-inflammatory 3E0T33Z
Destructive Agent 3E0T3TZ
Nose 3E09
Analgesics 3E09
Anesthetic Agent 3E09
Anti-infective 3E09
Anti-inflammatory 3E09
Antineoplastic 3E09
Destructive Agent 3E09
Diagnostic Substance, Other 3E09
Hypnotics 3E09
Radioactive Substance 3E09
Sedatives 3E09
Serum 3E09
Toxoid 3E09
Vaccine 3E09
Pancreatic Tract 3E0J
Analgesics 3E0J
Anesthetic Agent 3E0J
Anti-infective 3E0J
Anti-inflammatory 3E0J
Antineoplastic 3E0J0
Destructive Agent 3E0J
Diagnostic Substance, Other 3E0J
Electrolytic Substance 3E0J
Gas 3E0J
Hypnotics 3E0J
Islet Cells, Pancreatic 3E0JU
Nutritional Substance 3E0J
Radioactive Substance 3E0J
Sedatives 3E0J
Water Balance Substance 3E0J
Pericardial Cavity 3E0Y
Analgesics 3E0Y3NZ
Anesthetic Agent 3E0Y3BZ
Anti-infective 3E0Y32
Anti-inflammatory 3E0Y33Z
Antineoplastic 3E0Y
Destructive Agent 3E0Y3TZ
Diagnostic Substance, Other 3E0Y3KZ
Electrolytic Substance 3E0Y37Z
Gas 3E0Y
Hypnotics 3E0Y3NZ
Nutritional Substance 3E0Y36Z
Radioactive Substance 3E0Y3HZ

Introduction of substance in or on (continued)
Pericardial Cavity (continued)
Sedatives 3E0Y3NZ
Water Balance Substance 3E0Y37Z
Peritoneal Cavity 3E0M
Adhesion Barrier 3E0M
Analgesics 3E0M3NZ
Anesthetic Agent 3E0M3BZ
Anti-infective 3E0M32
Anti-inflammatory 3E0M33Z
Antineoplastic 3E0M
Destructive Agent 3E0M3TZ
Diagnostic Substance, Other 3E0M3KZ
Electrolytic Substance 3E0M37Z
Gas 3E0M
Hypnotics 3E0M3NZ
Nutritional Substance 3E0M36Z
Radioactive Substance 3E0M3HZ
Sedatives 3E0M3NZ
Water Balance Substance 3E0M37Z
Pharynx 3E0D
Analgesics 3E0D
Anesthetic Agent 3E0D
Anti-infective 3E0D
Anti-inflammatory 3E0D
Antiarrhythmic 3E0D
Antineoplastic 3E0D
Destructive Agent 3E0D
Diagnostic Substance, Other 3E0D
Electrolytic Substance 3E0D
Hypnotics 3E0D
Nutritional Substance 3E0D
Radioactive Substance 3E0D
Sedatives 3E0D
Serum 3E0D
Toxoid 3E0D
Vaccine 3E0D
Water Balance Substance 3E0D
Pleural Cavity 3E0L
Adhesion Barrier 3E0L
Analgesics 3E0L3NZ
Anesthetic Agent 3E0L3BZ
Anti-infective 3E0L32
Anti-inflammatory 3E0L33Z
Antineoplastic 3E0L
Destructive Agent 3E0L3TZ
Diagnostic Substance, Other 3E0L3KZ
Electrolytic Substance 3E0L37Z
Gas 3E0L
Hypnotics 3E0L3NZ
Nutritional Substance 3E0L36Z
Radioactive Substance 3E0L3HZ
Sedatives 3E0L3NZ
Water Balance Substance 3E0L37Z
Products of Conception 3E0E
Analgesics 3E0E
Anesthetic Agent 3E0E
Anti-infective 3E0E2
Anti-inflammatory 3E0E
Antineoplastic 3E0E0
Destructive Agent 3E0E
Diagnostic Substance, Other 3E0E
Electrolytic Substance 3E0E
Gas 3E0E
Hypnotics 3E0E
Nutritional Substance 3E0E
Radioactive Substance 3E0E
Sedatives 3E0E
Water Balance Substance 3E0E

Introduction of substance in or on (continued)
Reproductive
Female 3E0P
Adhesion Barrier 3E0P0
Analgesics 3E0P
Anesthetic Agent 3E0P
Anti-infective 3E0P
Anti-inflammatory 3E0P
Antineoplastic 3E0P
Destructive Agent 3E0P
Diagnostic Substance, Other 3E0P
Electrolytic Substance 3E0P
Gas 3E0P
Hormone 3E0P
Hypnotics 3E0P
Nutritional Substance 3E0P
Ovum, Fertilized 3E0P
Radioactive Substance 3E0P
Sedatives 3E0P
Sperm 3E0P
Water Balance Substance 3E0P
Male 3E0N
Analgesics 3E0N
Anesthetic Agent 3E0N
Anti-infective 3E0N
Anti-inflammatory 3E0N
Antineoplastic 3E0N0
Destructive Agent 3E0N
Diagnostic Substance, Other 3E0N
Electrolytic Substance 3E0N
Gas 3E0N
Hypnotics 3E0N
Nutritional Substance 3E0N
Radioactive Substance 3E0N
Sedatives 3E0N
Water Balance Substance 3E0N
Respiratory Tract 3E0F
Analgesics 3E0F
Anesthetic Agent 3E0F
Anti-infective 3E0F
Anti-inflammatory 3E0F
Antineoplastic 3E0F
Destructive Agent 3E0F
Diagnostic Substance, Other 3E0F
Electrolytic Substance 3E0F
Gas 3E0F
Hypnotics 3E0F
Nutritional Substance 3E0F
Radioactive Substance 3E0F
Sedatives 3E0F
Water Balance Substance 3E0F
Skin 3E00XGC
Analgesics 3E00XNZ
Anesthetic Agent 3E00XBZ
Anti-infective 3E00X2
Anti-inflammatory 3E00X3Z
Antineoplastic 3E00X0
Destructive Agent 3E00XTZ
Diagnostic Substance, Other 3E00XKZ
Hypnotics 3E00XNZ
Pigment 3E00XMZ
Sedatives 3E00XNZ
Serum 3E00X4Z
Toxoid 3E00X4Z
Vaccine 3E00X4Z
Spinal Canal 3E0R3GC
Analgesics 3E0R3NZ
Anesthetic Agent 3E0R3BZ
Anti-infective 3E0R32
Anti-inflammatory 3E0R33Z
Antineoplastic 3E0R30
Destructive Agent 3E0R3TZ

Introduction of substance in or on (continued)
Spinal Canal (continued)
Diagnostic Substance, Other 3E0R3KZ
Electrolytic Substance 3E0R37Z
Gas 3E0R
Hypnotics 3E0R3NZ
Nutritional Substance 3E0R36Z
Radioactive Substance 3E0R3HZ
Sedatives 3E0R3NZ
Stem Cells
Embryonic 3E0R
Somatic 3E0R
Water Balance Substance 3E0R37Z
Subcutaneous Tissue 3E013GC
Analgesics 3E013NZ
Anesthetic Agent 3E013BZ
Anti-infective 3E01
Anti-inflammatory 3E0133Z
Antineoplastic 3E0130
Destructive Agent 3E013TZ
Diagnostic Substance, Other 3E013KZ
Electrolytic Substance 3E0137Z
Hormone 3E013V
Hypnotics 3E013NZ
Nutritional Substance 3E0136Z
Radioactive Substance 3E013HZ
Sedatives 3E013NZ
Serum 3E0134Z
Toxoid 3E0134Z
Vaccine 3E0134Z
Water Balance Substance 3E0137Z
Vein
Central 3E04
Analgesics 3E04
Anesthetic, Intracirculatory 3E04
Anti-infective 3E04
Anti-inflammatory 3E04
Antiarrhythmic 3E04
Antineoplastic 3E04
Destructive Agent 3E04
Diagnostic Substance, Other 3E04
Electrolytic Substance 3E04
Hormone 3E04
Hypnotics 3E04
Immunotherapeutic 3E04
Nutritional Substance 3E04
Platelet Inhibitor 3E04
Radioactive Substance 3E04
Sedatives 3E04
Serum 3E04
Thrombolytic 3E04
Toxoid 3E04
Vaccine 3E04
Vasopressor 3E04
Water Balance Substance 3E04
Peripheral 3E03
Analgesics 3E03
Anesthetic, Intracirculatory 3E03
Anti-infective 3E03
Anti-inflammatory 3E03
Antiarrhythmic 3E03
Antineoplastic 3E03
Destructive Agent 3E03
Diagnostic Substance, Other 3E03
Electrolytic Substance 3E03
Hormone 3E03
Hypnotics 3E03
Immunotherapeutic 3E03

Introduction of substance in or on *(continued)*
Vein *(continued)*
Peripheral *(continued)*
Islet Cells, Pancreatic 3E03
Nutritional Substance 3E03
Platelet Inhibitor 3E03
Radioactive Substance 3E03
Sedatives 3E03
Serum 3E03
Thrombolytic 3E03
Toxoid 3E03
Vaccine 3E03
Vasopressor 3E03
Water Balance Substance 3E03
Intubation
Airway
see Insertion of device in, Esophagus 0DH5
see Insertion of device in, Mouth and Throat 0CHY
see Insertion of device in, Trachea 0BH1
Drainage device
see Drainage
Feeding Device
see Insertion of device in, Gastrointestinal System 0DH
INTUITY Elite valve system, EDWARDS
use Zooplastic Tissue, Rapid Deployment Technique in New Technology
IPPB (intermittent positive pressure breathing)
see Assistance, Respiratory 5A09
IRE (Irreversible Electroporation)
see Destruction, Hepatobiliary System and Pancreas 0F5
Iridectomy
see Excision, Eye 08B
see Resection, Eye 08T
Iridoplasty
see Repair, Eye 08Q
see Replacement, Eye 08R
see Supplement, Eye 08U
Iridotomy
see Drainage, Eye 089
Irreversible Electroporation (IRE)
see Destruction, Hepatobiliary System and Pancreas 0F5
Irrigation
Biliary Tract, Irrigating Substance 3E1J
Brain, Irrigating Substance 3E1Q38Z
Cranial Cavity, Irrigating Substance 3E1Q38Z
Ear, Irrigating Substance 3E1B
Epidural Space, Irrigating Substance 3E1S38Z
Eye, Irrigating Substance 3E1C
Gastrointestinal Tract
Lower, Irrigating Substance 3E1H
Upper, Irrigating Substance 3E1G
Genitourinary Tract, Irrigating Substance 3E1K
Irrigating Substance 3C1ZX8Z
Joint, Irrigating Substance 3E1U38Z
Mucous Membrane, Irrigating Substance 3E10
Nose, Irrigating Substance 3E19
Pancreatic Tract, Irrigating Substance 3E1J
Pericardial Cavity, Irrigating Substance 3E1Y38Z
Irrigation *(continued)*
Peritoneal Cavity
Dialysate 3E1M39Z
Irrigating Substance 3E1M38Z
Pleural Cavity, Irrigating Substance 3E1L38Z
Reproductive
Female, Irrigating Substance 3E1P
Male, Irrigating Substance 3E1N
Respiratory Tract, Irrigating Substance 3E1F
Skin, Irrigating Substance 3E10
Spinal Canal, Irrigating Substance 3E1R38Z
Isavuconazole Anti-infective XW0
Ischiatic nerve
use Nerve, Sciatic
Ischiocavernosus muscle
use Muscle, Perineum
Ischiofemoral ligament
use Bursa and Ligament, Hip, Left
use Bursa and Ligament, Hip, Right
Ischium
use Bone, Pelvic, Left
use Bone, Pelvic, Right
Isolation 8E0ZXY6
Isotope Administration, Whole Body DWY5G
Itrel (3)(4) neurostimulator
use Stimulator Generator, Single Array in 0JH

J

Jejunal artery
use Artery, Superior Mesenteric
Jejunectomy
see Excision, Jejunum 0DBA
see Resection, Jejunum 0DTA
Jejunocolostomy
see Bypass, Gastrointestinal System 0D1
see Drainage, Gastrointestinal System 0D9
Jejunopexy
see Repair, Jejunum 0DQA
see Reposition, Jejunum 0DSA
Jejunostomy
see Bypass, Jejunum 0D1A
see Drainage, Jejunum 0D9A
Jejunotomy
see Drainage, Jejunum 0D9A
Joint fixation plate
use Internal Fixation Device in Lower Joints
use Internal Fixation Device in Upper Joints
Joint liner (insert)
use Liner in Lower Joints
Joint spacer (antibiotic)
use Spacer in Lower Joints
use Spacer in Upper Joints
Jugular body
use Glomus Jugulare
Jugular lymph node
use Lymphatic, Neck, Left
use Lymphatic, Neck, Right

K

Kappa
use Pacemaker, Dual Chamber in 0JH
Kcentra
use 4-Factor Prothrombin Complex Concentrate
Keratectomy, kerectomy
see Excision, Eye 08B
see Resection, Eye 08T
Keratocentesis
see Drainage, Eye 089
Keratoplasty
see Repair, Eye 08Q
see Replacement, Eye 08R
see Supplement, Eye 08U
Keratotomy
see Drainage, Eye 089
see Repair, Eye 08Q
Kirschner wire (K-wire)
use Internal Fixation Device in Head and Facial Bones
use Internal Fixation Device in Lower Bones
use Internal Fixation Device in Lower Joints
use Internal Fixation Device in Upper Bones
use Internal Fixation Device in Upper Joints
Knee (implant) insert
use Liner in Lower Joints
KUB x-ray
see Plain Radiography, Kidney, Ureter and Bladder BT04
Kuntscher nail
use Internal Fixation Device, Intramedullary in Lower Bones
use Internal Fixation Device, Intramedullary in Upper Bones
KYMRIAH
use Engineered Autologous Chimeric Antigen Receptor T-cell Immunotherapy

L

Labia majora
use Vulva
Labia minora
use Vulva
Labial gland
use Lip, Lower
use Lip, Upper
Labiectomy
see Excision, Female Reproductive System 0UB
see Resection, Female Reproductive System 0UT
see Release, Central Nervous System 00N
see Release, Peripheral Nervous System 01N
Lacrimal canaliculus
use Duct, Lacrimal, Left
use Duct, Lacrimal, Right
Lacrimal punctum
use Duct, Lacrimal, Left
use Duct, Lacrimal, Right
Lacrimal sac
use Duct, Lacrimal, Left
use Duct, Lacrimal, Right
LAGB (laparoscopic adjustable gastric banding)
Initial procedure 0DV64CZ
Surgical correction
see Revision of device in, Stomach 0DW6
Laminectomy
see Excision, Lower Bones 0QB
see Excision, Upper Bones 0PB
see Release, Central Nervous System and Cranial Nerves 00N
see Release, Peripheral Nervous System 01N
Laminotomy
see Drainage, Lower Bones 0Q9
see Drainage, Upper Bones 0P9
Laminotomy *(continued)*
see Excision, Lower Bones 0QB
see Excision, Upper Bones 0PB
see Release, Central Nervous System and Cranial Nerves 00
see Release, Lower Bones 0QN
see Release, Peripheral Nervous System 01N
see Release, Upper Bones 0PN
LAP-BAND® adjustable gastric banding system
use Extraluminal Device
Laparoscopic-assisted transanal pull-through
see Excision, Gastrointestinal System 0DB
see Resection, Gastrointestinal System 0DT
Laparoscopy
see Inspection
Laparotomy
Drainage
see Drainage, Peritoneal Cavity 0W9G
Exploratory
see Inspection, Peritoneal Cavity 0WJG
Laryngectomy
see Excision, Larynx 0CBS
see Resection, Larynx 0CTS
Laryngocentesis
see Drainage, Larynx 0C9S
Laryngogram
see Fluoroscopy, Larynx B91J
Laryngopexy
see Repair, Larynx 0CQS
Laryngopharynx
use Pharynx
Laryngoplasty
see Repair, Larynx 0CQS
see Replacement, Larynx 0CRS
see Supplement, Larynx 0CUS
Laryngorrhaphy
see Repair, Larynx 0CQS
Laryngoscopy 0CJS8ZZ
Laryngotomy
see Drainage, Larynx 0C9S
Laser Interstitial Thermal Therapy
Adrenal Gland DGY2KZZ
Anus DDY8KZZ
Bile Ducts DFY2KZZ
Brain D0Y0KZZ
Brain Stem D0Y1KZZ
Breast
Left DMY0KZZ
Right DMY1KZZ
Bronchus DBY1KZZ
Chest Wall DBY7KZZ
Colon DDY5KZZ
Diaphragm DBY8KZZ
Duodenum DDY2KZZ
Esophagus DDY0KZZ
Gallbladder DFY1KZZ
Gland
Adrenal DGY2KZZ
Parathyroid DGY4KZZ
Pituitary DGY0KZZ
Thyroid DGY5KZZ
Ileum DDY4KZZ
Jejunum DDY3KZZ
Liver DFY0KZZ
Lung DBY2KZZ
Mediastinum DBY6KZZ
Nerve, Peripheral D0Y7KZZ
Pancreas DFY3KZZ
Parathyroid Gland DGY4KZZ
Pineal Body DGY1KZZ
Pituitary Gland DGY0KZZ
Pleura DBY5KZZ
Prostate DVY0KZZ

Laser Interstitial Thermal Therapy *(continued)*
Rectum DDY7KZZ
Spinal Cord D0Y6KZZ
Stomach DDY1KZZ
Thyroid Gland DGY5KZZ
Trachea DBY0KZZ
Lateral (brachial) lymph node
use Lymphatic, Axillary, Left
use Lymphatic, Axillary, Right
Lateral canthus
use Eyelid, Upper, Left
use Eyelid, Upper, Right
Lateral collateral ligament (LCL)
use Bursa and Ligament, Knee, Left
use Bursa and Ligament, Knee, Right
Lateral condyle of femur
use Femur, Lower, Left
use Femur, Lower, Right
Lateral condyle of tibia
use Tibia, Left
use Tibia, Right
Lateral cuneiform bone
use Tarsal, Left
use Tarsal, Right
Lateral epicondyle of femur
use Femur, Lower, Left
use Femur, Lower, Right
Lateral epicondyle of humerus
use Humeral Shaft, Left
use Humeral Shaft, Right
Lateral femoral cutaneous nerve
use Nerve, Lumbar Plexus
Lateral malleolus
use Fibula, Left
use Fibula, Right
Lateral meniscus
use Joint, Knee, Left
use Joint, Knee, Right
Lateral nasal cartilage
use Nasal Mucosa and Soft Tissue
Lateral plantar artery
use Artery, Foot, Left
use Artery, Foot, Right
Lateral plantar nerve
use Nerve, Tibial
Lateral rectus muscle
use Muscle, Extraocular, Left
use Muscle, Extraocular, Right
Lateral sacral artery
use Artery, Internal Iliac, Left
use Artery, Internal Iliac, Right
Lateral sacral vein
use Vein, Hypogastric, Left
use Vein, Hypogastric, Right
Lateral sural cutaneous nerve
use Nerve, Peroneal
Lateral tarsal artery
use Artery, Foot, Left
use Artery, Foot, Right
Lateral temporomandibular ligament
use Bursa and Ligament, Head and Neck
Lateral thoracic artery
use Artery, Axillary, Left
use Artery, Axillary, Right
Latissimus dorsi muscle
use Muscle, Trunk, Left
use Muscle, Trunk, Right
Latissimus Dorsi Myocutaneous Flap
Replacement
Bilateral 0HRV075
Left 0HRU075
Right 0HRT075
Transfer
Left 0KXG
Right 0KXF
Lavage
see Irrigation
Bronchial alveolar, diagnostic
see Drainage, Respiratory System 0B9
Least splanchnic nerve
use Nerve, Thoracic Sympathetic
Left ascending lumbar vein
use Vein, Hemiazygos
Left atrioventricular valve
use Valve, Mitral
Left auricular appendix
use Atrium, Left
Left colic vein
use Vein, Colic
Left coronary sulcus
use Heart, Left
Left gastric artery
use Artery, Gastric
Left gastroepiploic artery
use Artery, Splenic
Left gastroepiploic vein
use Vein, Splenic
Left inferior phrenic vein
use Vein, Renal, Left
Left inferior pulmonary vein
use Vein, Pulmonary, Left
Left jugular trunk
use Lymphatic, Thoracic Duct
Left lateral ventricle
use Cerebral Ventricle
Left ovarian vein
use Vein, Renal, Left
Left second lumbar vein
use Vein, Renal, Left
Left subclavian trunk
use Lymphatic, Thoracic Duct
Left subcostal vein
use Vein, Hemiazygos
Left superior pulmonary vein
use Vein, Pulmonary, Left
Left suprarenal vein
use Vein, Renal, Left
Left testicular vein
use Vein, Renal, Left
Lengthening
Bone, with device
see Insertion of Limb Lengthening Device
Muscle, by incision
see Division, Muscles 0K8
Tendon, by incision
see Division, Tendons 0L8
Leptomeninges, intracranial
use Cerebral Meninges
Leptomeninges, spinal
use Spinal Meninges
Lesser alar cartilage
use Nasal Mucosa and Soft Tissue
Lesser occipital nerve
use Nerve, Cervical Plexus
Lesser Omentum
use Omentum
Lesser saphenous vein
use Saphenous Vein, Left
use Saphenous Vein, Right
Lesser splanchnic nerve
use Nerve, Thoracic Sympathetic
Lesser trochanter
use Femur, Upper, Left
use Femur, Upper, Right
Lesser tuberosity
use Humeral Head, Left
use Humeral Head, Right
Lesser wing
use Bone, Sphenoid
Leukopheresis, therapeutic
see Pheresis, Circulatory 6A55
Levator anguli oris muscle
use Muscle, Facial
Levator ani muscle
use Perineum Muscle
Levator labii superioris alaeque nasi muscle
use Muscle, Facial
Levator labii superioris muscle
use Muscle, Facial
Levator palpebrae superioris muscle
use Eyelid, Upper, Left
use Eyelid, Upper, Right
Levator scapulae muscle
use Muscle, Neck, Left
use Muscle, Neck, Right
Levator veli palatini muscle
use Muscle, Tongue, Palate, Pharynx
Levatores costarum muscle
use Muscle, Thorax, Left
use Muscle, Thorax, Right
LifeStent® (Flexstar)(XL) Vascular Stent System
use Intraluminal Device
Ligament of head of fibula
use Bursa and Ligament, Knee, Left
use Bursa and Ligament, Knee, Right
Ligament of the lateral malleolus
use Bursa and Ligament, Ankle, Left
use Bursa and Ligament, Ankle, Right
Ligamentum flavum, cervical
use Head and Neck Bursa and Ligament
Ligamentum flavum, lumbar
use Lower Spine Bursa and Ligament
Ligamentum flavum, thoracic
use Upper Spine Bursa and Ligament
Ligation
see Occlusion
Ligation, hemorrhoid
see Occlusion, Lower Veins, Hemorrhoidal Plexus
Light Therapy GZJZZZZ
Liner
Removal of device from
Hip
Left 0SPB09Z
Right 0SP909Z
Knee
Left 0SPD09Z
Right 0SPC09Z
Revision of device in
Hip
Left 0SWB09Z
Right 0SW909Z
Knee
Left 0SWD09Z
Right 0SWC09Z
Supplement
Hip
Left 0SUB09Z
Acetabular Surface 0SUE09Z
Femoral Surface 0SUS09Z
Right 0SU909Z
Acetabular Surface 0SUA09Z
Femoral Surface 0SUR09Z
Knee
Left 0SUD09
Femoral Surface 0SUU09Z
Tibial Surface 0SUW09Z
Right 0SUC09
Femoral Surface 0SUT09Z
Tibial Surface 0SUV09Z
Lingual artery
use Artery, External Carotid, Left
use Artery, External Carotid, Right
Lingual tonsil
use Pharynx
Lingulectomy, lung
see Excision, Lung Lingula 0BBH
see Resection, Lung Lingula 0BTH
Lithotripsy
see Fragmentation
With removal of fragments
see Extirpation
LITT (laser interstitial thermal therapy)
see Laser Interstitial Thermal Therapy
LIVIAN™ CRT-D
use Cardiac Resynchronization Defibrillator Pulse Generator in 0JH
Lobectomy
see Excision, Central Nervous System and Cranial Nerves 00B
see Excision, Endocrine System 0GB
see Excision, Hepatobiliary System and Pancreas 0FB
see Excision, Respiratory System 0BB
see Resection, Endocrine System 0GT
see Resection, Hepatobiliary System and Pancreas 0FT
see Resection, Respiratory System 0BT
Lobotomy
see Division, Brain 0080
Localization
see Map
see Imaging
Locus ceruleus
use Pons
Long thoracic nerve
use Nerve, Brachial Plexus
Loop ileostomy
see Bypass, Ileum 0D1B
Loop recorder, implantable
use Monitoring Device
Lower GI series
see Fluoroscopy, Colon BD14
Lumbar artery
use Aorta, Abdominal
Lumbar facet joint
use Joint, Lumbar Vertebral
Lumbar ganglion
use Nerve, Lumbar Sympathetic
Lumbar lymph node
use Lymphatic, Aortic
Lumbar lymphatic trunk
use Cisterna Chyli
Lumbar splanchnic nerve
use Nerve, Lumbar Sympathetic
Lumbosacral facet joint
use Joint, Lumbosacral
Lumbosacral trunk
use Nerve, Lumbar
Lumpectomy
see Excision
Lunate bone
use Carpal, Left
use Carpal, Right
Lunotriquetral ligament
use Bursa and Ligament, Hand, Left
use Bursa and Ligament, Hand, Right
Lymphadenectomy
see Excision, Lymphatic and Hemic Systems 07B
see Resection, Lymphatic and Hemic Systems 07T

- **Lymphadenotomy**
  - *see* Drainage, Lymphatic and Hemic Systems 079
- **Lymphangiectomy**
  - *see* Excision, Lymphatic and Hemic Systems 07B
  - *see* Resection, Lymphatic and Hemic Systems 07T
- **Lymphangiogram**
  - *see* Plain Radiography, Lymphatic System B70
- **Lymphangioplasty**
  - *see* Repair, Lymphatic and Hemic Systems 07Q
  - *see* Supplement, Lymphatic and Hemic Systems 07U
- **Lymphangiorrhaphy**
  - *see* Repair, Lymphatic and Hemic Systems 07Q
- **Lymphangiotomy**
  - *see* Drainage, Lymphatic and Hemic Systems 079
- **Lysis**
  - *see* Release

M

- **Macula**
  - *use* Retina, Left
  - *use* Retina, Right
- **MAGEC® Spinal Bracing and Distraction System**
  - *use* Magnetically Controlled Growth Rod(s) in New Technology
- **Magnet extraction, ocular foreign body**
  - *see* Extirpation, Eye 08C
- **Magnetic Resonance Imaging (MRI)**
  - Abdomen BW30
  - Ankle
    - Left BQ3H
    - Right BQ3G
  - Aorta
    - Abdominal B430
    - Thoracic B330
  - Arm
    - Left BP3F
    - Right BP3E
  - Artery
    - Celiac B431
    - Cervico-Cerebral Arch B33Q
    - Common Carotid, Bilateral B335
    - Coronary
      - Bypass Graft, Multiple B233
      - Multiple B231
    - Internal Carotid, Bilateral B338
    - Intracranial B33R
    - Lower Extremity
      - Bilateral B43H
      - Left B43G
      - Right B43F
    - Pelvic B43C
    - Renal, Bilateral B438
    - Spinal B33M
    - Superior Mesenteric B434
    - Upper Extremity
      - Bilateral B33K
      - Left B33J
      - Right B33H
    - Vertebral, Bilateral B33G
  - Bladder BT30
  - Brachial Plexus BW3P
  - Brain B030
  - Breast
    - Bilateral BH32
    - Left BH31
    - Right BH30

- **Magnetic Resonance Imaging (MRI)** *(continued)*
  - Calcaneus
    - Left BQ3K
    - Right BQ3J
  - Chest BW33Y
  - Coccyx BR3F
  - Connective Tissue
    - Lower Extremity BL31
    - Upper Extremity BL30
  - Corpora Cavernosa BV30
  - Disc
    - Cervical BR31
    - Lumbar BR33
    - Thoracic BR32
  - Ear B930
  - Elbow
    - Left BP3H
    - Right BP3G
  - Eye
    - Bilateral B837
    - Left B836
    - Right B835
  - Femur
    - Left BQ34
    - Right BQ33
  - Fetal Abdomen BY33
  - Fetal Extremity BY35
  - Fetal Head BY30
  - Fetal Heart BY31
  - Fetal Spine BY34
  - Fetal Thorax BY32
  - Fetus, Whole BY36
  - Foot
    - Left BQ3M
    - Right BQ3L
  - Forearm
    - Left BP3K
    - Right BP3J
  - Gland
    - Adrenal, Bilateral BG32
    - Parathyroid BG33
    - Parotid, Bilateral B936
    - Salivary, Bilateral B93D
    - Submandibular, Bilateral B939
    - Thyroid BG34
  - Head BW38
  - Heart, Right and Left B236
  - Hip
    - Left BQ31
    - Right BQ30
  - Intracranial Sinus B532
  - Joint
    - Finger
      - Left BP3D
      - Right BP3C
    - Hand
      - Left BP3D
      - Right BP3C
    - Temporomandibular, Bilateral BN39
  - Kidney
    - Bilateral BT33
    - Left BT32
    - Right BT31
    - Transplant BT39
  - Knee
    - Left BQ38
    - Right BQ37
  - Larynx B93J
  - Leg
    - Left BQ3F
    - Right BQ3D
  - Liver BF35
  - Liver and Spleen BF36
  - Lung Apices BB3G
  - Nasopharynx B93F
  - Neck BW3F
  - Nerve
    - Acoustic B03C
    - Brachial Plexus BW3P

- **Magnetic Resonance Imaging (MRI)** *(continued)*
  - Oropharynx B93F
  - Ovary
    - Bilateral BU35
    - Left BU34
    - Right BU33
  - Ovary and Uterus BU3C
  - Pancreas BF37
  - Patella
    - Left BQ3W
    - Right BQ3V
  - Pelvic Region BW3G
  - Pelvis BR3C
  - Pituitary Gland B039
  - Plexus, Brachial BW3P
  - Prostate BV33
  - Retroperitoneum BW3H
  - Sacrum BR3F
  - Scrotum BV34
  - Sella Turcica B039
  - Shoulder
    - Left BP39
    - Right BP38
  - Sinus
    - Intracranial B532
    - Paranasal B932
  - Spinal Cord B03B
  - Spine
    - Cervical BR30
    - Lumbar BR39
    - Thoracic BR37
  - Spleen and Liver BF36
  - Subcutaneous Tissue
    - Abdomen BH3H
    - Extremity
      - Lower BH3J
      - Upper BH3F
    - Head BH3D
    - Neck BH3D
    - Pelvis BH3H
    - Thorax BH3G
  - Tendon
    - Lower Extremity BL33
    - Upper Extremity BL32
  - Testicle
    - Bilateral BV37
    - Left BV36
    - Right BV35
  - Toe
    - Left BQ3Q
    - Right BQ3P
  - Uterus BU36
    - Pregnant BU3B
  - Uterus and Ovary BU3C
  - Vagina BU39
  - Vein
    - Cerebellar B531
    - Cerebral B531
    - Jugular, Bilateral B535
    - Lower Extremity
      - Bilateral B53D
      - Left B53C
      - Right B53B
    - Other B53V
    - Pelvic (Iliac) Bilateral B53H
    - Portal B53T
    - Pulmonary, Bilateral B53S
    - Renal, Bilateral B53L
    - Spanchnic B53T
    - Upper Extremity
      - Bilateral B53P
      - Left B53N
      - Right B53M
  - Vena Cava
    - Inferior B539
    - Superior B538
  - Wrist
    - Left BP3M
    - Right BP3L

- **Magnetically Controlled Growth Rod(s)**
  - Cervical XNS3
  - Lumbar XNS0
  - Thoracic XNS4
- **Malleotomy**
  - *see* Drainage, Ear, Nose, Sinus 099
- **Malleus**
  - *use* Auditory Ossicle, Left
  - *use* Auditory Ossicle, Right
- **Mammaplasty, mammoplasty**
  - *see* Alteration, Skin and Breast 0H0
  - *see* Repair, Skin and Breast 0HQ
  - *see* Replacement, Skin and Breast 0HR
  - *see* Supplement, Skin and Breast 0HU
- **Mammary duct**
  - *use* Breast, Bilateral
  - *use* Breast, Left
  - *use* Breast, Right
- **Mammary gland**
  - *use* Breast, Bilateral
  - *use* Breast, Left
  - *use* Breast, Right
- **Mammectomy**
  - *see* Excision, Skin and Breast 0HE
  - *see* Resection, Skin and Breast 0H
- **Mammillary body**
  - *use* Hypothalamus
- **Mammography**
  - *see* Plain Radiography, Skin, Subcutaneous Tissue and Brea BH0
- **Mammotomy**
  - *see* Drainage, Skin and Breast 0H
- **Mandibular nerve**
  - *use* Nerve, Trigeminal
- **Mandibular notch**
  - *use* Mandible, Left
  - *use* Mandible, Right
- **Mandibulectomy**
  - *see* Excision, Head and Facial Bones 0NB
  - *see* Resection, Head and Facial Bones 0NT
- **Manipulation**
  - Adhesions
    - *see* Release
  - Chiropractic
    - *see* Chiropractic Manipulation
- **Manual removal, retained placenta**
  - *see* Extraction, Products of Conception, Retained 10I
- **Manubrium**
  - *use* Sternum
- **Map**
  - Basal Ganglia 00K8
  - Brain 00K0
  - Cerebellum 00KC
  - Cerebral Hemisphere 00K7
  - Conduction Mechanism 02K8
  - Hypothalamus 00KA
  - Medulla Oblongata 00KD
  - Pons 00KB
  - Thalamus 00K9
- **Mapping**
  - Doppler ultrasound
    - *see* Ultrasonography
  - Electrocardiogram only
    - *see* Measurement, Cardiac 4A02
- **Mark IV Breathing Pacemaker System**
  - *use* Stimulator Generator in Subcutaneous Tissue and Fas
- **Marsupialization**
  - *see* Drainage
  - *see* Excision

Massage, cardiac
External 5A12012
Open 02QA0ZZ
Masseter muscle
use Muscle, Head
Masseteric fascia
use Subcutaneous Tissue and Fascia, Face
Mastectomy
see Excision, Skin and Breast 0HB
see Resection, Skin and Breast 0HT
Mastoid (postauricular) lymph node
use Lymphatic, Neck, Left
use Lymphatic, Neck, Right
Mastoid air cells
use Sinus, Mastoid, Left
use Sinus, Mastoid, Right
Mastoid process
use Bone, Temporal, Left
use Bone, Temporal, Right
Mastoidectomy
see Excision, Ear, Nose, Sinus 09B
see Resection, Ear, Nose, Sinus 09T
Mastoidotomy
see Drainage, Ear, Nose, Sinus 099
Mastopexy
see Repair, Skin and Breast 0HQ
see Reposition, Skin and Breast 0HS
Mastorrhaphy
see Repair, Skin and Breast 0HQ
Mastotomy
see Drainage, Skin and Breast 0H9
Maxillary artery
use Artery, External Carotid, Left
use Artery, External Carotid, Right
Maxillary nerve
use Nerve, Trigeminal
Maximo II DR (VR)
use Defibrillator Generator in 0JH
Maximo II DR CRT-D
use Cardiac Resynchronization Defibrillator Pulse Generator in 0JH
Measurement
Arterial
Flow
Coronary 4A03
Peripheral 4A03
Pulmonary 4A03
Pressure
Coronary 4A03
Peripheral 4A03
Pulmonary 4A03
Thoracic, Other 4A03
Pulse
Coronary 4A03
Peripheral 4A03
Pulmonary 4A03
Saturation, Peripheral 4A03
Sound, Peripheral 4A03
Biliary
Flow 4A0C
Pressure 4A0C
Cardiac
Action Currents 4A02
Defibrillator 4B02XTZ
Electrical Activity 4A02
Guidance 4A02X4A
No Qualifier 4A02X4Z
Output 4A02
Pacemaker 4B02XSZ
Rate 4A02
Rhythm 4A02
Sampling and Pressure
Bilateral 4A02
Left Heart 4A02
Right Heart 4A02
Sound 4A02
Total Activity, Stress 4A02XM4
Measurement *(continued)*
Central Nervous
Conductivity 4A00
Electrical Activity 4A00
Pressure 4A000BZ
Intracranial 4A00
Saturation, Intracranial 4A00
Stimulator 4B00XVZ
Temperature, Intracranial 4A00
Circulatory, Volume 4A05XLZ
Gastrointestinal
Motility 4A0B
Pressure 4A0B
Secretion 4A0B
Lymphatic
Flow 4A06
Pressure 4A06
Metabolism 4A0Z
Musculoskeletal
Contractility 4A0F
Stimulator 4B0FXVZ
Olfactory, Acuity 4A08X0Z
Peripheral Nervous
Conductivity
Motor 4A01
Sensory 4A01
Electrical Activity 4A01
Stimulator 4B01XVZ
Products of Conception
Cardiac
Electrical Activity 4A0H
Rate 4A0H
Rhythm 4A0H
Sound 4A0HH
Nervous
Conductivity 4A0J
Electrical Activity 4A0J
Pressure 4A0J
Respiratory
Capacity 4A09
Flow 4A09
Pacemaker 4B09X
Rate 4A09
Resistance 4A09
Total Activity 4A09
Volume 4A09
Sleep 4A0ZXQZ
Temperature 4A0Z
Urinary
Contractility 4A0D
Flow 4A0D
Pressure 4A0D
Resistance 4A0D
Volume 4A0D
Venous
Flow
Central 4A04
Peripheral 4A04
Portal 4A04
Pulmonary 4A04
Pressure
Central 4A04
Peripheral 4A04
Portal 4A04
Pulmonary 4A04
Pulse
Central 4A04
Peripheral 4A04
Portal 4A04
Pulmonary 4A04
Saturation, Peripheral 4A04
Visual
Acuity 4A07X0Z
Mobility 4A07X7Z
Pressure 4A07XBZ
Meatoplasty, urethra
see Repair, Urethra 0TQD
Meatotomy
see Drainage, Urinary System 0T9
Mechanical ventilation
see Performance, Respiratory 5A19
Medial canthus
use Eyelid, Lower, Left
use Eyelid, Lower, Right
Medial collateral ligament (MCL)
use Bursa and Ligament, Knee, Left
use Bursa and Ligament, Knee, Right
Medial condyle of femur
use Femur, Lower, Left
use Femur, Lower, Right
Medial condyle of tibia
use Tibia, Left
use Tibia, Right
Medial cuneiform bone
use Tarsal, Left
use Tarsal, Right
Medial epicondyle of femur
use Femur, Lower, Left
use Femur, Lower, Right
Medial epicondyle of humerus
use Humeral Shaft, Left
use Humeral Shaft, Right
Medial malleolus
use Tibia, Left
use Tibia, Right
Medial meniscus
use Joint, Knee, Left
use Joint, Knee, Right
Medial plantar artery
use Artery, Foot, Left
use Artery, Foot, Right
Medial plantar nerve
use Nerve, Tibial
Medial popliteal nerve
use Nerve, Tibial
Medial rectus muscle
use Muscle, Extraocular, Left
use Muscle, Extraocular, Right
Medial sural cutaneous nerve
use Nerve, Tibial
Median antebrachial vein
use Vein, Basilic, Left
use Vein, Basilic, Right
Median cubital vein
use Vein, Basilic, Left
use Vein, Basilic, Right
Median sacral artery
use Aorta, Abdominal
Mediastinal cavity
use Mediastinum
Mediastinal lymph node
use Lymphatic, Thorax
Mediastinal space
use Mediastinum
Mediastinoscopy 0WJC4ZZ
Medication Management GZ3ZZZZ
for substance abuse
Antabuse HZ83ZZZ
Bupropion HZ87ZZZ
Clonidine HZ86ZZZ
Levo-alpha-acetyl-methadol (LAAM) HZ82ZZZ
Methadone Maintenance HZ81ZZZ
Naloxone HZ85ZZZ
Naltrexone HZ84ZZZ
Nicotine Replacement HZ80ZZZ
Other Replacement Medication HZ89ZZZ
Psychiatric Medication HZ88ZZZ
Meditation 8E0ZXY5
Medtronic Endurant® II AAA stent graft system
use Intraluminal Device
Meissner's (submucous) plexus
use Nerve, Abdominal Sympathetic
Melody® transcatheter pulmonary valve
use Zooplastic Tissue in Heart and Great Vessels
Membranous urethra
use Urethra
Meningeorrhaphy
see Repair, Cerebral Meninges 00Q1
see Repair, Spinal Meninges 00QT
Meniscectomy, knee
see Excision, Joint, Knee, Left 0SBD
see Excision, Joint, Knee, Right 0SBC
Mental foramen
use Mandible, Left
use Mandible, Right
Mentalis muscle
use Muscle, Facial
Mentoplasty
see Alteration, Jaw, Lower 0W05
Mesenterectomy
see Excision, Mesentery 0DBV
Mesenteriorrhaphy, mesenterorrhaphy
see Repair, Mesentery 0DQV
Mesenteriplication
see Repair, Mesentery 0DQV
Mesoappendix
use Mesentery
Mesocolon
use Mesentery
Metacarpal ligament
use Bursa and Ligament, Hand, Left
use Bursa and Ligament, Hand, Right
Metacarpophalangeal ligament
use Bursa and Ligament, Hand, Left
use Bursa and Ligament, Hand, Right
Metal on metal bearing surface
use Synthetic Substitute, Metal in 0SR
Metatarsal ligament
use Bursa and Ligament, Foot, Left
use Bursa and Ligament, Foot, Right
Metatarsectomy
see Excision, Lower Bones 0QB
see Resection, Lower Bones 0QT
Metatarsophalangeal (MTP) joint
use Joint, Metatarsal-Phalangeal, Left
use Joint, Metatarsal-Phalangeal, Right
Metatarsophalangeal ligament
use Bursa and Ligament, Foot, Left
use Bursa and Ligament, Foot, Right
Metathalamus
use Thalamus
Micro-Driver stent (RX) (OTW)
use Intraluminal Device
MicroMed HeartAssist
use Implantable Heart Assist System in Heart and Great Vessels
Micrus CERECYTE microcoil
use Intraluminal Device, Bioactive in Upper Arteries
Midcarpal joint
use Joint, Carpal, Left
use Joint, Carpal, Right
Middle cardiac nerve
use Nerve, Thoracic Sympathetic
Middle cerebral artery
use Artery, Intracranial
Middle cerebral vein
use Vein, Intracranial

Middle colic vein
use Vein, Colic
Middle genicular artery
use Artery, Popliteal, Left
use Artery, Popliteal, Right
Middle hemorrhoidal vein
use Vein, Hypogastric, Left
use Vein, Hypogastric, Right
Middle rectal artery
use Artery, Internal Iliac, Left
use Artery, Internal Iliac, Right
Middle suprarenal artery
use Aorta, Abdominal
Middle temporal artery
use Artery, Temporal, Left
use Artery, Temporal, Right
Middle turbinate
use Turbinate, Nasal
MIRODERM™ Biologic Wound Matrix
use Skin Substitute, Porcine Liver Derived in New Technology
MitraClip valve repair system
use Synthetic Substitute
Mitral annulus
use Valve, Mitral
Mitroflow® Aortic Pericardial Heart Valve
use Zooplastic Tissue in Heart and Great Vessels
Mobilization, adhesions
see Release
Molar gland
use Buccal Mucosa
Monitoring
Arterial
Flow
Coronary 4A13
Peripheral 4A13
Pulmonary 4A13
Pressure
Coronary 4A13
Peripheral 4A13
Pulmonary 4A13
Pulse
Coronary 4A13
Peripheral 4A13
Pulmonary 4A13
Saturation, Peripheral 4A13
Sound, Peripheral 4A13
Cardiac
Electrical Activity 4A12
Ambulatory 4A12X45
No Qualifier 4A12X4Z
Output 4A12
Rate 4A12
Rhythm 4A12
Sound 4A12
Total Activity, Stress 4A12XM4
Vascular Perfusion, Indocyanine Green Dye 4A12XSH
Central Nervous
Conductivity 4A10
Electrical Activity
Intraoperative 4A10
No Qualifier 4A10
Pressure 4A100BZ
Intracranial 4A10
Saturation, Intracranial 4A10
Temperature, Intracranial 4A10
Gastrointestinal
Motility 4A1B
Pressure 4A1B
Secretion 4A1B
Vascular Perfusion, Indocyanine Green Dye 4A1BXSH
Intraopertive Knee Replacement Sensor XR2
Monitoring *(continued)*
Lymphatic
Flow 4A16
Pressure 4A16
Peripheral Nervous
Conductivity
Motor 4A11
Sensory 4A11
Electrical Activity
Intraoperative 4A11
No Qualifier 4A11
Products of Conception
Cardiac
Electrical Activity 4A1H
Rate 4A1H
Rhythm 4A1H
Sound 4A1H
Nervous
Conductivity 4A1J
Electrical Activity 4A1J
Pressure 4A1J
Respiratory
Capacity 4A19
Flow 4A19
Rate 4A19
Resistance 4A19
Volume 4A19
Skin and Breast
Vascular Perfusion, Indocyanine Green Dye 4A1GXSH
Sleep 4A1ZXQZ
Temperature 4A1Z
Urinary
Contractility 4A1D
Flow 4A1D
Pressure 4A1D
Resistance 4A1D
Volume 4A1D
Venous
Flow
Central 4A14
Peripheral 4A14
Portal 4A14
Pulmonary 4A14
Pressure
Central 4A14
Peripheral 4A14
Portal 4A14
Pulmonary 4A14
Pulse
Central 4A14
Peripheral 4A14
Portal 4A14
Pulmonary 4A14
Saturation
Central 4A14
Portal 4A14
Pulmonary 4A14
Monitoring Device, Hemodynamic
Abdomen 0JH8
Chest 0JH6
Mosaic Bioprosthesis (aortic) (mitral) valve
use Zooplastic Tissue in Heart and Great Vessels
Motor Function Assessment F01
Motor Treatment F07
MR Angiography
see Magnetic Resonance Imaging (MRI), Heart B23
see Magnetic Resonance Imaging (MRI), Lower Arteries B43
see Magnetic Resonance Imaging (MRI), Upper Arteries B33
MULTI-LINK (VISION)(MINI-VISION)(ULTRA) Coronary Stent System
use Intraluminal Device
Multiple sleep latency test 4A0ZXQZ
Musculocutaneous nerve
use Nerve, Brachial Plexus
Musculopexy
see Repair, Muscles 0KQ
see Reposition, Muscles 0KS
Musculophrenic artery
use Artery, Internal Mammary, Left
use Artery, Internal Mammary, Right
Musculoplasty
see Repair, Muscles 0KQ
see Supplement, Muscles 0KU
Musculorrhaphy
see Repair, Muscles 0KQ
Musculospiral nerve
use Nerve, Radial
Myectomy
see Excision, Muscles 0KB
see Resection, Muscles 0KT
Myelencephalon
use Medulla Oblongata
Myelogram
CT
see Computerized Tomography (CT Scan), Central Nervous System B02
MRI
see Magnetic Resonance Imaging (MRI), Central Nervous System B03
Myenteric (Auerbach's) plexus
use Nerve, Abdominal Sympathetic
Myocardial Bridge Release
see Release, Artery, Coronary
Myomectomy
see Excision, Female Reproductive System 0UB
Myometrium
use Uterus
Myopexy
see Repair, Muscles 0KQ
see Reposition, Muscles 0KS
Myoplasty
see Repair, Muscles 0KQ
see Supplement, Muscles 0KU
Myorrhaphy
see Repair, Muscles 0KQ
Myoscopy
see Inspection, Muscles 0KJ
Myotomy
see Division, Muscles 0K8
see Drainage, Muscles 0K9
Myringectomy
see Excision, Ear, Nose, Sinus 09B
see Resection, Ear, Nose, Sinus 09T
Myringoplasty
see Repair, Ear, Nose, Sinus 09Q
see Replacement, Ear, Nose, Sinus 09R
see Supplement, Ear, Nose, Sinus 09U
Myringostomy
see Drainage, Ear, Nose, Sinus 099
Myringotomy
see Drainage, Ear, Nose, Sinus 099

N

Nail bed
use Finger Nail
use Toe Nail
Nail plate
use Finger Nail
use Toe Nail
nanoLOCK™ interbody fusion device
use Interbody Fusion Device, Nanotextured Surface in New Technology
Narcosynthesis GZGZZZZ
Nasal cavity
use Nasal Mucosa and Soft Tissue
Nasal concha
use Turbinate, Nasal
Nasalis muscle
use Muscle, Facial
Nasolacrimal duct
use Duct, Lacrimal, Left
use Duct, Lacrimal, Right
Nasopharyngeal airway (NPA)
use Intraluminal Device, Airway in Ear, Nose, Sinus
Navicular bone
use Tarsal, Left
use Tarsal, Right
Near Infrared Spectroscopy, Circulatory System 8E023DZ
Neck of femur
use Femur, Upper, Left
use Femur, Upper, Right
Neck of humerus (anatomical) (surgical)
use Humeral Head, Left
use Humeral Head, Right
Nephrectomy
see Excision, Urinary System 0TB
see Resection, Urinary System 0T
Nephrolithotomy
see Extirpation, Urinary System 0TC
Nephrolysis
see Release, Urinary System 0TN
Nephropexy
see Repair, Urinary System 0TQ
see Reposition, Urinary System 0T
Nephroplasty
see Repair, Urinary System 0TQ
see Supplement, Urinary System 0TU
Nephropyeloureterostomy
see Bypass, Urinary System 0T1
see Drainage, Urinary System 0T9
Nephrorrhaphy
see Repair, Urinary System 0TQ
Nephroscopy, transurethral 0TJ58ZZ
Nephrostomy
see Bypass, Urinary System 0T1
see Drainage, Urinary System 0T9
Nephrotomography
see Fluoroscopy, Urinary System BT1
see Plain Radiography, Urinary System BT0
Nephrotomy
see Division, Urinary System 0T8
see Drainage, Urinary System 0T9
Nerve conduction study
see Measurement, Central Nervou 4A00
see Measurement, Peripheral Nervous 4A01
Nerve Function Assessment F01
Nerve to the stapedius
use Nerve, Facial
Nesiritide
use Human B-type Natriuretic Peptide
Neurectomy
see Excision, Central Nervous System and Cranial Nerves 00
see Excision, Peripheral Nervous System 01B
Neurexeresis
see Extraction, Central Nervous System and Cranial Nerves 00D
see Extraction, Peripheral Nervou System 01D
Neurohypophysis
use Gland, Pituitary

eurolysis
- *see* Release, Central Nervous System and Cranial Nerves 00N
- *see* Release, Peripheral Nervous System 01N

euromuscular electrical stimulation (NEMS) lead
- *use* Stimulator Lead in Muscles

europhysiologic monitoring
- *see* Monitoring, Central Nervous 4A10

europlasty
- *see* Repair, Central Nervous System and Cranial Nerves 00Q
- *see* Repair, Peripheral Nervous System 01Q
- *see* Supplement, Central Nervous System and Cranial Nerves 00U
- *see* Supplement, Peripheral Nervous System 01U

eurorrhaphy
- *see* Repair, Central Nervous System and Cranial Nerves 00Q
- *see* Repair, Peripheral Nervous System 01Q

eurostimulator Generator
- Insertion of device in, Skull 0NH00NZ
- Removal of device from, Skull 0NP00NZ
- Revision of device in, Skull 0NW00NZ

eurostimulator generator, multiple channel
- *use* Stimulator Generator, Multiple Array in 0JH

eurostimulator generator, multiple channel rechargeable
- *use* Stimulator Generator, Multiple Array Rechargeable in 0JH

eurostimulator generator, single channel
- *use* Stimulator Generator, Single Array in 0JH

eurostimulator generator, single channel rechargeable
- *use* Stimulator Generator, Single Array Rechargeable in 0JH

eurostimulator Lead
- Insertion of device in
  - Brain 00H0
  - Cerebral Ventricle 00H6
  - Nerve
    - Cranial 00HE
    - Peripheral 01HY
  - Spinal Canal 00HU
  - Spinal Cord 00HV
  - Vein
    - Azygos 05H0
    - Innominate
      - Left 05H4
      - Right 05H3
- Removal of device from
  - Brain 00P0
  - Cerebral Ventricle 00P6
  - Nerve
    - Cranial 00PE
    - Peripheral 01PY
  - Spinal Canal 00PU
  - Spinal Cord 00PV
  - Vein
    - Azygos 05P0
    - Innominate
      - Left 05P4
      - Right 05HP3
- Revision of device in
  - Brain 00W0
  - Cerebral Ventricle 00W6

Neurostimulator Lead *(continued)*
- Revision of device in *(continued)*
  - Nerve
    - Cranial 00WE
    - Peripheral 01WY
  - Spinal Canal 00WU
  - Spinal Cord 00WV
  - Vein
    - Azygos 05W0
    - Innominate
      - Left 05W4
      - Right 05HW3

Neurotomy
- *see* Division, Central Nervous System and Cranial Nerves 008
- *see* Division, Peripheral Nervous System and Cranial Nerves 018

Neurotripsy
- *see* Destruction, Central Nervous System and Cranial Nerves 005
- *see* Destruction, Peripheral Nervous System 015

Neutralization plate
- *use* Internal Fixation Device in Head and Facial Bones
- *use* Internal Fixation Device in Lower Bones
- *use* Internal Fixation Device in Upper Bones

New Technology
- Andexanet alfa, Factor Xa Inhibitor Reversal Agent XW0
- Bezlotoxumab Monoclonal Antibody XW0
- Blinatumomab Antineoplastic Immunotherapy XW0
- Ceftazidime-Avibactam Anti0infective XW0
- Cerebral Embolic Filtration, Dual Filter X2A5312
- Concentrated Bone Marrow Aspirate XK02303
- Cytarabine and Daunorubicin Liposome Antineoplastic XW0
- Defibrotide Sodium Anticoagulant XW0
- Destruction, Prostate, Robotic Waterjet Ablation XV508A4
- Endothelial Damage Inhibitor XY0VX83
- Engineered Autologous Chimeric Antigen Receptor T-cell Immunotherapy XW0
- Fusion
  - Cervical Vertebral
    - 2 or more
      - Nanotextured Surface XRG2092
      - Radiolucent Porous XRG20F3
    - Interbody Fusion Device
      - Nanotextured Surface XRG1092
      - Radiolucent Porous XRG10F3
  - Cervicothoracic Vertebral
    - Nanotextured Surface XRG4092
    - Radiolucent Porous XRG40F3
  - Lumbar Vertebral
    - 2 or more
      - Nanotextured Surface XRGC092
      - Radiolucent Porous XRGC0F3
    - Interbody Fusion Device
      - Nanotextured Surface XRGB092
      - Radiolucent Porous XRGB0F3

New Technology *(continued)*
- Fusion *(continued)*
  - Lumbosacral
    - Nanotextured Surface XRGD092
    - Radiolucent Porous XRGD0F3
  - Occipital-cervical
    - Nanotextured Surface XRG0092
    - Radiolucent Porous XRG00F3
  - Thoracic Vertebral
    - 2 to 7
      - Nanotextured Surface XRG7092
      - Radiolucent Porous XRG70F3
    - 8 or more
      - Nanotextured Surface XRG8092
      - Radiolucent Porous XRG80F3
    - Interbody Fusion Device
      - Nanotextured Surface XRG6092
      - Radiolucent Porous XRG60F3
  - Thoracolumbar Vertebral
    - Nanotextured Surface XRGA092
    - Radiolucent Porous XRGA0F3
- Idarucizumab, Dabigatran Reversal Agent XW0
- Intraoperative Knee Replacement Sensor XR2
- Isavuconazole Anti-infective XW0
- Orbital Atherectomy Technology X2C
- Other New Technology Therapeutic Substance XW0
- Plazomicin Anti-infective XW0
- Replacement
  - Skin Substitute, Porcine Liver Derived XHRPXL2
  - Zooplastic Tissue, Rapid Deployment Technique X2RF
- Reposition
  - Cervical, Magnetically Controlled Growth Rod(s) XNS3
  - Lumbar, Magnetically Controlled Growth Rod(s) XNS0
  - Thoracic, Magnetically Controlled Growth Rod(s) XNS4
- Synthetic Human Angiotensin II XW0
- Uridine Triacetate XW0DX82

Ninth cranial nerve
- *use* Nerve, Glossopharyngeal

Nitinol framed polymer mesh
- *use* Synthetic Substitute

Non-tunneled central venous catheter
- *use* Infusion Device

Nonimaging Nuclear Medicine Assay
- Bladder, Kidneys and Ureters CT63
- Blood C763
- Kidneys, Ureters and Bladder CT63
- Lymphatics and Hematologic System C76YYZZ
- Ureters, Kidneys and Bladder CT63
- Urinary System CT6YYZZ

Nonimaging Nuclear Medicine Probe
- Abdomen CW50
- Abdomen and Chest CW54
- Abdomen and Pelvis CW51
- Brain C050
- Central Nervous System C05YYZZ
- Chest CW53ZZ
- Chest and Abdomen CW54

Nonimaging Nuclear Medicine Probe *(continued)*
- Chest and Neck CW56
- Extremity
  - Lower CP5PZZZ
  - Upper CP5NZZZ
- Head and Neck CW5B
- Heart C25YYZZ
  - Right and Left C256
- Lymphatics
  - Head C75J
  - Head and Neck C755
  - Lower Extremity C75P
  - Neck C75K
  - Pelvic C75D
  - Trunk C75M
  - Upper Chest C75L
  - Upper Extremity C75N
- Lymphatics and Hematologic System C75YYZZ
- Musculoskeletal System, Other CP5YYZZ
- Neck and Chest CW56
- Neck and Head CW5B
- Pelvic Region CW5J
- Pelvis and Abdomen CW51
- Spine CP55ZZZ

Nonimaging Nuclear Medicine Uptake
- Endocrine System CG4YYZZ
- Gland, Thyroid CG42

Nostril
- *use* Nasal Mucosa and Soft Tissue

Novacor Left Ventricular Assist Device
- *use* Implantable Heart Assist System in Heart and Great Vessels

Novation® Ceramic AHS® (Articulation Hip System)
- *use* Synthetic Substitute, Ceramic in 0SR

Nuclear medicine
- *see* Nonimaging Nuclear Medicine Assay
- *see* Nonimaging Nuclear Medicine Probe
- *see* Nonimaging Nuclear Medicine Uptake
- *see* Planar Nuclear Medicine Imaging
- *see* Positron Emission Tomographic (PET) Imaging
- *see* Systemic Nuclear Medicine Therapy
- *see* Tomographic (Tomo) Nuclear Medicine Imaging

Nuclear scintigraphy
- *see* Nuclear Medicine

Nutrition, concentrated substances
- Enteral infusion 3E0G36Z
- Parenteral (peripheral) infusion
  - *see* Introduction of Nutritional Substance

O

Obliteration
- *see* Destruction

Obturator artery
- *use* Artery, Internal Iliac, Left
- *use* Artery, Internal Iliac, Right

Obturator lymph node
- *use* Lymphatic, Pelvis

Obturator muscle
- *use* Muscle, Hip, Left
- *use* Muscle, Hip, Right

Obturator nerve
- *use* Nerve, Lumbar Plexus

Obturator vein
- *use* Vein, Hypogastric, Left
- *use* Vein, Hypogastric, Right

Obtuse margin
- *use* Heart, Left

Occipital artery
- *use* Artery, External Carotid, Left
- *use* Artery, External Carotid, Right

Occipital lobe
- *use* Cerebral Hemisphere

Occipital lymph node
- *use* Lymphatic, Neck, Left
- *use* Lymphatic, Neck, Right

Occipitofrontalis muscle
- *use* Muscle, Facial

Occlusion
- Ampulla of Vater 0FLC
- Anus 0DLQ
- Aorta
  - Abdominal 04L0
  - Thoracic, Descending 02LW3DJ
- Artery
  - Anterior Tibial
    - Left 04LQ
    - Right 04LP
  - Axillary
    - Left 03L6
    - Right 03L5
  - Brachial
    - Left 03L8
    - Right 03L7
  - Celiac 04L1
  - Colic
    - Left 04L7
    - Middle 04L8
    - Right 04L6
  - Common Carotid
    - Left 03LJ
    - Right 03LH
  - Common Iliac
    - Left 04LD
    - Right 04LC
  - External Carotid
    - Left 03LN
    - Right 03LM
  - External Iliac
    - Left 04LJ
    - Right 04LH
  - Face 03LR
  - Femoral
    - Left 04LL
    - Right 04LK
  - Foot
    - Left 04LW
    - Right 04LV
  - Gastric 04L2
  - Hand
    - Left 03LF
    - Right 03LD
  - Hepatic 04L3
  - Inferior Mesenteric 04LB
  - Innominate 03L2
  - Internal Carotid
    - Left 03LL
    - Right 03LK
  - Internal Iliac
    - Left 04LF
    - Right 04LE
  - Internal Mammary
    - Left 03L1
    - Right 03L0
  - Intracranial 03LG
  - Lower 04LY
  - Peroneal
    - Left 04LU
    - Right 04LT
  - Popliteal
    - Left 04LN
    - Right 04LM
  - Posterior Tibial
    - Left 04LS
    - Right 04LR

Occlusion *(continued)*
- Artery *(continued)*
  - Pulmonary
    - Left 02LR
    - Right 02LQ
  - Pulmonary Trunk 02LP
  - Radial
    - Left 03LC
    - Right 03LB
  - Renal
    - Left 04LA
    - Right 04L9
  - Splenic 04L4
  - Subclavian
    - Left 03L4
    - Right 03L3
  - Superior Mesenteric 04L5
  - Temporal
    - Left 03LT
    - Right 03LS
  - Thyroid
    - Left 03LV
    - Right 03LU
  - Ulnar
    - Left 03LA
    - Right 03L9
  - Upper 03LY
  - Vertebral
    - Left 03LQ
    - Right 03LP
- Atrium, Left 02L7
- Bladder 0TLB
- Bladder Neck 0TLC
- Bronchus
  - Lingula 0BL9
  - Lower Lobe
    - Left 0BLB
    - Right 0BL6
  - Main
    - Left 0BL7
    - Right 0BL3
  - Middle Lobe, Right 0BL5
  - Upper Lobe
    - Left 0BL8
    - Right 0BL4
- Carina 0BL2
- Cecum 0DLH
- Cisterna Chyli 07LL
- Colon
  - Ascending 0DLK
  - Descending 0DLM
  - Sigmoid 0DLN
  - Transverse 0DLL
- Cord
  - Bilateral 0VLH
  - Left 0VLG
  - Right 0VLF
- Cul-de-sac 0ULF
- Duct
  - Common Bile 0FL9
  - Cystic 0FL8
  - Hepatic
    - Common 0FL7
    - Left 0FL6
    - Right 0FL5
  - Lacrimal
    - Left 08LY
    - Right 08LX
  - Pancreatic 0FLD
    - Accessory 0FLF
  - Parotid
    - Left 0CLC
    - Right 0CLB
- Duodenum 0DL9
- Esophagogastric Junction 0DL4
- Esophagus 0DL5
  - Lower 0DL3
  - Middle 0DL2
  - Upper 0DL1

Occlusion *(continued)*
- Fallopian Tube
  - Left 0UL6
  - Right 0UL5
- Fallopian Tubes, Bilateral 0UL7
- Ileocecal Valve 0DLC
- Ileum 0DLB
- Intestine
  - Large 0DLE
    - Left 0DLG
    - Right 0DLF
  - Small 0DL8
- Jejunum 0DLA
- Kidney Pelvis
  - Left 0TL4
  - Right 0TL3
- Left atrial appendage (LAA)
  - *see* Occlusion, Atrium, Left 02L7
- Lymphatic
  - Aortic 07LD
  - Axillary
    - Left 07L6
    - Right 07L5
  - Head 07L0
  - Inguinal
    - Left 07LJ
    - Right 07LH
  - Internal Mammary
    - Left 07L9
    - Right 07L8
  - Lower Extremity
    - Left 07LG
    - Right 07LF
  - Mesenteric 07LB
  - Neck
    - Left 07L2
    - Right 07L1
  - Pelvis 07LC
  - Thoracic Duct 07LK
  - Thorax 07L7
  - Upper Extremity
    - Left 07L4
    - Right 07L3
- Rectum 0DLP
- Stomach 0DL6
  - Pylorus 0DL7
- Trachea 0BL1
- Ureter
  - Left 0TL7
  - Right 0TL6
- Urethra 0TLD
- Vagina 0ULG
- Valve, Pulmonary 02LH
- Vas Deferens
  - Bilateral 0VLQ
  - Left 0VLP
  - Right 0VLN
- Vein
  - Axillary
    - Left 05L8
    - Right 05L7
  - Azygos 05L0
  - Basilic
    - Left 05LC
    - Right 05LB
  - Brachial
    - Left 05LA
    - Right 05L9
  - Cephalic
    - Left 05LF
    - Right 05LD
  - Colic 06L7
  - Common Iliac
    - Left 06LD
    - Right 06LC
  - Esophageal 06L3
  - External Iliac
    - Left 06LG
    - Right 06LF

Occlusion *(continued)*
- Vein *(continued)*
  - External Jugular
    - Left 05LQ
    - Right 05LP
  - Face
    - Left 05LV
    - Right 05LT
  - Femoral
    - Left 06LN
    - Right 06LM
  - Foot
    - Left 06LV
    - Right 06LT
  - Gastric 06L2
  - Hand
    - Left 05LH
    - Right 05LG
  - Hemiazygos 05L1
  - Hepatic 06L4
  - Hypogastric
    - Left 06LJ
    - Right 06LH
  - Inferior Mesenteric 06L6
  - Innominate
    - Left 05L4
    - Right 05L3
  - Internal Jugular
    - Left 05LN
    - Right 05LM
  - Intracranial 05LL
  - Lower 06LY
  - Portal 06L8
  - Pulmonary
    - Left 02LT
    - Right 02LS
  - Renal
    - Left 06LB
    - Right 06L9
  - Saphenous
    - Left 06LQ
    - Right 06LP
  - Splenic 06L1
  - Subclavian
    - Left 05L6
    - Right 05L5
  - Superior Mesenteric 06L5
  - Upper 05LY
  - Vertebral
    - Left 05LS
    - Right 05LR
- Vena Cava
  - Inferior 06L0
  - Superior 02LV

Occlusion, REBOA (resuscitative endovascular balloon occlusion of the aorta)
- 02LW3DJ
- 04L03DJ

Occupational therapy
- *see* Activities of Daily Living Treatment, Rehabilitation F08

Odentectomy
- *see* Excision, Mouth and Throat 0C
- *see* Resection, Mouth and Throat 0C

Odontoid process
- *use* Cervical Vertebra

Olecranon bursa
- *use* Bursa and Ligament, Elbow, L
- *use* Bursa and Ligament, Elbow, Ri

Olecranon process
- *use* Ulna, Left
- *use* Ulna, Right

Olfactory bulb
- *use* Nerve, Olfactory

Omentectomy, omentumectomy
- *see* Excision, Gastrointestinal System 0DB
- *see* Resection, Gastrointestinal System 0DT

entofixation
see Repair, Gastrointestinal System 0DQ
entoplasty
see Repair, Gastrointestinal System 0DQ
see Replacement, Gastrointestinal System 0DR
see Supplement, Gastrointestinal System 0DU
entorrhaphy
see Repair, Gastrointestinal System 0DQ
entotomy
see Drainage, Gastrointestinal System 0D9
nilink Elite Vascular Balloon Expandable Stent System
use Intraluminal Device
ychectomy
see Excision, Skin and Breast 0HB
see Resection, Skin and Breast 0HT
ychoplasty
see Repair, Skin and Breast 0HQ
see Replacement, Skin and Breast 0HR
ychotomy
see Drainage, Skin and Breast 0H9
phorectomy
see Excision, Female Reproductive System 0UB
see Resection, Female Reproductive System 0UT
phoropexy
see Repair, Female Reproductive System 0UQ
see Reposition, Female Reproductive System 0US
phoroplasty
see Repair, Female Reproductive System 0UQ
see Supplement, Female Reproductive System 0UU
phororrhaphy
see Repair, Female Reproductive System 0UQ
phorostomy
see Drainage, Female Reproductive System 0U9
phorotomy
see Drainage, Female Reproductive System 0U9
see Division, Female Reproductive System 0U8
phorrhaphy
see Repair, Female Reproductive System 0UQ
en Pivot (mechanical) valve
use Synthetic Substitute
en Pivot Aortic Valve Graft (AVG)
use Synthetic Substitute
hthalmic artery
use Intracranial Artery
hthalmic nerve
use Nerve, Trigeminal
hthalmic vein
use Vein, Intracranial
ponensplasty
Tendon replacement
see Replacement, Tendons 0LR
Tendon transfer
see Transfer, Tendons 0LX
ic chiasma
use Nerve, Optic
ic disc
use Retina, Left
use Retina, Right
ic foramen
use Bone, Sphenoid
Optical coherence tomography, intravascular
see Computerized Tomography (CT Scan)
Optimizer™ III implantable pulse generator
use Contractility Modulation Device in 0JH
Orbicularis oculi muscle
use Eyelid, Upper, Left
use Eyelid, Upper, Right
Orbicularis oris muscle
use Muscle, Facial
Orbital Atherectomy Technology X2C
Orbital fascia
use Subcutaneous Tissue and Fascia, Face
Orbital portion of ethmoid bone
use Orbit, Left
use Orbit, Right
Orbital portion of frontal bone
use Orbit, Left
use Orbit, Right
Orbital portion of lacrimal bone
use Orbit, Left
use Orbit, Right
Orbital portion of maxilla
use Orbit, Left
use Orbit, Right
Orbital portion of palatine bone
use Orbit, Left
use Orbit, Right
Orbital portion of sphenoid bone
use Orbit, Left
use Orbit, Right
Orbital portion of zygomatic bone
use Orbit, Left
use Orbit, Right
Orchectomy, orchidectomy, orchiectomy
see Excision, Male Reproductive System 0VB
see Resection, Male Reproductive System 0VT
Orchidoplasty, orchioplasty
see Repair, Male Reproductive System 0VQ
see Replacement, Male Reproductive System 0VR
see Supplement, Male Reproductive System 0VU
Orchidorrhaphy, orchiorrhaphy
see Repair, Male Reproductive System 0VQ
Orchidotomy, orchiotomy, orchotomy
see Drainage, Male Reproductive System 0V9
Orchiopexy
see Repair, Male Reproductive System 0VQ
see Reposition, Male Reproductive System 0VS
Oropharyngeal airway (OPA)
use Intraluminal Device, Airway in Mouth and Throat
Oropharynx
use Pharynx
Ossiculectomy
see Excision, Ear, Nose, Sinus 09B
see Resection, Ear, Nose, Sinus 09T
Ossiculotomy
see Drainage, Ear, Nose, Sinus 099
Ostectomy
see Excision, Head and Facial Bones 0NB
see Excision, Lower Bones 0QB
see Excision, Upper Bones 0PB
see Resection, Head and Facial Bones 0NT
Ostectomy *(continued)*
see Resection, Lower Bones 0QT
see Resection, Upper Bones 0PT
Osteoclasis
see Division, Head and Facial Bones 0N8
see Division, Lower Bones 0Q8
see Division, Upper Bones 0P8
Osteolysis
see Release, Head and Facial Bones 0NN
see Release, Lower Bones 0QN
see Release, Upper Bones 0PN
Osteopathic Treatment
Abdomen 7W09X
Cervical 7W01X
Extremity
Lower 7W06X
Upper 7W07X
Head 7W00X
Lumbar 7W03X
Pelvis 7W05X
Rib Cage 7W08X
Sacrum 7W04X
Thoracic 7W02X
Osteopexy
see Repair, Head and Facial Bones 0NQ
see Repair, Lower Bones 0QQ
see Repair, Upper Bones 0PQ
see Reposition, Head and Facial Bones 0NS
see Reposition, Lower Bones 0QS
see Reposition, Upper Bones 0PS
Osteoplasty
see Repair, Head and Facial Bones 0NQ
see Repair, Lower Bones 0QQ
see Repair, Upper Bones 0PQ
see Replacement, Head and Facial Bones 0NR
see Replacement, Lower Bones 0QR
see Replacement, Upper Bones 0PR
see Supplement, Head and Facial Bones 0NU
see Supplement, Lower Bones 0QU
see Supplement, Upper Bones 0PU
Osteorrhaphy
see Repair, Head and Facial Bones 0NQ
see Repair, Lower Bones 0QQ
see Repair, Upper Bones 0PQ
Osteotomy, ostotomy
see Division, Head and Facial Bones 0N8
see Division, Lower Bones 0Q8
see Division, Upper Bones 0P8
see Drainage, Head and Facial Bones 0N9
see Drainage, Lower Bones 0Q9
see Drainage, Upper Bones 0P9
Otic ganglion
use Nerve, Head and Neck Sympathetic
Otoplasty
see Repair, Ear, Nose, Sinus 09Q
see Replacement, Ear, Nose, Sinus 09R
see Supplement, Ear, Nose, Sinus 09U
Otoscopy
see Inspection, Ear, Nose, Sinus 09J
Oval window
use Ear, Middle, Left
use Ear, Middle, Right
Ovarian artery
use Aorta, Abdominal
Ovarian ligament
use Uterine Supporting Structure
Ovariectomy
see Excision, Female Reproductive System 0UB
see Resection, Female Reproductive System 0UT
Ovariocentesis
see Drainage, Female Reproductive System 0U9
Ovariopexy
see Repair, Female Reproductive System 0UQ
see Reposition, Female Reproductive System 0US
Ovariotomy
see Division, Female Reproductive System 0U8
see Drainage, Female Reproductive System 0U9
Ovatio™ CRT-D
use Cardiac Resynchronization Defibrillator Pulse Generator in 0JH
Oversewing
Gastrointestinal ulcer
see Repair, Gastrointestinal System 0DQ
Pleural bleb
see Repair, Respiratory System 0BQ
Oviduct
use Fallopian Tube, Left
use Fallopian Tube, Right
Oximetry, Fetal pulse 10H073Z
OXINIUM
use Synthetic Substitute, Oxidized Zirconium on Polyethylene in 0SR
Oxygenation
Extracorporeal membrane (ECMO)
see Performance, Circulatory 5A15
Hyperbaric
see Assistance, Circulatory 5A05
Supersaturated
see Assistance, Circulatory 5A05

P

Pacemaker
Dual Chamber
Abdomen 0JH8
Chest 0JH6
Intracardiac
Insertion of device in
Atrium
Left 02H7
Right 02H6
Vein, Coronary 02H4
Ventricle
Left 02HL
Right 02HK
Removal of device from
Heart 02PA
Revision of device in
Heart 02WA
Single Chamber
Abdomen 0JH8
Chest 0JH6
Single Chamber Rate Responsive
Abdomen 0JH8
Chest 0JH6
Packing
Abdominal Wall 2W43X5Z
Anorectal 2Y43X5Z
Arm
Lower
Left 2W4DX5Z
Right 2W4CX5Z

Packing *(continued)*
- Arm *(continued)*
  - Upper
    - Left 2W4BX5Z
    - Right 2W4AX5Z
- Back 2W45X5Z
- Chest Wall 2W44X5Z
- Ear 2Y42X5Z
- Extremity
  - Lower
    - Left 2W4MX5Z
    - Right 2W4LX5Z
  - Upper
    - Left 2W49X5Z
    - Right 2W48X5Z
- Face 2W41X5Z
- Finger
  - Left 2W4KX5Z
  - Right 2W4JX5Z
- Foot
  - Left 2W4TX5Z
  - Right 2W4SX5Z
- Genital Tract, Female 2Y44X5Z
- Hand
  - Left 2W4FX5Z
  - Right 2W4EX5Z
- Head 2W40X5Z
- Inguinal Region
  - Left 2W47X5Z
  - Right 2W46X5Z
- Leg
  - Lower
    - Left 2W4RX5Z
    - Right 2W4QX5Z
  - Upper
    - Left 2W4PX5Z
    - Right 2W4NX5Z
- Mouth and Pharynx 2Y40X5Z
- Nasal 2Y41X5Z
- Neck 2W42X5Z
- Thumb
  - Left 2W4HX5Z
  - Right 2W4GX5Z
- Toe
  - Left 2W4VX5Z
  - Right 2W4UX5Z
- Urethra 2Y45X5Z

Paclitaxel-eluting coronary stent
- *use* Intraluminal Device, Drug-eluting in Heart and Great Vessels

Paclitaxel-eluting peripheral stent
- *use* Intraluminal Device, Drug-eluting in Lower Arteries
- *use* Intraluminal Device, Drug-eluting in Upper Arteries

Palatine gland
- *use* Buccal Mucosa

Palatine tonsil
- *use* Tonsils

Palatine uvula
- *use* Uvula

Palatoglossal muscle
- *use* Muscle, Tongue, Palate, Pharynx

Palatopharyngeal muscle
- *use* Muscle, Tongue, Palate, Pharynx

Palatoplasty
- *see* Repair, Mouth and Throat 0CQ
- *see* Replacement, Mouth and Throat 0CR
- *see* Supplement, Mouth and Throat 0CU

Palatorrhaphy
- *see* Repair, Mouth and Throat 0CQ

Palmar (volar) digital vein
- *use* Vein, Hand, Left
- *use* Vein, Hand, Right

Palmar (volar) metacarpal vein
- *use* Vein, Hand, Left
- *use* Vein, Hand, Right

Palmar cutaneous nerve
- *use* Nerve, Median
- *use* Nerve, Radial

Palmar fascia (aponeurosis)
- *use* Subcutaneous Tissue and Fascia, Hand, Left
- *use* Subcutaneous Tissue and Fascia, Hand, Right

Palmar interosseous muscle
- *use* Muscle, Hand, Left
- *use* Muscle, Hand, Right

Palmar ulnocarpal ligament
- *use* Bursa and Ligament, Wrist, Left
- *use* Bursa and Ligament, Wrist, Right

Palmaris longus muscle
- *use* Muscle, Lower Arm and Wrist, Left
- *use* Muscle, Lower Arm and Wrist, Right

Pancreatectomy
- *see* Excision, Pancreas 0FBG
- *see* Resection, Pancreas 0FTG

Pancreatic artery
- *use* Artery, Splenic

Pancreatic plexus
- *use* Nerve, Abdominal Sympathetic

Pancreatic vein
- *use* Vein, Splenic

Pancreaticoduodenostomy
- *see* Bypass, Hepatobiliary System and Pancreas 0F1

Pancreaticosplenic lymph node
- *use* Lymphatic, Aortic

Pancreatogram, endoscopic retrograde
- *see* Fluoroscopy, Pancreatic Duct BF18

Pancreatolithotomy
- *see* Extirpation, Pancreas 0FCG

Pancreatotomy
- *see* Division, Pancreas 0F8G
- *see* Drainage, Pancreas 0F9G

Panniculectomy
- *see* Excision, Abdominal Wall 0WBF
- *see* Excision, Skin, Abdomen 0HB7

Paraaortic lymph node
- *use* Lymphatic, Aortic

Paracentesis
- Eye
  - *see* Drainage, Eye 089
- Peritoneal Cavity
  - *see* Drainage, Peritoneal Cavity 0W9G
- Tympanum
  - *see* Drainage, Ear, Nose, Sinus 099

Pararectal lymph node
- *use* Lymphatic, Mesenteric

Parasternal lymph node
- *use* Lymphatic, Thorax

Parathyroidectomy
- *see* Excision, Endocrine System 0GB
- *see* Resection, Endocrine System 0GT

Paratracheal lymph node
- *use* Lymphatic, Thorax

Paraurethral (Skene's) gland
- *use* Gland, Vestibular

Parenteral nutrition, total
- *see* Introduction of Nutritional Substance

Parietal lobe
- *use* Cerebral Hemisphere

Parotid lymph node
- *use* Lymphatic, Head

Parotid plexus
- *use* Nerve, Facial

Parotidectomy
- *see* Excision, Mouth and Throat 0CB
- *see* Resection, Mouth and Throat 0CT

Pars flaccida
- *use* Tympanic Membrane, Left
- *use* Tympanic Membrane, Right

Partial joint replacement
- Hip
  - *see* Replacement, Lower Joints 0SR
- Knee
  - *see* Replacement, Lower Joints 0SR
- Shoulder
  - *see* Replacement, Upper Joints 0RR

Partially absorbable mesh
- *use* Synthetic Substitute

Patch, blood, spinal 3E0R3GC

Patellapexy
- *see* Repair, Lower Bones 0QQ
- *see* Reposition, Lower Bones 0QS

Patellaplasty
- *see* Repair, Lower Bones 0QQ
- *see* Replacement, Lower Bones 0QR
- *see* Supplement, Lower Bones 0QU

Patellar ligament
- *use* Bursa and Ligament, Knee, Left
- *use* Bursa and Ligament, Knee, Right

Patellar tendon
- *use* Tendon, Knee, Left
- *use* Tendon, Knee, Right

Patellectomy
- *see* Excision, Lower Bones 0QB
- *see* Resection, Lower Bones 0QT

Patellofemoral joint
- *use* Joint, Knee, Left
- *use* Joint, Knee, Left, Femoral Surface
- *use* Joint, Knee, Right
- *use* Joint, Knee, Right, Femoral Surface

Pectineus muscle
- *use* Muscle, Upper Leg, Left
- *use* Muscle, Upper Leg, Right

Pectoral (anterior) lymph node
- *use* Lymphatic, Axillary, Left
- *use* Lymphatic, Axillary, Right

Pectoral fascia
- *use* Subcutaneous Tissue and Fascia, Chest

Pectoralis major muscle
- *use* Muscle, Thorax, Left
- *use* Muscle, Thorax, Right

Pectoralis minor muscle
- *use* Muscle, Thorax, Left
- *use* Muscle, Thorax, Right

Pedicle-based dynamic stabilization device
- *use* Spinal Stabilization Device, Pedicle-Based in 0RH
- *use* Spinal Stabilization Device, Pedicle-Based in 0SH

PEEP (positive end expiratory pressure)
- *see* Assistance, Respiratory 5A09

PEG (percutaneous endoscopic gastrostomy) 0DH63UZ

PEJ (percutaneous endoscopic jejunostomy) 0DHA3UZ

Pelvic splanchnic nerve
- *use* Nerve, Abdominal Sympathetic
- *use* Nerve, Sacral Sympathetic

Penectomy
- *see* Excision, Male Reproductive System 0VB
- *see* Resection, Male Reproductive System 0VT

Penile urethra
- *use* Urethra

Perceval sutureless valve
- *use* Zooplastic Tissue, Rapid Deployment Technique in Ne[w] Technology

Percutaneous endoscopic gastrojejunostomy (PEG/J) tube
- *use* Feeding Device in Gastrointestinal System

Percutaneous endoscopic gastrosto[my] (PEG) tube
- *use* Feeding Device in Gastrointestinal System

Percutaneous nephrostomy catheter
- *use* Drainage Device

Percutaneous transluminal corona[ry] angioplasty (PTCA)
- *see* Dilation, Heart and Great Vessels 027

Performance
- Biliary
  - Multiple, Filtration 5A1C60Z
  - Single, Filtration 5A1C00Z
- Cardiac
  - Continuous
    - Output 5A1221Z
    - Pacing 5A1223Z
  - Intermittent, Pacing 5A1213Z
  - Single, Output, Manual 5A12012
- Circulatory
  - Central Membrane 5A1522F
  - Peripheral Veno-arterial Membrane 5A1522G
  - Peripheral Veno-venous Membrane 5A1522H
- Respiratory
  - 24-96 Consecutive Hours, Ventilation 5A1945Z
  - Greater than 96 Consecutive Hours, Ventilation 5A1955Z
  - Less than 24 Consecutive Ho[urs,] Ventilation 5A1935Z
  - Single, Ventilation, Nonmechanical5A19054
- Urinary
  - Continuous, Greater than 18 hours per day, Filtration 5A1D90Z
  - Intermittent, Less than 6 hour[s] per day, Filtration 5A1D7[0Z]
  - Prolonged Intermittent, 6-18 hours per day, Filtration 5A1D80Z

Perfusion
- *see* Introduction of substance in or on

Perfusion, donor organ
- Heart 6AB50BZ
- Kidney(s) 6ABT0BZ
- Liver 6ABF0BZ
- Lung(s) 6ABB0BZ

Pericardiectomy
- *see* Excision, Pericardium 02BN
- *see* Resection, Pericardium 02TN

Pericardiocentesis
- *see* Drainage, Pericardial Cavity 0W9D

Pericardiolysis
- *see* Release, Pericardium 02NN

ericardiophrenic artery
use Artery, Internal Mammary, Left
use Artery, Internal Mammary, Right
ericardioplasty
see Repair, Pericardium 02QN
see Replacement, Pericardium 02RN
see Supplement, Pericardium 02UN
ericardiorrhaphy
see Repair, Pericardium 02QN
ericardiostomy
see Drainage, Pericardial Cavity 0W9D
ericardiotomy
see Drainage, Pericardial Cavity 0W9D
erimetrium
use Uterus
ripheral parenteral nutrition
see Introduction of Nutritional Substance
eripherally inserted central catheter (PICC)
use Infusion Device
ritoneal dialysis 3E1M39Z
ritoneocentesis
see Drainage, Peritoneal Cavity 0W9G
see Drainage, Peritoneum 0D9W
ritoneoplasty
see Repair, Peritoneum 0DQW
see Replacement, Peritoneum 0DRW
see Supplement, Peritoneum 0DUW
ritoneoscopy 0DJW4ZZ
ritoneotomy
see Drainage, Peritoneum 0D9W
ritoneumectomy
see Excision, Peritoneum 0DBW
roneus brevis muscle
use Muscle, Lower Leg, Left
use Muscle, Lower Leg, Right
roneus longus muscle
use Muscle, Lower Leg, Left
use Muscle, Lower Leg, Right
ssary ring
use Intraluminal Device, Pessary in Female Reproductive System
T scan
see Positron Emission Tomographic (PET) Imaging
trous part of temporal bone
use Bone, Temporal, Left
use Bone, Temporal, Right
acoemulsification, lens
With IOL implant
see Replacement, Eye 08R
Without IOL implant
see Extraction, Eye 08D
alangectomy
see Excision, Lower Bones 0QB
see Excision, Upper Bones 0PB
see Resection, Lower Bones 0QT
see Resection, Upper Bones 0PT
allectomy
see Excision, Penis 0VBS
see Resection, Penis 0VTS
alloplasty
see Repair, Penis 0VQS
see Supplement, Penis 0VUS
allotomy
see Drainage, Penis 0V9S
armacotherapy, for substance abuse
Antabuse HZ93ZZZ
Bupropion HZ97ZZZ
Clonidine HZ96ZZZ
Levo-alpha-acetyl-methadol (LAAM) HZ92ZZZ
Methadone Maintenance HZ91ZZZ
Naloxone HZ95ZZZ
Naltrexone HZ94ZZZ
Pharmacotherapy, for substance abuse *(continued)*
Nicotine Replacement HZ90ZZZ
Psychiatric Medication HZ98ZZZ
Replacement Medication, Other HZ99ZZZ
Pharyngeal constrictor muscle
use Muscle, Tongue, Palate, Pharynx
Pharyngeal plexus
use Nerve, Vagus
Pharyngeal recess
use Nasopharynx
Pharyngeal tonsil
use Adenoids
Pharyngogram
see Fluoroscopy, Pharynx B91G
Pharyngoplasty
see Repair, Mouth and Throat 0CQ
see Replacement, Mouth and Throat 0CR
see Supplement, Mouth and Throat 0CU
Pharyngorrhaphy
see Repair, Mouth and Throat 0CQ
Pharyngotomy
see Drainage, Mouth and Throat 0C9
Pharyngotympanic tube
use Eustachian Tube, Left
use Eustachian Tube, Right
Pheresis
Erythrocytes 6A55
Leukocytes 6A55
Plasma 6A55
Platelets 6A55
Stem Cells
Cord Blood 6A55
Hematopoietic 6A55
Phlebectomy
see Excision, Lower Veins 06B
see Excision, Upper Veins 05B
see Extraction, Lower Veins 06D
see Extraction, Upper Veins 05D
Phlebography
see Plain Radiography, Veins B50
Impedance 4A04X51
Phleborrhaphy
see Repair, Lower Veins 06Q
see Repair, Upper Veins 05Q
Phlebotomy
see Drainage, Lower Veins 069
see Drainage, Upper Veins 059
Photocoagulation
For Destruction
see Destruction
For Repair
see Repair
Photopheresis, therapeutic
see Phototherapy, Circulatory 6A65
Phototherapy
Circulatory 6A65
Skin 6A60
Ultraviolet light
see Ultraviolet Light Therapy, Physiological Systems 6A8
Phrenectomy, phrenoneurectomy
see Excision, Nerve, Phrenic 01B2
Phrenemphraxis
see Destruction, Nerve, Phrenic 0152
Phrenic nerve stimulator generator
use Stimulator Generator in Subcutaneous Tissue and Fascia
Phrenic nerve stimulator lead
use Diaphragmatic Pacemaker Lead in Respiratory System
Phreniclasis
see Destruction, Nerve, Phrenic 0152
Phrenicoexeresis
see Extraction, Nerve, Phrenic 01D2
Phrenicotomy
see Division, Nerve, Phrenic 0182
Phrenicotripsy
see Destruction, Nerve, Phrenic 0152
Phrenoplasty
see Repair, Respiratory System 0BQ
see Supplement, Respiratory System 0BU
Phrenotomy
see Drainage, Respiratory System 0B9
Physiatry
see Motor Treatment, Rehabilitation F07
Physical medicine
see Motor Treatment, Rehabilitation F07
Physical therapy
see Motor Treatment, Rehabilitation F07
PHYSIOMESH™ Flexible Composite Mesh
use Synthetic Substitute
Pia mater, intracranial
use Cerebral Meninges
Pia mater, spinal
use Spinal Meninges
Pinealectomy
see Excision, Pineal Body 0GB1
see Resection, Pineal Body 0GT1
Pinealoscopy 0GJ14ZZ
Pinealotomy
see Drainage, Pineal Body 0G91
Pinna
use Ear, External, Bilateral
use Ear, External, Left
use Ear, External, Right
Pipeline™ Embolization device (PED)
use Intraluminal Device
Piriform recess (sinus)
use Pharynx
Piriformis muscle
use Muscle, Hip, Right
use Muscle, Hip, Left
PIRRT (Prolonged intermittent renal replacement therapy) 5A1D80Z
Pisiform bone
use Carpal, Left
use Carpal, Right
Pisohamate ligament
use Bursa and Ligament, Hand, Left
use Bursa and Ligament, Hand, Right
Pisometacarpal ligament
use Bursa and Ligament, Hand, Left
use Bursa and Ligament, Hand, Right
Pituitectomy
see Excision, Gland, Pituitary 0GB0
see Resection, Gland, Pituitary 0GT0
Plain film radiology
see Plain Radiography
Plain Radiography
Abdomen BW00ZZZ
Abdomen and Pelvis BW01ZZZ
Abdominal Lymphatic
Bilateral B701
Unilateral B700
Airway, Upper BB0DZZZ
Ankle
Left BQ0H
Right BQ0G
Aorta
Abdominal B400
Thoracic B300
Thoraco-Abdominal B30P
Plain Radiography *(continued)*
Aorta and Bilateral Lower Extremity Arteries B40D
Arch
Bilateral BN0DZZZ
Left BN0CZZZ
Right BN0BZZZ
Arm
Left BP0FZZZ
Right BP0EZZZ
Artery
Brachiocephalic-Subclavian, Right B301
Bronchial B30L
Bypass Graft, Other B20F
Cervico-Cerebral Arch B30Q
Common Carotid
Bilateral B305
Left B304
Right B303
Coronary
Bypass Graft
Multiple B203
Single B202
Multiple B201
Single B200
External Carotid
Bilateral B30C
Left B30B
Right B309
Hepatic B402
Inferior Mesenteric B405
Intercostal B30L
Internal Carotid
Bilateral B308
Left B307
Right B306
Internal Mammary Bypass Graft
Left B208
Right B207
Intra-Abdominal, Other B40B
Intracranial B30R
Lower, Other B40J
Lower Extremity
Bilateral and Aorta B40D
Left B40G
Right B40F
Lumbar B409
Pelvic B40C
Pulmonary
Left B30T
Right B30S
Renal
Bilateral B408
Left B407
Right B406
Transplant B40M
Spinal B30M
Splenic B403
Subclavian, Left B302
Superior Mesenteric B404
Upper, Other B30N
Upper Extremity
Bilateral B30K
Left B30J
Right B30H
Vertebral
Bilateral B30G
Left B30F
Right B30D
Bile Duct BF00
Bile Duct and Gallbladder BF03
Bladder BT00
Kidney and Ureter BT04
Bladder and Urethra BT0B
Bone
Facial BN05ZZZ
Nasal BN04ZZZ
Bones, Long, All BW0BZZZ

Plain Radiography *(continued)*
- Breast
  - Bilateral BH02ZZZ
  - Left BH01ZZZ
  - Right BH00ZZZ
- Calcaneus
  - Left BQ0KZZZ
  - Right BQ0JZZZ
- Chest BW03ZZZ
- Clavicle
  - Left BP05ZZZ
  - Right BP04ZZZ
- Coccyx BR0FZZZ
- Corpora Cavernosa BV00
- Dialysis Fistula B50W
- Dialysis Shunt B50W
- Disc
  - Cervical BR01
  - Lumbar BR03
  - Thoracic BR02
- Duct
  - Lacrimal
    - Bilateral B802
    - Left B801
    - Right B800
  - Mammary
    - Multiple
      - Left BH06
      - Right BH05
    - Single
      - Left BH04
      - Right BH03
- Elbow
  - Left BP0H
  - Right BP0G
- Epididymis
  - Left BV02
  - Right BV01
- Extremity
  - Lower BW0CZZZ
  - Upper BW0JZZZ
- Eye
  - Bilateral B807ZZZ
  - Left B806ZZZ
  - Right B805ZZZ
- Facet Joint
  - Cervical BR04
  - Lumbar BR06
  - Thoracic BR05
- Fallopian Tube
  - Bilateral BU02
  - Left BU01
  - Right BU00
- Fallopian Tube and Uterus BU08
- Femur
  - Left, Densitometry BQ04ZZ1
  - Right, Densitometry BQ03ZZ1
- Finger
  - Left BP0SZZZ
  - Right BP0RZZZ
- Foot
  - Left BQ0MZZZ
  - Right BQ0LZZZ
- Forearm
  - Left BP0KZZZ
  - Right BP0JZZZ
- Gallbladder and Bile Duct BF03
- Gland
  - Parotid
    - Bilateral B906
    - Left B905
    - Right B904
  - Salivary
    - Bilateral B90D
    - Left B90C
    - Right B90B
  - Submandibular
    - Bilateral B909
    - Left B908
    - Right B907

Plain Radiography *(continued)*
- Hand
  - Left BP0PZZZ
  - Right BP0NZZZ
- Heart
  - Left B205
  - Right B204
  - Right and Left B206
- Hepatobiliary System, All BF0C
- Hip
  - Left BQ01
    - Densitometry BQ01ZZ1
  - Right BQ00
    - Densitometry BQ00ZZ1
- Humerus
  - Left BP0BZZZ
  - Right BP0AZZZ
- Ileal Diversion Loop BT0C
- Intracranial Sinus B502
- Joint
  - Acromioclavicular, Bilateral BP03ZZZ
  - Finger
    - Left BP0D
    - Right BP0C
  - Foot
    - Left BQ0Y
    - Right BQ0X
  - Hand
    - Left BP0D
    - Right BP0C
  - Lumbosacral BR0BZZZ
  - Sacroiliac BR0D
  - Sternoclavicular
    - Bilateral BP02ZZZ
    - Left BP01ZZZ
    - Right BP00ZZZ
  - Temporomandibular
    - Bilateral BN09
    - Left BN08
    - Right BN07
  - Thoracolumbar BR08ZZZ
  - Toe
    - Left BQ0Y
    - Right BQ0X
- Kidney
  - Bilateral BT03
  - Left BT02
  - Right BT01
  - Ureter and Bladder BT04
- Knee
  - Left BQ08
  - Right BQ07
- Leg
  - Left BQ0FZZZ
  - Right BQ0DZZZ
- Lymphatic
  - Head B704
  - Lower Extremity
    - Bilateral B70B
    - Left B709
    - Right B708
  - Neck B704
  - Pelvic B70C
  - Upper Extremity
    - Bilateral B707
    - Left B706
    - Right B705
- Mandible BN06ZZZ
- Mastoid B90HZZZ
- Nasopharynx B90FZZZ
- Optic Foramina
  - Left B804ZZZ
  - Right B803ZZZ
- Orbit
  - Bilateral BN03ZZZ
  - Left BN02ZZZ
  - Right BN01ZZZ
- Oropharynx B90FZZZ

Plain Radiography *(continued)*
- Patella
  - Left BQ0WZZZ
  - Right BQ0VZZZ
- Pelvis BR0CZZZ
- Pelvis and Abdomen BW01ZZZ
- Prostate BV03
- Retroperitoneal Lymphatic
  - Bilateral B701
  - Unilateral B700
- Ribs
  - Left BP0YZZZ
  - Right BP0XZZZ
- Sacrum BR0FZZZ
- Scapula
  - Left BP07ZZZ
  - Right BP06ZZZ
- Shoulder
  - Left BP09
  - Right BP08
- Sinus
  - Intracranial B502
  - Paranasal B902ZZZ
- Skull BN00ZZZ
- Spinal Cord B00B
- Spine
  - Cervical, Densitometry BR00ZZ1
  - Lumbar, Densitometry BR09ZZ1
  - Thoracic, Densitometry BR07ZZ1
  - Whole, Densitometry BR0GZZ1
- Sternum BR0HZZZ
- Teeth
  - All BN0JZZZ
  - Multiple BN0HZZZ
- Testicle
  - Left BV06
  - Right BV05
- Toe
  - Left BQ0QZZZ
  - Right BQ0PZZZ
- Tooth, Single BN0GZZZ
- Tracheobronchial Tree
  - Bilateral BB09YZZ
  - Left BB08Y
  - Right BB07Y
- Ureter
  - Bilateral BT08
  - Kidney and Bladder BT04
  - Left BT07
  - Right BT06
- Urethra BT05
- Urethra and Bladder BT0B
- Uterus BU06
- Uterus and Fallopian Tube BU08
- Vagina BU09
- Vasa Vasorum BV08
- Vein
  - Cerebellar B501
  - Cerebral B501
  - Epidural B500
  - Jugular
    - Bilateral B505
    - Left B504
    - Right B503
  - Lower Extremity
    - Bilateral B50D
    - Left B50C
    - Right B50B
  - Other B50V
  - Pelvic (Iliac)
    - Left B50G
    - Right B50F
  - Pelvic (Iliac) Bilateral B50H
  - Portal B50T
  - Pulmonary
    - Bilateral B50S
    - Left B50R

Plain Radiography *(continued)*
- Vein *(continued)*
  - Pulmonary *(continued)*
    - Right B50Q
  - Renal
    - Bilateral B50L
    - Left B50K
    - Right B50J
  - Spanchnic B50T
  - Subclavian
    - Left B507
    - Right B506
  - Upper Extremity
    - Bilateral B50P
    - Left B50N
    - Right B50M
- Vena Cava
  - Inferior B509
  - Superior B508
- Whole Body BW0KZZZ
  - Infant BW0MZZZ
- Whole Skeleton BW0LZZZ
- Wrist
  - Left BP0M
  - Right BP0L

Planar Nuclear Medicine Imaging
- Abdomen CW10
- Abdomen and Chest CW14
- Abdomen and Pelvis CW11
- Anatomical Regions, Multiple CW1YYZZ
- Anatomical Region, Other CW1ZZZZ
- Bladder, Kidneys and Ureters CT1
- Bladder and Ureters CT1H
- Blood C713
- Bone Marrow C710
- Brain C010
- Breast CH1YYZZ
  - Bilateral CH12
  - Left CH11
  - Right CH10
- Bronchi and Lungs CB12
- Central Nervous System C01YYZ
- Cerebrospinal Fluid C015
- Chest CW13
- Chest and Abdomen CW14
- Chest and Neck CW16
- Digestive System CD1YYZZ
- Ducts, Lacrimal, Bilateral C819
- Ear, Nose, Mouth and Throat C91YYZZ
- Endocrine System CG1YYZZ
- Extremity
  - Lower CW1D
    - Bilateral CP1F
    - Left CP1D
    - Right CP1C
  - Upper CW1M
    - Bilateral CP1B
    - Left CP19
    - Right CP18
- Eye C81YYZZ
- Gallbladder CF14
- Gastrointestinal Tract CD17
  - Upper CD15
- Gland
  - Adrenal, Bilateral CG14
  - Parathyroid CG11
  - Thyroid CG12
- Glands, Salivary, Bilateral C91B
- Head and Neck CW1B
- Heart C21YYZZ
  - Right and Left C216
- Hepatobiliary System, All CF1C
- Hepatobiliary System and Pancrea
  CF1YYZZ
- Kidneys, Ureters and Bladder CT
- Liver CF15
- Liver and Spleen CF16

- **Planar Nuclear Medicine Imaging** *(continued)*
  - Lungs and Bronchi CB12
  - Lymphatics
    - Head C71J
    - Head and Neck C715
    - Lower Extremity C71P
    - Neck C71K
    - Pelvic C71D
    - Trunk C71M
    - Upper Chest C71L
    - Upper Extremity C71N
  - Lymphatics and Hematologic System C71YYZZ
  - Musculoskeletal System
    - All CP1Z
    - Other CP1YYZZ
  - Myocardium C21G
  - Neck and Chest CW16
  - Neck and Head CW1B
  - Pancreas and Hepatobiliary System CF1YYZZ
  - Pelvic Region CW1J
  - Pelvis CP16
  - Pelvis and Abdomen CW11
  - Pelvis and Spine CP17
  - Reproductive System, Male CV1YYZZ
  - Respiratory System CB1YYZZ
  - Skin CH1YYZZ
  - Skull CP11
  - Spine CP15
  - Spine and Pelvis CP17
  - Spleen C712
  - Spleen and Liver CF16
  - Subcutaneous Tissue CH1YYZZ
  - Testicles, Bilateral CV19
  - Thorax CP14
  - Ureters, Kidneys and Bladder CT13
  - Ureters and Bladder CT1H
  - Urinary System CT1YYZZ
  - Veins C51YYZZ
    - Central C51R
    - Lower Extremity
      - Bilateral C51D
      - Left C51C
      - Right C51B
    - Upper Extremity
      - Bilateral C51Q
      - Left C51P
      - Right C51N
  - Whole Body CW1N
- **Plantar digital vein**
  - *use* Vein, Foot, Left
  - *use* Vein, Foot, Right
- **Plantar fascia (aponeurosis)**
  - *use* Subcutaneous Tissue and Fascia, Foot, Left
  - *use* Subcutaneous Tissue and Fascia, Foot, Right
- **Plantar metatarsal vein**
  - *use* Vein, Foot, Left
  - *use* Vein, Foot, Right
- **Plantar venous arch**
  - *use* Vein, Foot, Left
  - *use* Vein, Foot, Right
- **Plaque Radiation**
  - Abdomen DWY3FZZ
  - Adrenal Gland DGY2FZZ
  - Anus DDY8FZZ
  - Bile Ducts DFY2FZZ
  - Bladder DTY2FZZ
  - Bone, Other DPYCFZZ
  - Bone Marrow D7Y0FZZ
  - Brain D0Y0FZZ
  - Brain Stem D0Y1FZZ
  - Breast
    - Left DMY0FZZ
    - Right DMY1FZZ
  - Bronchus DBY1FZZ
- **Plaque Radiation** *(continued)*
  - Cervix DUY1FZZ
  - Chest DWY2FZZ
  - Chest Wall DBY7FZZ
  - Colon DDY5FZZ
  - Diaphragm DBY8FZZ
  - Duodenum DDY2FZZ
  - Ear D9Y0FZZ
  - Esophagus DDY0FZZ
  - Eye D8Y0FZZ
  - Femur DPY9FZZ
  - Fibula DPYBFZZ
  - Gallbladder DFY1FZZ
  - Gland
    - Adrenal DGY2FZZ
    - Parathyroid DGY4FZZ
    - Pituitary DGY0FZZ
    - Thyroid DGY5FZZ
  - Glands, Salivary D9Y6FZZ
  - Head and Neck DWY1FZZ
  - Hemibody DWY4FZZ
  - Humerus DPY6FZZ
  - Ileum DDY4FZZ
  - Jejunum DDY3FZZ
  - Kidney DTY0FZZ
  - Larynx D9YBFZZ
  - Liver DFY0FZZ
  - Lung DBY2FZZ
  - Lymphatics
    - Abdomen D7Y6FZZ
    - Axillary D7Y4FZZ
    - Inguinal D7Y8FZZ
    - Neck D7Y3FZZ
    - Pelvis D7Y7FZZ
    - Thorax D7Y5FZZ
  - Mandible DPY3FZZ
  - Maxilla DPY2FZZ
  - Mediastinum DBY6FZZ
  - Mouth D9Y4FZZ
  - Nasopharynx D9YDFZZ
  - Neck and Head DWY1FZZ
  - Nerve, Peripheral D0Y7FZZ
  - Nose D9Y1FZZ
  - Ovary DUY0FZZ
  - Palate
    - Hard D9Y8FZZ
    - Soft D9Y9FZZ
  - Pancreas DFY3FZZ
  - Parathyroid Gland DGY4FZZ
  - Pelvic Bones DPY8FZZ
  - Pelvic Region DWY6FZZ
  - Pharynx D9YCFZZ
  - Pineal Body DGY1FZZ
  - Pituitary Gland DGY0FZZ
  - Pleura DBY5FZZ
  - Prostate DVY0FZZ
  - Radius DPY7FZZ
  - Rectum DDY7FZZ
  - Rib DPY5FZZ
  - Sinuses D9Y7FZZ
  - Skin
    - Abdomen DHY8FZZ
    - Arm DHY4FZZ
    - Back DHY7FZZ
    - Buttock DHY9FZZ
    - Chest DHY6FZZ
    - Face DHY2FZZ
    - Foot DHYCFZZ
    - Hand DHY5FZZ
    - Leg DHYBFZZ
    - Neck DHY3FZZ
  - Skull DPY0FZZ
  - Spinal Cord D0Y6FZZ
  - Spleen D7Y2FZZ
  - Sternum DPY4FZZ
  - Stomach DDY1FZZ
  - Testis DVY1FZZ
  - Thymus D7Y1FZZ
  - Thyroid Gland DGY5FZZ
  - Tibia DPYBFZZ
- **Plaque Radiation** *(continued)*
  - Tongue D9Y5FZZ
  - Trachea DBY0FZZ
  - Ulna DPY7FZZ
  - Ureter DTY1FZZ
  - Urethra DTY3FZZ
  - Uterus DUY2FZZ
  - Whole Body DWY5FZZ
- **Plasmapheresis, therapeutic**
  - *see* Pheresis, Physiological Systems 6A5
- **Plateletpheresis, therapeutic**
  - *see* Pheresis, Physiological Systems 6A5
- **Platysma muscle**
  - *use* Muscle, Neck, Left
  - *use* Muscle, Neck, Right
- **Plazomicin Anti-infective** XW0
- **Pleurectomy**
  - *see* Excision, Respiratory System 0BB
  - *see* Resection, Respiratory System 0BT
- **Pleurocentesis**
  - *see* Drainage, Anatomical Regions, General 0W9
- **Pleurodesis, pleurosclerosis**
  - Chemical injection
    - *see* Introduction of substance in or on, Pleural Cavity 3E0L
  - Surgical
    - *see* Destruction, Respiratory System 0B5
- **Pleurolysis**
  - *see* Release, Respiratory System 0BN
- **Pleuroscopy** 0BJQ4ZZ
- **Pleurotomy**
  - *see* Drainage, Respiratory System 0B9
- **Plica semilunaris**
  - *use* Conjunctiva, Left
  - *use* Conjunctiva, Right
- **Plication**
  - *see* Restriction
- **Pneumectomy**
  - *see* Excision, Respiratory System 0BB
  - *see* Resection, Respiratory System 0BT
- **Pneumocentesis**
  - *see* Drainage, Respiratory System 0B9
- **Pneumogastric nerve**
  - *use* Nerve, Vagus
- **Pneumolysis**
  - *see* Release, Respiratory System 0BN
- **Pneumonectomy**
  - *see* Resection, Respiratory System 0BT
- **Pneumonolysis**
  - *see* Release, Respiratory System 0BN
- **Pneumonopexy**
  - *see* Repair, Respiratory System 0BQ
  - *see* Reposition, Respiratory System 0BS
- **Pneumonorrhaphy**
  - *see* Repair, Respiratory System 0BQ
- **Pneumonotomy**
  - *see* Drainage, Respiratory System 0B9
- **Pneumotaxic center**
  - *use* Pons
- **Pneumotomy**
  - *see* Drainage, Respiratory System 0B9
- **Pollicization**
  - *see* Transfer, Anatomical Regions, Upper Extremities 0XX
- **Polyethylene socket**
  - *use* Synthetic Substitute, Polyethylene in 0SR
- **Polymethylmethacrylate (PMMA)**
  - *use* Synthetic Substitute
- **Polypectomy, gastrointestinal**
  - *see* Excision, Gastrointestinal System 0DB
- **Polypropylene mesh**
  - *use* Synthetic Substitute
- **Polysomnogram** 4A1ZXQZ
- **Pontine tegmentum**
  - *use* Pons
- **Popliteal ligament**
  - *use* Bursa and Ligament, Knee, Left
  - *use* Bursa and Ligament, Knee, Right
- **Popliteal lymph node**
  - *use* Lymphatic, Lower Extremity, Left
  - *use* Lymphatic, Lower Extremity, Right
- **Popliteal vein**
  - *use* Vein, Femoral, Left
  - *use* Vein, Femoral, Right
- **Popliteus muscle**
  - *use* Muscle, Lower Leg, Left
  - *use* Muscle, Lower Leg, Right
- **Porcine (bioprosthetic) valve**
  - *use* Zooplastic Tissue in Heart and Great Vessels
- **Positive end expiratory pressure**
  - *see* Performance, Respiratory 5A19
- **Positron Emission Tomographic (PET) Imaging**
  - Brain C030
  - Bronchi and Lungs CB32
  - Central Nervous System C03YYZZ
  - Heart C23YYZZ
  - Lungs and Bronchi CB32
  - Myocardium C23G
  - Respiratory System CB3YYZZ
  - Whole Body CW3NYZZ
- **Positron emission tomography**
  - *see* Positron Emission Tomographic (PET) Imaging
- **Postauricular (mastoid) lymph node**
  - *use* Lymphatic, Neck, Left
  - *use* Lymphatic, Neck, Right
- **Postcava**
  - *use* Vena Cava, Inferior
- **Posterior (subscapular) lymph node**
  - *use* Lymphatic, Axillary, Left
  - *use* Lymphatic, Axillary, Right
- **Posterior auricular artery**
  - *use* Artery, External Carotid, Left
  - *use* Artery, External Carotid, Right
- **Posterior auricular nerve**
  - *use* Nerve, Facial
- **Posterior auricular vein**
  - *use* Vein, External Jugular, Left
  - *use* Vein, External Jugular, Right
- **Posterior cerebral artery**
  - *use* Artery, Intracranial
- **Posterior chamber**
  - *use* Eye, Left
  - *use* Eye, Right
- **Posterior circumflex humeral artery**
  - *use* Artery, Axillary, Left
  - *use* Artery, Axillary, Right
- **Posterior communicating artery**
  - *use* Artery, Intracranial
- **Posterior cruciate ligament (PCL)**
  - *use* Bursa and Ligament, Knee, Left
  - *use* Bursa and Ligament, Knee, Right

Posterior facial (retromandibular) vein
use Vein, Face, Left
use Vein, Face, Right
Posterior femoral cutaneous nerve
use Nerve, Sacral Plexus
Posterior inferior cerebellar artery (PICA)
use Artery, Intracranial
Posterior interosseous nerve
use Nerve, Radial
Posterior labial nerve
use Nerve, Pudendal
Posterior scrotal nerve
use Nerve, Pudendal
Posterior spinal artery
use Artery, Vertebral, Left
use Artery, Vertebral, Right
Posterior tibial recurrent artery
use Artery, Anterior Tibial, Left
use Artery, Anterior Tibial, Right
Posterior ulnar recurrent artery
use Artery, Ulnar, Left
use Artery, Ulnar, Right
Posterior vagal trunk
use Nerve, Vagus
PPN (peripheral parenteral nutrition)
see Introduction of Nutritional Substance
Preauricular lymph node
use Lymphatic, Head
Precava
use Vena Cava, Superior
Prepatellar bursa
use Bursa and Ligament, Knee, Left
use Bursa and Ligament, Knee, Right
Preputiotomy
see Drainage, Male Reproductive System 0V9
Pressure support ventilation
see Performance, Respiratory 5A19
PRESTIGE® Cervical Disc
use Synthetic Substitute
Pretracheal fascia
use Subcutaneous Tissue and Fascia, Neck, Left
use Subcutaneous Tissue and Fascia, Neck, Right
Prevertebral fascia
use Subcutaneous Tissue and Fascia, Neck, Left
use Subcutaneous Tissue and Fascia, Neck, Right
PrimeAdvanced neurostimulator (SureScan)(MRI Safe)
use Stimulator Generator, Multiple Array in 0JH
Princeps pollicis artery
use Artery, Hand, Left
use Artery, Hand, Right
Probing, duct
Diagnostic
see Inspection
Dilation
see Dilation
PROCEED™ Ventral Patch
use Synthetic Substitute
Procerus muscle
use Muscle, Facial
Proctectomy
see Excision, Rectum 0DBP
see Resection, Rectum 0DTP
Proctoclysis
see Introduction of substance in or on, Gastrointestinal Tract, Lower 3E0H
Proctocolectomy
see Excision, Gastrointestinal System 0DB
Proctocolectomy *(continued)*
see Resection, Gastrointestinal System 0DT
Proctocolpoplasty
see Repair, Gastrointestinal System 0DQ
see Supplement, Gastrointestinal System 0DU
Proctoperineoplasty
see Repair, Gastrointestinal System 0DQ
see Supplement, Gastrointestinal System 0DU
Proctoperineorrhaphy
see Repair, Gastrointestinal System 0DQ
Proctopexy
see Repair, Rectum 0DQP
see Reposition, Rectum 0DSP
Proctoplasty
see Repair, Rectum 0DQP
see Supplement, Rectum 0DUP
Proctorrhaphy
see Repair, Rectum 0DQP
Proctoscopy 0DJD8ZZ
Proctosigmoidectomy
see Excision, Gastrointestinal System 0DB
see Resection, Gastrointestinal System 0DT
Proctosigmoidoscopy 0DJD8ZZ
Proctostomy
see Drainage, Rectum 0D9P
Proctotomy
see Drainage, Rectum 0D9P
Prodisc-C
use Synthetic Substitute
Prodisc-L
use Synthetic Substitute
Production, atrial septal defect
see Excision, Septum, Atrial 02B5
Profunda brachii
use Artery, Brachial, Left
use Artery, Brachial, Right
Profunda femoris (deep femoral) vein
use Vein, Femoral, Left
use Vein, Femoral, Right
PROLENE Polypropylene Hernia System (PHS)
use Synthetic Substitute
Prolonged intermittent renal replacement therapy (PIRRT) 5A1D80Z
Pronator quadratus muscle
use Muscle, Lower Arm and Wrist, Left
use Muscle, Lower Arm and Wrist, Right
Pronator teres muscle
use Muscle, Lower Arm and Wrist, Left
use Muscle, Lower Arm and Wrist, Right
Prostatectomy
see Excision, Prostate 0VB0
see Resection, Prostate 0VT0
Prostatic urethra
use Urethra
Prostatomy, prostatotomy
see Drainage, Prostate 0V90
Protecta XT CRT-D
use Cardiac Resynchronization Defibrillator Pulse Generator in 0JH
Protecta XT DR (XT VR)
use Defibrillator Generator in 0JH
Protégé® RX Carotid Stent System
use Intraluminal Device
Proximal radioulnar joint
use Joint, Elbow, Left
use Joint, Elbow, Right
Psoas muscle
use Muscle, Hip, Left
use Muscle, Hip, Right
PSV (pressure support ventilation)
see Performance, Respiratory 5A19
Psychoanalysis GZ54ZZZ
Psychological Tests
Cognitive Status GZ14ZZZ
Developmental GZ10ZZZ
Intellectual and Psychoeducational GZ12ZZZ
Neurobehavioral Status GZ14ZZZ
Neuropsychological GZ13ZZZ
Personality and Behavioral GZ11ZZZ
Psychotherapy
Family, Mental Health Services GZ72ZZZ
Group
GZHZZZZ
Mental Health Services GZHZZZZ
Individual
see Psychotherapy, Individual, Mental Health Services
for substance abuse
12-Step HZ53ZZZ
Behavioral HZ51ZZZ
Cognitive HZ50ZZZ
Cognitive-Behavioral HZ52ZZZ
Confrontational HZ58ZZZ
Interactive HZ55ZZZ
Interpersonal HZ54ZZZ
Motivational Enhancement HZ57ZZZ
Psychoanalysis HZ5BZZZ
Psychodynamic HZ5CZZZ
Psychoeducation HZ56ZZZ
Psychophysiological HZ5DZZZ
Supportive HZ59ZZZ
Mental Health Services
Behavioral GZ51ZZZ
Cognitive GZ52ZZZ
Cognitive-Behavioral GZ58ZZZ
Interactive GZ50ZZZ
Interpersonal GZ53ZZZ
Psychoanalysis GZ54ZZZ
Psychodynamic GZ55ZZZ
Psychophysiological GZ59ZZZ
Supportive GZ56ZZZ
PTCA (percutaneous transluminal coronary angioplasty)
see Dilation, Heart and Great Vessels 027
Pterygoid muscle
use Muscle, Head
Pterygoid process
use Bone, Sphenoid
Pterygopalatine (sphenopalatine) ganglion
use Nerve, Head and Neck Sympathetic
Pubis
use Bone, Pelvic, Left
use Bone, Pelvic, Right
Pubofemoral ligament
use Bursa and Ligament, Hip, Left
use Bursa and Ligament, Hip, Right
Pudendal nerve
use Nerve, Sacral Plexus
Pull-through, laparoscopic-assisted transanal
see Excision, Gastrointestinal System 0DB
see Resection, Gastrointestinal System 0DT
Pull-through, rectal
see Resection, Rectum 0DTP
Pulmoaortic canal
use Artery, Pulmonary, Left
Pulmonary annulus
use Valve, Pulmonary
Pulmonary artery wedge monitoring
see Monitoring, Arterial 4A13
Pulmonary plexus
use Nerve, Thoracic Sympathetic
use Nerve, Vagus
Pulmonic valve
use Valve, Pulmonary
Pulpectomy
see Excision, Mouth and Throat 0CB
Pulverization
see Fragmentation
Pulvinar
use Thalamus
Pump reservoir
use Infusion Device, Pump in Subcutaneous Tissue and Fasc
Punch biopsy
see Excision with qualifier Diagnostic
Puncture
see Drainage
Puncture, lumbar
see Drainage, Spinal Canal 009U
Pyelography
see Fluoroscopy, Urinary System BT1
see Plain Radiography, Urinary System BT0
Pyeloileostomy, urinary diversion
see Bypass, Urinary System 0T1
Pyeloplasty
see Repair, Urinary System 0TQ
see Replacement, Urinary System 0TR
see Supplement, Urinary System 0T
Pyelorrhaphy
see Repair, Urinary System 0TQ
Pyeloscopy 0TJ58ZZ
Pyelostomy
see Drainage, Urinary System 0T9
see Bypass, Urinary System 0T1
Pyelotomy
see Drainage, Urinary System 0T9
Pylorectomy
see Excision, Stomach, Pylorus 0D
see Resection, Stomach, Pylorus 0DT7
Pyloric antrum
use Stomach, Pylorus
Pyloric canal
use Stomach, Pylorus
Pyloric sphincter
use Stomach, Pylorus
Pylorodiosis
see Dilation, Stomach, Pylorus 0D
Pylorogastrectomy
see Excision, Gastrointestinal System 0DB
see Resection, Gastrointestinal System 0DT
Pyloroplasty
see Repair, Stomach, Pylorus 0DQ
see Supplement, Stomach, Pyloru 0DU7
Pyloroscopy 0DJ68ZZ
Pylorotomy
see Drainage, Stomach, Pylorus 0D

Pyramidalis muscle
  use Muscle, Abdomen, Left
  use Muscle, Abdomen, Right

Q

Quadrangular cartilage
  use Septum, Nasal
Quadrant resection of breast
  see Excision, Skin and Breast 0HB
Quadrate lobe
  use Liver
Quadratus femoris muscle
  use Muscle, Hip, Left
  use Muscle, Hip, Right
Quadratus lumborum muscle
  use Muscle, Trunk, Left
  use Muscle, Trunk, Right
Quadratus plantae muscle
  use Muscle, Foot, Left
  use Muscle, Foot, Right
Quadriceps (femoris)
  use Muscle, Upper Leg, Left
  use Muscle, Upper Leg, Right
Quarantine 8E0ZXY6

R

Radial collateral carpal ligament
  use Bursa and Ligament, Wrist, Left
  use Bursa and Ligament, Wrist, Right
Radial collateral ligament
  use Bursa and Ligament, Elbow, Left
  use Bursa and Ligament, Elbow, Right
Radial notch
  use Ulna, Left
  use Ulna, Right
Radial recurrent artery
  use Artery, Radial, Left
  use Artery, Radial, Right
Radial vein
  use Vein, Brachial, Left
  use Vein, Brachial, Right
Radialis indicis
  use Artery, Hand, Left
  use Artery, Hand, Right
Radiation Therapy
  see Beam Radiation
  see Brachytherapy
  see Stereotactic Radiosurgery
Radiation treatment
  see Radiation Therapy
Radiocarpal joint
  use Joint, Wrist, Left
  use Joint, Wrist, Right
Radiocarpal ligament
  use Bursa and Ligament, Wrist, Left
  use Bursa and Ligament, Wrist, Right
Radiography
  see Plain Radiography
Radiology, analog
  see Plain Radiography
Radiology, diagnostic
  see Imaging, Diagnostic
Radioulnar ligament
  use Bursa and Ligament, Wrist, Left
  use Bursa and Ligament, Wrist, Right
Range of motion testing
  see Motor Function Assessment, Rehabilitation F01
REALIZE® Adjustable Gastric Band
  use Extraluminal Device
Reattachment
  Abdominal Wall 0WMF0ZZ
  Ampulla of Vater 0FMC
  Ankle Region
    Left 0YML0ZZ
    Right 0YMK0ZZ
  Arm
    Lower
      Left 0XMF0ZZ
      Right 0XMD0ZZ
    Upper
      Left 0XM90ZZ
      Right 0XM80ZZ
  Axilla
    Left 0XM50ZZ
    Right 0XM40ZZ
  Back
    Lower 0WML0ZZ
    Upper 0WMK0ZZ
  Bladder 0TMB
  Bladder Neck 0TMC
  Breast
    Bilateral 0HMVXZZ
    Left 0HMUXZZ
    Right 0HMTXZZ
  Bronchus
    Lingula 0BM90ZZ
    Lower Lobe
      Left 0BMB0ZZ
      Right 0BM60ZZ
    Main
      Left 0BM70ZZ
      Right 0BM30ZZ
    Middle Lobe, Right 0BM50ZZ
    Upper Lobe
      Left 0BM80ZZ
      Right 0BM40ZZ
  Bursa and Ligament
    Abdomen
      Left 0MMJ
      Right 0MMH
    Ankle
      Left 0MMR
      Right 0MMQ
    Elbow
      Left 0MM4
      Right 0MM3
    Foot
      Left 0MMT
      Right 0MMS
    Hand
      Left 0MM8
      Right 0MM7
    Head and Neck 0MM0
    Hip
      Left 0MMM
      Right 0MML
    Knee
      Left 0MMP
      Right 0MMN
    Lower Extremity
      Left 0MMW
      Right 0MMV
    Perineum 0MMK
    Rib(s) 0MMG
    Shoulder
      Left 0MM2
      Right 0MM1
    Spine
      Lower 0MMD
      Upper 0MMC
    Sternum 0MMF
    Upper Extremity
      Left 0MMB
      Right 0MM9
    Wrist
      Left 0MM6
      Right 0MM5
  Buttock
    Left 0YM10ZZ
    Right 0YM00ZZ
  Carina 0BM20ZZ

Reattachment *(continued)*
  Cecum 0DMH
  Cervix 0UMC
  Chest Wall 0WM80ZZ
  Clitoris 0UMJXZZ
  Colon
    Ascending 0DMK
    Descending 0DMM
    Sigmoid 0DMN
    Transverse 0DML
  Cord
    Bilateral 0VMH
    Left 0VMG
    Right 0VMF
  Cul-de-sac 0UMF
  Diaphragm 0BMT0ZZ
  Duct
    Common Bile 0FM9
    Cystic 0FM8
    Hepatic
      Common 0FM7
      Left 0FM6
      Right 0FM5
    Pancreatic 0FMD
      Accessory 0FMF
  Duodenum 0DM9
  Ear
    Left 09M1XZZ
    Right 09M0XZZ
  Elbow Region
    Left 0XMC0ZZ
    Right 0XMB0ZZ
  Esophagus 0DM5
  Extremity
    Lower
      Left 0YMB0ZZ
      Right 0YM90ZZ
    Upper
      Left 0XM70ZZ
      Right 0XM60ZZ
  Eyelid
    Lower
      Left 08MRXZZ
      Right 08MQXZZ
    Upper
      Left 08MPXZZ
      Right 08MNXZZ
  Face 0WM20ZZ
  Fallopian Tube
    Left 0UM6
    Right 0UM5
  Fallopian Tubes, Bilateral 0UM7
  Femoral Region
    Left 0YM80ZZ
    Right 0YM70ZZ
  Finger
    Index
      Left 0XMP0ZZ
      Right 0XMN0ZZ
    Little
      Left 0XMW0ZZ
      Right 0XMV0ZZ
    Middle
      Left 0XMR0ZZ
      Right 0XMQ0ZZ
    Ring
      Left 0XMT0ZZ
      Right 0XMS0ZZ
  Foot
    Left 0YMN0ZZ
    Right 0YMM0ZZ
  Forequarter
    Left 0XM10ZZ
    Right 0XM00ZZ
  Gallbladder 0FM4
  Gland
    Left 0GM2
    Right 0GM3
  Hand
    Left 0XMK0ZZ

Reattachment *(continued)*
  Hand *(continued)*
    Right 0XMJ0ZZ
  Hindquarter
    Bilateral 0YM40ZZ
    Left 0YM30ZZ
    Right 0YM20ZZ
  Hymen 0UMK
  Ileum 0DMB
  Inguinal Region
    Left 0YM60ZZ
    Right 0YM50ZZ
  Intestine
    Large 0DME
      Left 0DMG
      Right 0DMF
    Small 0DM8
  Jaw
    Lower 0WM50ZZ
    Upper 0WM40ZZ
  Jejunum 0DMA
  Kidney
    Left 0TM1
    Right 0TM0
  Kidney Pelvis
    Left 0TM4
    Right 0TM3
  Kidneys, Bilateral 0TM2
  Knee Region
    Left 0YMG0ZZ
    Right 0YMF0ZZ
  Leg
    Lower
      Left 0YMJ0ZZ
      Right 0YMH0ZZ
    Upper
      Left 0YMD0ZZ
      Right 0YMC0ZZ
  Lip
    Lower 0CM10ZZ
    Upper 0CM00ZZ
  Liver 0FM0
    Left Lobe 0FM2
    Right Lobe 0FM1
  Lung
    Left 0BML0ZZ
    Lower Lobe
      Left 0BMJ0ZZ
      Right 0BMF0ZZ
    Middle Lobe, Right 0BMD0ZZ
    Right 0BMK0ZZ
    Upper Lobe
      Left 0BMG0ZZ
      Right 0BMC0ZZ
  Lung Lingula 0BMH0ZZ
  Muscle
    Abdomen
      Left 0KML
      Right 0KMK
    Facial 0KM1
    Foot
      Left 0KMW
      Right 0KMV
    Hand
      Left 0KMD
      Right 0KMC
    Head 0KM0
    Hip
      Left 0KMP
      Right 0KMN
    Lower Arm and Wrist
      Left 0KMB
      Right 0KM9
    Lower Leg
      Left 0KMT
      Right 0KMS
    Neck
      Left 0KM3
      Right 0KM2
    Perineum 0KMM

Reattachment *(continued)*
- Muscle *(continued)*
  - Shoulder
    - Left 0KM6
    - Right 0KM5
  - Thorax
    - Left 0KMJ
    - Right 0KMH
  - Tongue, Palate, Pharynx 0KM4
  - Trunk
    - Left 0KMG
    - Right 0KMF
  - Upper Arm
    - Left 0KM8
    - Right 0KM7
  - Upper Leg
    - Left 0KMR
    - Right 0KMQ
- Nasal Mucosa and Soft Tissue 09MKXZZ
- Neck 0WM60ZZ
- Nipple
  - Left 0HMXXZZ
  - Right 0HMWXZZ
- Ovary
  - Bilateral 0UM2
  - Left 0UM1
  - Right 0UM0
- Palate, Soft 0CM30ZZ
- Pancreas 0FMG
- Parathyroid Gland 0GMR
  - Inferior
    - Left 0GMP
    - Right 0GMN
  - Multiple 0GMQ
  - Superior
    - Left 0GMM
    - Right 0GML
- Penis 0VMSXZZ
- Perineum
  - Female 0WMN0ZZ
  - Male 0WMM0ZZ
- Rectum 0DMP
- Scrotum 0VM5XZZ
- Shoulder Region
  - Left 0XM30ZZ
  - Right 0XM20ZZ
- Skin
  - Abdomen 0HM7XZZ
  - Back 0HM6XZZ
  - Buttock 0HM8XZZ
  - Chest 0HM5XZZ
  - Ear
    - Left 0HM3XZZ
    - Right 0HM2XZZ
  - Face 0HM1XZZ
  - Foot
    - Left 0HMNXZZ
    - Right 0HMMXZZ
  - Hand
    - Left 0HMGXZZ
    - Right 0HMFXZZ
  - Inguinal 0HMAXZZ
  - Lower Arm
    - Left 0HMEXZZ
    - Right 0HMDXZZ
  - Lower Leg
    - Left 0HMLXZZ
    - Right 0HMKXZZ
  - Neck 0HM4XZZ
  - Perineum 0HM9XZZ
  - Scalp 0HM0XZZ
  - Upper Arm
    - Left 0HMCXZZ
    - Right 0HMBXZZ
  - Upper Leg
    - Left 0HMJXZZ
    - Right 0HMHXZZ
- Stomach 0DM6

Reattachment *(continued)*
- Tendon
  - Abdomen
    - Left 0LMG
    - Right 0LMF
  - Ankle
    - Left 0LMT
    - Right 0LMS
  - Foot
    - Left 0LMW
    - Right 0LMV
  - Hand
    - Left 0LM8
    - Right 0LM7
  - Head and Neck 0LM0
  - Hip
    - Left 0LMK
    - Right 0LMJ
  - Knee
    - Left 0LMR
    - Right 0LMQ
  - Lower Arm and Wrist
    - Left 0LM6
    - Right 0LM5
  - Lower Leg
    - Left 0LMP
    - Right 0LMN
  - Perineum 0LMH
  - Shoulder
    - Left 0LM2
    - Right 0LM1
  - Thorax
    - Left 0LMD
    - Right 0LMC
  - Trunk
    - Left 0LMB
    - Right 0LM9
  - Upper Arm
    - Left 0LM4
    - Right 0LM3
  - Upper Leg
    - Left 0LMM
    - Right 0LML
- Testis
  - Bilateral 0VMC
  - Left 0VMB
  - Right 0VM9
- Thumb
  - Left 0XMM0ZZ
  - Right 0XML0ZZ
- Thyroid Gland
  - Left Lobe 0GMG
  - Right Lobe 0GMH
- Toe
  - 1st
    - Left 0YMQ0ZZ
    - Right 0YMP0ZZ
  - 2nd
    - Left 0YMS0ZZ
    - Right 0YMR0ZZ
  - 3rd
    - Left 0YMU0ZZ
    - Right 0YMT0ZZ
  - 4th
    - Left 0YMW0ZZ
    - Right 0YMV0ZZ
  - 5th
    - Left 0YMY0ZZ
    - Right 0YMX0ZZ
- Tongue 0CM70ZZ
- Tooth
  - Lower 0CMX
  - Upper 0CMW
- Trachea 0BM10ZZ
- Tunica Vaginalis
  - Left 0VM7
  - Right 0VM6
- Ureter
  - Left 0TM7

Reattachment *(continued)*
- Ureter *(continued)*
  - Right 0TM6
- Ureters, Bilateral 0TM8
- Urethra 0TMD
- Uterine Supporting Structure 0UM4
- Uterus 0UM9
- Uvula 0CMN0ZZ
- Vagina 0UMG
- Vulva 0UMMXZZ
- Wrist Region
  - Left 0XMH0ZZ
  - Right 0XMG0ZZ

REBOA (resuscitative endovascular balloon occlusion of the aorta) 02LW3DJ 04L03DJ

Rebound HRD® (Hernia Repair Device)
- *use* Synthetic Substitute

Recession
- *see* Repair
- *see* Reposition

Reclosure, disrupted abdominal wall 0WQFXZZ

Reconstruction
- *see* Repair
- *see* Replacement
- *see* Supplement

Rectectomy
- *see* Excision, Rectum 0DBP
- *see* Resection, Rectum 0DTP

Rectocele repair
- *see* Repair, Subcutaneous Tissue and Fascia, Pelvic Region 0JQC

Rectopexy
- *see* Repair, Gastrointestinal System 0DQ
- *see* Reposition, Gastrointestinal System 0DS

Rectoplasty
- *see* Repair, Gastrointestinal System 0DQ
- *see* Supplement, Gastrointestinal System 0DU

Rectorrhaphy
- *see* Repair, Gastrointestinal System 0DQ

Rectoscopy 0DJD8ZZ

Rectosigmoid junction
- *use* Colon, Sigmoid

Rectosigmoidectomy
- *see* Excision, Gastrointestinal System 0DB
- *see* Resection, Gastrointestinal System 0DT

Rectostomy
- *see* Drainage, Rectum 0D9P

Rectotomy
- *see* Drainage, Rectum 0D9P

Rectus abdominis muscle
- *use* Muscle, Abdomen, Left
- *use* Muscle, Abdomen, Right

Rectus femoris muscle
- *use* Muscle, Upper Leg, Left
- *use* Muscle, Upper Leg, Right

Recurrent laryngeal nerve
- *use* Nerve, Vagus

Reduction
- Dislocation
  - *see* Reposition
- Fracture
  - *see* Reposition
- Intussusception, intestinal
  - *see* Reposition, Gastrointestinal System 0DS
- Mammoplasty
  - *see* Excision, Skin and Breast 0HB

Reduction *(continued)*
- Prolapse
  - *see* Reposition
- Torsion
  - *see* Reposition
- Volvulus, gastrointestinal
  - *see* Reposition, Gastrointestinal System 0DS

Refusion
- *see* Fusion

Rehabilitation
- *see* Activities of Daily Living Assessment, Rehabilitation F02
- *see* Activities of Daily Living Treatment, Rehabilitation F08
- *see* Caregiver Training, Rehabilitation F0F
- *see* Cochlear Implant Treatment, Rehabilitation F0B
- *see* Device Fitting, Rehabilitation F0D
- *see* Hearing Treatment, Rehabilitation F09
- *see* Motor Function Assessment, Rehabilitation F01
- *see* Motor Treatment, Rehabilitation F07
- *see* Speech Assessment, Rehabilitation F00
- *see* Speech Treatment, Rehabilitation F06
- *see* Vestibular Treatment, Rehabilitation F0C

Reimplantation
- *see* Reattachment
- *see* Reposition
- *see* Transfer

Reinforcement
- *see* Repair
- *see* Supplement

Relaxation, scar tissue
- *see* Release

Release
- Acetabulum
  - Left 0QN5
  - Right 0QN4
- Adenoids 0CNQ
- Ampulla of Vater 0FNC
- Anal Sphincter 0DNR
- Anterior Chamber
  - Left 08N33ZZ
  - Right 08N23ZZ
- Anus 0DNQ
- Aorta
  - Abdominal 04N0
  - Thoracic
    - Ascending/Arch 02NX
    - Descending 02NW
- Aortic Body 0GND
- Appendix 0DNJ
- Artery
  - Anterior Tibial
    - Left 04NQ
    - Right 04NP
  - Axillary
    - Left 03N6
    - Right 03N5
  - Brachial
    - Left 03N8
    - Right 03N7
  - Celiac 04N1
  - Colic
    - Left 04N7
    - Middle 04N8
    - Right 04N6
  - Common Carotid
    - Left 03NJ
    - Right 03NH
  - Common Iliac
    - Left 04ND

Release *(continued)*
- Artery *(continued)*
  - Common Iliac *(continued)*
    - Right 04NC
  - Coronary
    - Four or More Arteries 02N3
    - One Artery 02N0
    - Three Arteries 02N2
    - Two Arteries 02N1
  - External Carotid
    - Left 03NN
    - Right 03NM
  - External Iliac
    - Left 04NJ
    - Right 04NH
  - Face 03NR
  - Femoral
    - Left 04NL
    - Right 04NK
  - Foot
    - Left 04NW
    - Right 04NV
  - Gastric 04N2
  - Hand
    - Left 03NF
    - Right 03ND
  - Hepatic 04N3
  - Inferior Mesenteric 04NB
  - Innominate 03N2
  - Internal Carotid
    - Left 03NL
    - Right 03NK
  - Internal Iliac
    - Left 04NF
    - Right 04NE
  - Internal Mammary
    - Left 03N1
    - Right 03N0
  - Intracranial 03NG
  - Lower 04NY
  - Peroneal
    - Left 04NU
    - Right 04NT
  - Popliteal
    - Left 04NN
    - Right 04NM
  - Posterior Tibial
    - Left 04NS
    - Right 04NR
  - Pulmonary
    - Left 02NR
    - Right 02NQ
  - Pulmonary Trunk 02NP
  - Radial
    - Left 03NC
    - Right 03NB
  - Renal
    - Left 04NA
    - Right 04N9
  - Splenic 04N4
  - Subclavian
    - Left 03N4
    - Right 03N3
  - Superior Mesenteric 04N5
  - Temporal
    - Left 03NT
    - Right 03NS
  - Thyroid
    - Left 03NV
    - Right 03NU
  - Ulnar
    - Left 03NA
    - Right 03N9
  - Upper 03NY
  - Vertebral
    - Left 03NQ
    - Right 03NP
- Atrium
  - Left 02N7
  - Right 02N6

Release *(continued)*
- Auditory Ossicle
  - Left 09NA
  - Right 09N9
- Basal Ganglia 00N8
- Bladder 0TNB
- Bladder Neck 0TNC
- Bone
  - Ethmoid
    - Left 0NNG
    - Right 0NNF
  - Frontal 0NN1
  - Hyoid 0NNX
  - Lacrimal
    - Left 0NNJ
    - Right 0NNH
  - Nasal 0NNB
  - Occipital 0NN7
  - Palatine
    - Left 0NNL
    - Right 0NNK
  - Parietal
    - Left 0NN4
    - Right 0NN3
  - Pelvic
    - Left 0QN3
    - Right 0QN2
  - Sphenoid 0NNC
  - Temporal
    - Left 0NN6
    - Right 0NN5
  - Zygomatic
    - Left 0NNN
    - Right 0NNM
- Brain 00N0
- Breast
  - Bilateral 0HNV
  - Left 0HNU
  - Right 0HNT
- Bronchus
  - Lingula 0BN9
  - Lower Lobe
    - Left 0BNB
    - Right 0BN6
  - Main
    - Left 0BN7
    - Right 0BN3
  - Middle Lobe, Right 0BN5
  - Upper Lobe
    - Left 0BN8
    - Right 0BN4
- Buccal Mucosa 0CN4
- Bursa and Ligament
  - Abdomen
    - Left 0MNJ
    - Right 0MNH
  - Ankle
    - Left 0MNR
    - Right 0MNQ
  - Elbow
    - Left 0MN4
    - Right 0MN3
  - Foot
    - Left 0MNT
    - Right 0MNS
  - Hand
    - Left 0MN8
    - Right 0MN7
  - Head and Neck 0MN0
  - Hip
    - Left 0MNM
    - Right 0MNL
  - Knee
    - Left 0MNP
    - Right 0MNN
  - Lower Extremity
    - Left 0MNW
    - Right 0MNV
  - Perineum 0MNK
  - Rib(s) 0MNG

Release *(continued)*
- Bursa and Ligament *(continued)*
  - Shoulder
    - Left 0MN2
    - Right 0MN1
  - Spine
    - Lower 0MND
    - Upper 0MNC
  - Sternum 0MNF
  - Upper Extremity
    - Left 0MNB
    - Right 0MN9
  - Wrist
    - Left 0MN6
    - Right 0MN5
- Carina 0BN2
- Carotid Bodies, Bilateral 0GN8
- Carotid Body
  - Left 0GN6
  - Right 0GN7
- Carpal
  - Left 0PNN
  - Right 0PNM
- Cecum 0DNH
- Cerebellum 00NC
- Cerebral Hemisphere 00N7
- Cerebral Meninges 00N1
- Cerebral Ventricle 00N6
- Cervix 0UNC
- Chordae Tendineae 02N9
- Choroid
  - Left 08NB
  - Right 08NA
- Cisterna Chyli 07NL
- Clavicle
  - Left 0PNB
  - Right 0PN9
- Clitoris 0UNJ
- Coccygeal Glomus 0GNB
- Coccyx 0QNS
- Colon
  - Ascending 0DNK
  - Descending 0DNM
  - Sigmoid 0DNN
  - Transverse 0DNL
- Conduction Mechanism 02N8
- Conjunctiva
  - Left 08NTXZZ
  - Right 08NSXZZ
- Cord
  - Bilateral 0VNH
  - Left 0VNG
  - Right 0VNF
- Cornea
  - Left 08N9XZZ
  - Right 08N8XZZ
- Cul-de-sac 0UNF
- Diaphragm 0BNT
- Disc
  - Cervical Vertebral 0RN3
  - Cervicothoracic Vertebral 0RN5
  - Lumbar Vertebral 0SN2
  - Lumbosacral 0SN4
  - Thoracic Vertebral 0RN9
  - Thoracolumbar Vertebral 0RNB
- Duct
  - Common Bile 0FN9
  - Cystic 0FN8
  - Hepatic
    - Common 0FN7
    - Left 0FN6
    - Right 0FN5
  - Lacrimal
    - Left 08NY
    - Right 08NX
  - Pancreatic 0FND
    - Accessory 0FNF
  - Parotid
    - Left 0CNC
    - Right 0CNB

Release *(continued)*
- Duodenum 0DN9
- Dura Mater 00N2
- Ear
  - External
    - Left 09N1
    - Right 09N0
  - External Auditory Canal
    - Left 09N4
    - Right 09N3
  - Inner
    - Left 09NE
    - Right 09ND
  - Middle
    - Left 09N6
    - Right 09N5
- Epididymis
  - Bilateral 0VNL
  - Left 0VNK
  - Right 0VNJ
- Epiglottis 0CNR
- Esophagogastric Junction 0DN4
- Esophagus 0DN5
  - Lower 0DN3
  - Middle 0DN2
  - Upper 0DN1
- Eustachian Tube
  - Left 09NG
  - Right 09NF
- Eye
  - Left 08N1XZZ
  - Right 08N0XZZ
- Eyelid
  - Lower
    - Left 08NR
    - Right 08NQ
  - Upper
    - Left 08NP
    - Right 08NN
- Fallopian Tube
  - Left 0UN6
  - Right 0UN5
- Fallopian Tubes, Bilateral 0UN7
- Femoral Shaft
  - Left 0QN9
  - Right 0QN8
- Femur
  - Lower
    - Left 0QNC
    - Right 0QNB
  - Upper
    - Left 0QN7
    - Right 0QN6
- Fibula
  - Left 0QNK
  - Right 0QNJ
- Finger Nail 0HNQXZZ
- Gallbladder 0FN4
- Gingiva
  - Lower 0CN6
  - Upper 0CN5
- Gland
  - Adrenal
    - Bilateral 0GN4
    - Left 0GN2
    - Right 0GN3
  - Lacrimal
    - Left 08NW
    - Right 08NV
  - Minor Salivary 0CNJ
  - Parotid
    - Left 0CN9
    - Right 0CN8
  - Pituitary 0GN0
  - Sublingual
    - Left 0CNF
    - Right 0CND
  - Submaxillary
    - Left 0CNH
    - Right 0CNG
  - Vestibular 0UNL

Release *(continued)*
- Glenoid Cavity
  - Left 0PN8
  - Right 0PN7
- Glomus Jugulare 0GNC
- Humeral Head
  - Left 0PND
  - Right 0PNC
- Humeral Shaft
  - Left 0PNG
  - Right 0PNF
- Hymen 0UNK
- Hypothalamus 00NA
- Ileocecal Valve 0DNC
- Ileum 0DNB
- Intestine
  - Large 0DNE
    - Left 0DNG
    - Right 0DNF
  - Small 0DN8
- Iris
  - Left 08ND3
  - Right 08NC3
- Jejunum 0DNA
- Joint
  - Acromioclavicular
    - Left 0RNH
    - Right 0RNG
  - Ankle
    - Left 0SNG
    - Right 0SNF
  - Carpal
    - Left 0RNR
    - Right 0RNQ
  - Carpometacarpal
    - Left 0RNT
    - Right 0RNS
  - Cervical Vertebral 0RN1
  - Cervicothoracic Vertebral 0RN4
  - Coccygeal 0SN6
  - Elbow
    - Left 0RNM
    - Right 0RNL
  - Finger Phalangeal
    - Left 0RNX
    - Right 0RNW
  - Hip
    - Left 0SNB
    - Right 0SN9
  - Knee
    - Left 0SND
    - Right 0SNC
  - Lumbar Vertebral 0SN0
  - Lumbosacral 0SN3
  - Metacarpophalangeal
    - Left 0RNV
    - Right 0RNU
  - Metatarsal-Phalangeal
    - Left 0SNN
    - Right 0SNM
  - Occipital-cervical 0RN0
  - Sacrococcygeal 0SN5
  - Sacroiliac
    - Left 0SN8
    - Right 0SN7
  - Shoulder
    - Left 0RNK
    - Right 0RNJ
  - Sternoclavicular
    - Left 0RNF
    - Right 0RNE
  - Tarsal
    - Left 0SNJ
    - Right 0SNH
  - Tarsometatarsal
    - Left 0SNL
    - Right 0SNK
  - Temporomandibular
    - Left 0RND
    - Right 0RNC

Release *(continued)*
- Joint *(continued)*
  - Thoracic Vertebral 0RN6
  - Thoracolumbar Vertebral 0RNA
  - Toe Phalangeal
    - Left 0SNQ
    - Right 0SNP
  - Wrist
    - Left 0RNP
    - Right 0RNN
- Kidney
  - Left 0TN1
  - Right 0TN0
- Kidney Pelvis
  - Left 0TN4
  - Right 0TN3
- Larynx 0CNS
- Lens
  - Left 08NK3ZZ
  - Right 08NJ3ZZ
- Lip
  - Lower 0CN1
  - Upper 0CN0
- Liver 0FN0
  - Left Lobe 0FN2
  - Right Lobe 0FN1
- Lung
  - Bilateral 0BNM
  - Left 0BNL
  - Lower Lobe
    - Left 0BNJ
    - Right 0BNF
  - Middle Lobe, Right 0BND
  - Right 0BNK
  - Upper Lobe
    - Left 0BNG
    - Right 0BNC
- Lung Lingula 0BNH
- Lymphatic
  - Aortic 07ND
  - Axillary
    - Left 07N6
    - Right 07N5
  - Head 07N0
  - Inguinal
    - Left 07NJ
    - Right 07NH
  - Internal Mammary
    - Left 07N9
    - Right 07N8
  - Lower Extremity
    - Left 07NG
    - Right 07NF
  - Mesenteric 07NB
  - Neck
    - Left 07N2
    - Right 07N1
  - Pelvis 07NC
  - Thoracic Duct 07NK
  - Thorax 07N7
  - Upper Extremity
    - Left 07N4
    - Right 07N3
- Mandible
  - Left 0NNV
  - Right 0NNT
- Maxilla 0NNR
- Medulla Oblongata 00ND
- Mesentery 0DNV
- Metacarpal
  - Left 0PNQ
  - Right 0PNP
- Metatarsal
  - Left 0QNP
  - Right 0QNN
- Muscle
  - Abdomen
    - Left 0KNL
    - Right 0KNK

Release *(continued)*
- Muscle *(continued)*
  - Extraocular
    - Left 08NM
    - Right 08NL
  - Facial 0KN1
  - Foot
    - Left 0KNW
    - Right 0KNV
  - Hand
    - Left 0KND
    - Right 0KNC
  - Head 0KN0
  - Hip
    - Left 0KNP
    - Right 0KNN
  - Lower Arm and Wrist
    - Left 0KNB
    - Right 0KN9
  - Lower Leg
    - Left 0KNT
    - Right 0KNS
  - Neck
    - Left 0KN3
    - Right 0KN2
  - Papillary 02ND
  - Perineum 0KNM
  - Shoulder
    - Left 0KN6
    - Right 0KN5
  - Thorax
    - Left 0KNJ
    - Right 0KNH
  - Tongue, Palate, Pharynx 0KN4
  - Trunk
    - Left 0KNG
    - Right 0KNF
  - Upper Arm
    - Left 0KN8
    - Right 0KN7
  - Upper Leg
    - Left 0KNR
    - Right 0KNQ
- Myocardial Bridge
  - *see* Release, Artery, Coronary
- Nasal Mucosa and Soft Tissue 09NK
- Nasopharynx 09NN
- Nerve
  - Abdominal Sympathetic 01NM
  - Abducens 00NL
  - Accessory 00NR
  - Acoustic 00NN
  - Brachial Plexus 01N3
  - Cervical 01N1
  - Cervical Plexus 01N0
  - Facial 00NM
  - Femoral 01ND
  - Glossopharyngeal 00NP
  - Head and Neck Sympathetic 01NK
  - Hypoglossal 00NS
  - Lumbar 01NB
  - Lumbar Plexus 01N9
  - Lumbar Sympathetic 01NN
  - Lumbosacral Plexus 01NA
  - Median 01N5
  - Oculomotor 00NH
  - Olfactory 00NF
  - Optic 00NG
  - Peroneal 01NH
  - Phrenic 01N2
  - Pudendal 01NC
  - Radial 01N6
  - Sacral 01NR
  - Sacral Plexus 01NQ
  - Sacral Sympathetic 01NP
  - Sciatic 01NF

Release *(continued)*
- Nerve *(continued)*
  - Thoracic 01N8
  - Thoracic Sympathetic 01NL
  - Tibial 01NG
  - Trigeminal 00NK
  - Trochlear 00NJ
  - Ulnar 01N4
  - Vagus 00NQ
- Nipple
  - Left 0HNX
  - Right 0HNW
- Nose 09NKZZ
- Omentum 0DNU
- Orbit
  - Left 0NNQ
  - Right 0NNP
- Ovary
  - Bilateral 0UN2
  - Left 0UN1
  - Right 0UN0
- Palate
  - Hard 0CN2
  - Soft 0CN3
- Pancreas 0FNG
- Para-aortic Body 0GN9
- Paraganglion Extremity 0GNF
- Parathyroid Gland 0GNR
  - Inferior
    - Left 0GNP
    - Right 0GNN
  - Multiple 0GNQ
  - Superior
    - Left 0GNM
    - Right 0GNL
- Patella
  - Left 0QNF
  - Right 0QND
- Penis 0VNSZZ
- Pericardium 02NN
- Peritoneum 0DNW
- Phalanx
  - Finger
    - Left 0PNV
    - Right 0PNT
  - Thumb
    - Left 0PNS
    - Right 0PNR
  - Toe
    - Left 0QNR
    - Right 0QNQ
- Pharynx 0CNM
- Pineal Body 0GN1
- Pleura
  - Left 0BNP
  - Right 0BNN
- Pons 00NB
- Prepuce 0VNT
- Prostate 0VN0
- Radius
  - Left 0PNJ
  - Right 0PNH
- Rectum 0DNP
- Retina
  - Left 08NF3ZZ
  - Right 08NE3ZZ
- Retinal Vessel
  - Left 08NH3ZZ
  - Right 08NG3ZZ
- Ribs
  - 1 to 2 0PN1
  - 3 or More 0PN2
- Sacrum 0QN1
- Scapula
  - Left 0PN6
  - Right 0PN5
- Sclera
  - Left 08N7XZZ
  - Right 08N6XZZ
- Scrotum 0VN5

elease *(continued)*
Septum
Atrial 02N5
Nasal 09NM
Ventricular 02NM
Sinus
Accessory 09NP
Ethmoid
Left 09NV
Right 09NU
Frontal
Left 09NT
Right 09NS
Mastoid
Left 09NC
Right 09NB
Maxillary
Left 09NR
Right 09NQ
Sphenoid
Left 09NX
Right 09NW
Skin
Abdomen 0HN7XZZ
Back 0HN6XZZ
Buttock 0HN8XZZ
Chest 0HN5XZZ
Ear
Left 0HN3XZZ
Right 0HN2XZZ
Face 0HN1XZZ
Foot
Left 0HNNXZZ
Right 0HNMXZZ
Hand
Left 0HNGXZZ
Right 0HNFXZZ
Inguinal 0HNAXZZ
Lower Arm
Left 0HNEXZZ
Right 0HNDXZZ
Lower Leg
Left 0HNLXZZ
Right 0HNKXZZ
Neck 0HN4XZZ
Perineum 0HN9XZZ
Scalp 0HN0XZZ
Upper Arm
Left 0HNCXZZ
Right 0HNBXZZ
Upper Leg
Left 0HNJXZZ
Right 0HNHXZZ
Spinal Cord
Cervical 00NW
Lumbar 00NY
Thoracic 00NX
Spinal Meninges 00NT
Spleen 07NP
Sternum 0PN0
Stomach 0DN6
Pylorus 0DN7
Subcutaneous Tissue and Fascia
Abdomen 0JN8
Back 0JN7
Buttock 0JN9
Chest 0JN6
Face 0JN1
Foot
Left 0JNR
Right 0JNQ
Hand
Left 0JNK
Right 0JNJ
Lower Arm
Left 0JNH
Right 0JNG
Lower Leg
Left 0JNP
Right 0JNN

Release *(continued)*
Subcutaneous Tissue and Fascia *(continued)*
Neck
Left 0JN5
Right 0JN4
Pelvic Region 0JNC
Perineum 0JNB
Scalp 0JN0
Upper Arm
Left 0JNF
Right 0JND
Upper Leg
Left 0JNM
Right 0JNL
Tarsal
Left 0QNM
Right 0QNL
Tendon
Abdomen
Left 0LNG
Right 0LNF
Ankle
Left 0LNT
Right 0LNS
Foot
Left 0LNW
Right 0LNV
Hand
Left 0LN8
Right 0LN7
Head and Neck 0LN0
Hip
Left 0LNK
Right 0LNJ
Knee
Left 0LNR
Right 0LNQ
Lower Arm and Wrist
Left 0LN6
Right 0LN5
Lower Leg
Left 0LNP
Right 0LNN
Perineum 0LNH
Shoulder
Left 0LN2
Right 0LN1
Thorax
Left 0LND
Right 0LNC
Trunk
Left 0LNB
Right 0LN9
Upper Arm
Left 0LN4
Right 0LN3
Upper Leg
Left 0LNM
Right 0LNL
Testis
Bilateral 0VNC
Left 0VNB
Right 0VN9
Thalamus 00N9
Thymus 07NM
Thyroid Gland 0GNK
Left Lobe 0GNG
Right Lobe 0GNH
Tibia
Left 0QNH
Right 0QNG
Toe Nail 0HNRXZZ
Tongue 0CN7
Tonsils 0CNP
Tooth
Lower 0CNX
Upper 0CNW
Trachea 0BN1

Release *(continued)*
Tunica Vaginalis
Left 0VN7
Right 0VN6
Turbinate, Nasal 09NL
Tympanic Membrane
Left 09N8
Right 09N7
Ulna
Left 0PNL
Right 0PNK
Ureter
Left 0TN7
Right 0TN6
Urethra 0TND
Uterine Supporting Structure 0UN4
Uterus 0UN9
Uvula 0CNN
Vagina 0UNG
Valve
Aortic 02NF
Mitral 02NG
Pulmonary 02NH
Tricuspid 02NJ
Vas Deferens
Bilateral 0VNQ
Left 0VNP
Right 0VNN
Vein
Axillary
Left 05N8
Right 05N7
Azygos 05N0
Basilic
Left 05NC
Right 05NB
Brachial
Left 05NA
Right 05N9
Cephalic
Left 05NF
Right 05ND
Colic 06N7
Common Iliac
Left 06ND
Right 06NC
Coronary 02N4
Esophageal 06N3
External Iliac
Left 06NG
Right 06NF
External Jugular
Left 05NQ
Right 05NP
Face
Left 05NV
Right 05NT
Femoral
Left 06NN
Right 06NM
Foot
Left 06NV
Right 06NT
Gastric 06N2
Hand
Left 05NH
Right 05NG
Hemiazygos 05N1
Hepatic 06N4
Hypogastric
Left 06NJ
Right 06NH
Inferior Mesenteric 06N6
Innominate
Left 05N4
Right 05N3
Internal Jugular
Left 05NN
Right 05NM
Intracranial 05NL
Lower 06NY

Release *(continued)*
Vein *(continued)*
Portal 06N8
Pulmonary
Left 02NT
Right 02NS
Renal
Left 06NB
Right 06N9
Saphenous
Left 06NQ
Right 06NP
Splenic 06N1
Subclavian
Left 05N6
Right 05N5
Superior Mesenteric 06N5
Upper 05NY
Vertebral
Left 05NS
Right 05NR
Vena Cava
Inferior 06N0
Superior 02NV
Ventricle
Left 02NL
Right 02NK
Vertebra
Cervical 0PN3
Lumbar 0QN0
Thoracic 0PN4
Vesicle
Bilateral 0VN3
Left 0VN2
Right 0VN1
Vitreous
Left 08N53ZZ
Right 08N43ZZ
Vocal Cord
Left 0CNV
Right 0CNT
Vulva 0UNM
Relocation
see Reposition
Removal
Abdominal Wall 2W53X
Anorectal 2Y53X5
Arm
Lower
Left 2W5DX
Right 2W5CX
Upper
Left 2W5BX
Right 2W5AX
Back 2W55X
Chest Wall 2W54X
Ear 2Y52X5Z
Extremity
Lower
Left 2W5MX
Right 2W5LX
Upper
Left 2W59X
Right 2W58X
Face 2W51X
Finger
Left 2W5KX
Right 2W5JX
Foot
Left 2W5TX
Right 2W5SX
Genital Tract, Female 2Y54X5Z
Hand
Left 2W5FX
Right 2W5EX
Head 2W50X
Inguinal Region
Left 2W57X
Right 2W56X

Removal *(continued)*
- Leg
  - Lower
    - Left 2W5RX
    - Right 2W5QX
  - Upper
    - Left 2W5PX
    - Right 2W5NX
- Mouth and Pharynx 2Y50X5Z
- Nasal 2Y51X5Z
- Neck 2W52X
- Thumb
  - Left 2W5HX
  - Right 2W5GX
- Toe
  - Left 2W5VX
  - Right 2W5UX
- Urethra 2Y55X5Z

Removal of device from
- Abdominal Wall 0WPF
- Acetabulum
  - Left 0QP5
  - Right 0QP4
- Anal Sphincter 0DPR
- Anus 0DPQ
- Artery
  - Lower 04PY
  - Upper 03PY
- Back
  - Lower 0WPL
  - Upper 0WPK
- Bladder 0TPB
- Bone
  - Facial 0NPW
  - Lower 0QPY
  - Nasal 0NPB
  - Pelvic
    - Left 0QP3
    - Right 0QP2
  - Upper 0PPY
- Bone Marrow 07PT
- Brain 00P0
- Breast
  - Left 0HPU
  - Right 0HPT
- Bursa and Ligament
  - Lower 0MPY
  - Upper 0MPX
- Carpal
  - Left 0PPN
  - Right 0PPM
- Cavity, Cranial 0WP1
- Cerebral Ventricle 00P6
- Chest Wall 0WP8
- Cisterna Chyli 07PL
- Clavicle
  - Left 0PPB
  - Right 0PP9
- Coccyx 0QPS
- Diaphragm 0BPT
- Disc
  - Cervical Vertebral 0RP3
  - Cervicothoracic Vertebral 0RP5
  - Lumbar Vertebral 0SP2
  - Lumbosacral 0SP4
  - Thoracic Vertebral 0RP9
  - Thoracolumbar Vertebral 0RPB
- Duct
  - Hepatobiliary 0FPB
  - Pancreatic 0FPD
- Ear
  - Inner
    - Left 09PE
    - Right 09PD
  - Left 09PJ
  - Right 09PH
- Epididymis and Spermatic Cord 0VPM
- Esophagus 0DP5

Removal of device from *(continued)*
- Extremity
  - Lower
    - Left 0YPB
    - Right 0YP9
  - Upper
    - Left 0XP7
    - Right 0XP6
- Eye
  - Left 08P1
  - Right 08P0
- Face 0WP2
- Fallopian Tube 0UP8
- Femoral Shaft
  - Left 0QP9
  - Right 0QP8
- Femur
  - Lower
    - Left 0QPC
    - Right 0QPB
  - Upper
    - Left 0QP7
    - Right 0QP6
- Fibula
  - Left 0QPK
  - Right 0QPJ
- Finger Nail 0HPQX
- Gallbladder 0FP4
- Gastrointestinal Tract 0WPP
- Genitourinary Tract 0WPR
- Gland
  - Adrenal 0GP5
  - Endocrine 0GPS
  - Pituitary 0GP0
  - Salivary 0CPA
- Glenoid Cavity
  - Left 0PP8
  - Right 0PP7
- Great Vessel 02PY
- Hair 0HPSX
- Head 0WP0
- Heart 02PA
- Humeral Head
  - Left 0PPD
  - Right 0PPC
- Humeral Shaft
  - Left 0PPG
  - Right 0PPF
- Intestinal Tract
  - Lower 0DPD
  - Upper 0DP0
- Jaw
  - Lower 0WP5
  - Upper 0WP4
- Joint
  - Acromioclavicular
    - Left 0RPH
    - Right 0RPG
  - Ankle
    - Left 0SPG
    - Right 0SPF
  - Carpal
    - Left 0RPR
    - Right 0RPQ
  - Carpometacarpal
    - Left 0RPT
    - Right 0RPS
  - Cervical Vertebral 0RP1
  - Cervicothoracic Vertebral 0RP4
  - Coccygeal 0SP6
  - Elbow
    - Left 0RPM
    - Right 0RPL
  - Finger Phalangeal
    - Left 0RPX
    - Right 0RPW
  - Hip
    - Left 0SPB
      - Acetabular Surface 0SPE

Removal of device from *(continued)*
- Joint *(continued)*
  - Hip *(continued)*
    - Left *(continued)*
      - Femoral Surface 0SPS
    - Right 0SP9
      - Acetabular Surface 0SPA
      - Femoral Surface 0SPR
  - Knee
    - Left 0SPD
      - Femoral Surface 0SPU
      - Tibial Surface 0SPW
    - Right 0SPC
      - Femoral Surface 0SPT
      - Tibial Surface 0SPV
  - Lumbar Vertebral 0SP0
  - Lumbosacral 0SP3
  - Metacarpophalangeal
    - Left 0RPV
    - Right 0RPU
  - Metatarsal-Phalangeal
    - Left 0SPN
    - Right 0SPM
  - Occipital-cervical 0RP0
  - Sacrococcygeal 0SP5
  - Sacroiliac
    - Left 0SP8
    - Right 0SP7
  - Shoulder
    - Left 0RPK
    - Right 0RPJ
  - Sternoclavicular
    - Left 0RPF
    - Right 0RPE
  - Tarsal
    - Left 0SPJ
    - Right 0SPH
  - Tarsometatarsal
    - Left 0SPL
    - Right 0SPK
  - Temporomandibular
    - Left 0RPD
    - Right 0RPC
  - Thoracic Vertebral 0RP6
  - Thoracolumbar Vertebral 0RPA
  - Toe Phalangeal
    - Left 0SPQ
    - Right 0SPP
  - Wrist
    - Left 0RPP
    - Right 0RPN
- Kidney 0TP5
- Larynx 0CPS
- Lens
  - Left 08PK3
  - Right 08PJ3
- Liver 0FP0
- Lung
  - Left 0BPL
  - Right 0BPK
- Lymphatic 07PN
  - Thoracic Duct 07PK
- Mediastinum 0WPC
- Mesentery 0DPV
- Metacarpal
  - Left 0PPQ
  - Right 0PPP
- Metatarsal
  - Left 0QPP
  - Right 0QPN
- Mouth and Throat 0CPY
- Muscle
  - Extraocular
    - Left 08PM
    - Right 08PL
  - Lower 0KPY
  - Upper 0KPX
- Nasal Mucosa and Soft Tissue 09PK
- Neck 0WP6

Removal of device from *(continued)*
- Nerve
  - Cranial 00PE
  - Peripheral 01PY
- Omentum 0DPU
- Ovary 0UP3
- Pancreas 0FPGZ
- Parathyroid Gland 0GPR0
- Patella
  - Left 0QPF
  - Right 0QPD
- Pelvic Cavity 0WPJ
- Penis 0VPS
- Pericardial Cavity 0WPD
- Perineum
  - Female 0WPN
  - Male 0WPM
- Peritoneal Cavity 0WPG
- Peritoneum 0DPW
- Phalanx
  - Finger
    - Left 0PPV
    - Right 0PPT
  - Thumb
    - Left 0PPS
    - Right 0PPR
  - Toe
    - Left 0QPR
    - Right 0QPQ
- Pineal Body 0GP10
- Pleura 0BPQ
- Pleural Cavity
  - Left 0WPB
  - Right 0WP9
- Products of Conception 10P0
- Prostate and Seminal Vesicles 0VP4
- Radius
  - Left 0PPJ
  - Right 0PPH
- Rectum 0DPP1
- Respiratory Tract 0WPQZ
- Retroperitoneum 0WPH
- Ribs
  - 1 to 2 0PP1
  - 3 or More 0PP2
- Sacrum 0QP1
- Scapula
  - Left 0PP6
  - Right 0PP5
- Scrotum and Tunica Vaginalis 0VP8
- Sinus 09PY0
- Skin 0HPPX
- Skull 0NP0
- Spinal Canal 00PU
- Spinal Cord 00PV
- Spleen 07PP
- Sternum 0PP0
- Stomach 0DP6
- Subcutaneous Tissue and Fascia
  - Head and Neck 0JPS
  - Lower Extremity 0JPW
  - Trunk 0JPT
  - Upper Extremity 0JPV
- Tarsal
  - Left 0QPM
  - Right 0QPL
- Tendon
  - Lower 0LPY
  - Upper 0LPX
- Testis 0VPD
- Thymus 07PM
- Thyroid Gland 0GPK0
- Tibia
  - Left 0QPH
  - Right 0QPG
- Toe Nail 0HPRXZ
- Trachea 0BP1
- Tracheobronchial Tree 0BP0

emoval of device from *(continued)*
  Tympanic Membrane
    Left 09P80
    Right 09P70
  Ulna
    Left 0PPL
    Right 0PPK
  Ureter 0TP9
  Urethra 0TPD
  Uterus and Cervix 0UPD
  Vagina and Cul-de-sac 0UPH
  Vas Deferens 0VPR
  Vein
    Azygos 05P0
    Innominate
      Left 05P4
      Right 05P3
    Lower 06PY
    Upper 05PY
  Vertebra
    Cervical 0PP3
    Lumbar 0QP0
    Thoracic 0PP4
  Vulva 0UPM
enal calyx
  use Kidney
  use Kidneys, Bilateral
  use Kidney, Left
  use Kidney, Right
enal capsule
  use Kidney
  use Kidneys, Bilateral
  use Kidney, Left
  use Kidney, Right
enal cortex
  use Kidney
  use Kidneys, Bilateral
  use Kidney, Left
  use Kidney, Right
enal dialysis
  see Performance, Urinary 5A1D
enal plexus
  use Nerve, Abdominal Sympathetic
enal segment
  use Kidney
  use Kidneys, Bilateral
  use Kidney, Left
  use Kidney, Right
enal segmental artery
  use Artery, Renal, Left
  use Artery, Renal, Right
eopening, operative site
  Control of bleeding
    see Control bleeding in
  Inspection only
    see Inspection
epair
  Abdominal Wall 0WQF
  Acetabulum
    Left 0QQ5
    Right 0QQ4
  Adenoids 0CQQ
  Ampulla of Vater 0FQC
  Anal Sphincter 0DQR
  Ankle Region
    Left 0YQL
    Right 0YQK
  Anterior Chamber
    Left 08Q33
    Right 08Q23
  Anus 0DQQ
  Aorta
    Abdominal 04Q0
    Thoracic
      Ascending/Arch 02QX
      Descending 02QW
  Aortic Body 0GQD
  Appendix 0DQJ
Repair *(continued)*
  Arm
    Lower
      Left 0XQF
      Right 0XQD
    Upper
      Left 0XQ9
      Right 0XQ8
  Artery
    Anterior Tibial
      Left 04QQ
      Right 04QP
    Axillary
      Left 03Q6
      Right 03Q5
    Brachial
      Left 03Q8
      Right 03Q7
    Celiac 04Q1
    Colic
      Left 04Q7
      Middle 04Q8
      Right 04Q6
    Common Carotid
      Left 03QJ
      Right 03QH
    Common Iliac
      Left 04QD
      Right 04QC
    Coronary
      Four or More Arteries 02Q3
      One Artery 02Q0
      Three Arteries 02Q2
      Two Arteries 02Q1
    External Carotid
      Left 03QN
      Right 03QM
    External Iliac
      Left 04QJ
      Right 04QH
    Face 03QR
    Femoral
      Left 04QL
      Right 04QK
    Foot
      Left 04QW
      Right 04QV
    Gastric 04Q2
    Hand
      Left 03QF
      Right 03QD
    Hepatic 04Q3
    Inferior Mesenteric 04QB
    Innominate 03Q2
    Internal Carotid
      Left 03QL
      Right 03QK
    Internal Iliac
      Left 04QF
      Right 04QE
    Internal Mammary
      Left 03Q1
      Right 03Q0
    Intracranial 03QG
    Lower 04QY
    Peroneal
      Left 04QU
      Right 04QT
    Popliteal
      Left 04QN
      Right 04QM
    Posterior Tibial
      Left 04QS
      Right 04QR
    Pulmonary
      Left 02QR
      Right 02QQ
Repair *(continued)*
  Artery *(continued)*
    Pulmonary Trunk 02QP
    Radial
      Left 03QC
      Right 03QB
    Renal
      Left 04QA
      Right 04Q9
    Splenic 04Q4
    Subclavian
      Left 03Q4
      Right 03Q3
    Superior Mesenteric 04Q5
    Temporal
      Left 03QT
      Right 03QS
    Thyroid
      Left 03QV
      Right 03QU
    Ulnar
      Left 03QA
      Right 03Q9
    Upper 03QY
    Vertebral
      Left 03QQ
      Right 03QP
  Atrium
    Left 02Q7
    Right 02Q6
  Auditory Ossicle
    Left 09QA
    Right 09Q9
  Axilla
    Left 0XQ5
    Right 0XQ4
  Back
    Lower 0WQL
    Upper 0WQK
  Basal Ganglia 00Q8
  Bladder 0TQB
  Bladder Neck 0TQC
  Bone
    Ethmoid
      Left 0NQG
      Right 0NQF
    Frontal 0NQ1
    Hyoid 0NQX
    Lacrimal
      Left 0NQJ
      Right 0NQH
    Nasal 0NQB
    Occipital 0NQ7
    Palatine
      Left 0NQL
      Right 0NQK
    Parietal
      Left 0NQ4
      Right 0NQ3
    Pelvic
      Left 0QQ3
      Right 0QQ2
    Sphenoid 0NQC
    Temporal
      Left 0NQ6
      Right 0NQ
    Zygomatic
      Left 0NQN
      Right 0NQM
  Brain 00Q0
  Breast
    Bilateral 0HQV
    Left 0HQU
    Right 0HQT
    Supernumerary 0HQY
  Bronchus
    Lingula 0BQ9
Repair *(continued)*
  Bronchus *(continued)*
    Lower Lobe
      Left 0BQB
      Right 0BQ6
    Main
      Left 0BQ7
      Right 0BQ3
    Middle Lobe, Right 0BQ5
    Upper Lobe
      Left 0BQ8
      Right 0BQ4
  Buccal Mucosa 0CQ4
  Bursa and Ligament
    Abdomen
      Left 0MQJ
      Right 0MQH
    Ankle
      Left 0MQR
      Right 0MQQ
    Elbow
      Left 0MQ4
      Right 0MQ3
    Foot
      Left 0MQT
      Right 0MQS
    Hand
      Left 0MQ8
      Right 0MQ7
    Head and Neck 0MQ0
    Hip
      Left 0MQM
      Right 0MQL
    Knee
      Left 0MQP
      Right 0MQN
    Lower Extremity
      Left 0MQW
      Right 0MQV
    Perineum 0MQK
    Rib(s) 0MQG
    Shoulder
      Left 0MQ2
      Right 0MQ1
    Spine
      Lower 0MQD
      Upper 0MQC
    Sternum 0MQF
    Upper Extremity
      Left 0MQB
      Right 0MQ9
    Wrist
      Left 0MQ6
      Right 0MQ5
  Buttock
    Left 0YQ1
    Right 0YQ0
  Carina 0BQ2
  Carotid Bodies, Bilateral 0GQ8
  Carotid Body
    Left 0GQ6
    Right 0GQ7
  Carpal
    Left 0PQN
    Right 0PQM
  Cecum 0DQH
  Cerebellum 00QC
  Cerebral Hemisphere 00Q7
  Cerebral Meninges 00Q1
  Cerebral Ventricle 00Q6
  Cervix 0UQC
  Chest Wall 0WQ8
  Chordae Tendineae 02Q9
  Choroid
    Left 08QB
    Right 08QA
  Cisterna Chyli 07QL
  Clavicle
    Left 0PQB
    Right 0PQ9

Repair *(continued)*
- Clitoris 0UQJ
- Coccygeal Glomus 0GQB
- Coccyx 0QQS
- Colon
  - Ascending 0DQK
  - Descending 0DQM
  - Sigmoid 0DQN
  - Transverse 0DQL
- Conduction Mechanism 02Q8
- Conjunctiva
  - Left 08QTXZZ
  - Right 08QSXZZ
- Cord
  - Bilateral 0VQH
  - Left 0VQG
  - Right 0VQF
- Cornea
  - Left 08Q9XZZ
  - Right 08Q8XZZ
- Cul-de-sac 0UQF
- Diaphragm 0BQT
- Disc
  - Cervical Vertebral 0RQ3
  - Cervicothoracic Vertebral 0RQ5
  - Lumbar Vertebral 0SQ2
  - Lumbosacral 0SQ4
  - Thoracic Vertebral 0RQ9
  - Thoracolumbar Vertebral 0RQB
- Duct
  - Common Bile 0FQ9
  - Cystic 0FQ8
  - Hepatic
    - Common 0FQ7
    - Left 0FQ6
    - Right 0FQ5
  - Lacrimal
    - Left 08QY
    - Right 08QX
  - Pancreatic 0FQD
    - Accessory 0FQF
  - Parotid
    - Left 0CQC
    - Right 0CQB
- Duodenum 0DQ9
- Dura Mater 00Q2
- Ear
  - External
    - Bilateral 09Q2
    - Left 09Q1
    - Right 09Q0
  - External Auditory Canal
    - Left 09Q4
    - Right 09Q3
  - Inner
    - Left 09QE
    - Right 09QD
  - Middle
    - Left 09Q6
    - Right 09Q5
- Elbow Region
  - Left 0XQC
  - Right 0XQB
- Epididymis
  - Bilateral 0VQL
  - Left 0VQK
  - Right 0VQJ
- Epiglottis 0CQR
- Esophagogastric Junction 0DQ4
- Esophagus 0DQ5
  - Lower 0DQ3
  - Middle 0DQ2
  - Upper 0DQ1
- Eustachian Tube
  - Left 09QG
  - Right 09QF
- Extremity
  - Lower
    - Left 0YQB
    - Right 0YQ9

Repair *(continued)*
- Extremity *(continued)*
  - Upper
    - Left 0XQ7
    - Right 0XQ6
- Eye
  - Left 08Q1XZZ
  - Right 08Q0XZZ
- Eyelid
  - Lower
    - Left 08QR
    - Right 08QQ
  - Upper
    - Left 08QP
    - Right 08QN
- Face 0WQ2
- Fallopian Tube
  - Left 0UQ6
  - Right 0UQ5
- Fallopian Tubes, Bilateral 0UQ7
- Femoral Region
  - Bilateral 0YQE
  - Left 0YQ8
  - Right 0YQ7
- Femoral Shaft
  - Left 0QQ9
  - Right 0QQ8
- Femur
  - Lower
    - Left 0QQC
    - Right 0QQB
  - Upper
    - Left 0QQ7
    - Right 0QQ6
- Fibula
  - Left 0QQK
  - Right 0QQJ
- Finger
  - Index
    - Left 0XQP
    - Right 0XQN
  - Little
    - Left 0XQW
    - Right 0XQV
  - Middle
    - Left 0XQR
    - Right 0XQQ
  - Ring
    - Left 0XQT
    - Right 0XQS
- Finger Nail 0HQQXZZ
- Floor of mouth
  - *see* Repair, Oral Cavity and Throat 0WQ3
- Foot
  - Left 0YQN
  - Right 0YQM
- Gallbladder 0FQ4
- Gingiva
  - Lower 0CQ6
  - Upper 0CQ5
- Gland
  - Adrenal
    - Bilateral 0GQ4
    - Left 0GQ2
    - Right 0GQ3
  - Lacrimal
    - Left 08QW
    - Right 08QV
  - Minor Salivary 0CQJ
  - Parotid
    - Left 0CQ9
    - Right 0CQ8
  - Pituitary 0GQ0
  - Sublingual
    - Left 0CQF
    - Right 0CQD
  - Submaxillary
    - Left 0CQH
    - Right 0CQG

Repair *(continued)*
- Gland *(continued)*
  - Vestibular 0UQL
- Glenoid Cavity
  - Left 0PQ8
  - Right 0PQ7
- Glomus Jugulare 0GQC
- Hand
  - Left 0XQK
  - Right 0XQJ
- Head 0WQ0
- Heart 02QA
  - Left 02QC
  - Right 02QB
- Humeral Head
  - Left 0PQD
  - Right 0PQC
- Humeral Shaft
  - Left 0PQG
  - Right 0PQF
- Hymen 0UQK
- Hypothalamus 00QA
- Ileocecal Valve 0DQC
- Ileum 0DQB
- Inguinal Region
  - Bilateral 0YQA
  - Left 0YQ6
  - Right 0YQ5
- Intestine
  - Large 0DQE
    - Left 0DQG
    - Right 0DQF
  - Small 0DQ8
- Iris
  - Left 08QD3ZZ
  - Right 08QC3ZZ
- Jaw
  - Lower 0WQ5
  - Upper 0WQ4
- Jejunum 0DQA
- Joint
  - Acromioclavicular
    - Left 0RQH
    - Right 0RQG
  - Ankle
    - Left 0SQG
    - Right 0SQF
  - Carpal
    - Left 0RQR
    - Right 0RQQ
  - Carpometacarpal
    - Left 0RQT
    - Right 0RQS
  - Cervical Vertebral 0RQ1
  - Cervicothoracic Vertebral 0RQ4
  - Coccygeal 0SQ6
  - Elbow
    - Left 0RQM
    - Right 0RQL
  - Finger Phalangeal
    - Left 0RQX
    - Right 0RQW
  - Hip
    - Left 0SQB
    - Right 0SQ9
  - Knee
    - Left 0SQD
    - Right 0SQC
  - Lumbar Vertebral 0SQ0
  - Lumbosacral 0SQ3
  - Metacarpophalangeal
    - Left 0RQV
    - Right 0RQU
  - Metatarsal-Phalangeal
    - Left 0SQN
    - Right 0SQM
  - Occipital-cervical 0RQ0
  - Sacrococcygeal 0SQ5

Repair *(continued)*
- Joint *(continued)*
  - Sacroiliac
    - Left 0SQ8
    - Right 0SQ7
  - Shoulder
    - Left 0RQK
    - Right 0RQJ
  - Sternoclavicular
    - Left 0RQF
    - Right 0RQE
  - Tarsal
    - Left 0SQJ
    - Right 0SQH
  - Tarsometatarsal
    - Left 0SQL
    - Right 0SQK
  - Temporomandibular
    - Left 0RQD
    - Right 0RQC
  - Thoracic Vertebral 0RQ6
  - Thoracolumbar Vertebral 0RQ
  - Toe Phalangeal
    - Left 0SQQ
    - Right 0SQP
  - Wrist
    - Left 0RQP
    - Right 0RQN
- Kidney
  - Left 0TQ1
  - Right 0TQ0
- Kidney Pelvis
  - Left 0TQ4
  - Right 0TQ3
- Knee Region
  - Left 0YQG
  - Right 0YQF
- Larynx 0CQS
- Leg
  - Lower
    - Left 0YQJ
    - Right 0YQH
  - Upper
    - Left 0YQD
    - Right 0YQC
- Lens
  - Left 08QK3ZZ
  - Right 08QJ3ZZ
- Lip
  - Lower 0CQ1
  - Upper 0CQ0
- Liver 0FQ0
  - Left Lobe 0FQ2
  - Right Lobe 0FQ1
- Lung
  - Bilateral 0BQM
  - Left 0BQL
  - Lower Lobe
    - Left 0BQJ
    - Right 0BQF
  - Middle Lobe, Right 0BQD
  - Right 0BQK
  - Upper Lobe
    - Left 0BQG
    - Right 0BQC
- Lung Lingula 0BQH
- Lymphatic
  - Aortic 07QD
  - Axillary
    - Left 07Q6
    - Right 07Q5
  - Head 07Q0
  - Inguinal
    - Left 07QJ
    - Right 07QH
  - Internal Mammary
    - Left 07Q9
    - Right 07Q8
  - Lower Extremity
    - Left 07QG

Repair *(continued)*
- Lymphatic *(continued)*
  - Lower Extremity *(continued)*
    - Right 07QF
  - Mesenteric 07QB
  - Neck
    - Left 07Q2
    - Right 07Q1
  - Pelvis 07QC
  - Thoracic Duct 07QK
  - Thorax 07Q7
  - Upper Extremity
    - Left 07Q4
    - Right 07Q3
- Mandible
  - Left 0NQV
  - Right 0NQT
- Maxilla 0NQR
- Mediastinum 0WQC
- Medulla Oblongata 00QD
- Mesentery 0DQV
- Metacarpal
  - Left 0PQQ
  - Right 0PQP
- Metatarsal
  - Left 0QQP
  - Right 0QQN
- Muscle
  - Abdomen
    - Left 0KQL
    - Right 0KQK
  - Extraocular
    - Left 08QM
    - Right 08QL
  - Facial 0KQ1
  - Foot
    - Left 0KQW
    - Right 0KQV
  - Hand
    - Left 0KQD
- Right 0KQC
  - Head 0KQ0
  - Hip
    - Left 0KQP
    - Right 0KQN
  - Lower Arm and Wrist
    - Left 0KQB
    - Right 0KQ9
  - Lower Leg
    - Left 0KQT
    - Right 0KQS
  - Neck
    - Left 0KQ3
    - Right 0KQ2
  - Papillary 02QD
  - Perineum 0KQM
  - Shoulder
    - Left 0KQ6
    - Right 0KQ5
  - Thorax
    - Left 0KQJ
    - Right 0KQH
  - Tongue, Palate, Pharynx 0KQ4
  - Trunk
    - Left 0KQG
    - Right 0KQF
  - Upper Arm
    - Left 0KQ8
    - Right 0KQ7
  - Upper Leg
    - Left 0KQR
    - Right 0KQQ
- Nasal Mucosa and Soft Tissue 09QK
- Nasopharynx 09QN
- Neck 0WQ6
- Nerve
  - Abdominal Sympathetic 01QM
  - Abducens 00QL

Repair *(continued)*
- Nerve *(continued)*
  - Accessory 00QR
  - Acoustic 00QN
  - Brachial Plexus 01Q3
  - Cervical 01Q1
  - Cervical Plexus 01Q0
  - Facial 00QM
  - Femoral 01QD
  - Glossopharyngeal 00QP
  - Head and Neck Sympathetic 01QK
  - Hypoglossal 00QS
  - Lumbar 01QB
  - Lumbar Plexus 01Q9
  - Lumbar Sympathetic 01QN
  - Lumbosacral Plexus 01QA
  - Median 01Q5
  - Oculomotor 00QH
  - Olfactory 00QF
  - Optic 00QG
  - Peroneal 01QH
  - Phrenic 01Q2
  - Pudendal 01QC
  - Radial 01Q6
  - Sacral 01QR
  - Sacral Plexus 01QQ
  - Sacral Sympathetic 01QP
  - Sciatic 01QF
  - Thoracic 01Q8
  - Thoracic Sympathetic 01QL
  - Tibial 01QG
  - Trigeminal 00QK
  - Trochlear 00QJ
  - Ulnar 01Q4
  - Vagus 00QQ
- Nipple
  - Left 0HQX
  - Right 0HQW
- Omentum 0DQU
- Oral Cavity and Throat 0WQ3
- Orbit
  - Left 0NQQ
  - Right 0NQP
- Ovary
  - Bilateral 0UQ2
  - Left 0UQ1
  - Right 0UQ0
- Palate
  - Hard 0CQ2
  - Soft 0CQ3
- Pancreas 0FQG
- Para-aortic Body 0GQ9
- Paraganglion Extremity 0GQF
- Parathyroid Gland 0GQR
  - Inferior
    - Left 0GQP
    - Right 0GQN
  - Multiple 0GQQ
  - Superior
    - Left 0GQM
    - Right 0GQL
- Patella
  - Left 0QQF
  - Right 0QQD
- Penis 0VQS
- Pericardium 02QN
- Perineum
  - Female 0WQN
  - Male 0WQM
- Peritoneum 0DQW
- Phalanx
  - Finger
    - Left 0PQV
    - Right 0PQT
  - Thumb
    - Left 0PQS
    - Right 0PQR

Repair *(continued)*
- Phalanx *(continued)*
  - Toe
    - Left 0QQR
    - Right 0QQQ
- Pharynx 0CQM
- Pineal Body 0GQ1
- Pleura
  - Left 0BQP
  - Right 0BQN
- Pons 00QB
- Prepuce 0VQT
- Products of Conception 10Q0
- Prostate 0VQ0
- Radius
  - Left 0PQJ
  - Right 0PQH
- Rectum 0DQP
- Retina
  - Left 08QF3ZZ
  - Right 08QE3ZZ
- Retinal Vessel
  - Left 08QH3ZZ
  - Right 08QG3ZZ
- Ribs
  - 1 to 2 0PQ1
  - 3 or More 0PQ2
- Sacrum 0QQ1
- Scapula
  - Left 0PQ6
  - Right 0PQ5
- Sclera
  - Left 08Q7XZZ
  - Right 08Q6XZZ
- Scrotum 0VQ5
- Septum
  - Atrial 02Q5
  - Nasal 09QM
  - Ventricular 02QM
- Shoulder Region
  - Left 0XQ3
  - Right 0XQ2
- Sinus
  - Accessory 09QP
  - Ethmoid
    - Left 09QV
    - Right 09QU
  - Frontal
    - Left 09QT
    - Right 09QS
  - Mastoid
    - Left 09QC
    - Right 09QB
  - Maxillary
    - Left 09QR
    - Right 09QQ
  - Sphenoid
    - Left 09QX
    - Right 09QW
- Skin
  - Abdomen 0HQ7XZZ
  - Back 0HQ6XZZ
  - Buttock 0HQ8XZZ
  - Chest 0HQ5XZZ
  - Ear
    - Left 0HQ3XZZ
    - Right 0HQ2XZZ
  - Face 0HQ1XZZ
  - Foot
    - Left 0HQNXZZ
    - Right 0HQMXZZ
  - Hand
    - Left 0HQGXZZ
    - Right 0HQFXZZ
  - Inguinal 0HQAXZZ
  - Lower Arm
    - Left 0HQEXZZ
    - Right 0HQDXZZ

Repair *(continued)*
- Skin *(continued)*
  - Lower Leg
    - Left 0HQLXZZ
    - Right 0HQKXZZ
  - Neck 0HQ4XZZ
  - Perineum 0HQ9XZZ
  - Scalp 0HQ0XZZ
  - Upper Arm
    - Left 0HQCXZZ
    - Right 0HQBXZZ
  - Upper Leg
    - Left 0HQJXZZ
    - Right 0HQHXZZ
- Skull 0NQ0
- Spinal Cord
  - Cervical 00QW
  - Lumbar 00QY
  - Thoracic 00QX
- Spinal Meninges 00QT
- Spleen 07QP
- Sternum 0PQ0
- Stomach 0DQ6
  - Pylorus 0DQ7
- Subcutaneous Tissue and Fascia
  - Abdomen 0JQ8
  - Back 0JQ7
  - Buttock 0JQ9
  - Chest 0JQ6
  - Face 0JQ1
  - Foot
    - Left 0JQR
    - Right 0JQQ
  - Hand
    - Left 0JQK
    - Right 0JQJ
  - Lower Arm
    - Left 0JQH
    - Right 0JQG
  - Lower Leg
    - Left 0JQP
    - Right 0JQN
  - Neck
    - Left 0JQ5
    - Right 0JQ4
  - Pelvic Region 0JQC
  - Perineum 0JQB
  - Scalp 0JQ0
  - Upper Arm
    - Left 0JQF
    - Right 0JQD
  - Upper Leg
    - Left 0JQM
    - Right 0JQL
- Tarsal
  - Left 0QQM
  - Right 0QQL
- Tendon
  - Abdomen
    - Left 0LQG
    - Right 0LQF
  - Ankle
    - Left 0LQT
    - Right 0LQS
  - Foot
    - Left 0LQW
    - Right 0LQV
  - Hand
    - Left 0LQ8
    - Right 0LQ7
  - Head and Neck 0LQ0
  - Hip
    - Left 0LQK
    - Right 0LQJ
  - Knee
    - Left 0LQR
    - Right 0LQQ
  - Lower Arm and Wrist
    - Left 0LQ6
    - Right 0LQ5

Repair *(continued)*
Tendon *(continued)*
Lower Leg
Left 0LQP
Right 0LQN
Perineum 0LQH
Shoulder
Left 0LQ2
Right 0LQ1
Thorax
Left 0LQD
Right 0LQC
Trunk
Left 0LQB
Right 0LQ9
Upper Arm
Left 0LQ4
Right 0LQ3
Upper Leg
Left 0LQM
Right 0LQL
Testis
Bilateral 0VQC
Left 0VQB
Right 0VQ9
Thalamus 00Q9
Thumb
Left 0XQM
Right 0XQL
Thymus 07QM
Thyroid Gland 0GQK
Left Lobe 0GQG
Right Lobe 0GQH
Thyroid Gland Isthmus
0GQJ
Tibia
Left 0QQH
Right 0QQG
Toe
1st
Left 0YQQ
Right 0YQP
2nd
Left 0YQS
Right 0YQR
3rd
Left 0YQU
Right 0YQT
4th
Left 0YQW
Right 0YQV
5th
Left 0YQY
Right 0YQX
Toe Nail 0HQRXZZ
Tongue 0CQ7
Tonsils 0CQP
Tooth
Lower 0CQX
Upper 0CQW
Trachea 0BQ1
Tunica Vaginalis
Left 0VQ7
Right 0VQ6
Turbinate, Nasal 09QL
Tympanic Membrane
Left 09Q8
Right 09Q7
Ulna
Left 0PQL
Right 0PQK
Ureter
Left 0TQ7
Right 0TQ6
Urethra 0TQD
Uterine Supporting Structure
0UQ4
Uterus 0UQ9
Uvula 0CQN
Vagina 0UQG

Repair *(continued)*
Valve
Aortic 02QF
Mitral 02QG
Pulmonary 02QH
Tricuspid 02QJ
Vas Deferens
Bilateral 0VQQ
Left 0VQP
Right 0VQN
Vein
Axillary
Left 05Q8
Right 05Q7
Azygos 05Q0
Basilic
Left 05QC
Right 05QB
Brachial
Left 05QA
Right 05Q9
Cephalic
Left 05QF
Right 05QD
Colic 06Q7
Common Iliac
Left 06QD
Right 06QC
Coronary 02Q4
Esophageal 06Q3
External Iliac
Left 06QG
Right 06QF
External Jugular
Left 05QQ
Right 05QP
Face
Left 05QV
Right 05QT
Femoral
Left 06QN
Right 06QM
Foot
Left 06QV
Right 06QT
Gastric 06Q2
Hand
Left 05QH
Right 05QG
Hemiazygos 05Q1
Hepatic 06Q4
Hypogastric
Left 06QJ
Right 06QH
Inferior Mesenteric
06Q6
Innominate
Left 05Q4
Right 05Q3
Internal Jugular
Left 05QN
Right 05QM
Intracranial 05QL
Lower 06QY
Portal 06Q8
Pulmonary
Left 02QT
Right 02QS
Renal
Left 06QB
Right 06Q9
Saphenous
Left 06QQ
Right 06QP
Splenic 06Q1
Subclavian
Left 05Q6
Right 05Q5
Superior Mesenteric
06Q5

Repair *(continued)*
Vein *(continued)*
Upper 05QY
Vertebral
Left 05QS
Right 05QR
Vena Cava
Inferior 06Q0
Superior 02QV
Ventricle
Left 02QL
Right 02QK
Vertebra
Cervical 0PQ3
Lumbar 0QQ0
Thoracic 0PQ4
Vesicle
Bilateral 0VQ3
Left 0VQ2
Right 0VQ1
Vitreous
Left 08Q53ZZ
Right 08Q43ZZ
Vocal Cord
Left 0CQV
Right 0CQT
Vulva 0UQM
Wrist Region
Left 0XQH
Right 0XQG
Repair, obstetric laceration, periurethral
0UQMXZZ
Replacement
Acetabulum
Left 0QR5
Right 0QR4
Ampulla of Vater 0FRC
Anal Sphincter 0DRR
Aorta
Abdominal 04R0
Thoracic
Ascending/Arch
02RX
Descending 02RW
Artery
Anterior Tibial
Left 04RQ
Right 04RP
Axillary
Left 03R6
Right 03R5
Brachial
Left 03R8
Right 03R7
Celiac 04R1
Colic
Left 04R7
Middle 04R8
Right 04R6
Common Carotid
Left 03RJ
Right 03RH
Common Iliac
Left 04RD
Right 04RC
External Carotid
Left 03RN
Right 03RM
External Iliac
Left 04RJ
Right 04RH
Face 03RR
Femoral
Left 04RL
Right 04RK
Foot
Left 04RW
Right 04RV
Gastric 04R2

Replacement *(continued)*
Artery *(continued)*
Hand
Left 03RF
Right 03RD
Hepatic 04R3
Inferior Mesenteric
04R B
Innominate 03R2
Internal Carotid
Left 03RL
Right 03RK
Internal Iliac
Left 04RF
Right 04RE
Internal Mammary
Left 03R1
Right 03R0
Intracranial 03RG
Lower 04RY
Peroneal
Left 04RU
Right 04RT
Popliteal
Left 04RN
Right 04RM
Posterior Tibial
Left 04RS
Right 04RR
Pulmonary
Left 02RR
Right 02RQ
Pulmonary Trunk
02RP
Radial
Left 03RC
Right 03RB
Renal
Left 04RA
Right 04R9
Splenic 04R4
Subclavian
Left 03R4
Right 03R3
Superior Mesenteric 04R5
Temporal
Left 03RT
Right 03RS
Thyroid
Left 03RV
Right 03RU
Ulnar
Left 03RA
Right 03R9
Upper 03RY
Vertebral
Left 03RQ
Right 03RP
Atrium
Left 02R
Right 02R6
Auditory Ossicle
Left 09RA0
Right 09R90
Bladder 0TRB
Bladder Neck 0TRC
Bone
Ethmoid
Left 0NRG
Right 0NRF
Frontal 0NR1
Hyoid 0NRX
Lacrimal
Left 0NRJ
Right 0NRH
Nasal 0NRB
Occipital 0NR7
Palatine
Left 0NRL
Right 0NRK

Replacement *(continued)*
- Bone *(continued)*
  - Parietal
    - Left 0NR4
    - Right 0NR3
  - Pelvic
    - Left 0QR3
    - Right 0QR2
  - Sphenoid 0NRC
  - Temporal
    - Left 0NR6
    - Right 0NR5
  - Zygomatic
    - Left 0NRN
    - Right 0NRM
- Breast
  - Bilateral 0HRV
  - Left 0HRU
  - Right 0HRT
- Bronchus
  - Lingula 0BR9
  - Lower Lobe
    - Left 0BRB
    - Right 0BR6
  - Main
    - Left 0BR7
    - Right 0BR3
  - Middle Lobe, Right 0BR5
  - Upper Lobe
    - Left 0BR8
    - Right 0BR4
- Buccal Mucosa 0CR4
- Bursa and Ligament
  - Abdomen
    - Left 0MRJ
    - Right 0MRH
  - Ankle
    - Left 0MRR
    - Right 0MRQ
  - Elbow
    - Left 0MR4
    - Right 0MR3
  - Foot
    - Left 0MRT
    - Right 0MRS
  - Hand
    - Left 0MR8
    - Right 0MR7
  - Head and Neck 0MR0
  - Hip
    - Left 0MRM
    - Right 0MRL
  - Knee
    - Left 0MRP
    - Right 0MRN
  - Lower Extremity
    - Left 0MRW
    - Right 0MRV
  - Perineum 0MRK
  - Rib(s) 0MRG
  - Shoulder
    - Left 0MR2
    - Right 0MR1
  - Spine
    - Lower 0MRD
    - Upper 0MRC
  - Sternum 0MRF
  - Upper Extremity
    - Left 0MRB
    - Right 0MR9
  - Wrist
    - Left 0MR6
    - Right 0MR5
- Carina 0BR2
- Carpal
  - Left 0PRN
  - Right 0PRM
- Cerebral Meninges 00R1
- Cerebral Ventricle 00R6
- Chordae Tendineae 02R9

Replacement *(continued)*
- Choroid
  - Left 08RB
  - Right 08RA
- Clavicle
  - Left 0PRB
  - Right 0PR9
- Coccyx 0QRS
- Conjunctiva
  - Left 08RTX
  - Right 08RSX
- Cornea
  - Left 08R9
  - Right 08R8
- Diaphragm 0BRT
- Disc
  - Cervical Vertebral 0RR30
  - Cervicothoracic Vertebral 0RR50
  - Lumbar Vertebral 0SR20
  - Lumbosacral 0SR40
  - Thoracic Vertebral 0RR90
  - Thoracolumbar Vertebral 0RRB0
- Duct
  - Common Bile 0FR9
  - Cystic 0FR8
  - Hepatic
    - Common 0FR7
    - Left 0FR6
    - Right 0FR5
  - Lacrimal
    - Left 08RY
    - Right 08RX
  - Pancreatic 0FRD
    - Accessory 0FRF
  - Parotid
    - Left 0CRC
    - Right 0CRB
- Dura Mater 00R2
- Ear
  - External
    - Bilateral 09R2
    - Left 09R1
    - Right 09R0
  - Inner
    - Left 09RE0
    - Right 09RD0
  - Middle
    - Left 09R60
    - Right 09R50
- Epiglottis 0CRR
- Esophagus 0DR5
- Eye
  - Left 08R1
  - Right 08R0
- Eyelid
  - Lower
    - Left 08RR
    - Right 08RQ
  - Upper
    - Left 08RP
    - Right 08RN
- Femoral Shaft
  - Left 0QR9
  - Right 0QR8
- Femur
  - Lower
    - Left 0QRC
    - Right 0QRB
  - Upper
    - Left 0QR7
    - Right 0QR6
- Fibula
  - Left 0QRK
  - Right 0QRJ
- Finger Nail 0HRQX
- Gingiva
  - Lower 0CR6
  - Upper 0CR5

Replacement *(continued)*
- Glenoid Cavity
  - Left 0PR8
  - Right 0PR7
- Hair 0HRSX
- Humeral Head
  - Left 0PRD
  - Right 0PRC
- Humeral Shaft
  - Left 0PRG
  - Right 0PRF
- Iris
  - Left 08RD3
  - Right 08RC3
- Joint
  - Acromioclavicular
    - Left 0RRH0
    - Right 0RRG0
  - Ankle
    - Left 0SRG
    - Right 0SRF
  - Carpal
    - Left 0RRR0
    - Right 0RRQ0
  - Carpometacarpal
    - Left 0RRT0
    - Right 0RRS0
  - Cervical Vertebral 0RR10
  - Cervicothoracic Vertebral 0RR40
  - Coccygeal 0SR60
  - Elbow
    - Left 0RRM0
    - Right 0RRL0
  - Finger Phalangeal
    - Left 0RRX0
    - Right 0RRW0
  - Hip
    - Left 0SRB
      - Acetabular Surface 0SRE
      - Femoral Surface 0SRS
    - Right 0SR9
      - Acetabular Surface 0SRA
      - Femoral Surface 0SRR
  - Knee
    - Left 0SRD
      - Femoral Surface 0SRU
      - Tibial Surface 0SRW
    - Right 0SRC
      - Femoral Surface 0SRT
      - Tibial Surface 0SRV
  - Lumbar Vertebral 0SR00
  - Lumbosacral 0SR30
  - Metacarpophalangeal
    - Left 0RRV0
    - Right 0RRU0
  - Metatarsal-Phalangeal
    - Left 0SRN0
    - Right 0SRM0
  - Occipital-cervical 0RR00
  - Sacrococcygeal 0SR50
  - Sacroiliac
    - Left 0SR80
    - Right 0SR70
  - Shoulder
    - Left 0RRK
    - Right 0RRJ
  - Sternoclavicular
    - Left 0RRF0
    - Right 0RRE0
  - Tarsal
    - Left 0SRJ0
    - Right 0SRH0
  - Tarsometatarsal
    - Left 0SRL0
    - Right 0SRK0
  - Temporomandibular
    - Left 0RRD0
    - Right 0RRC0

Replacement *(continued)*
- Joint *(continued)*
  - Thoracic Vertebral 0RR60
  - Thoracolumbar Vertebral 0RRA0
  - Toe Phalangeal
    - Left 0SRQ0
    - Right 0SRP0
  - Wrist
    - Left 0RRP0
    - Right 0RRN0
- Kidney Pelvis
  - Left 0TR4
  - Right 0TR3
- Larynx 0CRS
- Lens
  - Left 08RK30Z
  - Right 08RJ30Z
- Lip
  - Lower 0CR1
  - Upper 0CR0
- Mandible
  - Left 0NRV
  - Right 0NRT
- Maxilla 0NRR
- Mesentery 0DRV
- Metacarpal
  - Left 0PRQ
  - Right 0PRP
- Metatarsal
  - Left 0QRP
  - Right 0QR
- Muscle
  - Abdomen
    - Left 0KRL
    - Right 0KRK
  - Facial 0KR1
  - Foot
    - Left 0KRW
    - Right 0KRV
  - Hand
    - Left 0KRD
    - Right 0KRC
  - Head 0KR0
  - Hip
    - Left 0KRP
    - Right 0KRN
  - Lower Arm and Wrist
    - Left 0KRB
    - Right 0KR9
  - Lower Leg
    - Left 0KRT
    - Right 0KRS
  - Neck
    - Left 0KR3
    - Right 0KR2
  - Papillary 02RD
  - Perineum 0KRM
  - Shoulder
    - Left 0KR6
    - Right 0KR5
  - Thorax
    - Left 0KRJ
    - Right 0KRH
  - Tongue, Palate, Pharynx 0KR4
  - Trunk
    - Left 0KRG
    - Right 0KRF
  - Upper Arm
    - Left 0KR8
    - Right 0KR7
  - Upper Leg
    - Left 0KRR
    - Right 0KRQ
- Nasal Mucosa and Soft Tissue 09RK
- Nasopharynx 09RN
- Nerve
  - Abducens 00RL
  - Accessory 00RR
  - Acoustic 00RN

- **Replacement** *(continued)*
  - Nerve *(continued)*
    - Cervical 01R1
    - Facial 00RM
    - Femoral 01RD
    - Glossopharyngeal 00RP
    - Hypoglossal 00RS
    - Lumbar 01RB
    - Median 01R5
    - Oculomotor 00RH
    - Olfactory 00RF
    - Optic 00RG
    - Peroneal 01RH
    - Phrenic 01R2
    - Pudendal 01RC
    - Radial 01R6
    - Sacral 01RR
    - Sciatic 01RF
    - Thoracic 01R8
    - Tibial 01RG
    - Trigeminal 00RK
    - Trochlear 00RJ
    - Ulnar 01R4
    - Vagus 00RQ
  - Nipple
    - Left 0HRX
    - Right 0HRW
  - Omentum 0DRU
  - Orbit
    - Left 0NRQ
    - Right 0NRP
  - Palate
    - Hard 0CR2
    - Soft 0CR3
  - Patella
    - Left 0QRF
    - Right 0QRD
  - Pericardium 02RN
  - Peritoneum 0DRW
  - Phalanx
    - Finger
      - Left 0PRV
      - Right 0PRT
    - Thumb
      - Left 0PRS
      - Right 0PRR
    - Toe
      - Left 0QRR
      - Right 0QRQ
  - Pharynx 0CRM
  - Radius
    - Left 0PRJ
    - Right 0PRH
  - Retinal Vessel
    - Left 08RH3
    - Right 08RG3
  - Ribs
    - 1 to 2 0PR1
    - 3 or More 0PR2
  - Sacrum 0QR1
  - Scapula
    - Left 0PR6
    - Right 0PR5
  - Sclera
    - Left 08R7X
    - Right 08R6X
  - Septum
    - Atrial 02R5
    - Nasal 09RM
    - Ventricular 02RM
  - Skin
    - Abdomen 0HR7
    - Back 0HR6
    - Buttock 0HR8
    - Chest 0HR5
    - Ear
      - Left 0HR3
      - Right 0HR2
    - Face 0HR1
    - Foot
      - Left 0HRN
      - Right 0HRM
    - Hand
      - Left 0HRG
      - Right 0HRF
    - Inguinal 0HRA
    - Lower Arm
      - Left 0HRE
      - Right 0HRD
    - Lower Leg
      - Left 0HRL
      - Right 0HRK
    - Neck 0HR4
    - Perineum 0HR9
    - Scalp 0HR0
    - Upper Arm
      - Left 0HRC
      - Right 0HRB
    - Upper Leg
      - Left 0HRJ
      - Right 0HRH
  - Skin Substitute, Porcine Liver Derived XHRPL2
  - Skull 0NR0
  - Spinal Meninges 00RT
  - Sternum 0PR0
  - Subcutaneous Tissue and Fascia
    - Abdomen 0JR8
    - Back 0JR7
    - Buttock 0JR9
    - Chest 0JR6
    - Face 0JR1
    - Foot
      - Left 0JRR
      - Right 0JRQ
    - Hand
      - Left 0JRK
      - Right 0JRJ
    - Lower Arm
      - Left 0JRH
      - Right 0JRG
    - Lower Leg
      - Left 0JRP
      - Right 0JRN
    - Neck
      - Left 0JR5
      - Right 0JR4
    - Pelvic Region 0JRC
    - Perineum 0JRB
    - Scalp 0JR0
    - Upper Arm
      - Left 0JRF
      - Right 0JRD
    - Upper Leg
      - Left 0JRM
      - Right 0JRL
  - Tarsal
    - Left 0QRM
    - Right 0QRL
  - Tendon
    - Abdomen
      - Left 0LRG
      - Right 0LRF
    - Ankle
      - Left 0LRT
      - Right 0LRS
    - Foot
      - Left 0LRW
      - Right 0LRV
    - Hand
      - Left 0LR8
      - Right 0LR7
    - Head and Neck 0LR0
    - Hip
      - Left 0LRK
      - Right 0LRJ
    - Knee
      - Left 0LRR
      - Right 0LRQ
    - Lower Arm and Wrist
      - Left 0LR6
      - Right 0LR5
    - Lower Leg
      - Left 0LRP
      - Right 0LRN
    - Perineum 0LRH
    - Shoulder
      - Left 0LR2
      - Right 0LR1
    - Thorax
      - Left 0LRD
      - Right 0LRC
    - Trunk
      - Left 0LRB
      - Right 0LR9
    - Upper Arm
      - Left 0LR4
      - Right 0LR3
    - Upper Leg
      - Left 0LRM
      - Right 0LRL
  - Testis
    - Bilateral 0VRC0J
    - Left 0VRB0J
    - Right 0VR90J
  - Thumb
    - Left 0XRM
    - Right 0XRL
  - Tibia
    - Left 0QRH
    - Right 0QRG
  - Toe Nail 0HRRX
  - Tongue 0CR7
  - Tooth
    - Lower 0CRX
    - Upper 0CRW
  - Trachea 0BR1
  - Turbinate, Nasal 09RL
  - Tympanic Membrane
    - Left 09R8
    - Right 09R7
  - Ulna
    - Left 0PRL
    - Right 0PRK
  - Ureter
    - Left 0TR7
    - Right 0TR6
  - Urethra 0TRD
  - Uvula 0CRN
  - Valve
    - Aortic 02RF
    - Mitral 02RG
    - Pulmonary 02RH
    - Tricuspid 02RJ
  - Vein
    - Axillary
      - Left 05R8
      - Right 05R7
    - Azygos 05R0
    - Basilic
      - Left 05RC
      - Right 05RB
    - Brachial
      - Left 05RA
      - Right 05R9
    - Cephalic
      - Left 05RF
      - Right 05RD
    - Colic 06R7
    - Common Iliac
      - Left 06RD
      - Right 06RC
    - Esophageal 06R3
    - External Iliac
      - Left 06RG
      - Right 06RF
    - External Jugular
      - Left 05RQ
      - Right 05RP
    - Face
      - Left 05RV
      - Right 05RT
    - Femoral
      - Left 06RN
      - Right 06RM
    - Foot
      - Left 06RV
      - Right 06RT
    - Gastric 06R2
    - Hand
      - Left 05RH
      - Right 05RG
    - Hemiazygos 05R1
    - Hepatic 06R4
    - Hypogastric
      - Left 06RJ
      - Right 06RH
    - Inferior Mesenteric 06R6
    - Innominate
      - Left 05R4
      - Right 05R3
    - Internal Jugular
      - Left 05RN
      - Right 05RM
    - Intracranial 05RL
    - Lower 06RY
    - Portal 06R8
    - Pulmonary
      - Left 02RT
      - Right 02RS
    - Renal
      - Left 06RB
      - Right 06R9
    - Saphenous
      - Left 06RQ
      - Right 06RP
    - Splenic 06R1
    - Subclavian
      - Left 05R6
      - Right 05R5
    - Superior Mesenteric 06R5
    - Upper 05RY
    - Vertebral
      - Left 05RS
      - Right 05RR
  - Vena Cava
    - Inferior 06R0
    - Superior 02RV
  - Ventricle
    - Left 02RL
    - Right 02RK
  - Vertebra
    - Cervical 0PR3
    - Lumbar 0QR0
    - Thoracic 0PR4
  - Vitreous
    - Left 08R53
    - Right 08R43
  - Vocal Cord
    - Left 0CRV
    - Right 0CRT
  - Zooplastic Tissue, Rapid Deployment Technique X2RF
- **Replacement, hip**
  - Partial or total
    - *see* Replacement, Lower Joints 0SR
  - Resurfacing only
    - *see* Supplement, Lower Joints 0SU

Replantation
- *see* Reposition

Replantation, scalp
- *see* Reattachment, Skin, Scalp 0HM0

Reposition
- Acetabulum
  - Left 0QS5
  - Right 0QS4
- Ampulla of Vater 0FSC
- Anus 0DSQ
- Aorta
  - Abdominal 04S0
  - Thoracic
    - Ascending/Arch 02SX0ZZ
    - Descending 02SW0ZZ
- Artery
  - Anterior Tibial
    - Left 04SQ
    - Right 04SP
  - Axillary
    - Left 03S6
    - Right 03S5
  - Brachial
    - Left 03S8
    - Right 03S7
  - Celiac 04S1
  - Colic
    - Left 04S7
    - Middle 04S8
    - Right 04S6
  - Common Carotid
    - Left 03SJ
    - Right 03SH
  - Common Iliac
    - Left 04SD
    - Right 04SC
  - Coronary
    - One Artery 02S00ZZ
    - Two Arteries 02S10ZZ
  - External Carotid
    - Left 03SN
    - Right 03SM
  - External Iliac
    - Left 04SJ
    - Right 04SH
  - Face 03SR
  - Femoral
    - Left 04SL
    - Right 04SK
  - Foot
    - Left 04SW
    - Right 04SV
  - Gastric 04S2
  - Hand
    - Left 03SF
    - Right 03SD
  - Hepatic 04S3
  - Inferior Mesenteric 04SB
  - Innominate 03S2
  - Internal Carotid
    - Left 03SL
    - Right 03SK
  - Internal Iliac
    - Left 04SF
    - Right 04SE
  - Internal Mammary
    - Left 03S1
    - Right 03S0
  - Intracranial 03SG
  - Lower 04SY
  - Peroneal
    - Left 04SU
    - Right 04ST
  - Popliteal
    - Left 04SN
    - Right 04SM
  - Posterior Tibial
    - Left 04SS

Reposition *(continued)*
- Artery *(continued)*
  - Posterior Tibial *(continued)*
    - Right 04SR
  - Pulmonary
    - Left 02SR0ZZ
    - Right 02SQ0ZZ
  - Pulmonary Trunk 02SP0ZZ
  - Radial
    - Left 03SC
    - Right 03SB
  - Renal
    - Left 04SA
    - Right 04S9
  - Splenic 04S4
  - Subclavian
    - Left 03S4
    - Right 03S3
  - Superior Mesenteric 04S5
  - Temporal
    - Left 03ST
    - Right 03SS
  - Thyroid
    - Left 03SV
    - Right 03SU
  - Ulnar
    - Left 03SA
    - Right 03S9
  - Upper 03SY
  - Vertebral
    - Left 03SQ
    - Right 03SP
- Auditory Ossicle
  - Left 09SA
  - Right 09S9
- Bladder 0TSB
- Bladder Neck 0TSC
- Bone
  - Ethmoid
    - Left 0NSG
    - Right 0NSF
  - Frontal 0NS1
  - Hyoid 0NSX
  - Lacrimal
    - Left 0NSJ
    - Right 0NSH
  - Nasal 0NSB
  - Occipital 0NS7
  - Palatine
    - Left 0NSL
    - Right 0NSK
  - Parietal
    - Left 0NS4
    - Right 0NS3
  - Pelvic
    - Left 0QS3
    - Right 0QS2
  - Sphenoid 0NSC
  - Temporal
    - Left 0NS6
    - Right 0NS5
  - Zygomatic
    - Left 0NSN
    - Right 0NSM
- Breast
  - Bilateral 0HSV0ZZ
  - Left 0HSU0ZZ
  - Right 0HST0ZZ
- Bronchus
  - Lingula 0BS90ZZ
  - Lower Lobe
    - Left 0BSB0ZZ
    - Right 0BS60ZZ
  - Main
    - Left 0BS70ZZ
    - Right 0BS30ZZ
  - Middle Lobe, Right 0BS50ZZ

Reposition *(continued)*
- Bronchus *(continued)*
  - Upper Lobe
    - Left 0BS80ZZ
    - Right 0BS40ZZ
- Bursa and Ligament
  - Abdomen
    - Left 0MSJ
    - Right 0MSH
  - Ankle
    - Left 0MSR
    - Right 0MSQ
  - Elbow
    - Left 0MS4
    - Right 0MS3
  - Foot
    - Left 0MST
    - Right 0MSS
  - Hand
    - Left 0MS8
    - Right 0MS7
  - Head and Neck 0MS0
  - Hip
    - Left 0MSM
    - Right 0MSL
  - Knee
    - Left 0MSP
    - Right 0MSN
  - Lower Extremity
    - Left 0MSW
    - Right 0MSV
  - Perineum 0MSK
  - Rib(s) 0MSG
  - Shoulder
    - Left 0MS2
    - Right 0MS1
  - Spine
    - Lower 0MSD
    - Upper 0MSC
  - Sternum 0MSF
  - Upper Extremity
    - Left 0MSB
    - Right 0MS9
  - Wrist
    - Left 0MS6
    - Right 0MS5
- Carina 0BS20ZZ
- Carpal
  - Left 0PSN
  - Right 0PSM
- Cecum 0DSH
- Cervix 0USC
- Clavicle
  - Left 0PSB
  - Right 0PS9
- Coccyx 0QSS
- Colon
  - Ascending 0DSK
  - Descending 0DSM
  - Sigmoid 0DSN
  - Transverse 0DSL
- Cord
  - Bilateral 0VSH
  - Left 0VSG
  - Right 0VSF
- Cul-de-sac 0USF
- Diaphragm 0BST0ZZ
- Duct
  - Common Bile 0FS9
  - Cystic 0FS8
  - Hepatic
    - Common 0FS7
    - Left 0FS6
    - Right 0FS5
  - Lacrimal
    - Left 08SY
    - Right 08SX
  - Pancreatic 0FSD
    - Accessory 0FSF

Reposition *(continued)*
- Duct *(continued)*
  - Parotid
    - Left 0CSC
    - Right 0CSB
- Duodenum 0DS9ZZ
- Ear
  - Bilateral 09S2ZZ
  - Left 09S1ZZ
  - Right 09S0ZZ
- Epiglottis 0CSR
- Esophagus 0DS5ZZ
- Eustachian Tube
  - Left 09SG
  - Right 09SF
- Eyelid
  - Lower
    - Left 08SR
    - Right 08SQ
  - Upper
    - Left 08SP
    - Right 08SN
- Fallopian Tube
  - Left 0US6
  - Right 0US5
- Fallopian Tubes, Bilateral 0US7
- Femoral Shaft
  - Left 0QS9
  - Right 0QS8
- Femur
  - Lower
    - Left 0QSC
    - Right 0QSB
  - Upper
    - Left 0QS7
    - Right 0QS6
- Fibula
  - Left 0QSK
  - Right 0QSJ
- Gallbladder 0FS4
- Gland
  - Adrenal
    - Left 0GS2
    - Right 0GS3
  - Lacrimal
    - Left 08SW
    - Right 08SV
- Glenoid Cavity
  - Left 0PS8
  - Right 0PS7
- Hair 0HSSXZZ
- Humeral Head
  - Left 0PSD
  - Right 0PSC
- Humeral Shaft
  - Left 0PSG
  - Right 0PSF
- Ileum 0DSB
- Intestine
  - Large 0DSE
  - Small 0DS8
- Iris
  - Left 08SD3ZZ
  - Right 08SC3ZZ
- Jejunum 0DSAZZ
- Joint
  - Acromioclavicular
    - Left 0RSHZ
    - Right 0RSGZ
  - Ankle
    - Left 0SSG
    - Right 0SSF
  - Carpal
    - Left 0RSR
    - Right 0RSQ
  - Carpometacarpal
    - Left 0RST
    - Right 0RSS
  - Cervical Vertebral 0RS1

- **Reposition** *(continued)*
  - Joint *(continued)*
    - Cervicothoracic Vertebral 0RS4
    - Coccygeal 0SS6
    - Elbow
      - Left 0RSM
      - Right 0RSL
    - Finger Phalangeal
      - Left 0RSX
      - Right 0RSW
    - Hip
      - Left 0SSB
      - Right 0SS9
    - Knee
      - Left 0SSD
      - Right 0SSC
    - Lumbar Vertebral 0SS0
    - Lumbosacral 0SS3
    - Metacarpophalangeal
      - Left 0RSV
      - Right 0RSU
    - Metatarsal-Phalangeal
      - Left 0SSN
      - Right 0SSM
    - Occipital-cervical 0RS0
    - Sacrococcygeal 0SS5
    - Sacroiliac
      - Left 0SS8
      - Right 0SS7
    - Shoulder
      - Left 0RSK
      - Right 0RSJ
    - Sternoclavicular
      - Left 0RSF
      - Right 0RSE
    - Tarsal
      - Left 0SSJ
      - Right 0SSH
    - Tarsometatarsal
      - Left 0SSL
      - Right 0SSK
    - Temporomandibular
      - Left 0RSD
      - Right 0RSC
    - Thoracic Vertebral 0RS6
    - Thoracolumbar Vertebral 0RSA
    - Toe Phalangeal
      - Left 0SSQ
      - Right 0SSP
    - Wrist
      - Left 0RSP
      - Right 0RSN
  - Kidney
    - Left 0TS1
    - Right 0TS0
  - Kidney Pelvis
    - Left 0TS4
    - Right 0TS3
  - Kidneys, Bilateral 0TS2
  - Lens
    - Left 08SK3ZZ
    - Right 08SJ3ZZ
  - Lip
    - Lower 0CS1
    - Upper 0CS0
  - Liver 0FS0
  - Lung
    - Left 0BSL0ZZ
    - Lower Lobe
      - Left 0BSJ0ZZ
      - Right 0BSF0ZZ
    - Middle Lobe, Right 0BSD0ZZ
    - Right 0BSK0ZZ
    - Upper Lobe
      - Left 0BSG0ZZ
      - Right 0BSC0ZZ
  - Lung Lingula 0BSH0ZZ
  - Mandible
    - Left 0NSV
    - Right 0NST

- **Reposition** *(continued)*
  - Maxilla 0NSR
  - Metacarpal
    - Left 0PSQ
    - Right 0PSP
  - Metatarsal
    - Left 0QSP
    - Right 0QSN
  - Muscle
    - Abdomen
      - Left 0KSL
      - Right 0KSK
    - Extraocular
      - Left 08SM
      - Right 08SL
    - Facial 0KS1
    - Foot
      - Left 0KSW
      - Right 0KSV
    - Hand
      - Left 0KSD
      - Right 0KSC
    - Head 0KS0
    - Hip
      - Left 0KSP
      - Right 0KSN
    - Lower Arm and Wrist
      - Left 0KSB
      - Right 0KS9
    - Lower Leg
      - Left 0KST
      - Right 0KSS
    - Neck
      - Left 0KS3
      - Right 0KS2
    - Perineum 0KSM
    - Shoulder
      - Left 0KS6
      - Right 0KS5
    - Thorax
      - Left 0KSJ
      - Right 0KSH
    - Tongue, Palate, Pharynx 0KS4
    - Trunk
      - Left 0KSG
      - Right 0KSF
    - Upper Arm
      - Left 0KS8
      - Right 0KS7
    - Upper Leg
      - Left 0KSR
      - Right 0KSQ
  - Nasal Mucosa and Soft Tissue 09SK
  - Nerve
    - Abducens 00SL
    - Accessory 00SR
    - Acoustic 00SN
    - Brachial Plexus 01S3
    - Cervical 01S1
    - Cervical Plexus 01S0
    - Facial 00SM
    - Femoral 01SD
    - Glossopharyngeal 00SP
    - Hypoglossal 00SS
    - Lumbar 01SB
    - Lumbar Plexus 01S9
    - Lumbosacral Plexus 01SA
    - Median 01S5
    - Oculomotor 00SH
    - Olfactory 00SF
    - Optic 00SG
    - Peroneal 01SH
    - Phrenic 01S2
    - Pudendal 01SC
    - Radial 01S6
    - Sacral 01SR
    - Sacral Plexus 01SQ
    - Sciatic 01SF
    - Thoracic 01S8
    - Tibial 01SG

- **Reposition** *(continued)*
  - Nerve *(continued)*
    - Trigeminal 00SK
    - Trochlear 00SJ
    - Ulnar 01S4
    - Vagus 00SQ
  - Nipple
    - Left 0HSXXZZ
    - Right 0HSWXZZ
  - Orbit
    - Left 0NSQ
    - Right 0NSP
  - Ovary
    - Bilateral 0US2
    - Left 0US1
    - Right 0US0
  - Palate
    - Hard 0CS2
    - Soft 0CS3
  - Pancreas 0FSG
  - Parathyroid Gland 0GSR
    - Inferior
      - Left 0GSP
      - Right 0GSN
    - Multiple 0GSQ
    - Superior
      - Left 0GSM
      - Right 0GSL
  - Patella
    - Left 0QSF
    - Right 0QSD
  - Phalanx
    - Finger
      - Left 0PSV
      - Right 0PST
    - Thumb
      - Left 0PSS
      - Right 0PSR
    - Toe
      - Left 0QSR
      - Right 0QSQ
  - Products of Conception 10S0
    - Ectopic 10S2
  - Radius
    - Left 0PSJ
    - Right 0PSH
  - Rectum 0DSP
  - Retinal Vessel
    - Left 08SH3ZZ
    - Right 08SG3ZZ
  - Ribs
    - 1 to 2 0PS1
    - 3 or More 0PS2
  - Sacrum 0QS1
  - Scapula
    - Left 0PS6
    - Right 0PS5
  - Septum, Nasal 09SM
  - Sesamoid Bone(s) 1st Toe
    - *see* Reposition, Metatarsal, Right 0QSN
    - *see* Reposition, Metatarsal, Left 0QSP
  - Skull 0NS0
  - Spinal Cord
    - Cervical 00SW
    - Lumbar 00SY
    - Thoracic 00SX
  - Spleen 07SP0ZZ
  - Sternum 0PS0
  - Stomach 0DS6
  - Tarsal
    - Left 0QSM
    - Right 0QSL
  - Tendon
    - Abdomen
      - Left 0LSG
      - Right 0LSF
    - Ankle
      - Left 0LST

- **Reposition** *(continued)*
  - Tendon *(continued)*
    - Ankle *(continued)*
      - Right 0LSS
    - Foot
      - Left 0LSW
      - Right 0LSV
    - Hand
      - Left 0LS8
      - Right 0LS7
    - Head and Neck 0LS0
    - Hip
      - Left 0LSK
      - Right 0LSJ
    - Knee
      - Left 0LSR
      - Right 0LSQ
    - Lower Arm and Wrist
      - Left 0LS6
      - Right 0LS5
    - Lower Leg
      - Left 0LSP
      - Right 0LSN
    - Perineum 0LSH
    - Shoulder
      - Left 0LS2
      - Right 0LS1
    - Thorax
      - Left 0LSD
      - Right 0LSC
    - Trunk
      - Left 0LSB
      - Right 0LS9
    - Upper Arm
      - Left 0LS4
      - Right 0LS3
    - Upper Leg
      - Left 0LSM
      - Right 0LSL
  - Testis
    - Bilateral 0VSC
    - Left 0VSB
    - Right 0VS9
  - Thymus 07SM0ZZ
  - Thyroid Gland
    - Left Lobe 0GSG
    - Right Lobe 0GSH
  - Tibia
    - Left 0QSH
    - Right 0QSG
  - Tongue 0CS7
  - Tooth
    - Lower 0CSX
    - Upper 0CSW
  - Trachea 0BS10ZZ
  - Turbinate, Nasal 09SL
  - Tympanic Membrane
    - Left 09S8
    - Right 09S7
  - Ulna
    - Left 0PSL
    - Right 0PSK
  - Ureter
    - Left 0TS7
    - Right 0TS6
  - Ureters, Bilateral 0TS8
  - Urethra 0TSD
  - Uterine Supporting Structure 0US
  - Uterus 0US9
  - Uvula 0CSN
  - Vagina 0USG
  - Vein
    - Axillary
      - Left 05S8
      - Right 05S7
    - Azygos 05S0
    - Basilic
      - Left 05SC
      - Right 05SB

Reposition *(continued)*
Vein *(continued)*
Brachial
Left 05SA
Right 05S9
Cephalic
Left 05SF
Right 05SD
Colic 06S7
Common Iliac
Left 06SD
Right 06SC
Esophageal 06S3
External Iliac
Left 06SG
Right 06SF
External Jugular
Left 05SQ
Right 05SP
Face
Left 05SV
Right 05ST
Femoral
Left 06SN
Right 06SM
Foot
Left 06SV
Right 06ST
Gastric 06S2
Hand
Left 05SH
Right 05SG
Hemiazygos 05S1
Hepatic 06S4
Hypogastric
Left 06SJ
Right 06SH
Inferior Mesenteric 06S6
Innominate
Left 05S4
Right 05S3
Internal Jugular
Left 05SN
Right 05SM
Intracranial 05SL
Lower 06SY
Portal 06S8
Pulmonary
Left 02ST0ZZ
Right 02SS0ZZ
Renal
Left 06SB
Right 06S9
Saphenous
Left 06SQ
Right 06SP
Splenic 06S1
Subclavian
Left 05S6
Right 05S5
Superior Mesenteric 06S5
Upper 05SY
Vertebral
Left 05SS
Right 05SR
Vena Cava
Inferior 06S0
Superior 02SV0ZZ
Vertebra
Cervical 0PS3
Magnetically Controlled Growth Rod(s) XNS3
Lumbar 0QS0
Magnetically Controlled Growth Rod(s) XNS0
Thoracic 0PS4
Magnetically Controlled Growth Rod(s) XNS4
Vocal Cord
Left 0CSV
Right 0CST

Resection
Acetabulum
Left 0QT50ZZ
Right 0QT40ZZ
Adenoids 0CTQ
Ampulla of Vater 0FTC
Anal Sphincter 0DTR
Anus 0DTQ
Aortic Body 0GTD
Appendix 0DTJ
Auditory Ossicle
Left 09TA
Right 09T9
Bladder 0TTB
Bladder Neck 0TTC
Bone
Ethmoid
Left 0NTG0ZZ
Right 0NTF0ZZ
Frontal 0NT10ZZ
Hyoid 0NTX0ZZ
Lacrimal
Left 0NTJ0ZZ
Right 0NTH0ZZ
Nasal 0NTB0ZZ
Occipital 0NT70ZZ
Palatine
Left 0NTL0ZZ
Right 0NTK0ZZ
Parietal
Left 0NT40ZZ
Right 0NT30ZZ
Pelvic
Left 0QT30ZZ
Right 0QT20ZZ
Sphenoid 0NTC0ZZ
Temporal
Left 0NT60ZZ
Right 0NT50ZZ
Zygomatic
Left 0NTN0ZZ
Right 0NTM0ZZ
Breast
Bilateral 0HTV0ZZ
Left 0HTU0ZZ
Right 0HTT0ZZ
Supernumerary 0HTY0ZZ
Bronchus
Lingula 0BT9
Lower Lobe
Left 0BTB
Right 0BT6
Main
Left 0BT7
Right 0BT3
Middle Lobe, Right 0BT5
Upper Lobe
Left 0BT8
Right 0BT4
Bursa and Ligament
Abdomen
Left 0MTJ
Right 0MTH
Ankle
Left 0MTR
Right 0MTQ
Elbow
Left 0MT4
Right 0MT3
Foot
Left 0MTT
Right 0MTS
Hand
Left 0MT8
Right 0MT7
Head and Neck 0MT0
Hip
Left 0MTM
Right 0MTL

Resection *(continued)*
Bursa and Ligament *(continued)*
Knee
Left 0MTP
Right 0MTN
Lower Extremity
Left 0MTW
Right 0MTV
Perineum 0MTK
Rib(s) 0MTG
Shoulder
Left 0MT2
Right 0MT1
Spine
Lower 0MTD
Upper 0MTC
Sternum 0MTF
Upper Extremity
Left 0MTB
Right 0MT9
Wrist
Left 0MT6
Right 0MT5
Carina 0BT2
Carotid Bodies, Bilateral 0GT8
Carotid Body
Left 0GT6
Right 0GT7
Carpal
Left 0PTN0ZZ
Right 0PTM0ZZ
Cecum 0DTH
Cerebral Hemisphere 00T7
Cervix 0UTC
Chordae Tendineae 02T9
Cisterna Chyli 07TL
Clavicle
Left 0PTB0ZZ
Right 0PT90ZZ
Clitoris 0UTJ
Coccygeal Glomus 0GTB
Coccyx 0QTS0ZZ
Colon
Ascending 0DTK
Descending 0DTM
Sigmoid 0DTN
Transverse 0DTL
Conduction Mechanism 02T8
Cord
Bilateral 0VTH
Left 0VTG
Right 0VTF
Cornea
Left 08T9XZZ
Right 08T8XZZ
Cul-de-sac 0UTF
Diaphragm 0BTT
Disc
Cervical Vertebral 0RT30ZZ
Cervicothoracic Vertebral 0RT50ZZ
Lumbar Vertebral 0ST20ZZ
Lumbosacral 0ST40ZZ
Thoracic Vertebral 0RT90ZZ
Thoracolumbar Vertebral 0RTB0ZZ
Duct
Common Bile 0FT9
Cystic 0FT8
Hepatic
Common 0FT7
Left 0FT6
Right 0FT5
Lacrimal
Left 08TY
Right 08TX
Pancreatic 0FTD
Accessory 0FTF

Resection *(continued)*
Duct *(continued)*
Parotid
Left 0CTC0ZZ
Right 0CTB0ZZ
Duodenum 0DT9
Ear
External
Left 09T1
Right 09T0
Inner
Left 09TE
Right 09TD
Middle
Left 09T6
Right 09T5
Epididymis
Bilateral 0VTL
Left 0VTK
Right 0VTJ
Epiglottis 0CTR
Esophagogastric Junction 0DT4
Esophagus 0DT5
Lower 0DT3
Middle 0DT2
Upper 0DT1
Eustachian Tube
Left 09TG
Right 09TF
Eye
Left 08T1XZZ
Right 08T0XZZ
Eyelid
Lower
Left 08TR
Right 08TQ
Upper
Left 08TP
Right 08TN
Fallopian Tube
Left 0UT6
Right 0UT5
Fallopian Tubes, Bilateral 0UT7
Femoral Shaft
Left 0QT90ZZ
Right 0QT80ZZ
Femur
Lower
Left 0QTC0ZZ
Right 0QTB0ZZ
Upper
Left 0QT70ZZ
Right 0QT60ZZ
Fibula
Left 0QTK0ZZ
Right 0QTJ0ZZ
Finger Nail 0HTQXZZ
Gallbladder 0FT4
Gland
Adrenal
Bilateral 0GT4
Left 0GT2
Right 0GT3
Lacrimal
Left 08TW
Right 08TV
Minor Salivary 0CTJ0ZZ
Parotid
Left 0CT90ZZ
Right 0CT80ZZ
Pituitary 0GT0
Sublingual
Left 0CTF0ZZ
Right 0CTD0ZZ
Submaxillary
Left 0CTH0ZZ
Right 0CTG0ZZ
Vestibular 0UTL
Glenoid Cavity
Left 0PT80ZZ
Right 0PT70ZZ

Resection *(continued)*
Glomus Jugulare 0GTC
Humeral Head
Left 0PTD0ZZ
Right 0PTC0ZZ
Humeral Shaft
Left 0PTG0ZZ
Right 0PTF0ZZ
Hymen 0UTK
Ileocecal Valve 0DTC
Ileum 0DTB
Intestine
Large 0DTE
Left 0DTG
Right 0DTF
Small 0DT8
Iris
Left 08TD3ZZ
Right 08TC3ZZ
Jejunum 0DTA
Joint
Acromioclavicular
Left 0RTH0ZZ
Right 0RTG0ZZ
Ankle
Left 0STG0ZZ
Right 0STF0ZZ
Carpal
Left 0RTR0ZZ
Right 0RTQ0ZZ
Carpometacarpal
Left 0RTT0ZZ
Right 0RTS0ZZ
Cervicothoracic Vertebral
0RT40ZZ
Coccygeal 0ST60ZZ
Elbow
Left 0RTM0ZZ
Right 0RTL0ZZ
Finger Phalangeal
Left 0RTX0ZZ
Right 0RTW0ZZ
Hip
Left 0STB0ZZ
Right 0ST90ZZ
Knee
Left 0STD0ZZ
Right 0STC0ZZ
Metacarpophalangeal
Left 0RTV0ZZ
Right 0RTU0ZZ
Metatarsal-Phalangeal
Left 0STN0ZZ
Right 0STM0ZZ
Sacrococcygeal
0ST50ZZ
Sacroiliac
Left 0ST80ZZ
Right 0ST70ZZ
Shoulder
Left 0RTK0ZZ
Right 0RTJ0ZZ
Sternoclavicular
Left 0RTF0ZZ
Right 0RTE0ZZ
Tarsal
Left 0STJ0ZZ
Right 0STH0ZZ
Tarsometatarsal
Left 0STL0ZZ
Right 0STK0ZZ
Temporomandibular
Left 0RTD0ZZ
Right 0RTC0ZZ
Toe Phalangeal
Left 0STQ0ZZ
Right 0STP0ZZ
Wrist
Left 0RTP0ZZ
Right 0RTN0ZZ

Resection *(continued)*
Kidney
Left 0TT1
Right 0TT0
Kidney Pelvis
Left 0TT4
Right 0TT3
Kidneys, Bilateral 0TT2
Larynx 0CTS
Lens
Left 08TK3ZZ
Right 08TJ3ZZ
Lip
Lower 0CT1
Upper 0CT0
Liver 0FT0
Left Lobe 0FT2
Right Lobe 0FT1
Lung
Bilateral 0BTM
Left 0BTL
Lower Lobe
Left 0BTJ
Right 0BTF
Middle Lobe, Right 0BTD
Right 0BTK
Upper Lobe
Left 0BTG
Right 0BTC
Lung Lingula 0BTH
Lymphatic
Aortic 07TD
Axillary
Left 07T6
Right 07T5
Head 07T0
Inguinal
Left 07TJ
Right 07TH
Internal Mammary
Left 07T9
Right 07T8
Lower Extremity
Left 07TG
Right 07TF
Mesenteric 07TB
Neck
Left 07T2
Right 07T1
Pelvis 07TC
Thoracic Duct 07TK
Thorax 07T7
Upper Extremity
Left 07T4
Right 07T3
Mandible
Left 0NTV0ZZ
Right 0NTT0ZZ
Maxilla 0NTR0ZZ
Metacarpal
Left 0PTQ0ZZ
Right 0PTP0ZZ
Metatarsal
Left 0QTP0ZZ
Right 0QTN0ZZ
Muscle
Abdomen
Left 0KTL
Right 0KTK
Extraocular
Left 08TM
Right 08TL
Facial 0KT1
Foot
Left 0KTW
Right 0KTV
Hand
Left 0KTD
Right 0KTC
Head 0KT0

Resection *(continued)*
Muscle *(continued)*
Hip
Left 0KTP
Right 0KTN
Lower Arm and Wrist
Left 0KTB
Right 0KT9
Lower Leg
Left 0KTT
Right 0KTS
Neck
Left 0KT3
Right 0KT2
Papillary 02TD
Perineum 0KTM
Shoulder
Left 0KT6
Right 0KT5
Thorax
Left 0KTJ
Right 0KTH
Tongue, Palate, Pharynx 0KT4
Trunk
Left 0KTG
Right 0KTF
Upper Arm
Left 0KT8
Right 0KT7
Upper Leg
Left 0KTR
Right 0KTQ
Nasal Mucosa and Soft Tissue
09TK
Nasopharynx 09TN
Nipple
Left 0HTXXZZ
Right 0HTWXZZ
Omentum 0DTU
Orbit
Left 0NTQ0ZZ
Right 0NTP0ZZ
Ovary
Bilateral 0UT2
Left 0UT1
Right 0UT0
Palate
Hard 0CT2
Soft 0CT3
Pancreas 0FTG
Para-aortic Body 0GT9
Paraganglion Extremity 0GTF
Parathyroid Gland 0GTR
Inferior
Left 0GTP
Right 0GTN
Multiple 0GTQ
Superior
Left 0GTM
Right 0GTL
Patella
Left 0QTF0ZZ
Right 0QTD0ZZ
Penis 0VTS
Pericardium 02TN
Phalanx
Finger
Left 0PTV0ZZ
Right 0PTT0ZZ
Thumb
Left 0PTS0ZZ
Right 0PTR0ZZ
Toe
Left 0QTR0ZZ
Right 0QTQ0ZZ
Pharynx 0CTM
Pineal Body 0GT1
Prepuce 0VTT
Products of Conception, Ectopic
10T2

Resection *(continued)*
Prostate 0VT0
Radius
Left 0PTJ0ZZ
Right 0PTH0ZZ
Rectum 0DTP
Ribs
1 to 2 0PT10ZZ
3 or More 0PT20ZZ
Scapula
Left 0PT60ZZ
Right 0PT50ZZ
Scrotum 0VT5
Septum
Atrial 02T5
Nasal 09TM
Ventricular 02TM
Sinus
Accessory 09TP
Ethmoid
Left 09TV
Right 09TU
Frontal
Left 09TT
Right 09TS
Mastoid
Left 09TC
Right 09TB
Maxillary
Left 09TR
Right 09TQ
Sphenoid
Left 09TX
Right 09TW
Spleen 07TP
Sternum 0PT00ZZ
Stomach 0DT6
Pylorus 0DT7
Tarsal
Left 0QTM0ZZ
Right 0QTL0ZZ
Tendon
Abdomen
Left 0LTG
Right 0LTF
Ankle
Left 0LTT
Right 0LTS
Foot
Left 0LTW
Right 0LTV
Hand
Left 0LT8
Right 0LT7
Head and Neck 0LT0
Hip
Left 0LTK
Right 0LTJ
Knee
Left 0LTR
Right 0LTQ
Lower Arm and Wrist
Left 0LT6
Right 0LT5
Lower Leg
Left 0LTP
Right 0LTN
Perineum 0LTH
Shoulder
Left 0LT2
Right 0LT1
Thorax
Left 0LTD
Right 0LTC
Trunk
Left 0LTB
Right 0LT9
Upper Arm
Left 0LT4
Right 0LT3

Resection *(continued)*
- Tendon *(continued)*
  - Upper Leg
    - Left 0LTM
    - Right 0LTL
- Testis
  - Bilateral 0VTC
  - Left 0VTB
  - Right 0VT9
- Thymus 07TM
- Thyroid Gland 0GTK
  - Left Lobe 0GTG
  - Right Lobe 0GTH
- Thyroid Gland Isthmus 0GTJ
- Tibia
  - Left 0QTH0ZZ
  - Right 0QTG0ZZ
- Toe Nail 0HTRXZZ
- Tongue 0CT7
- Tonsils 0CTP
- Tooth
  - Lower 0CTX0Z
  - Upper 0CTW0Z
- Trachea 0BT1
- Tunica Vaginalis
  - Left 0VT7
  - Right 0VT6
- Turbinate, Nasal 09TL
- Tympanic Membrane
  - Left 09T8
  - Right 09T7
- Ulna
  - Left 0PTL0ZZ
  - Right 0PTK0ZZ
- Ureter
  - Left 0TT7
  - Right 0TT6
- Urethra 0TTD
- Uterine Supporting Structure 0UT4
- Uterus 0UT9
- Uvula 0CTN
- Vagina 0UTG
- Valve, Pulmonary 02TH
- Vas Deferens
  - Bilateral 0VTQ
  - Left 0VTP
  - Right 0VTN
- Vesicle
  - Bilateral 0VT3
  - Left 0VT2
  - Right 0VT1
- Vitreous
  - Left 08T53ZZ
  - Right 08T43ZZ
- Vocal Cord
  - Left 0CTV
  - Right 0CTT
- Vulva 0UTM

Resection, Left ventricular outflow tract obstruction (LVOT)
- *see* Dilation, Ventricle, Left 027L

Resection, Subaortic membrane (Left ventricular outflow tract obstruction)
- *see* Dilation, Ventricle, Left 027L

Restoration, Cardiac, Single, Rhythm 5A2204Z

RestoreAdvanced neurostimulator (SureScan)(MRI Safe)
- *use* Stimulator Generator, Multiple Array Rechargeable in 0JH

RestoreSensor neurostimulator (SureScan)(MRI Safe)
- *use* Stimulator Generator, Multiple Array Rechargeable in 0JH

RestoreUltra neurostimulator (SureScan)(MRI Safe)
- *use* Stimulator Generator, Multiple Array Rechargeable in 0JH

Restriction
- Ampulla of Vater 0FVC
- Anus 0DVQ
- Aorta
  - Abdominal 04V0
    - Intraluminal Device, Branched or Fenestrated 04V0
  - Thoracic
    - Ascending/Arch, Intraluminal Device, Branched or Fenestrated 02VX
    - Descending, Intraluminal Device, Branched or Fenestrated 02VW
- Artery
  - Anterior Tibial
    - Left 04VQ
    - Right 04VP
  - Axillary
    - Left 03V6
    - Right 03V5
  - Brachial
    - Left 03V8
    - Right 03V7
  - Celiac 04V1
  - Colic
    - Left 04V7
    - Middle 04V8
    - Right 04V6
  - Common Carotid
    - Left 03VJ
    - Right 03VH
  - Common Iliac
    - Left 04VD
    - Right 04VC
  - External Carotid
    - Left 03VN
    - Right 03VM
  - External Iliac
    - Left 04VJ
    - Right, 04VHZ
  - Face 03VR
  - Femoral
    - Left 04VL
    - Right 04VK
  - Foot
    - Left 04VW
    - Right 04VV
  - Gastric 04V2
  - Hand
    - Left 03VF
    - Right 03VD
  - Hepatic 04V3
  - Inferior Mesenteric 04VB
  - Innominate 03V2
  - Internal Carotid
    - Left 03VL
    - Right 03VK
  - Internal Iliac
    - Left 04VF
    - Right 04VE
  - Internal Mammary
    - Left 03V1
    - Right 03V0
  - Intracranial 03VG
  - Lower 04VY
  - Peroneal
    - Left 04VU
    - Right 04VT
  - Popliteal
    - Left 04VN
    - Right 04VM
  - Posterior Tibial
    - Left 04VS
    - Right 04VR
  - Pulmonary
    - Left 02VR
    - Right 02VQ
  - Pulmonary Trunk 02VP

Restriction *(continued)*
- Artery *(continued)*
  - Radial
    - Left 03VC
    - Right 03VB
  - Renal
    - Left 04VA
    - Right 04V9
  - Splenic 04V4
  - Subclavian
    - Left 03V4
    - Right 03V3
  - Superior Mesenteric 04V5
  - Temporal
    - Left 03VT
    - Right 03VS
  - Thyroid
    - Left 03VV
    - Right 03VU
  - Ulnar
    - Left 03VA
    - Right 03V9
  - Upper 03VY
  - Vertebral
    - Left 03VQ
    - Right 03VP
- Bladder 0TVB
- Bladder Neck 0TVC
- Bronchus
  - Lingula 0BV9
  - Lower Lobe
    - Left 0BVB
    - Right 0BV6
  - Main
    - Left 0BV7
    - Right 0BV3
  - Middle Lobe, Right 0BV5
  - Upper Lobe
    - Left 0BV8
    - Right 0BV4
- Carina 0BV2
- Cecum 0DVH
- Cervix 0UVC
- Cisterna Chyli 07VL
- Colon
  - Ascending 0DVK
  - Descending 0DVM
  - Sigmoid 0DVN
  - Transverse 0DVL
- Duct
  - Common Bile 0FV9
  - Cystic 0FV8
  - Hepatic
    - Common 0FV7
    - Left 0FV6
    - Right 0FV5
  - Lacrimal
    - Left 08VY
    - Right 08VX
  - Pancreatic 0FVD
    - Accessory 0FVF
  - Parotid
    - Left 0CVC
    - Right 0CVB
- Duodenum 0DV9
- Esophagogastric Junction 0DV4
- Esophagus 0DV5
  - Lower 0DV3
  - Middle 0DV2
  - Upper 0DV1
- Heart 02VA
- Ileocecal Valve 0DVC
- Ileum 0DVB
- Intestine
  - Large 0DVE
    - Left 0DVG
    - Right 0DVF
  - Small 0DV8
- Jejunum 0DVA

Restriction *(continued)*
- Kidney Pelvis
  - Left 0TV4
  - Right 0TV3
- Lymphatic
  - Aortic 07VD
  - Axillary
    - Left 07V6
    - Right 07V5
  - Head 07V0
  - Inguinal
    - Left 07VJ
    - Right 07VH
  - Internal Mammary
    - Left 07V9
    - Right 07V8
  - Lower Extremity
    - Left 07VG
    - Right 07VF
  - Mesenteric 07VB
  - Neck
    - Left 07V2
    - Right 07V1
  - Pelvis 07VC
  - Thoracic Duct 07VK
  - Thorax 07V7
  - Upper Extremity
    - Left 07V4
    - Right 07V3
- Rectum 0DVP
- Stomach 0DV6
  - Pylorus 0DV7
- Trachea 0BV1
- Ureter
  - Left 0TV7
  - Right 0TV6
- Urethra 0TVD
- Valve, Mitral 02VG
- Vein
  - Axillary
    - Left 05V8
    - Right 05V7
  - Azygos 05V0
  - Basilic
    - Left 05VC
    - Right 05VB
  - Brachial
    - Left 05VA
    - Right 05V9
  - Cephalic
    - Left 05VF
    - Right 05VD
  - Colic 06V7Z
  - Common Iliac
    - Left 06VD
    - Right 06VC
  - Esophageal 06V3
  - External Iliac
    - Left 06VG
    - Right 06VF
  - External Jugular
    - Left 05VQ
    - Right 05VP
  - Face
    - Left 05VV
    - Right 05VT
  - Femoral
    - Left 06VN
    - Right 06VM
  - Foot
    - Left 06VV
    - Right 06VT
  - Gastric 06V2
  - Hand
    - Left 05VH
    - Right 05VG
  - Hemiazygos 05V1
  - Hepatic 06V4
  - Hypogastric
    - Left 06VJ

Restriction *(continued)*
Vein *(continued)*
Hypogastric *(continued)*
Right 06VH
Inferior Mesenteric 06V6
Innominate
Left 05V4
Right 05V3
Internal Jugular
Left 05VN
Right 05VM
Intracranial 05VL
Lower 06VY
Portal 06V8
Pulmonary
Left 02VT
Right 02VS
Renal
Left 06VB
Right 06V9
Saphenous
Left 06VQ
Right 06VP
Splenic 06V1
Subclavian
Left 05V6
Right 05V5
Superior Mesenteric 06V5
Upper 05VY
Vertebral
Left 05VS
Right 05VR
Vena Cava
Inferior 06V0
Superior 02VV
Resurfacing Device
Removal of device from
Left 0SPB0BZ
Right 0SP90BZ
Revision of device in
Left 0SWB0BZ
Right 0SW90BZ
Supplement
Left 0SUB0BZ
Acetabular Surface 0SUE0BZ
Femoral Surface 0SUS0BZ
Right 0SU90BZ
Acetabular Surface 0SUA0BZ
Femoral Surface 0SUR0BZ
Resuscitation
Cardiopulmonary
see Assistance, Cardiac 5A02
Cardioversion 5A2204Z
Defibrillation 5A2204Z
Endotracheal intubation
see Insertion of device in, Trachea 0BH1
External chest compression 5A12012
Pulmonary 5A19054
Resuscitative endovascular balloon occlusion of the aorta (REBOA)
02LW3DJ
04L03DJ
Resuture, Heart valve prosthesis
see Revision of device in, Heart and Great Vessels 02W
Retained placenta, manual removal
see Extraction, Products of Conception, Retained 10D1
Retraining
Cardiac
see Motor Treatment, Rehabilitation F07
Vocational
see Activities of Daily Living Treatment, Rehabilitation F08
Retrogasserian rhizotomy
see Division, Nerve, Trigeminal 008K
Retroperitoneal cavity
use Retroperitoneum
Retroperitoneal lymph node
use Lymphatic, Aortic
Retroperitoneal space
use Retroperitoneum
Retropharyngeal lymph node
use Lymphatic, Neck, Left
use Lymphatic, Neck, Right
Retropubic space
use Pelvic Cavity
Reveal (DX)(XT)
use Monitoring Device
Reverse® Shoulder Prosthesis
use Synthetic Substitute, Reverse Ball and Socket in 0RR
Reverse total shoulder replacement
see Replacement, Upper Joints 0RR
Revision
Correcting a portion of existing device
see Revision of device in
Removal of device without replacement
see Removal of device from
Replacement of existing device
see Removal of device from
see Root operation to place new device, e.g., Insertion, Replacement, Supplement
Revision of device in
Abdominal Wall 0WWF
Acetabulum
Left 0QW5
Right 0QW4
Anal Sphincter 0DWR
Anus 0DWQ
Artery
Lower 04WY
Upper 03WYM
Auditory Ossicle
Left 09WA
Right 09W9
Back
Lower 0WWL
Upper 0WWK
Bladder 0TWB
Bone
Facial 0NWW
Lower 0QWY
Nasal 0NWB
Pelvic
Left 0QW3
Right 0QW2
Upper 0PWY
Bone Marrow 07WT
Brain 00W0
Breast
Left 0HWU
Right 0HWT
Bursa and Ligament
Lower 0MWY
Upper 0MWX
Carpal
Left 0PWN
Right 0PWM
Cavity, Cranial 0WW1
Cerebral Ventricle 00W6
Chest Wall 0WW8
Cisterna Chyli 07WL
Clavicle
Left 0PWB
Right 0PW9
Coccyx 0QWS
Diaphragm 0BWTM
Disc
Cervical Vertebral 0RW3
Cervicothoracic Vertebral 0RW5
Lumbar Vertebral 0SW2
Lumbosacral 0SW4
Revision of device in *(continued)*
Disc *(continued)*
Thoracic Vertebral 0RW9
Thoracolumbar Vertebral 0RWB
Duct
Hepatobiliary 0FWB
Pancreatic 0FWD
Ear
Inner
Left 09WE
Right 09WD
Left 09WJ
Right 09WH
Epididymis and Spermatic Cord 0VWM
Esophagus 0DW5D
Extremity
Lower
Left 0YWB
Right 0YW9
Upper
Left 0XW7
Right 0XW6
Eye
Left 08W1
Right 08W0
Face 0WW2
Fallopian Tube 0UW8
Femoral Shaft
Left 0QW9
Right 0QW8
Femur
Lower
Left 0QWC
Right 0QWB
Upper
Left 0QW7
Right 0QW6
Fibula
Left 0QWK
Right 0QWJ
Finger Nail 0HWQX
Gallbladder 0FW4
Gastrointestinal Tract 0WWP
Genitourinary Tract 0WWR
Gland
Adrenal 0GW50
Endocrine 0GWS
Pituitary 0GW00
Salivary 0CWA
Glenoid Cavity
Left 0PW8
Right 0PW7
Great Vessel 02WY
Hair 0HWSX
Head 0WW0
Heart 02WA
Humeral Head
Left 0PWD
Right 0PWC
Humeral Shaft
Left 0PWG
Right 0PWF
Intestinal Tract
Lower 0DWD
Upper 0DW0
Intestine
Large 0DWE
Small 0DW8
Jaw
Lower 0WW5
Upper 0WW4
Joint
Acromioclavicular
Left 0RWH
Right 0RWG
Ankle
Left 0SWG
Right 0SWF
Revision of device in *(continued)*
Joint *(continued)*
Carpal
Left 0RWR
Right 0RWQ
Carpometacarpal
Left 0RWT
Right 0RWS
Cervical Vertebral 0RW1
Cervicothoracic Vertebral 0RW
Coccygeal 0SW6
Elbow
Left 0RWM
Right 0RWL
Finger Phalangeal
Left 0RWX
Right 0RWW
Hip
Left 0SWB
Acetabluar Surface 0S
Femoral Surface 0SW
Right 0SW9
Acetabluar Surface 0S
Femoral Surface 0SW
Knee
Left 0SWD
Femoral Surface 0SW
Tibial Surface 0SWW
Right 0SWC
Femoral Surface 0SW
Tibial Surface 0SWV
Lumbar Vertebral 0SW0
Lumbosacral 0SW3
Metacarpophalangeal
Left 0RWV
Right 0RWU
Metatarsal-Phalangeal
Left 0SWN
Right 0SWM
Occipital-cervical 0RW0
Sacrococcygeal 0SW5
Sacroiliac
Left 0SW8
Right 0SW7
Shoulder
Left 0RWK
Right 0RWJ
Sternoclavicular
Left 0RWF
Right 0RWE
Tarsal
Left 0SWJ
Right 0SWH
Tarsometatarsal
Left 0SWL
Right 0SWK
Temporomandibular
Left 0RWD
Right 0RWC
Thoracic Vertebral 0RW6
Thoracolumbar Vertebral 0RWA
Toe Phalangeal
Left 0SWQ
Right 0SWP
Wrist
Left 0RWP
Right 0RWN
Kidney 0TW5
Larynx 0CWS
Lens
Left 08WKJ
Right 08WJ
Liver 0FW0
Lung
Left 0BWL
Right 0BWK
Lymphatic 07WN
Thoracic Duct 07WK
Mediastinum 0WWC
Mesentery 0DWV

- **Revision of device in** *(continued)*
  - Metacarpal
    - Left 0PWQ
    - Right 0PWP
  - Metatarsal
    - Left 0QWP
    - Right 0QWN
  - Mouth and Throat 0CWY
  - Muscle
    - Extraocular
      - Left 08WM
      - Right 08WL
    - Lower 0KWY
    - Upper 0KWX
  - Nasal Mucosa and Soft Tissue 09WK
  - Neck 0WW6
  - Nerve
    - Cranial 00WE
    - Peripheral 01WY
  - Omentum 0DWU
  - Ovary 0UW3
  - Pancreas 0FWG
  - Parathyroid Gland 0GWR
  - Patella
    - Left 0QWF
    - Right 0QWD
  - Pelvic Cavity 0WWJ
  - Penis 0VWS
  - Pericardial Cavity 0WWD
  - Perineum
    - Female 0WWN
    - Male 0WWM
  - Peritoneal Cavity 0WWG
  - Peritoneum 0DWW
  - Phalanx
    - Finger
      - Left 0PWV
      - Right 0PWT
    - Thumb
      - Left 0PWS
      - Right 0PWR
    - Toe
      - Left 0QWR
      - Right 0QWQ
  - Pineal Body 0GW10
  - Pleura 0BWQ
  - Pleural Cavity
    - Left 0WWB
    - Right 0WW9
  - Prostate and Seminal Vesicles 0VW4
  - Radius
    - Left 0PWJ
    - Right 0PWH
  - Respiratory Tract 0WWQ
  - Retroperitoneum 0WWH
  - Ribs
    - 1 to 2 0PW1
    - 3 or More 0PW2
  - Sacrum 0QW1
  - Scapula
    - Left 0PW6
    - Right 0PW5
  - Scrotum and Tunica Vaginalis 0VW8
  - Septum
    - Atrial 02W5
    - Ventricular 02WM
  - Sinus 09WY0
  - Skin 0HWPX
  - Skull 0NW0
  - Spinal Canal 00WU
  - Spinal Cord 00WV
  - Spleen 07WP
  - Sternum 0PW0
  - Stomach 0DW6
  - Subcutaneous Tissue and Fascia
    - Head and Neck 0JWS
- **Revision of device in** *(continued)*
  - Subcutaneous Tissue and Fascia *(continued)*
    - Lower Extremity 0JWW
    - Trunk 0JWT
    - Upper Extremity 0JWV
  - Tarsal
    - Left 0QWM
    - Right 0QWL
  - Tendon
    - Lower 0LWY
    - Upper 0LWX
  - Testis 0VWD
  - Thymus 07WM
  - Thyroid Gland 0GWK0
  - Tibia
    - Left 0QWH
    - Right 0QWG
  - Toe Nail 0HWRX
  - Trachea 0BW1F
  - Tracheobronchial Tree 0BW0
  - Tympanic Membrane
    - Left 09W8
    - Right 09W7
  - Ulna
    - Left 0PWL
    - Right 0PWK
  - Ureter 0TW9M
  - Urethra 0TWD
  - Uterus and Cervix 0UWD
  - Vagina and Cul-de-sac 0UWH
  - Valve
    - Aortic 02WF
    - Mitral 02WG
    - Pulmonary 02WH
    - Tricuspid 02WJ
  - Vas Deferens 0VWR
  - Vein
    - Azygos 05W0
    - Innominate
      - Left 05W4
      - Right 05W3
    - Lower 06WY
    - Upper 05WY
  - Vertebra
    - Cervical 0PW3
    - Lumbar 0QW0
    - Thoracic 0PW4
  - Vulva 0UWM
- **Revo MRI™ SureScan® pacemaker**
  - *use* Pacemaker, Dual Chamber in 0JH
- **rhBMP-2**
  - *use* Recombinant Bone Morphogenetic Protein
- **Rheos® System device**
  - *use* Stimulator Generator in Subcutaneous Tissue and Fascia
- **Rheos® System lead**
  - *use* Stimulator Lead in Upper Arteries
- **Rhinopharynx**
  - *use* Nasopharynx
- **Rhinoplasty**
  - *see* Alteration, Nasal Mucosa and Soft Tissue 090K
  - *see* Repair, Nasal Mucosa and Soft Tissue 09QK
  - *see* Replacement, Nasal Mucosa and Soft Tissue 09RK
  - *see* Supplement, Nasal Mucosa and Soft Tissue 09UK
- **Rhinorrhaphy**
  - *see* Repair, Nasal Mucosa and Soft Tissue 09QK
- **Rhinoscopy** 09JKXZZ
- **Rhizotomy**
  - *see* Division, Central Nervous System and Cranial Nerves 008
  - *see* Division, Peripheral Nervous System 018
- **Rhomboid major muscle**
  - *use* Muscle, Trunk, Left
  - *use* Muscle, Trunk, Right
- **Rhomboid minor muscle**
  - *use* Muscle, Trunk, Left
  - *use* Muscle, Trunk, Right
- **Rhythm electrocardiogram**
  - *see* Measurement, Cardiac 4A02
- **Rhytidectomy**
  - *see* Alteration, Face 0W02
- **Right ascending lumbar vein**
  - *use* Vein, Azygos
- **Right atrioventricular valve**
  - *use* Valve, Tricuspid
- **Right auricular appendix**
  - *use* Atrium, Right
- **Right colic vein**
  - *use* Vein, Colic
- **Right coronary sulcus**
  - *use* Heart, Right
- **Right gastric artery**
  - *use* Artery, Gastric
- **Right gastroepiploic vein**
  - *use* Vein, Superior Mesenteric
- **Right inferior phrenic vein**
  - *use* Vena Cava, Inferior
- **Right inferior pulmonary vein**
  - *use* Vein, Pulmonary, Right
- **Right jugular trunk**
  - *use* Lymphatic, Neck, Right
- **Right lateral ventricle**
  - *use* Cerebral Ventricle
- **Right lymphatic duct**
  - *use* Lymphatic, Neck, Right
- **Right ovarian vein**
  - *use* Vena Cava, Inferior
- **Right second lumbar vein**
  - *use* Vena Cava, Inferior
- **Right subclavian trunk**
  - *use* Lymphatic, Neck, Right
- **Right subcostal vein**
  - *use* Vein, Azygos
- **Right superior pulmonary vein**
  - *use* Vein, Pulmonary, Right
- **Right suprarenal vein**
  - *use* Vena Cava, Inferior
- **Right testicular vein**
  - *use* Vena Cava, Inferior
- **Rima glottidis**
  - *use* Larynx
- **Risorius muscle**
  - *use* Muscle, Facial
- **RNS System lead**
  - *use* Neurostimulator Lead in Central Nervous System and Cranial Nerves
- **RNS system neurostimulator generator**
  - *use* Neurostimulator Generator in Head and Facial Bones
- **Robotic Assisted Procedure**
  - Extremity
    - Lower 8E0Y
    - Upper 8E0X
  - Head and Neck Region 8E09
  - Trunk Region 8E0W
- **Robotic Waterjet Ablation, Destruction, Prostate** XV508A4
- **Rotation of fetal head**
  - Forceps 10S07ZZ
  - Manual 10S0XZZ
- **Round ligament of uterus**
  - *use* Uterine Supporting Structure
- **Round window**
  - *use* Ear, Inner, Left
  - *use* Ear, Inner, Right
- **Roux-en-Y operation**
  - *see* Bypass, Gastrointestinal System 0D1
- **Roux-en-Y operation***(continued)*
  - *see* Bypass, Hepatobiliary System and Pancreas 0F1
- **Rupture**
  - Adhesions
    - *see* Release
  - Fluid collection
    - *see* Drainage

S

- **Sacral ganglion**
  - *use* Nerve, Sacral Sympathetic
- **Sacral lymph node**
  - *use* Lymphatic, Pelvis
- **Sacral nerve modulation (SNM) lead**
  - *use* Stimulator Lead in Urinary System
- **Sacral neuromodulation lead**
  - *use* Stimulator Lead in Urinary System
- **Sacral splanchnic nerve**
  - *use* Nerve, Sacral Sympathetic
- **Sacrectomy**
  - *see* Excision, Lower Bones 0QB
- **Sacrococcygeal ligament**
  - *use* Bursa and Ligament, Lower Spine
- **Sacrococcygeal symphysis**
  - *use* Joint, Sacrococcygeal
- **Sacroiliac ligament**
  - *use* Bursa and Ligament, Lower Spine
- **Sacrospinous ligament**
  - *use* Bursa and Ligament, Lower Spine
- **Sacrotuberous ligament**
  - *use* Bursa and Ligament, Lower Spine
- **Salpingectomy**
  - *see* Excision, Female Reproductive System 0UB
  - *see* Resection, Female Reproductive System 0UT
- **Salpingolysis**
  - *see* Release, Female Reproductive System 0UN
- **Salpingopexy**
  - *see* Repair, Female Reproductive System 0UQ
  - *see* Reposition, Female Reproductive System 0US
- **Salpingopharyngeus muscle**
  - *use* Muscle, Tongue, Palate, Pharynx
- **Salpingoplasty**
  - *see* Repair, Female Reproductive System 0UQ
  - *see* Supplement, Female Reproductive System 0UU
- **Salpingorrhaphy**
  - *see* Repair, Female Reproductive System 0UQ
- **Salpingoscopy** 0UJ88ZZ
- **Salpingostomy**
  - *see* Drainage, Female Reproductive System 0U9
- **Salpingotomy**
  - *see* Drainage, Female Reproductive System 0U9
- **Salpinx**
  - *use* Fallopian Tube, Left
  - *use* Fallopian Tube, Right
- **Saphenous nerve**
  - *use* Nerve, Femoral
- **SAPIEN transcatheter aortic valve**
  - *use* Zooplastic Tissue in Heart and Great Vessels
- **Sartorius muscle**
  - *use* Muscle, Upper Leg, Left
  - *use* Muscle, Upper Leg, Right

Scalene muscle
use Muscle, Neck, Left
use Muscle, Neck, Right
Scan
Computerized Tomography (CT)
see Computerized Tomography (CT Scan)
Radioisotope
see Planar Nuclear Medicine Imaging
Scaphoid bone
use Carpal, Left
use Carpal, Right
Scapholunate ligament
use Bursa and Ligament, Hand, Left
use Bursa and Ligament, Hand, Right
Scaphotrapezium ligament
use Bursa and Ligament, Hand, Left
use Bursa and Ligament, Hand, Right
Scapulectomy
see Excision, Upper Bones 0PB
see Resection, Upper Bones 0PT
Scapulopexy
see Repair, Upper Bones 0PQ
see Reposition, Upper Bones 0PS
Scarpa's (vestibular) ganglion
use Nerve, Acoustic
Sclerectomy
see Excision, Eye 08B
Sclerotherapy, mechanical
see Destruction
Sclerotherapy, via injection of sclerosing agent
see Introduction, Destructive Agent
Sclerotomy
see Drainage, Eye 089
Scrotectomy
see Excision, Male Reproductive System 0VB
see Resection, Male Reproductive System 0VT
Scrotoplasty
see Repair, Male Reproductive System 0VQ
see Supplement, Male Reproductive System 0VU
Scrotorrhaphy
see Repair, Male Reproductive System 0VQ
Scrototomy
see Drainage, Male Reproductive System 0V9
Sebaceous gland
use Skin
Second cranial nerve
use Nerve, Optic
Section, cesarean
see Extraction, Pregnancy 10D
Secura (DR) (VR)
use Defibrillator Generator in 0JH
Sella Turcica
use Bone, Sphenoid
Semicircular canal
use Ear, Inner, Left
use Ear, Inner, Right
Semimembranosus muscle
use Muscle, Upper Leg, Left
use Muscle, Upper Leg, Right
Semitendinosus muscle
use Muscle, Upper Leg, Left
use Muscle, Upper Leg, Right
Seprafilm
use Adhesion Barrier
Septal cartilage
use Septum, Nasal
Septectomy
see Excision, Ear, Nose, Sinus 09B
see Excision, Heart and Great Vessels 02B
see Resection, Ear, Nose, Sinus 09T
Septectomy *(continued)*
see Resection, Heart and Great Vessels 02T
Septoplasty
see Repair, Ear, Nose, Sinus 09Q
see Repair, Heart and Great Vessels 02Q
see Replacement, Ear, Nose, Sinus 09R
see Replacement, Heart and Great Vessels 02R
see Reposition, Ear, Nose, Sinus 09S
see Supplement, Ear, Nose, Sinus 09U
see Supplement, Heart and Great Vessels 02U
Septostomy, balloon atrial 02163Z7
Septotomy
see Drainage, Ear, Nose, Sinus 099
Sequestrectomy, bone
see Extirpation
Serratus anterior muscle
use Muscle, Thorax, Left
use Muscle, Thorax, Right
Serratus posterior muscle
use Muscle, Trunk, Left
use Muscle, Trunk, Right
Seventh cranial nerve
use Nerve, Facial
Sheffield hybrid external fixator
use External Fixation Device, Hybrid in 0PH
use External Fixation Device, Hybrid in 0PS
use External Fixation Device, Hybrid in 0QH
use External Fixation Device, Hybrid in 0QS
Sheffield ring external fixator
use External Fixation Device, Ring in 0PH
use External Fixation Device, Ring in 0PS
use External Fixation Device, Ring in 0QH
use External Fixation Device, Ring in 0QS
Shirodkar cervical cerclage 0UVC7ZZ
Shock Wave Therapy, Musculoskeletal 6A93
Short gastric artery
use Artery, Splenic
Shortening
see Excision
see Repair
see Reposition
Shunt creation
see Bypass
Sialoadenectomy
Complete
see Resection, Mouth and Throat 0CT
Partial
see Excision, Mouth and Throat 0CB
Sialodochoplasty
see Repair, Mouth and Throat 0CQ
see Replacement, Mouth and Throat 0CR
see Supplement, Mouth and Throat 0CU
Sialoectomy
see Excision, Mouth and Throat 0CB
see Resection, Mouth and Throat 0CT
Sialography
see Plain Radiography, Ear, Nose, Mouth and Throat B90
Sialolithotomy
see Extirpation, Mouth and Throat 0CC
Sigmoid artery
use Artery, Inferior Mesenteric
Sigmoid flexure
use Colon, Sigmoid
Sigmoid vein
use Vein, Inferior Mesenteric
Sigmoidectomy
see Excision, Gastrointestinal System 0DB
see Resection, Gastrointestinal System 0DT
Sigmoidorrhaphy
see Repair, Gastrointestinal System 0DQ
Sigmoidoscopy 0DJD8ZZ
Sigmoidotomy
see Drainage, Gastrointestinal System 0D9
Single lead pacemaker (atrium) (ventricle)
use Pacemaker, Single Chamber in 0JH
Single lead rate responsive pacemaker (atrium)(ventricle)
use Pacemaker, Single Chamber Rate Responsive in 0JH
Sinoatrial node
use Conduction Mechanism
Sinogram
Abdominal Wall
see Fluoroscopy, Abdomen and Pelvis BW11
Chest Wall
see Plain Radiography, Chest BW03
Retroperitoneum
see Fluoroscopy, Abdomen and Pelvis BW11
Sinusectomy
see Excision, Ear, Nose, Sinus 09B
see Resection, Ear, Nose, Sinus 09T
Sinusoscopy 09JY4ZZ
Sinusotomy
see Drainage, Ear, Nose, Sinus 099
Sinus venosus
use Atrium, Right
Sirolimus-eluting coronary stent
use Intraluminal Device, Drug-eluting in Heart and Great Vessels
Sixth cranial nerve
use Nerve, Abducens
Size reduction, breast
see Excision, Skin and Breast 0HB
SJM Biocor® Stented Valve System
use Zooplastic Tissue in Heart and Great Vessels
Skene's (paraurethral) gland
use Gland, Vestibular
Skin Substitute, Porcine Liver Derived, Replacement XHRPXL2
Sling
Fascial, orbicularis muscle (mouth)
see Supplement, Muscle, Facial 0KU1
Levator muscle, for urethral suspension
see Reposition, Bladder Neck 0TSC
Pubococcygeal, for urethral suspension
see Reposition, Bladder Neck 0TSC
Rectum
see Reposition, Rectum 0DSP
Small bowel series
see Fluoroscopy, Bowel, Small BD1
Small saphenous vein
use Vein, Saphenous, Left
use Vein, Saphenous, Right
Snaring, polyp, colon
see Excision, Gastrointestinal System 0DB
Solar (celiac) plexus
use Nerve, Abdominal Sympathetic
Soleus muscle
use Muscle, Lower Leg, Left
use Muscle, Lower Leg, Right
Spacer
Insertion of device in
Disc
Lumbar Vertebral 0SH2
Lumbosacral 0SH4
Joint
Acromioclavicular
Left 0RHH
Right 0RHG
Ankle
Left 0SHG
Right 0SHF
Carpal
Left 0RHR
Right 0RHQ
Carpometacarpal
Left 0RHT
Right 0RHS
Cervical Vertebral 0RH1
Cervicothoracic Vertebral 0RH4
Coccygeal 0SH6
Elbow
Left 0RHM
Right 0RHL
Finger Phalangeal
Left 0RHX
Right 0RHW
Hip
Left 0SHB
Right 0SH9
Knee
Left 0SHD
Right 0SHC
Lumbar Vertebral 0SH0
Lumbosacral 0SH3
Metacarpophalangeal
Left 0RHV
Right 0RHU
Metatarsal-Phalangeal
Left 0SHN
Right 0SHM
Occipital-cervical 0RH0
Sacrococcygeal 0SH5
Sacroiliac
Left 0SH8
Right 0SH7
Shoulder
Left 0RHK
Right 0RHJ
Sternoclavicular
Left 0RHF
Right 0RHE
Tarsal
Left 0SHJ
Right 0SHH
Tarsometatarsal
Left 0SHL
Right 0SHK
Temporomandibular
Left 0RHD
Right 0RHC
Thoracic Vertebral 0RH6
Thoracolumbar Vertebral 0RHA
Toe Phalangeal
Left 0SHQ
Right 0SHP

pacer *(continued)*
Insertion of device in *(continued)*
Joint *(continued)*
Wrist
Left 0RHP
Right 0RHN
Removal of device from
Acromioclavicular
Left 0RPH
Right 0RPG
Ankle
Left 0SPG
Right 0SPF
Carpal
Left 0RPR
Right 0RPQ
Carpometacarpal
Left 0RPT
Right 0RPS
Cervical Vertebral 0RP1
Cervicothoracic Vertebral 0RP4
Coccygeal 0SP6
Elbow
Left 0RPM
Right 0RPL
Finger Phalangeal
Left 0RPX
Right 0RPW
Hip
Left 0SPB
Right 0SP9
Knee
Left 0SPD
Right 0SPC
Lumbar Vertebral 0SP0
Lumbosacral 0SP3
Metacarpophalangeal
Left 0RPV
Right 0RPU
Metatarsal-Phalangeal
Left 0SPN
Right 0SPM
Occipital-cervical 0RP0
Sacrococcygeal 0SP5
Sacroiliac
Left 0SP8
Right 0SP7
Shoulder
Left 0RPK
Right 0RPJ
Sternoclavicular
Left 0RPF
Right 0RPE
Tarsal
Left 0SPJ
Right 0SPH
Tarsometatarsal
Left 0SPL
Right 0SPK
Temporomandibular
Left 0RPD
Right 0RPC
Thoracic Vertebral 0RP6
Thoracolumbar Vertebral 0RPA
Toe Phalangeal
Left 0SPQ
Right 0SPP
Wrist
Left 0RPP
Right 0RPN
Revision of device in
Acromioclavicular
Left 0RWH
Right 0RWG
Ankle
Left 0SWG
Right 0SWF
Carpal
Left 0RWR
Right 0RWQ

Spacer *(continued)*
Revision of device in *(continued)*
Carpometacarpal
Left 0RWT
Right 0RWS
Cervical Vertebral 0RW1
Cervicothoracic Vertebral 0RW4
Coccygeal 0SW6
Elbow
Left 0RWM
Right 0RWL
Finger Phalangeal
Left 0RWX
Right 0RWW
Hip
Left 0SWB
Right 0SW9
Knee
Left 0SWD
Right 0SWC
Lumbar Vertebral 0SW0
Lumbosacral 0SW3
Metacarpophalangeal
Left 0RWV
Right 0RWU
Metatarsal-Phalangeal
Left 0SWN
Right 0SWM
Occipital-cervical 0RW0
Sacrococcygeal 0SW5
Sacroiliac
Left 0SW8
Right 0SW7
Shoulder
Left 0RWK
Right 0RWJ
Sternoclavicular
Left 0RWF
Right 0RWE
Tarsal
Left 0SWJ
Right 0SWH
Tarsometatarsal
Left 0SWL
Right 0SWK
Temporomandibular
Left 0RWD
Right 0RWC
Thoracic Vertebral 0RW6
Thoracolumbar Vertebral 0RWA
Toe Phalangeal
Left 0SWQ
Right 0SWP
Wrist
Left 0RWP
Right 0RWN
Spacer, Articulating (Antibiotic)
use Articulating Spacer in Lower Joints
Spacer, Static (Antibiotic)
use Spacer in Lower Joints
Spectroscopy
Intravascular 8E023DZ
Near infrared 8E023DZ
Speech Assessment F00
Speech therapy
see Speech Treatment, Rehabilitation F06
Speech Treatment F06
Sphenoidectomy
see Excision, Ear, Nose, Sinus 09B
see Excision, Head and Facial Bones 0NB
see Resection, Ear, Nose, Sinus 09T
see Resection, Head and Facial Bones 0NT
Sphenoidotomy
see Drainage, Ear, Nose, Sinus 099
Sphenomandibular ligament
use Bursa and Ligament, Head and Neck

Sphenopalatine (pterygopalatine) ganglion
use Nerve, Head and Neck Sympathetic
Sphincterorrhaphy, anal
see Repair, Anal Sphincter 0DQR
Sphincterotomy, anal
see Division, Anal Sphincter 0D8R
see Drainage, Anal Sphincter 0D9R
Spinal cord neurostimulator lead
use Neurostimulator Lead in Central Nervous System and Cranial Nerves
Spinal growth rod(s), magnetically controlled
use Magnetically Controlled Growth Rod(s) in New Technology
Spinal nerve, cervical
use Nerve, Cervical
Spinal nerve, lumbar
use Nerve, Lumbar
Spinal nerve, sacral
use Nerve, Sacral
Spinal nerve, thoracic
use Nerve, Thoracic
Spinal Stabilization Device
Facet Replacement
Cervical Vertebral 0RH1
Cervicothoracic Vertebral 0RH4
Lumbar Vertebral 0SH0
Lumbosacral 0SH3
Occipital-cervical 0RH0
Thoracic Vertebral 0RH6
Thoracolumbar Vertebral 0RHA
Interspinous Process
Cervical Vertebral 0RH1
Cervicothoracic Vertebral 0RH4
Lumbar Vertebral 0SH0
Lumbosacral 0SH3
Occipital-cervical 0RH0
Thoracic Vertebral 0RH6
Thoracolumbar Vertebral 0RHA
Pedicle-Based
Cervical Vertebral 0RH1
Cervicothoracic Vertebral 0RH4
Lumbar Vertebral 0SH0
Lumbosacral 0SH3
Occipital-cervical 0RH0
Thoracic Vertebral 0RH6
Thoracolumbar Vertebral 0RHA
Spinous process
use Vertebra, Cervical
use Vertebra, Lumbar
use Vertebra, Thoracic
Spiral ganglion
use Nerve, Acoustic
Spiration IBV™ Valve System
use Intraluminal Device, Endobronchial Valve in Respiratory System
Splenectomy
see Excision, Lymphatic and Hemic Systems 07B
see Resection, Lymphatic and Hemic Systems 07T
Splenic flexure
use Colon, Transverse
Splenic plexus
use Nerve, Abdominal Sympathetic
Splenius capitis muscle
use Muscle, Head
Splenius cervicis muscle
use Muscle, Neck, Left
use Muscle, Neck, Right
Splenolysis
see Release, Lymphatic and Hemic Systems 07N
Splenopexy
see Repair, Lymphatic and Hemic Systems 07Q

Splenopexy *(continued)*
see Reposition, Lymphatic and Hemic Systems 07S
Splenoplasty
see Repair, Lymphatic and Hemic Systems 07Q
Splenorrhaphy
see Repair, Lymphatic and Hemic Systems 07Q
Splenotomy
see Drainage, Lymphatic and Hemic Systems 079
Splinting, musculoskeletal
see Immobilization, Anatomical Regions 2W3
SPY system intravascular fluorescence angiography
see Monitoring, Physiological Systems 4A1
Stapedectomy
see Excision, Ear, Nose, Sinus 09B
see Resection, Ear, Nose, Sinus 09T
Stapediolysis
see Release, Ear, Nose, Sinus 09N
Stapedioplasty
see Repair, Ear, Nose, Sinus 09Q
see Replacement, Ear, Nose, Sinus 09R
see Supplement, Ear, Nose, Sinus 09U
Stapedotomy
see Drainage, Ear, Nose, Sinus 099
Stapes
use Auditory Ossicle, Left
use Auditory Ossicle, Right
Static Spacer (Antibiotic)
use Spacer in Lower Joints
STELARA®
use Other New Technology Therapeutic Substance
Stellate ganglion
use Nerve, Head and Neck Sympathetic
Stem cell transplant
see Transfusion, Circulatory 302
Stensen's duct
use Duct, Parotid, Left
use Duct, Parotid, Right
Stent retriever thrombectomy
see Extirpation, Upper Arteries 03C
Stent, intraluminal (cardiovascular) (gastrointestinal) (hepatobiliary)(urinary)
use Intraluminal Device
Stented tissue valve
use Zooplastic Tissue in Heart and Great Vessels
Stereotactic Radiosurgery
Abdomen DW23
Adrenal Gland DG22
Bile Ducts DF22
Bladder DT22
Bone Marrow D720
Brain D020
Brain Stem D021
Breast
Left DM20
Right DM21
Bronchus DB21
Cervix DU21
Chest DW22
Chest Wall DB27
Colon DD25
Diaphragm DB28
Duodenum DD22
Ear D920
Esophagus DD20
Eye D820
Gallbladder DF21
Gamma Beam
Abdomen DW23JZZ

Stereotactic Radiosurgery *(continued)*
Gamma Beam *(continued)*
Adrenal Gland DG22JZZ
Bile Ducts DF22JZZ
Bladder DT22JZZ
Bone Marrow D720JZZ
Brain D020JZZ
Brain Stem D021JZZ
Breast
Left DM20JZZ
Right DM21JZZ
Bronchus DB21JZZ
Cervix DU21JZZ
Chest DW22JZZ
Chest Wall DB27JZZ
Colon DD25JZZ
Diaphragm DB28JZZ
Duodenum DD22JZZ
Ear D920JZZ
Esophagus DD20JZZ
Eye D820JZZ
Gallbladder DF21JZZ
Gland
Adrenal DG22JZZ
Parathyroid DG24JZZ
Pituitary DG20JZZ
Thyroid DG25JZZ
Glands, Salivary D926JZZ
Head and Neck DW21JZZ
Ileum DD24JZZ
Jejunum DD23JZZ
Kidney DT20JZZ
Larynx D92BJZZ
Liver DF20JZZ
Lung DB22JZZ
Lymphatics
Abdomen D726JZZ
Axillary D724JZZ
Inguinal D728JZZ
Neck D723JZZ
Pelvis D727JZZ
Thorax D725JZZ
Mediastinum DB26JZZ
Mouth D924JZZ
Nasopharynx D92DJZZ
Neck and Head DW21JZZ
Nerve, Peripheral D027JZZ
Nose D921JZZ
Ovary DU20JZZ
Palate
Hard D928JZZ
Soft D929JZZ
Pancreas DF23JZZ
Parathyroid Gland DG24JZZ
Pelvic Region DW26JZZ
Pharynx D92CJZZ
Pineal Body DG21JZZ
Pituitary Gland DG20JZZ
Pleura DB25JZZ
Prostate DV20JZZ
Rectum DD27JZZ
Sinuses D927JZZ
Spinal Cord D026JZZ
Spleen D722JZZ
Stomach DD21JZZ
Testis DV21JZZ
Thymus D721JZZ
Thyroid Gland DG25JZZ
Tongue D925JZZ
Trachea DB20JZZ
Ureter DT21JZZ
Urethra DT23JZZ
Uterus DU22JZZ
Gland
Adrenal DG22
Parathyroid DG24
Pituitary DG20
Thyroid DG25
Glands, Salivary D926
Head and Neck DW21

Stereotactic Radiosurgery *(continued)*
Ileum DD24
Jejunum DD23
Kidney DT20
Larynx D92B
Liver DF20
Lung DB22
Lymphatics
Abdomen D726
Axillary D724
Inguinal D728
Neck D723
Pelvis D727
Thorax D725
Mediastinum DB26
Mouth D924
Nasopharynx D92D
Neck and Head DW21
Nerve, Peripheral D027
Nose D921
Other Photon
Abdomen DW23DZZ
Adrenal Gland DG22DZZ
Bile Ducts DF22DZZ
Bladder DT22DZZ
Bone Marrow D720DZZ
Brain D020DZZ
Brain Stem D021DZZ
Breast
Left DM20DZZ
Right DM21DZZ
Bronchus DB21DZZ
Cervix DU21DZZ
Chest DW22DZZ
Chest Wall DB27DZZ
Colon DD25DZZ
Diaphragm DB28DZZ
Duodenum DD22DZZ
Ear D920DZZ
Esophagus DD20DZZ
Eye D820DZZ
Gallbladder DF21DZZ
Gland
Adrenal DG22DZZ
Parathyroid DG24DZZ
Pituitary DG20DZZ
Thyroid DG25DZZ
Glands, Salivary D926DZZ
Head and Neck DW21DZZ
Ileum DD24DZZ
Jejunum DD23DZZ
Kidney DT20DZZ
Larynx D92BDZZ
Liver DF20DZZ
Lung DB22DZZ
Lymphatics
Abdomen D726DZZ
Axillary D724DZZ
Inguinal D728DZZ
Neck D723DZZ
Pelvis D727DZZ
Thorax D725DZZ
Mediastinum DB26DZZ
Mouth D924DZZ
Nasopharynx D92DDZZ
Neck and Head DW21DZZ
Nerve, Peripheral D027DZZ
Nose D921DZZ
Ovary DU20DZZ
Palate
Hard D928DZZ
Soft D929DZZ
Pancreas DF23DZZ
Parathyroid Gland DG24DZZ
Pelvic Region DW26DZZ
Pharynx D92CDZZ
Pineal Body DG21DZZ

Stereotactic Radiosurgery *(continued)*
Other Photon *(continued)*
Pituitary Gland DG20DZZ
Pleura DB25DZZ
Prostate DV20DZZ
Rectum DD27DZZ
Sinuses D927DZZ
Spinal Cord D026DZZ
Spleen D722DZZ
Stomach DD21DZZ
Testis DV21DZZ
Thymus D721DZZ
Thyroid Gland DG25DZZ
Tongue D925DZZ
Trachea DB20DZZ
Ureter DT21DZZ
Urethra DT23DZZ
Uterus DU22DZZ
Ovary DU20
Palate
Hard D928
Soft D929
Pancreas DF23
Parathyroid Gland DG24
Particulate
Abdomen DW23HZZ
Adrenal Gland DG22HZZ
Bile Ducts DF22HZZ
Bladder DT22HZZ
Bone Marrow D720HZZ
Brain D020HZZ
Brain Stem D021HZZ
Breast
Left DM20HZZ
Right DM21HZZ
Bronchus DB21HZZ
Cervix DU21HZZ
Chest DW22HZZ
Chest Wall DB27HZZ
Colon DD25HZZ
Diaphragm DB28HZZ
Duodenum DD22HZZ
Ear D920HZZ
Esophagus DD20HZZ
Eye D820HZZ
Gallbladder DF21HZZ
Gland
Adrenal DG22HZZ
Parathyroid DG24HZZ
Pituitary DG20HZZ
Thyroid DG25HZZ
Glands, Salivary D926HZZ
Head and Neck DW21HZZ
Ileum DD24HZZ
Jejunum DD23HZZ
Kidney DT20HZZ
Larynx D92BHZZ
Liver DF20HZZ
Lung DB22HZZ
Lymphatics
Abdomen D726HZZ
Axillary D724HZZ
Inguinal D728HZZ
Neck D723HZZ
Pelvis D727HZZ
Thorax D725HZZ
Mediastinum DB26HZZ
Mouth D924HZZ
Nasopharynx D92DHZZ
Neck and Head DW21HZZ
Nerve, Peripheral D027HZZ
Nose D921HZZ
Ovary DU20HZZ
Palate
Hard D928HZZ
Soft D929HZZ
Pancreas DF23HZZ
Parathyroid Gland DG24HZZ
Pelvic Region DW26HZZ
Pharynx D92CHZZ

Stereotactic Radiosurgery *(continue*
Particulate *(continued)*
Pineal Body DG21HZZ
Pituitary Gland DG20HZZ
Pleura DB25HZZ
Prostate DV20HZZ
Rectum DD27HZZ
Sinuses D927HZZ
Spinal Cord D026HZZ
Spleen D722HZZ
Stomach DD21HZZ
Testis DV21HZZ
Thymus D721HZZ
Thyroid Gland DG25HZZ
Tongue D925HZZ
Trachea DB20HZZ
Ureter DT21HZZ
Urethra DT23HZZ
Uterus DU22HZZ
Pelvic Region DW26
Pharynx D92C
Pineal Body DG21
Pituitary Gland DG20
Pleura DB25
Prostate DV20
Rectum DD27
Sinuses D927
Spinal Cord D026
Spleen D722
Stomach DD21
Testis DV21
Thymus D721
Thyroid Gland DG25
Tongue D925
Trachea SB20
Ureter DT21
Urethra DT23
Uterus DU22
Sternoclavicular ligament
use Bursa and Ligament, Shoulde
Right
Sternocleidomastoid artery
use Artery, Thyroid, Left
use Artery, Thyroid, Right
Sternocleidomastoid muscle
use Muscle, Neck, Left
use Muscle, Neck, Right
Sternocostal ligament
use Sternum Bursa and Ligament
Sternotomy
see Division, Sternum 0P80
see Drainage, Sternum 0P90
Stimulation, cardiac
Cardioversion 5A2204Z
Electrophysiologic testing
see Measurement, Cardiac 4A02
Stimulator Generator
Insertion of device in
Abdomen 0JH8
Back 0JH7
Chest 0JH6
Multiple Array
Abdomen 0JH8
Back 0JH7
Chest 0JH6
Multiple Array Rechargeable
Abdomen 0JH8
Back 0JH7
Chest 0JH6
Removal of device from, Subcutaneous Tissue and Fas
Trunk 0JPT
Revision of device in, Subcutane
Tissue and Fascia, Trunk 0JW
Single Array
Abdomen 0JH8
Back 0JH7
Chest 0JH6

Stimulator Generator *(continued)*
Single Array Rechargeable
Abdomen 0JH8
Back 0JH7
Chest 0JH6
Stimulator Lead
Insertion of device in
Anal Sphincter 0DHR
Artery
Left 03HL
Right 03HK
Bladder 0THB
Muscle
Lower 0KHY
Upper 0KHX
Stomach 0DH6
Ureter 0TH9
Removal of device from
Anal Sphincter 0DPR
Artery, Upper 03PY
Bladder 0TPB
Muscle
Lower 0KPY
Upper 0KPX
Stomach 0DP6
Ureter 0TP9
Revision of device in
Anal Sphincter 0DWR
Artery, Upper 03WY
Bladder 0TWB
Muscle
Lower 0KWY
Upper 0KWX
Stomach 0DW6
Ureter 0TW9
toma
Excision
Abdominal Wall 0WBFXZ2
Neck 0WB6XZ2
Repair
Abdominal Wall 0WQFXZ2
Neck 0WQ6XZ2
tomatoplasty
see Repair, Mouth and Throat 0CQ
see Replacement, Mouth and Throat 0CR
see Supplement, Mouth and Throat 0CU
tomatorrhaphy
see Repair, Mouth and Throat 0CQ
tratos LV
use Cardiac Resynchronization Pacemaker Pulse Generator in 0JH
tress test
4A02XM4
4A12XM4
tripping
see Extraction
tudy
Electrophysiologic stimulation, cardiac
see Measurement, Cardiac 4A02
Ocular motility 4A07X7Z
Pulmonary airway flow measurement
see Measurement, Respiratory 4A09
Visual acuity 4A07X0Z
yloglossus muscle
use Muscle, Tongue, Palate, Pharynx
ylomandibular ligament
use Bursa and Ligament, Head and Neck
ylopharyngeus muscle
use Muscle, Tongue, Palate, Pharynx
ıbacromial bursa
use Bursa and Ligament, Shoulder, Left
use Bursa and Ligament, Shoulder, Right
Subaortic (common iliac) lymph node
use Lymphatic, Pelvis
Subarachnoid space, spinal
use Spinal Canal
Subclavicular (apical) lymph node
use Lymphatic, Axillary, Left
use Lymphatic, Axillary, Right
Subclavius muscle
use Muscle, Thorax, Left
use Muscle, Thorax, Right
Subclavius nerve
use Nerve, Brachial Plexus
Subcostal artery
use Upper Artery
Subcostal muscle
use Muscle, Thorax, Left
use Muscle, Thorax, Right
Subcostal nerve
use Nerve, Thoracic
Subcutaneous injection reservoir, port
use Vascular Access Device, Totally Implantable in Subcutaneous Tissue and Fascia
Subcutaneous injection reservoir, pump
use Infusion Device, Pump in Subcutaneous Tissue and Fascia
Subdermal progesterone implant
use Contraceptive Device in Subcutaneous Tissue and Fascia
Subdural space, spinal
use Spinal Canal
Submandibular ganglion
use Nerve, Facial
use Nerve, Head and Neck Sympathetic
Submandibular gland
use Gland, Submaxillary, Left
use Gland, Submaxillary, Right
Submandibular lymph node
use Lymphatic, Head
Submaxillary ganglion
use Nerve, Head and Neck Sympathetic
Submaxillary lymph node
use Lymphatic, Head
Submental artery
use Artery, Face
Submental lymph node
use Lymphatic, Head
Submucous (Meissner's) plexus
use Nerve, Abdominal Sympathetic
Suboccipital nerve
use Nerve, Cervical
Suboccipital venous plexus
use Vein, Vertebral, Left
use Vein, Vertebral, Right
Subparotid lymph node
use Lymphatic, Head
Subscapular (posterior) lymph node
use Lymphatic, Axillary, Left
use Lymphatic, Axillary, Right
Subscapular aponeurosis
use Subcutaneous Tissue and Fascia, Upper Arm, Left
use Subcutaneous Tissue and Fascia, Upper Arm, Right
Subscapular artery
use Artery, Axillary, Left
use Artery, Axillary, Right
Subscapularis muscle
use Muscle, Shoulder, Left
use Muscle, Shoulder, Right
Substance Abuse Treatment
Counseling
Family, for substance abuse, Other Family Counseling HZ63ZZZ
Group
12-Step HZ43ZZZ
Substance Abuse Treatment *(continued)*
Counseling *(continued)*
Group *(continued)*
Behavioral HZ41ZZZ
Cognitive HZ40ZZZ
Cognitive-Behavioral HZ42ZZZ
Confrontational HZ48ZZZ
Continuing Care HZ49ZZZ
Infectious Disease
Post-Test HZ4CZZZ
Pre-Test HZ4CZZZ
Interpersonal HZ44ZZZ
Motivational Enhancement HZ47ZZZ
Psychoeducation HZ46ZZZ
Spiritual HZ4BZZZ
Vocational HZ45ZZZ
Individual
12-Step HZ33ZZZ
Behavioral HZ31ZZZ
Cognitive HZ30ZZZ
Cognitive-Behavioral HZ32ZZZ
Confrontational HZ38ZZZ
Continuing Care HZ39ZZZ
Infectious Disease
Post-Test HZ3CZZZ
Pre-Test HZ3CZZZ
Interpersonal HZ34ZZZ
Motivational Enhancement HZ37ZZZ
Psychoeducation HZ36ZZZ
Spiritual HZ3BZZZ
Vocational HZ35ZZZ
Detoxification Services, for substance abuse HZ2ZZZZ
Medication Management
Antabuse HZ83ZZZ
Bupropion HZ87ZZZ
Clonidine HZ86ZZZ
Levo-alpha-acetyl-methadol (LAAM) HZ82ZZZ
Methadone Maintenance HZ81ZZZ
Naloxone HZ85ZZZ
Naltrexone HZ84ZZZ
Nicotine Replacement HZ80ZZZ
Other Replacement Medication HZ89ZZZ
Psychiatric Medication HZ88ZZZ
Pharmacotherapy
Antabuse HZ93ZZZ
Bupropion HZ97ZZZ
Clonidine HZ96ZZZ
Levo-alpha-acetyl-methadol (LAAM) HZ92ZZZ
Methadone Maintenance HZ91ZZZ
Naloxone HZ95ZZZ
Naltrexone HZ94ZZZ
Nicotine Replacement HZ90ZZZ
Psychiatric Medication HZ98ZZZ
Replacement Medication, Other HZ99ZZZ
Psychotherapy
12-Step HZ53ZZZ
Behavioral HZ51ZZZ
Cognitive HZ50ZZZ
Cognitive-Behavioral HZ52ZZZ
Confrontational HZ58ZZZ
Interactive HZ55ZZZ
Interpersonal HZ54ZZZ
Motivational Enhancement HZ57ZZZ
Substance Abuse Treatment *(continued)*
Psychotherapy *(continued)*
Psychoanalysis HZ5BZZZ
Psychodynamic HZ5CZZZ
Psychoeducation HZ56ZZZ
Psychophysiological HZ5DZZZ
Supportive HZ59ZZZ
Substantia nigra
use Basal Ganglia
Subtalar (talocalcaneal) joint
use Joint, Tarsal, Left
use Joint, Tarsal, Right
Subtalar ligament
use Bursa and Ligament, Foot, Left
use Bursa and Ligament, Foot, Right
Subthalamic nucleus
use Basal Ganglia
Suction curettage (D&C), nonobstetric
see Extraction, Endometrium 0UDB
Suction curettage, obstetric post-delivery
see Extraction, Products of Conception, Retained 10D1
Superficial circumflex iliac vein
use Vein, Saphenous, Left
use Vein, Saphenous, Right
Superficial epigastric artery
use Artery, Femoral, Left
use Artery, Femoral, Right
Superficial epigastric vein
use Vein, Saphenous, Left
use Vein, Saphenous, Right
Superficial Inferior Epigastric Artery Flap
Replacement
Bilateral 0HRV078
Left 0HRU078
Right 0HRT078
Transfer
Left 0KXG
Right 0KXF
Superficial palmar arch
use Artery, Hand, Left
use Artery, Hand, Right
Superficial palmar venous arch
use Vein, Hand, Left
use Vein, Hand, Right
Superficial temporal artery
use Artery, Temporal, Left
use Artery, Temporal, Right
Superficial transverse perineal muscle
use Muscle, Perineum
Superior cardiac nerve
use Nerve, Thoracic Sympathetic
Superior cerebellar vein
use Vein, Intracranial
Superior cerebral vein
use Vein, Intracranial
Superior clunic (cluneal) nerve
use Nerve, Lumbar
Superior epigastric artery
use Artery, Internal Mammary, Left
use Artery, Internal Mammary, Right
Superior genicular artery
use Artery, Popliteal, Left
use Artery, Popliteal, Right
Superior gluteal artery
use Artery, Internal Iliac, Left
use Artery, Internal Iliac, Right
Superior gluteal nerve
use Nerve, Lumbar Plexus
Superior hypogastric plexus
use Nerve, Abdominal Sympathetic
Superior labial artery
use Artery, Face
Superior laryngeal artery
use Artery, Thyroid, Left
use Artery, Thyroid, Right

Superior laryngeal nerve
use Nerve, Vagus
Superior longitudinal muscle
use Muscle, Tongue, Palate, Pharynx
Superior mesenteric ganglion
use Nerve, Abdominal Sympathetic
Superior mesenteric lymph node
use Lymphatic, Mesenteric
Superior mesenteric plexus
use Nerve, Abdominal Sympathetic
Superior oblique muscle
use Muscle, Extraocular, Left
use Muscle, Extraocular, Right
Superior olivary nucleus
use Pons
Superior rectal artery
use Artery, Inferior Mesenteric
Superior rectal vein
use Vein, Inferior Mesenteric
Superior rectus muscle
use Muscle, Extraocular, Left
use Muscle, Extraocular, Right
Superior tarsal plate
use Eyelid, Upper, Left
use Eyelid, Upper, Right
Superior thoracic artery
use Artery, Axillary, Left
use Artery, Axillary, Right
Superior thyroid artery
use External Carotid Artery, Left
use External Carotid Artery, Right
use Thyroid, Left
use Thyroid, Right
Superior turbinate
use Turbinate, Nasal
Superior ulnar collateral artery
use Artery, Brachial, Left
use Artery, Brachial, Right
Supersaturated Oxygen therapy
5A0512C
5A0522C
Supplement
Abdominal Wall 0WUF
Acetabulum
Left 0QU5
Right 0QU4
Ampulla of Vater 0FUC
Anal Sphincter 0DUR
Ankle Region
Left 0YUL
Right 0YUK
Anus 0DUQ
Aorta
Abdominal 04U0
Thoracic
Ascending/Arch 02UX
Descending 02UW
Arm
Lower
Left 0XUF
Right 0XUD
Upper
Left 0XU9
Right 0XU8
Artery
Anterior Tibial
Left 04UQ
Right 04UP
Axillary
Left 03U6
Right 03U5
Brachial
Left 03U8
Right 03U7
Celiac 04U1
Colic
Left 04U7
Middle 04U8
Right 04U6
Supplement *(continued)*
Artery *(continued)*
Common Carotid
Left 03UJ
Right 03UH
Common Iliac
Left 04UD
Right 04UC
External Carotid
Left 03UN
Right 03UM
External Iliac
Left 04UJ
Right 04UH
Face 03UR
Femoral
Left 04UL
Right 04UK
Foot
Left 04UW
Right 04UV
Gastric 04U2
Hand
Left 03UF
Right 03UD
Hepatic 04U3
Inferior Mesenteric 04UB
Innominate 03U2
Internal Carotid
Left 03UL
Right 03UK
Internal Iliac
Left 04UF
Right 04UE
Internal Mammary
Left 03U1
Right 03U0
Intracranial 03UG
Lower 04UY
Peroneal
Left 04UU
Right 04UT
Popliteal
Left 04UN
Right 04UM
Posterior Tibial
Left 04US
Right 04UR
Pulmonary
Left 02UR
Right 02UQ
Pulmonary Trunk 02UP
Radial
Left 03UC
Right 03UB
Renal
Left 04UA
Right 04U9
Splenic 04U4
Subclavian
Left 03U4
Right 03U3
Superior Mesenteric 04U5
Temporal
Left 03UT
Right 03US
Thyroid
Left 03UV
Right 03UU
Ulnar
Left 03UA
Right 03U9
Upper 03UY
Vertebral
Left 03UQ
Right 03UP
Atrium
Left 02U7
Right 02U6
Supplement *(continued)*
Auditory Ossicle
Left 09UA
Right 09U9
Axilla
Left 0XU5
Right 0XU4
Back
Lower 0WUL
Upper 0WUK
Bladder 0TUB
Bladder Neck 0TUC
Bone
Ethmoid
Left 0NUG
Right 0NUF
Frontal 0NU1
Hyoid 0NUX
Lacrimal
Left 0NUJ
Right 0NUH
Nasal 0NUB
Occipital 0NU7
Palatine
Left 0NUL
Right 0NUK
Parietal
Left 0NU4
Right 0NU3
Pelvic
Left 0QU3
Right 0QU2
Sphenoid 0NUC
Temporal
Left 0NU6
Right 0NU5
Zygomatic
Left 0NUN
Right 0NUM
Breast
Bilateral 0HUV
Left 0HUU
Right 0HUT
Bronchus
Lingula 0BU9
Lower Lobe
Left 0BUB
Right 0BU6
Main
Left 0BU7
Right 0BU3
Middle Lobe, Right 0BU5
Upper Lobe
Left 0BU8
Right 0BU4
Buccal Mucosa 0CU4
Bursa and Ligament
Abdomen
Left 0MUJ
Right 0MUH
Ankle
Left 0MUR
Right 0MUQ
Elbow
Left 0MU4
Right 0MU3
Foot
Left 0MUT
Right 0MUS
Hand
Left 0MU8
Right 0MU7
Head and Neck 0MU0
Hip
Left 0MUM
Right 0MUL
Knee
Left 0MUP
Right 0MUN
Supplement *(continued)*
Bursa and Ligament *(continued)*
Lower Extremity
Left 0MUW
Right 0MUV
Perineum 0MUK
Rib(s) 0MUC
Shoulder
Left 0MU2
Right 0MU1
Spine
Lower 0MUD
Upper 0MUC
Sternum 0MUF
Upper Extremity
Left 0MUB
Right 0MU9
Wrist
Left 0MU6
Right 0MU5
Buttock
Left 0YU1
Right 0YU0
Carina 0BU2
Carpal
Left 0PUN
Right 0PUM
Cecum 0DUH
Cerebral Meninges 00U1
Cerebral Ventricle 00U6
Chest Wall 0WU8
Chordae Tendineae 02U9
Cisterna Chyli 07UL
Clavicle
Left 0PUB
Right 0PU9
Clitoris 0UUJ
Coccyx 0QUS
Colon
Ascending 0DUK
Descending 0DUM
Sigmoid 0DUN
Transverse 0DUL
Cord
Bilateral 0VUH
Left 0VUG
Right 0VUF
Cornea
Left 08U9
Right 08U8
Cul-de-sac 0UUF
Diaphragm 0BUT
Disc
Cervical Vertebral 0RU3
Cervicothoracic Vertebral 0RU
Lumbar Vertebral 0SU2
Lumbosacral 0SU4
Thoracic Vertebral 0RU9
Thoracolumbar Vertebral 0RU
Duct
Common Bile 0FU9
Cystic 0FU8
Hepatic
Common 0FU7
Left 0FU6
Right 0FU5
Lacrimal
Left 08UY
Right 08UX
Pancreatic 0FUD
Accessory 0FUF
Duodenum 0DU9
Dura Mater 00U2
Ear
External
Bilateral 09U2
Left 09U1
Right 09U0
Inner
Left 09UE
Right 09UD

upplement *(continued)*
- Ear *(continued)*
  - Middle
    - Left 09U6
    - Right 09U5
- Elbow Region
  - Left 0XUC
  - Right 0XUB
- Epididymis
  - Bilateral 0VUL
  - Left 0VUK
  - Right 0VUJ
- Epiglottis 0CUR
- Esophagogastric Junction 0DU4
- Esophagus 0DU5
  - Lower 0DU3
  - Middle 0DU2
  - Upper 0DU1
- Extremity
  - Lower
    - Left 0YUB
    - Right 0YU9
  - Upper
    - Left 0XU7
    - Right 0XU6
- Eye
  - Left 08U1
  - Right 08U0
- Eyelid
  - Lower
    - Left 08UR
    - Right 08UQ
  - Upper
    - Left 08UP
    - Right 08UN
- Face 0WU2
- Fallopian Tube
  - Left 0UU6
  - Right 0UU5
- Fallopian Tubes, Bilateral 0UU7
- Femoral Region
  - Bilateral 0YUE
  - Left 0YU8
  - Right 0YU7
- Femoral Shaft
  - Left 0QU9
  - Right 0QU8
- Femur
  - Lower
    - Left 0QUC
    - Right 0QUB
  - Upper
    - Left 0QU7
    - Right 0QU6
- Fibula
  - Left 0QUK
  - Right 0QUJ
- Finger
  - Index
    - Left 0XUP
    - Right 0XUN
  - Little
    - Left 0XUW
    - Right 0XUV
  - Middle
    - Left 0XUR
    - Right 0XUQ
  - Ring
    - Left 0XUT
    - Right 0XUS
- Foot
  - Left 0YUN
  - Right 0YUM
- Gingiva
  - Lower 0CU6
  - Upper 0CU5
- Glenoid Cavity
  - Left 0PU8
  - Right 0PU7
- Hand
  - Left 0XUK

Supplement *(continued)*
- Hand *(continued)*
  - Right 0XUJ
- Head 0WU0
- Heart 02UA
- Humeral Head
  - Left 0PUD
  - Right 0PUC
- Humeral Shaft
  - Left 0PUG
  - Right 0PUF
- Hymen 0UUK
- Ileocecal Valve 0DUC
- Ileum 0DUB
- Inguinal Region
  - Bilateral 0YUA
  - Left 0YU6
  - Right 0YU5
- Intestine
  - Large 0DUE
    - Left 0DUG
    - Right 0DUF
  - Small 0DU8
- Iris
  - Left 08UD
  - Right 08UC
- Jaw
  - Lower 0WU5
  - Upper 0WU4
- Jejunum 0DUA
- Joint
  - Acromioclavicular
    - Left 0RUH
    - Right 0RUG
  - Ankle
    - Left 0SUG
    - Right 0SUF
  - Carpal
    - Left 0RUR
    - Right 0RUQ
  - Carpometacarpal
    - Left 0RUT
    - Right 0RUS
  - Cervical Vertebral 0RU1
  - Cervicothoracic Vertebral 0RU4
  - Coccygeal 0SU6
  - Elbow
    - Left 0RUM
    - Right 0RUL
  - Finger Phalangeal
    - Left 0RUX
    - Right 0RUW
  - Hip
    - Left 0SUB
      - Acetabular Surface 0SUE
      - Femoral Surface 0SUS
    - Right 0SU9
      - Acetabular Surface 0SUA
      - Femoral Surface 0SUR
  - Knee
    - Left 0SUD
      - Femoral Surface 0SUU09Z
      - Tibial Surface 0SUW09Z
    - Right 0SUC
      - Femoral Surface 0SUT09Z
      - Tibial Surface 0SUV09Z
  - Lumbar Vertebral 0SU0
  - Lumbosacral 0SU3
  - Metacarpophalangeal
    - Left 0RUV
    - Right 0RUU
  - Metatarsal-Phalangeal
    - Left 0SUN
    - Right 0SUM
  - Occipital-cervical 0RU0
  - Sacrococcygeal 0SU5

Supplement *(continued)*
- Joint *(continued)*
  - Sacroiliac
    - Left 0SU8
    - Right 0SU7
  - Shoulder
    - Left 0RUK
    - Right 0RUJ
  - Sternoclavicular
    - Left 0RUF
    - Right 0RUE
  - Tarsal
    - Left 0SUJ
    - Right 0SUH
  - Tarsometatarsal
    - Left 0SUL
    - Right 0SUK
  - Temporomandibular
    - Left 0RUD
    - Right 0RUC
  - Thoracic Vertebral 0RU6
  - Thoracolumbar Vertebral 0RUA
  - Toe Phalangeal
    - Left 0SUQ
    - Right 0SUP
  - Wrist
    - Left 0RUP
    - Right 0RUN
- Kidney Pelvis
  - Left 0TU4
  - Right 0TU3
- Knee Region
  - Left 0YUG
  - Right 0YUF
- Larynx 0CUS
- Leg
  - Lower
    - Left 0YUJ
    - Right 0YUH
  - Upper
    - Left 0YUD
    - Right 0YUC
- Lip
  - Lower 0CU1
  - Upper 0CU0
- Lymphatic
  - Aortic 07UD
  - Axillary
    - Left 07U6
    - Right 07U5
  - Head 07U0
  - Inguinal
    - Left 07UJ
    - Right 07UH
  - Internal Mammary
    - Left 07U9
    - Right 07U8
  - Lower Extremity
    - Left 07UG
    - Right 07UF
  - Mesenteric 07UB
  - Neck
    - Left 07U2
    - Right 07U1
  - Pelvis 07UC
  - Thoracic Duct 07UK
  - Thorax 07U7
  - Upper Extremity
    - Left 07U4
    - Right 07U3
- Mandible
  - Left 0NUV
  - Right 0NUT
- Maxilla 0NUR
- Mediastinum 0WUC
- Mesentery 0DUV
- Metacarpal
  - Left 0PUQ
  - Right 0PUP
- Metatarsal
  - Left 0QUP

Supplement *(continued)*
- Metatarsal *(continued)*
  - Right 0QUN
- Muscle
  - Abdomen
    - Left 0KUL
    - Right 0KUK
  - Extraocular
    - Left 08UM
    - Right 08UL
  - Facial 0KU1
  - Foot
    - Left 0KUW
    - Right 0KUV
  - Hand
    - Left 0KUD
    - Right 0KUC
  - Head 0KU0
  - Hip
    - Left 0KUP
    - Right 0KUN
  - Lower Arm and Wrist
    - Left 0KUB
    - Right 0KU9
  - Lower Leg
    - Left 0KUT
    - Right 0KUS
  - Neck
    - Left 0KU3
    - Right 0KU2
  - Papillary 02UD
  - Perineum 0KUM
  - Shoulder
    - Left 0KU6
    - Right 0KU5
  - Thorax
    - Left 0KUJ
    - Right 0KUH
  - Tongue, Palate, Pharynx 0KU4
  - Trunk
    - Left 0KUG
    - Right 0KUF
  - Upper Arm
    - Left 0KU8
    - Right 0KU7
  - Upper Leg
    - Left 0KUR
    - Right 0KUQ
- Nasal Mucosa and Soft Tissue 09UK
- Nasopharynx 09UN
- Neck 0WU6
- Nerve
  - Abducens 00UL
  - Accessory 00UR
  - Acoustic 00UN
  - Cervical 01U1
  - Facial 00UM
  - Femoral 01UD
  - Glossopharyngeal 00UP
  - Hypoglossal 00US
  - Lumbar 01UB
  - Median 01U5
  - Oculomotor 00UH
  - Olfactory 00UF
  - Optic 00UG
  - Peroneal 01UH
  - Phrenic 01U2
  - Pudendal 01UC
  - Radial 01U6
  - Sacral 01UR
  - Sciatic 01UF
  - Thoracic 01U8
  - Tibial 01UG
  - Trigeminal 00UK
  - Trochlear 00UJ
  - Ulnar 01U4
  - Vagus 00UQ
- Nipple
  - Left 0HUX
  - Right 0HUW
- Omentum 0DUU

Supplement *(continued)*
Orbit
Left 0NUQ
Right 0NUP
Palate
Hard 0CU2
Soft 0CU3
Patella
Left 0QUF
Right 0QUD
Penis 0VUS
Pericardium 02UN
Perineum
Female 0WUN
Male 0WUM
Peritoneum 0DUW
Phalanx
Finger
Left 0PUV
Right 0PUT
Thumb
Left 0PUS
Right 0PUR
Toe
Left 0QUR
Right 0QUQ
Pharynx 0CUM
Prepuce 0VUT
Radius
Left 0PUJ
Right 0PUH
Rectum 0DUP
Retina
Left 08UF
Right 08UE
Retinal Vessel
Left 08UH
Right 08UG
Ribs
1 to 2 0PU1
3 or More 0PU2
Sacrum 0QU1
Scapula
Left 0PU6
Right 0PU5
Scrotum 0VU5
Septum
Atrial 02U5
Nasal 09UM
Ventricular 02UM
Shoulder Region
Left 0XU3
Right 0XU2
Skull 0NU0
Spinal Meninges 00UT
Sternum 0PU0
Stomach 0DU6
Pylorus 0DU7
Subcutaneous Tissue and Fascia
Abdomen 0JU8
Back 0JU7
Buttock 0JU9
Chest 0JU6
Face 0JU1
Foot
Left 0JUR
Right 0JUQ
Hand
Left 0JUK
Right 0JUJ
Lower Arm
Left 0JUH
Right 0JUG
Lower Leg
Left 0JUP
Right 0JUN
Neck
Left 0JU5
Right 0JU4
Pelvic Region 0JUC

Supplement *(continued)*
Subcutaneous Tissue and Fascia *(continued)*
Perineum 0JUB
Scalp 0JU0
Upper Arm
Left 0JUF
Right 0JUD
Upper Leg
Left 0JUM
Right 0JUL
Tarsal
Left 0QUM
Right 0QUL
Tendon
Abdomen
Left 0LUG
Right 0LUF
Ankle
Left 0LUT
Right 0LUS
Foot
Left 0LUW
Right 0LUV
Hand
Left 0LU8
Right 0LU7
Head and Neck 0LU0
Hip
Left 0LUK
Right 0LUJ
Knee
Left 0LUR
Right 0LUQ
Lower Arm and Wrist
Left 0LU6
Right 0LU5
Lower Leg
Left 0LUP
Right 0LUN
Perineum 0LUH
Shoulder
Left 0LU2
Right 0LU1
Thorax
Left 0LUD
Right 0LUC
Trunk
Left 0LUB
Right 0LU9
Upper Arm
Left 0LU4
Right 0LU3
Upper Leg
Left 0LUM
Right 0LUL
Testis
Bilateral 0VUC0
Left 0VUB0
Right 0VU90
Thumb
Left 0XUM
Right 0XUL
Tibia
Left 0QUH
Right 0QUG
Toe
1st
Left 0YUQ
Right 0YUP
2nd
Left 0YUS
Right 0YUR
3rd
Left 0YUU
Right 0YUT
4th
Left 0YUW
Right 0YUV

Supplement *(continued)*
Toe *(continued)*
5th
Left 0YUY
Right 0YUX
Tongue 0CU7
Trachea 0BU1
Tunica Vaginalis
Left 0VU7
Right 0VU6
Turbinate, Nasal 09UL
Tympanic Membrane
Left 09U8
Right 09U7
Ulna
Left 0PUL
Right 0PUK
Ureter
Left 0TU7
Right 0TU6
Urethra 0TUD
Uterine Supporting Structure 0UU4
Uvula 0CUN
Vagina 0UUG
Valve
Aortic 02UF
Mitral 02UG
Pulmonary 02UH
Tricuspid 02UJ
Vas Deferens
Bilateral 0VUQ
Left 0VUP
Right 0VUN
Vein
Axillary
Left 05U8
Right 05U7
Azygos 05U0
Basilic
Left 05UC
Right 05UB
Brachial
Left 05UA
Right 05U9
Cephalic
Left 05UF
Right 05UD
Colic 06U7
Common Iliac
Left 06UD
Right 06UC
Esophageal 06U3
External Iliac
Left 06UG
Right 06UF
External Jugular
Left 05UQ
Right 05UP
Face
Left 05UV
Right 05UT
Femoral
Left 06UN
Right 06UM
Foot
Left 06UV
Right 06UT
Gastric 06U2
Hand
Left 05UH
Right 05UG
Hemiazygos 05U1
Hepatic 06U4
Hypogastric
Left 06UJ
Right 06UH
Inferior Mesenteric 06U6
Innominate
Left 05U4
Right 05U3

Supplement *(continued)*
Vein *(continued)*
Internal Jugular
Left 05UN
Right 05UM
Intracranial 05UL
Lower 06UY
Portal 06U8
Pulmonary
Left 02UT
Right 02US
Renal
Left 06UB
Right 06U9
Saphenous
Left 06UQ
Right 06UP
Splenic 06U1
Subclavian
Left 05U6
Right 05U5
Superior Mesenteric 06U5
Upper 05UY
Vertebral
Left 05US
Right 05UR
Vena Cava
Inferior 06U0
Superior 02UV
Ventricle
Left 02UL
Right 02UK
Vertebra
Cervical 0PU3
Lumbar 0QU0
Thoracic 0PU4
Vesicle
Bilateral 0VU3
Left 0VU2
Right 0VU1
Vocal Cord
Left 0CUV
Right 0CUT
Vulva 0UUM
Wrist Region
Left 0XUH
Right 0XUG

Supraclavicular (Virchow's) lymph node
use Lymphatic, Neck, Left
use Lymphatic, Neck, Right
Supraclavicular nerve
use Nerve, Cervical Plexus
Suprahyoid lymph node
use Lymphatic, Head
Suprahyoid muscle
use Muscle, Neck, Left
use Muscle, Neck, Right
Suprainguinal lymph node
use Lymphatic, Pelvis
Supraorbital vein
use Vein, Face, Left
use Vein, Face, Right
Suprarenal gland
use Gland, Adrenal
use Gland, Adrenal, Bilateral
use Gland, Adrenal, Left
use Gland, Adrenal, Right
Suprarenal plexus
use Nerve, Abdominal Sympathe
Suprascapular nerve
use Nerve, Brachial Plexus
Supraspinatus fascia
use Subcutaneous Tissue and Fas Upper Arm, Left
use Subcutaneous Tissue and Fas Upper Arm, Right
Supraspinatus muscle
use Muscle, Shoulder, Left
use Muscle, Shoulder, Right

upraspinous ligament
use Bursa and Ligament, Lower Spine
use Bursa and Ligament, Upper Spine
uprasternal notch
use Sternum
upratrochlear lymph node
use Lymphatic, Upper Extremity, Left
use Lymphatic, Upper Extremity, Right
ural artery
use Artery, Popliteal, Left
use Artery, Popliteal, Right
uspension
Bladder Neck
see Reposition, Bladder Neck 0TSC
Kidney
see Reposition, Urinary System 0TS
Urethra
see Reposition, Urinary System 0TS
Urethrovesical
see Reposition, Bladder Neck 0TSC
Uterus
see Reposition, Uterus 0US9
Vagina
see Reposition, Vagina 0USG
uture
Laceration repair
see Repair
Ligation
see Occlusion
uture Removal
Extremity
Lower 8E0YXY8
Upper 8E0XXY8
Head and Neck Region 8E09XY8
Trunk Region 8E0WXY8
utureless valve, Perceval
use Zooplastic Tissue, Rapid Deployment Technique in New Technology
weat gland
use Skin
ympathectomy
see Excision, Peripheral Nervous System 01B
ynCardia Total Artificial Heart
use Synthetic Substitute
ynchra CRT-P
use Cardiac Resynchronization Pacemaker Pulse Generator in 0JH
ynchroMed pump
use Infusion Device, Pump in Subcutaneous Tissue and Fascia
nechiotomy, iris
see Release, Eye 08N
novectomy
Lower joint
see Excision, Lower Joints 0SB
Upper joint
see Excision, Upper Joints 0RB
stemic Nuclear Medicine Therapy
Abdomen CW70
Anatomical Regions, Multiple CW7YYZZ
Chest CW73
Thyroid CW7G
Whole Body CW7N
nthetic Human Angiotensin II XW0

kedown
Arteriovenous shunt
see Removal of device from, Upper Arteries 03P
Takedown *(continued)*
Arteriovenous shunt, with creation of new shunt
see Bypass, Upper Arteries 031
Stoma
see Excision
see Reposition
Talent® Converter
use Intraluminal Device
Talent® Occluder
use Intraluminal Device
Talent® Stent Graft (abdominal) (thoracic)
use Intraluminal Device
Talocalcaneal (subtalar) joint
use Joint, Tarsal, Left
use Joint, Tarsal, Right
Talocalcaneal ligament
use Bursa and Ligament, Foot, Left
use Bursa and Ligament, Foot, Right
Talocalcaneonavicular joint
use Joint, Tarsal, Left
use Joint, Tarsal, Right
Talocalcaneonavicular ligament
use Bursa and Ligament, Foot, Left
use Bursa and Ligament, Foot, Right
Talocrural joint
use Joint, Ankle, Left
use Joint, Ankle, Right
Talofibular ligament
use Bursa and Ligament, Ankle, Left
use Bursa and Ligament, Ankle, Right
Talus bone
use Tarsal, Left
use Tarsal, Right
TandemHeart® System
use Short-term External Heart Assist System in Heart and Great Vessels
Tarsectomy
see Excision, Lower Bones 0QB
see Resection, Lower Bones 0QT
Tarsometatarsal ligament
use Bursa and Ligament, Foot, Left
use Bursa and Ligament, Foot, Right
Tarsorrhaphy
see Repair, Eye 08Q
Tattooing
Cornea 3E0CXMZ
Skin
see Introduction of substance in or on, Skin 3E00
TAXUS® Liberté® Paclitaxel-eluting Coronary Stent System
use Intraluminal Device, Drug-eluting in Heart and Great Vessels
TBNA (transbronchial needle aspiration)
Fluid or gas
see Drainage, Respiratory System 0B9
Tissue biopsy
see Extraction, Respiratory System 0BD
Telemetry 4A12X4Z
Ambulatory 4A12X45
Temperature gradient study 4A0ZXKZ
Temporal lobe
use Cerebral Hemisphere
Temporalis muscle
use Muscle, Head
Temporoparietalis muscle
use Muscle, Head
Tendolysis
see Release, Tendons 0LN
Tendonectomy
see Excision, Tendons 0LB
see Resection, Tendons 0LT
Tendonoplasty, tenoplasty
see Repair, Tendons 0LQ
see Replacement, Tendons 0LR
see Supplement, Tendons 0LU
Tendorrhaphy
see Repair, Tendons 0LQ
Tendototomy
see Division, Tendons 0L8
see Drainage, Tendons 0L9
Tenectomy, tenonectomy
see Excision, Tendons 0LB
see Resection, Tendons 0LT
Tenolysis
see Release, Tendons 0LN
Tenontorrhaphy
see Repair, Tendons 0LQ
Tenontotomy
see Division, Tendons 0L8
see Drainage, Tendons 0L9
Tenorrhaphy
see Repair, Tendons 0LQ
Tenosynovectomy
see Excision, Tendons 0LB
see Resection, Tendons 0LT
Tenotomy
see Division, Tendons 0L8
see Drainage, Tendons 0L9
Tensor fasciae latae muscle
use Muscle, Hip, Left
use Muscle, Hip, Right
Tensor veli palatini muscle
use Muscle, Tongue, Palate, Pharynx
Tenth cranial nerve
use Nerve, Vagus
Tentorium cerebelli
use Dura Mater
Teres major muscle
use Muscle, Shoulder, Left
use Muscle, Shoulder, Right
Teres minor muscle
use Muscle, Shoulder, Left
use Muscle, Shoulder, Right
Termination of pregnancy
Aspiration curettage 10A07ZZ
Dilation and curettage 10A07ZZ
Hysterotomy 10A00ZZ
Intra-amniotic injection 10A03ZZ
Laminaria 10A07ZW
Vacuum 10A07Z6
Testectomy
see Excision, Male Reproductive System 0VB
see Resection, Male Reproductive System 0VT
Testicular artery
use Aorta, Abdominal
Testing
Glaucoma 4A07XBZ
Hearing
see Hearing Assessment, Diagnostic Audiology F13
Mental health
see Psychological Tests
Muscle function, electromyography (EMG)
see Measurement, Musculoskeletal 4A0F
Muscle function, manual
see Motor Function Assessment, Rehabilitation F01
Neurophysiologic monitoring, intra-operative
see Monitoring, Physiological Systems 4A1
Range of motion
see Motor Function Assessment, Rehabilitation F01
Vestibular function
see Vestibular Assessment, Diagnostic Audiology F15
Thalamectomy
see Excision, Thalamus 00B9
Thalamotomy
see Drainage, Thalamus 0099
Thenar muscle
use Muscle, Hand, Left
use Muscle, Hand, Right
Therapeutic Massage
Musculoskeletal System 8E0KX1Z
Reproductive System
Prostate 8E0VX1C
Rectum 8E0VX1D
Therapeutic occlusion coil(s)
use Intraluminal Device
Thermography 4A0ZXKZ
Thermotherapy, prostate
see Destruction, Prostate 0V50
Third cranial nerve
use Nerve, Oculomotor
Third occipital nerve
use Nerve, Cervical
Third ventricle
use Cerebral Ventricle
Thoracectomy
see Excision, Anatomical Regions, General 0WB
Thoracentesis
see Drainage, Anatomical Regions, General 0W9
Thoracic aortic plexus
use Nerve, Thoracic Sympathetic
Thoracic esophagus
use Esophagus, Middle
Thoracic facet joint
use Joint, Thoracic Vertebral
Thoracic ganglion
use Nerve, Thoracic Sympathetic
Thoracoacromial artery
use Artery, Axillary, Left
use Artery, Axillary, Right
Thoracocentesis
see Drainage, Anatomical Regions, General 0W9
Thoracolumbar facet joint
use Joint, Thoracolumbar Vertebral
Thoracoplasty
see Repair, Anatomical Regions, General 0WQ
see Supplement, Anatomical Regions, General 0WU
Thoracostomy tube
use Drainage Device
Thoracostomy, for lung collapse
see Drainage, Respiratory System 0B9
Thoracotomy
see Drainage, Anatomical Regions, General 0W9
Thoratec IVAD (Implantable Ventricular Assist Device)
use Implantable Heart Assist System in Heart and Great Vessels
Thoratec Paracorporeal Ventricular Assist Device
use Short-term External Heart Assist System in Heart and Great Vessels
Thrombectomy
see Extirpation
Thymectomy
see Excision, Lymphatic and Hemic Systems 07B
see Resection, Lymphatic and Hemic Systems 07T
Thymopexy
see Repair, Lymphatic and Hemic Systems 07Q
see Reposition, Lymphatic and Hemic Systems 07S
Thymus gland
use Thymus

Thyroarytenoid muscle
- *use* Muscle, Neck, Left
- *use* Muscle, Neck, Right

Thyrocervical trunk
- *use* Artery, Thyroid, Left
- *use* Artery, Thyroid, Right

Thyroid cartilage
- *use* Larynx

Thyroidectomy
- *see* Excision, Endocrine System 0GB
- *see* Resection, Endocrine System 0GT

Thyroidorrhaphy
- *see* Repair, Endocrine System 0GQ

Thyroidoscopy 0GJK4ZZ

Thyroidotomy
- *see* Drainage, Endocrine System 0G9

Tibial insert
- *use* Liner in Lower Joints

Tibialis anterior muscle
- *use* Muscle, Lower Leg, Left
- *use* Muscle, Lower Leg, Right

Tibialis posterior muscle
- *use* Muscle, Lower Leg, Left
- *use* Muscle, Lower Leg, Right

Tibiofemoral joint
- *use* Joint, Knee, Left
- *use* Joint, Knee, Left, Tibial Surface
- *use* Joint, Knee, Right
- *use* Joint, Knee, Right, Tibial Surface

Tisagenlecleucel
- *use* Engineered Autologous Chimeric Antigen Receptor T-cell Immunotherapy

Tissue bank graft
- *use* Nonautologous Tissue Substitute

Tissue Expander
- Insertion of device in
  - Breast
    - Bilateral 0HHV
    - Left 0HHU
    - Right 0HHT
  - Nipple
    - Left 0HHX
    - Right 0HHW
  - Subcutaneous Tissue and Fascia
    - Abdomen 0JH8
    - Back 0JH7
    - Buttock 0JH9
    - Chest 0JH6
    - Face 0JH1
    - Foot
      - Left 0JHR
      - Right 0JHQ
    - Hand
      - Left 0JHK
      - Right 0JHJ
    - Lower Arm
      - Left 0JHH
      - Right 0JHG
    - Lower Leg
      - Left 0JHP
      - Right 0JHN
    - Neck
      - Left 0JH5
      - Right 0JH4
    - Pelvic Region 0JHC
    - Perineum 0JHB
    - Scalp 0JH0
    - Upper Arm
      - Left 0JHF
      - Right 0JHD
    - Upper Leg
      - Left 0JHM
      - Right 0JHL
- Removal of device from
  - Breast
    - Left 0HPU
    - Right 0HPT

Tissue Expander *(continued)*
- Removal of device from *(continued)*
  - Subcutaneous Tissue and Fascia
    - Head and Neck 0JPS
    - Lower Extremity 0JPW
    - Trunk 0JPT
    - Upper Extremity 0JPV
- Revision of device in
  - Breast
    - Left 0HWU
    - Right 0HWT
  - Subcutaneous Tissue and Fascia
    - Head and Neck 0JWS
    - Lower Extremity 0JWW
    - Trunk 0JWT
    - Upper Extremity 0JWV

Tissue expander (inflatable)(injectable)
- *use* Tissue Expander in Skin and Breast
- *use* Tissue Expander in Subcutaneous Tissue and Fascia

Tissue Plasminogen Activator (tPA) (r-tPA)
- *use* Thrombolytic Other

Titanium Sternal Fixation System (TSFS)
- *use* Internal Fixation Device, Rigid Plate in 0PS
- *use* Internal Fixation Device, Rigid Plate in 0PH

Tomographic (Tomo) Nuclear Medicine Imaging
- Abdomen CW20
- Abdomen and Chest CW24
- Abdomen and Pelvis CW21
- Anatomical Regions, Multiple CW2YYZZ
- Bladder, Kidneys and Ureters CT23
- Brain C020
- Breast CH2YYZZ
  - Bilateral CH22
  - Left CH21
  - Right CH20
- Bronchi and Lungs CB22
- Central Nervous System C02YYZZ
- Cerebrospinal Fluid C025
- Chest CW23
- Chest and Abdomen CW24
- Chest and Neck CW26
- Digestive System CD2YYZZ
- Endocrine System CG2YYZZ
- Extremity
  - Lower CW2D
    - Bilateral CP2F
    - Left CP2D
    - Right CP2C
  - Upper CW2M
    - Bilateral CP2B
    - Left CP29
    - Right CP28
- Gallbladder CF24
- Gastrointestinal Tract CD27
- Gland, Parathyroid CG21
- Head and Neck CW2B
- Heart C22YYZZ
  - Right and Left C226
- Hepatobiliary System and Pancreas CF2YYZZ
- Kidneys, Ureters and Bladder CT23
- Liver CF25
- Liver and Spleen CF26
- Lungs and Bronchi CB22
- Lymphatics and Hematologic System C72YYZZ
- Musculoskeletal System, Other CP2YYZZ
- Myocardium C22G
- Neck and Chest CW26
- Neck and Head CW2B

Tomographic (Tomo) Nuclear Medicine Imaging *(continued)*
- Pancreas and Hepatobiliary System CF2YYZZ
- Pelvic Region CW2J
- Pelvis CP26
- Pelvis and Abdomen CW21
- Pelvis and Spine CP27
- Respiratory System CB2YYZZ
- Skin CH2YYZZ
- Skull CP21
- Skull and Cervical Spine CP23
- Spine
  - Cervical CP22
  - Cervical and Skull CP23
  - Lumbar CP2H
  - Thoracic CP2G
  - Thoracolumbar CP2J
- Spine and Pelvis CP27
- Spleen C722
- Spleen and Liver CF26
- Subcutaneous Tissue CH2YYZZ
- Thorax CP24
- Ureters, Kidneys and Bladder CT23
- Urinary System CT2YYZZ

Tomography, computerized
- *see* Computerized Tomography (CT Scan)

Tongue, base of
- *use* Pharynx

Tonometry 4A07XBZ

Tonsillectomy
- *see* Excision, Mouth and Throat 0CB
- *see* Resection, Mouth and Throat 0CT

Tonsillotomy
- *see* Drainage, Mouth and Throat 0C9

Total Anomalous Pulmonary Venous Return (TAPVR) repair
- *see* Bypass, Atrium, Left 0217
- *see* Bypass, Vena Cava, Superior 021V

Total artificial (replacement) heart
- *use* Synthetic Substitute

Total parenteral nutrition (TPN)
- *see* Introduction of Nutritional Substance

Trachectomy
- *see* Excision, Trachea 0BB1
- *see* Resection, Trachea 0BT1

Trachelectomy
- *see* Excision, Cervix 0UBC
- *see* Resection, Cervix 0UTC

Trachelopexy
- *see* Repair, Cervix 0UQC
- *see* Reposition, Cervix 0USC

Tracheloplasty
- *see* Repair, Cervix 0UQC

Trachelorrhaphy
- *see* Repair, Cervix 0UQC

Trachelotomy
- *see* Drainage, Cervix 0U9C

Tracheobronchial lymph node
- *use* Lymphatic, Thorax

Tracheoesophageal fistulization 0B110D6

Tracheolysis
- *see* Release, Respiratory System 0BN

Tracheoplasty
- *see* Repair, Respiratory System 0BQ
- *see* Supplement, Respiratory System 0BU

Tracheorrhaphy
- *see* Repair, Respiratory System 0BQ

Tracheoscopy 0BJ18ZZ

Tracheostomy
- *see* Bypass, Respiratory System 0B1

Tracheostomy Device
- Bypass, Trachea 0B11
- Change device in, Trachea 0B21XFZ
- Removal of device from, Trachea 0BP1
- Revision of device in, Trachea 0BW

Tracheostomy tube
- *use* Tracheostomy Device in Respiratory System

Tracheotomy
- *see* Drainage, Respiratory System 0B9

Traction
- Abdominal Wall 2W63X
- Arm
  - Lower
    - Left 2W6DX
    - Right 2W6CX
  - Upper
    - Left 2W6BX
    - Right 2W6AX
- Back 2W65X
- Chest Wall 2W64X
- Extremity
  - Lower
    - Left 2W6MX
    - Right 2W6LX
  - Upper
    - Left 2W69X
    - Right 2W68X
- Face 2W61X
- Finger
  - Left 2W6KX
  - Right 2W6JX
- Foot
  - Left 2W6TX
  - Right 2W6SX
- Hand
  - Left 2W6FXZ
  - Right 2W6EXZ
- Head 2W60X
- Inguinal Region
  - Left 2W67X
  - Right 2W66X
- Leg
  - Lower
    - Left 2W6RX
    - Right 2W6QX
  - Upper
    - Left 2W6PX
    - Right 2W6NX
- Neck 2W62X
- Thumb
  - Left 2W6HX
  - Right 2W6GX
- Toe
  - Left 2W6VX
  - Right 2W6UX

Tractotomy
- *see* Division, Central Nervous System and Cranial Nerves 0C

Tragus
- *use* Ear, External, Bilateral
- *use* Ear, External, Left
- *use* Ear, External, Right

Training, caregiver
- *see* Caregiver Training

TRAM (transverse rectus abdomin myocutaneous) flap reconstruction
- Free
  - *see* Replacement, Skin and Breast 0HR
- Pedicled
  - *see* Transfer, Muscles 0KX

Transection
- *see* Division

Transfer
- Buccal Mucosa 0CX4

Transfer *(continued)*
- Bursa and Ligament
  - Abdomen
    - Left 0MXJ
    - Right 0MXH
  - Ankle
    - Left 0MXR
    - Right 0MXQ
  - Elbow
    - Left 0MX4
    - Right 0MX3
  - Foot
    - Left 0MXT
    - Right 0MXS
  - Hand
    - Left 0MX8
    - Right 0MX7
  - Head and Neck 0MX0
  - Hip
    - Left 0MXM
    - Right 0MXL
  - Knee
    - Left 0MXP
    - Right 0MXN
  - Lower Extremity
    - Left 0MXW
    - Right 0MXV
  - Perineum 0MXK
  - Rib(s) 0MXG
  - Shoulder
    - Left 0MX2
    - Right 0MX1
  - Spine
    - Lower 0MXD
    - Upper 0MXC
  - Sternum 0MXF
  - Upper Extremity
    - Left 0MXB
    - Right 0MX9
  - Wrist
    - Left 0MX6
    - Right 0MX5
- Finger
  - Left 0XXP0ZM
  - Right 0XXN0ZL
- Gingiva
  - Lower 0CX6
  - Upper 0CX5
- Intestine
  - Large 0DXE
  - Small 0DX8
- Lip
  - Lower 0CX1
  - Upper 0CX0
- Muscle
  - Abdomen
    - Left 0KXL
    - Right 0KXK
  - Extraocular
    - Left 08XM
    - Right 08XL
  - Facial 0KX1
  - Foot
    - Left 0KXW
    - Right 0KXV
  - Hand
    - Left 0KXD
    - Right 0KXC
  - Head 0KX0
  - Hip
    - Left 0KXP
    - Right 0KXN
  - Lower Arm and Wrist
    - Left 0KXB
    - Right 0KX9
  - Lower Leg
    - Left 0KXT
    - Right 0KXS
  - Neck
    - Left 0KX3
    - Right 0KX2

Transfer *(continued)*
- Muscle *(continued)*
  - Perineum 0KXM
  - Shoulder
    - Left 0KX6
    - Right 0KX5
  - Thorax
    - Left 0KXJ
    - Right 0KXH
  - Tongue, Palate, Pharynx 0KX4
  - Trunk
    - Left 0KXG
    - Right 0KXF
  - Upper Arm
    - Left 0KX8
    - Right 0KX7
  - Upper Leg
    - Left 0KXR
    - Right 0KXQ
- Nerve
  - Abducens 00XL
  - Accessory 00XR
  - Acoustic 00XN
  - Cervical 01X1
  - Facial 00XM
  - Femoral 01XD
  - Glossopharyngeal 00XP
  - Hypoglossal 00XS
  - Lumbar 01XB
  - Median 01X5
  - Oculomotor 00XH
  - Olfactory 00XF
  - Optic 00XG
  - Peroneal 01XH
  - Phrenic 01X2
  - Pudendal 01XC
  - Radial 01X6
  - Sciatic 01XF
  - Thoracic 01X8
  - Tibial 01XG
  - Trigeminal 00XK
  - Trochlear 00XJ
  - Ulnar 01X4
  - Vagus 00XQ
- Palate, Soft 0CX3
- Prepuce 0VXT
- Skin
  - Abdomen 0HX7XZZ
  - Back 0HX6XZZ
  - Buttock 0HX8XZZ
  - Chest 0HX5XZZ
  - Ear
    - Left 0HX3XZZ
    - Right 0HX2XZZ
  - Face 0HX1XZZ
  - Foot
    - Left 0HXNXZZ
    - Right 0HXMXZZ
  - Hand
    - Left 0HXGXZZ
    - Right 0HXFXZZ
  - Inguinal 0HXAXZZ
  - Lower Arm
    - Left 0HXEXZZ
    - Right 0HXDXZZ
  - Lower Leg
    - Left 0HXLXZZ
    - Right 0HXKXZZ
  - Neck 0HX4XZZ
  - Perineum 0HX9XZZ
  - Scalp 0HX0XZZ
  - Upper Arm
    - Left 0HXCXZZ
    - Right 0HXBXZZ
  - Upper Leg
    - Left 0HXJXZZ
    - Right 0HXHXZZ
- Stomach 0DX6
- Subcutaneous Tissue and Fascia
  - Abdomen 0JX8
  - Back 0JX7

Transfer *(continued)*
- Subcutaneous Tissue and Fascia *(continued)*
  - Buttock 0JX9
  - Chest 0JX6
  - Face 0JX1
  - Foot
    - Left 0JXR
    - Right 0JXQ
  - Hand
    - Left 0JXK
    - Right 0JXJ
  - Lower Arm
    - Left 0JXH
    - Right 0JXG
  - Lower Leg
    - Left 0JXP
    - Right 0JXN
  - Neck
    - Left 0JX5
    - Right 0JX4
  - Pelvic Region 0JXC
  - Perineum 0JXB
  - Scalp 0JX0
  - Upper Arm
    - Left 0JXF
    - Right 0JXD
  - Upper Leg
    - Left 0JXM
    - Right 0JXL
- Tendon
  - Abdomen
    - Left 0LXG
    - Right 0LXF
  - Ankle
    - Left 0LXT
    - Right 0LXS
  - Foot
    - Left 0LXW
    - Right 0LXV
  - Hand
    - Left 0LX8
    - Right 0LX7
  - Head and Neck 0LX0
  - Hip
    - Left 0LXK
    - Right 0LXJ
  - Knee
    - Left 0LXR
    - Right 0LXQ
  - Lower Arm and Wrist
    - Left 0LX6
    - Right 0LX5
  - Lower Leg
    - Left 0LXP
    - Right 0LXN
  - Perineum 0LXH
  - Shoulder
    - Left 0LX2
    - Right 0LX1
  - Thorax
    - Left 0LXD
    - Right 0LXC
  - Trunk
    - Left 0LXB
    - Right 0LX9
  - Upper Arm
    - Left 0LX4
    - Right 0LX3
  - Upper Leg
    - Left 0LXM
    - Right 0LXL
- Tongue 0CX7

Transfusion
- Artery
  - Central
    - Antihemophilic Factors 3026
    - Blood
      - Platelets 3026
      - Red Cells 3026

Transfusion *(continued)*
- Artery *(continued)*
  - Central *(continued)*
    - Blood *(continued)*
      - Red Cells *(continued)*
        - Frozen 3026
      - White Cells 3026
      - Whole 3026
    - Bone Marrow 3026
    - Factor IX 3026
    - Fibrinogen 3026
    - Globulin 3026
    - Plasma
      - Fresh 3026
      - Frozen 3026
    - Plasma Cryoprecipitate 3026
    - Serum Albumin 3026
    - Stem Cells
      - Cord Blood 3026
      - Hematopoietic 3026
  - Peripheral
    - Antihemophilic Factors 3025
    - Blood
      - Platelets 3025
      - Red Cells 3025
      - Frozen 3025
      - White Cells 3025
      - Whole 3025
    - Bone Marrow 3025
    - Factor IX 3025
    - Fibrinogen 3025
    - Globulin 3025
    - Plasma
      - Fresh 3025
      - Frozen 3025
    - Plasma Cryoprecipitate 3025
    - Serum Albumin 3025
    - Stem Cells
      - Cord Blood 3025
      - Hematopoietic 3025
- Products of Conception
  - Antihemophilic Factors 3027
  - Blood
    - Platelets 3027
    - Red Cells 3027
      - Frozen 3027
    - White Cells 3027
    - Whole 3027
  - Factor IX 3027
  - Fibrinogen 3027
  - Globulin 3027
  - Plasma
    - Fresh 3027
    - Frozen 3027
  - Plasma Cryoprecipitate 3027
  - Serum Albumin 3027
- Vein
  - 4-Factor Prothrombin Complex Concentrate 3028
  - Central
    - Antihemophilic Factors 3024
    - Blood
      - Platelets 3024
      - Red Cells 3024
      - Frozen 3024
      - White Cells 3024
      - Whole 3024
    - Bone Marrow 3024
    - Factor IX 3024
    - Fibrinogen 3024
    - Globulin 3024
    - Plasma
      - Fresh 3024
      - Frozen 3024
    - Plasma Cryoprecipitate 3024
    - Serum Albumin 3024
    - Stem Cells
      - Cord Blood 3024
      - Embryonic 3024
      - Hematopoietic 3024

- **Transfusion** *(continued)*
  - Vein *(continued)*
    - Peripheral
      - Antihemophilic Factors 3023
      - Blood
        - Platelets 3023
        - Red Cells 3023
        - Frozen 3023
        - White Cells 3023
        - Whole 3023
      - Bone Marrow 3023
      - Factor IX 3023
      - Fibrinogen 3023
      - Globulin 3023
      - Plasma
        - Fresh 3023
        - Frozen 3023
      - Plasma Cryoprecipitate 3023
      - Serum Albumin 3023
      - Stem Cells
        - Cord Blood 3023X
        - Embryonic 3023
        - Hematopoietic 3023
- **Transplant**
  - *see* Transplantation
- **Transplantation**
  - Bone marrow
    - *see* Transfusion, Circulatory 302
  - Esophagus 0DY50Z
  - Face 0WY20Z
  - Hand
    - Left 0XYK0Z
    - Right 0XYJ0Z
  - Heart 02YA0Z
  - Hematopoietic cell
    - *see* Transfusion, Circulatory 302
  - Intestine
    - Large 0DYE0Z
    - Small 0DY80Z
  - Kidney
    - Left 0TY10Z
    - Right 0TY00Z
  - Liver 0FY00Z
  - Lung
    - Bilateral 0BYM0Z
    - Left 0BYL0Z
    - Lower Lobe
      - Left 0BYJ0Z
      - Right 0BYF0Z
    - Middle Lobe, Right 0BYD0Z
    - Right 0BYK0Z
    - Upper Lobe
      - Left 0BYG0Z
      - Right 0BYC0Z
  - Lung Lingula 0BYH0Z
  - Ovary
    - Left 0UY10Z
    - Right 0UY00Z
  - Pancreas 0FYG0Z
  - Products of Conception 10Y0
  - Spleen 07YP0Z
  - Stem cell
    - *see* Transfusion, Circulatory 302
  - Stomach 0DY60Z
  - Thymus 07YM0Z
  - Uterus 0UY90Z
- **Transposition**
  - *see* Bypass
  - *see* Reposition
  - *see* Transfer
- **Transversalis fascia**
  - *use* Subcutaneous Tissue and Fascia, Trunk
- **Transverse acetabular ligament**
  - *use* Bursa and Ligament, Hip, Left
  - *use* Bursa and Ligament, Hip, Right
- **Transverse (cutaneous) cervical nerve**
  - *use* Nerve, Cervical Plexus
- **Transverse facial artery**
  - *use* Artery, Temporal, Left
  - *use* Artery, Temporal, Right
- **Transverse foramen**
  - *use* Cervical Vertebra
- **Transverse humeral ligament**
  - *use* Bursa and Ligament, Shoulder, Left
  - *use* Bursa and Ligament, Shoulder, Right
- **Transverse ligament of atlas**
  - *use* Bursa and Ligament, Head and Neck
- **Transverse process**
  - *use* Cervical Vertebra
  - *use* Thoracic Vertebra
  - *use* Lumbar Vertebra
- **Transverse Rectus Abdominis Myocutaneous Flap**
  - Replacement
    - Bilateral 0HRV076
    - Left 0HRU076
    - Right 0HRT076
  - Transfer
    - Left 0KXL
    - Right 0KXK
- **Transverse scapular ligament**
  - *use* Bursa and Ligament, Shoulder, Left
  - *use* Bursa and Ligament, Shoulder, Right
- **Transverse thoracis muscle**
  - *use* Muscle, Thorax, Left
  - *use* Muscle, Thorax, Right
- **Transversospinalis muscle**
  - *use* Muscle, Trunk, Left
  - *use* Muscle, Trunk, Right
- **Transversus abdominis muscle**
  - *use* Muscle, Abdomen, Left
  - *use* Muscle, Abdomen, Right
- **Trapezium bone**
  - *use* Carpal, Left
  - *use* Carpal, Right
- **Trapezius muscle**
  - *use* Muscle, Trunk, Left
  - *use* Muscle, Trunk, Right
- **Trapezoid bone**
  - *use* Carpal, Left
  - *use* Carpal, Right
- **Triceps brachii muscle**
  - *use* Muscle, Upper Arm, Left
  - *use* Muscle, Upper Arm, Right
- **Tricuspid annulus**
  - *use* Valve, Tricuspid
- **Trifacial nerve**
  - *use* Nerve, Trigeminal
- **Trifecta™ Valve (aortic)**
  - *use* Zooplastic Tissue in Heart and Great Vessels
- **Trigone of bladder**
  - *use* Bladder
- **Trimming, excisional**
  - *see* Excision
- **Triquetral bone**
  - *use* Carpal, Left
  - *use* Carpal, Right
- **Trochanteric bursa**
  - *use* Bursa and Ligament, Hip, Left
  - *use* Bursa and Ligament, Hip, Right
- **TUMT (Transurethral microwave thermotherapy of prostate)** 0V507ZZ
- **TUNA (transurethral needle ablation of prostate)** 0V507ZZ
- **Tunneled central venous catheter**
  - *use* Vascular Access Device Tunneled in Subcutaneous Tissue and Fascia
- **Tunneled spinal (intrathecal) catheter**
  - *use* Infusion Device
- **Turbinectomy**
  - *see* Excision, Ear, Nose, Sinus 09B
  - *see* Resection, Ear, Nose, Sinus 09T
- **Turbinoplasty**
  - *see* Repair, Ear, Nose, Sinus 09Q
  - *see* Replacement, Ear, Nose, Sinus 09R
  - *see* Supplement, Ear, Nose, Sinus 09U
- **Turbinotomy**
  - *see* Division, Ear, Nose, Sinus 098
  - *see* Drainage, Ear, Nose, Sinus 099
- **TURP (transurethral resection of prostate)**
  - *see* Excision, Prostate 0VB0
  - *see* Resection, Prostate 0VT0
- **Twelfth cranial nerve**
  - *use* Nerve, Hypoglossal
- **Two lead pacemaker**
  - *use* Pacemaker, Dual Chamber in 0JH
- **Tympanic cavity**
  - *use* Ear, Middle, Left
  - *use* Ear, Middle, Right
- **Tympanic nerve**
  - *use* Nerve, Glossopharyngeal
- **Tympanic part of temoporal bone**
  - *use* Bone, Temporal, Left
  - *use* Bone, Temporal, Right
- **Tympanogram**
  - *see* Hearing Assessment, Diagnostic Audiology F13
- **Tympanoplasty**
  - *see* Repair, Ear, Nose, Sinus 09Q
  - *see* Replacement, Ear, Nose, Sinus 09R
  - *see* Supplement, Ear, Nose, Sinus 09U
- **Tympanosympathectomy**
  - *see* Excision, Nerve, Head and Neck Sympathetic 01BK
- **Tympanotomy**
  - *see* Drainage, Ear, Nose, Sinus 099

U

- **Ulnar collateral carpal ligament**
  - *use* Bursa and Ligament, Wrist, Left
  - *use* Bursa and Ligament, Wrist, Right
- **Ulnar collateral ligament**
  - *use* Bursa and Ligament, Elbow, Left
  - *use* Bursa and Ligament, Elbow, Right
- **Ulnar notch**
  - *use* Radius, Left
  - *use* Radius, Right
- **Ulnar vein**
  - *use* Vein, Brachial, Left
  - *use* Vein, Brachial, Right
- **Ultrafiltration**
  - Hemodialysis
    - *see* Performance, Urinary 5A1D
  - Therapeutic plasmapheresis
    - *see* Pheresis, Circulatory 6A55
- **Ultraflex™ Precision Colonic Stent System**
  - *use* Intraluminal Device
- **ULTRAPRO Hernia System (UHS)**
  - *use* Synthetic Substitute
- **ULTRAPRO Partially Absorbable Lightweight Mesh**
  - *use* Synthetic Substitute
- **ULTRAPRO Plug**
  - *use* Synthetic Substitute
- **Ultrasonic osteogenic stimulator**
  - *use* Bone Growth Stimulator in Head and Facial Bones
  - *use* Bone Growth Stimulator in Lower Bones
- **Ultrasonic osteogenic stimulator** *(continued)*
  - *use* Bone Growth Stimulator in Upper Bones
- **Ultrasonography**
  - Abdomen BW40ZZZ
  - Abdomen and Pelvis BW41ZZZ
  - Abdominal Wall BH49ZZZ
  - Aorta
    - Abdominal, Intravascular B440ZZ3
    - Thoracic, Intravascular B340ZZ3
  - Appendix BD48ZZZ
  - Artery
    - Brachiocephalic-Subclavian, Right, Intravascular B341ZZ3
    - Celiac and Mesenteric, Intravascular B44KZZ3
    - Common Carotid
      - Bilateral, Intravascular B345ZZ3
      - Left, Intravascular B344Z
      - Right, Intravascular B343ZZ3
    - Coronary
      - Multiple B241YZZ
        - Intravascular B241ZZ
        - Transesophageal B241ZZ4
      - Single B240YZZ
        - Intravascular B240ZZ
        - Transesophageal B240ZZ4
    - Femoral, Intravascular B44LZZ3
    - Inferior Mesenteric, Intravascular B445ZZ3
    - Internal Carotid
      - Bilateral, Intravascular B348ZZ3
      - Left, Intravascular B347Z
      - Right, Intravascular B346ZZ3
    - Intra-Abdominal, Other, Intravascular B44BZZ3
    - Intracranial, Intravascular B34RZZ3
    - Lower Extremity
      - Bilateral, Intravascular B44HZZ3
      - Left, Intravascular B44G
      - Right, Intravascular B44FZZ3
    - Mesenteric and Celiac, Intravascular B44KZZ3
    - Ophthalmic, Intravascular B34VZZ3
    - Penile, Intravascular B44NZ
    - Pulmonary
      - Left, Intravascular B34T
      - Right, Intravascular B34SZZ3
    - Renal
      - Bilateral, Intravascular B448ZZ3
      - Left, Intravascular B447
      - Right, Intravascular B446ZZ3
    - Subclavian, Left, Intravascul B342ZZ3
    - Superior Mesenteric, Intravascular B444ZZ3
    - Upper Extremity
      - Bilateral, Intravascular B34KZZ3
      - Left, Intravascular B34J
      - Right, Intravascular B34HZZ3

Ultrasonography *(continued)*
Bile Duct BF40ZZZ
Bile Duct and Gallbladder BF43ZZZ
Bladder BT40ZZZ
and Kidney BT4JZZZ
Brain B040ZZZ
Breast
Bilateral BH42ZZZ
Left BH41ZZZ
Right BH40ZZZ
Chest Wall BH4BZZZ
Coccyx BR4FZZZ
Connective Tissue
Lower Extremity BL41ZZZ
Upper Extremity BL40ZZZ
Duodenum BD49ZZZ
Elbow
Left, Densitometry BP4HZZ1
Right, Densitometry BP4GZZ1
Esophagus BD41ZZZ
Extremity
Lower BH48ZZZ
Upper BH47ZZZ
Eye
Bilateral B847ZZZ
Left B846ZZZ
Right B845ZZZ
Fallopian Tube
Bilateral BU42
Left BU41
Right BU40
Fetal Umbilical Cord BY47ZZZ
Fetus
First Trimester, Multiple Gestation BY4BZZZ
Second Trimester, Multiple Gestation BY4DZZZ
Single
First Trimester BY49ZZZ
Second Trimester BY4CZZZ
Third Trimester BY4FZZZ
Third Trimester, Multiple Gestation BY4GZZZ
Gallbladder BF42ZZZ
Gallbladder and Bile Duct BF43ZZZ
Gastrointestinal Tract BD47ZZZ
Gland
Adrenal
Bilateral BG42ZZZ
Left BG41ZZZ
Right BG40ZZZ
Parathyroid BG43ZZZ
Thyroid BG44ZZZ
Hand
Left, Densitometry BP4PZZ1
Right, Densitometry BP4NZZ1
Head and Neck BH4CZZZ
Heart
Left B245YZZ
Intravascular B245ZZ3
Transesophageal B245ZZ4
Pediatric B24DYZZ
Intravascular B24DZZ3
Transesophageal B24DZZ4
Right B244YZZ
Intravascular B244ZZ3
Transesophageal B244ZZ4
Right and Left B246YZZ
Intravascular B246ZZ3
Transesophageal B246ZZ4
Heart with Aorta B24BYZZ
Intravascular B24BZZ3
Transesophageal B24BZZ4
Hepatobiliary System, All BF4CZZZ
Hip
Bilateral BQ42ZZZ
Left BQ41ZZZ
Right BQ40ZZZ

Ultrasonography *(continued)*
Kidney
and Bladder BT4JZZZ
Bilateral BT43ZZZ
Left BT42ZZZ
Right BT41ZZZ
Transplant BT49ZZZ
Knee
Bilateral BQ49ZZZ
Left BQ48ZZZ
Right BQ47ZZZ
Liver BF45ZZZ
Liver and Spleen BF46ZZZ
Mediastinum BB4CZZZ
Neck BW4FZZZ
Ovary
Bilateral BU45
Left BU44
Right BU43
Ovary and Uterus BU4C
Pancreas BF47ZZZ
Pelvic Region BW4GZZZ
Pelvis and Abdomen BW41ZZZ
Penis BV4BZZZ
Pericardium B24CYZZ
Intravascular B24CZZ3
Transesophageal B24CZZ4
Placenta BY48ZZZ
Pleura BB4BZZZ
Prostate and Seminal Vesicle BV49ZZZ
Rectum BD4CZZZ
Sacrum BR4FZZZ
Scrotum BV44ZZZ
Seminal Vesicle and Prostate BV49ZZZ
Shoulder
Left, Densitometry BP49ZZ1
Right, Densitometry BP48ZZ1
Spinal Cord B04BZZZ
Spine
Cervical BR40ZZZ
Lumbar BR49ZZZ
Thoracic BR47ZZZ
Spleen and Liver BF46ZZZ
Stomach BD42ZZZ
Tendon
Lower Extremity BL43ZZZ
Upper Extremity BL42ZZZ
Ureter
Bilateral BT48ZZZ
Left BT47ZZZ
Right BT46ZZZ
Urethra BT45ZZZ
Uterus BU46
Uterus and Ovary BU4C
Vein
Jugular
Left, Intravascular B544ZZ3
Right, Intravascular B543ZZ3
Lower Extremity
Bilateral, Intravascular B54DZZ3
Left, Intravascular B54CZZ3
Right, Intravascular B54BZZ3
Portal, Intravascular B54TZZ3
Renal
Bilateral, Intravascular B54LZZ3
Left, Intravascular B54KZZ3
Right, Intravascular B54JZZ3
Spanchnic, Intravascular B54TZZ3
Subclavian
Left, Intravascular B547ZZ3
Right, Intravascular B546ZZ3

Ultrasonography *(continued)*
Vein *(continued)*
Upper Extremity
Bilateral, Intravascular B54PZZ3
Left, Intravascular B54NZZ3
Right, Intravascular B54MZZ3
Vena Cava
Inferior, Intravascular B549ZZ3
Superior, Intravascular B548ZZ3
Wrist
Left, Densitometry BP4MZZ1
Right, Densitometry BP4LZZ1
Ultrasound bone healing system
use Bone Growth Stimulator in Head and Facial Bones
use Bone Growth Stimulator in Lower Bones
use Bone Growth Stimulator in Upper Bones
Ultrasound Therapy
Heart 6A75
No Qualifier 6A75
Vessels
Head and Neck 6A75
Other 6A75
Peripheral 6A75
Ultraviolet Light Therapy, Skin 6A80
Umbilical artery
use Artery, Internal Iliac, Left
use Artery, Internal Iliac, Right
use Artery, Lower
Uniplanar external fixator
use External Fixation Device, Monoplanar in 0PH
use External Fixation Device, Monoplanar in 0PS
use External Fixation Device, Monoplanar in 0QH
use External Fixation Device, Monoplanar in 0QS
Upper GI series
see Fluoroscopy, Gastrointestinal, Upper BD15
Ureteral orifice
use Ureter
use Ureter, Left
use Ureter, Right
use Ureters, Bilateral
Ureterectomy
see Excision, Urinary System 0TB
see Resection, Urinary System 0TT
Ureterocolostomy
see Bypass, Urinary System 0T1
Ureterocystostomy
see Bypass, Urinary System 0T1
Ureteroenterostomy
see Bypass, Urinary System 0T1
Ureteroileostomy
see Bypass, Urinary System 0T1
Ureterolithotomy
see Extirpation, Urinary System 0TC
Ureterolysis
see Release, Urinary System 0TN
Ureteroneocystostomy
see Bypass, Urinary System 0T1
see Reposition, Urinary System 0TS
Ureteropelvic junction (UPJ)
use Kidney Pelvis, Left
use Kidney Pelvis, Right
Ureteropexy
see Repair, Urinary System 0TQ
see Reposition, Urinary System 0TS

Ureteroplasty
see Repair, Urinary System 0TQ
see Replacement, Urinary System 0TR
see Supplement, Urinary System 0TU
Ureteroplication
see Restriction, Urinary System 0TV
Ureteropyelography
see Fluoroscopy, Urinary System BT1
Ureterorrhaphy
see Repair, Urinary System 0TQ
Ureteroscopy 0TJ98ZZ
Ureterostomy
see Bypass, Urinary System 0T1
see Drainage, Urinary System 0T9
Ureterotomy
see Drainage, Urinary System 0T9
Ureteroureterostomy
see Bypass, Urinary System 0T1
Ureterovesical orifice
use Ureter
use Ureters, Bilateral
use Ureter, Left
use Ureter, Right
Urethral catheterization, indwelling 0T9B70Z
Urethrectomy
see Excision, Urethra 0TBD
see Resection, Urethra 0TTD
Urethrolithotomy
see Extirpation, Urethra 0TCD
Urethrolysis
see Release, Urethra 0TND
Urethropexy
see Repair, Urethra 0TQD
see Reposition, Urethra 0TSD
Urethroplasty
see Repair, Urethra 0TQD
see Replacement, Urethra 0TRD
see Supplement, Urethra 0TUD
Urethrorrhaphy
see Repair, Urethra 0TQD
Urethroscopy 0TJD8ZZ
Urethrotomy
see Drainage, Urethra 0T9D
Uridine Triacetate XW0DX82
Urinary incontinence stimulator lead
use Stimulator Lead in Urinary System
Urography
see Fluoroscopy, Urinary System BT1
Ustekinumab
use Other New Technology Therapeutic Substance
Uterine Artery
use Artery, Internal Iliac, Left
use Artery, Internal Iliac, Right
Uterine artery embolization (UAE)
see Occlusion, Lower Arteries 04L
Uterine cornu
use Uterus
Uterine tube
use Fallopian Tube, Left
use Fallopian Tube, Right
Uterine vein
use Vein, Hypogastric, Left
use Vein, Hypogastric, Right
Uvulectomy
see Excision, Uvula 0CBN
see Resection, Uvula 0CTN
Uvulorrhaphy
see Repair, Uvula 0CQN
Uvulotomy
see Drainage, Uvula 0C9N

V

Vaccination
see Introduction of Serum, Toxoid, and Vaccine
Vacuum extraction, obstetric 10D07Z6
Vaginal artery
use Artery, Internal Iliac, Left
use Artery, Internal Iliac, Right
Vaginal pessary
use Intraluminal Device, Pessary in Female Reproductive System
Vaginal vein
use Vein, Hypogastric, Left
use Vein, Hypogastric, Right
Vaginectomy
see Excision, Vagina 0UBG
see Resection, Vagina 0UTG
Vaginofixation
see Repair, Vagina 0UQG
see Reposition, Vagina 0USG
Vaginoplasty
see Repair, Vagina 0UQG
see Supplement, Vagina 0UUG
Vaginorrhaphy
see Repair, Vagina 0UQG
Vaginoscopy 0UJH8ZZ
Vaginotomy
see Drainage, Female Reproductive System 0U9
Vagotomy
see Division, Nerve, Vagus 008Q
Valiant Thoracic Stent Graft
use Intraluminal Device
Valvotomy, valvulotomy
see Division, Heart and Great Vessels 028
see Release, Heart and Great Vessels 02N
Valvuloplasty
see Repair, Heart and Great Vessels 02Q
see Replacement, Heart and Great Vessels 02R
see Supplement, Heart and Great Vessels 02U
Valvuloplasty, Alfieri Stitch
see Restriction, Valve, Mitral 02VG
Vascular Access Device
Totally Implantable
Insertion of device in
Abdomen 0JH8
Chest 0JH6
Lower Arm
Left 0JHH
Right 0JHG
Lower Leg
Left 0JHP
Right 0JHN
Upper Arm
Left 0JHF
Right 0JHD
Upper Leg
Left 0JHM
Right 0JHL
Removal of device from
Lower Extremity 0JPW
Trunk 0JPT
Upper Extremity 0JPV
Revision of device in
Lower Extremity 0JWW
Trunk 0JWT
Upper Extremity 0JWV
Tunneled
Insertion of device in
Abdomen 0JH8
Chest 0JH6
Vascular Access Device *(continued)*
Tunneled *(continued)*
Insertion of device in *(continued)*
Lower Arm
Left 0JHH
Right 0JHG
Lower Leg
Left 0JHP
Right 0JHN
Upper Arm
Left 0JHF
Right 0JHD
Upper Leg
Left 0JHM
Right 0JHL
Removal of device from
Lower Extremity 0JPW
Trunk 0JPT
Upper Extremity 0JPV
Revision of device in
Lower Extremity 0JWW
Trunk 0JWT
Upper Extremity 0JWV
Vasectomy
see Excision, Male Reproductive System 0VB
Vasography
see Fluoroscopy, Male Reproductive System BV1
see Plain Radiography, Male Reproductive System BV0
Vasoligation
see Occlusion, Male Reproductive System 0VL
Vasorrhaphy
see Repair, Male Reproductive System 0VQ
Vasostomy
see Bypass, Male Reproductive System 0V1
Vasotomy
Drainage
see Drainage, Male Reproductive System 0V9
see Occlusion, Male Reproductive System 0VL
With ligation
Vasovasostomy
see Repair, Male Reproductive System 0VQ
Vastus intermedius muscle
use Muscle, Upper Leg, Left
use Muscle, Upper Leg, Right
Vastus lateralis muscle
use Muscle, Upper Leg, Left
use Muscle, Upper Leg, Right
Vastus medialis muscle
use Muscle, Upper Leg, Left
use Muscle, Upper Leg, Right
VCG (vectorcardiogram)
see Measurement, Cardiac 4A02
Vectra® Vascular Access Graft
use Vascular Access Device, Tunneled in Subcutaneous Tissue and Fascia
Venectomy
see Excision, Lower Veins 06B
see Excision, Upper Veins 05B
Venography
see Fluoroscopy, Veins B51
see Plain Radiography, Veins B50
Venorrhaphy
see Repair, Lower Veins 06Q
see Repair, Upper Veins 05Q
Venotripsy
see Occlusion, Lower Veins 06L
see Occlusion, Upper Veins 05L
Ventricular fold
use Larynx
Ventriculoatriostomy
see Bypass, Central Nervous System and Cranial Nerves 001
Ventriculocisternostomy
see Bypass, Central Nervous System and Cranial Nerves 001
Ventriculogram, cardiac
Combined left and right heart
see Fluoroscopy, Heart, Right and Left B216
Left ventricle
see Fluoroscopy, Heart, Left B215
Right ventricle
see Fluoroscopy, Heart, Right B214
Ventriculopuncture, through previously implanted catheter 8C01X6J
Ventriculoscopy 00J04ZZ
Ventriculostomy
External drainage
see Drainage, Cerebral Ventricle 0096
Internal shunt
see Bypass, Cerebral Ventricle 0016
Ventriculovenostomy
see Bypass, Cerebral Ventricle 0016
Ventrio™ Hernia Patch
use Synthetic Substitute
VEP (visual evoked potential) 4A07X0Z
Vermiform appendix
use Appendix
Vermilion border
use Lip, Lower
use Lip, Upper
Versa
use Pacemaker, Dual Chamber in 0JH
Version, obstetric
External 10S0XZZ
Internal 10S07ZZ
Vertebral arch
use Vertebra, Cervical
use Vertebra, Lumbar
use Vertebra, Thoracic
Vertebral body
use Cervical Vertebra
use Thoracic Vertebra
use Lumbar Vertebra
Vertebral canal
use Spinal Canal
Vertebral foramen
use Vertebra, Cervical
use Vertebra, Lumbar
use Vertebra, Thoracic
Vertebral lamina
use Vertebra, Cervical
use Vertebra, Lumbar
use Vertebra, Thoracic
Vertebral pedicle
use Vertebra, Cervical
use Vertebra, Lumbar
use Vertebra, Thoracic
Vesical vein
use Vein, Hypogastric, Left
use Vein, Hypogastric, Right
Vesicotomy
see Drainage, Urinary System 0T9
Vesiculectomy
see Excision, Male Reproductive System 0VB
see Resection, Male Reproductive System 0VT
Vesiculogram, seminal
see Plain Radiography, Male Reproductive System BV0
Vesiculotomy
see Drainage, Male Reproductive System 0V9
Vestibular (Scarpa's) ganglion
use Nerve, Acoustic
Vestibular Assessment F15Z
Vestibular nerve
use Nerve, Acoustic
Vestibular Treatment F0C
Vestibulocochlear nerve
use Nerve, Acoustic
VH-IVUS (virtual histology intravascular ultrasound)
see Ultrasonography, Heart B24
Virchow's (supraclavicular) lymph node
use Lymphatic, Neck, Left
use Lymphatic, Neck, Right
Virtuoso (II) (DR) (VR)
use Defibrillator Generator in 0JH
Vistogard®
use Uridine Triacetate
Vitrectomy
see Excision, Eye 08B
see Resection, Eye 08T
Vitreous body
use Vitreous, Left
use Vitreous, Right
Viva (XT)(S)
use Cardiac Resynchronization Defibrillator Pulse Generator in 0JH
Vocal fold
use Vocal Cord, Left
use Vocal Cord, Right
Vocational
Assessment
Retraining
see Activities of Daily Living Assessment, Rehabilitatic F02
see Activities of Daily Living Treatment, Rehabilitation F08
Volar (palmar) digital vein
use Vein, Hand, Left
use Vein, Hand, Right
Volar (palmar) metacarpal vein
use Vein, Hand, Left
use Vein, Hand, Right
Vomer bone
use Septum, Nasal
Vomer of nasal septum
use Bone, Nasal
Voraxaze
Glucarpidase
Vulvectomy
see Excision, Female Reproducti System 0UB
see Resection, Female Reproducti System 0UT
VYXEOS™
use Cytarabine and Daunorubici Liposome Antineoplastic

W

WALLSTENT® Endoprosthesis
use Intraluminal Device
Washing
see Irrigation
Wedge resection, pulmonary
see Excision, Respiratory System 0BB
Window
see Drainage
Wiring, dental 2W31X9Z

ray
see Plain Radiography
STOP® Spacer
use Spinal Stabilization Device, Interspinous Process in 0RH
use Spinal Stabilization Device, Interspinous Process in 0SH
ct Carotid Stent System
use Intraluminal Device
nograft
use Zooplastic Tissue in Heart and Great Vessels
ENCE Everolimus Eluting Coronary Stent System
use Intraluminal Device, Drug-eluting in Heart and Great Vessels
phoid process
use Sternum
XLIF® System
use Interbody Fusion Device in Lower Joints

Y

Yoga Therapy 8E0ZXY4

Z

Z-plasty, skin for scar contracture
see Release, Skin and Breast 0HN
Zenith AAA Endovascular Graft
use Intraluminal Device
use Intraluminal Device, Branched or Fenestrated, One or Two Arteries in 04V
use Intraluminal Device, Branched or Fenestrated, Three or More Arteries in 04V
Zenith Flex® AAA Endovascular Graft
use Intraluminal Device
Zenith TX2® TAA Endovascular Graft
use Intraluminal Device
Zenith® Renu™ AAA Ancillary Graft
use Intraluminal Device
Zilver® PTX® (paclitaxel) Drug-Eluting Peripheral Stent
use Intraluminal Device, Drug-eluting in Lower Arteries
use Intraluminal Device, Drug-eluting in Upper Arteries
Zimmer® NexGen® LPS Mobile Bearing Knee
use Synthetic Substitute
Zimmer® NexGen® LPS-Flex Mobile Knee
use Synthetic Substitute
ZINPLAVA™
use Bezlotoxumab Monoclonal AntibodyZonule of Zinn
Zonule of Zinn
use Lens, Left
use Lens, Right
Zooplastic Tissue, Rapid Deployment Technique, Replacement X2RF
Zotarolimus-eluting coronary stent
use Intraluminal Device, Drug-eluting in Heart and Great Vessels
Zygomatic process of frontal bone
use Bone, Frontal
Zygomatic process of temporal bone
use Bone, Temporal, Left
use Bone, Temporal, Right
Zygomaticus muscle
use Muscle, Facial
Zyvox
use Oxazolidinones

Medical and Surgical (001–0YW)

Within each section of ICD-10-PCS the characters have different meanings. The seven character meanings for the Medical and Surgi section are illustrated here through the procedure example of *Percutaneous needle core biopsy of the right kidney.*

Section	Body System	Root Operation	Body Part	Approach	Device	Qualifier
Med/Surg	Urinary	Excision	Kidney, Right	Percutaneous	None	Diagnostic
0	T	B	0	3	Z	X

Section (Character 1)

All Medical and Surgical procedure codes have a first character value of 0.

Body System (Character 2)

The alphanumeric character for the body system is placed in the second position. The following are the body systems applicable to Medical and Surgical section.

Character Value	Character Value Description
0	Central Nervous System and Cranial Nerves
1	Peripheral Nervous System
2	Heart and Great Vessels
3	Upper Arteries
4	Lower Arteries
5	Upper Veins
6	Lower Veins
7	Lymphatic and Hemic Systems
8	Eye
9	Ear, Nose, Sinus
B	Respiratory System
C	Mouth and Throat
D	Gastrointestinal System
F	Hepatobiliary System and Pancreas
G	Endocrine System
H	Skin and Breast
J	Subcutaneous Tissue and Fascia
K	Muscles
L	Tendons
M	Bursae and Ligaments
N	Head and Facial Bones
P	Upper Bones
Q	Lower Bones
R	Upper Joints
S	Lower Joints
T	Urinary System
U	Female Reproductive System
V	Male Reproductive System
W	Anatomical Regions, General
X	Anatomical Regions, Upper Extremities
Y	Anatomical Regions, Lower Extremities

ot Operations (Character 3)

e alphanumeric character value for root operations is placed in the third position. Listed below are the root operations applicable to the edical and Surgical section with their associated meaning.

haracter Value	Root Operation	Root Operation Definition
0	Alteration	Modifying the anatomic structure of a body part without affecting the function of the body part
1	Bypass	Altering the route of passage of the contents of a tubular body part
2	Change	Taking out or off a device from a body part and putting back an identical or similar device in or on the same body part without cutting or puncturing the skin or a mucous membrane
3	Control	Stopping, or attempting to stop, postprocedural bleeding
4	Creation	Making a new genital structure that does not take over the function of a body part
5	Destruction	Physical eradication of all or a portion of a body part by the direct use of energy, force, or a destructive agent
6	Detachment	Cutting off all or a portion of the upper or lower extremities
7	Dilation	Expanding an orifice or the lumen of a tubular body part
8	Division	Cutting into a body part, without draining fluids and/or gases from the body part, in order to separate or transect a body part
9	Drainage	Taking or letting out fluids and/or gases from a body part
B	Excision	Cutting out or off, without replacement, a portion of a body part
C	Extirpation	Taking or cutting out solid matter from a body part
D	Extraction	Pulling or stripping out or off all or a portion of a body part by the use of force
F	Fragmentation	Breaking solid matter in a body part into pieces
G	Fusion	Joining together portions of an articular body part rendering the articular body part immobile
H	Insertion	Putting in a nonbiological appliance that monitors, assists, performs, or prevents a physiological function but does not physically take the place of a body part
J	Inspection	Visually and/or manually exploring a body part
K	Map	Locating the route of passage of electrical impulses and/or locating functional areas in a body part
L	Occlusion	Completely closing an orifice or the lumen of a tubular body part
M	Reattachment	Putting back in or on all or a portion of a separated body part to its normal location or other suitable location
N	Release	Freeing a body part from an abnormal physical constraint by cutting or by the use of force
P	Removal	Taking out or off a device from a body part
Q	Repair	Restoring, to the extent possible, a body part to its normal anatomic structure and function
R	Replacement	Putting in or on biological or synthetic material that physically takes the place and/or function of all or a portion of a body part
S	Reposition	Moving to its normal location, or other suitable location, all or a portion of a body part
T	Resection	Cutting out or off, without replacement, all of a body part
V	Restriction	Partially closing an orifice or the lumen of a tubular body part
W	Revision	Correcting, to the extent possible, a portion of a malfunctioning device or the position of a displaced device
U	Supplement	Putting in or on biological or synthetic material that physically reinforces and/or augments the function of a portion of a body part
X	Transfer	Moving, without taking out, all or a portion of a body part to another location to take over the function of all or a portion of a body part
Y	Transplantation	Putting in or on all or a portion of a living body part taken from another individual or animal to physically take the place and/or function of all or a portion of a similar body part

ody Part (Character 4)

r each body system the applicable body part character values will be available for procedure code construction. An example of a body rt for this section is the Large Intestines.

Approach (Character 5)

The approach is the technique used to reach the procedure site. The following are the approach character values for the Medical Surgical section with the associated definitions.

Character Value	Approach	Approach Definition
0	Open	Cutting through the skin or mucous membrane and any other body layers necessary to expo the site of the procedure
3	Percutaneous	Entry, by puncture or minor incision, of instrumentation through the skin or mucous membrane and any other body layers necessary to reach the site of the procedure
4	Percutaneous Endoscopic	Entry, by puncture or minor incision, of instrumentation through the skin or mucous membran and any other body layers necessary to reach and visualize the site of the procedure
7	Via Natural or Artificial Opening	Entry of instrumentation through a natural or artificial external opening to reach the site of the procedure
8	Via Natural or Artificial Opening Endoscopic	Entry of instrumentation through a natural or artificial external opening to reach and visuali the site of the procedure
F	Via Natural or Artificial Opening Percutaneous Endoscopic	Entry of instrumentation through a natural or artificial external opening to reach and visuali the site of the procedure, and entry, by puncture or minor incision, of instrumentation throug the skin or mucous membrane and any other body layers necessary to aid in the performanc of the procedure
X	External	Procedures performed directly on the skin or mucous membrane and procedures performed indirectly by the application of external force through the skin or mucous membrane

Device (Character 6)

Depending on the procedure performed there may or may not be a device used. There are several types of devices included in the Medi and Surgical section that fall into one of the four following categories.

- Electronic Appliances
- Grafts and Prostheses
- Implants
- Simple or Mechanical Appliances

When a device is not utilized during the procedure, the character value of Z should be reported.

If a coder is unsure of which option to select for the device utilized during the procedure, Appendix E can be used to guide the selecti For example, if the coder is in Table 02R (replacement of heart and great vessels) the coder can locate the device categories in Appendi (Autologous Tissue Substitute, Zooplastic Tissue, Synthetic Substitute, and Nonautologous Tissue Substitue). For each of these catego brand name devices and other devices are listed. The coder should select the category in which the device utilized during the procedure is lis

Qualifier (Character 7)

The qualifier represents an additional attribute for the procedure when applicable. In the preceding example of *Percutaneous needle c biopsy of the right kidney*, the qualifier of X was used to report that the biopsy procedure was diagnostic in nature. If there is no quali for a procedure, the Z character value should be reported.

Important Definitions for the Medical and Surgical Section

Medical Surgical Root Operation	Qualifier	Definition
Detachment of Upper and Lower Extremities (0X6 and 0Y6) Arms and Legs	1 – High	Amputation at the proximal portion of the shaft of the humerus or femur
	2 – Mid	Amputation at the middle portion of the shaft of the humerus or femur
	3 – Low	Amputation at the distal portion of the shaft of the humerus or femur
Detachment of Upper and Lower Extremities (0X6 and 0Y6) Fingers, Thumbs, and Toes	0 – Complete	Amputation at the metacarpophalangeal/metatarsal-phalangeal joint
	1 – High	Amputation anywhere along the proximal phalanx
	2 – Mid	Amputation through the proximal interphalangeal joint or anywhere along the midd phalanx
	3 – Low	Amputation through the distal interphalangeal joint or anywhere along the distal phalan
Transplantation	0 – Allogeneic	Being genetically different although belonging to or obtained from the same species
	1 – Syngeneic	Genetically identical or closely related, so as to allow tissue transplant; immunologically compatible*
	2 – Zooplastic	Surgical transfer of tissue from an animal to a human*

*Taken from The Free Dictionary by Farlex at www.thefreedictionary.com

fficial Coding Guidelines for the Medical and Surgical Section

edical and Surgical Section Guidelines (section 0)

. Body System

neral guidelines

.1a The procedure codes in the general anatomical regions body systems can be used when the procedure is performed on an anatomical ion rather than a specific body part (e.g., root operations Control and Detachment, Drainage of a body cavity) or on the rare occasion en no information is available to support assignment of a code to a specific body part.

amples: Control of postoperative hemorrhage is coded to the root operation Control found in the general anatomical regions body stems. Chest tube drainage of the pleural cavity is coded to the root operation Drainage found in the general anatomical regions body stems. Suture repair of the abdominal wall is coded to the root operation Repair in the general anatomical regions body system.

.1b Where the general body part values "upper" and "lower" are provided as an option in the Upper Arteries, Lower Arteries, Upper ins, Lower Veins, Muscles and Tendons body systems, "upper" or "lower" specifies body parts located above or below the diaphragm pectively.

ample: Vein body parts above the diaphragm are found in the Upper Veins body system; vein body parts below the diaphragm are found the Lower Veins body system.

. Root Operation

neral guidelines

.1a In order to determine the appropriate root operation, the full definition of the root operation as contained in the PCS Tables must applied.

.1b Components of a procedure specified in the root operation definition and explanation are not coded separately. Procedural steps cessary to reach the operative site and close the operative site, including anastomosis of a tubular body part, are also not coded separately.

amples: Resection of a joint as part of a joint replacement procedure is included in the root operation definition of Replacement and not coded separately. Laparotomy performed to reach the site of an open liver biopsy is not coded separately. In a resection of sigmoid lon with anastomosis of descending colon to rectum, the anastomosis is not coded separately. Excision of lesion in the ascending colon d excision of lesion in the transverse colon are coded separately.

ultiple procedures

.2 During the same operative episode, multiple procedures are coded if:

- **a.** The same root operation is performed on different body parts as defined by distinct values of the body part character.

  Examples: Diagnostic excision of liver and pancreas are coded separately. Excision of lesion in the ascending colon and excision of lesion in the transverse colon are coded separately.
- **b.** The same root operation is repeated at different body sites that are included in the same body part value.

  Examples: Excision of the sartorius muscle and excision of the gracilis muscle are both included in the upper leg muscle body part value, and multiple procedures are coded. Extraction of multiple toenails are coded separately.
- **c.** Multiple root operations with distinct objectives are performed on the same body part.

  Example: Destruction of sigmoid lesion and bypass of sigmoid colon are coded separately.
- **d.** The intended root operation is attempted using one approach, but is converted to a different approach.

  Example: Laparoscopic cholecystectomy converted to an open cholecystectomy is coded as percutaneous endoscopic Inspection and open Resection.

iscontinued or incomplete procedures

.3 If the intended procedure is discontinued or otherwise not complete, code the procedure to the root operation performed. If a ocedure is discontinued before any other root operation is performed, code the root operation Inspection of the body part or anatomical gion inspected.

ample: A planned aortic valve replacement procedure is discontinued after the initial thoracotomy and before any incision is made in heart muscle, when the patient becomes hemodynamically unstable. This procedure is coded as an open Inspection of the mediastinum.

opsy procedures

.4a Biopsy procedures are coded using the root operations Excision, Extraction, or Drainage and the qualifier Diagnostic.

amples: Fine needle aspiration biopsy of lung is coded to the root operation Drainage with the qualifier Diagnostic. Biopsy of bone arrow is coded to the root operation Extraction with the qualifier Diagnostic. Lymph node sampling for biopsy is coded to the root eration Excision with the qualifier Diagnostic.

Biopsy followed by more definitive treatment

B3.4b If a diagnostic Excision, Extraction, or Drainage procedure (biopsy) is followed by a more definitive procedure, such as Destruct Excision or Resection at the same procedure site, both the biopsy and the more definitive treatment are coded.

Example: Biopsy of breast followed by partial mastectomy at the same procedure site, both the biopsy and the partial mastectc procedure are coded.

Overlapping body layers

B3.5 If the root operations Excision, Repair or Inspection are performed on overlapping layers of the musculoskeletal system, the b part specifying the deepest layer is coded.

Example: Excisional debridement that includes skin and subcutaneous tissue and muscle is coded to the muscle body part.

Bypass procedures

B3.6a Bypass procedures are coded by identifying the body part bypassed "from" and the body part bypassed "to." The fourth chara body part specifies the body part bypassed from, and the qualifier specifies the body part bypassed to.

Example: Bypass from stomach to jejunum, stomach is the body part and jejunum is the qualifier.

B3.6b Coronary artery bypass procedures are coded differently than other bypass procedures as described in the previous guidel Rather than identifying the body part bypassed from, the body part identifies the number of coronary artery sites bypassed to, and qualifier specifies the vessel bypassed from.

Example: Aortocoronary artery bypass of the left anterior descending coronary artery and the obtuse marginal coronary artery is classi in the body part axis of classification as two coronary arteries and the qualifier specifies the aorta as the body part bypassed from.

B3.6c If multiple coronary arteries are bypassed, a separate procedure is coded for each coronary artery that uses a different device a or qualifier.

Example: Aortocoronary artery bypass and internal mammary coronary artery bypass are coded separately.

Control vs. more definitive root operations

B3.7 The root operation Control is defined as, "Stopping, or attempting to stop, postprocedural or other acute bleeding." If an atte to stop postprocedural or other acute bleeding is initially unsuccessful, and to stop the bleeding requires performing a more defini root operation, such as Bypass, Detachment, Excision, Extraction, Reposition, Replacement, or Resection, then the more definitive operation is coded instead of Control.

Example: Resection of spleen to stop bleeding is coded to Resection instead of Control.

Excision vs. Resection

B3.8 PCS contains specific body parts for anatomical subdivisions of a body part, such as lobes of the lungs or liver and regions of intestine. Resection of the specific body part is coded whenever all of the body part is cut out or off, rather than coding Excision of a specific body part.

Example: Left upper lung lobectomy is coded to Resection of Upper Lung Lobe, Left rather than Excision of Lung, Left.

Excision for graft

B3.9 If an autograft is obtained from a different procedure site in order to complete the objective of the procedure, a separate procedur coded.

Example: Coronary bypass with excision of saphenous vein graft, excision of saphenous vein is coded separately.

Fusion procedures of the spine

B3.10a The body part coded for a spinal vertebral joint(s) rendered immobile by a spinal fusion procedure is classified by the level of spine (e.g. thoracic). There are distinct body part values for a single vertebral joint and for multiple vertebral joints at each spinal leve

Example: Body part values specify Lumbar Vertebral Joint, Lumbar Vertebral Joints, 2 or More and Lumbosacral Vertebral Joint.

B3.10b If multiple vertebral joints are fused, a separate procedure is coded for each vertebral joint that uses a different device and/or quali

Example: Fusion of lumbar vertebral joint, posterior approach, anterior column and fusion of lumbar vertebral joint, posterior appro posterior column are coded separately.

B3.10c Combinations of devices and materials are often used on a vertebral joint to render the joint immobile. When combination devices are used on the same vertebral joint, the device value coded for the procedure is as follows:

- If an interbody fusion device is used to render the joint immobile (alone or containing other material like bone graft), the procedure is coded with the device value Interbody Fusion Device

- If bone graft is the only device used to render the joint immobile, the procedure is coded with the device value Nonautologous Tissue Substitute or Autologous Tissue Substitute
- If a mixture of autologous and nonautologous bone graft (with or without biological or synthetic extenders or binders) is used to render the joint immobile, code the procedure with the device value Autologous Tissue Substitute

mples: Fusion of a vertebral joint using a cage style interbody fusion device containing morsellized bone graft is coded to the device erbody Fusion Device. Fusion of a vertebral joint using a bone dowel interbody fusion device made of cadaver bone and packed with ixture of local morsellized bone and demineralized bone matrix is coded to the device Interbody Fusion Device. Fusion of a vertebral nt using both autologous bone graft and bone bank bone graft is coded to the device Autologous Tissue Substitute.

pection procedures

.11a Inspection of a body part(s) performed in order to achieve the objective of a procedure is not coded separately.

mple: Fiberoptic bronchoscopy performed for irrigation of bronchus, only the irrigation procedure is coded.

.11b If multiple tubular body parts are inspected, the most distal body part inspected is coded. If multiple non-tubular body parts in a ion are inspected, the body part that specifies the entire area inspected is coded.

amples: Cystoureteroscopy with inspection of bladder and ureters is coded to the ureter body part value. Exploratory laparotomy with eral inspection of abdominal contents is coded to the peritoneal cavity body part value.

.11c When both an Inspection procedure and another procedure are performed on the same body part during the same episode, if the pection procedure is performed using a different approach than the other procedure, the Inspection procedure is coded separately.

ample: Endoscopic Inspection of the duodenum is coded separately when open Excision of the duodenum is performed during the same cedural episode.

clusion vs. Restriction for vessel embolization procedures

.12 If the objective of an embolization procedure is to completely close a vessel, the root operation Occlusion is coded. If the objective an embolization procedure is to narrow the lumen of a vessel, the root operation Restriction is coded.

amples: Tumor embolization is coded to the root operation Occlusion, because the objective of the procedure is to cut off the od supply to the vessel. Embolization of a cerebral aneurysm is coded to the root operation Restriction, because the objective of procedure is not to close off the vessel entirely, but to narrow the lumen of the vessel at the site of the aneurysm where it is abnormally de.

lease procedures

.13 In the root operation Release, the body part value coded is the body part being freed and not the tissue being manipulated or cut to e the body part.

ample: Lysis of intestinal adhesions is coded to the specific intestine body part value.

lease vs. Division

.14 If the sole objective of the procedure is freeing a body part without cutting the body part, the root operation is Release. If the sole ective of the procedure is separating or transecting a body part, the root operation is Division.

ample: Freeing a nerve root from surrounding scar tissue to relieve pain is coded to the root operation Release. Severing a nerve root relieve pain is coded to the root operation Division.

position for fracture treatment

.15 Reduction of a displaced fracture is coded to the root operation Reposition and the application of a cast or splint in conjunction with Reposition procedure is not coded separately. Treatment of a nondisplaced fracture is coded to the procedure performed.

amples: Putting a pin in a nondisplaced fracture is coded to the root operation Insertion. Casting of a nondisplaced fracture is coded to root operation Immobilization in the Placement section.

ansplantation vs. Administration

.16 Putting in a mature and functioning living body part taken from another individual or animal is coded to the root operation ansplantation. Putting in autologous or nonautologous cells is coded to the Administration section.

ample: Putting in autologous or nonautologous bone marrow, pancreatic islet cells or stem cells is coded to the Administration section.

ansfer procedures using multiple tissue layers

.17 The root operation Transfer contains qualifiers that can be used to specify when a transfer flap is composed of more than one tissue yer, such as a musculocutaneous flap. For procedures involving transfer of multiple tissue layers including skin, subcutaneous tissue, fascia or muscle, the procedure is coded to the body part value that describes the deepest tissue layer in the flap, and the qualifier ca used to describe the other tissue layer(s) in the transfer flap.

Example: A musculocutaneous flap transfer is coded to the appropriate body part value in the body system Muscles, and the qualifie used to describe the additional tissue layer(s) in the transfer flap.

B4. Body Part

General guidelines

B4.1a If a procedure is performed on a portion of a body part that does not have a separate body part value, code the body part va corresponding to the whole body part.

Example: A procedure performed on the alveolar process of the mandible is coded to the mandible body part.

B4.1b If the prefix "peri" is combined with a body part to identify the site of the procedure, and the site of the procedure is not further specif then the procedure is coded to the body part named. This guideline applies only when a more specific body part value is not available.

Examples: A procedure site identified as perirenal is coded to the kidney body part when the site of the procedure is not further specif A procedure site described in the documentation as peri-urethral tissue, and the documentation also indicates that it is the vulvar tis and not the urethral tissue that is the site of the procedure, then the procedure is coded to the vulva body part.

B4.1c If a procedure is performed on a continuous section of a tubular body part, code the body part value corresponding to the furth anatomical site from the point of entry.

Example: A procedure performed on a continuous section of artery from the femoral artery to the external iliac artery with the poin entry at the femoral artery is coded to the external iliac body part.

Branches of body parts

B4.2 Where a specific branch of a body part does not have its own body part value in PCS, the body part is typically coded to the clo proximal branch that has a specific body part value. In the cardiovascular body systems, if a general body part is available in the cor root operation table, and coding to a proximal branch would require assigning a code in a different body system, the procedure is co using the general body part value.

Examples: A procedure performed on the mandibular branch of the trigeminal nerve is coded to the trigeminal nerve body part va Occlusion of the bronchial artery is coded to the body part value Upper Artery in the body system Upper Arteries, and not to the body p value Thoracic Aorta, Descending in the body system Heart and Great Vessels.

Bilateral body part values

B4.3 Bilateral body part values are available for a limited number of body parts. If the identical procedure is performed on contralat body parts, and a bilateral body part value exists for that body part, a single procedure is coded using the bilateral body part value. If bilateral body part value exists, each procedure is coded separately using the appropriate body part value.

Examples: The identical procedure performed on both fallopian tubes is coded once using the body part value Fallopian Tube, Bilate The identical procedure performed on both knee joints is coded twice using the body part values Knee Joint, Right and Knee Joint, L

Coronary arteries

B4.4 The coronary arteries are classified as a single body part that is further specified by number of arteries treated. One procedure c specifying multiple arteries is used when the same procedure is performed, including the same device and qualifier values.

Examples: Angioplasty of two distinct coronary arteries with placement of two stents is coded as Dilation of Coronary Artery, T Arteries, with Two Intraluminal Devices. Angioplasty of two distinct coronary arteries, one with stent placed and one without, is co separately as Dilation of Coronary Artery, One Artery with Intraluminal Device, and Dilation of Coronary Artery, One Artery with device.

Tendons, ligaments, bursae and fascia near a joint

B4.5 Procedures performed on tendons, ligaments, bursae and fascia supporting a joint are coded to the body part in the respective b system that is the focus of the procedure. Procedures performed on joint structures themselves are coded to the body part in the joint b systems.

Examples: Repair of the anterior cruciate ligament of the knee is coded to the knee bursae and ligament body part in the Bursae Ligaments body system. Knee arthroscopy with shaving of articular cartilage is coded to the knee joint body part in the Lower Joints b system.

Skin, subcutaneous tissue and fascia overlying a joint

B4.6 If a procedure is performed on the skin, subcutaneous tissue or fascia overlying a joint, the procedure is coded to the following body p

- Shoulder is coded to Upper Arm
- Elbow is coded to Lower Arm

- Wrist is coded to Lower Arm
- Hip is coded to Upper Leg
- Knee is coded to Lower Leg
- Ankle is coded to Foot

ngers and toes

4.7 If a body system does not contain a separate body part value for fingers, procedures performed on the fingers are coded to the body rt value for the hand. If a body system does not contain a separate body part value for toes, procedures performed on the toes are coded the body part value for the foot.

ample: Excision of finger muscle is coded to one of the hand muscle body part values in the Muscles body system.

pper and lower intestinal tract

4.8 In the Gastrointestinal body system, the general body part values Upper Intestinal Tract and Lower Intestinal Tract are provided as an tion for the root operations Change, Inspection, Removal and Revision. Upper Intestinal Tract includes the portion of the gastrointestinal ct from the esophagus down to and including the duodenum, and Lower Intestinal Tract includes the portion of the gastrointestinal tract om the jejunum down to and including the rectum and anus.

ample: In the root operation Change table, change of a device in the jejunum is coded using the body part Lower Intestinal Tract.

5. Approach

pen approach with percutaneous endoscopic assistance

5.2 Procedures performed using the open approach with percutaneous endoscopic assistance are coded to the approach Open.

ample: Laparoscopic-assisted sigmoidectomy is coded to the approach Open.

xternal approach

5.3a Procedures performed within an orifice on structures that are visible without the aid of any instrumentation are coded to the proach External.

xample: Resection of tonsils is coded to the approach External.

5.3b Procedures performed indirectly by the application of external force through the intervening body layers are coded to the approach xternal.

xample: Closed reduction of fracture is coded to the approach External.

ercutaneous procedure via device

5.4 Procedures performed percutaneously via a device placed for the procedure are coded to the approach Percutaneous.

xample: Fragmentation of kidney stone performed via percutaneous nephrostomy is coded to the approach Percutaneous.

6. Device

eneral guidelines

6.1a A device is coded only if a device remains after the procedure is completed. If no device remains, the device value No Device is oded. In limited root operations, the classification provides the qualifier values Temporary and Intraoperative, for specific procedures volving clinically significant devices, where the purpose of the device is to be utilized for a brief duration during the procedure or current patient stay. If a device that is intended to remain after the procedure is completed requires removal before the end of the operative oisode in which it was inserted (for example, the device size is inadequate or a complication occurs), both the insertion and removal of e device should be coded.

6.1b Materials such as sutures, ligatures, radiological markers and temporary post-operative wound drains are considered integral to the erformance of a procedure and are not coded as devices.

6.1c Procedures performed on a device only and not on a body part are specified in the root operations Change, Irrigation, Removal and evision, and are coded to the procedure performed.

xample: Irrigation of percutaneous nephrostomy tube is coded to the root operation Irrigation of indwelling device in the Administration ection.

rainage device

6.2 A separate procedure to put in a drainage device is coded to the root operation Drainage with the device value Drainage Device.

Coding Guidelines Reference

Coding Guidelines References

The tables below link ICD-10-PCS coding guidelines to Medical and Surgical section root operations, specific body system tables, a body systems. The guidelines identified in each table are provided in order to remind users to reference the coding guidelines prior code reporting. The tables provide coding guideline references at the body system and root operation level. It is imperative to review ICD-10-PCS coding guidelines to ensure the procedure code being reported is accurate and complete.

Root Operation References

Root Operation	Character Value	Coding Guideline(s)
Bypass	1	B3.6a
Change	2	B6.1c
Control	3	B3.7
Division	8	B3.14
Drainage	9	B3.4a, B3.4b, B6.2
Excision	B	B3.4a, B3.4b, B3.8, B3.9
Extraction	D	B3.4a, B3.4b
Inspection	J	B3.11a, B3.11b, B3.11c
Occlusion	L	B3.12
Release	N	B3.13, B3.14
Removal	P	B6.1c
Resection	T	B3.8
Restriction	V	B3.12
Revision	W	B6.1c
Transplantation	Y	B3.16

Table References

Table	Body System	Root Operation	Coding Guideline(s)
021	Heart and Great Vessels	Bypass	B3.6b, B3.6c, B4.4
027	Heart and Great Vessels	Dilation	B4.4
02C	Heart and Great Vessels	Extirpation	B4.4
02Q	Heart and Great Vessels	Repair	B4.4
0HB	Skin and Breast	Excision	B3.5
0HJ	Skin and Breast	Inspection	B3.5
0HQ	Skin and Breast	Repair	B3.5
0HX	Skin and Breast	Transfer	B3.17
0JB	Subcutaneous Tissue and Fascia	Excision	B3.5
0JJ	Subcutaneous Tissue and Fascia	Inspection	B3.5
0JQ	Subcutaneous Tissue and Fascia	Repair	B3.5
0JX	Subcutaneous Tissue and Fascia	Transfer	B3.17
0KB	Muscles	Excision	B3.5
0KJ	Muscles	Inspection	B3.5
0KQ	Muscles	Repair	B3.5
0KX	Muscles	Transfer	B3.17
0LB	Tendons	Excision	B3.5
0LJ	Tendons	Inspection	B3.5
0LQ	Tendons	Repair	B3.5
0MB	Bursae and Ligaments	Excision	B3.5

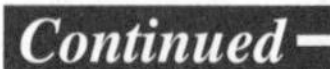
Continued

able	Body System	Root Operation	Coding Guideline(s)
MJ	Bursae and Ligaments	Inspection	B3.5
MQ	Bursae and Ligaments	Repair	B3.5
NB	Head and Facial Bones	Excision	B3.5
NJ	Head and Facial Bones	Inspection	B3.5
NQ	Head and Facial Bones	Repair	B3.5
NS	Head and Facial Bones	Reposition	B3.15
PB	Upper Bones	Excision	B3.5
PJ	Upper Bones	Inspection	B3.5
PQ	Upper Bones	Repair	B3.5
PS	Upper Bones	Reposition	B3.15
QB	Lower Bones	Excision	B3.5
QJ	Lower Bones	Inspection	B3.5
QQ	Lower Bones	Repair	B3.5
QS	Lower Bones	Reposition	B3.15
RB	Upper Joints	Excision	B3.5
RG	Upper Joints	Fusion	B3.10a, B3.10b, B3.10c
RJ	Upper Joints	Inspection	B3.5
RQ	Upper Joints	Repair	B3.5
SB	Lower Joints	Excision	B3.5
SG	Lower Joints	Fusion	B3.10a, B3.10b, B3.10c
SJ	Lower Joints	Inspection	B3.5
SQ	Lower Joints	Repair	B3.5
UD	Female Reproductive System	Extraction	C2

ody System References

ody System	Character Value	Coding Guideline(s)
Gastrointestinal System	D	B4.8
Subcutaneous Tissue and Fascia	J	B4.5, B4.6
Tendons	L	B4.5
Bursae and Ligaments	M	B4.5
Upper Joints	R	B4.5
Lower Joints	S	B4.5

Brain

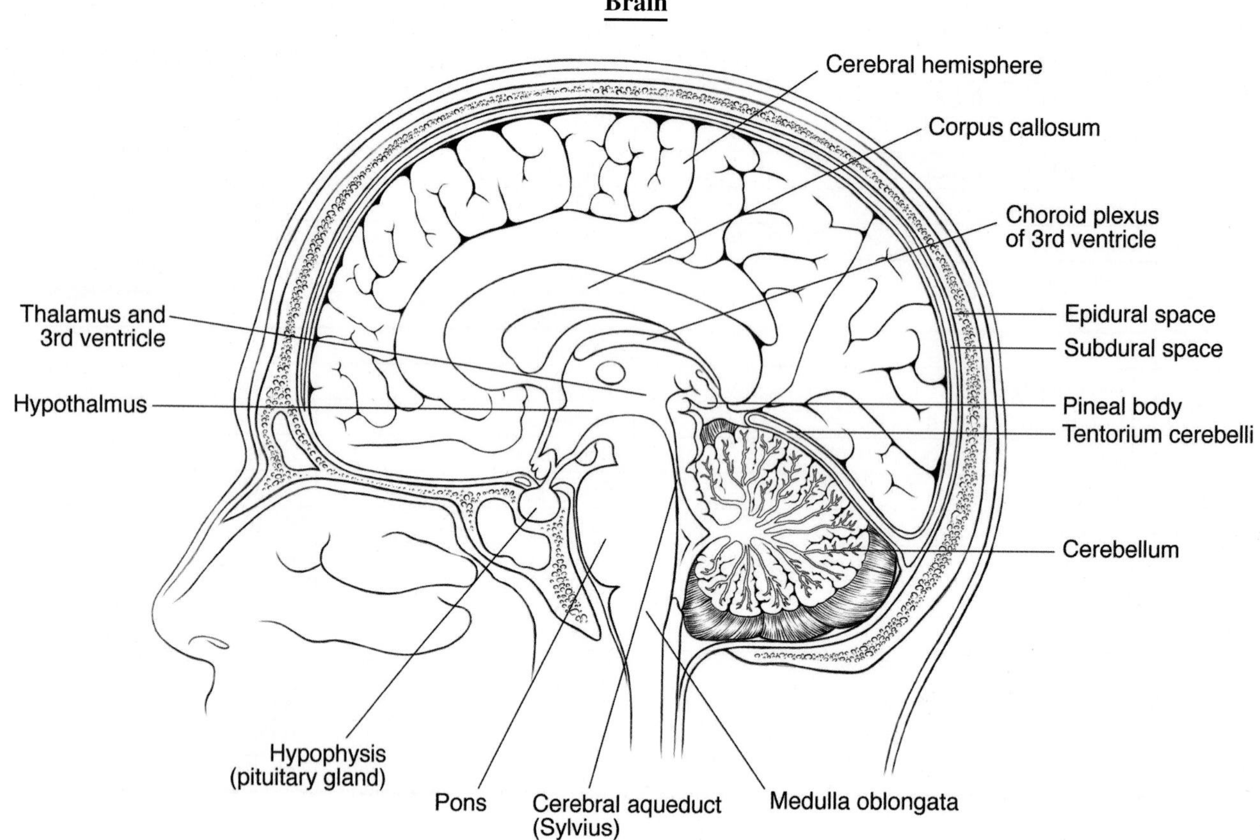

Cranial Nerves

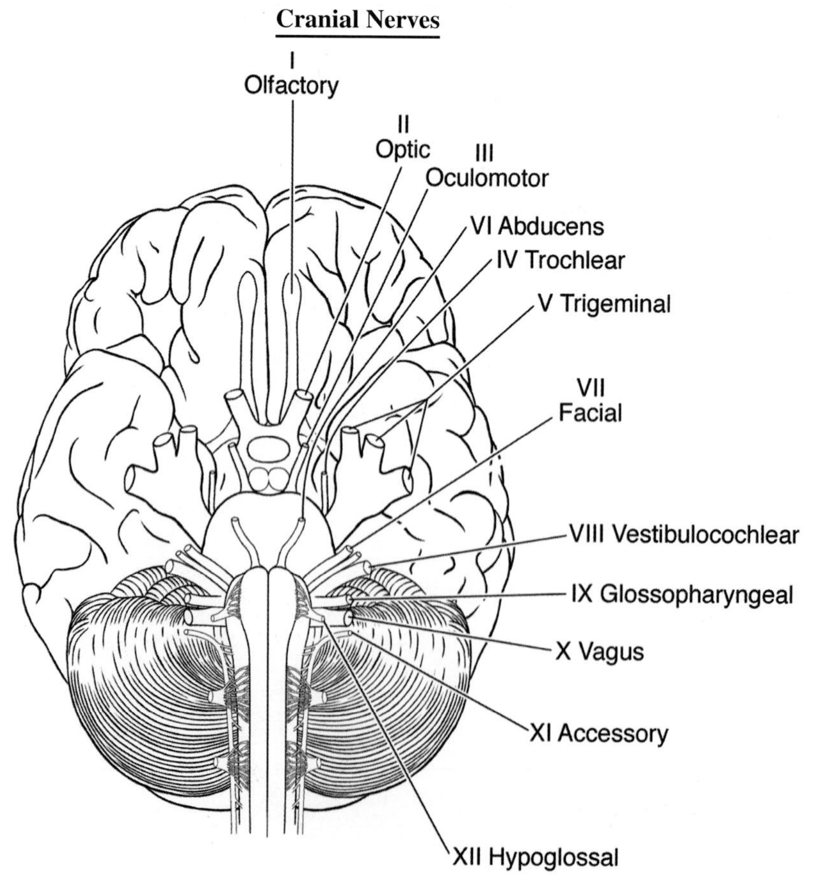

ction	0	**Medical and Surgical**
dy System	0	**Central Nervous System and Cranial Nerves**
eration	1	**Bypass:** Altering the route of passage of the contents of a tubular body part

Body Part (4th)	Approach (5th)	Device (6th)	Qualifier (7th)
Cerebral Ventricle	**0** Open **3** Percutaneous **4** Percutaneous Endoscopic	**7** Autologous Tissue Substitute **J** Synthetic Substitute **K** Nonautologous Tissue Substitute	**0** Nasopharynx **1** Mastoid Sinus **2** Atrium **3** Blood Vessel **4** Pleural Cavity **5** Intestine **6** Peritoneal Cavity **7** Urinary Tract **8** Bone Marrow **B** Cerebral Cisterns
Cerebral Ventricle	**0** Open **3** Percutaneous **4** Percutaneous Endoscopic	**Z** No Device	**B** Cerebral Cisterns
U Spinal Canal	**0** Open **3** Percutaneous **4** Percutaneous Endoscopic	**7** Autologous Tissue Substitute **J** Synthetic Substitute **K** Nonautologous Tissue Substitute	**2** Atrium **4** Pleural Cavity **6** Peritoneal Cavity **7** Urinary Tract **9** Fallopian Tube

ction	0	**Medical and Surgical**
dy System	0	**Central Nervous System and Cranial Nerves**
eration	2	**Change:** Taking out or off a device from a body part and putting back an identical or similar device in or on the same body part without cutting or puncturing the skin or a mucous membrane

Body Part (4th)	Approach (5th)	Device (6th)	Qualifier (7th)
Brain E Cranial Nerve U Spinal Canal	**X** External	**0** Drainage Device **Y** Other Device	**Z** No Qualifier

Section 0 **Medical and Surgical**
Body System 0 **Central Nervous System and Cranial Nerves**
Operation 5 **Destruction:** Physical eradication of all or a portion of a body part by the direct use of energy, force, or a destructive age

Body Part (4th)	Approach (5th)	Device (6th)	Qualifier (7th)
0 Brain 1 Cerebral Meninges 2 Dura Mater 6 Cerebral Ventricle 7 Cerebral Hemisphere 8 Basal Ganglia 9 Thalamus A Hypothalamus B Pons C Cerebellum D Medulla Oblongata F Olfactory Nerve G Optic Nerve H Oculomotor Nerve J Trochlear Nerve K Trigeminal Nerve L Abducens Nerve M Facial Nerve N Acoustic Nerve P Glossopharyngeal Nerve Q Vagus Nerve R Accessory Nerve S Hypoglossal Nerve T Spinal Meninges W Cervical Spinal Cord X Thoracic Spinal Cord Y Lumbar Spinal Cord	0 Open 3 Percutaneous 4 Percutaneous Endoscopic	Z No Device	Z No Qualifier

Section 0 **Medical and Surgical**
Body System 0 **Central Nervous System and Cranial Nerves**
Operation 7 **Dilation:** Expanding an orifice or the lumen of a tubular body part

Body Part (4th)	Approach (5th)	Device (6th)	Qualifier (7th)
6 Cerebral Ventricle	0 Open 3 Percutaneous 4 Percutaneous Endoscopic	Z No Device	Z No Qualifie

Section 0 **Medical and Surgical**
Body System 0 **Central Nervous System and Cranial Nerves**
Operation 8 **Division:** Cutting into a body part, without draining fluids and/or gases from the body part, in order to separate or transec body part

Body Part (4th)	Approach (5th)	Device (6th)	Qualifier (7th)
0 Brain 7 Cerebral Hemisphere 8 Basal Ganglia F Olfactory Nerve G Optic Nerve H Oculomotor Nerve J Trochlear Nerve K Trigeminal Nerve L Abducens Nerve M Facial Nerve N Acoustic Nerve P Glossopharyngeal Nerve Q Vagus Nerve R Accessory Nerve S Hypoglossal Nerve W Cervical Spinal Cord X Thoracic Spinal Cord Y Lumbar Spinal Cord	0 Open 3 Percutaneous 4 Percutaneous Endoscopic	Z No Device	Z No Qualifier

ction 0 **Medical and Surgical**
ody System 0 **Central Nervous System and Cranial Nerves**
peration 9 **Drainage:** Taking or letting out fluids and/or gases from a body part

Body Part (4th)	Approach (5th)	Device (6th)	Qualifier (7th)
0 Brain **1** Cerebral Meninges **2** Dura Mater **3** Epidural Space, Intracranial **4** Subdural Space, Intracranial **5** Subarachnoid Space, Intracranial **6** Cerebral Ventricle **7** Cerebral Hemisphere **8** Basal Ganglia **9** Thalamus **A** Hypothalamus **B** Pons **C** Cerebellum **D** Medulla Oblongata **F** Olfactory Nerve **G** Optic Nerve **H** Oculomotor Nerve **J** Trochlear Nerve **K** Trigeminal Nerve **L** Abducens Nerve **M** Facial Nerve **N** Acoustic Nerve **P** Glossopharyngeal Nerve **Q** Vagus Nerve **R** Accessory Nerve **S** Hypoglossal Nerve **T** Spinal Meninges **U** Spinal Canal **W** Cervical Spinal Cord **X** Thoracic Spinal Cord **Y** Lumbar Spinal Cord	**0** Open **3** Percutaneous **4** Percutaneous Endoscopic	**0** Drainage Device	**Z** No Qualifier
0 Brain **1** Cerebral Meninges **2** Dura Mater **3** Epidural Space, Intracranial **4** Subdural Space, Intracranial **5** Subarachnoid Space, Intracranial **6** Cerebral Ventricle **7** Cerebral Hemisphere **8** Basal Ganglia **9** Thalamus **A** Hypothalamus **B** Pons **C** Cerebellum **D** Medulla Oblongata **F** Olfactory Nerve **G** Optic Nerve **H** Oculomotor Nerve **J** Trochlear Nerve **K** Trigeminal Nerve **L** Abducens Nerve **M** Facial Nerve **N** Acoustic Nerve **P** Glossopharyngeal Nerve **Q** Vagus Nerve **R** Accessory Nerve **S** Hypoglossal Nerve **T** Spinal Meninges **U** Spinal Canal **W** Cervical Spinal Cord **X** Thoracic Spinal Cord **Y** Lumbar Spinal Cord	**0** Open **3** Percutaneous **4** Percutaneous Endoscopic	**Z** No Device	**X** Diagnostic **Z** No Qualifier

Section **0** **Medical and Surgical**
Body System **0** **Central Nervous System and Cranial Nerves**
Operation **B** **Excision:** Cutting out or off, without replacement, a portion of a body part

Body Part (4th)	Approach (5th)	Device (6th)	Qualifier (7th)
0 Brain **1** Cerebral Meninges **2** Dura Mater **6** Cerebral Ventricle **7** Cerebral Hemisphere **8** Basal Ganglia **9** Thalamus **A** Hypothalamus **B** Pons **C** Cerebellum **D** Medulla Oblongata **F** Olfactory Nerve **G** Optic Nerve **H** Oculomotor Nerve **J** Trochlear Nerve **K** Trigeminal Nerve **L** Abducens Nerve **M** Facial Nerve **N** Acoustic Nerve **P** Glossopharyngeal Nerve **Q** Vagus Nerve **R** Accessory Nerve **S** Hypoglossal Nerve **T** Spinal Meninges **W** Cervical Spinal Cord **X** Thoracic Spinal Cord **Y** Lumbar Spinal Cord	**0** Open **3** Percutaneous **4** Percutaneous Endoscopic	**Z** No Device	**X** Diagnostic **Z** No Qualifier

ction **0** **Medical and Surgical**
dy System **0** **Central Nervous System and Cranial Nerves**
eration **C** **Extirpation:** Taking or cutting out solid matter from a body part

Body Part (4th)	Approach (5th)	Device (6th)	Qualifier (7th)
0 Brain 1 Cerebral Meninges 2 Dura Mater 3 Epidural Space, Intracranial 4 Subdural Space, Intracranial 5 Subarachnoid Space, Intracranial 6 Cerebral Ventricle 7 Cerebral Hemisphere 8 Basal Ganglia 9 Thalamus A Hypothalamus B Pons C Cerebellum D Medulla Oblongata F Olfactory Nerve G Optic Nerve H Oculomotor Nerve J Trochlear Nerve K Trigeminal Nerve L Abducens Nerve M Facial Nerve N Acoustic Nerve P Glossopharyngeal Nerve Q Vagus Nerve R Accessory Nerve S Hypoglossal Nerve T Spinal Meninges U Spinal Canal W Cervical Spinal Cord X Thoracic Spinal Cord Y Lumbar Spinal Cord	**0** Open **3** Percutaneous **4** Percutaneous Endoscopic	**Z** No Device	**Z** No Qualifier

ction **0** **Medical and Surgical**
dy System **0** **Central Nervous System and Cranial Nerves**
peration **D** **Extraction:** Pulling or stripping out or off all or a portion of a body part by the use of force

Body Part (4th)	Approach (5th)	Device (6th)	Qualifier (7th)
1 Cerebral Meninges 2 Dura Mater F Olfactory Nerve G Optic Nerve H Oculomotor Nerve J Trochlear Nerve K Trigeminal Nerve L Abducens Nerve M Facial Nerve N Acoustic Nerve P Glossopharyngeal Nerve Q Vagus Nerve R Accessory Nerve S Hypoglossal Nerve T Spinal Meninges	**0** Open **3** Percutaneous **4** Percutaneous Endoscopic	**Z** No Device	**Z** No Qualifier

Section 0 **Medical and Surgical**
Body System 0 **Central Nervous System and Cranial Nerves**
Operation F **Fragmentation:** Breaking solid matter in a body part into pieces

Body Part (4th)	Approach (5th)	Device (6th)	Qualifier (7th)
3 Epidural Space, Intracranial **4** Subdural Space, Intracranial **5** Subarachnoid Space, Intracranial **6** Cerebral Ventricle **U** Spinal Canal	**0** Open **3** Percutaneous **4** Percutaneous Endoscopic **X** External	**Z** No Device	**Z** No Qualifier

Section 0 **Medical and Surgical**
Body System 0 **Central Nervous System and Cranial Nerves**
Operation H **Insertion:** Putting in a nonbiological appliance that monitors, assists, performs, or prevents a physiological function but does not physically take the place of a body part

Body Part (4th)	Approach (5th)	Device (6th)	Qualifier (7th)
0 Brain	**0** Open	**2** Monitoring Device **3** Infusion Device **4** Radioactive Element, Cesium-131 Collagen Implant **M** Neurostimulator Lead **Y** Other Device	**Z** No Qualifier
0 Brain	**3** Percutaneous **4** Percutaneous Endoscopic	**2** Monitoring Device **3** Infusion Device **M** Neurostimulator Lead **Y** Other Device	**Z** No Qualifier
6 Cerebral Ventricle **E** Cranial Nerve **U** Spinal Canal **V** Spinal Cord	**0** Open **3** Percutaneous **4** Percutaneous Endoscopic	**2** Monitoring Device **3** Infusion Device **M** Neurostimulator Lead **Y** Other Device	**Z** No Qualifier

Section 0 **Medical and Surgical**
Body System 0 **Central Nervous System and Cranial Nerves**
Operation J **Inspection:** Visually and/or manually exploring a body part

Body Part (4th)	Approach (5th)	Device (6th)	Qualifier (7th)
0 Brain **E** Cranial Nerve **U** Spinal Canal **V** Spinal Cord	**0** Open **3** Percutaneous **4** Percutaneous Endoscopic	**Z** No Device	**Z** No Qualifier

Section 0 **Medical and Surgical**
Body System 0 **Central Nervous System and Cranial Nerves**
Operation K **Map:** Locating the route of passage of electrical impulses and/or locating functional areas in a body part

Body Part (4th)	Approach (5th)	Device (6th)	Qualifier (7th)
0 Brain **7** Cerebral Hemisphere **8** Basal Ganglia **9** Thalamus **A** Hypothalamus **B** Pons **C** Cerebellum **D** Medulla Oblongata	**0** Open **3** Percutaneous **4** Percutaneous Endoscopic	**Z** No Device	**Z** No Qualifier

tion **0** **Medical and Surgical**
dy System **0** **Central Nervous System and Cranial Nerves**
eration **N** **Release:** Freeing a body part from an abnormal physical constraint by cutting or by the use of force

Body Part (4th)	Approach (5th)	Device (6th)	Qualifier (7th)
Brain Cerebral Meninges Dura Mater Cerebral Ventricle Cerebral Hemisphere Basal Ganglia Thalamus Hypothalamus Pons Cerebellum Medulla Oblongata Olfactory Nerve Optic Nerve Oculomotor Nerve Trochlear Nerve Trigeminal Nerve Abducens Nerve Facial Nerve Acoustic Nerve Glossopharyngeal Nerve Vagus Nerve Accessory Nerve Hypoglossal Nerve Spinal Meninges Cervical Spinal Cord Thoracic Spinal Cord Lumbar Spinal Cord	**0** Open **3** Percutaneous **4** Percutaneous Endoscopic	**Z** No Device	**Z** No Qualifier

ction **0** **Medical and Surgical**
dy System **0** **Central Nervous System and Cranial Nerves**
eration **P** **Removal:** Taking out or off a device from a body part

Body Part (4th)	Approach (5th)	Device (6th)	Qualifier (7th)
Brain Spinal Cord	**0** Open **3** Percutaneous **4** Percutaneous Endoscopic	**0** Drainage Device **2** Monitoring Device **3** Infusion Device **7** Autologous Tissue Substitute **J** Synthetic Substitute **K** Nonautologous Tissue Substitute **M** Neurostimulator Lead **Y** Other Device	**Z** No Qualifier
Brain Spinal Cord	**X** External	**0** Drainage Device **2** Monitoring Device **3** Infusion Device **M** Neurostimulator Lead	**Z** No Qualifier
Cerebral Ventricle Spinal Canal	**0** Open **3** Percutaneous **4** Percutaneous Endoscopic	**0** Drainage Device **2** Monitoring Device **3** Infusion Device **J** Synthetic Substitute **M** Neurostimulator Lead **Y** Other Device	**Z** No Qualifier
Cerebral Ventricle Spinal Canal	**X** External	**0** Drainage Device **2** Monitoring Device **3** Infusion Device **M** Neurostimulator Lead	**Z** No Qualifier

Continued →

00P Continu

Section 0 **Medical and Surgical**
Body System 0 **Central Nervous System and Cranial Nerves**
Operation P **Removal:** Taking out or off a device from a body part

Body Part (4th)	Approach (5th)	Device (6th)	Qualifier (7th)
E Cranial Nerve	**0** Open **3** Percutaneous **4** Percutaneous Endoscopic	**0** Drainage Device **2** Monitoring Device **3** Infusion Device **7** Autologous Tissue Substitute **M** Neurostimulator Lead **Y** Other Device	**Z** No Qualifier
E Cranial Nerve	**X** External	**0** Drainage Device **2** Monitoring Device **3** Infusion Device **M** Neurostimulator Lead	**Z** No Qualifier

Section 0 **Medical and Surgical**
Body System 0 **Central Nervous System and Cranial Nerves**
Operation Q **Repair:** Restoring, to the extent possible, a body part to its normal anatomic structure and function

Body Part (4th)	Approach (5th)	Device (6th)	Qualifier (7th)
0 Brain **1** Cerebral Meninges **2** Dura Mater **6** Cerebral Ventricle **7** Cerebral Hemisphere **8** Basal Ganglia **9** Thalamus **A** Hypothalamus **B** Pons **C** Cerebellum **D** Medulla Oblongata **F** Olfactory Nerve **G** Optic Nerve **H** Oculomotor Nerve **J** Trochlear Nerve **K** Trigeminal Nerve **L** Abducens Nerve **M** Facial Nerve **N** Acoustic Nerve **P** Glossopharyngeal Nerve **Q** Vagus Nerve **R** Accessory Nerve **S** Hypoglossal Nerve **T** Spinal Meninges **W** Cervical Spinal Cord **X** Thoracic Spinal Cord **Y** Lumbar Spinal Cord	**0** Open **3** Percutaneous **4** Percutaneous Endoscopic	**Z** No Device	**Z** No Qualifier

tion	**0**	**Medical and Surgical**
dy System	**0**	**Central Nervous System and Cranial Nerves**
eration	**R**	**Replacement:** Putting in or on biological or synthetic material that physically takes the place and/or function of all or a portion of a body part

Body Part (4th)	Approach (5th)	Device (6th)	Qualifier (7th)
Cerebral Meninges Dura Mater Cerebral Ventricle Olfactory Nerve Optic Nerve Oculomotor Nerve Trochlear Nerve Trigeminal Nerve Abducens Nerve Facial Nerve Acoustic Nerve Glossopharyngeal Nerve Vagus Nerve Accessory Nerve Hypoglossal Nerve Spinal Meninges	**0** Open **4** Percutaneous Endoscopic	**7** Autologous Tissue Substitute **J** Synthetic Substitute **K** Nonautologous Tissue Substitute	**Z** No Qualifier

ction	**0**	**Medical and Surgical**
dy System	**0**	**Central Nervous System and Cranial Nerves**
eration	**S**	**Reposition:** Moving to its normal location, or other suitable location, all or a portion of a body part

Body Part (4th)	Approach (5th)	Device (6th)	Qualifier (7th)
Olfactory Nerve Optic Nerve Oculomotor Nerve Trochlear Nerve Trigeminal Nerve Abducens Nerve Facial Nerve Acoustic Nerve Glossopharyngeal Nerve Vagus Nerve Accessory Nerve Hypoglossal Nerve Cervical Spinal Cord Thoracic Spinal Cord Lumbar Spinal Cord	**0** Open **3** Percutaneous **4** Percutaneous Endoscopic	**Z** No Device	**Z** No Qualifier

ction	**0**	**Medical and Surgical**
dy System	**0**	**Central Nervous System and Cranial Nerves**
eration	**T**	**Resection:** Cutting out or off, without replacement, all of a body part

Body Part (4th)	Approach (5th)	Device (6th)	Qualifier (7th)
Cerebral Hemisphere	**0** Open **3** Percutaneous **4** Percutaneous Endoscopic	**Z** No Device	**Z** No Qualifier

Section 0 **Medical and Surgical**
Body System 0 **Central Nervous System and Cranial Nerves**
Operation U **Supplement:** Putting in or on biological or synthetic material that physically reinforces and/or augments the function of a portion of a body part

Body Part (4th)	Approach (5th)	Device (6th)	Qualifier (7th)
1 Cerebral Meninges **2** Dura Mater **6** Cerebral Ventricle **F** Olfactory Nerve **G** Optic Nerve **H** Oculomotor Nerve **J** Trochlear Nerve **K** Trigeminal Nerve **L** Abducens Nerve **M** Facial Nerve **N** Acoustic Nerve **P** Glossopharyngeal Nerve **Q** Vagus Nerve **R** Accessory Nerve **S** Hypoglossal Nerve **T** Spinal Meninges	**0** Open **3** Percutaneous **4** Percutaneous Endoscopic	**7** Autologous Tissue Substitute **J** Synthetic Substitute **K** Nonautologous Tissue Substitute	**Z** No Qualifier

Section 0 **Medical and Surgical**
Body System 0 **Central Nervous System and Cranial Nerves**
Operation W **Revision:** Correcting, to the extent possible, a portion of a malfunctioning device or the position of a displaced device

Body Part (4th)	Approach (5th)	Device (6th)	Qualifier (7th)
0 Brain **V** Spinal Cord	**0** Open **3** Percutaneous **4** Percutaneous Endoscopic	**0** Drainage Device **2** Monitoring Device **3** Infusion Device **7** Autologous Tissue Substitute **J** Synthetic Substitute **K** Nonautologous Tissue Substitute **M** Neurostimulator Lead **Y** Other Device	**Z** No Qualifier
0 Brain **V** Spinal Cord	**X** External	**0** Drainage Device **2** Monitoring Device **3** Infusion Device **7** Autologous Tissue Substitute **J** Synthetic Substitute **K** Nonautologous Tissue Substitute **M** Neurostimulator Lead	**Z** No Qualifier
6 Cerebral Ventricle **U** Spinal Canal	**0** Open **3** Percutaneous **4** Percutaneous Endoscopic	**0** Drainage Device **2** Monitoring Device **3** Infusion Device **J** Synthetic Substitute **M** Neurostimulator Lead **Y** Other Device	**Z** No Qualifier
6 Cerebral Ventricle **U** Spinal Canal	**X** External	**0** Drainage Device **2** Monitoring Device **3** Infusion Device **J** Synthetic Substitute **M** Neurostimulator Lead	**Z** No Qualifier

Continued →

ction 0 **Medical and Surgical**
dy System 0 **Central Nervous System and Cranial Nerves**
peration W **Revision:** Correcting, to the extent possible, a portion of a malfunctioning device or the position of a displaced device

Body Part (4th)	Approach (5th)	Device (6th)	Qualifier (7th)
E Cranial Nerve	0 Open 3 Percutaneous 4 Percutaneous Endoscopic	0 Drainage Device 2 Monitoring Device 3 Infusion Device 7 Autologous Tissue Substitute M Neurostimulator Lead Y Other Device	Z No Qualifier
E Cranial Nerve	X External	0 Drainage Device 2 Monitoring Device 3 Infusion Device 7 Autologous Tissue Substitute M Neurostimulator Lead	Z No Qualifier

ction 0 **Medical and Surgical**
dy System 0 **Central Nervous System and Cranial Nerves**
peration X **Transfer:** Moving, without taking out, all or a portion of a body part to another location to take over the function of all or a portion of a body part

Body Part (4th)	Approach (5th)	Device (6th)	Qualifier (7th)
F Olfactory Nerve G Optic Nerve H Oculomotor Nerve J Trochlear Nerve K Trigeminal Nerve L Abducens Nerve M Facial Nerve N Acoustic Nerve P Glossopharyngeal Nerve Q Vagus Nerve R Accessory Nerve S Hypoglossal Nerve	0 Open 4 Percutaneous Endoscopic	Z No Device	F Olfactory Nerve G Optic Nerve H Oculomotor Nerve J Trochlear Nerve K Trigeminal Nerve L Abducens Nerve M Facial Nerve N Acoustic Nerve P Glossopharyngeal Nerve Q Vagus Nerve R Accessory Nerve S Hypoglossal Nerve

HA Coding Clinic

0163J6 Bypass Cerebral Ventricle to Peritoneal Cavity with Synthetic Substitute, Percutaneous Approach—AHA CC: 2Q, 2013, 36–37
0764AA Dilation of Cerebral Ventricle, Percutaneous Endoscopic Approach—AHA CC: 4Q, 2017, 40-41
09430Z Drainage of Intracranial Subdural Space with Drainage Device, Percutaneous Approach—AHA CC: 3Q, 2015, 11–12
09630Z Drainage of Cerebral Ventricle with Drainage Device, Percutaneous Approach—AHA CC: 3Q, 2015, 12–13
09U3ZX Drainage of Spinal Canal, Percutaneous Approach, Diagnostic—AHA CC: 1Q, 2014, 8
09W00Z Drainage of Cervical Spinal Cord with Drainage Device, Open Approach—AHA CC: 2Q, 2015, 30
0B00ZX Excision of Brain, Open Approach, Diagnostic—AHA CC: 1Q, 2015, 12–13
0B70ZZ Excision of Cerebral Hemisphere, Open Approach—AHA CC: 4Q, 2014, 34–35; 2Q, 2016, 18
0BM0ZZ Excision of Facial Nerve, Open Approach—AHA CC: 2Q, 2016, 12–14
0BR0ZZ Excision of Accessory Nerve, Open Approach—AHA CC: 2Q, 2016, 12–14
0BS0ZZ Excision of Hypoglossal Nerve, Open Approach—AHA CC: 2Q, 2016, 12–14
0BY0ZZ Excision of Lumbar Spinal Cord, Open Approach—AHA CC: 3Q, 2014, 24
0C00ZZ Extirpation of Matter from Brain, Open Approach—AHA CC: 1Q, 2015, 12–13; 4Q, 2016, 27–28
0C40ZZ Extirpation of Matter from Intracranial Subdural Space, Open Approach—AHA CC: 3Q, 2015, 10–11; 2Q, 2016, 29
0C74ZZ Extirpation of Matter from Cerebral Hemisphere, Percutaneous Endoscopic Approach—AHA CC: 3Q, 2015, 13
0CU0ZZ Extirpation of Matter from Spinal Canal, Open Approach—AHA CC: 4Q, 2017, 48
0D20ZZ Extraction of Dura Mater, Open Approach—AHA CC: 3Q, 2015, 13–14
0HU33Z Insertion of Infusion Device into Spinal Canal, Percutaneous Approach—AHA CC: 3Q, 2014, 19-20
0JU3ZZ Inspection of Spinal Canal, Percutaneous Approach—AHA CC: 1Q, 2017, 50

00N00ZZ Release Brain, Open Approach—AHA CC: 2Q, 2016, 29

00NC0ZZ Release Cerebellum, Open Approach—AHA CC: 3Q, 2017, 10-11

00NW0ZZ Release Cervical Spinal Cord, Open Approach—AHA CC: 2Q, 2015, 20–22; 2Q, 2017, 23–24

00NY0ZZ Release Lumbar Spinal Cord, Open Approach—AHA CC: 3Q, 2014, 24

00PU03Z Removal of Infusion Device from Spinal Canal, Open Approach—AHA CC: 3Q, 2014, 19–20

00Q20ZZ Repair Dura Mater, Open Approach—AHA CC: 3Q, 2013, 25; 3Q, 2014, 7–8

00SM0ZZ Reposition Facial Nerve, Open Approach—AHA CC: 4Q, 2014, 35

00U20KZ Supplement Dura Mater with Nonautologous Tissue Substitute, Open Approach—AHA CC: 3Q, 2017, 10-11; 1Q, 2018, 9

00UT0KZ Supplement Spinal Meninges with Nonautologous Tissue Substitute, Open Approach—AHA CC: 3Q, 2014, 24

Peripheral Nervous System

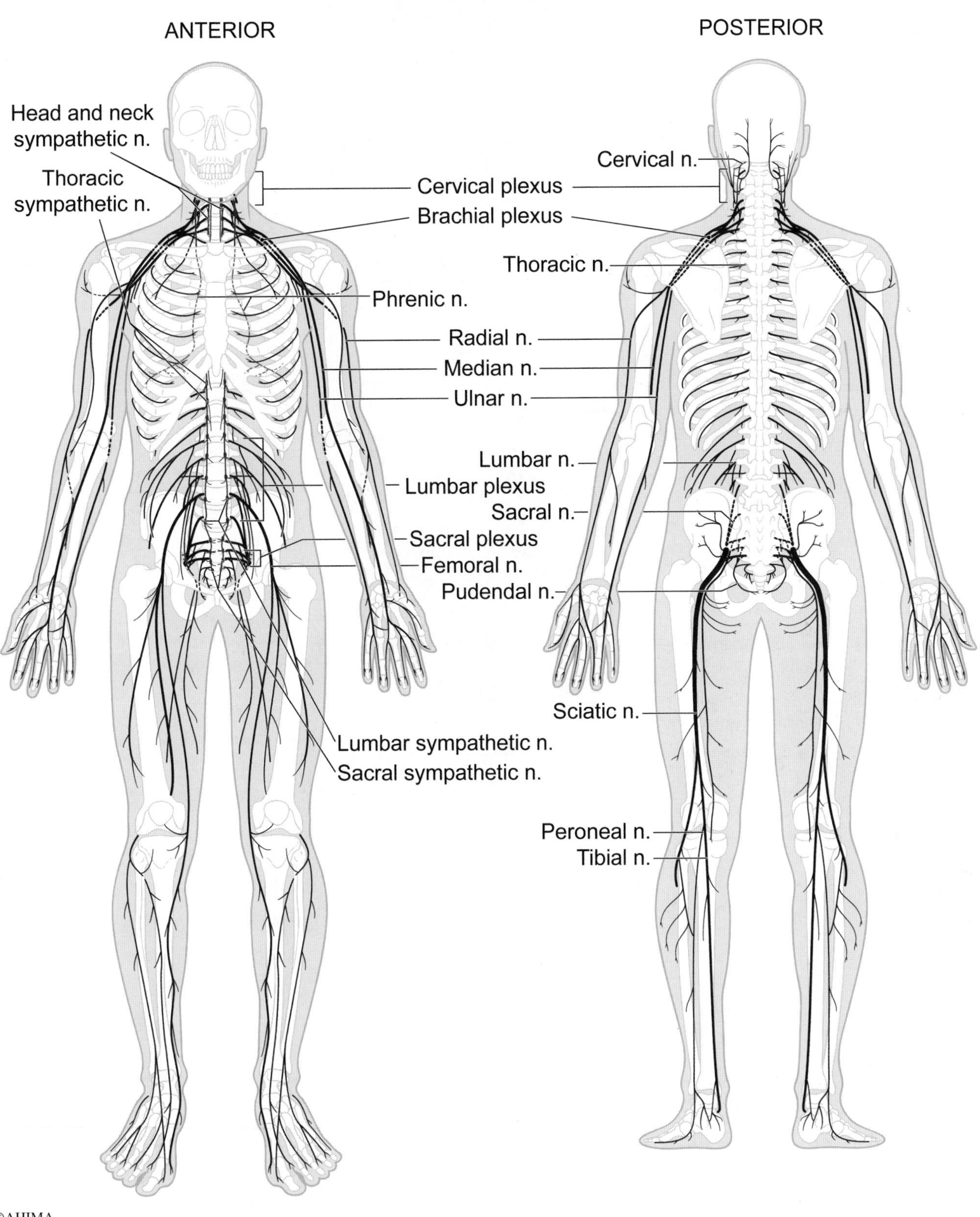

Spinal Column

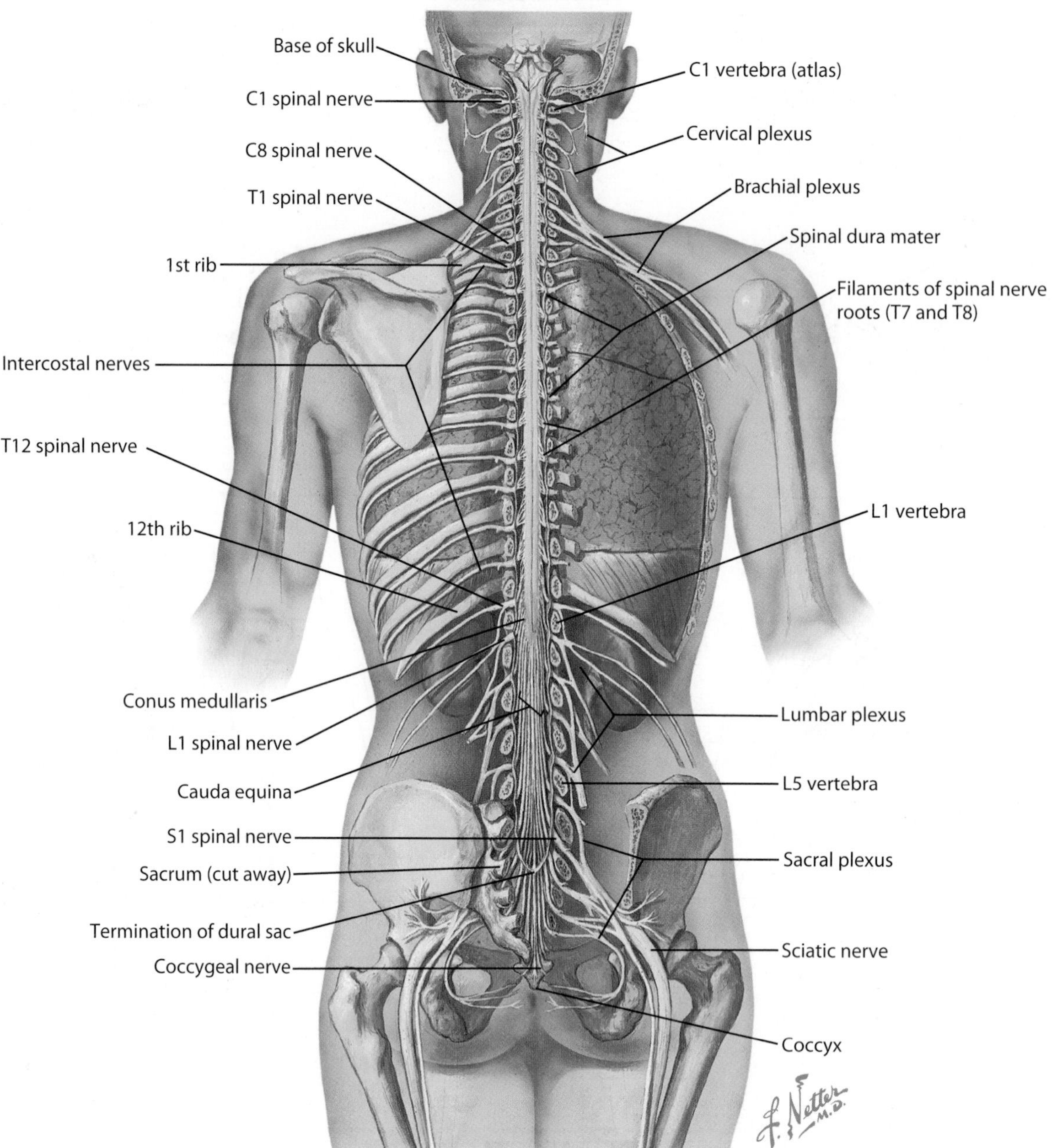

ripheral Nervous System Tables 012–01X

tion 0 **Medical and Surgical**
dy System 1 **Peripheral Nervous System**
eration 2 **Change:** Taking out or off a device from a body part and putting back an identical or similar device in or on the same body part without cutting or puncturing the skin or a mucous membrane

Body Part (4th)	Approach (5th)	Device (6th)	Qualifier (7th)
Peripheral Nerve	**X** External	**0** Drainage Device **Y** Other Device	**Z** No Qualifier

tion 0 **Medical and Surgical**
dy System 1 **Peripheral Nervous System**
eration 5 **Destruction:** Physical eradication of all or a portion of a body part by the direct use of energy, force, or a destructive agent

Body Part (4th)	Approach (5th)	Device (6th)	Qualifier (7th)
Cervical Plexus Cervical Nerve Phrenic Nerve Brachial Plexus Ulnar Nerve Median Nerve Radial Nerve Thoracic Nerve Lumbar Plexus Lumbosacral Plexus Lumbar Nerve Pudendal Nerve Femoral Nerve Sciatic Nerve Tibial Nerve Peroneal Nerve Head and Neck Sympathetic Nerve Thoracic Sympathetic Nerve Abdominal Sympathetic Nerve Lumbar Sympathetic Nerve Sacral Sympathetic Nerve Sacral Plexus Sacral Nerve	**0** Open **3** Percutaneous **4** Percutaneous Endoscopic	**Z** No Device	**Z** No Qualifier

Section 0 **Medical and Surgical**
Body System 1 **Peripheral Nervous System**
Operation 8 **Division:** Cutting into a body part, without draining fluids and/or gases from the body part, in order to separate or transe body part

Body Part (4th)	Approach (5th)	Device (6th)	Qualifier (7th)
0 Cervical Plexus **1** Cervical Nerve **2** Phrenic Nerve **3** Brachial Plexus **4** Ulnar Nerve **5** Median Nerve **6** Radial Nerve **8** Thoracic Nerve **9** Lumbar Plexus **A** Lumbosacral Plexus **B** Lumbar Nerve **C** Pudendal Nerve **D** Femoral Nerve **F** Sciatic Nerve **G** Tibial Nerve **H** Peroneal Nerve **K** Head and Neck Sympathetic Nerve **L** Thoracic Sympathetic Nerve **M** Abdominal Sympathetic Nerve **N** Lumbar Sympathetic Nerve **P** Sacral Sympathetic Nerve **Q** Sacral Plexus **R** Sacral Nerve	**0** Open **3** Percutaneous **4** Percutaneous Endoscopic	**Z** No Device	**Z** No Qualifier

Section 0 **Medical and Surgical**
Body System 1 **Peripheral Nervous System**
Operation 9 **Drainage:** Taking or letting out fluids and/or gases from a body part

Body Part (4th)	Approach (5th)	Device (6th)	Qualifier (7th)
0 Cervical Plexus **1** Cervical Nerve **2** Phrenic Nerve **3** Brachial Plexus **4** Ulnar Nerve **5** Median Nerve **6** Radial Nerve **8** Thoracic Nerve **9** Lumbar Plexus **A** Lumbosacral Plexus **B** Lumbar Nerve **C** Pudendal Nerve **D** Femoral Nerve **F** Sciatic Nerve **G** Tibial Nerve **H** Peroneal Nerve **K** Head and Neck Sympathetic Nerve **L** Thoracic Sympathetic Nerve **M** Abdominal Sympathetic Nerve **N** Lumbar Sympathetic Nerve **P** Sacral Sympathetic Nerve **Q** Sacral Plexus **R** Sacral Nerve	**0** Open **3** Percutaneous **4** Percutaneous Endoscopic	**0** Drainage Device	**Z** No Qualifier

Continued →

019 Continued

ction	**0**	**Medical and Surgical**
dy System	**1**	**Peripheral Nervous System**
eration	**9**	**Drainage:** Taking or letting out fluids and/or gases from a body part

Body Part (4th)	Approach (5th)	Device (6th)	Qualifier (7th)
0 Cervical Plexus **1** Cervical Nerve **2** Phrenic Nerve **3** Brachial Plexus **4** Ulnar Nerve **5** Median Nerve **6** Radial Nerve **8** Thoracic Nerve **9** Lumbar Plexus **A** Lumbosacral Plexus **B** Lumbar Nerve **C** Pudendal Nerve **D** Femoral Nerve **F** Sciatic Nerve **G** Tibial Nerve **H** Peroneal Nerve **K** Head and Neck Sympathetic Nerve **L** Thoracic Sympathetic Nerve **M** Abdominal Sympathetic Nerve **N** Lumbar Sympathetic Nerve **P** Sacral Sympathetic Nerve **Q** Sacral Plexus **R** Sacral Nerve	**0** Open **3** Percutaneous **4** Percutaneous Endoscopic	**Z** No Device	**X** Diagnostic **Z** No Qualifier

ction	**0**	**Medical and Surgical**
ody System	**1**	**Peripheral Nervous System**
peration	**B**	**Excision:** Cutting out or off, without replacement, a portion of a body part

Body Part (4th)	Approach (5th)	Device (6th)	Qualifier (7th)
0 Cervical Plexus **1** Cervical Nerve **2** Phrenic Nerve **3** Brachial Plexus **4** Ulnar Nerve **5** Median Nerve **6** Radial Nerve **8** Thoracic Nerve **9** Lumbar Plexus **A** Lumbosacral Plexus **B** Lumbar Nerve **C** Pudendal Nerve **D** Femoral Nerve **F** Sciatic Nerve **G** Tibial Nerve **H** Peroneal Nerve **K** Head and Neck Sympathetic Nerve **L** Thoracic Sympathetic Nerve **M** Abdominal Sympathetic Nerve **N** Lumbar Sympathetic Nerve **P** Sacral Sympathetic Nerve **Q** Sacral Plexus **R** Sacral Nerve	**0** Open **3** Percutaneous **4** Percutaneous Endoscopic	**Z** No Device	**X** Diagnostic **Z** No Qualifier

Section 0 **Medical and Surgical**
Body System 1 **Peripheral Nervous System**
Operation C **Extirpation:** Taking or cutting out solid matter from a body part

Body Part (4th)	Approach (5th)	Device (6th)	Qualifier (7th)
0 Cervical Plexus **1** Cervical Nerve **2** Phrenic Nerve **3** Brachial Plexus **4** Ulnar Nerve **5** Median Nerve **6** Radial Nerve **8** Thoracic Nerve **9** Lumbar Plexus **A** Lumbosacral Plexus **B** Lumbar Nerve **C** Pudendal Nerve **D** Femoral Nerve **F** Sciatic Nerve **G** Tibial Nerve **H** Peroneal Nerve **K** Head and Neck Sympathetic Nerve **L** Thoracic Sympathetic Nerve **M** Abdominal Sympathetic Nerve **N** Lumbar Sympathetic Nerve **P** Sacral Sympathetic Nerve **Q** Sacral Plexus **R** Sacral Nerve	**0** Open **3** Percutaneous **4** Percutaneous Endoscopic	**Z** No Device	**Z** No Qualifier

Section 0 **Medical and Surgical**
Body System 1 **Peripheral Nervous System**
Operation D **Extraction:** Pulling or stripping out or off all or a portion of a body part by the use of force

Body Part (4th)	Approach (5th)	Device (6th)	Qualifier (7th)
0 Cervical Plexus **1** Cervical Nerve **2** Phrenic Nerve **3** Brachial Plexus **4** Ulnar Nerve **5** Median Nerve **6** Radial Nerve **8** Thoracic Nerve **9** Lumbar Plexus **A** Lumbosacral Plexus **B** Lumbar Nerve **C** Pudendal Nerve **D** Femoral Nerve **F** Sciatic Nerve **G** Tibial Nerve **H** Peroneal Nerve **K** Head and Neck Sympathetic Nerve **L** Thoracic Sympathetic Nerve **M** Abdominal Sympathetic Nerve **N** Lumbar Sympathetic Nerve **P** Sacral Sympathetic Nerve **Q** Sacral Plexus **R** Sacral Nerve	**0** Open **3** Percutaneous **4** Percutaneous Endoscopic	**Z** No Device	**Z** No Qualifier

tion	0	**Medical and Surgical**
ly System	1	**Peripheral Nervous System**
eration	H	**Insertion:** Putting in a nonbiological appliance that monitors, assists, performs, or prevents a physiological function but does not physically take the place of a body part

Body Part (4th)	Approach (5th)	Device (6th)	Qualifier (7th)
Peripheral Nerve	**0** Open **3** Percutaneous **4** Percutaneous Endoscopic	**2** Monitoring Device **M** Neurostimulator Lead **Y** Other Device	**Z** No Qualifier

tion	0	**Medical and Surgical**
ly System	1	**Peripheral Nervous System**
eration	J	**Inspection:** Visually and/or manually exploring a body part

Body Part (4th)	Approach (5th)	Device (6th)	Qualifier (7th)
Peripheral Nerve	**0** Open **3** Percutaneous **4** Percutaneous Endoscopic	**Z** No Device	**Z** No Qualifier

tion	0	**Medical and Surgical**
ly System	1	**Peripheral Nervous System**
eration	N	**Release:** Freeing a body part from an abnormal physical constraint by cutting or by the use of force

Body Part (4th)	Approach (5th)	Device (6th)	Qualifier (7th)
Cervical Plexus Cervical Nerve Phrenic Nerve Brachial Plexus Ulnar Nerve Median Nerve Radial Nerve Thoracic Nerve Lumbar Plexus Lumbosacral Plexus Lumbar Nerve Pudendal Nerve Femoral Nerve Sciatic Nerve Tibial Nerve Peroneal Nerve Head and Neck Sympathetic Nerve Thoracic Sympathetic Nerve Abdominal Sympathetic Nerve Lumbar Sympathetic Nerve Sacral Sympathetic Nerve Sacral Plexus Sacral Nerve	**0** Open **3** Percutaneous **4** Percutaneous Endoscopic	**Z** No Device	**Z** No Qualifier

ction	0	**Medical and Surgical**
dy System	1	**Peripheral Nervous System**
eration	P	**Removal:** Taking out or off a device from a body part

Body Part (4th)	Approach (5th)	Device (6th)	Qualifier (7th)
Y Peripheral Nerve	**0** Open **3** Percutaneous **4** Percutaneous Endoscopic	**0** Drainage Device **2** Monitoring Device **7** Autologous Tissue Substitute **M** Neurostimulator Lead **Y** Other Device	**Z** No Qualifier
Y Peripheral Nerve	**X** External	**0** Drainage Device **2** Monitoring Device **M** Neurostimulator Lead	**Z** No Qualifier

Section 0 **Medical and Surgical**
Body System 1 **Peripheral Nervous System**
Operation Q **Repair:** Restoring, to the extent possible, a body part to its normal anatomic structure and function

Body Part (4th)	Approach (5th)	Device (6th)	Qualifier (7th)
0 Cervical Plexus **1** Cervical Nerve **2** Phrenic Nerve **3** Brachial Plexus **4** Ulnar Nerve **5** Median Nerve **6** Radial Nerve **8** Thoracic Nerve **9** Lumbar Plexus **A** Lumbosacral Plexus **B** Lumbar Nerve **C** Pudendal Nerve **D** Femoral Nerve **F** Sciatic Nerve **G** Tibial Nerve **H** Peroneal Nerve **K** Head and Neck Sympathetic Nerve **L** Thoracic Sympathetic Nerve **M** Abdominal Sympathetic Nerve **N** Lumbar Sympathetic Nerve **P** Sacral Sympathetic Nerve **Q** Sacral Plexus **R** Sacral Nerve	**0** Open **3** Percutaneous **4** Percutaneous Endoscopic	**Z** No Device	**Z** No Qualifier

Section 0 **Medical and Surgical**
Body System 1 **Peripheral Nervous System**
Operation R **Replacement:** Putting in or on biological or synthetic material that physically takes the place and/or function of all or a portion of a body part

Body Part (4th)	Approach (5th)	Device (6th)	Qualifier (7th)
1 Cervical Nerve **2** Phrenic Nerve **4** Ulnar Nerve **5** Median Nerve **6** Radial Nerve **8** Thoracic Nerve **B** Lumbar Nerve **C** Pudendal Nerve **D** Femoral Nerve **F** Sciatic Nerve **G** Tibial Nerve **H** Peroneal Nerve **R** Sacral Nerve	**0** Open **4** Percutaneous Endoscopic	**7** Autologous Tissue Substitute **J** Synthetic Substitute **K** Nonautologous Tissue Substitute	**Z** No Qualifier

ction **0** **Medical and Surgical**
dy System **1** **Peripheral Nervous System**
eration **S** **Reposition:** Moving to its normal location, or other suitable location, all or a portion of a body part

Body Part (4th)	Approach (5th)	Device (6th)	Qualifier (7th)
0 Cervical Plexus 1 Cervical Nerve 2 Phrenic Nerve 3 Brachial Plexus 4 Ulnar Nerve 5 Median Nerve 6 Radial Nerve 8 Thoracic Nerve 9 Lumbar Plexus A Lumbosacral Plexus B Lumbar Nerve C Pudendal Nerve D Femoral Nerve F Sciatic Nerve G Tibial Nerve H Peroneal Nerve Q Sacral Plexus R Sacral Nerve	**0** Open **3** Percutaneous **4** Percutaneous Endoscopic	**Z** No Device	**Z** No Qualifier

ction **0** **Medical and Surgical**
dy System **1** **Peripheral Nervous System**
eration **U** **Supplement:** Putting in or on biological or synthetic material that physically reinforces and/or augments the function of a portion of a body part

Body Part (4th)	Approach (5th)	Device (6th)	Qualifier (7th)
1 Cervical Nerve 2 Phrenic Nerve 4 Ulnar Nerve 5 Median Nerve 6 Radial Nerve 8 Thoracic Nerve B Lumbar Nerve C Pudendal Nerve D Femoral Nerve F Sciatic Nerve G Tibial Nerve H Peroneal Nerve R Sacral Nerve	**0** Open **3** Percutaneous **4** Percutaneous Endoscopic	**7** Autologous Tissue Substitute **J** Synthetic Substitute **K** Nonautologous Tissue Substitute	**Z** No Qualifier

ction **0** **Medical and Surgical**
dy System **1** **Peripheral Nervous System**
eration **W** **Revision:** Correcting, to the extent possible, a portion of a malfunctioning device or the position of a displaced device

Body Part (4th)	Approach (5th)	Device (6th)	Qualifier (7th)
Y Peripheral Nerve	**0** Open **3** Percutaneous **4** Percutaneous Endoscopic	**0** Drainage Device **2** Monitoring Device **7** Autologous Tissue Substitute **M** Neurostimulator Lead **Y** Other Device	**Z** No Qualifier
Y Peripheral Nerve	**X** External	**0** Drainage Device **2** Monitoring Device **7** Autologous Tissue Substitute **M** Neurostimulator Lead	**Z** No Qualifier

Section **0** **Medical and Surgical**
Body System **1** **Peripheral Nervous System**
Operation **X** **Transfer:** Moving, without taking out, all or a portion of a body part to another location to take over the function of all c portion of a body part

Body Part (4th)	Approach (5th)	Device (6th)	Qualifier (7th)
1 Cervical Nerve **2** Phrenic Nerve	**0** Open **4** Percutaneous Endoscopic	**Z** No Device	**1** Cervical Nerve **2** Phrenic Nerve
4 Ulnar Nerve **5** Median Nerve **6** Radial Nerve	**0** Open **4** Percutaneous Endoscopic	**Z** No Device	**4** Ulnar Nerve **5** Median Nerve **6** Radial Nerve
8 Thoracic Nerve	**0** Open **4** Percutaneous Endoscopic	**Z** No Device	**8** Thoracic Nerve
B Lumbar Nerve **C** Pudendal Nerve	**0** Open **4** Percutaneous Endoscopic	**Z** No Device	**B** Lumbar Nerve **C** Perineal Nerve
D Femoral Nerve **F** Sciatic Nerve **G** Tibial Nerve **H** Peroneal Nerve	**0** Open **4** Percutaneous Endoscopic	**Z** No Device	**D** Femoral Nerve **F** Sciatic Nerve **G** Tibial Nerve **H** Peroneal Nerve

AHA Coding Clinic

01BL0ZZ Excision of Thoracic Sympathetic Nerve, Open Approach—AHA CC: 2Q, 2017, 19-20
01N10ZZ Release Cervical Nerve, Open Approach—AHA CC: 2Q, 2016, 17
01N30ZZ Release Brachial Plexus, Open Approach—AHA CC: 2Q, 2016, 23
01N50ZZ Release Median Nerve, Open Approach—AHA CC: 3Q, 2014, 33-34
01NB0ZZ Release Lumbar Nerve, Open Approach—AHA CC: 2Q, 2015, 34; 2Q, 2016, 16; 2Q, 2018, 22-23
01U50KZ Supplement Median Nerve with Nonautologous Tissue Substitute, Open Approach—AHA CC: 4Q, 2017, 62

Heart

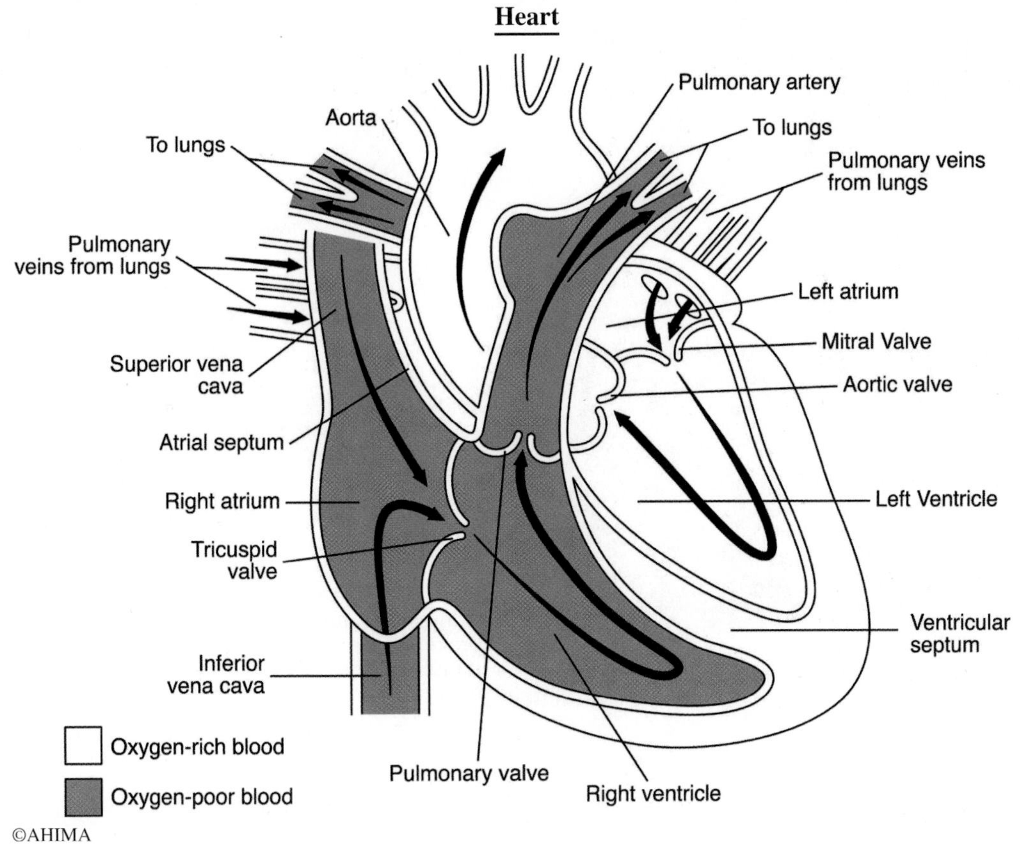

Great Vessels of Heart

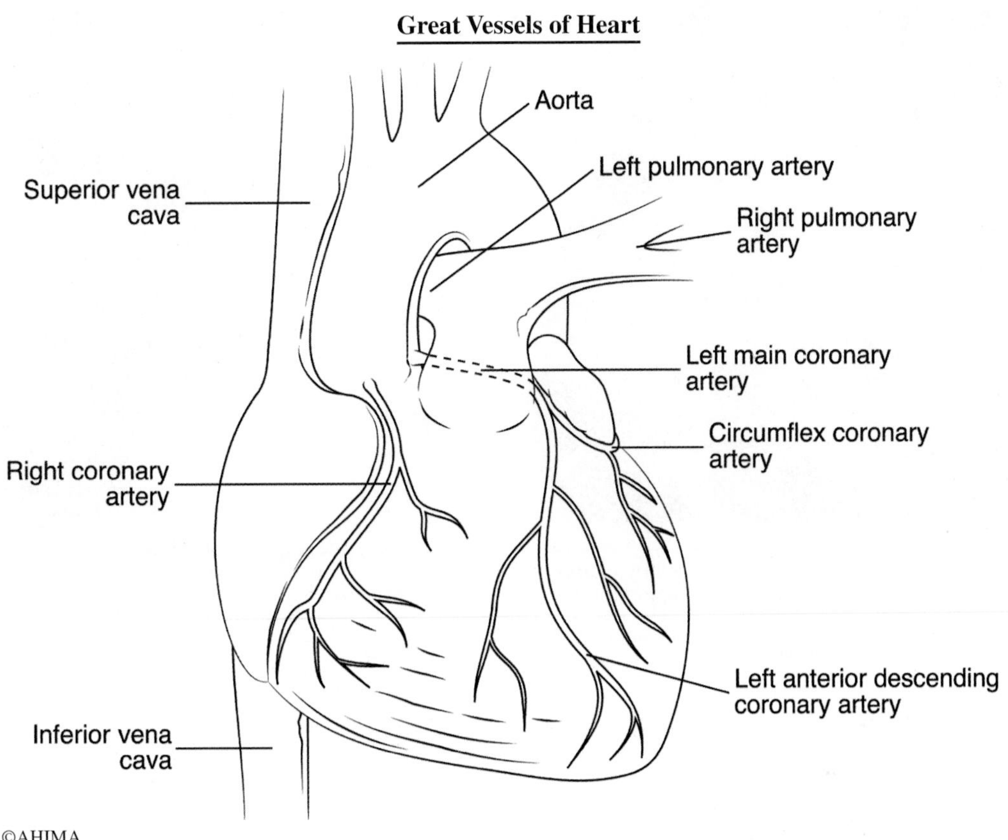

Right coronary-artery segmental replacement

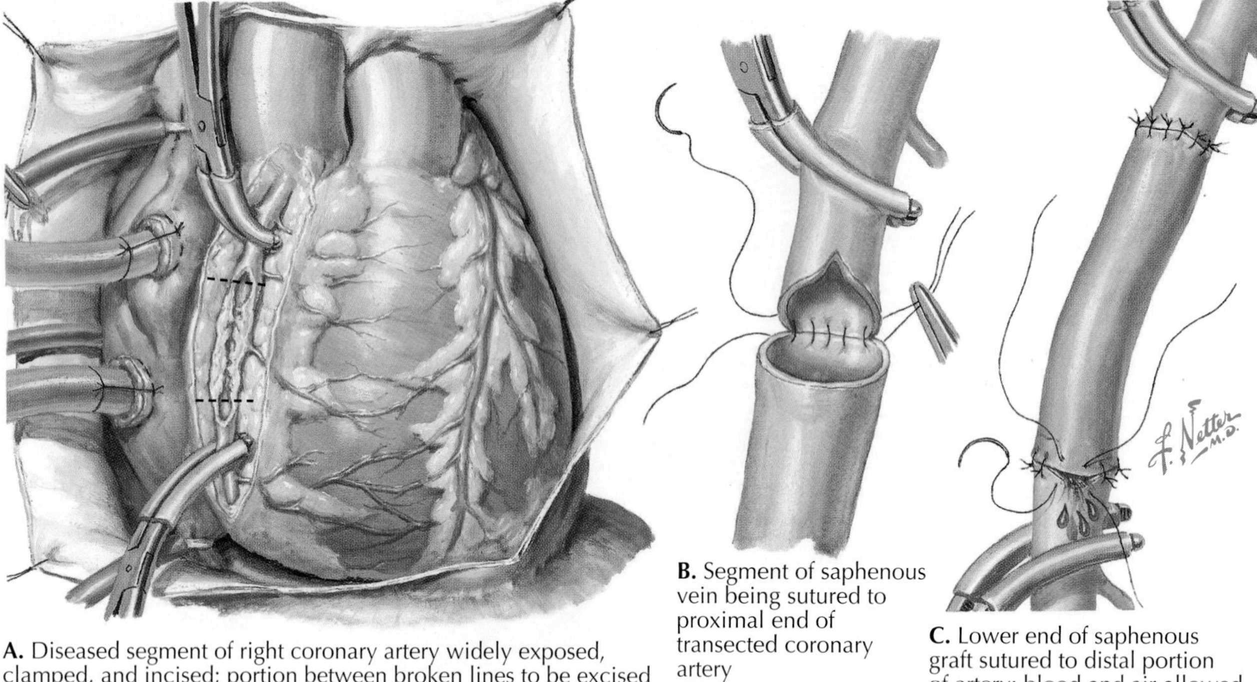

A. Diseased segment of right coronary artery widely exposed, clamped, and incised; portion between broken lines to be excised

B. Segment of saphenous vein being sutured to proximal end of transected coronary artery

C. Lower end of saphenous graft sutured to distal portion of artery; blood and air allowed to escape by loosening distal clamp prior to final closure

Right coronary-artery bypass

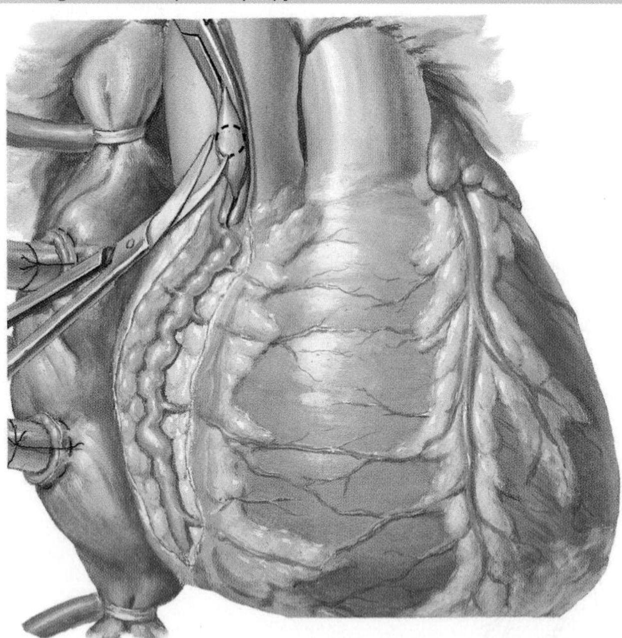

A′. Small area of aorta longitudinally isolated by clamp above right coronary orifice, and ostium created therein

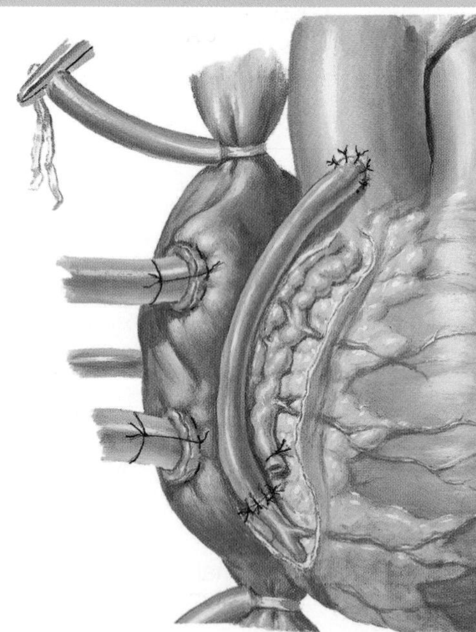

B′. Segment of saphenous vein implanted into new aortic ostium and anastomosed to end of divided right coronary artery distal to diseased area; proximal end of artery ligated

art and Great Vessels Tables 021–02Y

tion 0 **Medical and Surgical**
ly System 2 **Heart and Great Vessels**
eration 1 **Bypass:** Altering the route of passage of the contents of a tubular body part

Body Part (4th)	Approach (5th)	Device (6th)	Qualifier (7th)
Coronary Artery, One Artery Coronary Artery, Two Arteries Coronary Artery, Three Arteries Coronary Artery, Four or More Arteries	**0** Open	**8** Zooplastic Tissue **9** Autologous Venous Tissue **A** Autologous Arterial Tissue **J** Synthetic Substitute **K** Nonautologous Tissue Substitute	**3** Coronary Artery **8** Internal Mammary, Right **9** Internal Mammary, Left **C** Thoracic Artery **F** Abdominal Artery **W** Aorta
Coronary Artery, One Artery Coronary Artery, Two Arteries Coronary Artery, Three Arteries Coronary Artery, Four or More Arteries	**0** Open	**Z** No Device	**3** Coronary Artery **8** Internal Mammary, Right **9** Internal Mammary, Left **C** Thoracic Artery **F** Abdominal Artery
Coronary Artery, One Artery Coronary Artery, Two Arteries Coronary Artery, Three Arteries Coronary Artery, Four or More Arteries	**3** Percutaneous	**4** Intraluminal Device, Drug-eluting **D** Intraluminal Device	**4** Coronary Vein
Coronary Artery, One Artery Coronary Artery, Two Arteries Coronary Artery, Three Arteries Coronary Artery, Four or More Arteries	**4** Percutaneous Endoscopic	**4** Intraluminal Device, Drug-eluting **D** Intraluminal Device	**4** Coronary Vein
Coronary Artery, One Artery Coronary Artery, Two Arteries Coronary Artery, Three Arteries Coronary Artery, Four or More Arteries	**4** Percutaneous Endoscopic	**8** Zooplastic Tissue **9** Autologous Venous Tissue **A** Autologous Arterial Tissue **J** Synthetic Substitute **K** Nonautologous Tissue Substitute	**3** Coronary Artery **8** Internal Mammary, Right **9** Internal Mammary, Left **C** Thoracic Artery **F** Abdominal Artery **W** Aorta
Coronary Artery, One Artery Coronary Artery, Two Arteries Coronary Artery, Three Arteries Coronary Artery, Four or More Arteries	**4** Percutaneous Endoscopic	**Z** No Device	**3** Coronary Artery **8** Internal Mammary, Right **9** Internal Mammary, Left **C** Thoracic Artery **F** Abdominal Artery
Atrium, Right	**0** Open **4** Percutaneous Endoscopic	**8** Zooplastic Tissue **9** Autologous Venous Tissue **A** Autologous Arterial Tissue **J** Synthetic Substitute **K** Nonautologous Tissue Substitute	**P** Pulmonary Trunk **Q** Pulmonary Artery, Right **R** Pulmonary Artery, Left
Atrium, Right	**0** Open **4** Percutaneous Endoscopic	**Z** No Device	**7** Atrium, Left **P** Pulmonary Trunk **Q** Pulmonary Artery, Right **R** Pulmonary Artery, Left
Atrium, Right	**3** Percutaneous	**Z** No Device	**7** Atrium, Left
Atrium, Left Superior Vena Cava	**0** Open **4** Percutaneous Endoscopic	**8** Zooplastic Tissue **9** Autologous Venous Tissue **A** Autologous Arterial Tissue **J** Synthetic Substitute **K** Nonautologous Tissue Substitute **Z** No Device	**P** Pulmonary Trunk **Q** Pulmonary Artery, Right **R** Pulmonary Artery, Left **S** Pulmonary Vein, Right **T** Pulmonary Vein, Left **U** Pulmonary Vein, Confluence
Ventricle, Right Ventricle, Left	**0** Open **4** Percutaneous Endoscopic	**8** Zooplastic Tissue **9** Autologous Venous Tissue **A** Autologous Arterial Tissue **J** Synthetic Substitute **K** Nonautologous Tissue Substitute	**P** Pulmonary Trunk **Q** Pulmonary Artery, Right **R** Pulmonary Artery, Left

Continued →

Section 0 **Medical and Surgical**
Body System 2 **Heart and Great Vessels**
Operation 1 **Bypass:** Altering the route of passage of the contents of a tubular body part

021 Contin

Body Part (4th)	Approach (5th)	Device (6th)	Qualifier (7th)
K Ventricle, Right **L** Ventricle, Left	**0** Open **4** Percutaneous Endoscopic	**Z** No Device	**5** Coronary Circulation **8** Internal Mammary, Right **9** Internal Mammary, Left **C** Thoracic Artery **F** Abdominal Artery **P** Pulmonary Trunk **Q** Pulmonary Artery, Right **R** Pulmonary Artery, Left **W** Aorta
P Pulmonary Trunk **Q** Right Pulmonary Artery **R** Left Pulmonary Artery	**0** Open **4** Percutaneous Endoscopic	**8** Zooplastic Tissue **9** Autologous Venous Tissue **A** Autologous Arterial Tissue **J** Synthetic Substitute **K** Nonautologous Tissue Substitute	**A** Innominate Artery **B** Subclavin **D** Carotid
W Thoracic Aorta, Descending	**0** Open	**8** Zooplastic Tissue **9** Autologous Venous Tissue **A** Autologous Arterial Tissue **J** Synthetic Substitute **K** Nonautologous Tissue Substitute	**B** Subclavian **D** Carotid **F** Abdominal Artery **G** Axillary Artery **H** Brachial Artery **P** Pulmonary Trunk **Q** Pulmonary Artery, Right **R** Pulmonary Artery, Left **V** Lower Extremity Artery
W Thoracic Aorta, Descending	**0** Open	**Z** No Device	**B** Subclavian **D** Carotid **P** Pulmonary Trunk **Q** Pulmonary Artery, Right **R** Pulmonary Artery, Left
W Thoracic Aorta, Descending	**4** Percutaneous Endoscopic	**8** Zooplastic Tissue **9** Autologous Venous Tissue **A** Autologous Arterial Tissue **J** Synthetic Substitute **K** Nonautologous Tissue Substitute **Z** No Device	**B** Subclavian **D** Carotid **P** Pulmonary Trunk **Q** Pulmonary Artery, Right **R** Pulmonary Artery, Left
X Thoracic Aorta, Ascending/Arch	**0** Open **4** Percutaneous Endoscopic	**8** Zooplastic Tissue **9** Autologous Venous Tissue **A** Autologous Arterial Tissue **J** Synthetic Substitute **K** Nonautologous Tissue Substitute **Z** No Device	**B** Subclavian **D** Carotid **P** Pulmonary Trunk **Q** Pulmonary Artery, Right **R** Pulmonary Artery, Left

Section 0 **Medical and Surgical**
Body System 2 **Heart and Great Vessels**
Operation 4 **Creation:** Putting in or on biological or synthetic material to form a new body part that to the extent possible replicates anatomic structure or function of an absent body part

Body Part (4th)	Approach (5th)	Device (6th)	Qualifier (7th)
F Aortic Valve	**0** Open	**7** Autologous Tissue Substitute **8** Zooplastic Tissue **J** Synthetic Substitute **K** Nonautologous Tissue Substitute	**J** Truncal Valve
G Mitral Valve **J** Tricuspid Valve	**0** Open	**7** Autologous Tissue Substitute **8** Zooplastic Tissue **J** Synthetic Substitute **K** Nonautologous Tissue Substitute	**2** Common Atrioventricular Valve

tion	0	**Medical and Surgical**
dy System	2	**Heart and Great Vessels**
eration	5	**Destruction:** Physical eradication of all or a portion of a body part by the direct use of energy, force, or a destructive agent

Body Part (4th)	Approach (5th)	Device (6th)	Qualifier (7th)
Coronary Vein Atrial Septum Atrium, Right Conduction Mechanism Chordae Tendineae Papillary Muscle Aortic Valve Mitral Valve Pulmonary Valve Tricuspid Valve Ventricle, Right Ventricle, Left Ventricular Septum Pericardium Pulmonary Trunk Pulmonary Artery, Right Pulmonary Artery, Left Pulmonary Vein, Right Pulmonary Vein, Left Superior Vena Cava V Thoracic Aorta, Descending Thoracic Aorta, Ascending/Arch	**0** Open **3** Percutaneous **4** Percutaneous Endoscopic	**Z** No Device	**Z** No Qualifier
Atrium, Left	**0** Open **3** Percutaneous **4** Percutaneous Endoscopic	**Z** No Device	**K** Left Atrial Appendage **Z** No Qualifier

ction	0	**Medical and Surgical**
dy System	2	**Heart and Great Vessels**
eration	7	**Dilation:** Expanding an orifice or the lumen of a tubular body part

Body Part (4th)	Approach (5th)	Device (6th)	Qualifier (7th)
Coronary Artery, One Artery Coronary Artery, Two Arteries Coronary Artery, Three Arteries Coronary Artery, Four or More Arteries	**0** Open **3** Percutaneous **4** Percutaneous Endoscopic	**4** Intraluminal Device, Drug-eluting **5** Intraluminal Device, Drug-eluting, Two **6** Intraluminal Device, Drug-eluting, Three **7** Intraluminal Device, Drug-eluting, Four or More **D** Intraluminal Device **E** Intraluminal Devices, Two **F** Intraluminal Devices, Three **G** Intraluminal Devices, Four or More **T** Intraluminal Device, Radioactive **Z** No Device	**6** Bifurcation **Z** No Qualifier
F Aortic Valve **G** Mitral Valve **H** Pulmonary Valve **J** Tricuspid Valve **K** Ventricle, Right **L** Ventricle, Left **P** Pulmonary Trunk **Q** Pulmonary Artery, Right **S** Pulmonary Vein, Right **T** Pulmonary Vein, Left **V** Superior Vena Cava **W** Thoracic Aorta, Descending **X** Thoracic Aorta, Ascending/Arch	**0** Open **3** Percutaneous **4** Percutaneous Endoscopic	**4** Intraluminal Device, Drug-eluting **D** Intraluminal Device **Z** No Device	**Z** No Qualifier
R Pulmonary Artery, Left	**0** Open **3** Percutaneous **4** Percutaneous Endoscopic	**4** Intraluminal Device, Drug-eluting **D** Intraluminal Device **Z** No Device	**T** Ductus Arteriosus **Z** No Qualifier

Section 0 **Medical and Surgical**
Body System 2 **Heart and Great Vessels**
Operation 8 **Division:** Cutting into a body part, without draining fluids and/or gases from the body part, in order to separate or transe body part

Body Part (4th)	Approach (5th)	Device (6th)	Qualifier (7th)
8 Conduction Mechanism **9** Chordae Tendineae **D** Papillary Muscle	**0** Open **3** Percutaneous **4** Percutaneous Endoscopic	**Z** No Device	**Z** No Qualifier

Section 0 **Medical and Surgical**
Body System 2 **Heart and Great Vessels**
Operation B **Excision:** Cutting out or off, without replacement, a portion of a body part

Body Part (4th)	Approach (5th)	Device (6th)	Qualifier (7th)
4 Coronary Vein **5** Atrial Septum **6** Atrium, Right **8** Conduction Mechanism **9** Chordae Tendineae **D** Papillary Muscle **F** Aortic Valve **G** Mitral Valve **H** Pulmonary Valve **J** Tricuspid Valve **K** Ventricle, Right **L** Ventricle, Left **M** Ventricular Septum **N** Pericardium **P** Pulmonary Trunk **Q** Pulmonary Artery, Right **R** Pulmonary Artery, Left **S** Pulmonary Vein, Right **T** Pulmonary Vein, Left **V** Superior Vena Cava **W** Thoracic Aorta, Descending **X** Thoracic Aorta, Ascending/Arch	**0** Open **3** Percutaneous **4** Percutaneous Endoscopic	**Z** No Device	**X** Diagnostic **Z** No Qualifier
7 Atrium, Left	**0** Open **3** Percutaneous **4** Percutaneous Endoscopic	**Z** No Device	**K** Left Atrial Appendage **X** Diagnostic **Z** No Qualifier

Section 0 **Medical and Surgical**
Body System 2 **Heart and Great Vessels**
Operation C **Extirpation:** Taking or cutting out solid matter from a body part

Body Part (4th)	Approach (5th)	Device (6th)	Qualifier (7th)
0 Coronary Artery, One Artery **1** Coronary Artery, Two Arteries **2** Coronary Artery, Three Arteries **3** Coronary Artery, Four or More Arteries	**0** Open **3** Percutaneous **4** Percutaneous Endoscopic	**Z** No Device	**6** Bifurcation **Z** No Qualifier

Continued →

tion	0	**Medical and Surgical**
ly System	2	**Heart and Great Vessels**
eration	C	**Extirpation:** Taking or cutting out solid matter from a body part

Body Part (4th)	Approach (5th)	Device (6th)	Qualifier (7th)
Coronary Vein Atrial Septum Atrium, Right Atrium, Left Conduction Mechanism Chordae Tendineae Papillary Muscle Aortic Valve Mitral Valve Pulmonary Valve Tricuspid Valve Ventricle, Right Ventricle, Left Ventricular Septum Pericardium Pulmonary Trunk Pulmonary Artery, Right Pulmonary Artery, Left Pulmonary Vein, Right Pulmonary Vein, Left Superior Vena Cava Thoracic Aorta, Descending Thoracic Aorta, Ascending/Arch	**0** Open **3** Percutaneous **4** Percutaneous Endoscopic	**Z** No Device	**Z** No Qualifier

ction	0	**Medical and Surgical**
dy System	2	**Heart and Great Vessels**
eration	F	**Fragmentation:** Breaking solid matter in a body part into pieces

Body Part (4th)	Approach (5th)	Device (6th)	Qualifier (7th)
Pericardium	**0** Open **3** Percutaneous **4** Percutaneous Endoscopic **X** External	**Z** No Device	**Z** No Qualifier

ction	0	**Medical and Surgical**
dy System	2	**Heart and Great Vessels**
eration	H	**Insertion:** Putting in a nonbiological appliance that monitors, assists, performs, or prevents a physiological function but does not physically take the place of a body part

Body Part (4th)	Approach (5th)	Device (6th)	Qualifier (7th)
Coronary Vein Atrium, Right Atrium, Left Ventricle, Right Ventricle, Left	**0** Open **3** Percutaneous **4** Percutaneous Endoscopic	**0** Monitoring Device, Pressure Sensor **2** Monitoring Device **3** Infusion Device **D** Intraluminal Device **J** Cardiac Lead, Pacemaker **K** Cardiac Lead, Defibrillator **M** Cardiac Lead **N** Intracardiac Pacemaker **Y** Other Device	**Z** No Qualifier
Heart	**0** Open **3** Percutaneous **4** Percutaneous Endoscopic	**Q** Implantable Heart Assist System **Y** Other Device	**Z** No Qualifier
Heart	**0** Open **3** Percutaneous **4** Percutaneous Endoscopic	**R** Short-term External Heart Assist System	**J** Intraoperative **S** Biventricular **Z** No Qualifier

Continued →

Section 0 **Medical and Surgical**
Body System 2 **Heart and Great Vessels**
Operation H **Insertion:** Putting in a nonbiological appliance that monitors, assists, performs, or prevents a physiological function but does not physically take the place of a body part

Body Part (4th)	Approach (5th)	Device (6th)	Qualifier (7th)
N Pericardium	**0** Open **3** Percutaneous **4** Percutaneous Endoscopic	**0** Monitoring Device, Pressure Sensor **2** Monitoring Device **J** Cardiac Lead, Pacemaker **K** Cardiac Lead, Defibrillator **M** Cardiac Lead **Y** Other Device	**Z** No Qualifier
P Pulmonary Trunk **Q** Pulmonary Artery, Right **R** Pulmonary Artery, Left **S** Pulmonary Vein, Right **T** Pulmonary Vein, Left **V** Superior Vena Cava **W** Thoracic Aorta, Descending	**0** Open **3** Percutaneous **4** Percutaneous Endoscopic	**0** Monitoring Device, Pressure Sensor **2** Monitoring Device **3** Infusion Device **D** Intraluminal Device **Y** Other Device	**Z** No Qualifier
X Thoracic Aorta, Ascending/ Arch	**0** Open **3** Percutaneous **4** Percutaneous Endoscopic	**0** Monitoring Device, Pressure Sensor **2** Monitoring Device **3** Infusion Device **D** Intraluminal Device	**Z** No Qualifier

Section 0 **Medical and Surgical**
Body System 2 **Heart and Great Vessels**
Operation J **Inspection:** Visually and/or manually exploring a body part

Body Part (4th)	Approach (5th)	Device (6th)	Qualifier (7th)
A Heart **Y** Great Vessel	**0** Open **3** Percutaneous **4** Percutaneous Endoscopic	**Z** No Device	**Z** No Qualifier

Section 0 **Medical and Surgical**
Body System 2 **Heart and Great Vessels**
Operation K **Map:** Locating the route of passage of electrical impulses and/or locating functional areas in a body part

Body Part (4th)	Approach (5th)	Device (6th)	Qualifier (7th)
8 Conduction Mechanism	**0** Open **3** Percutaneous **4** Percutaneous Endoscopic	**Z** No Device	**Z** No Qualifier

Section 0 **Medical and Surgical**
Body System 2 **Heart and Great Vessels**
Operation L **Occlusion:** Completely closing an orifice or the lumen of a tubular body part

Body Part (4th)	Approach (5th)	Device (6th)	Qualifier (7th)
7 Atrium, Left	**0** Open **3** Percutaneous **4** Percutaneous Endoscopic	**C** Extraluminal Device **D** Intraluminal Device **Z** No Device	**K** Left Atrial Appendage
H Pulmonary Valve **P** Pulmonary Trunk **Q** Pulmonary Artery, Right **S** Pulmonary Vein, Right **T** Pulmonary Vein, Left **V** Superior Vena Cava	**0** Open **3** Percutaneous **4** Percutaneous Endoscopic	**C** Extraluminal Device **D** Intraluminal Device **Z** No Device	**Z** No Qualifier
R Pulmonary Artery, Left	**0** Open **3** Percutaneous **4** Percutaneous Endoscopic	**C** Extraluminal Device **D** Intraluminal Device **Z** No Device	**T** Ductus Arteriosus **Z** No Qualifier
W Thoracic Aorta, Descending	**3** Percutaneous	**D** Intraluminal Device	**J** Temporary

tion **0** **Medical and Surgical**
dy System **2** **Heart and Great Vessels**
eration **N** **Release:** Freeing a body part from an abnormal physical constraint by cutting or by the use of force

Body Part (4th)	Approach (5th)	Device (6th)	Qualifier (7th)
Coronary Artery, One Artery Coronary Artery, Two Arteries Coronary Artery, Three Arteries Coronary Artery, Four or More Arteries Coronary Vein Atrial Septum Atrium, Right Atrium, Left Conduction Mechanism Chordae Tendineae Papillary Muscle Aortic Valve Mitral Valve Pulmonary Valve Tricuspid Valve Ventricle, Right Ventricle, Left Ventricular Septum Pericardium Pulmonary Trunk Pulmonary Artery, Right Pulmonary Artery, Left Pulmonary Vein, Right Pulmonary Vein, Left Superior Vena Cava W Thoracic Aorta, Descending Thoracic Aorta, Ascending/ Arch	**0** Open **3** Percutaneous **4** Percutaneous Endoscopic	**Z** No Device	**Z** No Qualifier

ction **0** **Medical and Surgical**
dy System **2** **Heart and Great Vessels**
eration **P** **Removal:** Taking out or off a device from a body part

Body Part (4th)	Approach (5th)	Device (6th)	Qualifier (7th)
Heart	**0** Open **3** Percutaneous **4** Percutaneous Endoscopic	**2** Monitoring Device **3** Infusion Device **7** Autologous Tissue Substitute **8** Zooplastic Tissue **C** Extraluminal Device **D** Intraluminal Device **J** Synthetic Substitute **K** Nonautologous Tissue Substitute **M** Cardiac Lead **N** Intracardiac Pacemaker **Q** Implantable Heart Assist System **Y** Other Device	**Z** No Qualifier
Heart	**0** Open **3** Percutaneous **4** Percutaneous Endoscopic	**R** Short-term External Heart Assist System	**S** Biventricular **Z** No Qualifier
Heart	**X** External	**2** Monitoring Device **3** Infusion Device **D** Intraluminal Device **M** Cardiac Lead	**Z** No Qualifier

Continued →

02P Contin.

Section 0 **Medical and Surgical**
Body System 2 **Heart and Great Vessels**
Operation P **Removal:** Taking out or off a device from a body part

Body Part (4th)	Approach (5th)	Device (6th)	Qualifier (7th)
Y Great Vessel	**0** Open **3** Percutaneous **4** Percutaneous Endoscopic	**2** Monitoring Device **3** Infusion Device **7** Autologous Tissue Substitute **8** Zooplastic Tissue **C** Extraluminal Device **D** Intraluminal Device **J** Synthetic Substitute **K** Nonautologous Tissue Substitute **Y** Other Device	**Z** No Qualifier
Y Great Vessel	**X** External	**2** Monitoring Device **3** Infusion Device **D** Intraluminal Device	**Z** No Qualifier

Section 0 **Medical and Surgical**
Body System 2 **Heart and Great Vessels**
Operation Q **Repair:** Restoring, to the extent possible, a body part to its normal anatomic structure and function

Body Part (4th)	Approach (5th)	Device (6th)	Qualifier (7th)
0 Coronary Artery, One Artery **1** Coronary Artery, Two Arteries **2** Coronary Artery, Three Arteries **3** Coronary Artery, Four or More Arteries **4** Coronary Vein **5** Atrial Septum **6** Atrium, Right **7** Atrium, Left **8** Conduction Mechanism **9** Chordae Tendineae **A** Heart **B** Heart, Right **C** Heart, Left **D** Papillary Muscle **H** Pulmonary Valve **K** Ventricle, Right **L** Ventricle, Left **M** Ventricular Septum **N** Pericardium **P** Pulmonary Trunk **Q** Pulmonary Artery, Right **R** Pulmonary Artery, Left **S** Pulmonary Vein, Right **T** Pulmonary Vein, Left **V** Superior Vena Cava **W** Thoracic Aorta, Descending **X** Thoracic Aorta, Ascending/Arch	**0** Open **3** Percutaneous **4** Percutaneous Endoscopic	**Z** No Device	**Z** No Qualifier
F Aortic Valve	**0** Open **3** Percutaneous **4** Percutaneous Endoscopic	**Z** No Device	**J** Truncal Valve **Z** No Qualifier
G Mitral Valve	**0** Open **3** Percutaneous **4** Percutaneous Endoscopic	**Z** No Device	**E** Atrioventricular Valve, L **Z** No Qualifier
J Tricuspid Valve	**0** Open **3** Percutaneous **4** Percutaneous Endoscopic	**Z** No Device	**G** Atrioventricular Valve, Right **Z** No Qualifier

tion 0 **Medical and Surgical**
dy System 2 **Heart and Great Vessels**
eration R **Replacement:** Putting in or on biological or synthetic material that physically takes the place and/or function of all or a portion of a body part

Body Part (4th)	Approach (5th)	Device (6th)	Qualifier (7th)
Atrial Septum Atrium, Right Atrium, Left Chordae Tendineae D Papillary Muscle K Ventricle, Right L Ventricle, Left M Ventricular Septum N Pericardium P Pulmonary Trunk Q Pulmonary Artery, Right R Pulmonary Artery, Left S Pulmonary Vein, Right T Pulmonary Vein, Left V Superior Vena Cava W Thoracic Aorta, Descending X Thoracic Aorta, Ascending/Arch	**0** Open **4** Percutaneous Endoscopic	**7** Autologous Tissue Substitute **8** Zooplastic Tissue **J** Synthetic Substitute **K** Nonautologous Tissue Substitute	**Z** No Qualifier
Aortic Valve G Mitral Valve H Pulmonary Valve Tricuspid Valve	**0** Open **4** Percutaneous Endoscopic	**7** Autologous Tissue Substitute **8** Zooplastic Tissue **J** Synthetic Substitute **K** Nonautologous Tissue Substitute	**Z** No Qualifier
Aortic Valve G Mitral Valve H Pulmonary Valve J Tricuspid Valve	**3** Percutaneous	**7** Autologous Tissue Substitute **8** Zooplastic Tissue **J** Synthetic Substitute **K** Nonautologous Tissue Substitute	**H** Transapical **Z** No Qualifier

ction 0 **Medical and Surgical**
dy System 2 **Heart and Great Vessels**
eration S **Reposition:** Moving to its normal location, or other suitable location, all or a portion of a body part

Body Part (4th)	Approach (5th)	Device (6th)	Qualifier (7th)
Coronary Artery, One Artery Coronary Artery, Two Arteries P Pulmonary Trunk Q Pulmonary Artery, Right R Pulmonary Artery, Left S Pulmonary Vein, Right T Pulmonary Vein, Left V Superior Vena Cava W Thoracic Aorta, Descending X Thoracic Aorta, Ascending/Arch	**0** Open	**Z** No Device	**Z** No Qualifier

ction 0 **Medical and Surgical**
dy System 2 **Heart and Great Vessels**
eration T **Resection:** Cutting out or off, without replacement, all of a body part

Body Part (4th)	Approach (5th)	Device (6th)	Qualifier (7th)
5 Atrial Septum 8 Conduction Mechanism 9 Chordae Tendineae D Papillary Muscle H Pulmonary Valve M Ventricular Septum N Pericardium	**0** Open **3** Percutaneous **4** Percutaneous Endoscopic	**Z** No Device	**Z** No Qualifier

Section 0 **Medical and Surgical**
Body System 2 **Heart and Great Vessels**
Operation U **Supplement:** Putting in or on biological or synthetic material that physically reinforces and/or augments the function of a portion of a body part

Body Part (4th)	Approach (5th)	Device (6th)	Qualifier (7th)
5 Atrial Septum **6** Atrium, Right **7** Atrium, Left **9** Chordae Tendineae **A** Heart **D** Papillary Muscle **H** Pulmonary Valve **K** Ventricle, Right **L** Ventricle, Left **M** Ventricular Septum **N** Pericardium **P** Pulmonary Trunk **Q** Pulmonary Artery, Right **R** Pulmonary Artery, Left **S** Pulmonary Vein, Right **T** Pulmonary Vein, Left **V** Superior Vena Cava **W** Thoracic Aorta, Descending **X** Thoracic Aorta, Ascending/Arch	**0** Open **3** Percutaneous **4** Percutaneous Endoscopic	**7** Autologous Tissue Substitute **8** Zooplastic Tissue **J** Synthetic Substitute **K** Nonautologous Tissue Substitute	**Z** No Qualifier
F Aortic Valve	**0** Open **3** Percutaneous **4** Percutaneous Endoscopic	**7** Autologous Tissue Substitute **8** Zooplastic Tissue **J** Synthetic Substitute **K** Nonautologous Tissue Substitute	**J** Truncal Valve **Z** No Qualifier
G Mitral Valve	**0** Open **3** Percutaneous **4** Percutaneous Endoscopic	**7** Autologous Tissue Substitute **8** Zooplastic Tissue **J** Synthetic Substitute **K** Nonautologous Tissue Substitute	**E** Atrioventricular Valve, Left **Z** No Qualifier
J Tricuspid Valve	**0** Open **3** Percutaneous **4** Percutaneous Endoscopic	**7** Autologous Tissue Substitute **8** Zooplastic Tissue **J** Synthetic Substitute **K** Nonautologous Tissue Substitute	**G** Atrioventricular Valve, Right **Z** No Qualifier

Section 0 **Medical and Surgical**
Body System 2 **Heart and Great Vessels**
Operation V **Restriction:** Partially closing an orifice or the lumen of a tubular body part

Body Part (4th)	Approach (5th)	Device (6th)	Qualifier (7th)
A Heart	**0** Open **3** Percutaneous **4** Percutaneous Endoscopic	**C** Extraluminal Device **Z** No Device	**Z** No Qualifier
G Mitral Valve	**0** Open **3** Percutaneous **4** Percutaneous Endoscopic	**Z** No Device	**Z** No Qualifier
P Pulmonary Trunk **Q** Pulmonary Artery, Right **S** Pulmonary Vein, Right **T** Pulmonary Vein, Left **V** Superior Vena Cava	**0** Open **3** Percutaneous **4** Percutaneous Endoscopic	**C** Extraluminal Device **D** Intraluminal Device **Z** No Device	**Z** No Qualifier

Continued →

tion 0 **Medical and Surgical**
dy System 2 **Heart and Great Vessels**
eration V **Restriction:** Partially closing an orifice or the lumen of a tubular body part

Body Part (4th)	Approach (5th)	Device (6th)	Qualifier (7th)
R Pulmonary Artery, Left	**0** Open **3** Percutaneous **4** Percutaneous Endoscopic	**C** Extraluminal Device **D** Intraluminal Device **Z** No Device	**T** Ductus Arteriosus **Z** No Qualifier
W Thoracic Aorta, Descending **X** Thoracic Aorta, Ascending/ Arch	**0** Open **3** Percutaneous **4** Percutaneous Endoscopic	**C** Extraluminal Device **D** Intraluminal Device **E** Intraluminal Device, Branched or Fenestrated, One or Two Arteries **F** Intraluminal Device, Branched or Fenestrated, Three or More Arteries **Z** No Device	**Z** No Qualifier

ction 0 **Medical and Surgical**
dy System 2 **Heart and Great Vessels**
eration W **Revision:** Correcting, to the extent possible, a portion of a malfunctioning device or the position of a displaced device

Body Part (4th)	Approach (5th)	Device (6th)	Qualifier (7th)
5 Atrial Septum **M** Ventricular Septum	**0** Open **4** Percutaneous Endoscopic	**J** Synthetic Substitute	**Z** No Qualifier
A Heart	**0** Open **3** Percutaneous **4** Percutaneous Endoscopic	**2** Monitoring Device **3** Infusion Device **7** Autologous Tissue Substitute **8** Zooplastic Tissue **C** Extraluminal Device **D** Intraluminal Device **J** Synthetic Substitute **K** Nonautologous Tissue Substitute **M** Cardiac Lead **N** Intracardiac Pacemaker **Q** Implantable Heart Assist System **Y** Other Device	**Z** No Qualifier
A Heart	**0** Open **3** Percutaneous **4** Percutaneous Endoscopic	**R** Short-term External Heart Assist System	**S** Biventricular **Z** No Qualifier
A Heart	**X** External	**2** Monitoring Device **3** Infusion Device **7** Autologous Tissue Substitute **8** Zooplastic Tissue **C** Extraluminal Device **D** Intraluminal Device **J** Synthetic Substitute **K** Nonautologous Tissue Substitute **M** Cardiac Lead **N** Intracardiac Pacemaker **Q** Implantable Heart Assist System	**Z** No Qualifier
A Heart	**X** External	**R** Short-term External Heart Assist System	**S** Biventricular **Z** No Qualifier
F Aortic Valve **G** Mitral Valve **H** Pulmonary Valve **J** Tricuspid Valve	**0** Open **3** Percutaneous **4** Percutaneous Endoscopic	**7** Autologous Tissue Substitute **8** Zooplastic Tissue **J** Synthetic Substitute **K** Nonautologous Tissue Substitute	**Z** No Qualifier

Continued →

Section 0 **Medical and Surgical**
Body System 2 **Heart and Great Vessels**
Operation W **Revision:** Correcting, to the extent possible, a portion of a malfunctioning device or the position of a displaced device

Body Part (4th)	Approach (5th)	Device (6th)	Qualifier (7th)
Y Great Vessel	**0** Open **3** Percutaneous **4** Percutaneous Endoscopic	**2** Monitoring Device **3** Infusion Device **7** Autologous Tissue Substitute **8** Zooplastic Tissue **C** Extraluminal Device **D** Intraluminal Device **J** Synthetic Substitute **K** Nonautologous Tissue Substitute **Y** Other Device	**Z** No Qualifier
Y Great Vessel	**X** External	**2** Monitoring Device **3** Infusion Device **7** Autologous Tissue Substitute **8** Zooplastic Tissue **C** Extraluminal Device **D** Intraluminal Device **J** Synthetic Substitute **K** Nonautologous Tissue Substitute	**Z** No Qualifier

Section 0 **Medical and Surgical**
Body System 2 **Heart and Great Vessels**
Operation Y **Transplantation:** Putting in or on all or a portion of a living body part taken from another individual or animal to physically take the place and/or function of all or a portion of a similar body part

Body Part (4th)	Approach (5th)	Device (6th)	Qualifier (7th)
A Heart	**0** Open	**Z** No Device	**0** Allogeneic **1** Syngeneic **2** Zooplastic

AHA Coding Clinic

021009W Bypass Coronary Artery, One Artery from Aorta with Autologous Venous Tissue, Open Approach—AHA CC: 1Q, 2014, 10-

02100AW Bypass Coronary Artery, One Artery from Aorta with Autologous Arterial Tissue, Open Approach—AHA CC: 4Q, 2016, 83-

02100Z9 Bypass Coronary Artery, One Artery from Left Internal Mammary, Open Approach— AHA CC: 3Q, 2014, 8, 20-21; 1Q, 20 27-28; 4Q, 2016, 83-84

021109W Bypass Coronary Artery, Two Arteries from Aorta with Autologous VenousTissue, Open Approach—AHA CC: 3Q, 2014, 20- 4Q, 2016, 83-84

021209W Bypass Coronary Artery, Three Arteries from Aorta with Autologous Venous Tissue, Open Approach—AHA CC: 1Q, 2016, 27-

02160JQ Bypass Right Atrium to Right Pulmonary Artery with Synthetic Substitute, Open Approach—AHA CC: 3Q, 2014, 29

02163Z7 Bypass Right Atrium to Left Atrium, Percutaneous Approach—AHA CC: 4Q, 2017, 56

02170ZU Bypass Left Atrium to Pulmonary Vein Confluence, Open Approach—AHA CC: 4Q, 2016, 108-109

021K0JP Bypass Right Ventricle to Pulmonary Trunk with Synthetic Substitute, Open Approach—AHA CC: 1Q, 2017, 19-20

021K0JQ Bypass Right Ventricle to Right Pulmonary Artery with Synthetic Substitute, Open Approach—AHA CC: 3Q, 2014, 30

021K0KP Bypass Right Ventricle to Pulmonary Trunk with Nonautologous Tissue Substitute, Open Approach—AHA CC: 3Q, 2015, 17; 4Q, 2015. 22-23, 25

021V08S Bypass Superior Vena Cava to Right Pulmonary Vein with Zooplastic Tissue, Open Approach—AHA CC: 4Q, 2016, 145

021V09S Bypass Superior Vena Cava to Right Pulmonary Vein with Autologous Venous Tissue, Open Approach—AHA CC: 4Q, 2016,

021W0JQ Bypass Thoracic Aorta, Descending to Right Pulmonary Artery with Synthetic Substitute, Open Approach—AHA CC: 3 2014, 3

02570ZK Destruction of Left Atrial Appendage, Open Approach—AHA CC: 3Q, 2014, 20-21

02580ZZ Destruction of Conduction Mechanism, Open Approach—AHA CC: 3Q, 2016, 44

02583ZZ Destruction of Conduction Mechanism, Percutaneous Approach—AHA CC: 3Q, 2014, 19; 4Q, 2014, 47-48; 3Q, 2016, 43-4

025N0ZZ Destruction of Pericardium, Open Approach—AHA CC: 2Q, 2016, 17-18

70346 Dilation of Coronary Artery, One Artery, Bifurcation, with Drug-eluting Intraluminal Device, Percutaneous Approach—AHA CC: 2Q, 2015, 4-5; 4Q, 2016, 88

7034Z Dilation of Coronary Artery, One Artery with Drug-eluting Intraluminal Device, Percutaneous Approach—AHA CC: 2Q, 2014, 4; 2Q, 2015, 3-4; 4Q, 2015, 13-14

7037Z Dilation of Coronary Artery, One Artery with Four or More Drug-eluting Intraluminal Devices, Percutaneous Approach—AHA CC: 4Q, 2016, 85-86

703DZ Dilation of Coronary Artery, One Artery with Intraluminal Device, Percutaneous Approach—AHA CC: 2Q, 2015, 4

703EZ Dilation of Coronary Artery, One Artery with Two Intraluminal Devices, Percutaneous Approach—AHA CC: 4Q, 2016, 84-85

703ZZ Dilation of Coronary Artery, One Artery, Percutaneous Approach—AHA CC: 3Q, 2015, 10; 4Q, 2016, 88

7134Z Dilation of Coronary Artery, Two Arteries with Drug-eluting Intraluminal Device, Percutaneous Approach—AHA CC: 2Q, 2015, 5

71356 Dilation of Coronary Artery, Two Arteries, Bifurcation, with Two Drug-eluting Intraluminal Devices, Percutaneous Approach—AHA CC: 4Q, 2016, 87

7136Z Dilation of Coronary Artery, Two Arteries with Three Drug-eluting Intraluminal Devices, Percutaneous Approach—AHA CC: 4Q, 2016, 84-85

7234Z Dilation of Coronary Artery, Three Arteries with Drug-eluting Intraluminal Device, Percutaneous Approach—AHA CC: 2Q, 2015, 3

7H0ZZ Dilation of Pulmonary Valve, Open Approach—AHA CC: 1Q, 2016, 16-17

7L0ZZ Dilation of Left Ventricle, Open Approach—AHA CC: 4Q, 2017, 33

7Q0DZ Dilation of Right Pulmonary Artery with Intraluminal Device, Open Approach—AHA CC: 3Q, 2015, 16-17

BG0ZZ Excision of Mitral Valve, Open Approach—AHA CC: 2Q, 2015, 23-24

CG0ZZ Extirpation of Matter from Mitral Valve, Open Approach—AHA CC: 2Q, 2016, 24-25

H633Z Insertion of Infusion Device into Right Atrium, Percutaneous Approach—AHA CC: 2Q, 2016, 15-16; 2Q, 2017, 24-26

H63KZ Insertion of Cardiac Lead into Right Atrium, Percutaneous Approach—AHA CC: 2Q, 2018, 19

H73DZ Insertion of Intraluminal Device into Left Atrium, Percutaneous Approach—AHA CC: 4Q, 2017, 104-105

HA3RJ Insertion of Short-term External Heart Assist System into Heart, Intraoperative, Percutaneous Approach—AHA CC: 4Q, 2017, 43-44

HA3RS Insertion of Biventricular Short-term External Heart Assist System into Heart, Percutaneous Approach—AHA CC: 4Q, 2016, 138-139

HA3RZ Insertion of Short-term External Heart Assist System into Heart, Percutaneous Approach—AHA CC: 1Q, 2017, 11-12; 4Q, 2017, 44-45

HK3DZ Insertion of Intraluminal Device into Right Ventricle, Percutaneous Approach—AHA CC: 2Q, 2015, 31-32

HP32Z Insertion of Monitoring Device into Pulmonary Trunk, Percutaneous Approach—AHA CC: 3Q, 2015, 35

HV33Z Insertion of Infusion Device into Superior Vena Cava, Percutaneous Approach—AHA CC: 3Q, 2013, 18; 2Q, 2015, 33-34; 4Q, 2015, 14-15, 28-32; 4Q, 2017, 63-64

JA3ZZ Inspection of Heart, Percutaneous Approach—AHA CC: 3Q, 2015, 9

L70CK Occlusion of Left Atrial Appendage with Extraluminal Device, Open Approach—AHA CC: 3Q, 2014, 20-21

LQ3DZ Occlusion of Right Pulmonary Artery with Intraluminal Device, Percutaneous Approach—AHA CC: 4Q, 2017, 34

LR0ZT Occlusion of Ductus Arteriosus, Open Approach—AHA CC: 4Q, 2015, 23-24

LS3DZ Occlusion of Right Pulmonary Vein with Intraluminal Device, Percutaneous Approach—AHA CC: 2Q, 2016, 26; 4Q, 2017, 34

NK0ZZ Release Right Ventricle, Open Approach—AHA CC: 3Q, 2014, 16-17

PA0RZ Removal of Short-term External Heart Assist System from Heart, Open Approach—AHA CC: 1Q, 2017, 13-14

PA3DZ Removal of Intraluminal Device from Heart, Percutaneous Approach—AHA CC: 4Q, 2017, 104-105

PA3MZ Removal of Cardiac Lead from Heart, Percutaneous Approach—AHA CC: 3Q, 2015, 33

PA3NZ Removal of Intracardiac Pacemaker from Heart, Percutaneous Approach—AHA CC: 4Q, 2016, 96-97

PA3RZ Removal of Short-term External Heart Assist System from Heart, Percutaneous Approach—AHA CC: 4Q, 2016, 139; 1Q, 2017, 11-12; 4Q, 2017, 44-45

PY33Z Removal of Infusion Device from Great Vessel, Percutaneous Approach—AHA CC: 4Q, 2015, 31-32; 2Q, 2016, 15-16; 2Q, 2017, 24-26

PYX3Z Removal of Infusion Device from Great Vessel, External Approach—AHA CC: 3Q, 2016, 19

Q50ZZ Repair Atrial Septum, Open Approach—AHA CC: 4Q, 2015, 23-24

QS0ZZ Repair Right Pulmonary Vein, Open Approach—AHA CC: 1Q, 2017, 18-19

02QT0ZZ Repair Left Pulmonary Vein, Open Approach—AHA CC: 1Q, 2017, 18-19

02QW0ZZ Repair Thoracic Aorta, Descending, Open Approach—AHA CC: 3Q, 2015, 16

02RJ3JZ Replacement of Tricuspid Valve with Synthetic Substitute, Percutaneous Approach—AHA CC: 4Q, 2017, 56

02RJ48Z Replacement of Tricuspid Valve with Zooplastic Tissue, Percutaneous Endoscopic Approach—AHA CC: 3Q, 2016, 32

02RK0JZ Replacement of Right Ventricle with Synthetic Substitute, Open Approach—AHA CC: 1Q, 2017, 13-14

02RL0JZ Replacement of Left Ventricle with Synthetic Substitute, Open Approach—AHA CC: 1Q, 2017, 13-14

02RW0KZ Replacement of Thoracic Aorta, Descending with Nonautologous Tissue Substitute, Open Approach—AHA CC: 1Q, 20 10-11

02S10ZZ Reposition Coronary Artery, Two Arteries, Open Approach—AHA CC: 4Q, 2016, 103-104

02SP0ZZ Reposition Pulmonary Trunk, Open Approach—AHA CC: 4Q, 2015, 23-24; 4Q, 2016, 103-104

02SW0ZZ Reposition Thoracic Aorta, Descending, Open Approach—AHA CC: 4Q, 2015, 23-24

02SX0ZZ Reposition Thoracic Aorta, Ascending/Arch, Open Approach—AHA CC: 4Q, 2016, 103-104

02U607Z Supplement Right Atrium with Autologous Tissue Substitute, Open Approach—AHA CC: 3Q, 2017, 7-8

02U707Z Supplement Left Atrium with Autologous Tissue Substitute, Open Approach— AHA CC: 3Q, 2017, 7-8

02UF08Z Supplement Aortic Valve with Zooplastic Tissue, Open Approach—AHA CC: 4Q, 2015, 25

02UG08Z Supplement Mitral Valve with Zooplastic Tissue, Open Approach—AHA CC: 4Q, 2017, 36

02UG0JZ Supplement Mitral Valve with Synthetic Substitute, Open Approach—AHA CC: 2Q, 2015, 23-24

02UM08Z Supplement Ventricular Septum with Zooplastic Tissue, Open Approach—AHA CC: 4Q, 2015, 25

02UM0JZ Supplement Ventricular Septum with Synthetic Substitute, Open Approach—AHA CC: 3Q, 2014, 16-17; 4Q, 2015, 22-23

02UP07Z Supplement Pulmonary Trunk with Autologous Tissue Substitute, Open Approach—AHA CC: 2Q, 2016, 23-24

02UQ0KZ Supplement Right Pulmonary Artery with Nonautologous Tissue Substitute, Open Approach—AHA CC: 3Q, 2015, 16-17

02UR07Z Supplement Left Pulmonary Artery with Autologous Tissue Substitute, Open Approach—AHA CC: 2Q, 2016, 23-24

02UR0KZ Supplement Left Pulmonary Artery with Nonautologous Tissue Substitute, Open Approach—AHA CC: 3Q, 2015, 16-17

02UW07Z Supplement Thoracic Aorta, Descending with Autologous Tissue Substitute, Open Approach—AHA CC: 4Q, 2015, 23-24

02UW0JZ Supplement Thoracic Aorta, Descending with Synthetic Substitute, Open Approach—AHA CC: 2Q, 2016, 26-27

02UX0KZ Supplement Thoracic Aorta, Ascending/Arch with Nonautologous Tissue Substitute, Open Approach—AHA CC: 1Q, 20 19-20

02VG0ZZ Restriction of Mitral Valve, Open Approach—AHA CC: 4Q, 2017, 36

02VW3DZ Restriction of Thoracic Aorta, Descending with Intraluminal Device, Percutaneous Approach—AHA CC: 4Q, 2016, 92-93

02WA3JZ Revision of Synthetic Substitute in Heart, Percutaneous Approach—AHA CC: 3Q, 2014, 31-32

02WA3MZ Revision of Cardiac Lead in Heart, Percutaneous Approach—AHA CC: 3Q, 2015, 32

02WA3NZ Revision of Intracardiac Pacemaker in Heart, Percutaneous Approach—AHA CC: 4Q, 2016, 96

02WAXRZ Revision of Short-term External Heart Assist System in Heart, External Approach—AHA CC: 1Q, 2018, 17

02YA0Z0 Transplantation of Heart, Allogeneic, Open Approach—AHA CC: 3Q, 2013, 18-19

Arteries

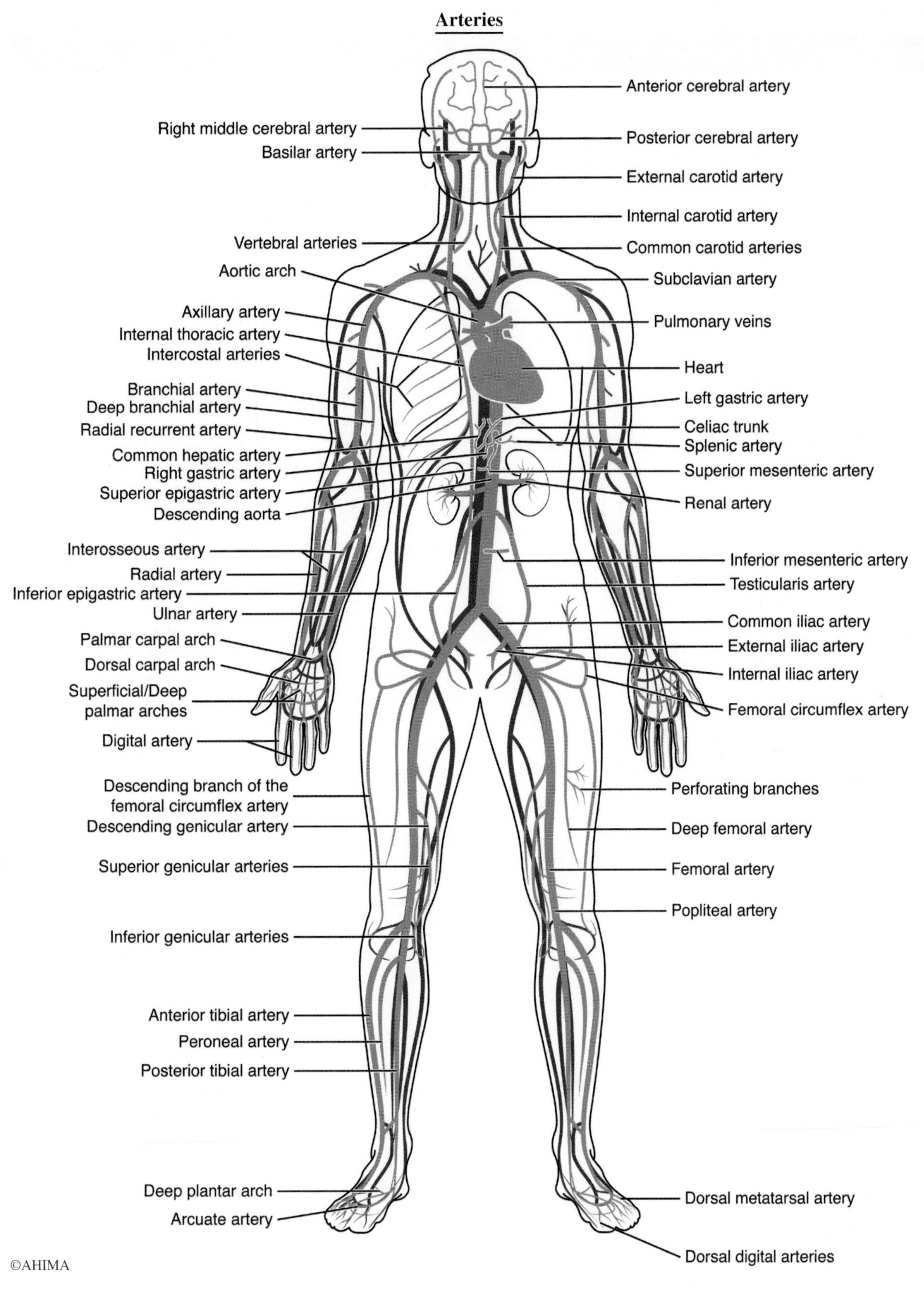
Anterior cerebral artery
Right middle cerebral artery
Posterior cerebral artery
Basilar artery
External carotid artery
Internal carotid artery
Vertebral arteries
Common carotid arteries
Aortic arch
Subclavian artery
Axillary artery
Pulmonary veins
Internal thoracic artery
Intercostal arteries
Heart
Branchial artery
Deep branchial artery
Left gastric artery
Radial recurrent artery
Celiac trunk
Splenic artery
Common hepatic artery
Right gastric artery
Superior mesenteric artery
Superior epigastric artery
Renal artery
Descending aorta
Interosseous artery
Inferior mesenteric artery
Radial artery
Testicularis artery
Inferior epigastric artery
Ulnar artery
Common iliac artery
Palmar carpal arch
External iliac artery
Dorsal carpal arch
Internal iliac artery
Superficial/Deep
palmar arches
Femoral circumflex artery
Digital artery
Descending branch of the
femoral circumflex artery
Perforating branches
Descending genicular artery
Deep femoral artery
Superior genicular arteries
Femoral artery
Popliteal artery
Inferior genicular arteries
Anterior tibial artery
Peroneal artery
Posterior tibial artery
Deep plantar arch
Dorsal metatarsal artery
Arcuate artery
Dorsal digital arteries

Section 0 **Medical and Surgical**
Body System 3 **Upper Arteries**
Operation 1 **Bypass:** Altering the route of passage of the contents of a tubular body part

Body Part (4th)	Approach (5th)	Device (6th)	Qualifier (7th)
2 Innominate Artery	**0** Open	**9** Autologous Venous Tissue **A** Autologous Arterial Tissue **J** Synthetic Substitute **K** Nonautologous Tissue Substitute **Z** No Device	**0** Upper Arm Artery, Right **1** Upper Arm Artery, Left **2** Upper Arm Artery, Bilateral **3** Lower Arm Artery, Right **4** Lower Arm Artery, Left **5** Lower Arm Artery, Bilateral **6** Upper Leg Artery, Right **7** Upper Leg Artery, Left **8** Upper Leg Artery, Bilateral **9** Lower Leg Artery, Right **B** Lower Leg Artery, Left **C** Lower Leg Artery, Bilateral **D** Upper Arm Vein **F** Lower Arm Vein **J** Extracranial Artery, Right **K** Extracranial Artery, Left
3 Subclavian Artery, Right **4** Subclavian Artery, Left	**0** Open	**9** Autologous Venous Tissue **A** Autologous Arterial Tissue **J** Synthetic Substitute **K** Nonautologous Tissue Substitute **Z** No Device	**0** Upper Arm Artery, Right **1** Upper Arm Artery, Left **2** Upper Arm Artery, Bilateral **3** Lower Arm Artery, Right **4** Lower Arm Artery, Left **5** Lower Arm Artery, Bilateral **6** Upper Leg Artery, Right **7** Upper Leg Artery, Left **8** Upper Leg Artery, Bilateral **9** Lower Leg Artery, Right **B** Lower Leg Artery, Left **C** Lower Leg Artery, Bilateral **D** Upper Arm Vein **F** Lower Arm Vein **J** Extracranial Artery, Right **K** Extracranial Artery, Left **M** Pulmonary Artery, Right **N** Pulmonary Artery, Left
5 Axillary Artery, Right **6** Axillary Artery, Left	**0** Open	**9** Autologous Venous Tissue **A** Autologous Arterial Tissue **J** Synthetic Substitute **K** Nonautologous Tissue Substitute **Z** No Device	**0** Upper Arm Artery, Right **1** Upper Arm Artery, Left **2** Upper Arm Artery, Bilateral **3** Lower Arm Artery, Right **4** Lower Arm Artery, Left **5** Lower Arm Artery, Bilateral **6** Upper Leg Artery, Right **7** Upper Leg Artery, Left **8** Upper Leg Artery, Bilateral **9** Lower Leg Artery, Right **B** Lower Leg Artery, Left **C** Lower Leg Artery, Bilateral **D** Upper Arm Vein **F** Lower Arm Vein **J** Extracranial Artery, Right **K** Extracranial Artery, Left **T** Abdominal Artery **V** Superior Vena Cava
7 Brachial Artery, Right	**0** Open	**9** Autologous Venous Tissue **A** Autologous Arterial Tissue **J** Synthetic Substitute **K** Nonautologous Tissue Substitute **Z** No Device	**0** Upper Arm Artery, Right **3** Lower Arm Artery, Right **D** Upper Arm Vein **F** Lower Arm Vein **V** Superior Vena Cava

Continued→

ction **0** **Medical and Surgical**
dy System **3** **Upper Arteries**
eration **1** **Bypass:** Altering the route of passage of the contents of a tubular body part

Body Part (4th)	Approach (5th)	Device (6th)	Qualifier (7th)
Brachial Artery, Left	**0** Open	**9** Autologous Venous Tissue **A** Autologous Arterial Tissue **J** Synthetic Substitute **K** Nonautologous Tissue Substitute **Z** No Device	**1** Upper Arm Artery, Left **4** Lower Arm Artery, Left **D** Upper Arm Vein **F** Lower Arm Vein **V** Superior Vena Cava
Ulnar Artery, Right Radial Artery, Right	**0** Open	**9** Autologous Venous Tissue **A** Autologous Arterial Tissue **J** Synthetic Substitute **K** Nonautologous Tissue Substitute **Z** No Device	**3** Lower Arm Artery, Right **F** Lower Arm Vein
Ulnar Artery, Left Radial Artery, Left	**0** Open	**9** Autologous Venous Tissue **A** Autologous Arterial Tissue **J** Synthetic Substitute **K** Nonautologous Tissue Substitute **Z** No Device	**4** Lower Arm Artery, Left **F** Lower Arm Vein
Intracranial Artery Temporal Artery, Right Temporal Artery, Left	**0** Open	**9** Autologous Venous Tissue **A** Autologous Arterial Tissue **J** Synthetic Substitute **K** Nonautologous Tissue Substitute **Z** No Device	**G** Intracranial Artery
Common Carotid Artery, Right Common Carotid Artery, Left	**0** Open	**9** Autologous Venous Tissue **A** Autologous Arterial Tissue **J** Synthetic Substitute **K** Nonautologous Tissue Substitute **Z** No Device	**G** Intracranial Artery **J** Extracranial Artery, Right **K** Extracranial Artery, Left **Y** Upper Artery
Internal Carotid Artery, Right Internal Carotid Artery, Left External Carotid Artery, Right External Carotid Artery, Left	**0** Open	**9** Autologous Venous Tissue **A** Autologous Arterial Tissue **J** Synthetic Substitute **K** Nonautologous Tissue Substitute **Z** No Device	**J** Extracranial Artery, Right **K** Extracranial Artery, Left

Section 0 **Medical and Surgical**
Body System 3 **Upper Arteries**
Operation 5 **Destruction:** Physical eradication of all or a portion of a body part by the direct use of energy, force, or a destructive ag

Body Part (4th)	Approach (5th)	Device (6th)	Qualifier (7th)
0 Internal Mammary Artery, Right **1** Internal Mammary Artery, Left **2** Innominate Artery **3** Subclavian Artery, Right **4** Subclavian Artery, Left **5** Axillary Artery, Right **6** Axillary Artery, Left **7** Brachial Artery, Right **8** Brachial Artery, Left **9** Ulnar Artery, Right **A** Ulnar Artery, Left **B** Radial Artery, Right **C** Radial Artery, Left **D** Hand Artery, Right **F** Hand Artery, Left **G** Intracranial Artery **H** Common Carotid Artery, Right **J** Common Carotid Artery, Left **K** Internal Carotid Artery, Right **L** Internal Carotid Artery, Left **M** External Carotid Artery, Right **N** External Carotid Artery, Left **P** Vertebral Artery, Right **Q** Vertebral Artery, Left **R** Face Artery **S** Temporal Artery, Right **T** Temporal Artery, Left **U** Thyroid Artery, Right **V** Thyroid Artery, Left **Y** Upper Artery	**0** Open **3** Percutaneous **4** Percutaneous Endoscopic	**Z** No Device	**Z** No Qualifier

tion **0 Medical and Surgical**
dy System **3 Upper Arteries**
eration **7 Dilation:** Expanding an orifice or the lumen of a tubular body part

Body Part (4th)	Approach (5th)	Device (6th)	Qualifier (7th)
0 Internal Mammary Artery, Right 1 Internal Mammary Artery, Left 2 Innominate Artery 3 Subclavian Artery, Right 4 Subclavian Artery, Left 5 Axillary Artery, Right 6 Axillary Artery, Left 7 Brachial Artery, Right 8 Brachial Artery, Left 9 Ulnar Artery, Right A Ulnar Artery, Left B Radial Artery, Right C Radial Artery, Left	**0** Open **3** Percutaneous **4** Percutaneous Endoscopic	**4** Intraluminal Device, Drug-eluting **5** Intraluminal Device, Drug-eluting, Two **6** Intraluminal Device, Drug-eluting, Three **7** Intraluminal Device, Drug-eluting, Four or More **E** Intraluminal Devices, Two **F** Intraluminal Devices, Three **G** Intraluminal Devices, Four or More	**6** Bifurcation **Z** No Qualifier
0 Internal Mammary Artery, Right 1 Internal Mammary Artery, Left 2 Innominate Artery 3 Subclavian Artery, Right 4 Subclavian Artery, Left 5 Axillary Artery, Right 6 Axillary Artery, Left 7 Brachial Artery, Right 8 Brachial Artery, Left 9 Ulnar Artery, Right A Ulnar Artery, Left B Radial Artery, Right C Radial Artery, Left	**0** Open **3** Percutaneous **4** Percutaneous Endoscopic	**D** Intraluminal Device **Z** No Device	**1** Drug-Coated Balloon **6** Bifurcation **Z** No Qualifier
D Hand Artery, Right F Hand Artery, Left G Intracranial Artery H Common Carotid Artery, Right J Common Carotid Artery, Left K Internal Carotid Artery, Right L Internal Carotid Artery, Left M External Carotid Artery, Right N External Carotid Artery, Left P Vertebral Artery, Right Q Vertebral Artery, Left R Face Artery S Temporal Artery, Right T Temporal Artery, Left U Thyroid Artery, Right V Thyroid Artery, Left Y Upper Artery	**0** Open **3** Percutaneous **4** Percutaneous Endoscopic	**4** Intraluminal Device, Drug-eluting **5** Intraluminal Device, Drug-eluting, Two **6** Intraluminal Device, Drug-eluting, Three **7** Intraluminal Device, Drug-eluting, Four or More **D** Intraluminal Device **E** Intraluminal Device, Two **F** Intraluminal Device, Three **G** Intraluminal Device, Four or More **Z** No Device	**6** Bifurcation **Z** No Qualifier

Section 0 **Medical and Surgical**
Body System 3 **Upper Arteries**
Operation 9 **Drainage:** Taking or letting out fluids and/or gases from a body part

Body Part (4th)	Approach (5th)	Device (6th)	Qualifier (7th)
0 Internal Mammary Artery, Right **1** Internal Mammary Artery, Left **2** Innominate Artery **3** Subclavian Artery, Right **4** Subclavian Artery, Left **5** Axillary Artery, Right **6** Axillary Artery, Left **7** Brachial Artery, Right **8** Brachial Artery, Left **9** Ulnar Artery, Right **A** Ulnar Artery, Left **B** Radial Artery, Right **C** Radial Artery, Left **D** Hand Artery, Right **F** Hand Artery, Left **G** Intracranial Artery **H** Common Carotid Artery, Right **J** Common Carotid Artery, Left **K** Internal Carotid Artery, Right **L** Internal Carotid Artery, Left **M** External Carotid Artery, Right **N** External Carotid Artery, Left **P** Vertebral Artery, Right **Q** Vertebral Artery, Left **R** Face Artery **S** Temporal Artery, Right **T** Temporal Artery, Left **U** Thyroid Artery, Right **V** Thyroid Artery, Left **Y** Upper Artery	**0** Open **3** Percutaneous **4** Percutaneous Endoscopic	**0** Drainage Device	**Z** No Qualifier
0 Internal Mammary Artery, Right **1** Internal Mammary Artery, Left **2** Innominate Artery **3** Subclavian Artery, Right **4** Subclavian Artery, Left **5** Axillary Artery, Right **6** Axillary Artery, Left **7** Brachial Artery, Right **8** Brachial Artery, Left **9** Ulnar Artery, Right **A** Ulnar Artery, Left **B** Radial Artery, Right **C** Radial Artery, Left **D** Hand Artery, Right **F** Hand Artery, Left **G** Intracranial Artery **H** Common Carotid Artery, Right **J** Common Carotid Artery, Left **K** Internal Carotid Artery, Right **L** Internal Carotid Artery, Left **M** External Carotid Artery, Right **N** External Carotid Artery, Left **P** Vertebral Artery, Right **Q** Vertebral Artery, Left **R** Face Artery **S** Temporal Artery, Right **T** Temporal Artery, Left **U** Thyroid Artery, Right **V** Thyroid Artery, Left **Y** Upper Artery	**0** Open **3** Percutaneous **4** Percutaneous Endoscopic	**Z** No Device	**X** Diagnostic **Z** No Qualifier

tion 0 **Medical and Surgical**
ly System 3 **Upper Arteries**
eration B **Excision:** Cutting out or off, without replacement, a portion of a body part

Body Part (4th)	Approach (5th)	Device (6th)	Qualifier (7th)
Internal Mammary Artery, Right Internal Mammary Artery, Left Innominate Artery Subclavian Artery, Right Subclavian Artery, Left Axillary Artery, Right Axillary Artery, Left Brachial Artery, Right Brachial Artery, Left Ulnar Artery, Right Ulnar Artery, Left Radial Artery, Right Radial Artery, Left Hand Artery, Right Hand Artery, Left Intracranial Artery Common Carotid Artery, Right Common Carotid Artery, Left Internal Carotid Artery, Right Internal Carotid Artery, Left External Carotid Artery, Right External Carotid Artery, Left Vertebral Artery, Right Vertebral Artery, Left Face Artery Temporal Artery, Right Temporal Artery, Left Thyroid Artery, Right Thyroid Artery, Left Upper Artery	**0** Open **3** Percutaneous **4** Percutaneous Endoscopic	**Z** No Device	**X** Diagnostic **Z** No Qualifier

tion 0 **Medical and Surgical**
dy System 3 **Upper Arteries**
eration C **Extirpation:** Taking or cutting out solid matter from a body part

Body Part (4th)	Approach (5th)	Device (6th)	Qualifier (7th)
Internal Mammary Artery, Right Internal Mammary Artery, Left Innominate Artery Subclavian Artery, Right Subclavian Artery, Left Axillary Artery, Right Axillary Artery, Left Brachial Artery, Right Brachial Artery, Left Ulnar Artery, Right Ulnar Artery, Left Radial Artery, Right Radial Artery, Left Hand Artery, Right Hand Artery, Left Face Artery Temporal Artery, Right Temporal Artery, Left Thyroid Artery, Right Thyroid Artery, Left Upper Artery	**0** Open **3** Percutaneous **4** Percutaneous Endoscopic	**Z** No Device	**6** Bifurcation **Z** No Qualifier

Continued →

Section 0 Medical and Surgical
Body System 3 Upper Arteries
Operation C Extirpation: Taking or cutting out solid matter from a body part

Body Part (4th)	Approach (5th)	Device (6th)	Qualifier (7th)
G Intracranial Artery H Common Carotid Artery, Right J Common Carotid Artery, Left K Internal Carotid Artery, Right L Internal Carotid Artery, Left M External Carotid Artery, Right N External Carotid Artery, Left P Vertebral Artery, Right Q Vertebral Artery, Left	0 Open 4 Percutaneous Endoscopic	Z No Device	**6** Bifurcation **Z** No Qualifier
G Intracranial Artery H Common Carotid Artery, Right J Common Carotid Artery, Left K Internal Carotid Artery, Right L Internal Carotid Artery, Left M External Carotid Artery, Right N External Carotid Artery, Left P Vertebral Artery, Right Q Vertebral Artery, Left	3 Percutaneous	Z No Device	**6** Bifurcation **7** Stent Retriever **Z** No Qualifier

Section 0 Medical and Surgical
Body System 3 Upper Arteries
Operation H Insertion: Putting in a nonbiological appliance that monitors, assists, performs, or prevents a physiological function but does not physically take the place of a body part

Body Part (4th)	Approach (5th)	Device (6th)	Qualifier (7th)
0 Internal Mammary Artery, Right **1** Internal Mammary Artery, Left **2** Innominate Artery **3** Subclavian Artery, Right **4** Subclavian Artery, Left **5** Axillary Artery, Right **6** Axillary Artery, Left **7** Brachial Artery, Right **8** Brachial Artery, Left **9** Ulnar Artery, Right **A** Ulnar Artery, Left **B** Radial Artery, Right **C** Radial Artery, Left **D** Hand Artery, Right **F** Hand Artery, Left **G** Intracranial Artery **H** Common Carotid Artery, Right **J** Common Carotid Artery, Left **M** External Carotid Artery, Right **N** External Carotid Artery, Left **P** Vertebral Artery, Right **Q** Vertebral Artery, Left **R** Face Artery **S** Temporal Artery, Right **T** Temporal Artery, Left **U** Thyroid Artery, Right **V** Thyroid Artery, Left	**0** Open **3** Percutaneous **4** Percutaneous Endoscopic	**3** Infusion Device **D** Intraluminal Device	**Z** No Qualifier
K Internal Carotid Artery, Right **L** Internal Carotid Artery, Left	**0** Open **3** Percutaneous **4** Percutaneous Endoscopic	**3** Infusion Device **D** Intraluminal Device **M** Stimulator Lead	**Z** No Qualifier
Y Upper Artery	**0** Open **3** Percutaneous **4** Percutaneous Endoscopic	**2** Monitoring Device **3** Infusion Device **D** Intraluminal Device **Y** Other Device	**Z** No Qualifier

ion 0 **Medical and Surgical**
y System 3 **Upper Arteries**
ration J **Inspection:** Visually and/or manually exploring a body part

Body Part (4th)	Approach (5th)	Device (6th)	Qualifier (7th)
Upper Artery	**0** Open **3** Percutaneous **4** Percutaneous Endoscopic **X** External	**Z** No Device	**Z** No Qualifier

tion 0 **Medical and Surgical**
y System 3 **Upper Arteries**
ration L **Occlusion:** Completely closing an orifice or the lumen of a tubular body part

Body Part (4th)	Approach (5th)	Device (6th)	Qualifier (7th)
Internal Mammary Artery, Right Internal Mammary Artery, Left Innominate Artery Subclavian Artery, Right Subclavian Artery, Left Axillary Artery, Right Axillary Artery, Left Brachial Artery, Right Brachial Artery, Left Ulnar Artery, Right Ulnar Artery, Left Radial Artery, Right Radial Artery, Left Hand Artery, Right Hand Artery, Left Face Artery Temporal Artery, Right Temporal Artery, Left Thyroid Artery, Right Thyroid Artery, Left Upper Artery	**0** Open **3** Percutaneous **4** Percutaneous Endoscopic	**C** Extraluminal Device **D** Intraluminal Device **Z** No Device	**Z** No Qualifier
Intracranial Artery Common Carotid Artery, Right Common Carotid Artery, Left Internal Carotid Artery, Right Internal Carotid Artery, Left External Carotid Artery, Right External Carotid Artery, Left Vertebral Artery, Right Vertebral Artery, Left	**0** Open **3** Percutaneous **4** Percutaneous Endoscopic	**B** Intraluminal Device, Bioactive **C** Extraluminal Device **D** Intraluminal Device **Z** No Device	**Z** No Qualifier

Section 0 **Medical and Surgical**
Body System 3 **Upper Arteries**
Operation N **Release:** Freeing a body part from an abnormal physical constraint by cutting or by the use of force

Body Part (4th)	Approach (5th)	Device (6th)	Qualifier (7th)
0 Internal Mammary Artery, Right **1** Internal Mammary Artery, Left **2** Innominate Artery **3** Subclavian Artery, Right **4** Subclavian Artery, Left **5** Axillary Artery, Right **6** Axillary Artery, Left **7** Brachial Artery, Right **8** Brachial Artery, Left **9** Ulnar Artery, Right **A** Ulnar Artery, Left **B** Radial Artery, Right **C** Radial Artery, Left **D** Hand Artery, Right **F** Hand Artery, Left **G** Intracranial Artery **H** Common Carotid Artery, Right **J** Common Carotid Artery, Left **K** Internal Carotid Artery, Right **L** Internal Carotid Artery, Left **M** External Carotid Artery, Right **N** External Carotid Artery, Left **P** Vertebral Artery, Right **Q** Vertebral Artery, Left **R** Face Artery **S** Temporal Artery, Right **T** Temporal Artery, Left **U** Thyroid Artery, Right **V** Thyroid Artery, Left **Y** Upper Artery	**0** Open **3** Percutaneous **4** Percutaneous Endoscopic	**Z** No Device	**Z** No Qualifier

Section 0 **Medical and Surgical**
Body System 3 **Upper Arteries**
Operation P **Removal:** Taking out or off a device from a body part

Body Part (4th)	Approach (5th)	Device (6th)	Qualifier (7th)
Y Upper Artery	**0** Open **3** Percutaneous **4** Percutaneous Endoscopic	**0** Drainage Device **2** Monitoring Device **3** Infusion Device **7** Autologous Tissue Substitute **C** Extraluminal Device **D** Intraluminal Device **J** Synthetic Substitute **K** Nonautologous Tissue Substitute **M** Stimulator Lead **Y** Other Device	**Z** No Qualifier
Y Upper Artery	**X** External	**0** Drainage Device **2** Monitoring Device **3** Infusion Device **D** Intraluminal Device **M** Stimulator Lead	**Z** No Qualifier

tion **0** **Medical and Surgical**
dy System **3** **Upper Arteries**
eration **Q** **Repair:** Restoring, to the extent possible, a body part to its normal anatomic structure and function

Body Part (4th)	Approach (5th)	Device (6th)	Qualifier (7th)
Internal Mammary Artery, Right Internal Mammary Artery, Left Innominate Artery Subclavian Artery, Right Subclavian Artery, Left Axillary Artery, Right Axillary Artery, Left Brachial Artery, Right Brachial Artery, Left Ulnar Artery, Right Ulnar Artery, Left Radial Artery, Right Radial Artery, Left Hand Artery, Right Hand Artery, Left Intracranial Artery Common Carotid Artery, Right Common Carotid Artery, Left Internal Carotid Artery, Right Internal Carotid Artery, Left External Carotid Artery, Right External Carotid Artery, Left Vertebral Artery, Right Vertebral Artery, Left Face Artery Temporal Artery, Right Temporal Artery, Left Thyroid Artery, Right Thyroid Artery, Left Upper Artery	**0** Open **3** Percutaneous **4** Percutaneous Endoscopic	**Z** No Device	**Z** No Qualifier

Section 0 **Medical and Surgical**
Body System 3 **Upper Arteries**
Operation R **Replacement:** Putting in or on biological or synthetic material that physically takes the place and/or function of all or a portion of a body part

Body Part (4th)	Approach (5th)	Device (6th)	Qualifier (7th)
0 Internal Mammary Artery, Right **1** Internal Mammary Artery, Left **2** Innominate Artery **3** Subclavian Artery, Right **4** Subclavian Artery, Left **5** Axillary Artery, Right **6** Axillary Artery, Left **7** Brachial Artery, Right **8** Brachial Artery, Left **9** Ulnar Artery, Right **A** Ulnar Artery, Left **B** Radial Artery, Right **C** Radial Artery, Left **D** Hand Artery, Right **F** Hand Artery, Left **G** Intracranial Artery **H** Common Carotid Artery, Right **J** Common Carotid Artery, Left **K** Internal Carotid Artery, Right **L** Internal Carotid Artery, Left **M** External Carotid Artery, Right **N** External Carotid Artery, Left **P** Vertebral Artery, Right **Q** Vertebral Artery, Left **R** Face Artery **S** Temporal Artery, Right **T** Temporal Artery, Left **U** Thyroid Artery, Right **V** Thyroid Artery, Left **Y** Upper Artery	**0** Open **4** Percutaneous Endoscopic	**7** Autologous Tissue Substitute **J** Synthetic Substitute **K** Nonautologous Tissue Substitute	**Z** No Qualifier

Section 0 **Medical and Surgical**
Body System 3 **Upper Arteries**
Operation S **Reposition:** Moving to its normal location, or other suitable location, all or a portion of a body part

Body Part (4th)	Approach (5th)	Device (6th)	Qualifier (7th)
0 Internal Mammary Artery, Right **1** Internal Mammary Artery, Left **2** Innominate Artery **3** Subclavian Artery, Right **4** Subclavian Artery, Left **5** Axillary Artery, Right **6** Axillary Artery, Left **7** Brachial Artery, Right **8** Brachial Artery, Left **9** Ulnar Artery, Right **A** Ulnar Artery, Left **B** Radial Artery, Right **C** Radial Artery, Left **D** Hand Artery, Right **F** Hand Artery, Left **G** Intracranial Artery **H** Common Carotid Artery, Right **J** Common Carotid Artery, Left **K** Internal Carotid Artery, Right **L** Internal Carotid Artery, Left **M** External Carotid Artery, Right **N** External Carotid Artery, Left **P** Vertebral Artery, Right **Q** Vertebral Artery, Left **R** Face Artery **S** Temporal Artery, Right **T** Temporal Artery, Left **U** Thyroid Artery, Right **V** Thyroid Artery, Left **Y** Upper Artery	**0** Open **3** Percutaneous **4** Percutaneous Endoscopic	**Z** No Device	**Z** No Qualifier

tion 0 **Medical and Surgical**
ly System 3 **Upper Arteries**
eration U **Supplement:** Putting in or on biological or synthetic material that physically reinforces and/or augments the function of a portion of a body part

Body Part (4th)	Approach (5th)	Device (6th)	Qualifier (7th)
Internal Mammary Artery, Right Internal Mammary Artery, Left Innominate Artery Subclavian Artery, Right Subclavian Artery, Left Axillary Artery, Right Axillary Artery, Left Brachial Artery, Right Brachial Artery, Left Ulnar Artery, Right Ulnar Artery, Left Radial Artery, Right Radial Artery, Left Hand Artery, Right Hand Artery, Left Intracranial Artery Common Carotid Artery, Right Common Carotid Artery, Left Internal Carotid Artery, Right Internal Carotid Artery, Left External Carotid Artery, Right External Carotid Artery, Left Vertebral Artery, Right Vertebral Artery, Left Face Artery Temporal Artery, Right Temporal Artery, Left Thyroid Artery, Right Thyroid Artery, Left Upper Artery	**0** Open **3** Percutaneous **4** Percutaneous Endoscopic	**7** Autologous Tissue Substitute **J** Synthetic Substitute **K** Nonautologous Tissue Substitute	**Z** No Qualifier

Section 0 **Medical and Surgical**
Body System 3 **Upper Arteries**
Operation V **Restriction:** Partially closing an orifice or the lumen of a tubular body part

Body Part (4th)	Approach (5th)	Device (6th)	Qualifier (7th)
0 Internal Mammary Artery, Right **1** Internal Mammary Artery, Left **2** Innominate Artery **3** Subclavian Artery, Right **4** Subclavian Artery, Left **5** Axillary Artery, Right **6** Axillary Artery, Left **7** Brachial Artery, Right **8** Brachial Artery, Left **9** Ulnar Artery, Right **A** Ulnar Artery, Left **B** Radial Artery, Right **C** Radial Artery, Left **D** Hand Artery, Right **F** Hand Artery, Left **R** Face Artery **S** Temporal Artery, Right **T** Temporal Artery, Left **U** Thyroid Artery, Right **V** Thyroid Artery, Left **Y** Upper Artery	**0** Open **3** Percutaneous **4** Percutaneous Endoscopic	**C** Extraluminal Device **D** Intraluminal Device **Z** No Device	**Z** No Qualifier
G Intracranial Artery **H** Common Carotid Artery, Right **J** Common Carotid Artery, Left **K** Internal Carotid Artery, Right **L** Internal Carotid Artery, Left **M** External Carotid Artery, Right **N** External Carotid Artery, Left **P** Vertebral Artery, Right **Q** Vertebral Artery, Left	**0** Open **3** Percutaneous **4** Percutaneous Endoscopic	**B** Intraluminal Device, Bioactive **C** Extraluminal Device **D** Intraluminal Device **Z** No Device	**Z** No Qualifier

Section 0 **Medical and Surgical**
Body System 3 **Upper Arteries**
Operation W **Revision:** Correcting, to the extent possible, a portion of a malfunctioning device or the position of a displaced device

Body Part (4th)	Approach (5th)	Device (6th)	Qualifier (7th)
Y Upper Artery	**0** Open **3** Percutaneous **4** Percutaneous Endoscopic	**0** Drainage Device **2** Monitoring Device **3** Infusion Device **7** Autologous Tissue Substitute **C** Extraluminal Device **D** Intraluminal Device **J** Synthetic Substitute **K** Nonautologous Tissue Substitute **M** Stimulator Lead **Y** Other Device	**Z** No Qualifier
Y Upper Artery	**X** External	**0** Drainage Device **2** Monitoring Device **3** Infusion Device **7** Autologous Tissue Substitute **C** Extraluminal Device **D** Intraluminal Device **J** Synthetic Substitute **K** Nonautologous Tissue Substitute **M** Neurostimulator Lead	**Z** No Qualifier

HA Coding Clinic

170ZD Bypass Right Brachial Artery to Upper Arm Vein, Open Approach—AHA CC: 4Q, 2013, 125-126

180JD Bypass Left Brachial Artery to Upper Arm Vein with Synthetic Substitute, Open Approach—AHA CC: 3Q, 2016, 37-38

1C0ZF Bypass Left Radial Artery to Lower Arm Vein, Open Approach—AHA CC: 1Q, 2013, 27-28

1J0JJ Bypass Left Common Carotid Artery to Right Extracranial Artery with Synthetic Substitute, Open Approach—AHA CC: 4Q, 17, 65

1J0ZK Bypass Left Common Carotid Artery to Left Extracranial Artery, Open Approach—AHA CC: 2Q, 2017, 22

BN0ZZ Excision of Left External Carotid Artery, Open Approach—AHA CC: 2Q, 2016, 12-14

CK0ZZ Extirpation of Matter from Right Internal Carotid Artery, Open Approach—AHA CC: 2Q, 2016, 11-12

CN0ZZ Extirpation of Matter from Left External Carotid Artery, Open Approach—AHA CC: 4Q, 2017, 65

HY32Z Insertion of Monitoring Device into Upper Artery, Percutaneous Approach—AHA CC: 2Q, 2016, 32-33

JY0ZZ Inspection of Upper Artery, Open Approach—AHA CC: 1Q, 2015, 29

LG0CZ Occlusion of Intracranial Artery with Extraluminal Device, Open Approach—AHA CC: 2Q, 2016, 30

LG3DZ Occlusion of Intracranial Artery with Intraluminal Device, Percutaneous Approach—AHA CC: 4Q, 2014, 37

QH0ZZ Repair Right Common Carotid Artery, Open Approach—AHA CC: 1Q, 2017, 31-32

SS0ZZ Reposition Right Temporal Artery, Open Approach—AHA CC: 3Q, 2015, 27-28

UK0JZ Supplement Right Internal Carotid Artery with Synthetic Substitute, Open Approach—AHA CC: 2Q, 2016, 11-12

VG3DZ Restriction of Intracranial Artery with Intraluminal Device, Percutaneous Approach—AHA CC: 1Q, 2016, 19-20

VM3DZ Restriction of Right External Carotid Artery with Intraluminal Device, Percutaneous Approach—AHA CC: 4Q, 2016, 26

WY0JZ Revision of Synthetic Substitute in Upper Artery, Open Approach—AHA CC: 3Q, 2016, 39-40

WY3DZ Revision of Intraluminal Device in Upper Artery, Percutaneous Approach—AHA CC: 1Q, 2015, 32-33

Arteries

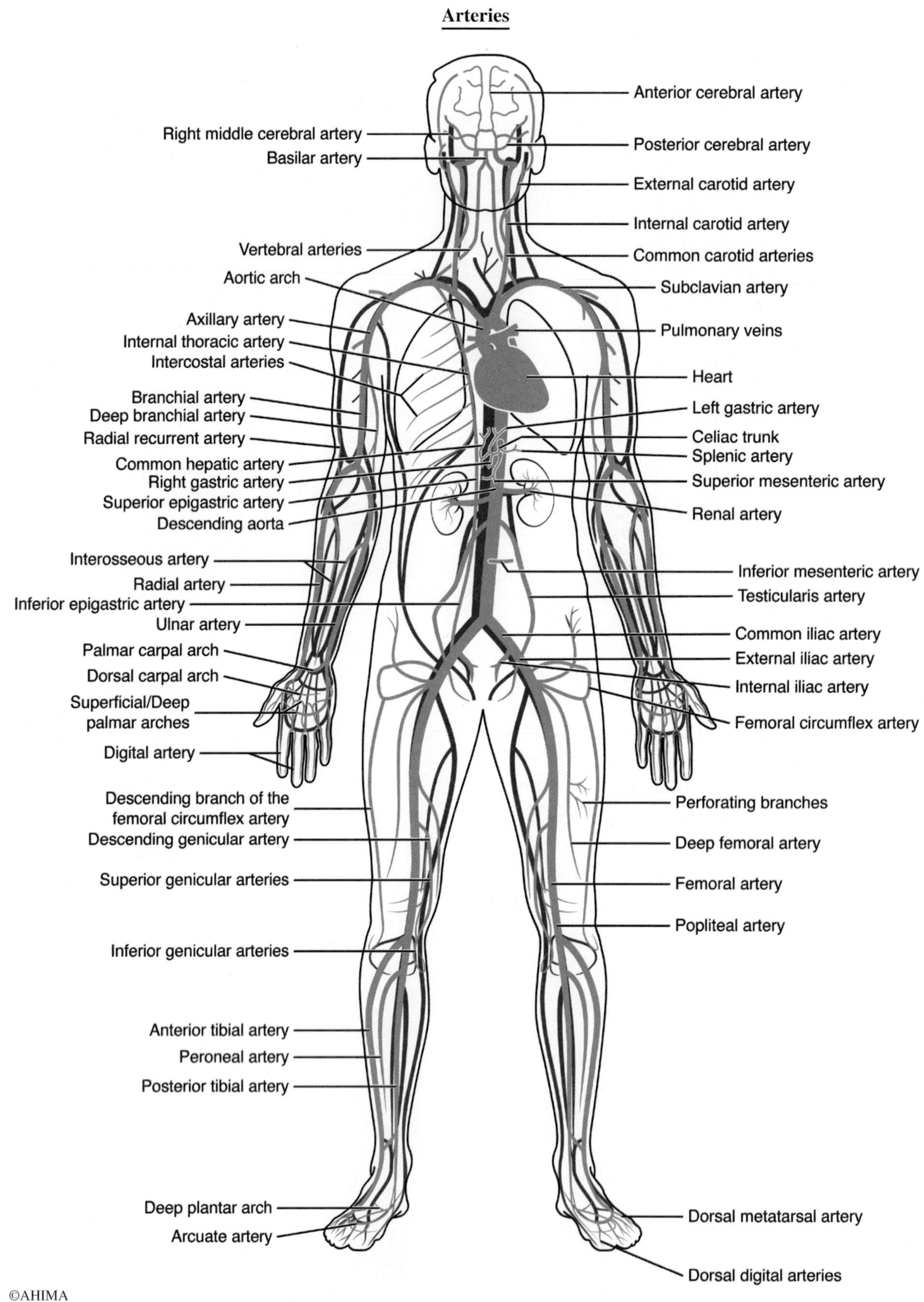

Anterior cerebral artery
Right middle cerebral artery
Posterior cerebral artery
Basilar artery
External carotid artery
Internal carotid artery
Vertebral arteries
Common carotid arteries
Aortic arch
Subclavian artery
Axillary artery
Pulmonary veins
Internal thoracic artery
Intercostal arteries
Heart
Branchial artery
Deep branchial artery
Left gastric artery
Radial recurrent artery
Celiac trunk
Splenic artery
Common hepatic artery
Right gastric artery
Superior mesenteric artery
Superior epigastric artery
Renal artery
Descending aorta
Interosseous artery
Inferior mesenteric artery
Radial artery
Testicularis artery
Inferior epigastric artery
Ulnar artery
Common iliac artery
Palmar carpal arch
External iliac artery
Dorsal carpal arch
Internal iliac artery
Superficial/Deep palmar arches
Femoral circumflex artery
Digital artery
Descending branch of the femoral circumflex artery
Perforating branches
Descending genicular artery
Deep femoral artery
Superior genicular arteries
Femoral artery
Popliteal artery
Inferior genicular arteries
Anterior tibial artery
Peroneal artery
Posterior tibial artery
Deep plantar arch
Dorsal metatarsal artery
Arcuate artery
Dorsal digital arteries

ction 0 **Medical and Surgical**
dy System 4 **Lower Arteries**
eration 1 **Bypass:** Altering the route of passage of the contents of a tubular body part

Body Part (4th)	Approach (5th)	Device (6th)	Qualifier (7th)
0 Abdominal Aorta **C** Common Iliac Artery, Right **D** Common Iliac Artery, Left	**0** Open **4** Percutaneous Endoscopic	**9** Autologous Venous Tissue **A** Autologous Arterial Tissue **J** Synthetic Substitute **K** Nonautologous Tissue Substitute **Z** No Device	**0** Abdominal Aorta **1** Celiac Artery **2** Mesenteric Artery **3** Renal Artery, Right **4** Renal Artery, Left **5** Renal Artery, Bilateral **6** Common Iliac Artery, Right **7** Common Iliac Artery, Left **8** Common Iliac Arteries, Bilateral **9** Internal Iliac Artery, Right **B** Internal Iliac Artery, Left **C** Internal Iliac Arteries, Bilateral **D** External Iliac Artery, Right **F** External Iliac Artery, Left **G** External Iliac Arteries, Bilateral **H** Femoral Artery, Right **J** Femoral Artery, Left **K** Femoral Arteries, Bilateral **Q** Lower Extremity Artery **R** Lower Artery
3 Hepatic Artery **4** Splenic Artery	**0** Open **4** Percutaneous Endoscopic	**9** Autologous Venous Tissue **A** Autologous Arterial Tissue **J** Synthetic Substitute **K** Nonautologous Tissue Substitute **Z** No Device	**3** Renal Artery, Right **4** Renal Artery, Left **5** Renal Artery, Bilateral
E Internal Iliac Artery, Right **F** Internal Iliac Artery, Left **H** External Iliac Artery, Right **J** External Iliac Artery, Left	**0** Open **4** Percutaneous Endoscopic	**9** Autologous Venous Tissue **A** Autologous Arterial Tissue **J** Synthetic Substitute **K** Nonautologous Tissue Substitute **Z** No Device	**9** Internal Iliac Artery, Right **B** Internal Iliac Artery, Left **C** Internal Iliac Arteries, Bilateral **D** External Iliac Artery, Right **F** External Iliac Artery, Left **G** External Iliac Arteries, Bilateral **H** Femoral Artery, Right **J** Femoral Artery, Left **K** Femoral Arteries, Bilateral **P** Foot Artery **Q** Lower Extremity Artery
K Femoral Artery, Right **L** Femoral Artery, Left	**0** Open **4** Percutaneous Endoscopic	**9** Autologous Venous Tissue **A** Autologous Arterial Tissue **J** Synthetic Substitute **K** Nonautologous Tissue Substitute **Z** No Device	**H** Femoral Artery, Right **J** Femoral Artery, Left **K** Femoral Arteries, Bilateral **L** Popliteal Artery **M** Peroneal Artery **N** Posterior Tibial Artery **P** Foot Artery **Q** Lower Extremity Artery **S** Lower Extremity Vein
K Femoral Artery, Right **L** Femoral Artery, Left	**3** Percutaneous	**J** Synthetic Substitute	**Q** Lower Extremity Artery **S** Lower Extremity Vein
M Popliteal Artery, Right **N** Popliteal Artery, Left	**0** Open **4** Percutaneous Endoscopic	**9** Autologous Venous Tissue **A** Autologous Arterial Tissue **J** Synthetic Substitute **K** Nonautologous Tissue Substitute **Z** No Device	**L** Popliteal Artery **M** Peroneal Artery **P** Foot Artery **Q** Lower Extremity Artery **S** Lower Extremity Vein

Continued →

041 Continued

Section 0 **Medical and Surgical**
Body System 4 **Lower Arteries**
Operation 1 **Bypass:** Altering the route of passage of the contents of a tubular body part

Body Part (4th)	Approach (5th)	Device (6th)	Qualifier (7th)
M Popliteal Artery, Right **N** Popliteal Artery, Left	**3** Percutaneous	**J** Synthetic Substitute	**Q** Lower Extremity Artery **S** Lower Extremity Vein
P Anterior Tibial Artery, Right **Q** Anterior Tibial Artery, Left **R** Posterior Tibial Artery, Right **S** Posterior Tibial Artery, Left	**0** Open **3** Percutaneou **4** Percutaneous Endoscopic	**J** Synthetic Substitute	**Q** Lower Extremity Artery **S** Lower Extremity Vein
T Peroneal Artery, Right **U** Peroneal Artery, Left **V** Foot Artery, Right **W** Foot Artery, Left	**0** Open **4** Percutaneous Endoscopic	**9** Autologous Venous Tissue **A** Autologous Arterial Tissue **J** Synthetic Substitute **K** Nonautologous Tissue Substitute **Z** No Device	**P** Foot Artery **Q** Lower Extremity Artery **S** Lower Extremity Vein
T Peroneal Artery, Right **U** Peroneal Artery, Left **V** Foot Artery, Right **W** Foot Artery, Left	**3** Percutaneous	**J** Synthetic Substitute	**Q** Lower Extremity Artery **S** Lower Extremity Vein

Section 0 **Medical and Surgical**
Body System 4 **Lower Arteries**
Operation 5 **Destruction:** Physical eradication of all or a portion of a body part by the direct use of energy, force, or a destructive agent

Body Part (4th)	Approach (5th)	Device (6th)	Qualifier (7th)
0 Abdominal Aorta **1** Celiac Artery **2** Gastric Artery **3** Hepatic Artery **4** Splenic Artery **5** Superior Mesenteric Artery **6** Colic Artery, Right **7** Colic Artery, Left **8** Colic Artery, Middle **9** Renal Artery, Right **A** Renal Artery, Left **B** Inferior Mesenteric Artery **C** Common Iliac Artery, Right **D** Common Iliac Artery, Left **E** Internal Iliac Artery, Right **F** Internal Iliac Artery, Left **H** External Iliac Artery, Right **J** External Iliac Artery, Left **K** Femoral Artery, Right **L** Femoral Artery, Left **M** Popliteal Artery, Right **N** Popliteal Artery, Left **P** Anterior Tibial Artery, Right **Q** Anterior Tibial Artery, Left **R** Posterior Tibial Artery, Right **S** Posterior Tibial Artery, Left **T** Peroneal Artery, Right **U** Peroneal Artery, Left **V** Foot Artery, Right **W** Foot Artery, Left **Y** Lower Artery	**0** Open **3** Percutaneous **4** Percutaneous Endoscopic	**Z** No Device	**Z** No Qualifier

tion **0** **Medical and Surgical**
ly System **4** **Lower Arteries**
eration **7** **Dilation:** Expanding an orifice or the lumen of a tubular body part

Body Part (4th)	Approach (5th)	Device (6th)	Qualifier (7th)
Abdominal Aorta Celiac Artery Gastric Artery Hepatic Artery Splenic Artery Superior Mesenteric Artery Colic Artery, Right Colic Artery, Left Colic Artery, Middle Renal Artery, Right Renal Artery, Left Inferior Mesenteric Artery Common Iliac Artery, Right Common Iliac Artery, Left Internal Iliac Artery, Right Internal Iliac Artery, Left External Iliac Artery, Right External Iliac Artery, Left Femoral Artery, Right Femoral Artery, Left Popliteal Artery, Right Popliteal Artery, Left Anterior Tibial Artery, Right Anterior Tibial Artery, Left Posterior Tibial Artery, Right Posterior Tibial Artery, Left Peroneal Artery, Right Peroneal Artery, Left Foot Artery, Right Foot Artery, Left Lower Artery	**0** Open **3** Percutaneous **4** Percutaneous Endoscopic	**4** Intraluminal Device, Drug-eluting **D** Intraluminal Device **Z** No Device	**1** Drug-Coated Balloon **6** Bifurcation **Z** No Qualifier
Abdominal Aorta Celiac Artery Gastric Artery Hepatic Artery Splenic Artery Superior Mesenteric Artery Colic Artery, Right Colic Artery, Left Colic Artery, Middle Renal Artery, Right Renal Artery, Left Inferior Mesenteric Artery Common Iliac Artery, Right Common Iliac Artery, Left Internal Iliac Artery, Right Internal Iliac Artery, Left External Iliac Artery, Right External Iliac Artery, Left Femoral Artery, Right Femoral Artery, Left Popliteal Artery, Right Popliteal Artery, Left Anterior Tibial Artery, Right Anterior Tibial Artery, Left Posterior Tibial Artery, Right Posterior Tibial Artery, Left Peroneal Artery, Right Peroneal Artery, Left Foot Artery, Right Foot Artery, Left Lower Artery	**0** Open **3** Percutaneous **4** Percutaneous Endoscopic	**5** Intraluminal Device, Drug-eluting, Two **6** Intraluminal Device, Drug-eluting, Three **7** Intraluminal Device, Drug-eluting, Four or More **E** Intraluminal Devices, Two **F** Intraluminal Devices, Three **G** Intraluminal Devices, Four or More	**6** Bifurcation **Z** No Qualifier

Section 0 **Medical and Surgical**
Body System 4 **Lower Arteries**
Operation 9 **Drainage:** Taking or letting out fluids and/or gases from a body part

Body Part (4th)	Approach (5th)	Device (6th)	Qualifier (7th)
0 Abdominal Aorta **1** Celiac Artery **2** Gastric Artery **3** Hepatic Artery **4** Splenic Artery **5** Superior Mesenteric Artery **6** Colic Artery, Right **7** Colic Artery, Left **8** Colic Artery, Middle **9** Renal Artery, Right **A** Renal Artery, Left **B** Inferior Mesenteric Artery **C** Common Iliac Artery, Right **D** Common Iliac Artery, Left **E** Internal Iliac Artery, Right **F** Internal Iliac Artery, Left **H** External Iliac Artery, Right **J** External Iliac Artery, Left **K** Femoral Artery, Right **L** Femoral Artery, Left **M** Popliteal Artery, Right **N** Popliteal Artery, Left **P** Anterior Tibial Artery, Right **Q** Anterior Tibial Artery, Left **R** Posterior Tibial Artery, Right **S** Posterior Tibial Artery, Left **T** Peroneal Artery, Right **U** Peroneal Artery, Left **V** Foot Artery, Right **W** Foot Artery, Left **Y** Lower Artery	**0** Open **3** Percutaneous **4** Percutaneous Endoscopic	**0** Drainage Device	**Z** No Qualifier
0 Abdominal Aorta **1** Celiac Artery **2** Gastric Artery **3** Hepatic Artery **4** Splenic Artery **5** Superior Mesenteric Artery **6** Colic Artery, Right **7** Colic Artery, Left **8** Colic Artery, Middle **9** Renal Artery, Right **A** Renal Artery, Left **B** Inferior Mesenteric Artery **C** Common Iliac Artery, Right **D** Common Iliac Artery, Left **E** Internal Iliac Artery, Right **F** Internal Iliac Artery, Left **H** External Iliac Artery, Right **J** External Iliac Artery, Left **K** Femoral Artery, Right **L** Femoral Artery, Left **M** Popliteal Artery, Right **N** Popliteal Artery, Left **P** Anterior Tibial Artery, Right **Q** Anterior Tibial Artery, Left **R** Posterior Tibial Artery, Right **S** Posterior Tibial Artery, Left **T** Peroneal Artery, Right **U** Peroneal Artery, Left **V** Foot Artery, Right **W** Foot Artery, Left **Y** Lower Artery	**0** Open **3** Percutaneous **4** Percutaneous Endoscopic	**Z** No Device	**X** Diagnostic **Z** No Qualifier

Section	**0**	**Medical and Surgical**
Body System	**4**	**Lower Arteries**
Operation	**B**	**Excision:** Cutting out or off, without replacement, a portion of a body part

Body Part (4th)	Approach (5th)	Device (6th)	Qualifier (7th)
0 Abdominal Aorta **1** Celiac Artery **2** Gastric Artery **3** Hepatic Artery **4** Splenic Artery **5** Superior Mesenteric Artery **6** Colic Artery, Right **7** Colic Artery, Left **8** Colic Artery, Middle **9** Renal Artery, Right **A** Renal Artery, Left **B** Inferior Mesenteric Artery **C** Common Iliac Artery, Right **D** Common Iliac Artery, Left **E** Internal Iliac Artery, Right **F** Internal Iliac Artery, Left **H** External Iliac Artery, Right **J** External Iliac Artery, Left **K** Femoral Artery, Right **L** Femoral Artery, Left **M** Popliteal Artery, Right **N** Popliteal Artery, Left **P** Anterior Tibial Artery, Right **Q** Anterior Tibial Artery, Left **R** Posterior Tibial Artery, Right **S** Posterior Tibial Artery, Left **T** Peroneal Artery, Right **U** Peroneal Artery, Left **V** Foot Artery, Right **W** Foot Artery, Left **Y** Lower Artery	**0** Open **3** Percutaneous **4** Percutaneous Endoscopic	**Z** No Device	**X** Diagnostic **Z** No Qualifier

Section 0 **Medical and Surgical**
Body System 4 **Lower Arteries**
Operation C **Extirpation:** Taking or cutting out solid matter from a body part

Body Part (4th)	Approach (5th)	Device (6th)	Qualifier (7th)
0 Abdominal Aorta **1** Celiac Artery **2** Gastric Artery **3** Hepatic Artery **4** Splenic Artery **5** Superior Mesenteric Artery **6** Colic Artery, Right **7** Colic Artery, Left **8** Colic Artery, Middle **9** Renal Artery, Right **A** Renal Artery, Left **B** Inferior Mesenteric Artery **C** Common Iliac Artery, Right **D** Common Iliac Artery, Left **E** Internal Iliac Artery, Right **F** Internal Iliac Artery, Left **H** External Iliac Artery, Right **J** External Iliac Artery, Left **K** Femoral Artery, Right **L** Femoral Artery, Left **M** Popliteal Artery, Right **N** Popliteal Artery, Left **P** Anterior Tibial Artery, Right **Q** Anterior Tibial Artery, Left **R** Posterior Tibial Artery, Right **S** Posterior Tibial Artery, Left **T** Peroneal Artery, Right **U** Peroneal Artery, Left **V** Foot Artery, Right **W** Foot Artery, Left **Y** Lower Artery	**0** Open **3** Percutaneous **4** Percutaneous Endoscopic	**Z** No Device	**6** Bifurcation **Z** No Qualifier

Section 0 **Medical and Surgical**
Body System 4 **Lower Arteries**
Operation H **Insertion:** Putting in a nonbiological appliance that monitors, assists, performs, or prevents a physiological function but does not physically take the place of a body part

Body Part (4th)	Approach (5th)	Device (6th)	Qualifier (7th)
0 Abdominal Aorta	**0** Open **3** Percutaneous **4** Percutaneous Endoscopic	**2** Monitoring Device **3** Infusion Device **D** Intraluminal Device	**Z** No Qualifier

Continued →

tion	**0**	**Medical and Surgical**
ly System	**4**	**Lower Arteries**
eration	**H**	**Insertion:** Putting in a nonbiological appliance that monitors, assists, performs, or prevents a physiological function but does not physically take the place of a body part

Body Part (4th)	Approach (5th)	Device (6th)	Qualifier (7th)
Celiac Artery Gastric Artery Hepatic Artery Splenic Artery Superior Mesenteric Artery Colic Artery, Right Colic Artery, Left Colic Artery, Middle Renal Artery, Right Renal Artery, Left Inferior Mesenteric Artery Common Iliac Artery, Right Common Iliac Artery, Left Internal Iliac Artery, Right Internal Iliac Artery, Left External Iliac Artery, Right External Iliac Artery, Left Femoral Artery, Right Femoral Artery, Left I Popliteal Artery, Right Popliteal Artery, Left Anterior Tibial Artery, Right Anterior Tibial Artery, Left Posterior Tibial Artery, Right Posterior Tibial Artery, Left Peroneal Artery, Right Peroneal Artery, Left Foot Artery, Right V Foot Artery, Left	**0** Open **3** Percutaneous **4** Percutaneous Endoscopic	**3** Infusion Device **D** Intraluminal Device	**Z** No Qualifier
Lower Artery	**0** Open **3** Percutaneous **4** Percutaneous Endoscopic	**2** Monitoring Device **3** Infusion Device **D** Intraluminal Device **Y** Other Device	**Z** No Qualifier

tion	**0**	**Medical and Surgical**
ly System	**4**	**Lower Arteries**
eration	**J**	**Inspection:** Visually and/or manually exploring a body part

Body Part (4th)	Approach (5th)	Device (6th)	Qualifier (7th)
Lower Artery	**0** Open **3** Percutaneous **4** Percutaneous Endoscopic **X** External	**Z** No Device	**Z** No Qualifier

Section 0 **Medical and Surgical**
Body System 4 **Lower Arteries**
Operation L **Occlusion:** Completely closing an orifice or the lumen of a tubular body part

Body Part (4th)	Approach (5th)	Device (6th)	Qualifier (7th)
0 Abdominal Aorta	**0** Open **4** Percutaneous Endoscopic	**C** Extraluminal Device **D** Intraluminal Device **Z** No Device	**Z** No Qualifier
0 Abdominal Aorta	**3** Percutaneous	**C** Extraluminal Device **Z** No Device	**Z** No Qualifier
0 Abdominal Aorta	**3** Percutaneous	**D** Intraluminal Device	**J** Temporary **Z** No Qualifier
1 Celiac Artery **2** Gastric Artery **3** Hepatic Artery **4** Splenic Artery **5** Superior Mesenteric Artery **6** Colic Artery, Right **7** Colic Artery, Left **8** Colic Artery, Middle **9** Renal Artery, Right **A** Renal Artery, Left **B** Inferior Mesenteric Artery **C** Common Iliac Artery, Right **D** Common Iliac Artery, Left **H** External Iliac Artery, Right **J** External Iliac Artery, Left **K** Femoral Artery, Right **L** Femoral Artery, Left **M** Popliteal Artery, Right **N** Popliteal Artery, Left **P** Anterior Tibial Artery, Right **Q** Anterior Tibial Artery, Left **R** Posterior Tibial Artery, Right **S** Posterior Tibial Artery, Left **T** Peroneal Artery, Right **U** Peroneal Artery, Left **V** Foot Artery, Right **W** Foot Artery, Left **Y** Lower Artery	**0** Open **3** Percutaneous **4** Percutaneous Endoscopic	**C** Extraluminal Device **D** Intraluminal Device **Z** No Device	**Z** No Qualifier
E Internal Iliac Artery, Right	**0** Open **3** Percutaneous **4** Percutaneous Endoscopic	**C** Extraluminal Device **D** Intraluminal Device **Z** No Device	**T** Uterine Artery, Right **Z** No Qualifier
F Internal Iliac Artery, Left	**0** Open **3** Percutaneous **4** Percutaneous Endoscopic	**C** Extraluminal Device **D** Intraluminal Device **Z** No Device	**U** Uterine Artery, Left **Z** No Qualifier

tion **0** **Medical and Surgical**
ly System **4** **Lower Arteries**
eration **N** **Release:** Freeing a body part from an abnormal physical constraint by cutting or by the use of force

Body Part (4th)	Approach (5th)	Device (6th)	Qualifier (7th)
Abdominal Aorta Celiac Artery Gastric Artery Hepatic Artery Splenic Artery Superior Mesenteric Artery Colic Artery, Right Colic Artery, Left Colic Artery, Middle Renal Artery, Right Renal Artery, Left Inferior Mesenteric Artery Common Iliac Artery, Right Common Iliac Artery, Left Internal Iliac Artery, Right Internal Iliac Artery, Left External Iliac Artery, Right External Iliac Artery, Left Femoral Artery, Right Femoral Artery, Left Popliteal Artery, Right Popliteal Artery, Left Anterior Tibial Artery, Right Anterior Tibial Artery, Left Posterior Tibial Artery, Right Posterior Tibial Artery, Left Peroneal Artery, Right Peroneal Artery, Left Foot Artery, Right Foot Artery, Left Lower Artery	**0** Open **3** Percutaneous **4** Percutaneous Endoscopic	**Z** No Device	**Z** No Qualifier

tion **0** **Medical and Surgical**
dy System **4** **Lower Arteries**
eration **P** **Removal:** Taking out or off a device from a body part

Body Part (4th)	Approach (5th)	Device (6th)	Qualifier (7th)
Lower Artery	**0** Open **3** Percutaneous **4** Percutaneous Endoscopic	**0** Drainage Device **2** Monitoring Device **3** Infusion Device **7** Autologous Tissue Substitute **C** Extraluminal Device **D** Intraluminal Device **J** Synthetic Substitute **K** Nonautologous Tissue Substitute **Y** Other Device	**Z** No Qualifier
Lower Artery	**X** External	**0** Drainage Device **1** Radioactive Element **2** Monitoring Device **3** Infusion Device **D** Intraluminal Device	**Z** No Qualifier

Section **0** **Medical and Surgical**
Body System **4** **Lower Arteries**
Operation **Q** **Repair:** Restoring, to the extent possible, a body part to its normal anatomic structure and function

Body Part (4th)	Approach (5th)	Device (6th)	Qualifier (7th)
0 Abdominal Aorta **1** Celiac Artery **2** Gastric Artery **3** Hepatic Artery **4** Splenic Artery **5** Superior Mesenteric Artery **6** Colic Artery, Right **7** Colic Artery, Left **8** Colic Artery, Middle **9** Renal Artery, Right **A** Renal Artery, Left **B** Inferior Mesenteric Artery **C** Common Iliac Artery, Right **D** Common Iliac Artery, Left **E** Internal Iliac Artery, Right **F** Internal Iliac Artery, Left **H** External Iliac Artery, Right **J** External Iliac Artery, Left **K** Femoral Artery, Right **L** Femoral Artery, Left **M** Popliteal Artery, Right **N** Popliteal Artery, Left **P** Anterior Tibial Artery, Right **Q** Anterior Tibial Artery, Left **R** Posterior Tibial Artery, Right **S** Posterior Tibial Artery, Left **T** Peroneal Artery, Right **U** Peroneal Artery, Left **V** Foot Artery, Right **W** Foot Artery, Left **Y** Lower Artery	**0** Open **3** Percutaneous **4** Percutaneous Endoscopic	**Z** No Device	**Z** No Qualifier

ction	**0**	**Medical and Surgical**
dy System	**4**	**Lower Arteries**
eration	**R**	**Replacement:** Putting in or on biological or synthetic material that physically takes the place and/or function of all or a portion of a body part

Body Part (4th)	Approach (5th)	Device (6th)	Qualifier (7th)
0 Abdominal Aorta **1** Celiac Artery **2** Gastric Artery **3** Hepatic Artery **4** Splenic Artery **5** Superior Mesenteric Artery **6** Colic Artery, Right **7** Colic Artery, Left **8** Colic Artery, Middle **9** Renal Artery, Right **A** Renal Artery, Left **B** Inferior Mesenteric Artery **C** Common Iliac Artery, Right **D** Common Iliac Artery, Left **E** Internal Iliac Artery, Right **F** Internal Iliac Artery, Left **H** External Iliac Artery, Right **J** External Iliac Artery, Left **K** Femoral Artery, Right **L** Femoral Artery, Left **M** Popliteal Artery, Right **N** Popliteal Artery, Left **P** Anterior Tibial Artery, Right **Q** Anterior Tibial Artery, Left **R** Posterior Tibial Artery, Right **S** Posterior Tibial Artery, Left **T** Peroneal Artery, Right **U** Peroneal Artery, Left **V** Foot Artery, Right **W** Foot Artery, Left **Y** Lower Artery	**0** Open **4** Percutaneous Endoscopic	**7** Autologous Tissue Substitute **J** Synthetic Substitute **K** Nonautologous Tissue Substitute	**Z** No Qualifier

Section **0** **Medical and Surgical**
Body System **4** **Lower Arteries**
Operation **S** **Reposition:** Moving to its normal location, or other suitable location, all or a portion of a body part

Body Part (4th)	Approach (5th)	Device (6th)	Qualifier (7th)
0 Abdominal Aorta **1** Celiac Artery **2** Gastric Artery **3** Hepatic Artery **4** Splenic Artery **5** Superior Mesenteric Artery **6** Colic Artery, Right **7** Colic Artery, Left **8** Colic Artery, Middle **9** Renal Artery, Right **A** Renal Artery, Left **B** Inferior Mesenteric Artery **C** Common Iliac Artery, Right **D** Common Iliac Artery, Left **E** Internal Iliac Artery, Right **F** Internal Iliac Artery, Left **H** External Iliac Artery, Right **J** External Iliac Artery, Left **K** Femoral Artery, Right **L** Femoral Artery, Left **M** Popliteal Artery, Right **N** Popliteal Artery, Left **P** Anterior Tibial Artery, Right **Q** Anterior Tibial Artery, Left **R** Posterior Tibial Artery, Right **S** Posterior Tibial Artery, Left **T** Peroneal Artery, Right **U** Peroneal Artery, Left **V** Foot Artery, Right **W** Foot Artery, Left **Y** Lower Artery	**0** Open **3** Percutaneous **4** Percutaneous Endoscopic	**Z** No Device	**Z** No Qualifier

tion 0 **Medical and Surgical**
ly System 4 **Lower Arteries**
ration U **Supplement:** Putting in or on biological or synthetic material that physically reinforces and/or augments the function of a portion of a body part

Body Part (4th)	Approach (5th)	Device (6th)	Qualifier (7th)
Abdominal Aorta Celiac Artery Gastric Artery Hepatic Artery Splenic Artery Superior Mesenteric Artery Colic Artery, Right Colic Artery, Left Colic Artery, Middle Renal Artery, Right Renal Artery, Left Inferior Mesenteric Artery Common Iliac Artery, Right Common Iliac Artery, Left Internal Iliac Artery, Right Internal Iliac Artery, Left External Iliac Artery, Right External Iliac Artery, Left Femoral Artery, Right Femoral Artery, Left Popliteal Artery, Right Popliteal Artery, Left Anterior Tibial Artery, Right Anterior Tibial Artery, Left Posterior Tibial Artery, Right Posterior Tibial Artery, Left Peroneal Artery, Right Peroneal Artery, Left Foot Artery, Right Foot Artery, Left Lower Artery	**0** Open **3** Percutaneous **4** Percutaneous Endoscopic	**7** Autologous Tissue Substitute **J** Synthetic Substitute **K** Nonautologous Tissue Substitute	**Z** No Qualifier

tion 0 **Medical and Surgical**
dy System 4 **Lower Arteries**
eration V **Restriction:** Partially closing an orifice or the lumen of a tubular body part

Body Part (4th)	Approach (5th)	Device (6th)	Qualifier (7th)
Abdominal Aorta	**0** Open **3** Percutaneous **4** Percutaneous Endoscopic	**C** Extraluminal Device **E** Intraluminal Device, Branched or Fenestrated, One or Two Arteries **F** Intraluminal Device, Branched or Fenestrated, Three or More Arteries **Z** No Device	**6** Bifurcation **Z** No Qualifier
Abdominal Aorta	**0** Open **3** Percutaneous **4** Percutaneous Endoscopic	**D** Intraluminal Device	**6** Bifurcation **J** Temporary **Z** No Qualifier

Continued →

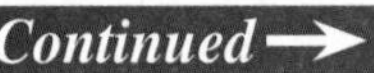

Section 0 **Medical and Surgical**
Body System 4 **Lower Arteries**
Operation V **Restriction:** Partially closing an orifice or the lumen of a tubular body part

Body Part (4th)	Approach (5th)	Device (6th)	Qualifier (7th)
1 Celiac Artery **2** Gastric Artery **3** Hepatic Artery **4** Splenic Artery **5** Superior Mesenteric Artery **6** Colic Artery, Right **7** Colic Artery, Left **8** Colic Artery, Middle **9** Renal Artery, Right **A** Renal Artery, Left **B** Inferior Mesenteric Artery **E** Internal Iliac Artery, Right **F** Internal Iliac Artery, Left **H** External Iliac Artery, Right **J** External Iliac Artery, Left **K** Femoral Artery, Right **L** Femoral Artery, Left **M** Popliteal Artery, Right **N** Popliteal Artery, Left **P** Anterior Tibial Artery, Right **Q** Anterior Tibial Artery, Left **R** Posterior Tibial Artery, Right **S** Posterior Tibial Artery, Left **T** Peroneal Artery, Right **U** Peroneal Artery, Left **V** Foot Artery, Right **W** Foot Artery, Left **Y** Lower Artery	**0** Open **3** Percutaneous **4** Percutaneous Endoscopic	**C** Extraluminal Device **D** Intraluminal Device **Z** No Device	**Z** No Qualifier
C Common Iliac Artery, Right **D** Common Iliac Artery, Left	**0** Open **3** Percutaneous **4** Percutaneous Endoscopic	**C** Extraluminal Device **D** Intraluminal Device **E** Intraluminal Device, Branched or Fenestrated, One or Two Arteries **Z** No Device	**Z** No Qualifier

Section 0 **Medical and Surgical**
Body System 4 **Lower Arteries**
Operation W **Revision:** Correcting, to the extent possible, a portion of a malfunctioning device or the position of a displaced device

Body Part (4th)	Approach (5th)	Device (6th)	Qualifier (7th)
Y Lower Artery	**0** Open **3** Percutaneous **4** Percutaneous Endoscopic	**0** Drainage Device **2** Monitoring Device **3** Infusion Device **7** Autologous Tissue Substitute **C** Extraluminal Device **D** Intraluminal Device **J** Synthetic Substitute **K** Nonautologous Tissue Substitute **Y** Other Device	**Z** No Qualifier
Y Lower Artery	**X** External	**0** Drainage Device **2** Monitoring Device **3** Infusion Device **7** Autologous Tissue Substitute **C** Extraluminal Device **D** Intraluminal Device **J** Synthetic Substitute **K** Nonautologus Tissue Substitute	**Z** No Qualifier

100Z3 Bypass Abdominal Aorta to Right Renal Artery, Open Approach—AHA CC: 3Q, 2015, 28

130Z3 Bypass Hepatic Artery to Right Renal Artery, Open Approach— AHA CC: 4Q, 2017, 47

140Z4 Bypass Splenic Artery to Left Renal Artery, Open Approach—AHA CC: 3Q, 2015, 28; 4Q, 2017, 47

1C0J2 Bypass Right Common Iliac Artery to Mesenteric Artery with Synthetic Substitute, Open Approach— AHA CC: 3Q, 2017, 16

1C0J5 Bypass Right Common Iliac Artery to Bilateral Renal Artery with Synthetic Substitute, Open Approach— AHA CC: 3Q, 2017, 16

1K09N Bypass Right Femoral Artery to Posterior Tibial Artery with Autologous Venous Tissue, Open Approach—AHA CC: 3Q, 2017, 5-6

1K0JN Bypass Right Femoral Artery to Posterior Tibial Artery with Synthetic Substitute, Open Approach—AHA CC: 2Q, 2016, 18-19;), 2017, 5-6

1M09P Bypass Right Popliteal Artery to Foot Artery with Autologous Venous Tissue, Open Approach—AHA CC: 1Q, 2017, 32-33

7K3D1 Dilation of Right Femoral Artery with Intraluminal Device, using Drug-Coated Balloon, Percutaneous Approach—AHA CC: 4Q, 2015, 7,15

7K3Z6 Dilation of Right Femoral Artery, Bifurcation, Percutaneous Approach—AHA CC: 4Q, 2016, 88-89

7L3Z1 Dilation of Left Femoral Artery using Drug-Coated Balloon, Percutaneous Approach—AHA CC: 4Q, 2015, 15

CJ0ZZ Extirpation of Matter from Left External Iliac Artery, Open Approach—AHA CC: 1Q, 2016, 31

CK3Z6 Extirpation of Matter from Right Femoral Artery, Bifurcation, Percutaneous Approach—AHA CC: 4Q, 2016, 88-89

CL3ZZ Extirpation of Matter from Left Femoral Artery, Percutaneous Approach—AHA CC: 1Q, 2015, 36

HY32Z Insertion of Monitoring Device into Lower Artery, Percutaneous Approach—AHA CC: 1Q, 2017, 30

L33DZ Occlusion of Hepatic Artery with Intraluminal Device, Percutaneous Approach—AHA CC: 3Q, 2014, 26-27

L73DZ Occlusion of Left Colic Artery with Intraluminal Device, Percutaneous Approach—AHA CC: 1Q, 2014, 24

LB3DZ Occlusion of Inferior Mesenteric Artery with Intraluminal Device, Percutaneous Approach—AHA CC: 1Q, 2014, 24

LE3DT Occlusion of Right Uterine Artery with Intraluminal Device, Percutaneous Approach—AHA CC: 2Q, 2015, 27

LH0CZ Occlusion of Right External Iliac Artery with Extraluminal Device, Open Approach—AHA CC: 2Q, 2018, 18-19

LJ0CZ Occlusion of Left External Iliac Artery with Extraluminal Device, Open Approach—AHA CC: 2Q, 2018, 18-19

N10ZZ Release Celiac Artery, Open Approach—AHA CC: 2Q, 2015, 28

QK0ZZ Repair Right Femoral Artery, Open Approach—AHA CC: 1Q, 2014, 21-22

R10JZ Replacement of Celiac Artery with Synthetic Substitute, Open Approach—AHA CC: 2Q, 2015, 28

UJ0KZ Supplement Left External Iliac Artery with Nonautologous Tissue Substitute, Open Approach—AHA CC: 1Q, 2016, 31

UK0KZ Supplement Right Femoral Artery with Nonautologous Tissue Substitute, Open Approach—AHA CC: 4Q, 2014, 37-38

UK3JZ Supplement Right Femoral Artery with Synthetic Substitute, Percutaneous Approach—AHA CC: 1Q, 2014, 22-23

UR07Z Supplement Right Posterior Tibial Artery with Autologous Tissue Substitute, Open Approach—AHA CC: 2Q, 2016, 18-19

V03DZ Restriction of Abdominal Aorta with Intraluminal Device, Percutaneous Approach—AHA CC: 1Q, 2014, 9; 3Q, 2016, 39

V03E6 Restriction of Abdominal Aorta, Bifurcation, with Branched or Fenestrated Intraluminal Device, One or Two Arteries, Percutaneous Approach—AHA CC: 4Q, 2016, 91-92

V03F6 Restriction of Abdominal Aorta, Bifurcation, with Branched or Fenestrated Intraluminal Device, Three or More Arteries, Percutaneous Approach—AHA CC: 4Q, 2016, 92-94

VC3EZ Restriction of Right Common Iliac Artery with Branched or Fenestrated Intraluminal Device, One or Two Arteries, Percutaneous Approach—AHA CC: 4Q, 2016, 93-94

VD3EZ Restriction of Left Common Iliac Artery with Branched or Fenestrated Intraluminal Device, One or Two Arteries, Percutaneous Approach—AHA CC: 4Q, 2016, 93-94

WY07Z Revision of Autologous Tissue Substitute in Lower Artery, Open Approach—AHA CC: 1Q, 2015, 36-37

WY37Z Revision of Autologous Tissue Substitute in Lower Artery, Percutaneous Approach—AHA CC: 1Q, 2014, 26

WY3DZ Revision of Intraluminal Device in Lower Artery, Percutaneous Approach—AHA CC: 1Q, 2014, 9-10

Veins

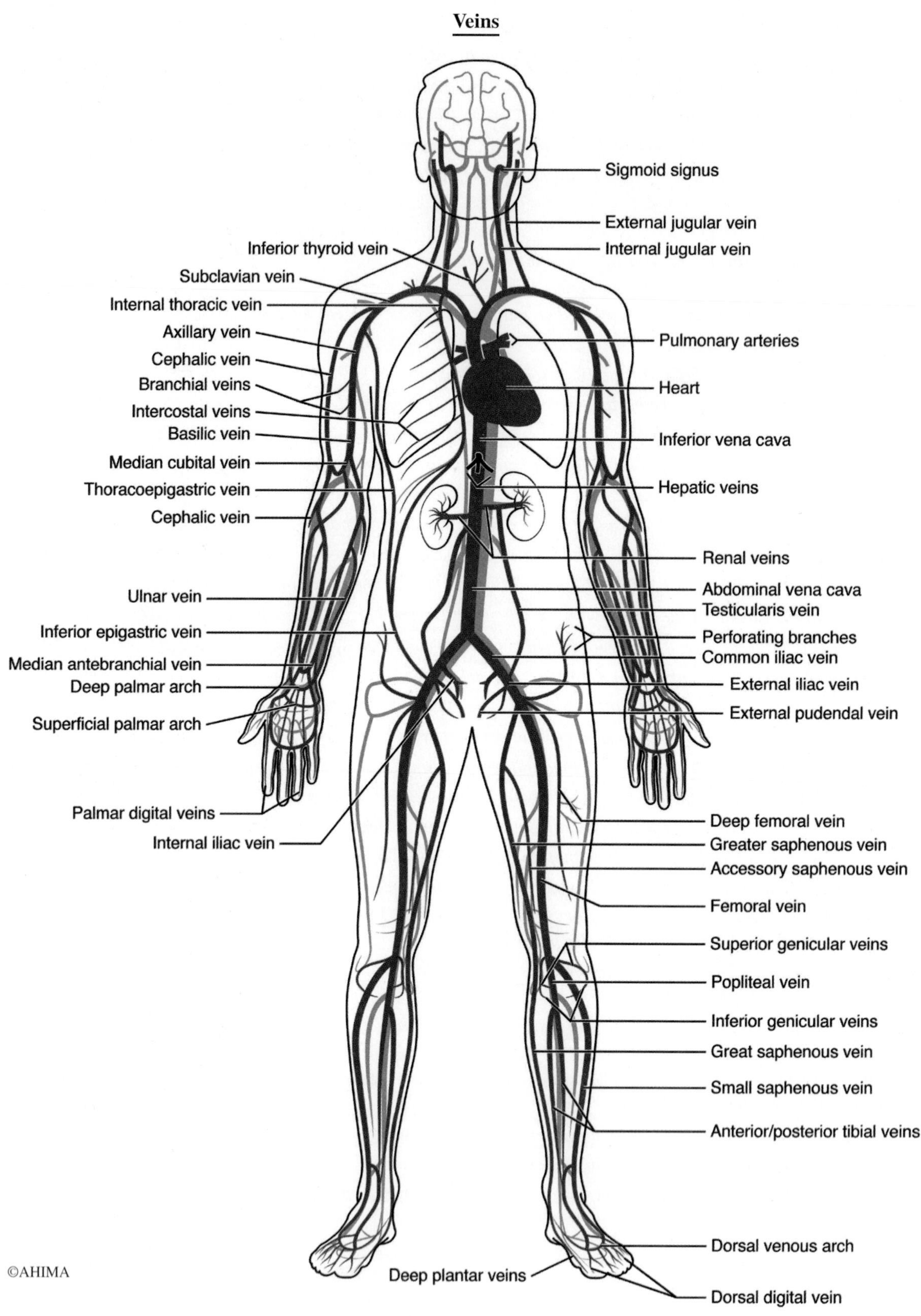
Sigmoid signus
External jugular vein
Internal jugular vein
Inferior thyroid vein
Subclavian vein
Internal thoracic vein
Axillary vein
Cephalic vein
Branchial veins
Intercostal veins
Basilic vein
Median cubital vein
Thoracoepigastric vein
Cephalic vein
Pulmonary arteries
Heart
Inferior vena cava
Hepatic veins
Renal veins
Abdominal vena cava
Testicularis vein
Perforating branches
Common iliac vein
External iliac vein
External pudendal vein
Ulnar vein
Inferior epigastric vein
Median antebranchial vein
Deep palmar arch
Superficial palmar arch
Palmar digital veins
Internal iliac vein
Deep femoral vein
Greater saphenous vein
Accessory saphenous vein
Femoral vein
Superior genicular veins
Popliteal vein
Inferior genicular veins
Great saphenous vein
Small saphenous vein
Anterior/posterior tibial veins
Dorsal venous arch
Deep plantar veins
Dorsal digital vein
©AHIMA

per Veins Tables 051–05W

ction **0** **Medical and Surgical**
dy System **5** **Upper Veins**
eration **1** **Bypass:** Altering the route of passage of the contents of a tubular body part

Body Part (4th)	Approach (5th)	Device (6th)	Qualifier (7th)
0 Azygos Vein 1 Hemiazygos Vein 3 Innominate Vein, Right 4 Innominate Vein, Left 5 Subclavian Vein, Right 6 Subclavian Vein, Left 7 Axillary Vein, Right 8 Axillary Vein, Left 9 Brachial Vein, Right A Brachial Vein, Left B Basilic Vein, Right C Basilic Vein, Left D Cephalic Vein, Right F Cephalic Vein, Left G Hand Vein, Right H Hand Vein, Left L Intracranial Vein M Internal Jugular Vein, Right N Internal Jugular Vein, Left P External Jugular Vein, Right Q External Jugular Vein, Left R Vertebral Vein, Right S Vertebral Vein, Left T Face Vein, Right V Face Vein, Left	**0** Open **4** Percutaneous Endoscopic	**7** Autologous Tissue Substitute **9** Autologous Venous Tissue **A** Autologous Arterial Tissue **J** Synthetic Substitute **K** Nonautologous Tissue Substitute **Z** No Device	**Y** Upper Vein

ction **0** **Medical and Surgical**
dy System **5** **Upper Veins**
peration **5** **Destruction:** Physical eradication of all or a portion of a body part by the direct use of energy, force, or a destructive agent

Body Part (4th)	Approach (5th)	Device (6th)	Qualifier (7th)
0 Azygos Vein 1 Hemiazygos Vein 3 Innominate Vein, Right 4 Innominate Vein, Left 5 Subclavian Vein, Right 6 Subclavian Vein, Left 7 Axillary Vein, Right 8 Axillary Vein, Left 9 Brachial Vein, Right A Brachial Vein, Left B Basilic Vein, Right C Basilic Vein, Left D Cephalic Vein, Right F Cephalic Vein, Left G Hand Vein, Right H Hand Vein, Left L Intracranial Vein M Internal Jugular Vein, Right N Internal Jugular Vein, Left P External Jugular Vein, Right Q External Jugular Vein, Left R Vertebral Vein, Right S Vertebral Vein, Left T Face Vein, Right V Face Vein, Left Y Upper Vein	**0** Open **3** Percutaneous **4** Percutaneous Endoscopic	**Z** No Device	**Z** No Qualifier

Section 0 **Medical and Surgical**
Body System 5 **Upper Veins**
Operation 7 **Dilation:** Expanding an orifice or the lumen of a tubular body part

Body Part (4th)	Approach (5th)	Device (6th)	Qualifier (7th)
0 Azygos Vein **1** Hemiazygos Vein **G** Hand Vein, Right **H** Hand Vein, Left **L** Intracranial Vein **M** Internal Jugular Vein, Right **N** Internal Jugular Vein, Left **P** External Jugular Vein, Right **Q** External Jugular Vein, Left **R** Vertebral Vein, Right **S** Vertebral Vein, Left **T** Face Vein, Right **V** Face Vein, Left **Y** Upper Vein	**0** Open **3** Percutaneous **4** Percutaneous Endoscopic	**D** Intraluminal Device **Z** No Device	**Z** No Qualifier
3 Innominate Vein, Right **4** Innominate Vein, Left **5** Subclavian Vein, Right **6** Subclavian Vein, Left **7** Axillary Vein, Right **8** Axillary Vein, Left **9** Brachial Vein, Right **A** Brachial Vein, Left **B** Basilic Vein, Right **C** Basilic Vein, Left **D** Cephalic Vein, Right **F** Cephalic Vein, Left	**0** Open **3** Percutaneous **4** Percutaneous Endoscopic	**D** Intraluminal Device **Z** No Device	**1** Drug-Coated Balloon **Z** No Qualifier

Section 0 **Medical and Surgical**
Body System 5 **Upper Veins**
Operation 9 **Drainage:** Taking or letting out fluids and/or gases from a body part

Body Part (4th)	Approach (5th)	Device (6th)	Qualifier (7th)
0 Azygos Vein **1** Hemiazygos Vein **3** Innominate Vein, Right **4** Innominate Vein, Left **5** Subclavian Vein, Right **6** Subclavian Vein, Left **7** Axillary Vein, Right **8** Axillary Vein, Left **9** Brachial Vein, Right **A** Brachial Vein, Left **B** Basilic Vein, Right **C** Basilic Vein, Left **D** Cephalic Vein, Right **F** Cephalic Vein, Left **G** Hand Vein, Right **H** Hand Vein, Left **L** Intracranial Vein **M** Internal Jugular Vein, Right **N** Internal Jugular Vein, Left **P** External Jugular Vein, Right **Q** External Jugular Vein, Left **R** Vertebral Vein, Right **S** Vertebral Vein, Left **T** Face Vein, Right **V** Face Vein, Left **Y** Upper Vein	**0** Open **3** Percutaneous **4** Percutaneous Endoscopic	**0** Drainage Device	**Z** No Qualifier

Continued →

ion	**0**	**Medical and Surgical**
y System	**5**	**Upper Veins**
ration	**9**	**Drainage:** Taking or letting out fluids and/or gases from a body part

Body Part (4th)	Approach (5th)	Device (6th)	Qualifier (7th)
Azygos Vein	**0** Open	**Z** No Device	**X** Diagnostic
Hemiazygos Vein	**3** Percutaneous		**Z** No Qualifier
Innominate Vein, Right	**4** Percutaneous Endoscopic		
Innominate Vein, Left			
Subclavian Vein, Right			
Subclavian Vein, Left			
Axillary Vein, Right			
Axillary Vein, Left			
Brachial Vein, Right			
Brachial Vein, Left			
Basilic Vein, Right			
Basilic Vein, Left			
Cephalic Vein, Right			
Cephalic Vein, Left			
Hand Vein, Right			
Hand Vein, Left			
Intracranial Vein			
Internal Jugular Vein, Right			
Internal Jugular Vein, Left			
External Jugular Vein, Right			
External Jugular Vein, Left			
Vertebral Vein, Right			
Vertebral Vein, Left			
Face Vein, Right			
Face Vein, Left			
Upper Vein			

tion	**0**	**Medical and Surgical**
ly System	**5**	**Upper Veins**
eration	**B**	**Excision:** Cutting out or off, without replacement, a portion of a body part

Body Part (4th)	Approach (5th)	Device (6th)	Qualifier (7th)
Azygos Vein	**0** Open	**Z** No Device	**X** Diagnostic
Hemiazygos Vein	**3** Percutaneous		**Z** No Qualifier
Innominate Vein, Right	**4** Percutaneous Endoscopic		
Innominate Vein, Left			
Subclavian Vein, Right			
Subclavian Vein, Left			
Axillary Vein, Right			
Axillary Vein, Left			
Brachial Vein, Right			
Brachial Vein, Left			
Basilic Vein, Right			
Basilic Vein, Left			
Cephalic Vein, Right			
Cephalic Vein, Left			
Hand Vein, Right			
Hand Vein, Left			
Intracranial Vein			
Internal Jugular Vein, Right			
Internal Jugular Vein, Left			
External Jugular Vein, Right			
External Jugular Vein, Left			
Vertebral Vein, Right			
Vertebral Vein, Left			
Face Vein, Right			
Face Vein, Left			
Upper Vein			

Section 0 **Medical and Surgical**
Body System 5 **Upper Veins**
Operation C **Extirpation:** Taking or cutting out solid matter from a body part

Body Part (4th)	Approach (5th)	Device (6th)	Qualifier (7th)
0 Azygos Vein **1** Hemiazygos Vein **3** Innominate Vein, Right **4** Innominate Vein, Left **5** Subclavian Vein, Right **6** Subclavian Vein, Left **7** Axillary Vein, Right **8** Axillary Vein, Left **9** Brachial Vein, Right **A** Brachial Vein, Left **B** Basilic Vein, Right **C** Basilic Vein, Left **D** Cephalic Vein, Right **F** Cephalic Vein, Left **G** Hand Vein, Right **H** Hand Vein, Left **L** Intracranial Vein **M** Internal Jugular Vein, Right **N** Internal Jugular Vein, Left **P** External Jugular Vein, Right **Q** External Jugular Vein, Left **R** Vertebral Vein, Right **S** Vertebral Vein, Left **T** Face Vein, Right **V** Face Vein, Left **Y** Upper Vein	**0** Open **3** Percutaneous **4** Percutaneous Endoscopic	**Z** No Device	**Z** No Qualifier

Section 0 **Medical and Surgical**
Body System 5 **Upper Veins**
Operation D **Extraction:** Pulling or stripping out or off all or a portion of a body part by the use of force

Body Part (4th)	Approach (5th)	Device (6th)	Qualifier (7th)
9 Brachial Vein, Right **A** Brachial Vein, Left **B** Basilic Vein, Right **C** Basilic Vein, Left **D** Cephalic Vein, Right **F** Cephalic Vein, Left **G** Hand Vein, Right **H** Hand Vein, Left **Y** Upper Vein	**0** Open **3** Percutaneous	**Z** No Device	**Z** No Qualifier

Section 0 **Medical and Surgical**
Body System 5 **Upper Veins**
Operation H **Insertion:** Putting in a nonbiological appliance that monitors, assists, performs, or prevents a physiological function but does not physically take the place of a body part

Body Part (4th)	Approach (5th)	Device (6th)	Qualifier (7th)
0 Azygos Vein	**0** Open **3** Percutaneous **4** Percutaneous Endoscopic	**2** Monitoring Device **3** Infusion Device **D** Intraluminal Device **M** Neurostimulator Lead	**Z** No Qualifier
1 Hemiazygos Vein **5** Subclavian Vein, Right **6** Subclavian Vein, Left **7** Axillary Vein, Right **8** Axillary Vein, Left **9** Brachial Vein, Right **A** Brachial Vein, Left **B** Basilic Vein, Right **C** Basilic Vein, Left **D** Cephalic Vein, Right **F** Cephalic Vein, Left **G** Hand Vein, Right **H** Hand Vein, Left **L** Intracranial Vein **M** Internal Jugular Vein, Right **N** Internal Jugular Vein, Left **P** External Jugular Vein, Right **Q** External Jugular Vein, Left **R** Vertebral Vein, Right **S** Vertebral Vein, Left **T** Face Vein, Right **V** Face Vein, Left	**0** Open **3** Percutaneous **4** Percutaneous Endoscopic	**3** Infusion Device **D** Intraluminal Device	**Z** No Qualifier
3 Innominate Vein, Right **4** Innominate Vein, Left	**0** Open **3** Percutaneous **4** Percutaneous Endoscopic	**3** Infusion Device **D** Intraluminal Device **M** Neurostimulator Lead	**Z** No Qualifier
Y Upper Vein	**0** Open **3** Percutaneous **4** Percutaneous Endoscopic	**2** Monitoring Device **3** Infusion Device **D** Intraluminal Device **Y** Other Device	**Z** No Qualifier

Section 0 **Medical and Surgical**
Body System 5 **Upper Veins**
Operation J **Inspection:** Visually and/or manually exploring a body part

Body Part (4th)	Approach (5th)	Device (6th)	Qualifier (7th)
Y Upper Vein	**0** Open **3** Percutaneous **4** Percutaneous Endoscopic **X** External	**Z** No Device	**Z** No Qualifier

Section 0 **Medical and Surgical**
Body System 5 **Upper Veins**
Operation L **Occlusion:** Completely closing an orifice or the lumen of a tubular body part

Body Part (4th)	Approach (5th)	Device (6th)	Qualifier (7th)
0 Azygos Vein **1** Hemiazygos Vein **3** Innominate Vein, Right **4** Innominate Vein, Left **5** Subclavian Vein, Right **6** Subclavian Vein, Left **7** Axillary Vein, Right **8** Axillary Vein, Left **9** Brachial Vein, Right **A** Brachial Vein, Left **B** Basilic Vein, Right **C** Basilic Vein, Left **D** Cephalic Vein, Right **F** Cephalic Vein, Left **G** Hand Vein, Right **H** Hand Vein, Left **L** Intracranial Vein **M** Internal Jugular Vein, Right **N** Internal Jugular Vein, Left **P** External Jugular Vein, Right **Q** External Jugular Vein, Left **R** Vertebral Vein, Right **S** Vertebral Vein, Left **T** Face Vein, Right **V** Face Vein, Left **Y** Upper Vein	**0** Open **3** Percutaneous **4** Percutaneous Endoscopic	**C** Extraluminal Device **D** Intraluminal Device **Z** No Device	**Z** No Qualifier

Section 0 **Medical and Surgical**
Body System 5 **Upper Veins**
Operation N **Release:** Freeing a body part from an abnormal physical constraint by cutting or by the use of force

Body Part (4th)	Approach (5th)	Device (6th)	Qualifier (7th)
0 Azygos Vein **1** Hemiazygos Vein **3** Innominate Vein, Right **4** Innominate Vein, Left **5** Subclavian Vein, Right **6** Subclavian Vein, Left **7** Axillary Vein, Right **8** Axillary Vein, Left **9** Brachial Vein, Right **A** Brachial Vein, Left **B** Basilic Vein, Right **C** Basilic Vein, Left **D** Cephalic Vein, Right **F** Cephalic Vein, Left **G** Hand Vein, Right **H** Hand Vein, Left **L** Intracranial Vein **M** Internal Jugular Vein, Right **N** Internal Jugular Vein, Left **P** External Jugular Vein, Right **Q** External Jugular Vein, Left **R** Vertebral Vein, Right **S** Vertebral Vein, Left **T** Face Vein, Right **V** Face Vein, Left **Y** Upper Vein	**0** Open **3** Percutaneous **4** Percutaneous Endoscopic	**Z** No Device	**Z** No Qualifier

tion **0** **Medical and Surgical**
ly System **5** **Upper Veins**
eration **P** **Removal:** Taking out or off a device from a body part

Body Part (4th)	Approach (5th)	Device (6th)	Qualifier (7th)
Azygos Vein	**0** Open **3** Percutaneous **4** Percutaneous Endoscopic **X** External	**2** Monitoring Device **M** Neurostimulator Lead	**Z** No Qualifier
Innominate Vein, Right Innominate Vein, Left	**0** Open **3** Percutaneous **4** Percutaneous Endoscopic **X** External	**M** Neurostimulator Lead	**Z** No Qualifier
Upper Vein	**0** Open **3** Percutaneous **4** Percutaneous Endoscopic	**0** Drainage Device **2** Monitoring Device **3** Infusion Device **7** Autologous Tissue Substitute **C** Extraluminal Device **D** Intraluminal Device **J** Synthetic Substitute **K** Nonautologous Tissue Substitute **Y** Other Device	**Z** No Qualifier
Upper Vein	**X** External	**0** Drainage Device **2** Monitoring Device **3** Infusion Device **D** Intraluminal Device	**Z** No Qualifier

tion **0** **Medical and Surgical**
ly System **5** **Upper Veins**
eration **Q** **Repair:** Restoring, to the extent possible, a body part to its normal anatomic structure and function

Body Part (4th)	Approach (5th)	Device (6th)	Qualifier (7th)
Azygos Vein Hemiazygos Vein Innominate Vein, Right Innominate Vein, Left Subclavian Vein, Right Subclavian Vein, Left Axillary Vein, Right Axillary Vein, Left Brachial Vein, Right Brachial Vein, Left Basilic Vein, Right Basilic Vein, Left Cephalic Vein, Right Cephalic Vein, Left Hand Vein, Right Hand Vein, Left Intracranial Vein Internal Jugular Vein, Right Internal Jugular Vein, Left External Jugular Vein, Right External Jugular Vein, Left Vertebral Vein, Right Vertebral Vein, Left Face Vein, Right Face Vein, Left Upper Vein	**0** Open **3** Percutaneous **4** Percutaneous Endoscopic	**Z** No Device	**Z** No Qualifier

Section 0 **Medical and Surgical**
Body System 5 **Upper Veins**
Operation R **Replacement:** Putting in or on biological or synthetic material that physically takes the place and/or function of all or a portion of a body part

Body Part (4th)	Approach (5th)	Device (6th)	Qualifier (7th)
0 Azygos Vein **1** Hemiazygos Vein **3** Innominate Vein, Right **4** Innominate Vein, Left **5** Subclavian Vein, Right **6** Subclavian Vein, Left **7** Axillary Vein, Right **8** Axillary Vein, Left **9** Brachial Vein, Right **A** Brachial Vein, Left **B** Basilic Vein, Right **C** Basilic Vein, Left **D** Cephalic Vein, Right **F** Cephalic Vein, Left **G** Hand Vein, Right **H** Hand Vein, Left **L** Intracranial Vein **M** Internal Jugular Vein, Right **N** Internal Jugular Vein, Left **P** External Jugular Vein, Right **Q** External Jugular Vein, Left **R** Vertebral Vein, Right **S** Vertebral Vein, Left **T** Face Vein, Right **V** Face Vein, Left **Y** Upper Vein	**0** Open **4** Percutaneous Endoscopic	**7** Autologous Tissue Substitute **J** Synthetic Substitute **K** Nonautologous Tissue Substitute	**Z** No Qualifier

Section 0 **Medical and Surgical**
Body System 5 **Upper Veins**
Operation S **Reposition:** Moving to its normal location, or other suitable location, all or a portion of a body part

Body Part (4th)	Approach (5th)	Device (6th)	Qualifier (7th)
0 Azygos Vein **1** Hemiazygos Vein **3** Innominate Vein, Right **4** Innominate Vein, Left **5** Subclavian Vein, Right **6** Subclavian Vein, Left **7** Axillary Vein, Right **8** Axillary Vein, Left **9** Brachial Vein, Right **A** Brachial Vein, Left **B** Basilic Vein, Right **C** Basilic Vein, Left **D** Cephalic Vein, Right **F** Cephalic Vein, Left **G** Hand Vein, Right **H** Hand Vein, Left **L** Intracranial Vein **M** Internal Jugular Vein, Right **N** Internal Jugular Vein, Left **P** External Jugular Vein, Right **Q** External Jugular Vein, Left **R** Vertebral Vein, Right **S** Vertebral Vein, Left **T** Face Vein, Right **V** Face Vein, Left **Y** Upper Vein	**0** Open **3** Percutaneous **4** Percutaneous Endoscopic	**Z** No Device	**Z** No Qualifier

tion 0 **Medical and Surgical**
ly System 5 **Upper Veins**
ration U **Supplement:** Putting in or on biological or synthetic material that physically reinforces and/or augments the function of a portion of a body part

Body Part (4th)	Approach (5th)	Device (6th)	Qualifier (7th)
Azygos Vein	**0** Open	**7** Autologous Tissue Substitute	**Z** No Qualifier
Hemiazygos Vein	**3** Percutaneous	**J** Synthetic Substitute	
Innominate Vein, Right	**4** Percutaneous Endoscopic	**K** Nonautologous Tissue Substitute	
Innominate Vein, Left			
Subclavian Vein, Right			
Subclavian Vein, Left			
Axillary Vein, Right			
Axillary Vein, Left			
Brachial Vein, Right			
Brachial Vein, Left			
Basilic Vein, Right			
Basilic Vein, Left			
Cephalic Vein, Right			
Cephalic Vein, Left			
Hand Vein, Right			
Hand Vein, Left			
Intracranial Vein			
Internal Jugular Vein, Right			
Internal Jugular Vein, Left			
External Jugular Vein, Right			
External Jugular Vein, Left			
Vertebral Vein, Right			
Vertebral Vein, Left			
Face Vein, Right			
Face Vein, Left			
Upper Vein			

tion 0 **Medical and Surgical**
ly System 5 **Upper Veins**
eration V **Restriction:** Partially closing an orifice or the lumen of a tubular body part

Body Part (4th)	Approach (5th)	Device (6th)	Qualifier (7th)
Azygos Vein	**0** Open	**C** Extraluminal Device	**Z** No Qualifier
Hemiazygos Vein	**3** Percutaneous	**D** Intraluminal Device	
Innominate Vein, Right	**4** Percutaneous Endoscopic	**Z** No Device	
Innominate Vein, Left			
Subclavian Vein, Right			
Subclavian Vein, Left			
Axillary Vein, Right			
Axillary Vein, Left			
Brachial Vein, Right			
Brachial Vein, Left			
Basilic Vein, Right			
Basilic Vein, Left			
Cephalic Vein, Right			
Cephalic Vein, Left			
Hand Vein, Right			
Hand Vein, Left			
Intracranial Vein			
Internal Jugular Vein, Right			
Internal Jugular Vein, Left			
External Jugular Vein, Right			
External Jugular Vein, Left			
Vertebral Vein, Right			
Vertebral Vein, Left			
Face Vein, Right			
Face Vein, Left			
Upper Vein			

Section 0 **Medical and Surgical**
Body System 5 **Upper Veins**
Operation W **Revision:** Correcting, to the extent possible, a portion of a malfunctioning device or the position of a displaced device

Body Part (4th)	Approach (5th)	Device (6th)	Qualifier (7th)
0 Azygos Vein	**0** Open **3** Percutaneous **4** Percutaneous Endoscopic **X** External	**2** Monitoring Device **M** Neurostimulator Lead	**Z** No Qualifier
3 Innominate Vein, Right **4** Innominate Vein, Left	**0** Open **3** Percutaneous **4** Percutaneous Endoscopic **X** External	**M** Neurostimulator Lead	**Z** No Qualifier
Y Upper Vein	**0** Open **3** Percutaneous **4** Percutaneous Endoscopic	**0** Drainage Device **2** Monitoring Device **3** Infusion Device **7** Autologous Tissue Substitute **C** Extraluminal Device **D** Intraluminal Device **J** Synthetic Substitute **K** Nonautologous Tissue Substitute **Y** Other Device	**Z** No Qualifier
Y Upper Vein	**X** External	**0** Drainage Device **2** Monitoring Device **3** Infusion Device **7** Autologous Tissue Substitute **C** Extraluminal Device **D** Intraluminal Device **J** Synthetic Substitute **K** Nonautologus Tissue Substitute	**Z** No Qualifier

AHA Coding Clinic

05BN0ZZ Excision of Left Internal Jugular Vein, Open Approach—AHA CC: 2Q, 2016, 12-14
05BQ0ZZ Excision of Left External Jugular Vein, Open Approach—AHA CC: 2Q, 2016, 12-14
05H032Z Insertion of Monitoring Device into Azygos Vein, Percutaneous Approach—AHA CC: 4Q, 2016, 98-99
05H43MZ Insertion of Neurostimulator Lead into Left Innominate Vein, Percutaneous Approach—AHA CC: 4Q, 2016, 98-99
05Q40ZZ Repair Left Innominate Vein, Open Approach—AHA CC: 3Q, 2017, 15-16
05SD0ZZ Reposition Right Cephalic Vein, Open Approach—AHA CC: 4Q, 2013, 125-126

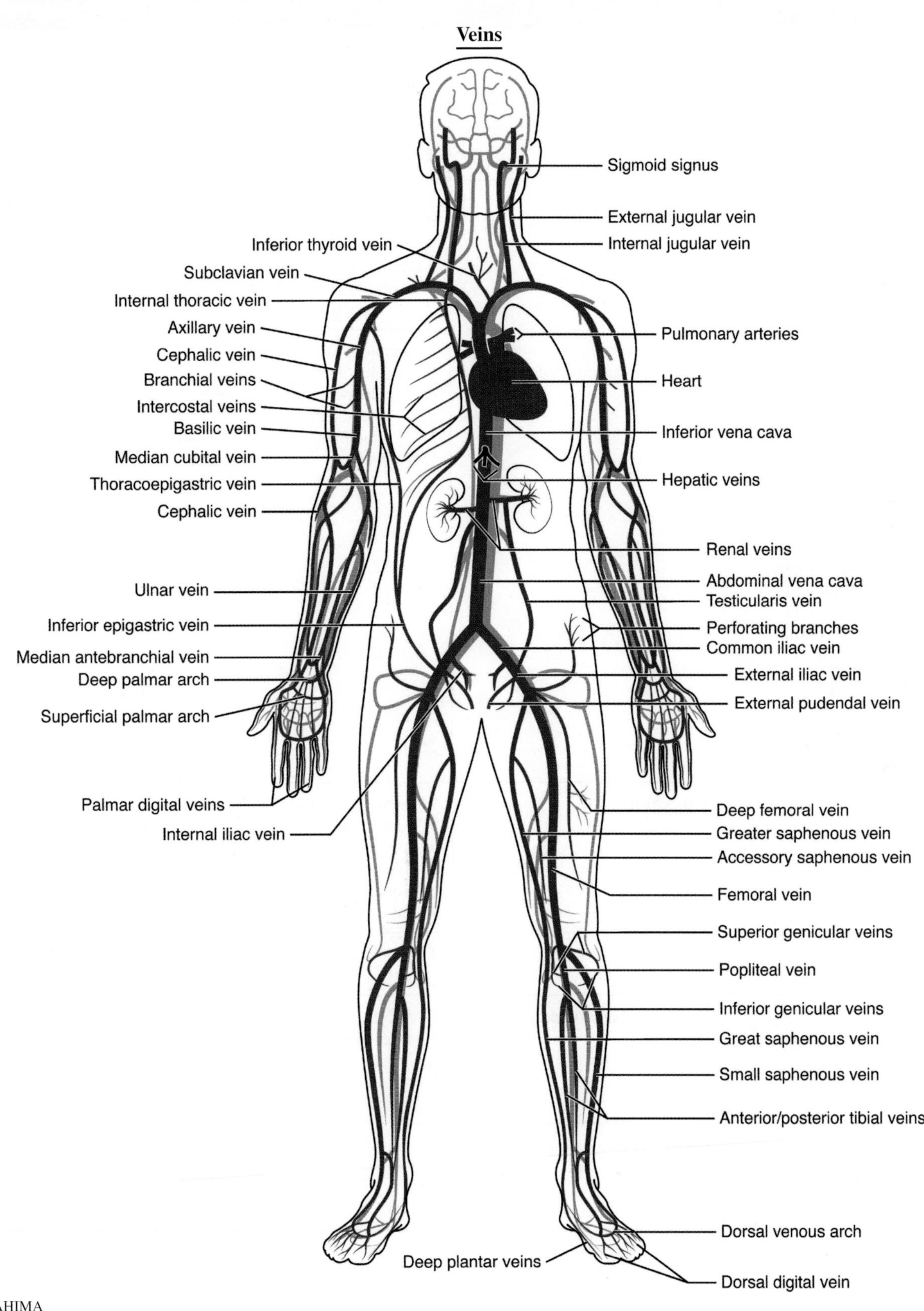
Veins
Sigmoid signus
External jugular vein
Internal jugular vein
Inferior thyroid vein
Subclavian vein
Internal thoracic vein
Axillary vein
Cephalic vein
Branchial veins
Intercostal veins
Basilic vein
Median cubital vein
Thoracoepigastric vein
Cephalic vein
Pulmonary arteries
Heart
Inferior vena cava
Hepatic veins
Renal veins
Abdominal vena cava
Testicularis vein
Perforating branches
Common iliac vein
External iliac vein
External pudendal vein
Ulnar vein
Inferior epigastric vein
Median antebranchial vein
Deep palmar arch
Superficial palmar arch
Palmar digital veins
Internal iliac vein
Deep femoral vein
Greater saphenous vein
Accessory saphenous vein
Femoral vein
Superior genicular veins
Popliteal vein
Inferior genicular veins
Great saphenous vein
Small saphenous vein
Anterior/posterior tibial veins
Dorsal venous arch
Deep plantar veins
Dorsal digital vein

Lower Veins Tables 061–06W

Section 0 **Medical and Surgical**
Body System 6 **Lower Veins**
Operation 1 **Bypass:** Altering the route of passage of the contents of a tubular body part

Body Part (4th)	Approach (5th)	Device (6th)	Qualifier (7th)
0 Inferior Vena Cava	**0** Open **4** Percutaneous Endoscopic	**7** Autologous Tissue Substitute **9** Autologous Venous Tissue **A** Autologous Arterial Tissue **J** Synthetic Substitute **K** Nonautologous Tissue Substitute **Z** No Device	**5** Superior Mesenteric Vein **6** Inferior Mesenteric Vein **P** Pulmonary Trunk **Q** Pulmonary Artery, Right **R** Pulmonary Artery, Left **Y** Lower Vein
1 Splenic Vein	**0** Open **4** Percutaneous Endoscopic	**7** Autologous Tissue Substitute **9** Autologous Venous Tissue **A** Autologous Arterial Tissue **J** Synthetic Substitute **K** Nonautologous Tissue Substitute **Z** No Device	**9** Renal Vein, Right **B** Renal Vein, Left **Y** Lower Vein
2 Gastric Vein **3** Esophageal Vein **4** Hepatic Vein **5** Superior Mesenteric Vein **6** Inferior Mesenteric Vein **7** Colic Vein **9** Renal Vein, Right **B** Renal Vein, Left **C** Common Iliac Vein, Right **D** Common Iliac Vein, Left **F** External Iliac Vein, Right **G** External Iliac Vein, Left **H** Hypogastric Vein, Right **J** Hypogastric Vein, Left **M** Femoral Vein, Right **N** Femoral Vein, Left **P** Saphenous Vein, Right **Q** Saphenous Vein, Left **T** Foot Vein, Right **V** Foot Vein, Left	**0** Open **4** Percutaneous Endoscopic	**7** Autologous Tissue Substitute **9** Autologous Venous Tissue **A** Autologous Arterial Tissue **J** Synthetic Substitute **K** Nonautologous Tissue Substitute **Z** No Device	**Y** Lower Vein
8 Portal Vein	**0** Open	**7** Autologous Tissue Substitute **9** Autologous Venous Tissue **A** Autologous Arterial Tissue **J** Synthetic Substitute **K** Nonautologous Tissue Substitute **Z** No Device	**9** Renal Vein, Right **B** Renal Vein, Left **Y** Lower Vein
8 Portal Vein	**3** Percutaneous	**J** Synthetic Substitute	**4** Hepatic Vein **Y** Lower Vein
8 Portal Vein	**4** Percutaneous Endoscopic	**7** Autologous Tissue Substitute **9** Autologous Venous Tissue **A** Autologous Arterial Tissue **K** Nonautologous Tissue Substitute **Z** No Device	**9** Renal Vein, Right **B** Renal Vein, Left **Y** Lower Vein
8 Portal Vein	**4** Percutaneous Endoscopic	**J** Synthetic Substitute	**4** Hepatic Vein **9** Renal Vein, Right **B** Renal Vein, Left **Y** Lower Vein

ion 0 **Medical and Surgical**
y System 6 **Lower Veins**
ration 5 **Destruction:** Physical eradication of all or a portion of a body part by the direct use of energy, force, or a destructive agent

Body Part (4th)	Approach (5th)	Device (6th)	Qualifier (7th)
Inferior Vena Cava Splenic Vein Gastric Vein Esophageal Vein Hepatic Vein Superior Mesenteric Vein Inferior Mesenteric Vein Colic Vein Portal Vein Renal Vein, Right Renal Vein, Left Common Iliac Vein, Right Common Iliac Vein, Left External Iliac Vein, Right External Iliac Vein, Left Hypogastric Vein, Right Hypogastric Vein, Left Femoral Vein, Right Femoral Vein, Left Saphenous Vein, Right Saphenous Vein, Left Foot Vein, Right Foot Vein, Left	**0** Open **3** Percutaneous **4** Percutaneous Endoscopic	**Z** No Device	**Z** No Qualifier
Lower Vein	**0** Open **3** Percutaneous **4** Percutaneous Endoscopic	**Z** No Device	**C** Hemorrhoidal Plexus **Z** No Qualifier

tion 0 **Medical and Surgical**
ly System 6 **Lower Veins**
eration 7 **Dilation:** Expanding an orifice or the lumen of a tubular body part

Body Part (4th)	Approach (5th)	Device (6th)	Qualifier (7th)
Inferior Vena Cava Splenic Vein Gastric Vein Esophageal Vein Hepatic Vein Superior Mesenteric Vein Inferior Mesenteric Vein Colic Vein Portal Vein Renal Vein, Right Renal Vein, Left Common Iliac Vein, Right Common Iliac Vein, Left External Iliac Vein, Right External Iliac Vein, Left Hypogastric Vein, Right Hypogastric Vein, Left Femoral Vein, Right Femoral Vein, Left Saphenous Vein, Right Saphenous Vein, Left Foot Vein, Right Foot Vein, Left Lower Vein	**0** Open **3** Percutaneous **4** Percutaneous Endoscopic	**D** Intraluminal Device **Z** No Device	**Z** No Qualifier

Section **0** **Medical and Surgical**
Body System **6** **Lower Veins**
Operation **9** **Drainage:** Taking or letting out fluids and/or gases from a body part

Body Part (4th)	Approach (5th)	Device (6th)	Qualifier (7th)
0 Inferior Vena Cava **1** Splenic Vein **2** Gastric Vein **3** Esophageal Vein **4** Hepatic Vein **5** Superior Mesenteric Vein **6** Inferior Mesenteric Vein **7** Colic Vein **8** Portal Vein **9** Renal Vein, Right **B** Renal Vein, Left **C** Common Iliac Vein, Right **D** Common Iliac Vein, Left **F** External Iliac Vein, Right **G** External Iliac Vein, Left **H** Hypogastric Vein, Right **J** Hypogastric Vein, Left **M** Femoral Vein, Right **N** Femoral Vein, Left **P** Saphenous Vein, Right **Q** Saphenous Vein, Left **T** Foot Vein, Right **V** Foot Vein, Left **Y** Lower Vein	**0** Open **3** Percutaneous **4** Percutaneous Endoscopic	**0** Drainage Device	**Z** No Qualifier
0 Inferior Vena Cava **1** Splenic Vein **2** Gastric Vein **3** Esophageal Vein **4** Hepatic Vein **5** Superior Mesenteric Vein **6** Inferior Mesenteric Vein **7** Colic Vein **8** Portal Vein **9** Renal Vein, Right **B** Renal Vein, Left **C** Common Iliac Vein, Right **D** Common Iliac Vein, Left **F** External Iliac Vein, Right **G** External Iliac Vein, Left **H** Hypogastric Vein, Right **J** Hypogastric Vein, Left **M** Femoral Vein, Right **N** Femoral Vein, Left **P** Saphenous Vein, Right **Q** Saphenous Vein, Left **T** Foot Vein, Right **V** Foot Vein, Left **Y** Lower Vein	**0** Open **3** Percutaneous **4** Percutaneous Endoscopic	**Z** No Device	**X** Diagnostic **Z** No Qualifier

ction **0** **Medical and Surgical**
dy System **6** **Lower Veins**
eration **B** **Excision:** Cutting out or off, without replacement, a portion of a body part

Body Part (4th)	Approach (5th)	Device (6th)	Qualifier (7th)
0 Inferior Vena Cava 1 Splenic Vein 2 Gastric Vein 3 Esophageal Vein 4 Hepatic Vein 5 Superior Mesenteric Vein 6 Inferior Mesenteric Vein 7 Colic Vein 8 Portal Vein 9 Renal Vein, Right B Renal Vein, Left C Common Iliac Vein, Right D Common Iliac Vein, Left F External Iliac Vein, Right G External Iliac Vein, Left H Hypogastric Vein, Right J Hypogastric Vein, Left M Femoral Vein, Right N Femoral Vein, Left P Saphenous Vein, Right Q Saphenous Vein, Left T Foot Vein, Right V Foot Vein, Left	0 Open 3 Percutaneous 4 Percutaneous Endoscopic	Z No Device	X Diagnostic Z No Qualifier
Y Lower Vein	0 Open 3 Percutaneous 4 Percutaneous Endoscopic	Z No Device	C Hemorrhoidal Plexus X Diagnostic Z No Qualifier

ction **0** **Medical and Surgical**
ody System **6** **Lower Veins**
peration **C** **Extirpation:** Taking or cutting out solid matter from a body part

Body Part (4th)	Approach (5th)	Device (6th)	Qualifier (7th)
0 Inferior Vena Cava 1 Splenic Vein 2 Gastric Vein 3 Esophageal Vein 4 Hepatic Vein 5 Superior Mesenteric Vein 6 Inferior Mesenteric Vein 7 Colic Vein 8 Portal Vein 9 Renal Vein, Right B Renal Vein, Left C Common Iliac Vein, Right D Common Iliac Vein, Left F External Iliac Vein, Right G External Iliac Vein, Left H Hypogastric Vein, Right J Hypogastric Vein, Left M Femoral Vein, Right N Femoral Vein, Left P Saphenous Vein, Right Q Saphenous Vein, Left T Foot Vein, Right V Foot Vein, Left Y Lower Vein	0 Open 3 Percutaneous 4 Percutaneous Endoscopic	Z No Device	Z No Qualifier

Section 0 **Medical and Surgical**
Body System 6 **Lower Veins**
Operation D **Extraction:** Pulling or stripping out or off all or a portion of a body part by the use of force

Body Part (4th)	Approach (5th)	Device (6th)	Qualifier (7th)
M Femoral Vein, Right **N** Femoral Vein, Left **P** Saphenous Vein, Right **Q** Saphenous Vein, Left **T** Foot Vein, Right **V** Foot Vein, Left **Y** Lower Vein	**0** Open **3** Percutaneous **4** Percutaneous Endoscopic	**Z** No Device	**Z** No Qualifier

Section 0 **Medical and Surgical**
Body System 6 **Lower Veins**
Operation H **Insertion:** Putting in a nonbiological appliance that monitors, assists, performs, or prevents a physiological function but does not physically take the place of a body part

Body Part (4th)	Approach (5th)	Device (6th)	Qualifier (7th)
0 Inferior Vena Cava	**0** Open **3** Percutaneous	**3** Infusion Device	**T** Via Umbilical Vein **Z** No Qualifier
0 Inferior Vena Cava	**0** Open **3** Percutaneous	**D** Intraluminal Device	**Z** No Qualifier
0 Inferior Vena Cava	**4** Percutaneous Endoscopic	**3** Infusion Device **D** Intraluminal Device	**Z** No Qualifier
1 Splenic Vein **2** Gastric Vein **3** Esophageal Vein **4** Hepatic Vein **5** Superior Mesenteric Vein **6** Inferior Mesenteric Vein **7** Colic Vein **8** Portal Vein **9** Renal Vein, Right **B** Renal Vein, Left **C** Common Iliac Vein, Right **D** Common Iliac Vein, Left **F** External Iliac Vein, Right **G** External Iliac Vein, Left **H** Hypogastric Vein, Right **J** Hypogastric Vein, Left **M** Femoral Vein, Right **N** Femoral Vein, Left **P** Saphenous Vein, Right **Q** Saphenous Vein, Left **T** Foot Vein, Right **V** Foot Vein, Left	**0** Open **3** Percutaneous **4** Percutaneous Endoscopic	**3** Infusion Device **D** Intraluminal Device	**Z** No Qualifier
Y Lower Vein	**0** Open **3** Percutaneous **4** Percutaneous Endoscopic	**2** Monitoring Device **3** Infusion Device **D** Intraluminal Device **Y** Other Device	**Z** No Qualifier

ction 0 Medical and Surgical
dy System 6 Lower Veins
peration J **Inspection:** Visually and/or manually exploring a body part

Body Part (4th)	Approach (5th)	Device (6th)	Qualifier (7th)
Y Lower Vein	0 Open 3 Percutaneous 4 Percutaneous Endoscopic X External	Z No Device	Z No Qualifier

ction 0 Medical and Surgical
dy System 6 Lower Veins
peration L **Occlusion:** Completely closing an orifice or the lumen of a tubular body part

Body Part (4th)	Approach (5th)	Device (6th)	Qualifier (7th)
0 Inferior Vena Cava 1 Splenic Vein 2 Gastric Vein 4 Hepatic Vein 5 Superior Mesenteric Vein 6 Inferior Mesenteric Vein 7 Colic Vein 8 Portal Vein 9 Renal Vein, Right B Renal Vein, Left C Common Iliac Vein, Right D Common Iliac Vein, Left F External Iliac Vein, Right G External Iliac Vein, Left H Hypogastric Vein, Right J Hypogastric Vein, Left M Femoral Vein, Right N Femoral Vein, Left P Saphenous Vein, Right Q Saphenous Vein, Left T Foot Vein, Right V Foot Vein, Left	0 Open 3 Percutaneous 4 Percutaneous Endoscopic	C Extraluminal Device D Intraluminal Device Z No Device	Z No Qualifier
3 Esophageal Vein	0 Open 3 Percutaneous 4 Percutaneous Endoscopic 7 Via Natural or Artificial Opening 8 Via Natural or Artificial Opening Endoscopic	C Extraluminal Device D Intraluminal Device Z No Device	Z No Qualifier
Y Lower Vein	0 Open 3 Percutaneous 4 Percutaneous Endoscopic	C Extraluminal Device D Intraluminal Device Z No Device	C Hemorrhoidal Plexus Z No Qualifier

Section 0 **Medical and Surgical**
Body System 6 **Lower Veins**
Operation N **Release:** Freeing a body part from an abnormal physical constraint by cutting or by the use of force

Body Part (4th)	Approach (5th)	Device (6th)	Qualifier (7th)
0 Inferior Vena Cava **1** Splenic Vein **2** Gastric Vein **3** Esophageal Vein **4** Hepatic Vein **5** Superior Mesenteric Vein **6** Inferior Mesenteric Vein **7** Colic Vein **8** Portal Vein **9** Renal Vein, Right **B** Renal Vein, Left **C** Common Iliac Vein, Right **D** Common Iliac Vein, Left **F** External Iliac Vein, Right **G** External Iliac Vein, Left **H** Hypogastric Vein, Right **J** Hypogastric Vein, Left **M** Femoral Vein, Right **N** Femoral Vein, Left **P** Saphenous Vein, Right **Q** Saphenous Vein, Left **T** Foot Vein, Right **V** Foot Vein, Left **Y** Lower Vein	**0** Open **3** Percutaneous **4** Percutaneous Endoscopic	**Z** No Device	**Z** No Qualifier

Section 0 **Medical and Surgical**
Body System 6 **Lower Veins**
Operation P **Removal:** Taking out or off a device from a body part

Body Part (4th)	Approach (5th)	Device (6th)	Qualifier (7th)
Y Lower Vein	**0** Open **3** Percutaneous **4** Percutaneous Endoscopic	**0** Drainage Device **2** Monitoring Device **3** Infusion Device **7** Autologous Tissue Substitute **C** Extraluminal Device **D** Intraluminal Device **J** Synthetic Substitute **K** Nonautologous Tissue Substitute **Y** Other Device	**Z** No Qualifier
Y Lower Vein	**X** External	**0** Drainage Device **2** Monitoring Device **3** Infusion Device **D** Intraluminal Device	**Z** No Qualifier

tion	**0**	**Medical and Surgical**
ly System	**6**	**Lower Veins**
eration	**Q**	**Repair:** Restoring, to the extent possible, a body part to its normal anatomic structure and function

Body Part (4th)	Approach (5th)	Device (6th)	Qualifier (7th)
Inferior Vena Cava Splenic Vein Gastric Vein Esophageal Vein Hepatic Vein Superior Mesenteric Vein Inferior Mesenteric Vein Colic Vein Portal Vein Renal Vein, Right Renal Vein, Left Common Iliac Vein, Right Common Iliac Vein, Left External Iliac Vein, Right External Iliac Vein, Left Hypogastric Vein, Right Hypogastric Vein, Left Femoral Vein, Right Femoral Vein, Left Saphenous Vein, Right Saphenous Vein, Left Foot Vein, Right Foot Vein, Left Lower Vein	**0** Open **3** Percutaneous **4** Percutaneous Endoscopic	**Z** No Device	**Z** No Qualifier

tion	**0**	**Medical and Surgical**
dy System	**6**	**Lower Veins**
eration	**R**	**Replacement:** Putting in or on biological or synthetic material that physically takes the place and/or function of all or a portion of a body part

Body Part (4th)	Approach (5th)	Device (6th)	Qualifier (7th)
Inferior Vena Cava Splenic Vein Gastric Vein Esophageal Vein Hepatic Vein Superior Mesenteric Vein Inferior Mesenteric Vein Colic Vein Portal Vein Renal Vein, Right Renal Vein, Left Common Iliac Vein, Right Common Iliac Vein, Left External Iliac Vein, Right External Iliac Vein, Left Hypogastric Vein, Right Hypogastric Vein, Left Femoral Vein, Right Femoral Vein, Left Saphenous Vein, Right Saphenous Vein, Left Foot Vein, Right Foot Vein, Left Lower Vein	**0** Open **4** Percutaneous Endoscopic	**7** Autologous Tissue Substitute **J** Synthetic Substitute **K** Nonautologous Tissue Substitute	**Z** No Qualifier

Section 0 **Medical and Surgical**
Body System 6 **Lower Veins**
Operation S **Reposition:** Moving to its normal location, or other suitable location, all or a portion of a body part

Body Part (4th)	Approach (5th)	Device (6th)	Qualifier (7th)
0 Inferior Vena Cava **1** Splenic Vein **2** Gastric Vein **3** Esophageal Vein **4** Hepatic Vein **5** Superior Mesenteric Vein **6** Inferior Mesenteric Vein **7** Colic Vein **8** Portal Vein **9** Renal Vein, Right **B** Renal Vein, Left **C** Common Iliac Vein, Right **D** Common Iliac Vein, Left **F** External Iliac Vein, Right **G** External Iliac Vein, Left **H** Hypogastric Vein, Right **J** Hypogastric Vein, Left **M** Femoral Vein, Right **N** Femoral Vein, Left **P** Saphenous Vein, Right **Q** Saphenous Vein, Left **T** Foot Vein, Right **V** Foot Vein, Left **Y** Lower Vein	**0** Open **3** Percutaneous **4** Percutaneous Endoscopic	**Z** No Device	**Z** No Qualifier

Section 0 **Medical and Surgical**
Body System 6 **Lower Veins**
Operation U **Supplement:** Putting in or on biological or synthetic material that physically reinforces and/or augments the function of portion of a body part

Body Part (4th)	Approach (5th)	Device (6th)	Qualifier (7th)
0 Inferior Vena Cava **1** Splenic Vein **2** Gastric Vein **3** Esophageal Vein **4** Hepatic Vein **5** Superior Mesenteric Vein **6** Inferior Mesenteric Vein **7** Colic Vein **8** Portal Vein **9** Renal Vein, Right **B** Renal Vein, Left **C** Common Iliac Vein, Right **D** Common Iliac Vein, Left **F** External Iliac Vein, Right **G** External Iliac Vein, Left **H** Hypogastric Vein, Right **J** Hypogastric Vein, Left **M** Femoral Vein, Right **N** Femoral Vein, Left **P** Saphenous Vein, Right **Q** Saphenous Vein, Left **T** Foot Vein, Right **V** Foot Vein, Left **Y** Lower Vein	**0** Open **3** Percutaneous **4** Percutaneous Endoscopic	**7** Autologous Tissue Substitute **J** Synthetic Substitute **K** Nonautologous Tissue Substitute	**Z** No Qualifier

Section 0 **Medical and Surgical**
Body System 6 **Lower Veins**
Operation V **Restriction:** Partially closing an orifice or the lumen of a tubular body part

Body Part (4th)	Approach (5th)	Device (6th)	Qualifier (7th)
0 Inferior Vena Cava **1** Splenic Vein **2** Gastric Vein **3** Esophageal Vein **4** Hepatic Vein **5** Superior Mesenteric Vein **6** Inferior Mesenteric Vein **7** Colic Vein **8** Portal Vein **9** Renal Vein, Right **B** Renal Vein, Left **C** Common Iliac Vein, Right **D** Common Iliac Vein, Left **F** External Iliac Vein, Right **G** External Iliac Vein, Left **H** Hypogastric Vein, Right **J** Hypogastric Vein, Left **M** Femoral Vein, Right **N** Femoral Vein, Left **P** Saphenous Vein, Right **Q** Saphenous Vein, Left **T** Foot Vein, Right **V** Foot Vein, Left **Y** Lower Vein	**0** Open **3** Percutaneous **4** Percutaneous Endoscopic	**C** Extraluminal Device **D** Intraluminal Device **Z** No Device	**Z** No Qualifier

Section 0 **Medical and Surgical**
Body System 6 **Lower Veins**
Operation W **Revision:** Correcting, to the extent possible, a portion of a malfunctioning device or the position of a displaced device

Body Part (4th)	Approach (5th)	Device (6th)	Qualifier (7th)
Y Lower Vein	**0** Open **3** Percutaneous **4** Percutaneous Endoscopic **X** External	**0** Drainage Device **2** Monitoring Device **3** Infusion Device **7** Autologous Tissue Substitute **C** Extraluminal Device **D** Intraluminal Device **J** Synthetic Substitute **K** Nonautologous Tissue Substitute **Y** Other Device	**Z** No Qualifier
Y Lower Vein	**X** External	**0** Drainage Device **2** Monitoring Device **3** Infusion Device **7** Autologous Tissue Substitute **C** Extraluminal Device **D** Intraluminal Device **J** Synthetic Substitute **K** Nonautologus Tissue Substitute	**Z** No Qualifier

AHA Coding Clinic

06100JP Bypass Inferior Vena Cava to Pulmonary Trunk with Synthetic Substitute, Open Approach—AHA CC: 4Q, 2017, 37-38

06BP0ZZ Excision of Right Saphenous Vein, Open Approach—AHA CC: 1Q, 2014, 10-11; 2Q, 2016, 18-19; 1Q, 2017, 31-32; 3Q. 20 5-6

06BP4ZZ Excision of Right Saphenous Vein, Percutaneous Endoscopic Approach—AHA CC: 3Q, 2014, 20-21

06BQ0ZZ Excision of Left Saphenous Vein, Open Approach—AHA CC: 1Q, 2017, 32-33

06BQ4ZZ Excision of Left Saphenous Vein, Percutaneous Endoscopic Approach—AHA CC: 3Q, 2014, 20-21; 1Q, 2016, 27-28

06H033T Insertion of Infusion Device, Via Umbilical Vein, into Inferior Vena Cava, Percutaneous Approach—AHA CC: 1Q, 2017, 31

06H033Z Insertion of Infusion Device into Inferior Vena Cava, Percutaneous Approach—AHA CC: 3Q, 2013, 18-19

06HY33Z Insertion of Infusion Device into Lower Vein, Percutaneous Approach—AHA CC: 1Q, 2017, 31

06L34CZ Occlusion of Esophageal Vein with Extraluminal Device, Percutaneous Endoscopic Approach—AHA CC: 4Q, 2013, 112-11

06L38CZ Occlusion of Esophageal Vein with Extraluminal Device, Via Natural or Artificial Opening Endoscopic—AHA CC: 4Q, 20 57-58

06LF0CZ Occlusion of Right External Iliac Vein with Extraluminal Device, Open Approach—AHA CC: 2Q, 2018, 18-19

06LG0CZ Occlusion of Left External Iliac Vein with Extraluminal Device, Open Approach—AHA CC: 2Q, 2018, 18-19

06WY3DZ Revision of Intraluminal Device in Lower Vein, Percutaneous Approach—AHA CC: 3Q, 2014, 25-26; 1Q, 2018, 10-11

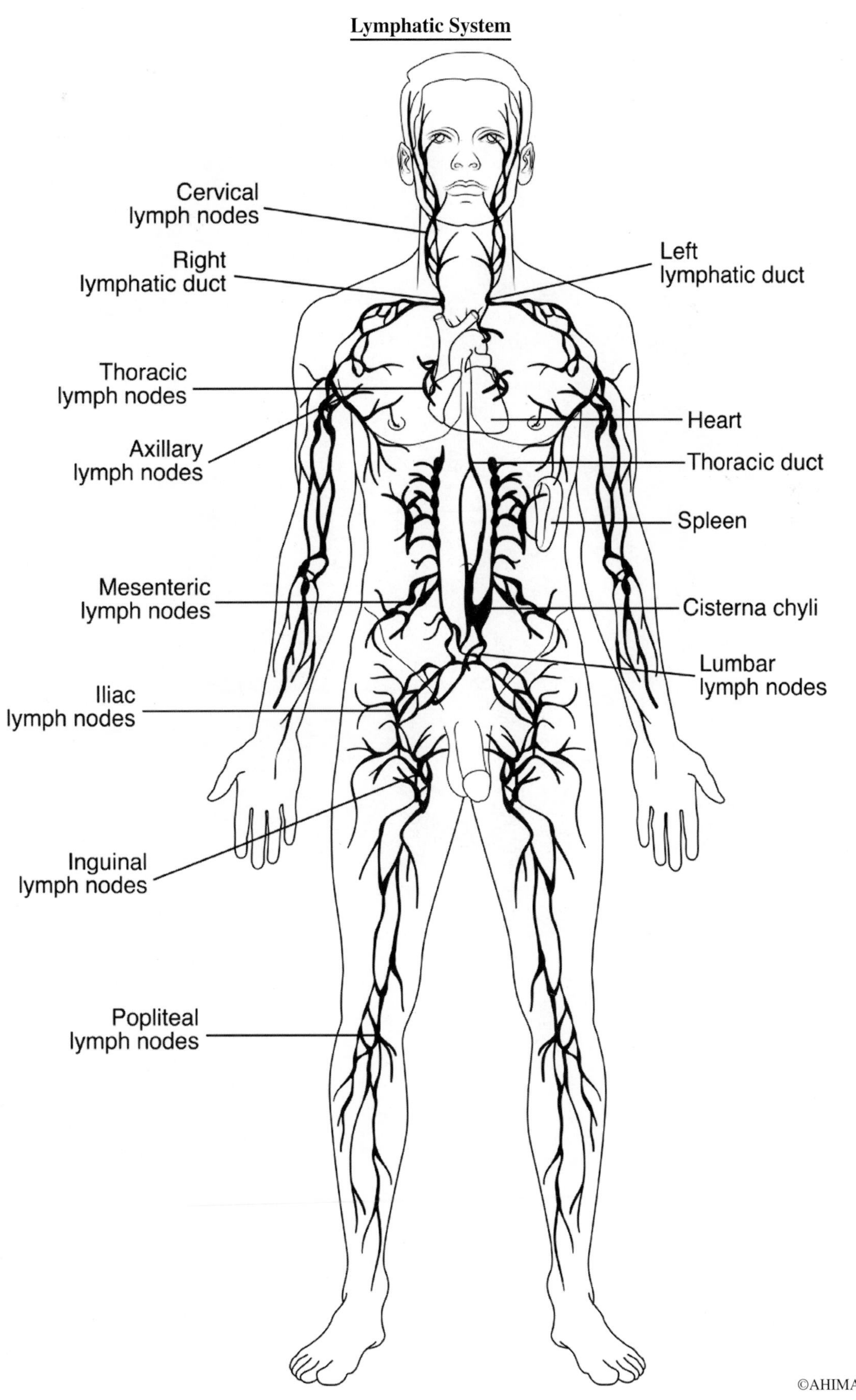
Lymphatic System
Cervical lymph nodes
Right lymphatic duct
Left lymphatic duct
Thoracic lymph nodes
Heart
Axillary lymph nodes
Thoracic duct
Spleen
Mesenteric lymph nodes
Cisterna chyli
Lumbar lymph nodes
Iliac lymph nodes
Inguinal lymph nodes
Popliteal lymph nodes

Lymph Vessels and Nodes of Mammary Gland Lymphatic Drainage

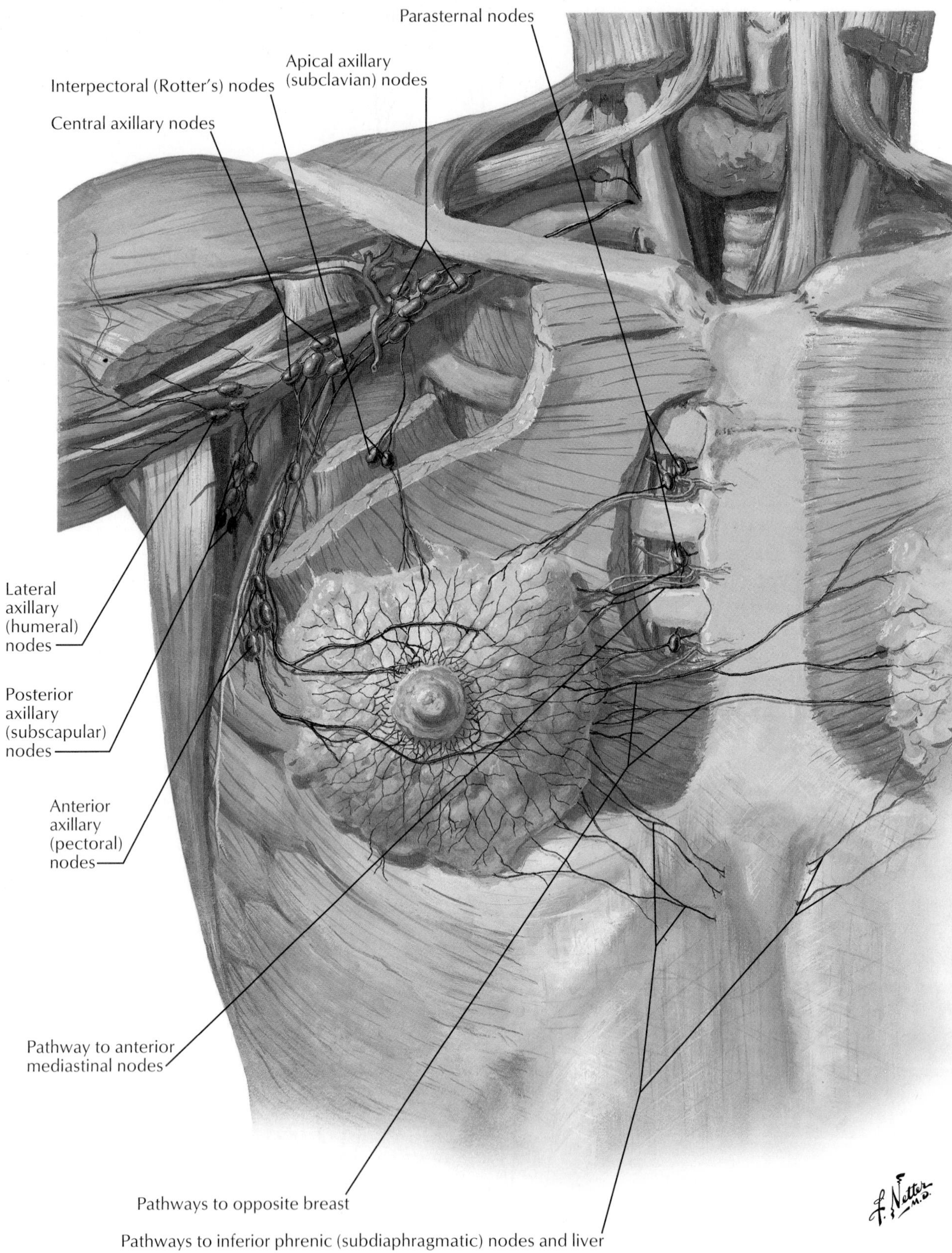

tion 0 **Medical and Surgical**
ly System 7 **Lymphatic and Hemic Systems**
eration 2 **Change:** Taking out or off a device from a body part and putting back an identical or similar device in or on the same body part without cutting or puncturing the skin or a mucous membrane

Body Part (4th)	Approach (5th)	Device (6th)	Qualifier (7th)
Thoracic Duct Cisterna Chyli Thymus Lymphatic Spleen Bone Marrow	**X** External	**0** Drainage Device **Y** Other Device	**Z** No Qualifier

tion 0 **Medical and Surgical**
ly System 7 **Lymphatic and Hemic Systems**
eration 5 **Destruction:** Physical eradication of all or a portion of a body part by the direct use of energy, force, or a destructive agent

Body Part (4th)	Approach (5th)	Device (6th)	Qualifier (7th)
Lymphatic, Head Lymphatic, Right Neck Lymphatic, Left Neck Lymphatic, Right Upper Extremity Lymphatic, Left Upper Extremity Lymphatic, Right Axillary Lymphatic, Left Axillary Lymphatic, Thorax Lymphatic, Internal Mammary, Right Lymphatic, Internal Mammary, Left Lymphatic, Mesenteric Lymphatic, Pelvis Lymphatic, Aortic Lymphatic, Right Lower Extremity Lymphatic, Left Lower Extremity Lymphatic, Right Inguinal Lymphatic, Left Inguinal Thoracic Duct Cisterna Chyli Thymus Spleen	**0** Open **3** Percutaneous **4** Percutaneous Endoscopic	**Z** No Device	**Z** No Qualifier

Section	**0**	**Medical and Surgical**
Body System	**7**	**Lymphatic and Hemic Systems**
Operation	**9**	**Drainage:** Taking or letting out fluids and/or gases from a body part

Body Part (4th)	Approach (5th)	Device (6th)	Qualifier (7th)
0 Lymphatic, Head **1** Lymphatic, Right Neck **2** Lymphatic, Left Neck **3** Lymphatic, Right Upper Extremity **4** Lymphatic, Left Upper Extremity **5** Lymphatic, Right Axillary **6** Lymphatic, Left Axillary **7** Lymphatic, Thorax **8** Lymphatic, Internal Mammary, Right **9** Lymphatic, Internal Mammary, Left **B** Lymphatic, Mesenteric **C** Lymphatic, Pelvis **D** Lymphatic, Aortic **F** Lymphatic, Right Lower Extremity **G** Lymphatic, Left Lower Extremity **H** Lymphatic, Right Inguinal **J** Lymphatic, Left Inguinal **K** Thoracic Duct **L** Cisterna Chyli	**0** Open **3** Percutaneous **4** Percutaneous Endoscopic **8** Via Natural or Artificial Opening Endoscopic	**0** Drainage Device	**Z** No Qualifier
0 Lymphatic, Head **1** Lymphatic, Right Neck **2** Lymphatic, Left Neck **3** Lymphatic, Right Upper Extremity **4** Lymphatic, Left Upper Extremity **5** Lymphatic, Right Axillary **6** Lymphatic, Left Axillary **7** Lymphatic, Thorax **8** Lymphatic, Internal Mammary, Right **9** Lymphatic, Internal Mammary, Left **B** Lymphatic, Mesenteric **C** Lymphatic, Pelvis **D** Lymphatic, Aortic **F** Lymphatic, Right Lower Extremity **G** Lymphatic, Left Lower Extremity **H** Lymphatic, Right Inguinal **J** Lymphatic, Left Inguinal **K** Thoracic Duct **L** Cisterna Chyli	**0** Open **3** Percutaneous **4** Percutaneous Endoscopic **8** Via Natural or Artificial Opening Endoscopic	**Z** No Device	**X** Diagnostic **Z** No Qualifier
M Thymus **P** Spleen **T** Bone Marrow	**0** Open **3** Percutaneous **4** Percutaneous Endoscopic	**0** Drainage Device	**Z** No Qualifier
M Thymus **P** Spleen **T** Bone Marrow	**0** Open **3** Percutaneous **4** Percutaneous Endoscopic	**Z** No Device	**X** No Diagnostic **Z** No Qualifier

ction **0** **Medical and Surgical**
dy System **7** **Lymphatic and Hemic Systems**
peration **B** **Excision:** Cutting out or off, without replacement, a portion of a body part

Body Part (4th)	Approach (5th)	Device (6th)	Qualifier (7th)
0 Lymphatic, Head	0 Open	Z No Device	X Diagnostic
1 Lymphatic, Right Neck	3 Percutaneous		Z No Qualifier
2 Lymphatic, Left Neck	4 Percutaneous Endoscopic		
3 Lymphatic, Right Upper Extremity			
4 Lymphatic, Left Upper Extremity			
5 Lymphatic, Right Axillary			
6 Lymphatic, Left Axillary			
7 Lymphatic, Thorax			
8 Lymphatic, Internal Mammary, Right			
9 Lymphatic, Internal Mammary, Left			
B Lymphatic, Mesenteric			
C Lymphatic, Pelvis			
D Lymphatic, Aortic			
F Lymphatic, Right Lower Extremity			
G Lymphatic, Left Lower Extremity			
H Lymphatic, Right Inguinal			
J Lymphatic, Left Inguinal			
K Thoracic Duct			
L Cisterna Chyli			
M Thymus			
P Spleen			

ction **0** **Medical and Surgical**
ody System **7** **Lymphatic and Hemic Systems**
peration **C** **Extirpation:** Taking or cutting out solid matter from a body part

Body Part (4th)	Approach (5th)	Device (6th)	Qualifier (7th)
0 Lymphatic, Head	0 Open	Z No Device	Z No Qualifier
1 Lymphatic, Right Neck	3 Percutaneous		
2 Lymphatic, Left Neck	4 Percutaneous Endoscopic		
3 Lymphatic, Right Upper Extremity			
4 Lymphatic, Left Upper Extremity			
5 Lymphatic, Right Axillary			
6 Lymphatic, Left Axillary			
7 Lymphatic, Thorax			
8 Lymphatic, Internal Mammary, Right			
9 Lymphatic, Internal Mammary, Left			
B Lymphatic, Mesenteric			
C Lymphatic, Pelvis			
D Lymphatic, Aortic			
F Lymphatic, Right Lower Extremity			
G Lymphatic, Left Lower Extremity			
H Lymphatic, Right Inguinal			
J Lymphatic, Left Inguinal			
K Thoracic Duct			
L Cisterna Chyli			
M Thymus			
P Spleen			

Section 0 **Medical and Surgical**
Body System 7 **Lymphatic and Hemic Systems**
Operation D **Extraction:** Pulling or stripping out or off all or a portion of a body part by the use of force

Body Part (4th)	Approach (5th)	Device (6th)	Qualifier (7th)
0 Lymphatic, Head **1** Lymphatic, Right Neck **2** Lymphatic, Left Neck **3** Lymphatic, Right Upper Extremity **4** Lymphatic, Left Upper Extremity **5** Lymphatic, Right Axillary **6** Lymphatic, Left Axillary **7** Lymphatic, Thorax **8** Lymphatic, Internal Mammary, Right **9** Lymphatic, Internal Mammary, Left **B** Lymphatic, Mesenteric **C** Lymphatic, Pelvis **D** Lymphatic, Aortic **F** Lymphatic, Right Lower Extremity **G** Lymphatic, Left Lower Extremity **H** Lymphatic, Right Inguinal **J** Lymphatic, Left Inguinal **K** Thoracic Duct **L** Cisterna Chyli	**3** Percutaneous **4** Percutaneous Endoscopic **8** Via Natural or Artificial Opening Endoscopic	**Z** No Device	**X** Diagnostic
M Thymus **P** Spleen	**3** Percutaneous **4** Percutaneous Endoscopic	**Z** No Device	**X** No Diagnostic
Q Bone Marrow, Sternum **R** Bone Marrow, Iliac **S** Bone Marrow, Vertebral	**0** Open **3** Percutaneous	**Z** No Device	**X** Diagnostic **Z** No Qualifier

Section 0 **Medical and Surgical**
Body System 7 **Lymphatic and Hemic Systems**
Operation H **Insertion:** Putting in a nonbiological appliance that monitors, assists, performs, or prevents a physiological function but does not physically take the place of a body part

Body Part (4th)	Approach (5th)	Device (6th)	Qualifier (7th)
K Thoracic Duct **L** Cisterna Chyli **M** Thymus **N** Lymphatic **P** Spleen	**0** Open **3** Percutaneous **4** Percutaneous Endoscopic	**3** Infusion Device **Y** Other Device	**Z** No Qualifier

Section 0 **Medical and Surgical**
Body System 7 **Lymphatic and Hemic Systems**
Operation J **Inspection:** Visually and/or manually exploring a body part

Body Part (4th)	Approach (5th)	Device (6th)	Qualifier (7th)
K Thoracic Duct **L** Cisterna Chyli **M** Thymus **T** Bone Marrow	**0** Open **3** Percutaneous **4** Percutaneous Endoscopic	**Z** No Device	**Z** No Qualifier
N Lymphatic	**0** Open **3** Percutaneous **4** Percutaneous Endoscopic **8** Via Natural or Artificial Opening Endoscopic **X** External	**Z** No Device	**Z** No Qualifier
P Spleen	**0** Open **3** Percutaneous **4** Percutaneous Endoscopic **X** External	**Z** No Device	**Z** No Qualifier

:ion	0	**Medical and Surgical**
y System	7	**Lymphatic and Hemic Systems**
:ration	L	**Occlusion:** Completely closing an orifice or the lumen of a tubular body part

Body Part (4th)	Approach (5th)	Device (6th)	Qualifier (7th)
Lymphatic, Head	**0** Open	**C** Extraluminal Device	**Z** No Qualifier
Lymphatic, Right Neck	**3** Percutaneous	**D** Intraluminal Device	
Lymphatic, Left Neck	**4** Percutaneous Endoscopic	**Z** No Device	
Lymphatic, Right Upper Extremity			
Lymphatic, Left Upper Extremity			
Lymphatic, Right Axillary			
Lymphatic, Left Axillary			
Lymphatic, Thorax			
Lymphatic, Internal Mammary, Right			
Lymphatic, Internal Mammary, Left			
Lymphatic, Mesenteric			
Lymphatic, Pelvis			
Lymphatic, Aortic			
Lymphatic, Right Lower Extremity			
Lymphatic, Left Lower Extremity			
Lymphatic, Right Inguinal			
Lymphatic, Left Inguinal			
Thoracic Duct			
Cisterna Chyli			

tion	0	**Medical and Surgical**
ly System	7	**Lymphatic and Hemic Systems**
eration	N	**Release:** Freeing a body part from an abnormal physical constraint by cutting or by the use of force

Body Part (4th)	Approach (5th)	Device (6th)	Qualifier (7th)
Lymphatic, Head	**0** Open	**Z** No Device	**Z** No Qualifier
Lymphatic, Right Neck	**3** Percutaneous		
Lymphatic, Left Neck	**4** Percutaneous Endoscopic		
Lymphatic, Right Upper Extremity			
Lymphatic, Left Upper Extremity			
Lymphatic, Right Axillary			
Lymphatic, Left Axillary			
Lymphatic, Thorax			
Lymphatic, Internal Mammary, Right			
Lymphatic, Internal Mammary, Left			
Lymphatic, Mesenteric			
Lymphatic, Pelvis			
Lymphatic, Aortic			
Lymphatic, Right Lower Extremity			
Lymphatic, Left Lower Extremity			
Lymphatic, Right Inguinal			
Lymphatic, Left Inguinal			
Thoracic Duct			
Cisterna Chyli			
Thymus			
Spleen			

Section 0 **Medical and Surgical**
Body System 7 **Lymphatic and Hemic Systems**
Operation P **Removal:** Taking out or off a device from a body part

Body Part (4th)	Approach (5th)	Device (6th)	Qualifier (7th)
K Thoracic Duct **L** Cisterna Chyli **N** Lymphatic	**0** Open **3** Percutaneous **4** Percutaneous Endoscopic	**0** Drainage Device **3** Infusion Device **7** Autologous Tissue Substitute **C** Extraluminal Device **D** Intraluminal Device **J** Synthetic Substitute **K** Nonautologous Tissue Substitute **Y** Other Device	**Z** No Qualifier
K Thoracic Duct **L** Cisterna Chyli **N** Lymphatic	**X** External	**0** Drainage Device **3** Infusion Device **D** Intraluminal Device	**Z** No Qualifier
M Thymus **P** Spleen	**0** Open **3** Percutaneous **4** Percutaneous Endoscopic	**0** Drainage Device **3** Infusion Device **Y** Other Device	**Z** No Qualifier
M Thymus **P** Spleen	**X** External	**0** Drainage Device **3** Infusion Device	**Z** No Qualifier
T Bone Marrow	**0** Open **3** Percutaneous **4** Percutaneous Endoscopic **X** External	**0** Drainage Device	**Z** No Qualifier

Section 0 **Medical and Surgical**
Body System 7 **Lymphatic and Hemic Systems**
Operation Q **Repair:** Restoring, to the extent possible, a body part to its normal anatomic structure and function

Body Part (4th)	Approach (5th)	Device (6th)	Qualifier (7th)
0 Lymphatic, Head **1** Lymphatic, Right Neck **2** Lymphatic, Left Neck **3** Lymphatic, Right Upper Extremity **4** Lymphatic, Left Upper Extremity **5** Lymphatic, Right Axillary **6** Lymphatic, Left Axillary **7** Lymphatic, Thorax **8** Lymphatic, Internal Mammary, Right **9** Lymphatic, Internal Mammary, Left **B** Lymphatic, Mesenteric **C** Lymphatic, Pelvis **D** Lymphatic, Aortic **F** Lymphatic, Right Lower Extremity **G** Lymphatic, Left Lower Extremity **H** Lymphatic, Right Inguinal **J** Lymphatic, Left Inguinal **K** Thoracic Duct **L** Cisterna Chyli	**0** Open **3** Percutaneous **4** Percutaneous Endoscopic **8** Via Natural or Artificial Opening Endoscopic	**Z** No Device	**Z** No Qualifier
M Thymus **P** Spleen	**0** Open **3** Percutaneous **4** Percutaneous Endoscopic	**Z** No Device	**Z** No Qualifier

ction 0 **Medical and Surgical**
dy System 7 **Lymphatic and Hemic Systems**
eration S **Reposition:** Moving to its normal location, or other suitable location, all or a portion of a body part

Body Part (4th)	Approach (5th)	Device (6th)	Qualifier (7th)
M Thymus P Spleen	0 Open	Z No Device	Z No Qualifier

ction 0 **Medical and Surgical**
dy System 7 **Lymphatic and Hemic Systems**
eration T **Resection:** Cutting out or off, without replacement, all of a body part

Body Part (4th)	Approach (5th)	Device (6th)	Qualifier (7th)
0 Lymphatic, Head 1 Lymphatic, Right Neck 2 Lymphatic, Left Neck 3 Lymphatic, Right Upper Extremity 4 Lymphatic, Left Upper Extremity 5 Lymphatic, Right Axillary 6 Lymphatic, Left Axillary 7 Lymphatic, Thorax 8 Lymphatic, Internal Mammary, Right 9 Lymphatic, Internal Mammary, Left B Lymphatic, Mesenteric C Lymphatic, Pelvis D Lymphatic, Aortic F Lymphatic, Right Lower Extremity G Lymphatic, Left Lower Extremity H Lymphatic, Right Inguinal J Lymphatic, Left Inguinal K Thoracic Duct L Cisterna Chyli M Thymus P Spleen	0 Open 4 Percutaneous Endoscopic	Z No Device	Z No Qualifier

ction 0 **Medical and Surgical**
dy System 7 **Lymphatic and Hemic Systems**
eration U **Supplement:** Putting in or on biological or synthetic material that physically reinforces and/or augments the function of a portion of a body part

Body Part (4th)	Approach (5th)	Device (6th)	Qualifier (7th)
0 Lymphatic, Head 1 Lymphatic, Right Neck 2 Lymphatic, Left Neck 3 Lymphatic, Right Upper Extremity 4 Lymphatic, Left Upper Extremity 5 Lymphatic, Right Axillary 6 Lymphatic, Left Axillary 7 Lymphatic, Thorax 8 Lymphatic, Internal Mammary, Right 9 Lymphatic, Internal Mammary, Left B Lymphatic, Mesenteric C Lymphatic, Pelvis D Lymphatic, Aortic F Lymphatic, Right Lower Extremity G Lymphatic, Left Lower Extremity H Lymphatic, Right Inguinal J Lymphatic, Left Inguinal K Thoracic Duct L Cisterna Chyli	0 Open 4 Percutaneous Endoscopic	7 Autologous Tissue Substitute J Synthetic Substitute K Nonautologous Tissue Substitute	Z No Qualifier

Section 0 **Medical and Surgical**
Body System 7 **Lymphatic and Hemic Systems**
Operation V **Restriction:** Partially closing an orifice or the lumen of a tubular body part

Body Part (4th)	Approach (5th)	Device (6th)	Qualifier (7th)
0 Lymphatic, Head **1** Lymphatic, Right Neck **2** Lymphatic, Left Neck **3** Lymphatic, Right Upper Extremity **4** Lymphatic, Left Upper Extremity **5** Lymphatic, Right Axillary **6** Lymphatic, Left Axillary **7** Lymphatic, Thorax **8** Lymphatic, Internal Mammary, Right **9** Lymphatic, Internal Mammary, Left **B** Lymphatic, Mesenteric **C** Lymphatic, Pelvis **D** Lymphatic, Aortic **F** Lymphatic, Right Lower Extremity **G** Lymphatic, Left Lower Extremity **H** Lymphatic, Right Inguinal **J** Lymphatic, Left Inguinal **K** Thoracic Duct **L** Cisterna Chyli	**0** Open **3** Percutaneous **4** Percutaneous Endoscopic	**C** Extraluminal Device **D** Intraluminal Device **Z** No Device	**Z** No Qualifier

Section 0 **Medical and Surgical**
Body System 7 **Lymphatic and Hemic Systems**
Operation W **Revision:** Correcting, to the extent possible, a portion of a malfunctioning device or the position of a displaced device

Body Part (4th)	Approach (5th)	Device (6th)	Qualifier (7th)
K Thoracic Duct **L** Cisterna Chyli **N** Lymphatic	**0** Open **3** Percutaneous **4** Percutaneous Endoscopic	**0** Drainage Device **3** Infusion Device **7** Autologous Tissue Substitute **C** Extraluminal Device **D** Intraluminal Device **J** Synthetic Substitute **K** Nonautologous Tissue Substitute **Y** Other Device	**Z** No Qualifier
K Thoracic Duct **L** Cisterna Chyli **N** Lymphatic	**X** External	**0** Drainage Device **3** Infusion Device **7** Autologous Tissue Substitute **C** Extraluminal Device **D** Intraluminal Device **J** Synthetic Substitute **K** Nonautologous Tissue Substitute	**Z** No Qualifier
M Thymus **P** Spleen	**0** Open **3** Percutaneous **4** Percutaneous Endoscopic	**0** Drainage Device **3** Infusion Device **Y** Other Device	**Z** No Qualifier
M Thymus **P** Spleen	**X** External	**0** Drainage Device **3** Infusion Device	**Z** No Qualifier
T Bone Marrow	**0** Open **3** Percutaneous **4** Percutaneous Endoscopic **X** External	**0** Drainage Device	**Z** No Qualifier

ction 0 **Medical and Surgical**
dy System 7 **Lymphatic and Hemic Systems**
eration Y **Transplantation:** Putting in or on all or a portion of a living body part taken from another individual or animal to physically take the place and/or function of all or a portion of a similar body part

Body Part (4th)	Approach (5th)	Device (6th)	Qualifier (7th)
M Thymus **P** Spleen	**0** Open	**Z** No Device	**0** Allogeneic **1** Syngeneic **2** Zooplastic

HA Coding Clinic

B74ZX Excision of Thorax Lymphatic, Percutaneous Endoscopic Approach, Diagnostic—AHA CC: 1Q, 2014, 20-21, 26; 3Q, 2014, 10-11

Q60ZZ Repair Left Axillary Lymphatic, Open Approach—AHA CC: 1Q, 2017, 34

T10ZZ Resection of Right Neck Lymphatic, Open Approach—AHA CC: 3Q, 2014, 9-10

T20ZZ Resection of Left Neck Lymphatic, Open Approach—AHA CC: 3Q, 2014, 9-10; 2Q, 2016, 12-14

T50ZZ Resection of Right Axillary Lymphatic, Open Approach AHA CC: 1Q, 2016, 30

TM0ZZ Resection of Thymus, Open Approach AHA CC: 3Q, 2014, 16-17

TP0ZZ Resection of Spleen, Open Approach AHA CC: 4Q, 2015, 13

Eye

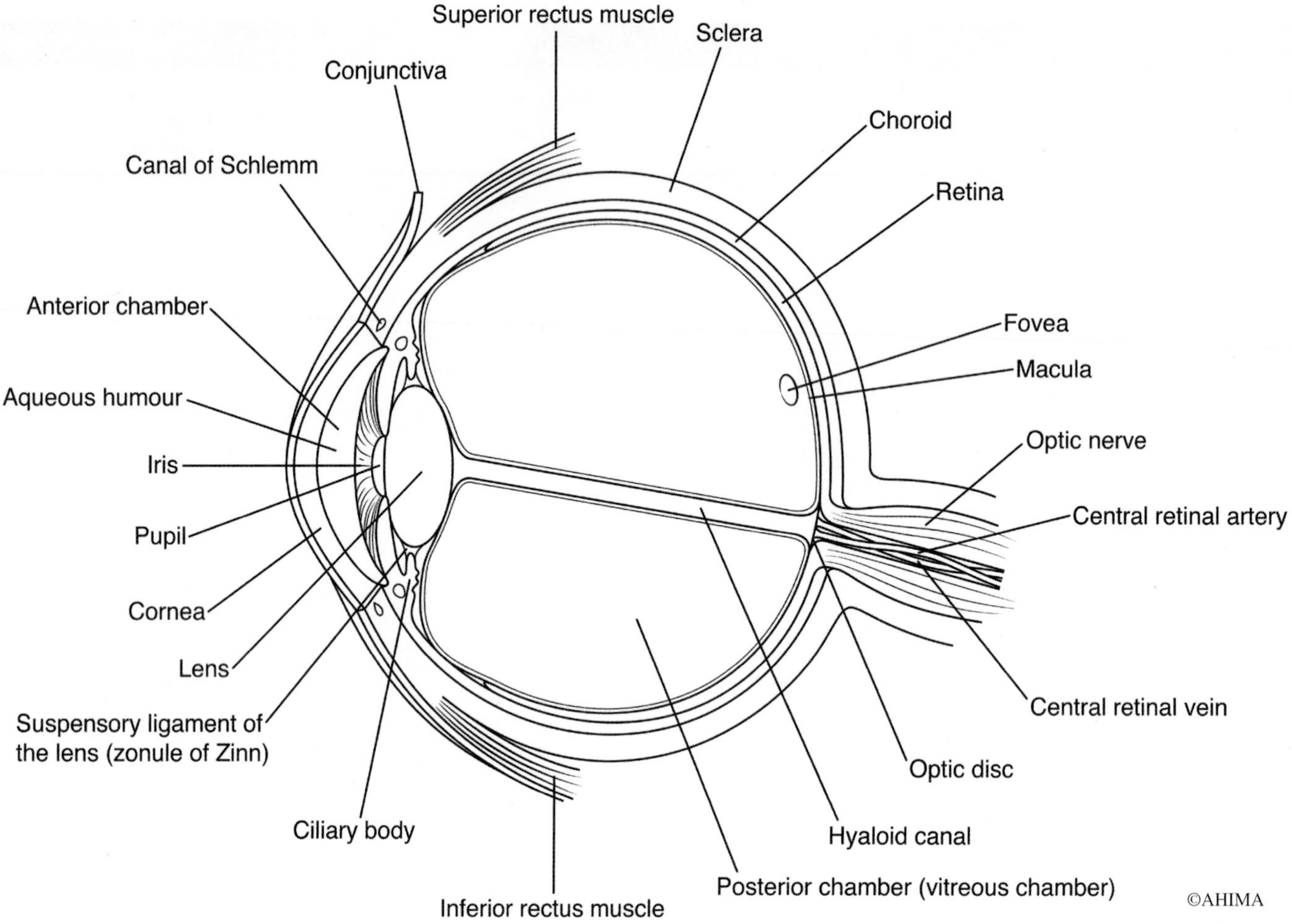

Superior rectus muscle
Sclera
Conjunctiva
Choroid
Canal of Schlemm
Retina
Anterior chamber
Fovea
Macula
Aqueous humour
Iris
Optic nerve
Central retinal artery
Pupil
Cornea
Lens
Central retinal vein
Suspensory ligament of
the lens (zonule of Zinn)
Optic disc
Ciliary body
Hyaloid canal
Posterior chamber (vitreous chamber)
Inferior rectus muscle

Upper eyelid
Lacrimal gland
Superior lacrimal canal
Lacrimal gland
ducts
Lacrimal sac
Sclera
Pupil
Lacrimal duct
Iris
Lower eyelid
Inferior lacrimal canal
Lacrimal puncta

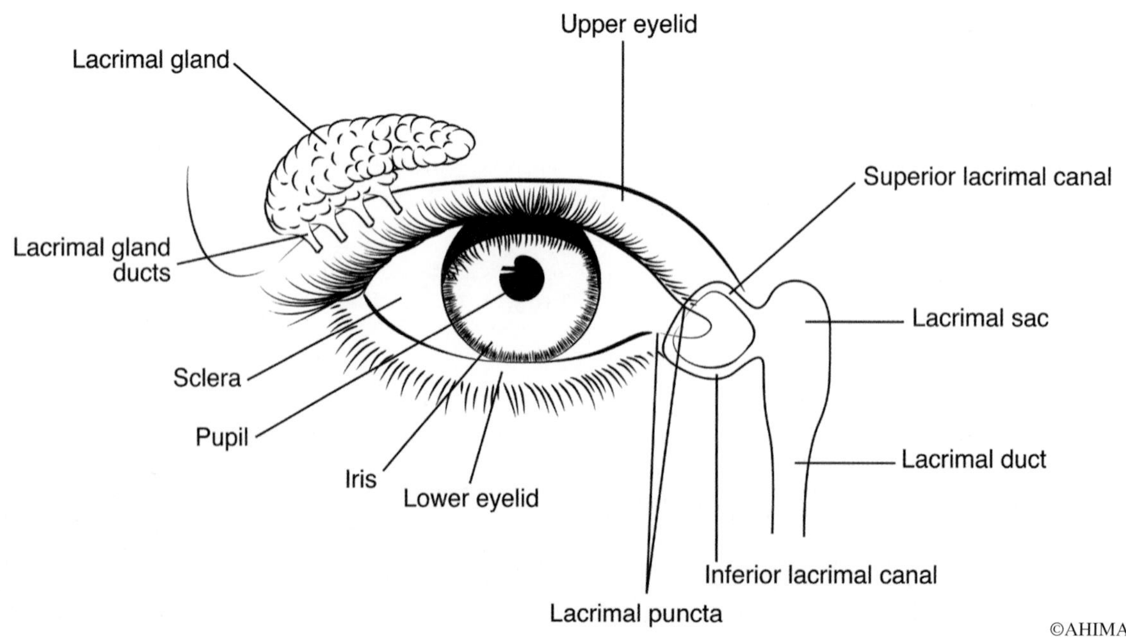

Eye Muscles

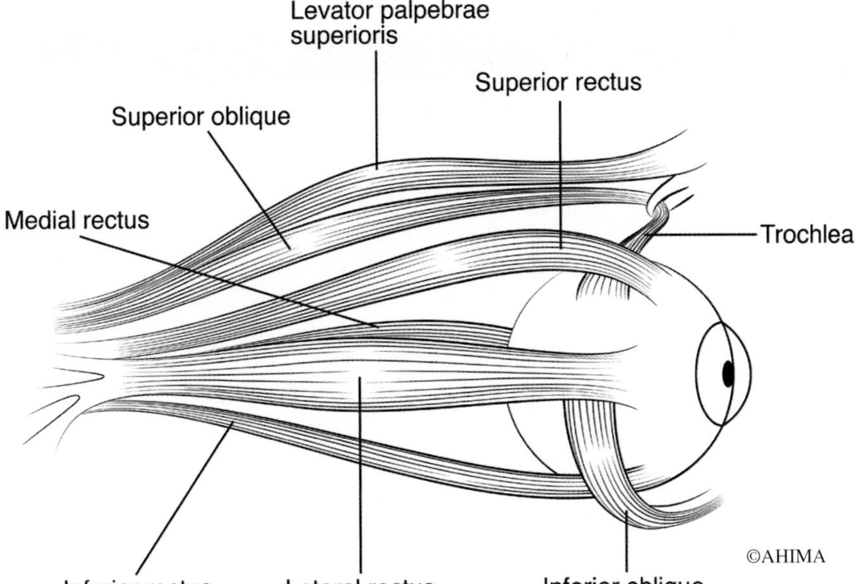

e Tables 080–08X

tion	0	**Medical and Surgical**
ly System	8	**Eye**
eration	0	**Alteration:** Modifying the anatomic structure of a body part without affecting the function of the body part

Body Part (4th)	Approach (5th)	Device (6th)	Qualifier (7th)
Upper Eyelid, Right Upper Eyelid, Left Lower Eyelid, Right Lower Eyelid, Left	**0** Open **3** Percutaneous **X** External	**7** Autologous Tissue Substitute **J** Synthetic Substitute **K** Nonautologous Tissue Substitute **Z** No Device	**Z** No Qualifier

tion	0	**Medical and Surgical**
dy System	8	**Eye**
eration	1	**Bypass:** Altering the route of passage of the contents of a tubular body part

Body Part (4th)	Approach (5th)	Device (6th)	Qualifier (7th)
Anterior Chamber, Right Anterior Chamber, Left	**3** Percutaneous	**J** Synthetic Substitute **K** Nonautologous Tissue Substitute **Z** No Device	**4** Sclera
Lacrimal Duct, Right Lacrimal Duct, Left	**0** Open **3** Percutaneous	**J** Synthetic Substitute **K** Nonautologous Tissue Substitute **Z** No Device	**3** Nasal Cavity

tion	0	**Medical and Surgical**
dy System	8	**Eye**
eration	2	**Change:** Taking out or off a device from a body part and putting back an identical or similar device in or on the same body part without cutting or puncturing the skin or a mucous membrane

Body Part (4th)	Approach (5th)	Device (6th)	Qualifier (7th)
Eye, Right Eye, Left	**X** External	**0** Drainage Device **Y** Other Device	**Z** No Qualifier

Section 0 **Medical and Surgical**
Body System 8 **Eye**
Operation 5 **Destruction:** Physical eradication of all or a portion of a body part by the direct use of energy, force, or a destructive ag

Body Part (4th)	Approach (5th)	Device (6th)	Qualifier (7th)
0 Eye, Right **1** Eye, Left **6** Sclera, Right **7** Sclera, Left **8** Cornea, Right **9** Cornea, Left **S** Conjunctiva, Right **T** Conjunctiva, Left	**X** External	**Z** No Device	**Z** No Qualifier
2 Anterior Chamber, Right **3** Anterior Chamber, Left **4** Vitreous, Right **5** Vitreous, Left **C** Iris, Right **D** Iris, Left **E** Retina, Right **F** Retina, Left **G** Retinal Vessel, Right **H** Retinal Vessel, Left **J** Lens, Right **K** Lens, Left	**3** Percutaneous	**Z** No Device	**Z** No Qualifier
A Choroid, Right **B** Choroid, Left **L** Extraocular Muscle, Right **M** Extraocular Muscle, Left **V** Lacrimal Gland, Right **W** Lacrimal Gland, Left	**0** Open **3** Percutaneous	**Z** No Device	**Z** No Qualifier
N Upper Eyelid, Right **P** Upper Eyelid, Left **Q** Lower Eyelid, Right **R** Lower Eyelid, Left	**0** Open **3** Percutaneous **X** External	**Z** No Device	**Z** No Qualifier
X Lacrimal Duct, Right **Y** Lacrimal Duct, Left	**0** Open **3** Percutaneous **7** Via Natural or Artificial Opening **8** Via Natural or Artificial Opening Endoscopic	**Z** No Device	**Z** No Qualifier

Section 0 **Medical and Surgical**
Body System 8 **Eye**
Operation 7 **Dilation:** Expanding an orifice or the lumen of a tubular body part

Body Part (4th)	Approach (5th)	Device (6th)	Qualifier (7th)
X Lacrimal Duct, Right **Y** Lacrimal Duct, Left	**0** Open **3** Percutaneous **7** Via Natural or Artificial Opening **8** Via Natural or Artificial Opening Endoscopic	**D** Intraluminal Device **Z** No Device	**Z** No Qualifier

tion **0** **Medical and Surgical**
dy System **8** **Eye**
eration **9** **Drainage:** Taking or letting out fluids and/or gases from a body part

Body Part (4th)	Approach (5th)	Device (6th)	Qualifier (7th)
Eye, Right Eye, Left Sclera, Right Sclera, Left Cornea, Right Cornea, Left Conjunctiva, Right Conjunctiva, Left	**X** External	**0** Drainage Device	**Z** No Qualifier
Eye, Right Eye, Left Sclera, Right Sclera, Left Cornea, Right Cornea, Left Conjunctiva, Right Conjunctiva, Left	**X** External	**Z** No Device	**X** Diagnostic **Z** No Qualifier
Anterior Chamber, Right Anterior Chamber, Left Vitreous, Right Vitreous, Left Iris, Right Iris, Left Retina, Right Retina, Left Retinal Vessel, Right Retinal Vessel, Left Lens, Right Lens, Left	**3** Percutaneous	**0** Drainage Device	**Z** No Qualifier
Anterior Chamber, Right Anterior Chamber, Left Vitreous, Right Vitreous, Left Iris, Right Iris, Left Retina, Right Retina, Left Retinal Vessel, Right Retinal Vessel, Left Lens, Right Lens, Left	**3** Percutaneous	**Z** No Device	**X** Diagnostic **Z** No Qualifier
Choroid, Right Choroid, Left Extraocular Muscle, Right **M** Extraocular Muscle, Left Lacrimal Gland, Right **W** Lacrimal Gland, Left	**0** Open **3** Percutaneous	**0** Drainage Device	**Z** No Qualifier
Choroid, Right Choroid, Left Extraocular Muscle, Right **M** Extraocular Muscle, Left Lacrimal Gland, Right **W** Lacrimal Gland, Left	**0** Open **3** Percutaneous	**Z** No Device	**X** Diagnostic **Z** No Qualifier
Upper Eyelid, Right Upper Eyelid, Left Lower Eyelid, Right Lower Eyelid, Left	**0** Open **3** Percutaneous **X** External	**0** Drainage Device	**Z** No Qualifier

Continued →

089 Continued

Section 0 **Medical and Surgical**
Body System 8 **Eye**
Operation 9 **Drainage:** Taking or letting out fluids and/or gases from a body part

Body Part (4th)	Approach (5th)	Device (6th)	Qualifier (7th)
N Upper Eyelid, Right **P** Upper Eyelid, Left **Q** Lower Eyelid, Right **R** Lower Eyelid, Left	**0** Open **3** Percutaneous **X** External	**Z** No Device	**X** Diagnostic **Z** No Qualifier
X Lacrimal Duct, Right **Y** Lacrimal Duct, Left	**0** Open **3** Percutaneous **7** Via Natural or Artificial Opening **8** Via Natural or Artificial Opening Endoscopic	**0** Drainage Device	**Z** No Qualifier
X Lacrimal Duct, Right **Y** Lacrimal Duct, Left	**0** Open **3** Percutaneous **7** Via Natural or Artificial Opening **8** Via Natural or Artificial Opening Endoscopic	**Z** No Device	**X** Diagnostic **Z** No Qualifier

Section 0 **Medical and Surgical**
Body System 8 **Eye**
Operation B **Excision:** Cutting out or off, without replacement, a portion of a body part

Body Part (4th)	Approach (5th)	Device (6th)	Qualifier (7th)
0 Eye, Right **1** Eye, Left **N** Upper Eyelid, Right **P** Upper Eyelid, Left **Q** Lower Eyelid, Right **R** Lower Eyelid, Left	**0** Open **3** Percutaneous **X** External	**Z** No Device	**X** Diagnostic **Z** No Qualifier
4 Vitreous, Right **5** Vitreous, Left **C** Iris, Right **D** Iris, Left **E** Retina, Right **F** Retina, Left **J** Lens, Right **K** Lens, Left	**3** Percutaneous	**Z** No Device	**X** Diagnostic **Z** No Qualifier
6 Sclera, Right **7** Sclera, Left **8** Cornea, Right **9** Cornea, Left **S** Conjunctiva, Right **T** Conjunctiva, Left	**X** External	**Z** No Device	**X** Diagnostic **Z** No Qualifier
A Choroid, Right **B** Choroid, Left **L** Extraocular Muscle, Right **M** Extraocular Muscle, Left **V** Lacrimal Gland, Right **W** Lacrimal Gland, Left	**0** Open **3** Percutaneous	**Z** No Device	**X** Diagnostic **Z** No Qualifier
X Lacrimal Duct, Right **Y** Lacrimal Duct, Left	**0** Open **3** Percutaneous **7** Via Natural or Artificial Opening **8** Via Natural or Artificial Opening Endoscopic	**Z** No Device	**X** Diagnostic **Z** No Qualifier

Section	**0**	**Medical and Surgical**
Body System	**8**	**Eye**
Operation	**C**	**Extirpation:** Taking or cutting out solid matter from a body part

Body Part (4th)	Approach (5th)	Device (6th)	Qualifier (7th)
0 Eye, Right **1** Eye, Left **6** Sclera, Right **7** Sclera, Left **8** Cornea, Right **9** Cornea, Left **S** Conjunctiva, Right **T** Conjunctiva, Left	**X** External	**Z** No Device	**Z** No Qualifier
2 Anterior Chamber, Right **3** Anterior Chamber, Left **4** Vitreous, Right **5** Vitreous, Left **C** Iris, Right **D** Iris, Left **E** Retina, Right **F** Retina, Left **G** Retinal Vessel, Right **H** Retinal Vessel, Left **J** Lens, Right **K** Lens, Left	**3** Percutaneous **X** External	**Z** No Device	**Z** No Qualifier
A Choroid, Right **B** Choroid, Left **L** Extraocular Muscle, Right **M** Extraocular Muscle, Left **N** Upper Eyelid, Right **P** Upper Eyelid, Left **Q** Lower Eyelid, Right **R** Lower Eyelid, Left **V** Lacrimal Gland, Right **W** Lacrimal Gland, Left	**0** Open **3** Percutaneous **X** External	**Z** No Device	**Z** No Qualifier
X Lacrimal Duct, Right **Y** Lacrimal Duct, Left	**0** Open **3** Percutaneous **7** Via Natural or Artificial Opening **8** Via Natural or Artificial Opening Endoscopic	**Z** No Device	**Z** No Qualifier

Section 0 **Medical and Surgical**
Body System 8 **Eye**
Operation D **Extraction:** Pulling or stripping out or off all or a portion of a body part by the use of force

Body Part (4th)	Approach (5th)	Device (6th)	Qualifier (7th)
8 Cornea, Right **9** Cornea, Left	**X** External	**Z** No Device	**X** Diagnostic **Z** No Qualifier
J Lens, Right **K** Lens, Left	**3** Percutaneous	**Z** No Device	**Z** No Qualifier

Section 0 **Medical and Surgical**
Body System 8 **Eye**
Operation F **Fragmentation:** Breaking solid matter in a body part into pieces

Body Part (4th)	Approach (5th)	Device (6th)	Qualifier (7th)
4 Vitreous, Right **5** Vitreous, Left	**3** Percutaneous **X** External	**Z** No Device	**Z** No Qualifier

Section 0 **Medical and Surgical**
Body System 8 **Eye**
Operation H **Insertion:** Putting in a nonbiological appliance that monitors, assists, performs, or prevents a physiological function but does not physically take the place of a body part

Body Part (4th)	Approach (5th)	Device (6th)	Qualifier (7th)
0 Eye, Right **1** Eye, Left	**0** Open	**5** Epiretinal Visual Prosthesis **Y** Other Device	**Z** No Qualifier
0 Eye, Right **1** Eye, Left	**3** Percutaneous	**1** Radioactive Element **3** Infusion Device **Y** Other Device	**Z** No Qualifier
0 Eye, Right **1** Eye, Left	**7** Via Natural or Artificial Opening **8** Via Natural or Artificial Opening Endoscopic	**Y** Other Device	**Z** No Qualifier
0 Eye, Right **1** Eye, Left	**X** External	**1** Radioactive Element **3** Infusion Device	**Z** No Qualifier

Section 0 **Medical and Surgical**
Body System 8 **Eye**
Operation J **Inspection:** Visually and/or manually exploring a body part

Body Part (4th)	Approach (5th)	Device (6th)	Qualifier (7th)
0 Eye, Right **1** Eye, Left **J** Lens, Right **K** Lens, Left	**X** External	**Z** No Device	**Z** No Qualifier
L Extraocular Muscle, Right **M** Extraocular Muscle, Left	**0** Open **X** External	**Z** No Device	**Z** No Qualifier

tion **0** **Medical and Surgical**
ly System **8** **Eye**
eration **L** **Occlusion:** Completely closing an orifice or the lumen of a tubular body part

Body Part (4th)	Approach (5th)	Device (6th)	Qualifier (7th)
Lacrimal Duct, Right Lacrimal Duct, Left	**0** Open **3** Percutaneous	**C** Extraluminal Device **D** Intraluminal Device **Z** No Device	**Z** No Qualifier
Lacrimal Duct, Right Lacrimal Duct, Left	**7** Via Natural or Artificial Opening **8** Via Natural or Artificial Opening Endoscopic	**D** Intraluminal Device **Z** No Device	**Z** No Qualifier

tion **0** **Medical and Surgical**
dy System **8** **Eye**
eration **M** **Reattachment:** Putting back in or on all or a portion of a separated body part to its normal location or other suitable location

Body Part (4th)	Approach (5th)	Device (6th)	Qualifier (7th)
Upper Eyelid, Right Upper Eyelid, Left Lower Eyelid, Right Lower Eyelid, Left	**X** External	**Z** No Device	**Z** No Qualifier

tion **0** **Medical and Surgical**
dy System **8** **Eye**
eration **N** **Release:** Freeing a body part from an abnormal physical constraint by cutting or by the use of force

Body Part (4th)	Approach (5th)	Device (6th)	Qualifier (7th)
Eye, Right Eye, Left Sclera, Right Sclera, Left Cornea, Right Cornea, Left Conjunctiva, Right Conjunctiva, Left	**X** External	**Z** No Device	**Z** No Qualifier
Anterior Chamber, Right Anterior Chamber, Left Vitreous, Right Vitreous, Left Iris, Right Iris, Left Retina, Right Retina, Left Retinal Vessel, Right Retinal Vessel, Left Lens, Right Lens, Left	**3** Percutaneous	**Z** No Device	**Z** No Qualifier
Choroid, Right Choroid, Left Extraocular Muscle, Right **M** Extraocular Muscle, Left **V** Lacrimal Gland, Right **W** Lacrimal Gland, Left	**0** Open **3** Percutaneous	**Z** No Device	**Z** No Qualifier
N Upper Eyelid, Right **P** Upper Eyelid, Left **Q** Lower Eyelid, Right **R** Lower Eyelid, Left	**0** Open **3** Percutaneous **X** External	**Z** No Device	**Z** No Qualifier
X Lacrimal Duct, Right **Y** Lacrimal Duct, Left	**0** Open **3** Percutaneous **7** Via Natural or Artificial Opening **8** Via Natural or Artificial Opening Endoscopic	**Z** No Device	**Z** No Qualifier

Section 0 **Medical and Surgical**
Body System 8 **Eye**
Operation P **Removal:** Taking out or off a device from a body part

Body Part (4th)	Approach (5th)	Device (6th)	Qualifier (7th)
0 Eye, Right **1** Eye, Left	**0** Open **3** Percutaneous **7** Via Natural or Artificial Opening **8** Via Natural or Artificial Opening Endoscopic	**0** Drainage Device **1** Radioactive Element **3** Infusion Device **7** Autologous Tissue Substitute **C** Extraluminal Device **D** Intraluminal Device **J** Synthetic Substitute **K** Nonautologous Tissue Substitute **Y** Other Device	**Z** No Qualifier
0 Eye, Right **1** Eye, Left	**X** External	**0** Drainage Device **1** Radioactive Element **3** Infusion Device **7** Autologous Tissue Substitute **C** Extraluminal Device **D** Intraluminal Device **J** Synthetic Substitute **K** Nonautologous Tissue Substitute	**Z** No Qualifier
J Lens, Right **K** Lens, Left	**3** Percutaneous	**J** Synthetic Substitute **Y** Other Device	**Z** No Qualifier
L Extraocular Muscle, Right **M** Extraocular Muscle, Left	**0** Open **3** Percutaneous	**0** Drainage Device **7** Autologous Tissue Substitute **J** Synthetic Substitute **K** Nonautologous Tissue Substitute **Y** Other Device	**Z** No Qualifier

Section 0 **Medical and Surgical**
Body System 8 **Eye**
Operation Q **Repair:** Restoring, to the extent possible, a body part to its normal anatomic structure and function

Body Part (4th)	Approach (5th)	Device (6th)	Qualifier (7th)
0 Eye, Right **1** Eye, Left **6** Sclera, Right **7** Sclera, Left **8** Cornea, Right **9** Cornea, Left **S** Conjunctiva, Right **T** Conjunctiva, Left	**X** External	**Z** No Device	**Z** No Qualifier
2 Anterior Chamber, Right **3** Anterior Chamber, Left **4** Vitreous, Right **5** Vitreous, Left **C** Iris, Right **D** Iris, Left **E** Retina, Right **F** Retina, Left **G** Retinal Vessel, Right **H** Retinal Vessel, Left **J** Lens, Right **K** Lens, Left	**3** Percutaneous	**Z** No Device	**Z** No Qualifier

Continued →

Section 0 Medical and Surgical
Body System 8 Eye
Operation Q **Repair:** Restoring, to the extent possible, a body part to its normal anatomic structure and function

Body Part (4th)	Approach (5th)	Device (6th)	Qualifier (7th)
A Choroid, Right **B** Choroid, Left **L** Extraocular Muscle, Right **M** Extraocular Muscle, Left **V** Lacrimal Gland, Right **W** Lacrimal Gland, Left	**0** Open **3** Percutaneous	**Z** No Device	**Z** No Qualifier
N Upper Eyelid, Right **P** Upper Eyelid, Left **Q** Lower Eyelid, Right **R** Lower Eyelid, Left	**0** Open **3** Percutaneous **X** External	**Z** No Device	**Z** No Qualifier
X Lacrimal Duct, Right **Y** Lacrimal Duct, Left	**0** Open **3** Percutaneous **7** Via Natural or Artificial Opening **8** Via Natural or Artificial Opening Endoscopic	**Z** No Device	**Z** No Qualifier

Section 0 Medical and Surgical
Body System 8 Eye
Operation R **Replacement:** Putting in or on biological or synthetic material that physically takes the place and/or function of all or a portion of a body part

Body Part (4th)	Approach (5th)	Device (6th)	Qualifier (7th)
0 Eye, Right **1** Eye, Left **A** Choroid, Right **B** Choroid, Left	**0** Open **3** Percutaneous	**7** Autologous Tissue Substitute **J** Synthetic Substitute **K** Nonautologous Tissue Substitute	**Z** No Qualifier
4 Vitreous, Right **5** Vitreous, Left **C** Iris, Right **D** Iris, Left **G** Retinal Vessel, Right **H** Retinal Vessel, Left	**3** Percutaneous	**7** Autologous Tissue Substitute **J** Synthetic Substitute **K** Nonautologous Tissue Substitute	**Z** No Qualifier
6 Sclera, Right **7** Sclera, Left **S** Conjunctiva, Right **T** Conjunctiva, Left	**X** External	**7** Autologous Tissue Substitute **J** Synthetic Substitute **K** Nonautologous Tissue Substitute	**Z** No Qualifier
8 Cornea, Right **9** Cornea, Left	**3** Percutaneous **X** External	**7** Autologous Tissue Substitute **J** Synthetic Substitute **K** Nonautologous Tissue Substitute	**Z** No Qualifier
J Lens, Right **K** Lens, Left	**3** Percutaneous	**0** Synthetic Substitute, Intraocular Telescope **7** Autologous Tissue Substitute **J** Synthetic Substitute **K** Nonautologous Tissue Substitute	**Z** No Qualifier
N Upper Eyelid, Right **P** Upper Eyelid, Left **Q** Lower Eyelid, Right **R** Lower Eyelid, Left	**0** Open **3** Percutaneous **X** External	**7** Autologous Tissue Substitute **J** Synthetic Substitute **K** Nonautologous Tissue Substitute	**Z** No Qualifier
X Lacrimal Duct, Right **Y** Lacrimal Duct, Left	**0** Open **3** Percutaneous **7** Via Natural or Artificial Opening **8** Via Natural or Artificial Opening Endoscopic	**7** Autologous Tissue Substitute **J** Synthetic Substitute **K** Nonautologous Tissue Substitute	**Z** No Qualifier

Section 0 **Medical and Surgical**
Body System 8 **Eye**
Operation S **Reposition:** Moving to its normal location, or other suitable location, all or a portion of a body part

Body Part (4th)	Approach (5th)	Device (6th)	Qualifier (7th)
C Iris, Right **D** Iris, Left **G** Retinal Vessel, Right **H** Retinal Vessel, Left **J** Lens, Right **K** Lens, Left	**3** Percutaneous	**Z** No Device	**Z** No Qualifier
L Extraocular Muscle, Right **M** Extraocular Muscle, Left **V** Lacrimal Gland, Right **W** Lacrimal Gland, Left	**0** Open **3** Percutaneous	**Z** No Device	**Z** No Qualifier
N Upper Eyelid, Right **P** Upper Eyelid, Left **Q** Lower Eyelid, Right **R** Lower Eyelid, Left	**0** Open **3** Percutaneous **X** External	**Z** No Device	**Z** No Qualifier
X Lacrimal Duct, Right **Y** Lacrimal Duct, Left	**0** Open **3** Percutaneous **7** Via Natural or Artificial Opening **8** Via Natural or Artificial Opening Endoscopic	**Z** No Device	**Z** No Qualifier

Section 0 **Medical and Surgical**
Body System 8 **Eye**
Operation T **Resection:** Cutting out or off, without replacement, all of a body part

Body Part (4th)	Approach (5th)	Device (6th)	Qualifier (7th)
0 Eye, Right **1** Eye, Left **8** Cornea, Right **9** Cornea, Left	**X** External	**Z** No Device	**Z** No Qualifier
4 Vitreous, Right **5** Vitreous, Left **C** Iris, Right **D** Iris, Left **J** Lens, Right **K** Lens, Left	**3** Percutaneous	**Z** No Device	**Z** No Qualifier
L Extraocular Muscle, Right **M** Extraocular Muscle, Left **V** Lacrimal Gland, Right **W** Lacrimal Gland, Left	**0** Open **3** Percutaneous	**Z** No Device	**Z** No Qualifier
N Upper Eyelid, Right **P** Upper Eyelid, Left **Q** Lower Eyelid, Right **R** Lower Eyelid, Left	**0** Open **X** External	**Z** No Device	**Z** No Qualifier
X Lacrimal Duct, Right **Y** Lacrimal Duct, Left	**0** Open **3** Percutaneous **7** Via Natural or Artificial Opening **8** Via Natural or Artificial Opening Endoscopic	**Z** No Device	**Z** No Qualifier

tion 0 **Medical and Surgical**
ly System 8 **Eye**
eration U **Supplement:** Putting in or on biological or synthetic material that physically reinforces and/or augments the function of a portion of a body part

Body Part (4th)	Approach (5th)	Device (6th)	Qualifier (7th)
Eye, Right Eye, Left Iris, Right Iris, Left Retina, Right Retina, Left Retinal Vessel, Right Retinal Vessel, Left Extraocular Muscle, Right Extraocular Muscle, Left	**0** Open **3** Percutaneous	**7** Autologous Tissue Substitute **J** Synthetic Substitute **K** Nonautologous Tissue Substitute	**Z** No Qualifier
Cornea, Right Cornea, Left Upper Eyelid, Right Upper Eyelid, Left Lower Eyelid, Right Lower Eyelid, Left	**0** Open **3** Percutaneous **X** External	**7** Autologous Tissue Substitute **J** Synthetic Substitute **K** Nonautologous Tissue Substitute	**Z** No Qualifier
Lacrimal Duct, Right Lacrimal Duct, Left	**0** Open **3** Percutaneous **7** Via Natural or Artificial Opening **8** Via Natural or Artificial Opening Endoscopic	**7** Autologous Tissue Substitute **J** Synthetic Substitute **K** Nonautologous Tissue Substitute	**Z** No Qualifier

tion 0 **Medical and Surgical**
dy System 8 **Eye**
eration V **Restriction:** Partially closing an orifice or the lumen of a tubular body part

Body Part (4th)	Approach (5th)	Device (6th)	Qualifier (7th)
Lacrimal Duct, Right Lacrimal Duct, Left	**0** Open **3** Percutaneous	**C** Extraluminal Device **D** Intraluminal Device **Z** No Device	**Z** No Qualifier
Lacrimal Duct, Right Lacrimal Duct, Left	**7** Via Natural or Artificial Opening **8** Via Natural or Artificial Opening Endoscopic	**D** Intraluminal Device **Z** No Device	**Z** No Qualifier

tion 0 **Medical and Surgical**
dy System 8 **Eye**
eration W **Revision:** Correcting, to the extent possible, a portion of a malfunctioning device or the position of a displaced device

Body Part (4th)	Approach (5th)	Device (6th)	Qualifier (7th)
Eye, Right Eye, Left	**0** Open **3** Percutaneous **7** Via Natural or Artificial Opening **8** Via Natural or Artificial Opening Endoscopic	**0** Drainage Device **3** Infusion Device **7** Autologous Tissue Substitute **C** Extraluminal Device **D** Intraluminal Device **J** Synthetic Substitute **K** Nonautologous Tissue Substitute **Y** Other Device	**Z** No Qualifier
Eye, Right Eye, Left	**X** External	**0** Drainage Device **3** Infusion Device **7** Autologous Tissue Substitute **C** Extraluminal Device **D** Intraluminal Device **J** Synthetic Substitute **K** Nonautologous Tissue Substitute	**Z** No Qualifier

Continued →

Section 0 Medical and Surgical
Body System 8 Eye
Operation W Revision: Correcting, to the extent possible, a portion of a malfunctioning device or the position of a displaced device

Body Part (4th)	Approach (5th)	Device (6th)	Qualifier (7th)
J Lens, Right **K** Lens, Left	**3** Percutaneous	**J** Synthetic Substitute **Y** Other Device	**Z** No Qualifier
J Lens, Right **K** Lens, Left	**X** External	**J** Synthetic Substitute	**Z** No Qualifier
L Extraocular Muscle, Right **M** Extraocular Muscle, Left	**0** Open **3** Percutaneous	**0** Drainage Device **7** Autologous Tissue Substitute **J** Synthetic Substitute **K** Nonautologous Tissue Substitute **Y** Other Device	**Z** No Qualifier

Section 0 Medical and Surgical
Body System 8 Eye
Operation X Transfer: Moving, without taking out, all or a portion of a body part to another location to take over the function of all or a portion of a body part

Body Part (4th)	Approach (5th)	Device (6th)	Qualifier (7th)
L Extraocular Muscle, Right **M** Extraocular Muscle, Left	**0** Open **3** Percutaneous	**Z** No Device	**Z** No Qualifier

AHA Coding Clinic

08923ZZ Drainage of Right Anterior Chamber, Percutaneous Approach—AHA CC: 2Q, 2016, 21-22

08B43ZZ Excision of Right Vitreous, Percutaneous Approach—AHA CC: 4Q, 2014, 36-37

08B53ZZ Excision of Left Vitreous, Percutaneous Approach—AHA CC: 4Q, 2014, 35-36

08J0XZZ Inspection of Right Eye, External Approach—AHA CC: 1Q, 2015, 35-36

08NC3ZZ Release Right Iris, Percutaneous Approach—AHA CC: 2Q, 2015, 24-25

08R8XKZ Replacement of Right Cornea with Nonautologous Tissue Substitute, External Approach—AHA CC: 2Q, 2015, 24-26

08T1XZZ Resection of Left Eye, External Approach—AHA CC: 2Q, 2015, 12-13

08TM0ZZ Resection of Left Extraocular Muscle, Open Approach—AHA CC: 2Q, 2015, 12-13

08TR0ZZ Resection of Left Lower Eyelid, Open Approach—AHA CC: 2Q, 2015, 12-13

08U9XKZ Supplement Left Cornea with Nonautologous Tissue Substitute, External Approach—AHA CC: 3Q, 2014, 31

Nose and Sinus

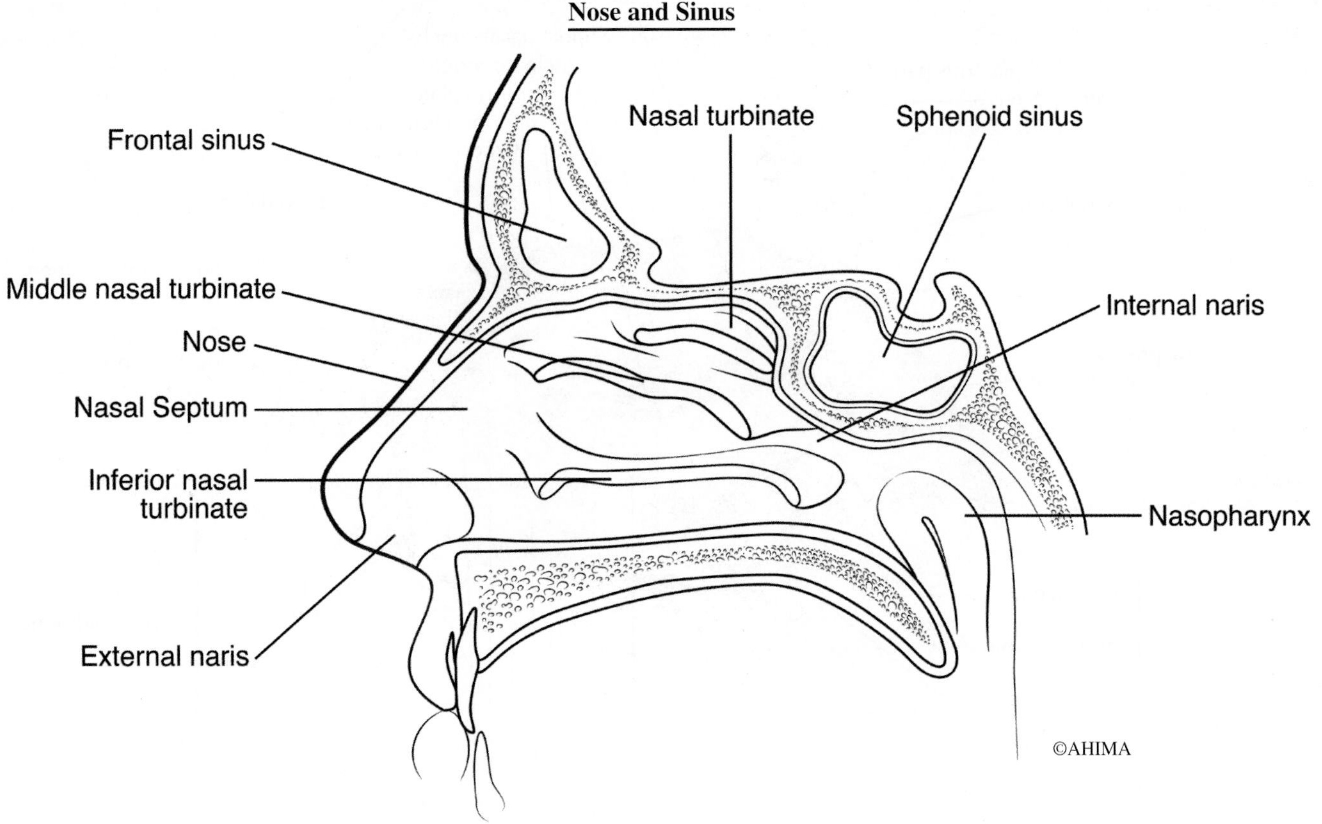

Lateral Wall of Nasal Cavity

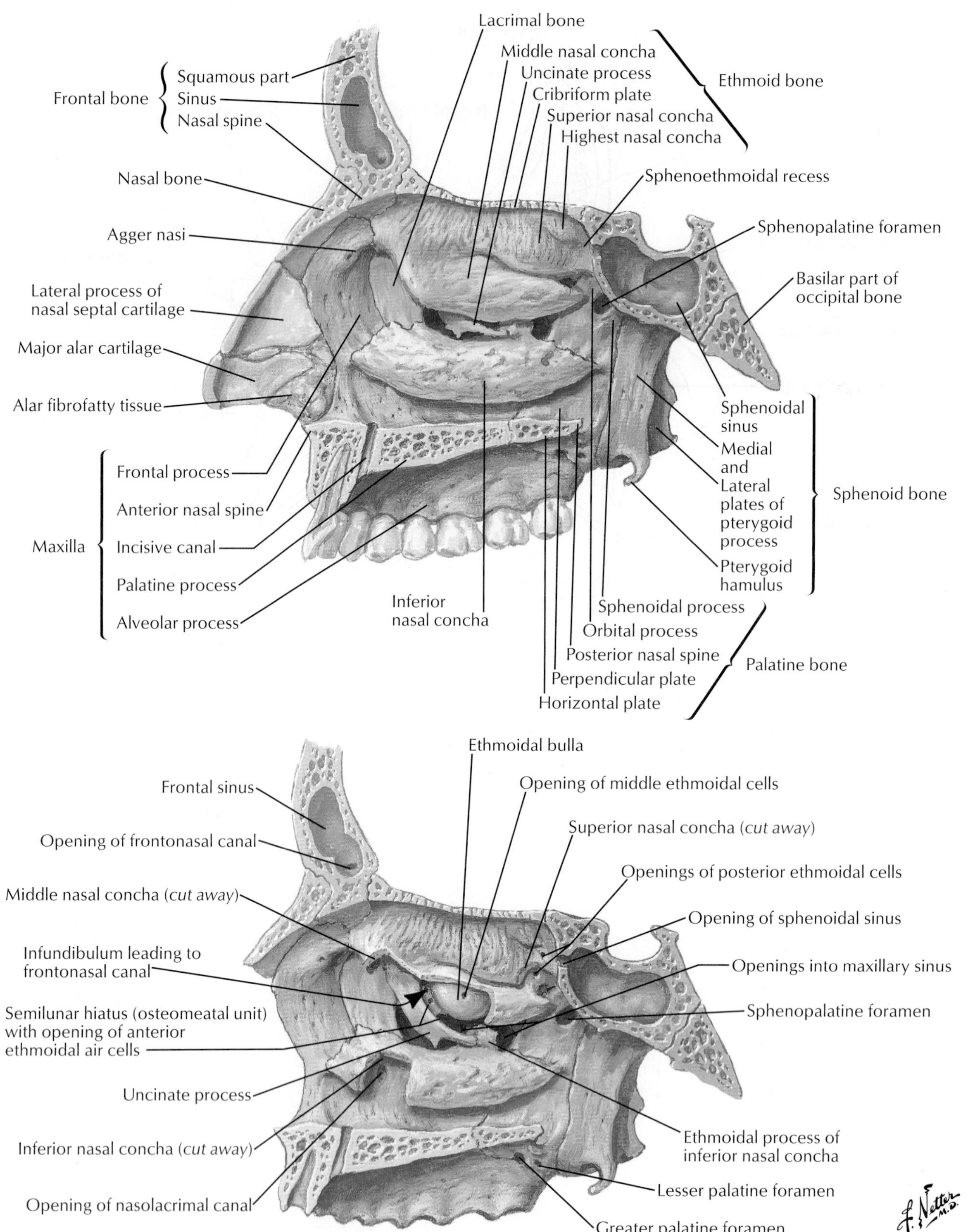

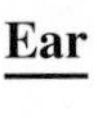

Ear

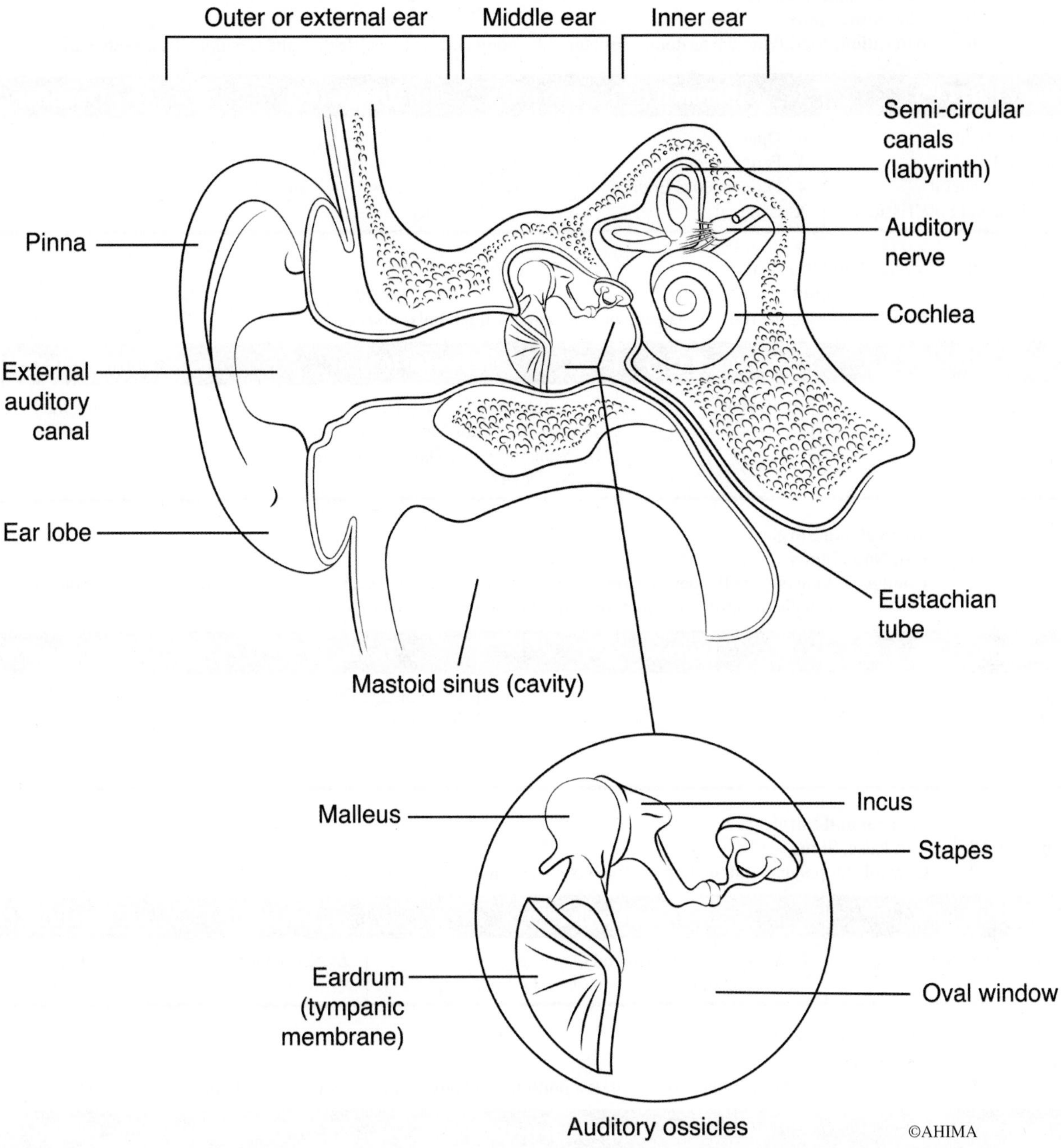

Outer or external ear
Middle ear
Inner ear
Semi-circular canals (labyrinth)
Pinna
Auditory nerve
Cochlea
External auditory canal
Ear lobe
Eustachian tube
Mastoid sinus (cavity)
Malleus
Incus
Stapes
Eardrum (tympanic membrane)
Oval window
Auditory ossicles
©AHIMA

Ear, Nose, Sinus Tables 090–09W

Section 0 **Medical and Surgical**
Body System 9 **Ear, Nose, Sinus**
Operation 0 **Alteration:** Modifying the anatomic structure of a body part without affecting the function of the body part

Body Part (4th)	Approach (5th)	Device (6th)	Qualifier (7th)
0 External Ear, Right **1** External Ear, Left **2** External Ear, Bilateral **K** Nasal Mucosa and Soft Tissue	**0** Open **3** Percutaneous **4** Percutaneous Endoscopic **X** External	**7** Autologous Tissue Substitute **J** Synthetic Substitute **K** Nonautologous Tissue Substitute **Z** No Device	**Z** No Qualifier

Section 0 **Medical and Surgical**
Body System 9 **Ear, Nose, Sinus**
Operation 1 **Bypass:** Altering the route of passage of the contents of a tubular body part

Body Part (4th)	Approach (5th)	Device (6th)	Qualifier (7th)
D Inner Ear, Right **E** Inner Ear, Left	**0** Open	**7** Autologous Tissue Substitute **J** Synthetic Substitute **K** Nonautologous Tissue Substitute **Z** No Device	**0** Endolymphatic

Section 0 **Medical and Surgical**
Body System 9 **Ear, Nose, Sinus**
Operation 2 **Change:** Taking out or off a device from a body part and putting back an identical or similar device in or on the same bo part without cutting or puncturing the skin or a mucous membrane

Body Part (4th)	Approach (5th)	Device (6th)	Qualifier (7th)
H Ear, Right **J** Ear, Left **K** Nasal Mucosa and Soft Tissue **Y** Sinus	**X** External	**0** Drainage Device **Y** Other Device	**Z** No Qualifier

Section 0 **Medical and Surgical**
Body System 9 **Ear, Nose, Sinus**
Operation 3 **Control:** Stopping, or attempting to stop, postprocedural or other acute bleeding

Body Part (4th)	Approach (5th)	Device (6th)	Qualifier (7th)
K Nasal Mucosa and Soft Tissue	**7** Via Natural or Artificial Opening **8** Via Natural or Artificial Opening Endoscopic	**Z** No Device	**Z** No Qualifier

Section 0 **Medical and Surgical**
Body System 9 **Ear, Nose, Sinus**
Operation 5 **Destruction:** Physical eradication of all or a portion of a body part by the direct use of energy, force, or a destructive age

Body Part (4th)	Approach (5th)	Device (6th)	Qualifier (7th)
0 External Ear, Right **1** External Ear, Left	**0** Open **3** Percutaneous **4** Percutaneous Endoscopic **X** External	**Z** No Device	**Z** No Qualifier
3 External Auditory Canal, Right **4** External Auditory Canal, Left	**0** Open **3** Percutaneous **4** Percutaneous Endoscopic **7** Via Natural or Artificial Opening **8** Via Natural or Artificial Opening Endoscopic **X** External	**Z** No Device	**Z** No Qualifier
5 Middle Ear, Right **6** Middle Ear, Left **9** Auditory Ossicle, Right **A** Auditory Ossicle, Left **D** Inner Ear, Right **E** Inner Ear, Left	**0** Open **8** Via Natural or Artificial Opening Endoscopic	**Z** No Device	**Z** No Qualifier

Continued →

095 Continued

tion 0 **Medical and Surgical**
ly System 9 **Ear, Nose, Sinus**
eration 5 **Destruction:** Physical eradication of all or a portion of a body part by the direct use of energy, force, or a destructive agent

Body Part (4th)	Approach (5th)	Device (6th)	Qualifier (7th)
Tympanic Membrane, Right Tympanic Membrane, Left Eustachian Tube, Right Eustachian Tube, Left Nasal Turbinate Nasopharynx	**0** Open **3** Percutaneous **4** Percutaneous Endoscopic **7** Via Natural or Artificial Opening **8** Via Natural or Artificial Opening Endoscopic	**Z** No Device	**Z** No Qualifier
Mastoid Sinus, Right Mastoid Sinus, Left Nasal Septum Accessory Sinus Maxillary Sinus, Right Maxillary Sinus, Left Frontal Sinus, Right Frontal Sinus, Left Ethmoid Sinus, Right Ethmoid Sinus, Left Sphenoid Sinus, Right Sphenoid Sinus, Left	**0** Open **3** Percutaneous **4** Percutaneous Endoscopic **8** Via Natural or Artificial Opening Endoscopic	**Z** No Device	**Z** No Qualifier
Nasal Mucosa and Soft Tissue	**0** Open **3** Percutaneous **4** Percutaneous Endoscopic **8** Via Natural or Artificial Opening Endoscopic **X** External	**Z** No Device	**Z** No Qualifier

tion 0 **Medical and Surgical**
dy System 9 **Ear, Nose, Sinus**
eration 7 **Dilation:** Expanding an orifice or the lumen of a tubular body part

Body Part (4th)	Approach (5th)	Device (6th)	Qualifier (7th)
Eustachian Tube, Right Eustachian Tube, Left	**0** Open **7** Via Natural or Artificial Opening **8** Via Natural or Artificial Opening Endoscopic	**D** Intraluminal Device **Z** No Device	**Z** No Qualifier
Eustachian Tube, Right Eustachian Tube, Left	**3** Percutaneous **4** Percutaneous Endoscopic	**Z** No Device	**Z** No Qualifier

ction 0 **Medical and Surgical**
dy System 9 **Ear, Nose, Sinus**
eration 8 **Division:** Cutting into a body part, without draining fluids and/or gases from the body part, in order to separate or transect a body part

Body Part (4th)	Approach (5th)	Device (6th)	Qualifier (7th)
Nasal Turbinate	**0** Open **3** Percutaneous **4** Percutaneous Endoscopic **7** Via Natural or Artificial Opening **8** Via Natural or Artificial Opening Endoscopic	**Z** No Device	**Z** No Qualifier

Section	**0**	**Medical and Surgical**
Body System	**9**	**Ear, Nose, Sinus**
Operation	**9**	**Drainage:** Taking or letting out fluids and/or gases from a body part

Body Part (4th)	Approach (5th)	Device (6th)	Qualifier (7th)
0 External Ear, Right **1** External Ear, Left	**0** Open **3** Percutaneous **4** Percutaneous Endoscopic **X** External	**0** Drainage Device	**Z** No Qualifier
0 External Ear, Right **1** External Ear, Left	**0** Open **3** Percutaneous **4** Percutaneous Endoscopic **X** External	**Z** No Device	**X** Diagnostic **Z** No Qualifier
3 External Auditory Canal, Right **4** External Auditory Canal, Left **K** Nasal Mucosa and Soft Tissue	**0** Open **3** Percutaneous **4** Percutaneous Endoscopic **7** Via Natural or Artificial Opening **8** Via Natural or Artificial Opening Endoscopic **X** External	**0** Drainage Device	**Z** No Qualifier
3 External Auditory Canal, Right **4** External Auditory Canal, Left **K** Nasal Mucosa and Soft Tissue	**0** Open **3** Percutaneous **4** Percutaneous Endoscopic **7** Via Natural or Artificial Opening **8** Via Natural or Artificial Opening Endoscopic **X** External	**Z** No Device	**X** Diagnostic **Z** No Qualifier
5 Middle Ear, Right **6** Middle Ear, Left **9** Auditory Ossicle, Right **A** Auditory Ossicle, Left **D** Inner Ear, Right **E** Inner Ear, Left	**0** Open **7** Via Natural or Artificial Opening **8** Via Natural or Artificial Opening Endoscopic	**0** Drainage Device	**Z** No Qualifier
5 Middle Ear, Right **6** Middle Ear, Left **9** Auditory Ossicle, Right **A** Auditory Ossicle, Left **D** Inner Ear, Right **E** Inner Ear, Left	**0** Open **7** Via Natural or Artificial Opening **8** Via Natural or Artificial Opening Endoscopic	**Z** No Device	**X** Diagnostic **Z** No Qualifier
7 Tympanic Membrane, Right **8** Tympanic Membrane, Left **B** Mastoid Sinus, Right **C** Mastoid Sinus, Left **F** Eustachian Tube, Right **G** Eustachian Tube, Left **L** Nasal Turbinate **M** Nasal Septum **N** Nasopharynx **P** Accessory Sinus **Q** Maxillary Sinus, Right **R** Maxillary Sinus, Left **S** Frontal Sinus, Right **T** Frontal Sinus, Left **U** Ethmoid Sinus, Right **V** Ethmoid Sinus, Left **W** Sphenoid Sinus, Right **X** Sphenoid Sinus, Left	**0** Open **3** Percutaneous **4** Percutaneous Endoscopic **7** Via Natural or Artificial Opening **8** Via Natural or Artificial Opening Endoscopic	**0** Drainage Device	**Z** No Qualifier

Continued →

Section 0 **Medical and Surgical**
Body System 9 **Ear, Nose, Sinus**
Operation 9 **Drainage:** Taking or letting out fluids and/or gases from a body part

Body Part (4th)	Approach (5th)	Device (6th)	Qualifier (7th)
7 Tympanic Membrane, Right 8 Tympanic Membrane, Left B Mastoid Sinus, Right C Mastoid Sinus, Left F Eustachian Tube, Right G Eustachian Tube, Left L Nasal Turbinate M Nasal Septum N Nasopharynx P Accessory Sinus Q Maxillary Sinus, Right R Maxillary Sinus, Left S Frontal Sinus, Right T Frontal Sinus, Left U Ethmoid Sinus, Right V Ethmoid Sinus, Left W Sphenoid Sinus, Right X Sphenoid Sinus, Left	**0** Open **3** Percutaneous **4** Percutaneous Endoscopic **7** Via Natural or Artificial Opening **8** Via Natural or Artificial Opening Endoscopic	**Z** No Device	**X** Diagnostic **Z** No Qualifier

Section 0 **Medical and Surgical**
Body System 9 **Ear, Nose, Sinus**
Operation B **Excision:** Cutting out or off, without replacement, a portion of a body part

Body Part (4th)	Approach (5th)	Device (6th)	Qualifier (7th)
0 External Ear, Right 1 External Ear, Left	**0** Open **3** Percutaneous **4** Percutaneous Endoscopic **X** External	**Z** No Device	**X** Diagnostic **Z** No Qualifier
3 External Auditory Canal, Right 4 External Auditory Canal, Left	**0** Open **3** Percutaneous **4** Percutaneous Endoscopic **7** Via Natural or Artificial Opening **8** Via Natural or Artificial Opening Endoscopic **X** External	**Z** No Device	**X** Diagnostic **Z** No Qualifier
5 Middle Ear, Right 6 Middle Ear, Left 9 Auditory Ossicle, Right A Auditory Ossicle, Left D Inner Ear, Right E Inner Ear, Left	**0** Open **8** Via Natural or Artificial Opening Endoscopic	**Z** No Device	**X** Diagnostic **Z** No Qualifier
7 Tympanic Membrane, Right 8 Tympanic Membrane, Left F Eustachian Tube, Right G Eustachian Tube, Left L Nasal Turbinate N Nasopharynx	**0** Open **3** Percutaneous **4** Percutaneous Endoscopic **7** Via Natural or Artificial Opening **8** Via Natural or Artificial Opening Endoscopic	**Z** No Device	**X** Diagnostic **Z** No Qualifier
B Mastoid Sinus, Right C Mastoid Sinus, Left M Nasal Septum P Accessory Sinus Q Maxillary Sinus, Right R Maxillary Sinus, Left S Frontal Sinus, Right T Frontal Sinus, Left U Ethmoid Sinus, Right V Ethmoid Sinus, Left W Sphenoid Sinus, Right X Sphenoid Sinus, Left	**0** Open **3** Percutaneous **4** Percutaneous Endoscopic **8** Via Natural or Artificial Opening Endoscopic	**Z** No Device	**X** Diagnostic **Z** No Qualifier

Continued →

09B Contin

Section 0 **Medical and Surgical**
Body System 9 **Ear, Nose, Sinus**
Operation B **Excision:** Cutting out or off, without replacement, a portion of a body part

Body Part (4th)	Approach (5th)	Device (6th)	Qualifier (7th)
K Nasal Mucosa and Soft Tissue	**0** Open **3** Percutaneous **4** Percutaneous Endoscopic **8** Via Natural or Artificial Opening Endoscopic **X** External	**Z** No Device	**X** Diagnostic **Z** No Qualifier

Section 0 **Medical and Surgical**
Body System 9 **Ear, Nose, Sinus**
Operation C **Extirpation:** Taking or cutting out solid matter from a body part

Body Part (4th)	Approach (5th)	Device (6th)	Qualifier (7th)
0 External Ear, Right **1** External Ear, Left	**0** Open **3** Percutaneous **4** Percutaneous Endoscopic **X** External	**Z** No Device	**Z** No Qualifier
3 External Auditory Canal, Right **4** External Auditory Canal, Left	**0** Open **3** Percutaneous **4** Percutaneous Endoscopic **7** Via Natural or Artificial Opening **8** Via Natural or Artificial Opening Endoscopic **X** External	**Z** No Device	**Z** No Qualifier
5 Middle Ear, Right **6** Middle Ear, Left **9** Auditory Ossicle, Right **A** Auditory Ossicle, Left **D** Inner Ear, Right **E** Inner Ear, Left	**0** Open **8** Via Natural or Artificial Opening Endoscopic	**Z** No Device	**Z** No Qualifier
7 Tympanic Membrane, Right **8** Tympanic Membrane, Left **F** Eustachian Tube, Right **G** Eustachian Tube, Left **L** Nasal Turbinate **N** Nasopharynx	**0** Open **3** Percutaneous **4** Percutaneous Endoscopic **7** Via Natural or Artificial Opening **8** Via Natural or Artificial Opening Endoscopic	**Z** No Device	**Z** No Qualifier
B Mastoid Sinus, Right **C** Mastoid Sinus, Left **M** Nasal Septum **P** Accessory Sinus **Q** Maxillary Sinus, Right **R** Maxillary Sinus, Left **S** Frontal Sinus, Right **T** Frontal Sinus, Left **U** Ethmoid Sinus, Right **V** Ethmoid Sinus, Left **W** Sphenoid Sinus, Right **X** Sphenoid Sinus, Left	**0** Open **3** Percutaneous **4** Percutaneous Endoscopic **8** Via Natural or Artificial Opening Endoscopic	**Z** No Device	**Z** No Qualifier
K Nasal Mucosa and Soft Tissue	**0** Open **3** Percutaneous **4** Percutaneous Endoscopic **8** Via Natural or Artificial Opening Endoscopic **X** External	**Z** No Device	**Z** No Qualifier

Section	**0**	**Medical and Surgical**
Body System	**9**	**Ear, Nose, Sinus**
Operation	**D**	**Extraction:** Pulling or stripping out or off all or a portion of a body part by the use of force

Body Part (4th)	Approach (5th)	Device (6th)	Qualifier (7th)
7 Tympanic Membrane, Right **8** Tympanic Membrane, Left **L** Nasal Turbinate	**0** Open **3** Percutaneous **4** Percutaneous Endoscopic **7** Via Natural or Artificial Opening **8** Via Natural or Artificial Opening Endoscopic	**Z** No Device	**Z** No Qualifier
9 Auditory Ossicle, Right **A** Auditory Ossicle, Left	**0** Open	**Z** No Device	**Z** No Qualifier
B Mastoid Sinus, Right **C** Mastoid Sinus, Left **M** Nasal Septum **P** Accessory Sinus **Q** Maxillary Sinus, Right **R** Maxillary Sinus, Left **S** Frontal Sinus, Right **T** Frontal Sinus, Left **U** Ethmoid Sinus, Right **V** Ethmoid Sinus, Left **W** Sphenoid Sinus, Right **X** Sphenoid Sinus, Left	**0** Open **3** Percutaneous **4** Percutaneous Endoscopic	**Z** No Device	**Z** No Qualifier

Section	**0**	**Medical and Surgical**
Body System	**9**	**Ear, Nose, Sinus**
Operation	**H**	**Insertion:** Putting in a nonbiological appliance that monitors, assists, performs, or prevents a physiological function but does not physically take the place of a body part

Body Part (4th)	Approach (5th)	Device (6th)	Qualifier (7th)
D Inner Ear, Right **E** Inner Ear, Left	**0** Open **3** Percutaneous **4** Percutaneous Endoscopic	**4** Hearing Device, Bone Conduction **5** Hearing Device, Single Channel Cochlear Prosthesis **6** Hearing Device, Multiple Channel Cochlear Prosthesis **S** Hearing Device	**Z** No Qualifier
H Ear, Right **J** Ear, Left **K** Nasal Mucosa and Soft Tissue **Y** Sinus	**0** Open **3** Percutaneous **4** Percutaneous Endoscopic **7** Via Natural or Artificial Opening **8** Via Natural or Artificial Opening Endoscopic	**Y** Other Device	**Z** No Qualifier
N Nasopharynx	**7** Via Natural or Artificial Opening **8** Via Natural or Artificial Opening Endoscopic	**B** Intraluminal Device, Airway	**Z** No Qualifier

Section	**0**	**Medical and Surgical**
Body System	**9**	**Ear, Nose, Sinus**
Operation	**J**	**Inspection:** Visually and/or manually exploring a body part

Body Part (4th)	Approach (5th)	Device (6th)	Qualifier (7th)
7 Tympanic Membrane, Right **8** Tympanic Membrane, Left **H** Ear, Right **J** Ear, Left	**0** Open **3** Percutaneous **4** Percutaneous Endoscopic **7** Via Natural or Artificial Opening **8** Via Natural or Artificial Opening Endoscopic **X** External	**Z** No Device	**Z** No Qualifier
D Inner Ear, Right **E** Inner Ear, Left **K** Nose **Y** Sinus	**0** Open **3** Percutaneous **4** Percutaneous Endoscopic **8** Via Natural or Artificial Opening Endoscopic **X** External	**Z** No Device	**Z** No Qualifier

Section 0 **Medical and Surgical**
Body System 9 **Ear, Nose, Sinus**
Operation M **Reattachment:** Putting back in or on all or a portion of a separated body part to its normal location or other suitable location

Body Part (4th)	Approach (5th)	Device (6th)	Qualifier (7th)
0 External Ear, Right **1** External Ear, Left **K** Nasal Mucosa and Soft Tissue	**X** External	**Z** No Device	**Z** No Qualifier

Section 0 **Medical and Surgical**
Body System 9 **Ear, Nose, Sinus**
Operation N **Release:** Freeing a body part from an abnormal physical constraint by cutting or by the use of force

Body Part (4th)	Approach (5th)	Device (6th)	Qualifier (7th)
0 External Ear, Right **1** External Ear, Left	**0** Open **3** Percutaneous **4** Percutaneous Endoscopic **X** External	**Z** No Device	**Z** No Qualifier
3 External Auditory Canal, Right **4** External Auditory Canal, Left	**0** Open **3** Percutaneous **4** Percutaneous Endoscopic **7** Via Natural or Artificial Opening **8** Via Natural or Artificial Opening Endoscopic **X** External	**Z** No Device	**Z** No Qualifier
5 Middle Ear, Right **6** Middle Ear, Left **9** Auditory Ossicle, Right **A** Auditory Ossicle, Left **D** Inner Ear, Right **E** Inner Ear, Left	**0** Open **8** Via Natural or Artificial Opening Endoscopic	**Z** No Device	**Z** No Qualifier
7 Tympanic Membrane, Right **8** Tympanic Membrane, Left **F** Eustachian Tube, Right **G** Eustachian Tube, Left **L** Nasal Turbinate **N** Nasopharynx	**0** Open **3** Percutaneous **4** Percutaneous Endoscopic **7** Via Natural or Artificial Opening **8** Via Natural or Artificial Opening Endoscopic	**Z** No Device	**Z** No Qualifier
B Mastoid Sinus, Right **C** Mastoid Sinus, Left **M** Nasal Septum **P** Accessory Sinus **Q** Maxillary Sinus, Right **R** Maxillary Sinus, Left **S** Frontal Sinus, Right **T** Frontal Sinus, Left **U** Ethmoid Sinus, Right **V** Ethmoid Sinus, Left **W** Sphenoid Sinus, Right **X** Sphenoid Sinus, Left	**0** Open **3** Percutaneous **4** Percutaneous Endoscopic **8** Via Natural or Artificial Opening Endoscopic	**Z** No Device	**Z** No Qualifier
K Nasal Mucosa and Soft Tissue	**0** Open **3** Percutaneous **4** Percutaneous Endoscopic **8** Via Natural or Artificial Opening Endoscopic **X** External	**Z** No Device	**Z** No Qualifier

tion 0 **Medical and Surgical**
dy System 9 **Ear, Nose, Sinus**
eration P **Removal:** Taking out or off a device from a body part

Body Part (4th)	Approach (5th)	Device (6th)	Qualifier (7th)
Tympanic Membrane, Right Tympanic Membrane, Left	**0** Open **7** Via Natural or Artificial Opening **8** Via Natural or Artificial Opening Endoscopic **X** External	**0** Drainage Device	**Z** No Qualifier
D Inner Ear, Right **E** Inner Ear, Left	**0** Open **7** Via Natural or Artificial Opening **8** Via Natural or Artificial Opening Endoscopic	**S** Hearing Device	**Z** No Qualifier
H Ear, Right Ear, Left **K** Nasal Mucosa and Soft Tissue	**0** Open **3** Percutaneous **4** Percutaneous Endoscopic **7** Via Natural or Artificial Opening **8** Via Natural or Artificial Opening Endoscopic	**0** Drainage Device **7** Autologous Tissue Substitute **D** Intraluminal Device **J** Synthetic Substitute **K** Nonautologous Tissue Substitute **Y** Other Device	**Z** No Qualifier
H Ear, Right **J** Ear, Left **K** Nasal Mucosa and Soft Tissue	**X** External	**0** Drainage Device **7** Autologous Tissue Substitute **D** Intraluminal Device **J** Synthetic Substitute **K** Nonautologous Tissue Substitute	**Z** No Qualifier
Y Sinus	**0** Open **3** Percutaneous **4** Percutaneous Endoscopic	**0** Drainage Device **Y** Other Device	**Z** No Qualifier
Y Sinus	**7** Via Natural or Artificial Opening **8** Via Natural or Artificial Opening Endoscopic	**Y** Other Device	**Z** No Qualifier
Y Sinus	**X** External	**0** Drainage Device	**Z** No Qualifier

ction 0 **Medical and Surgical**
dy System 9 **Ear, Nose, Sinus**
eration Q **Repair:** Restoring, to the extent possible, a body part to its normal anatomic structure and function

Body Part (4th)	Approach (5th)	Device (6th)	Qualifier (7th)
0 External Ear, Right **1** External Ear, Left **2** External Ear, Bilateral	**0** Open **3** Percutaneous **4** Percutaneous Endoscopic **X** External	**Z** No Device	**Z** No Qualifier
3 External Auditory Canal, Right **4** External Auditory Canal, Left **F** Eustachian Tube, Right **G** Eustachian Tube, Left	**0** Open **3** Percutaneous **4** Percutaneous Endoscopic **7** Via Natural or Artificial Opening **8** Via Natural or Artificial Opening Endoscopic **X** External	**Z** No Device	**Z** No Qualifier
5 Middle Ear, Right **6** Middle Ear, Left **9** Auditory Ossicle, Right **A** Auditory Ossicle, Left **D** Inner Ear, Right **E** Inner Ear, Left	**0** Open **8** Via Natural or Artificial Opening Endoscopic	**Z** No Device	**Z** No Qualifier
7 Tympanic Membrane, Right **8** Tympanic Membrane, Left **L** Nasal Turbinate **N** Nasopharynx	**0** Open **3** Percutaneous **4** Percutaneous Endoscopic **7** Via Natural or Artificial Opening **8** Via Natural or Artificial Opening Endoscopic	**Z** No Device	**Z** No Qualifier

Continued →

Section 0 **Medical and Surgical**
Body System 9 **Ear, Nose, Sinus**
Operation Q **Repair:** Restoring, to the extent possible, a body part to its normal anatomic structure and function

Body Part (4th)	Approach (5th)	Device (6th)	Qualifier (7th)
B Mastoid Sinus, Right **C** Mastoid Sinus, Left **M** Nasal Septum **P** Accessory Sinus **Q** Maxillary Sinus, Right **R** Maxillary Sinus, Left **S** Frontal Sinus, Right **T** Frontal Sinus, Left **U** Ethmoid Sinus, Right **V** Ethmoid Sinus, Left **W** Sphenoid Sinus, Right **X** Sphenoid Sinus, Left	**0** Open **3** Percutaneous **4** Percutaneous Endoscopic **8** Via Natural or Artificial Opening Endoscopic	**Z** No Device	**Z** No Qualifier
K Nasal Mucosa and Soft Tissue	**0** Open **3** Percutaneous **4** Percutaneous Endoscopic **8** Via Natural or Artificial Opening Endoscopic **X** External	**Z** No Device	**Z** No Qualifier

Section 0 **Medical and Surgical**
Body System 9 **Ear, Nose, Sinus**
Operation R **Replacement:** Putting in or on biological or synthetic material that physically takes the place and/or function of all or a portion of a body part

Body Part (4th)	Approach (5th)	Device (6th)	Qualifier (7th)
0 External Ear, Right **1** External Ear, Left **2** External Ear, Bilateral **K** Nasal Mucosa and Soft Tissue	**0** Open **X** External	**7** Autologous Tissue Substitute **J** Synthetic Substitute **K** Nonautologous Tissue Substitute	**Z** No Qualifier
5 Middle Ear, Right **6** Middle Ear, Left **9** Auditory Ossicle, Right **A** Auditory Ossicle, Left **D** Inner Ear, Right **E** Inner Ear, Left	**0** Open	**7** Autologous Tissue Substitute **J** Synthetic Substitute **K** Nonautologous Tissue Substitute	**Z** No Qualifier
7 Tympanic Membrane, Right **8** Tympanic Membrane, Left **N** Nasopharynx	**0** Open **7** Via Natural or Artificial Opening **8** Via Natural or Artificial Opening Endoscopic	**7** Autologous Tissue Substitute **J** Synthetic Substitute **K** Nonautologous Tissue Substitute	**Z** No Qualifier
L Nasal Turbinate	**0** Open **3** Percutaneous **4** Percutaneous Endoscopic **7** Via Natural or Artificial Opening **8** Via Natural or Artificial Opening Endoscopic	**7** Autologous Tissue Substitute **J** Synthetic Substitute **K** Nonautologous Tissue Substitute	**Z** No Qualifier
M Nasal Septum	**0** Open **3** Percutaneous **4** Percutaneous Endoscopic	**7** Autologous Tissue Substitute **J** Synthetic Substitute **K** Nonautologous Tissue Substitute	**Z** No Qualifier

Section 0 **Medical and Surgical**
Body System 9 **Ear, Nose, Sinus**
Operation S **Reposition:** Moving to its normal location, or other suitable location, all or a portion of a body part

Body Part (4th)	Approach (5th)	Device (6th)	Qualifier (7th)
0 External Ear, Right 1 External Ear, Left 2 External Ear, Bilateral K Nasal Mucosa and Soft Tissue	0 Open 4 Percutaneous Endoscopic X External	Z No Device	Z No Qualifier
7 Tympanic Membrane, Right 8 Tympanic Membrane, Left F Eustachian Tube, Right G Eustachian Tube, Left L Nasal Turbinate	0 Open 4 Percutaneous Endoscopic 7 Via Natural or Artificial Opening 8 Via Natural or Artificial Opening Endoscopic	Z No Device	Z No Qualifier
9 Auditory Ossicle, Right A Auditory Ossicle, Left M Nasal Septum	0 Open 4 Percutaneous Endoscopic	Z No Device	Z No Qualifier

Section 0 **Medical and Surgical**
Body System 9 **Ear, Nose, Sinus**
Operation T **Resection:** Cutting out or off, without replacement, all of a body part

Body Part (4th)	Approach (5th)	Device (6th)	Qualifier (7th)
0 External Ear, Right 1 External Ear, Left	0 Open 4 Percutaneous Endoscopic X External	Z No Device	Z No Qualifier
5 Middle Ear, Right 6 Middle Ear, Left 9 Auditory Ossicle, Right A Auditory Ossicle, Left D Inner Ear, Right E Inner Ear, Left	0 Open 8 Via Natural or Artificial Opening Endoscopic	Z No Device	Z No Qualifier
7 Tympanic Membrane, Right 8 Tympanic Membrane, Left F Eustachian Tube, Right G Eustachian Tube, Left L Nasal Turbinate N Nasopharynx	0 Open 4 Percutaneous Endoscopic 7 Via Natural or Artificial Opening 8 Via Natural or Artificial Opening Endoscopic	Z No Device	Z No Qualifier
B Mastoid Sinus, Right C Mastoid Sinus, Left M Nasal Septum P Accessory Sinus Q Maxillary Sinus, Right R Maxillary Sinus, Left S Frontal Sinus, Right T Frontal Sinus, Left U Ethmoid Sinus, Right V Ethmoid Sinus, Left W Sphenoid Sinus, Right X Sphenoid Sinus, Left	0 Open 4 Percutaneous Endoscopic 8 Via Natural or Artificial Opening Endoscopic	Z No Device	Z No Qualifier
K Nasal Mucosa and Soft Tissue	0 Open 4 Percutaneous Endoscopic 8 Via Natural or Artificial Opening Endoscopic X External	Z No Device	Z No Qualifier

Section 0 **Medical and Surgical**
Body System 9 **Ear, Nose, Sinus**
Operation U **Supplement:** Putting in or on biological or synthetic material that physically reinforces and/or augments the function of a portion of a body part

Body Part (4th)	Approach (5th)	Device (6th)	Qualifier (7th)
0 External Ear, Right **1** External Ear, Left **2** External Ear, Bilateral	**0** Open **X** External	**7** Autologous Tissue Substitute **J** Synthetic Substitute **K** Nonautologous Tissue Substitute	**Z** No Qualifier
5 Middle Ear, Right **6** Middle Ear, Left **9** Auditory Ossicle, Right **A** Auditory Ossicle, Left **D** Inner Ear, Right **E** Inner Ear, Left	**0** Open **8** Via Natural or Artificial Opening Endoscopic	**7** Autologous Tissue Substitute **J** Synthetic Substitute **K** Nonautologous Tissue Substitute	**Z** No Qualifier
7 Tympanic Membrane, Right **8** Tympanic Membrane, Left **N** Nasopharynx	**0** Open **7** Via Natural or Artificial Opening **8** Via Natural or Artificial Opening Endoscopic	**7** Autologous Tissue Substitute **J** Synthetic Substitute **K** Nonautologous Tissue Substitute	**Z** No Qualifier
K Nasal Mucosa and Soft Tissue	**0** Open **8** Via Natural or Artificial Opening Endoscopic **X** External	**7** Autologous Tissue Substitute **J** Synthetic Substitute **K** Nonautologous Tissue Substitute	**Z** No Qualifier
L Nasal Turbinate	**0** Open **3** Percutaneous **4** Percutaneous Endoscopic **7** Via Natural or Artificial Opening **8** Via Natural or Artificial Opening Endoscopic	**7** Autologous Tissue Substitute **J** Synthetic Substitute **K** Nonautologous Tissue Substitute	**Z** No Qualifier
M Nasal Septum	**0** Open **3** Percutaneous **4** Percutaneous Endoscopic **8** Via Natural or Artificial Opening Endoscopic	**7** Autologous Tissue Substitute **J** Synthetic Substitute **K** Nonautologous Tissue Substitute	**Z** No Qualifier

Section 0 **Medical and Surgical**
Body System 9 **Ear, Nose, Sinus**
Operation W **Revision:** Correcting, to the extent possible, a portion of a malfunctioning device or the position of a displaced device

Body Part (4th)	Approach (5th)	Device (6th)	Qualifier (7th)
7 Tympanic Membrane, Right **8** Tympanic Membrane, Left **9** Auditory Ossicle, Right **A** Auditory Ossicle, Left	**0** Open **7** Via Natural or Artificial Opening **8** Via Natural or Artificial Opening Endoscopic	**7** Autologous Tissue Substitute **J** Synthetic Substitute **K** Nonautologous Tissue Substitute	**Z** No Qualifier
D Inner Ear, Right **E** Inner Ear, Left	**0** Open **7** Via Natural or Artificial Opening **8** Via Natural or Artificial Opening Endoscopic	**S** Hearing Device	**Z** No Qualifier
H Ear, Right **J** Ear, Left **K** Nasal Mucosa and Soft Tissue	**0** Open **3** Percutaneous **4** Percutaneous Endoscopic **7** Via Natural or Artificial Opening **8** Via Natural or Artificial Opening Endoscopic	**0** Drainage Device **7** Autologous Tissue Substitute **D** Intraluminal Device **J** Synthetic Substitute **K** Nonautologous Tissue Substitute **Y** Other Device	**Z** No Qualifier

Continued →

tion 0 **Medical and Surgical**
dy System 9 **Ear, Nose, Sinus**
eration W **Revision:** Correcting, to the extent possible, a portion of a malfunctioning device or the position of a displaced device

Body Part (4th)	Approach (5th)	Device (6th)	Qualifier (7th)
Ear, Right Ear, Left Nasal Mucosa and Soft Tissue	**X** External	**0** Drainage Device **7** Autologous Tissue Substitute **D** Intraluminal Device **J** Synthetic Substitute **K** Nonautologous Tissue Substitute	**Z** No Qualifier
Sinus	**0** Open **3** Percutaneous **4** Percutaneous Endoscopic	**0** Drainage Device **Y** Other Device	**Z** No Qualifier
Sinus	**7** Via Natural or Artificial Opening **8** Via Natural or Artificial Opening Endoscopic	**Y** Other Device	**Z** No Qualifier
Sinus	**X** External	**0** Drainage Device	**Z** No Qualifier

IA Coding Clinic

QKXZZ Repair Nasal Mucosa and Soft Tissue, External Approach—AHA CC: 4Q, 2014, 20-21
QT4ZZ Repair Left Frontal Sinus, Percutaneous Endoscopic Approach—AHA CC: 4Q, 2013, 114
QW0ZZ Repair Right Sphenoid Sinus, Open Approach—AHA CC: 3Q, 2014, 22-23
QX0ZZ Repair Left Sphenoid Sinus, Open Approach—AHA CC: 3Q, 2014, 22-23

Lungs

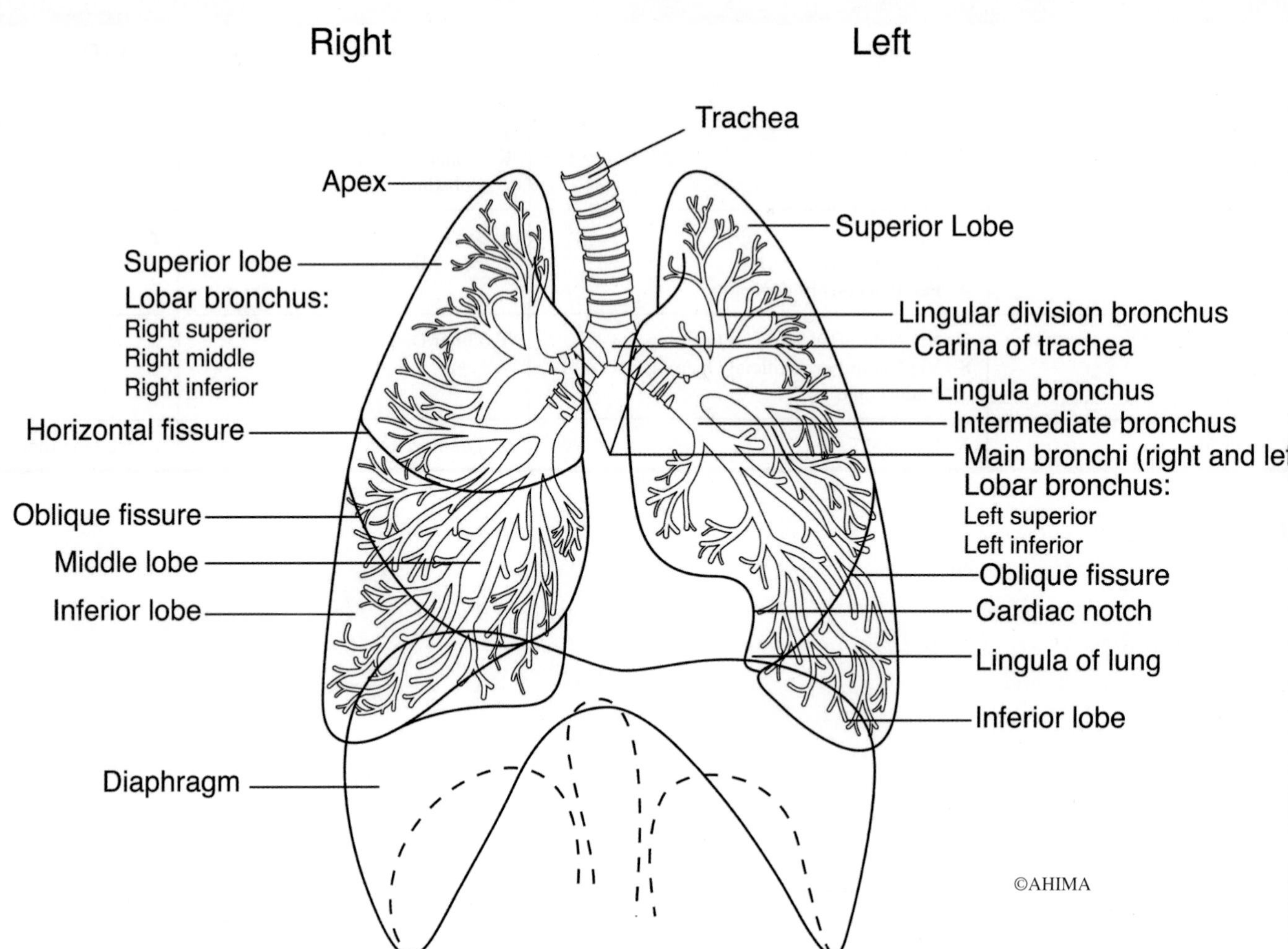
Right
Left
Trachea
Apex
Superior Lobe
Superior lobe
Lobar bronchus:
Right superior
Right middle
Right inferior
Lingular division bronchus
Carina of trachea
Lingula bronchus
Intermediate bronchus
Horizontal fissure
Main bronchi (right and lef
Lobar bronchus:
Left superior
Left inferior
Oblique fissure
Middle lobe
Inferior lobe
Oblique fissure
Cardiac notch
Lingula of lung
Inferior lobe
Diaphragm
©AHIMA

Structure of the Trachea and Major Bronchi

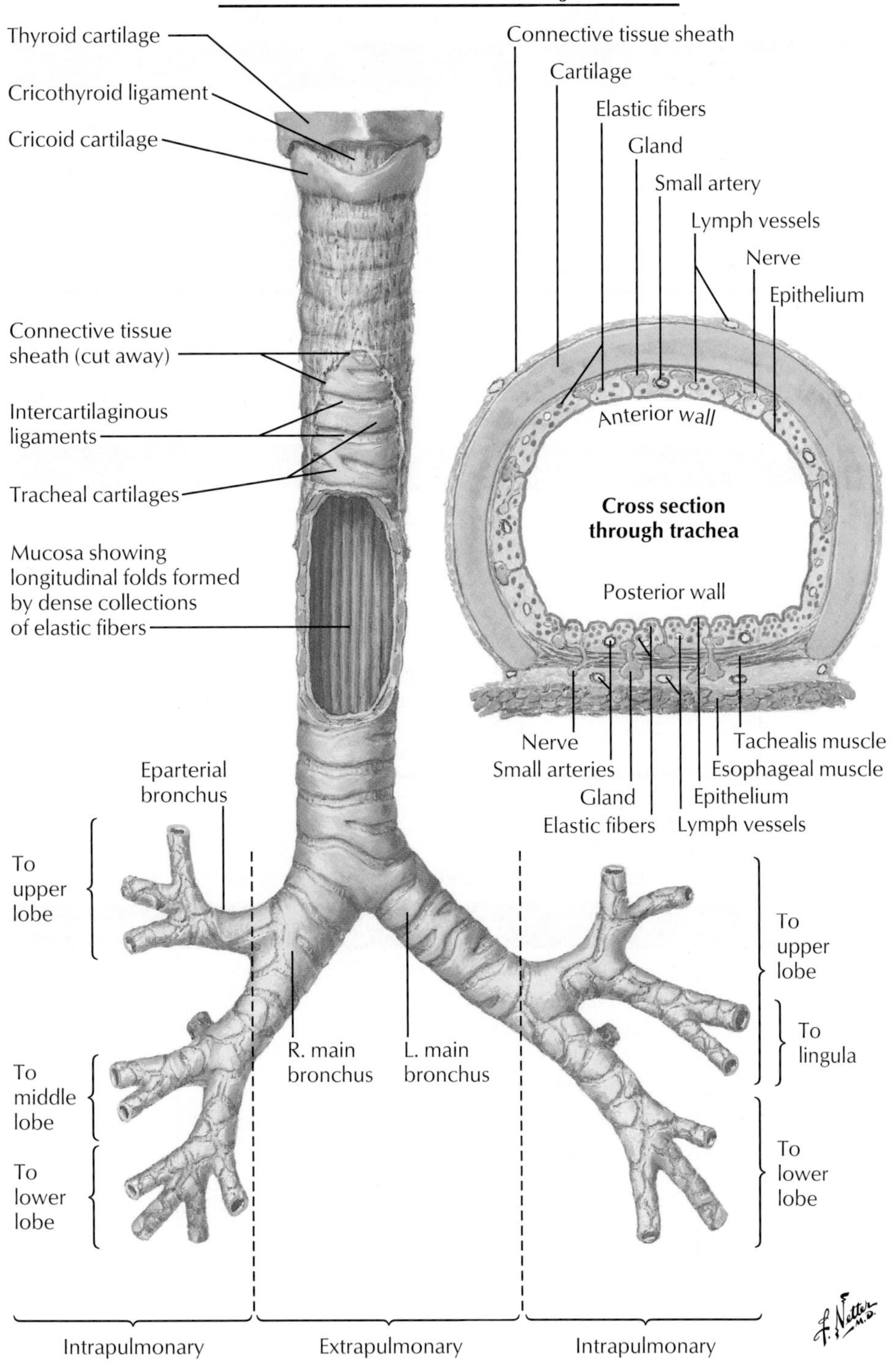

Respiratory System Tables 0B1–0BY

Section 0 **Medical and Surgical**
Body System B **Respiratory System**
Operation 1 **Bypass:** Altering the route of passage of the contents of a tubular body part

Body Part (4th)	Approach (5th)	Device (6th)	Qualifier (7th)
1 Trachea	**0** Open	**D** Intraluminal Device	**6** Esophagus
1 Trachea	**0** Open	**F** Tracheostomy Device **Z** No Device	**4** Cutaneous
1 Trachea	**3** Percutaneous **4** Percutaneous Endoscopic	**F** Tracheostomy Device **Z** No Device	**4** Cutaneous

Section 0 **Medical and Surgical**
Body System B **Respiratory System**
Operation 2 **Change:** Taking out or off a device from a body part and putting back an identical or similar device in or on the same bo part without cutting or puncturing the skin or a mucous membrane

Body Part (4th)	Approach (5th)	Device (6th)	Qualifier (7th)
0 Tracheobronchial Tree **K** Lung, Right **L** Lung, Left **Q** Pleura **T** Diaphragm	**X** External	**0** Drainage Device **Y** Other Device	**Z** No Qualifier
1 Trachea	**X** External	**0** Drainage Device **E** Intraluminal Device, Endotracheal Airway **F** Tracheostomy Device **Y** Other Device	**Z** No Qualifier

Section 0 **Medical and Surgical**
Body System B **Respiratory System**
Operation 5 **Destruction:** Physical eradication of all or a portion of a body part by the direct use of energy, force, or a destructive age

Body Part (4th)	Approach (5th)	Device (6th)	Qualifier (7th)
1 Trachea **2** Carina **3** Main Bronchus, Right **4** Upper Lobe Bronchus, Right **5** Middle Lobe Bronchus, Right **6** Lower Lobe Bronchus, Right **7** Main Bronchus, Left **8** Upper Lobe Bronchus, Left **9** Lingula Bronchus **B** Lower Lobe Bronchus, Left **C** Upper Lung Lobe, Right **D** Middle Lung Lobe, Right **F** Lower Lung Lobe, Right **G** Upper Lung Lobe, Left **H** Lung Lingula **J** Lower Lung Lobe, Left **K** Lung, Right **L** Lung, Left **M** Lungs, Bilateral	**0** Open **3** Percutaneous **4** Percutaneous Endoscopic **7** Via Natural or Artificial Opening **8** Via Natural or Artificial Opening Endoscopic	**Z** No Device	**Z** No Qualifier
N Pleura, Right **P** Pleura, Left **T** Diaphragm	**0** Open **3** Percutaneous **4** Percutaneous Endoscopic	**Z** No Device	**Z** No Qualifier

ction	**0**	**Medical and Surgical**
dy System	**B**	**Respiratory System**
eration	**7**	**Dilation:** Expanding an orifice or the lumen of a tubular body part

Body Part (4th)	Approach (5th)	Device (6th)	Qualifier (7th)
1 Trachea 2 Carina 3 Main Bronchus, Right 4 Upper Lobe Bronchus, Right 5 Middle Lobe Bronchus, Right 6 Lower Lobe Bronchus, Right 7 Main Bronchus, Left 8 Upper Lobe Bronchus, Left 9 Lingula Bronchus B Lower Lobe Bronchus, Left	**0** Open **3** Percutaneous **4** Percutaneous Endoscopic **7** Via Natural or Artificial Opening **8** Via Natural or Artificial Opening Endoscopic	**D** Intraluminal Device **Z** No Device	**Z** No Qualifier

ction	**0**	**Medical and Surgical**
dy System	**B**	**Respiratory System**
eration	**9**	**Drainage:** Taking or letting out fluids and/or gases from a body part

Body Part (4th)	Approach (5th)	Device (6th)	Qualifier (7th)
1 Trachea 2 Carina 3 Main Bronchus, Right 4 Upper Lobe Bronchus, Right 5 Middle Lobe Bronchus, Right 6 Lower Lobe Bronchus, Right 7 Main Bronchus, Left 8 Upper Lobe Bronchus, Left 9 Lingula Bronchus B Lower Lobe Bronchus, Left C Upper Lung Lobe, Right D Middle Lung Lobe, Right F Lower Lung Lobe, Right G Upper Lung Lobe, Left H Lung Lingula J Lower Lung Lobe, Left K Lung, Right L Lung, Left M Lungs, Bilateral	**0** Open **3** Percutaneous **4** Percutaneous Endoscopic **7** Via Natural or Artificial Opening **8** Via Natural or Artificial Opening Endoscopic	**0** Drainage Device	**Z** No Qualifier
1 Trachea 2 Carina 3 Main Bronchus, Right 4 Upper Lobe Bronchus, Right 5 Middle Lobe Bronchus, Right 6 Lower Lobe Bronchus, Right 7 Main Bronchus, Left 8 Upper Lobe Bronchus, Left 9 Lingula Bronchus B Lower Lobe Bronchus, Left C Upper Lung Lobe, Right D Middle Lung Lobe, Right F Lower Lung Lobe, Right G Upper Lung Lobe, Left H Lung Lingula J Lower Lung Lobe, Left K Lung, Right L Lung, Left M Lungs, Bilateral	**0** Open **3** Percutaneous **4** Percutaneous Endoscopic **7** Via Natural or Artificial Opening **8** Via Natural or Artificial Opening Endoscopic	**Z** No Device	**X** Diagnostic **Z** No Qualifier
N Pleura, Right P Pleura, Left	**0** Open **3** Percutaneous **4** Percutaneous Endoscopic **8** Via Natural or Artificial Opening Endoscopic	**0** Drainage Device	**Z** No Qualifier

Continued →

0B9 Continu

Section 0 **Medical and Surgical**
Body System B **Respiratory System**
Operation 9 **Drainage:** Taking or letting out fluids and/or gases from a body part

Body Part (4th)	Approach (5th)	Device (6th)	Qualifier (7th)
N Pleura, Right **P** Pleura, Left	**0** Open **3** Percutaneous **4** Percutaneous Endoscopic **8** Via Natural or Artificial Opening Endoscopic	**Z** No Device	**X** Diagnostic **Z** No Qualifier
T Diaphragm	**0** Open **3** Percutaneous **4** Percutaneous Endoscopic	**0** Drainage Device	**Z** No Qualifier
T Diaphragm	**0** Open **3** Percutaneous **4** Percutaneous Endoscopic	**Z** No Device	**X** Diagnostic **Z** No Qualifier

Section 0 **Medical and Surgical**
Body System B **Respiratory System**
Operation B **Excision:** Cutting out or off, without replacement, a portion of a body part

Body Part (4th)	Approach (5th)	Device (6th)	Qualifier (7th)
1 Trachea **2** Carina **3** Main Bronchus, Right **4** Upper Lobe Bronchus, Right **5** Middle Lobe Bronchus, Right **6** Lower Lobe Bronchus, Right **7** Main Bronchus, Left **8** Upper Lobe Bronchus, Left **9** Lingula Bronchus **B** Lower Lobe Bronchus, Left **C** Upper Lung Lobe, Right **D** Middle Lung Lobe, Right **F** Lower Lung Lobe, Right **G** Upper Lung Lobe, Left **H** Lung Lingula **J** Lower Lung Lobe, Left **K** Lung, Right **L** Lung, Left **M** Lungs, Bilateral	**0** Open **3** Percutaneous **4** Percutaneous Endoscopic **7** Via Natural or Artificial Opening **8** Via Natural or Artificial Opening Endoscopic	**Z** No Device	**X** Diagnostic **Z** No Qualifier
N Pleura, Right **P** Pleura, Left	**0** Open **3** Percutaneous **4** Percutaneous Endoscopic **8** Via Natural or Artificial Opening Endoscopic	**Z** No Device	**X** Diagnostic **Z** No Qualifier
T Diaphragm	**0** Open **3** Percutaneous **4** Percutaneous Endoscopic	**Z** No Device	**X** Diagnostic **Z** No Qualifier

tion 0 **Medical and Surgical**
ly System B **Respiratory System**
eration C **Extirpation:** Taking or cutting out solid matter from a body part

Body Part (4th)	Approach (5th)	Device (6th)	Qualifier (7th)
Trachea Carina Main Bronchus, Right Upper Lobe Bronchus, Right Middle Lobe Bronchus, Right Lower Lobe Bronchus, Right Main Bronchus, Left Upper Lobe Bronchus, Left Lingula Bronchus Lower Lobe Bronchus, Left Upper Lung Lobe, Right Middle Lung Lobe, Right Lower Lung Lobe, Right Upper Lung Lobe, Left Lung Lingula Lower Lung Lobe, Left Lung, Right Lung, Left Lungs, Bilateral	**0** Open **3** Percutaneous **4** Percutaneous Endoscopic **7** Via Natural or Artificial Opening **8** Via Natural or Artificial Opening Endoscopic	**Z** No Device	**Z** No Qualifier
Pleura, Right Pleura, Left Diaphragm	**0** Open **3** Percutaneous **4** Percutaneous Endoscopic	**Z** No Device	**Z** No Qualifier

tion 0 **Medical and Surgical**
dy System B **Respiratory System**
eration D **Extraction:** Pulling or stripping out or off all or a portion of a body part by the use of force

Body Part (4th)	Approach (5th)	Device (6th)	Qualifier (7th)
Trachea Carina Main Bronchus, Right Upper Lobe Bronchus, Right Middle Lobe Bronchus, Right Lower Lobe Bronchus, Right Main Bronchus, Left Upper Lobe Bronchus, Left Lingula Bronchus Lower Lobe Bronchus, Left Upper Lung Lobe, Right Middle Lung Lobe, Right Lower Lung Lobe, Right Upper Lung Lobe, Left Lung Lingula Lower Lung Lobe, Left Lung, Right Lung, Left Lung, Bilateral	**4** Percutaneous Endoscopic **8** Via Natural or Artificial Opening Endoscopic	**Z** No Device	**X** Diagnostic
Pleura, Right Pleura, Left	**0** Open **3** Percutaneous **4** Percutaneous Endoscopic	**Z** No Device	**X** Diagnostic **Z** No Qualifier

Section **0** **Medical and Surgical**
Body System **B** **Respiratory System**
Operation **F** **Fragmentation:** Breaking solid matter in a body part into pieces

Body Part (4th)	Approach (5th)	Device (6th)	Qualifier (7th)
1 Trachea **2** Carina **3** Main Bronchus, Right **4** Upper Lobe Bronchus, Right **5** Middle Lobe Bronchus, Right **6** Lower Lobe Bronchus, Right **7** Main Bronchus, Left **8** Upper Lobe Bronchus, Left **9** Lingula Bronchus **B** Lower Lobe Bronchus, Left	**0** Open **3** Percutaneous **4** Percutaneous Endoscopic **7** Via Natural or Artificial Opening **8** Via Natural or Artificial Opening Endoscopic **X** External	**Z** No Device	**Z** No Qualifier

Section **0** **Medical and Surgical**
Body System **B** **Respiratory System**
Operation **H** **Insertion:** Putting in a nonbiological appliance that monitors, assists, performs, or prevents a physiological function but does not physically take the place of a body part

Body Part (4th)	Approach (5th)	Device (6th)	Qualifier (7th)
0 Tracheobronchial Tree	**0** Open **3** Percutaneous **4** Percutaneous Endoscopic **7** Via Natural or Artificial Opening **8** Via Natural or Artificial Opening Endoscopic	**1** Radioactive Element **2** Monitoring Device **3** Infusion Device **D** Intraluminal Device **Y** Other Device	**Z** No Qualifier
1 Trachea	**0** Open	**2** Monitoring Device **D** Intraluminal Device **Y** Other Device	**Z** No Qualifier
1 Trachea	**3** Percutaneous	**D** Intraluminal Device **E** Intraluminal Device, Endotracheal Airway **Y** Other Device	**Z** No Qualifier
1 Trachea	**4** Percutaneous Endoscopic	**D** Intraluminal Device **Y** Other Device	**Z** No Qualifier
1 Trachea	**7** Via Natural or Artificial Opening **8** Via Natural or Artificial Opening Endoscopic	**2** Monitoring Device **D** Intraluminal Device **E** Intraluminal Device, Endotracheal Airway **Y** Other Device	**Z** No Qualifier
3 Main Bronchus, Right **4** Upper Lobe Bronchus, Right **5** Middle Lobe Bronchus, Right **6** Lower Lobe Bronchus, Right **7** Main Bronchus, Left **8** Upper Lobe Bronchus, Left **9** Lingula Bronchus **B** Lower Lobe Bronchus, Left	**0** Open **3** Percutaneous **4** Percutaneous Endoscopic **7** Via Natural or Artificial Opening **8** Via Natural or Artificial Opening Endoscopic	**G** Intraluminal Device, Endobronchial Valve	**Z** No Qualifier
K Lung, Right **L** Lung, Left	**0** Open **3** Percutaneous **4** Percutaneous Endoscopic **7** Via Natural or Artificial Opening **8** Via Natural or Artificial Opening Endoscopic	**1** Radioactive Element **2** Monitoring Device **3** Infusion Device **Y** Other Device	**Z** No Qualifier
Q Pleura	**0** Open **3** Percutaneous **4** Percutaneous Endoscopic **7** Via Natural or Artificial Opening **8** Via Natural or Artificial Opening Endoscopic	**Y** Other Device	**Z** No Qualifier

Continued

ction **0** **Medical and Surgical**
dy System **B** **Respiratory System**
eration **H** **Insertion:** Putting in a nonbiological appliance that monitors, assists, performs, or prevents a physiological function but does not physically take the place of a body part

Body Part (4th)	Approach (5th)	Device (6th)	Qualifier (7th)
T Diaphragm	**0** Open **3** Percutaneous **4** Percutaneous Endoscopic	**2** Monitoring Device **M** Diaphragmatic Pacemaker Lead **Y** Other Device	**Z** No Qualifier
T Diaphragm	**7** Via Natural or Artificial Opening **8** Via Natural or Artificial Opening Endoscopic	**Y** Other Device	**Z** No Qualifier

ction **0** **Medical and Surgical**
dy System **B** **Respiratory System**
eration **J** **Inspection:** Visually and/or manually exploring a body part

Body Part (4th)	Approach (5th)	Device (6th)	Qualifier (7th)
0 Tracheobronchial Tree **1** Trachea **K** Lung, Right **L** Lung, Left **Q** Pleura **T** Diaphragm	**0** Open **3** Percutaneous **4** Percutaneous Endoscopic **7** Via Natural or Artificial Opening **8** Via Natural or Artificial Opening Endoscopic **X** External	**Z** No Device	**Z** No Qualifier

ction **0** **Medical and Surgical**
dy System **B** **Respiratory System**
eration **L** **Occlusion:** Completely closing an orifice or the lumen of a tubular body part

Body Part (4th)	Approach (5th)	Device (6th)	Qualifier (7th)
1 Trachea **2** Carina **3** Main Bronchus, Right **4** Upper Lobe Bronchus, Right **5** Middle Lobe Bronchus, Right **6** Lower Lobe Bronchus, Right **7** Main Bronchus, Left **8** Upper Lobe Bronchus, Left **9** Lingula Bronchus **B** Lower Lobe Bronchus, Left	**0** Open **3** Percutaneous **4** Percutaneous Endoscopic	**C** Extraluminal Device **D** Intraluminal Device **Z** No Device	**Z** No Qualifier
1 Trachea **2** Carina **3** Main Bronchus, Right **4** Upper Lobe Bronchus, Right **5** Middle Lobe Bronchus, Right **6** Lower Lobe Bronchus, Right **7** Main Bronchus, Left **8** Upper Lobe Bronchus, Left **9** Lingula Bronchus **B** Lower Lobe Bronchus, Left	**7** Via Natural or Artificial Opening **8** Via Natural or Artificial Opening Endoscopic	**D** Intraluminal Device **Z** No Device	**Z** No Qualifier

Section 0 **Medical and Surgical**
Body System B **Respiratory System**
Operation M **Reattachment:** Putting back in or on all or a portion of a separated body part to its normal location or other suitable location

Body Part (4th)	Approach (5th)	Device (6th)	Qualifier (7th)
1 Trachea **2** Carina **3** Main Bronchus, Right **4** Upper Lobe Bronchus, Right **5** Middle Lobe Bronchus, Right **6** Lower Lobe Bronchus, Right **7** Main Bronchus, Left **8** Upper Lobe Bronchus, Left **9** Lingula Bronchus **B** Lower Lobe Bronchus, Left **C** Upper Lung Lobe, Right **D** Middle Lung Lobe, Right **F** Lower Lung Lobe, Right **G** Upper Lung Lobe, Left **H** Lung Lingula **J** Lower Lung Lobe, Left **K** Lung, Right **L** Lung, Left **T** Diaphragm	**0** Open	**Z** No Device	**Z** No Qualifier

Section 0 **Medical and Surgical**
Body System B **Respiratory System**
Operation N **Release:** Freeing a body part from an abnormal physical constraint by cutting or by the use of force

Body Part (4th)	Approach (5th)	Device (6th)	Qualifier (7th)
1 Trachea **2** Carina **3** Main Bronchus, Right **4** Upper Lobe Bronchus, Right **5** Middle Lobe Bronchus, Right **6** Lower Lobe Bronchus, Right **7** Main Bronchus, Left **8** Upper Lobe Bronchus, Left **9** Lingula Bronchus **B** Lower Lobe Bronchus, Left **C** Upper Lung Lobe, Right **D** Middle Lung Lobe, Right **F** Lower Lung Lobe, Right **G** Upper Lung Lobe, Left **H** Lung Lingula **J** Lower Lung Lobe, Left **K** Lung, Right **L** Lung, Left **M** Lungs, Bilateral	**0** Open **3** Percutaneous **4** Percutaneous Endoscopic **7** Via Natural or Artificial Opening **8** Via Natural or Artificial Opening Endoscopic	**Z** No Device	**Z** No Qualifier
N Pleura, Right **P** Pleura, Left **T** Diaphragm	**0** Open **3** Percutaneous **4** Percutaneous Endoscopic	**Z** No Device	**Z** No Qualifier

tion	0	**Medical and Surgical**
dy System	B	**Respiratory System**
eration	P	**Removal:** Taking out or off a device from a body part

Body Part (4th)	Approach (5th)	Device (6th)	Qualifier (7th)
Tracheobronchial Tree	**0** Open **3** Percutaneous **4** Percutaneous Endoscopic **7** Via Natural or Artificial Opening **8** Via Natural or Artificial Opening Endoscopic	**0** Drainage Device **1** Radioactive Element **2** Monitoring Device **3** Infusion Device **7** Autologous Tissue Substitute **C** Extraluminal Device **D** Intraluminal Device **J** Synthetic Substitute **K** Nonautologous Tissue Substitute **Y** Other Device	**Z** No Qualifier
Tracheobronchial Tree	**X** External	**0** Drainage Device **1** Radioactive Element **2** Monitoring Device **3** Infusion Device **D** Intraluminal Device	**Z** No Qualifier
Trachea	**0** Open **3** Percutaneous **4** Percutaneous Endoscopic **7** Via Natural or Artificial Opening **8** Via Natural or Artificial Opening Endoscopic	**0** Drainage Device **2** Monitoring Device **7** Autologous Tissue Substitute **C** Extraluminal Device **D** Intraluminal Device **F** Tracheostomy Device **J** Synthetic Substitute **K** Nonautologous Tissue Substitute	**Z** No Qualifier
Trachea	**X** External	**0** Drainage Device **2** Monitoring Device **D** Intraluminal Device **F** Tracheostomy Device	**Z** No Qualifier
K Lung, Right **L** Lung, Left	**0** Open **3** Percutaneous **4** Percutaneous Endoscopic **7** Via Natural or Artificial Opening **8** Via Natural or Artificial Opening Endoscopic	**0** Drainage Device **1** Radioactive Element **2** Monitoring Device **3** Infusion Device **Y** Other Device	**Z** No Qualifier
K Lung, Right **L** Lung, Left	**X** External	**0** Drainage Device **1** Radioactive Element **2** Monitoring Device **3** Infusion Device	**Z** No Qualifier
Q Pleura	**0** Open **3** Percutaneous **4** Percutaneous Endoscopic **7** Via Natural or Artificial Opening **8** Via Natural or Artificial Opening Endoscopic	**0** Drainage Device **1** Radioactive Element **2** Monitoring Device **Y** Other Device	**Z** No Qualifier
Q Pleura	**X** External	**0** Drainage Device **1** Radioactive Element **2** Monitoring Device	**Z** No Qualifier
T Diaphragm	**0** Open **3** Percutaneous **4** Percutaneous Endoscopic **7** Via Natural or Artificial Opening **8** Via Natural or Artificial Opening Endoscopic	**0** Drainage Device **2** Monitoring Device **7** Autologous Tissue Substitute **J** Synthetic Substitute **K** Nonautologous Tissue Substitute **M** Diaphragmatic Pacemaker Lead **Y** Other Device	**Z** No Qualifier
T Diaphragm	**X** External	**0** Drainage Device **2** Monitoring Device **M** Diaphragmatic Pacemaker Lead	**Z** No Qualifier

Section 0 **Medical and Surgical**
Body System B **Respiratory System**
Operation Q **Repair:** Restoring, to the extent possible, a body part to its normal anatomic structure and function

Body Part (4th)	Approach (5th)	Device (6th)	Qualifier (7th)
1 Trachea **2** Carina **3** Main Bronchus, Right **4** Upper Lobe Bronchus, Right **5** Middle Lobe Bronchus, Right **6** Lower Lobe Bronchus, Right **7** Main Bronchus, Left **8** Upper Lobe Bronchus, Left **9** Lingula Bronchus **B** Lower Lobe Bronchus, Left **C** Upper Lung Lobe, Right **D** Middle Lung Lobe, Right **F** Lower Lung Lobe, Right **G** Upper Lung Lobe, Left **H** Lung Lingula **J** Lower Lung Lobe, Left **K** Lung, Right **L** Lung, Left **M** Lungs, Bilateral	**0** Open **3** Percutaneous **4** Percutaneous Endoscopic **7** Via Natural or Artificial Opening **8** Via Natural or Artificial Opening Endoscopic	**Z** No Device	**Z** No Qualifier
N Pleura, Right **P** Pleura, Left **T** Diaphragm	**0** Open **3** Percutaneous **4** Percutaneous Endoscopic	**Z** No Device	**Z** No Qualifier

Section 0 **Medical and Surgical**
Body System B **Respiratory**
Operation R **Replacement:** Putting in or on biological or synthetic material that physically takes the place and/or function of all or a portion of a body part

Body Part (4th)	Approach (5th)	Device (6th)	Qualifier (7th)
1 Trachea **2** Carina **3** Main Bronchus, Right **4** Upper Lobe Bronchus, Right **5** Middle Lobe Bronchus, Right **6** Lower Lobe Bronchus, Right **7** Main Bronchus, Left **8** Upper Lobe Bronchus, Left **9** Lingula Bronchus **B** Lower Lobe Bronchus, Left **T** Diaphragm	**0** Open **4** Percutaneous Endoscopic	**7** Autologous Tissue Substitute **J** Synthetic Substitute **K** Nonautologous Tissue Substitute	**Z** No Qualifier

tion **0** **Medical and Surgical**
dy System **B** **Respiratory System**
eration **S** **Reposition:** Moving to its normal location, or other suitable location, all or a portion of a body part

Body Part (4th)	Approach (5th)	Device (6th)	Qualifier (7th)
Trachea	**0** Open	**Z** No Device	**Z** No Qualifier
Carina			
Main Bronchus, Right			
Upper Lobe Bronchus, Right			
Middle Lobe Bronchus, Right			
Lower Lobe Bronchus, Right			
Main Bronchus, Left			
Upper Lobe Bronchus, Left			
Lingula Bronchus			
Lower Lobe Bronchus, Left			
Upper Lung Lobe, Right			
Middle Lung Lobe, Right			
Lower Lung Lobe, Right			
Upper Lung Lobe, Left			
Lung Lingula			
Lower Lung Lobe, Left			
Lung, Right			
Lung, Left			
Diaphragm			

tion **0** **Medical and Surgical**
dy System **B** **Respiratory System**
eration **T** **Resection:** Cutting out or off, without replacement, all of a body part

Body Part (4th)	Approach (5th)	Device (6th)	Qualifier (7th)
Trachea	**0** Open	**Z** No Device	**Z** No Qualifier
Carina	**4** Percutaneous Endoscopic		
Main Bronchus, Right			
Upper Lobe Bronchus, Right			
Middle Lobe Bronchus, Right			
Lower Lobe Bronchus, Right			
Main Bronchus, Left			
Upper Lobe Bronchus, Left			
Lingula Bronchus			
Lower Lobe Bronchus, Left			
Upper Lung Lobe, Right			
Middle Lung Lobe, Right			
Lower Lung Lobe, Right			
Upper Lung Lobe, Left			
Lung Lingula			
Lower Lung Lobe, Left			
Lung, Right			
Lung, Left			
Lungs, Bilateral			
Diaphragm			

Section 0 **Medical and Surgical**
Body System B **Respiratory System**
Operation U **Supplement:** Putting in or on biological or synthetic material that physically reinforces and/or augments the function of portion of a body part

Body Part (4th)	Approach (5th)	Device (6th)	Qualifier (7th)
1 Trachea **2** Carina **3** Main Bronchus, Right **4** Upper Lobe Bronchus, Right **5** Middle Lobe Bronchus, Right **6** Lower Lobe Bronchus, Right **7** Main Bronchus, Left **8** Upper Lobe Bronchus, Left **9** Lingula Bronchus **B** Lower Lobe Bronchus, Left	**0** Open **4** Percutaneous Endoscopic **8** Via Natural or Artificial Opening Endoscopic	**7** Autologous Tissue Substitute **J** Synthetic Substitute **K** Nonautologous Tissue Substitute	**Z** No Qualifier
T Diaphragm	**0** Open **4** Percutaneous Endoscopic	**7** Autologous Tissue Substitute **J** Synthetic Substitute **K** Nonautologous Tissue Substitute	**Z** No Qualifier

Section 0 **Medical and Surgical**
Body System B **Respiratory System**
Operation V **Restriction:** Partially closing an orifice or the lumen of a tubular body part

Body Part (4th)	Approach (5th)	Device (6th)	Qualifier (7th)
1 Trachea **2** Carina **3** Main Bronchus, Right **4** Upper Lobe Bronchus, Right **5** Middle Lobe Bronchus, Right **6** Lower Lobe Bronchus, Right **7** Main Bronchus, Left **8** Upper Lobe Bronchus, Left **9** Lingula Bronchus **B** Lower Lobe Bronchus, Left	**0** Open **3** Percutaneous **4** Percutaneous Endoscopic	**C** Extraluminal Device **D** Intraluminal Device **Z** No Device	**Z** No Qualifier
1 Trachea **2** Carina **3** Main Bronchus, Right **4** Upper Lobe Bronchus, Right **5** Middle Lobe Bronchus, Right **6** Lower Lobe Bronchus, Right **7** Main Bronchus, Left **8** Upper Lobe Bronchus, Left **9** Lingula Bronchus **B** Lower Lobe Bronchus, Left	**7** Via Natural or Artificial Opening **8** Via Natural or Artificial Opening Endoscopic	**D** Intraluminal Device **Z** No Device	**Z** No Qualifier

Section 0 **Medical and Surgical**
Body System B **Respiratory System**
Operation W **Revision:** Correcting, to the extent possible, a portion of a malfunctioning device or the position of a displaced device

Body Part (4th)	Approach (5th)	Device (6th)	Qualifier (7th)
0 Tracheobronchial Tree	**0** Open **3** Percutaneous **4** Percutaneous Endoscopic **7** Via Natural or Artificial Opening **8** Via Natural or Artificial Opening Endoscopic	**0** Drainage Device **2** Monitoring Device **3** Infusion Device **7** Autologous Tissue Substitute **C** Extraluminal Device **D** Intraluminal Device **J** Synthetic Substitute **K** Nonautologous Tissue Substitute **Y** Other Device	**Z** No Qualifier

Continued →

ction	**0**	**Medical and Surgical**
dy System	**B**	**Respiratory System**
eration	**W**	**Revision:** Correcting, to the extent possible, a portion of a malfunctioning device or the position of a displaced device

Body Part (4th)	Approach (5th)	Device (6th)	Qualifier (7th)
Tracheobronchial Tree	**X** External	**0** Drainage Device **2** Monitoring Device **3** Infusion Device **7** Autologous Tissue Substitute **C** Extraluminal Device **D** Intraluminal Device **J** Synthetic Substitute **K** Nonautologous Tissue Substitute	**Z** No Qualifier
Trachea	**0** Open **3** Percutaneous **4** Percutaneous Endoscopic **7** Via Natural or Artificial Opening **8** Via Natural or Artificial Opening Endoscopic **X** External	**0** Drainage Device **2** Monitoring Device **7** Autologous Tissue Substitute **C** Extraluminal Device **D** Intraluminal Device **F** Tracheostomy Device **J** Synthetic Substitute **K** Nonautologous Tissue Substitute	**Z** No Qualifier
K Lung, Right **L** Lung, Left	**0** Open **3** Percutaneous **4** Percutaneous Endoscopic **7** Via Natural or Artificial Opening **8** Via Natural or Artificial Opening Endoscopic	**0** Drainage Device **2** Monitoring Device **3** Infusion Device **Y** Other Device	**Z** No Qualifier
K Lung, Right **L** Lung, Left	**X** External	**0** Drainage Device **2** Monitoring Device **3** Infusion Device	**Z** No Qualifier
Q Pleura	**0** Open **3** Percutaneous **4** Percutaneous Endoscopic **7** Via Natural or Artificial Opening **8** Via Natural or Artificial Opening Endoscopic	**0** Drainage Device **2** Monitoring Device **Y** Other Device	**Z** No Qualifier
Q Pleura	**X** External	**0** Drainage Device **2** Monitoring Device	**Z** No Qualifier
T Diaphragm	**0** Open **3** Percutaneous **4** Percutaneous Endoscopic **7** Via Natural or Artificial Opening **8** Via Natural or Artificial Opening Endoscopic	**0** Drainage Device **2** Monitoring Device **7** Autologous Tissue Substitute **J** Synthetic Substitute **K** Nonautologous Tissue Substitute **M** Diaphragmatic Pacemaker Lead **Y** Other Device	**Z** No Qualifier
T Diaphragm	**X** External	**0** Drainage Device **2** Monitoring Device **7** Autologous Tissue Substitute **J** Synthetic Substitute **K** Nonautologous Tissue Substitute **M** Diaphragmatic Pacemaker Lead	**Z** No Qualifier

Section **0** **Medical and Surgical**
Body System **B** **Respiratory System**
Operation **Y** **Transplantation:** Putting in or on all or a portion of a living body part taken from another individual or animal to physically take the place and/or function of all or a portion of a similar body part

Body Part (4th)	Approach (5th)	Device (6th)	Qualifier (7th)
C Upper Lung Lobe, Right **D** Middle Lung Lobe, Right **F** Lower Lung Lobe, Right **G** Upper Lung Lobe, Left **H** Lung Lingula **J** Lower Lung Lobe, Left **K** Lung, Right **L** Lung, Left **M** Lungs, Bilateral	**0** Open	**Z** No Device	**0** Allogeneic **1** Syngeneic **2** Zooplastic

AHA Coding Clinic

0B5P0ZZ Destruction of Left Pleura, Open Approach—AHA CC: 2Q, 2016, 17-18

0B948ZX Drainage of Right Upper Lobe Bronchus, Via Natural or Artificial Opening Endoscopic, Diagnostic—AHA CC: 1Q, 2016, 26-

0B988ZX Drainage of Left Upper Lobe Bronchus, Via Natural or Artificial Opening Endoscopic, Diagnostic—AHA CC: 1Q, 2016, 27

0B9J8ZX Drainage of Left Lower Lung Lobe, Via Natural or Artificial Opening Endoscopic, Diagnostic—AHA CC: 1Q, 2016, 26-27; 2017, 51

0B9M8ZZ Drainage of Bilateral Lungs, Via Natural or Artificial Opening Endoscopic—AHA CC: 3Q, 2017, 15

0BB10ZZ Excision of Trachea, Open Approach—AHA CC: 1Q, 2015, 15-16

0BB48ZX Excision of Right Upper Lobe Bronchus, Via Natural or Artificial Opening Endoscopic, Diagnostic—AHA CC: 1Q, 2016, 26-

0BB88ZX Excision of Left Upper Lobe Bronchus, Via Natural or Artificial Opening Endoscopic, Diagnostic—AHA CC: 1Q, 2016, 27

0BBC8ZX Excision of Right Upper Lung Lobe, Via Natural or Artificial Opening Endoscopic, Diagnostic—AHA CC: 1Q, 2016, 26-27

0BBK8ZX Excision of Right Lung, Via Natural or Artificial Opening Endoscopic, Diagnostic—AHA CC: 1Q, 2014, 20-21

0BC58ZZ Extirpation of Matter from Right Middle Lobe Bronchus, Via Natural or Artificial Opening Endoscopic—AHA CC: 3 2017, 14-15

0BH17EZ Insertion of Endotracheal Airway into Trachea, Via Natural or Artificial Opening—AHA CC: 4Q, 2014, 3-15

0BH18EZ Insertion of Endotracheal Airway into Trachea, Via Natural or Artificial Opening Endoscopic—AHA CC: 4Q, 2014, 3-15

0BJL8ZZ Inspection of Left Lung, Via Natural or Artificial Opening Endoscopic—AHA CC: 1Q, 2014, 20

0BJQ4ZZ Inspection of Pleura, Percutaneous Endoscopic Approach—AHA CC: 2Q, 2015, 31

0BN10ZZ Release Trachea, Open Approach—AHA CC: 3Q, 2015, 15-16

0BU307Z Supplement Right Main Bronchus with Autologous Tissue Substitute, Open Approach—AHA CC: 1Q, 2015, 28-29

Oral Cavity

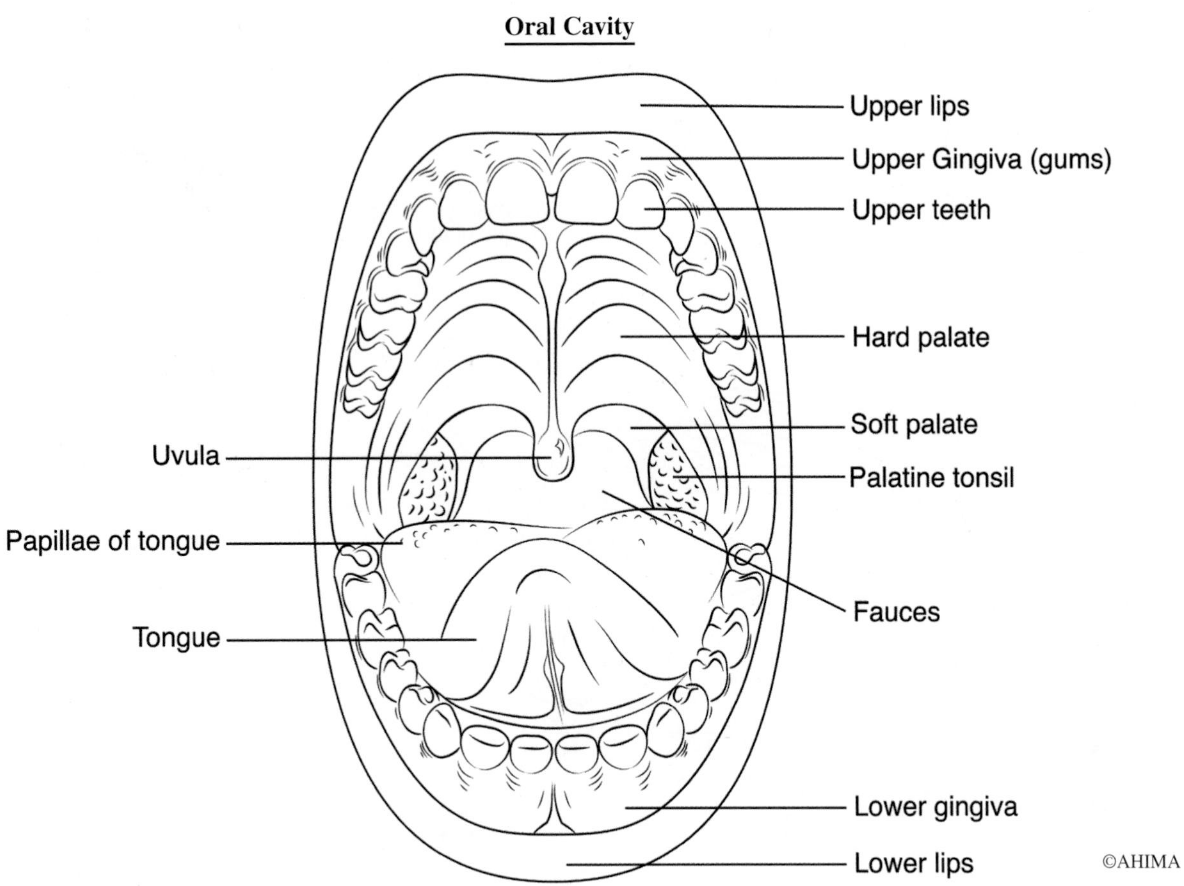
Upper lips
Upper Gingiva (gums)
Upper teeth
Hard palate
Soft palate
Palatine tonsil
Uvula
Papillae of tongue
Fauces
Tongue
Lower gingiva
Lower lips
©AHIMA

Glands of the Oral Cavity

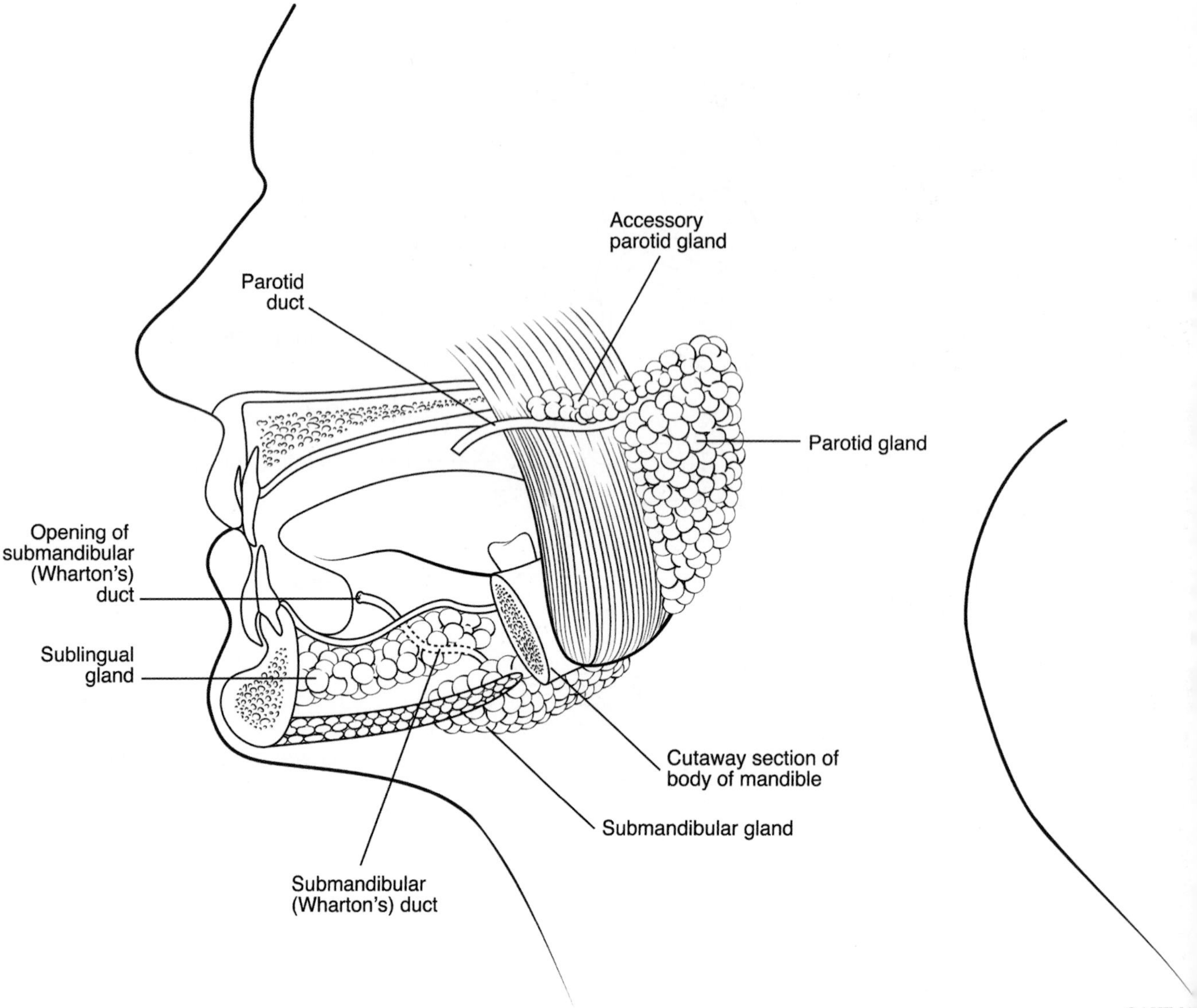

Accessory
parotid gland
Parotid
duct
Parotid gland
Opening of
submandibular
(Wharton's)
duct
Sublingual
gland
Cutaway section of
body of mandible
Submandibular gland
Submandibular
(Wharton's) duct

Throat

Tongue
Vocal cord
Epiglottis
Vestibular
fold
Pyriform
fossa
Esophagus
Trachea

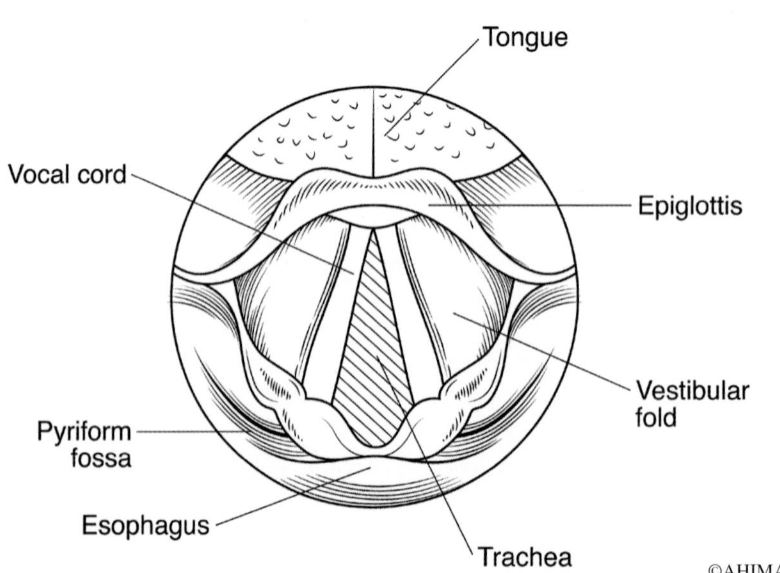

Section	0	Medical and Surgical
Body System	C	Mouth and Throat
Operation	0	**Alteration:** Modifying the anatomic structure of a body part without affecting the function of the body part

Body Part (4th)	Approach (5th)	Device (6th)	Qualifier (7th)
0 Upper Lip 1 Lower Lip	X External	7 Autologous Tissue Substitute J Synthetic Substitute K Nonautologous Tissue Substitute Z No Device	Z No Qualifier

Section	0	Medical and Surgical
Body System	C	Mouth and Throat
Operation	2	**Change:** Taking out or off a device from a body part and putting back an identical or similar device in or on the same body part without cutting or puncturing the skin or a mucous membrane

Body Part (4th)	Approach (5th)	Device (6th)	Qualifier (7th)
A Salivary Gland S Larynx Y Mouth and Throat	X External	0 Drainage Device Y Other Device	Z No Qualifier

Section	0	Medical and Surgical
Body System	C	Mouth and Throat
Operation	5	**Destruction:** Physical eradication of all or a portion of a body part by the direct use of energy, force, or a destructive agent

Body Part (4th)	Approach (5th)	Device (6th)	Qualifier (7th)
0 Upper Lip 1 Lower Lip 2 Hard Palate 3 Soft Palate 4 Buccal Mucosa 5 Upper Gingiva 6 Lower Gingiva 7 Tongue N Uvula P Tonsils Q Adenoids	0 Open 3 Percutaneous X External	Z No Device	Z No Qualifier
8 Parotid Gland, Right 9 Parotid Gland, Left B Parotid Duct, Right C Parotid Duct, Left D Sublingual Gland, Right F Sublingual Gland, Left G Submaxillary Gland, Right H Submaxillary Gland, Left J Minor Salivary Gland	0 Open 3 Percutaneous	Z No Device	Z No Qualifier
M Pharynx R Epiglottis S Larynx T Vocal Cord, Right V Vocal Cord, Left	0 Open 3 Percutaneous 4 Percutaneous Endoscopic 7 Via Natural or Artificial Opening 8 Via Natural or Artificial Opening Endoscopic	Z No Device	Z No Qualifier
W Upper Tooth X Lower Tooth	0 Open X External	Z No Device	0 Single 1 Multiple 2 All

Section 0 **Medical and Surgical**
Body System C **Mouth and Throat**
Operation 7 **Dilation:** Expanding an orifice or the lumen of a tubular body part

Body Part (4th)	Approach (5th)	Device (6th)	Qualifier (7th)
B Parotid Duct, Right **C** Parotid Duct, Left	**0** Open **3** Percutaneous **7** Via Natural or Artificial Opening	**D** Intraluminal Device **Z** No Device	**Z** No Qualifier
M Pharynx	**7** Via Natural or Artificial Opening **8** Via Natural or Artificial Opening Endoscopic	**D** Intraluminal Device **Z** No Device	**Z** No Qualifier
S Larynx	**0** Open **3** Percutaneous **4** Percutaneous Endoscopic **7** Via Natural or Artificial Opening **8** Via Natural or Artificial Opening Endoscopic	**D** Intraluminal Device **Z** No Device	**Z** No Qualifier

Section 0 **Medical and Surgical**
Body System C **Mouth and Throat**
Operation 9 **Drainage:** Taking or letting out fluids and/or gases from a body part

Body Part (4th)	Approach (5th)	Device (6th)	Qualifier (7th)
0 Upper Lip **1** Lower Lip **2** Hard Palate **3** Soft Palate **4** Buccal Mucosa **5** Upper Gingiva **6** Lower Gingiva **7** Tongue **N** Uvula **P** Tonsils **Q** Adenoids	**0** Open **3** Percutaneous **X** External	**0** Drainage Device	**Z** No Qualifier
0 Upper Lip **1** Lower Lip **2** Hard Palate **3** Soft Palate **4** Buccal Mucosa **5** Upper Gingiva **6** Lower Gingiva **7** Tongue **N** Uvula **P** Tonsils **Q** Adenoids	**0** Open **3** Percutaneous **X** External	**Z** No Device	**X** Diagnostic **Z** No Qualifier
8 Parotid Gland, Right **9** Parotid Gland, Left **B** Parotid Duct, Right **C** Parotid Duct, Left **D** Sublingual Gland, Right **F** Sublingual Gland, Left **G** Submaxillary Gland, Right **H** Submaxillary Gland, Left **J** Minor Salivary Gland	**0** Open **3** Percutaneous	**0** Drainage Device	**Z** No Qualifier
8 Parotid Gland, Right **9** Parotid Gland, Left **B** Parotid Duct, Right **C** Parotid Duct, Left **D** Sublingual Gland, Right **F** Sublingual Gland, Left **G** Submaxillary Gland, Right **H** Submaxillary Gland, Left **J** Minor Salivary Gland	**0** Open **3** Percutaneous	**Z** No Device	**X** Diagnostic **Z** No Qualifier

Continued →

ection **0** **Medical and Surgical**
ody System **C** **Mouth and Throat**
peration **9** **Drainage:** Taking or letting out fluids and/or gases from a body part

Body Part (4th)	Approach (5th)	Device (6th)	Qualifier (7th)
M Pharynx **R** Epiglottis **S** Larynx **T** Vocal Cord, Right **V** Vocal Cord, Left	**0** Open **3** Percutaneous **4** Percutaneous Endoscopic **7** Via Natural or Artificial Opening **8** Via Natural or Artificial Opening Endoscopic	**0** Drainage Device	**Z** No Qualifier
M Pharynx **R** Epiglottis **S** Larynx **T** Vocal Cord, Right **V** Vocal Cord, Left	**0** Open **3** Percutaneous **4** Percutaneous Endoscopic **7** Via Natural or Artificial Opening **8** Via Natural or Artificial Opening Endoscopic	**Z** No Device	**X** Diagnostic **Z** No Qualifier
W Upper Tooth **X** Lower Tooth	**0** Open **X** External	**0** Drainage Device **Z** No Device	**0** Single **1** Multiple **2** All

ection **0** **Medical and Surgical**
ody System **C** **Mouth and Throat**
peration **B** **Excision:** Cutting out or off, without replacement, a portion of a body part

Body Part (4th)	Approach (5th)	Device (6th)	Qualifier (7th)
0 Upper Lip **1** Lower Lip **2** Hard Palate **3** Soft Palate **4** Buccal Mucosa **5** Upper Gingiva **6** Lower Gingiva **7** Tongue **N** Uvula **P** Tonsils **Q** Adenoids	**0** Open **3** Percutaneous **X** External	**Z** No Device	**X** Diagnostic **Z** No Qualifier
8 Parotid Gland, Right **9** Parotid Gland, Left **B** Parotid Duct, Right **C** Parotid Duct, Left **D** Sublingual Gland, Right **F** Sublingual Gland, Left **G** Submaxillary Gland, Right **H** Submaxillary Gland, Left **J** Minor Salivary Gland	**0** Open **3** Percutaneous	**Z** No Device	**X** Diagnostic **Z** No Qualifier
M Pharynx **R** Epiglottis **S** Larynx **T** Vocal Cord, Right **V** Vocal Cord, Left	**0** Open **3** Percutaneous **4** Percutaneous Endoscopic **7** Via Natural or Artificial Opening **8** Via Natural or Artificial Opening Endoscopic	**Z** No Device	**X** Diagnostic **Z** No Qualifier
W Upper Tooth **X** Lower Tooth	**0** Open **X** External	**Z** No Device	**0** Single **1** Multiple **2** All

Section 0 **Medical and Surgical**
Body System C **Mouth and Throat**
Operation C **Extirpation:** Taking or cutting out solid matter from a body part

Body Part (4th)	Approach (5th)	Device (6th)	Qualifier (7th)
0 Upper Lip **1** Lower Lip **2** Hard Palate **3** Soft Palate **4** Buccal Mucosa **5** Upper Gingiva **6** Lower Gingiva **7** Tongue **N** Uvula **P** Tonsils **Q** Adenoids	**0** Open **3** Percutaneous **X** External	**Z** No Device	**Z** No Qualifier
8 Parotid Gland, Right **9** Parotid Gland, Left **B** Parotid Duct, Right **C** Parotid Duct, Left **D** Sublingual Gland, Right **F** Sublingual Gland, Left **G** Submaxillary Gland, Right **H** Submaxillary Gland, Left **J** Minor Salivary Gland	**0** Open **3** Percutaneous	**Z** No Device	**Z** No Qualifier
M Pharynx **R** Epiglottis **S** Larynx **T** Vocal Cord, Right **V** Vocal Cord, Left	**0** Open **3** Percutaneous **4** Percutaneous Endoscopic **7** Via Natural or Artificial Opening **8** Via Natural or Artificial Opening Endoscopic	**Z** No Device	**Z** No Qualifier
W Upper Tooth **X** Lower Tooth	**0** Open **X** External	**Z** No Device	**0** Single **1** Multiple **2** All

Section 0 **Medical and Surgical**
Body System C **Mouth and Throat**
Operation D **Extraction:** Pulling or stripping out or off all or a portion of a body part by the use of force

Body Part (4th)	Approach (5th)	Device (6th)	Qualifier (7th)
T Vocal Cord, Right **V** Vocal Cord, Left	**0** Open **3** Percutaneous **4** Percutaneous Endoscopic **7** Via Natural or Artificial Opening **8** Via Natural or Artificial Opening Endoscopic	**Z** No Device	**Z** No Qualifier
W Upper Tooth **X** Lower Tooth	**X** External	**Z** No Device	**0** Single **1** Multiple **2** All

Section 0 **Medical and Surgical**
Body System C **Mouth and Throat**
Operation F **Fragmentation:** Breaking solid matter in a body part into pieces

Body Part (4th)	Approach (5th)	Device (6th)	Qualifier (7th)
B Parotid Duct, Right **C** Parotid Duct, Left	**0** Open **3** Percutaneous **7** Via Natural or Artificial Opening **X** External	**Z** No Device	**Z** No Qualifier

tion 0 **Medical and Surgical**
y System C **Mouth and Throat**
ration H **Insertion:** Putting in a nonbiological appliance that monitors, assists, performs, or prevents a physiological function but does not physically take the place of a body part

Body Part (4th)	Approach (5th)	Device (6th)	Qualifier (7th)
Tongue	**0** Open **3** Percutaneous **X** External	**1** Radioactive Element	**Z** No Qualifier
Salivary Gland Larynx	**0** Open **3** Percutaneous **7** Via Natural or Artificial Opening **8** Via Natural or Artificial Opening Endoscopic	**Y** Other Device	**Z** No Qualifier
Mouth and Throat	**0** Open **3** Percutaneous	**Y** Other Device	**Z** No Qualifier
Mouth and Throat	**7** Via Natural or Artificial Opening **8** Via Natural or Artificial Opening Endoscopic	**Y** Other Device	**Z** No Qualifier

tion 0 **Medical and Surgical**
y System C **Mouth and Throat**
eration J **Inspection:** Visually and/or manually exploring a body part

Body Part (4th)	Approach (5th)	Device (6th)	Qualifier (7th)
SalivaryGland	**0** Open **3** Percutaneous **X** External	**Z** No Device	**Z** No Qualifier
Larynx Mouth and Throat	**0** Open **3** Percutaneous **4** Percutaneous Endoscopic **7** Via Natural or Artificial Opening **8** Via Natural or Artificial Opening Endoscopic **X** External	**Z** No Device	**Z** No Qualifier

tion 0 **Medical and Surgical**
ly System C **Mouth and Throat**
eration L **Occlusion:** Completely closing an orifice or the lumen of a tubular body part

Body Part (4th)	Approach (5th)	Device (6th)	Qualifier (7th)
Parotid Duct, Right Parotid Duct, Left	**0** Open **3** Percutaneous **4** Percutaneous Endoscopic	**C** Extraluminal Device **D** Intraluminal Device **Z** No Device	**Z** No Qualifier
Parotid Duct, Right Parotid Duct, Left	**7** Via Natural or Artificial Opening **8** Via Natural or Artificial Opening Endoscopic	**D** Intraluminal Device **Z** No Device	**Z** No Qualifier

tion 0 **Medical and Surgical**
dy System C **Mouth and Throat**
eration M **Reattachment:** Putting back in or on all or a portion of a separated body part to its normal location or other suitable location

Body Part (4th)	Approach (5th)	Device (6th)	Qualifier (7th)
Upper Lip Lower Lip Soft Palate Tongue Uvula	**0** Open	**Z** No Device	**Z** No Qualifier
Upper Tooth Lower Tooth	**0** Open **X** External	**Z** No Device	**0** Single **1** Multiple **2** All

Section **0** **Medical and Surgical**
Body System **C** **Mouth and Throat**
Operation **N** **Release:** Freeing a body part from an abnormal physical constraint by cutting or by the use of force

Body Part (4th)	Approach (5th)	Device (6th)	Qualifier (7th)
0 Upper Lip **1** Lower Lip **2** Hard Palate **3** Soft Palate **4** Buccal Mucosa **5** Upper Gingiva **6** Lower Gingiva **7** Tongue **N** Uvula **P** Tonsils **Q** Adenoids	**0** Open **3** Percutaneous **X** External	**Z** No Device	**Z** No Qualifier
8 Parotid Gland, Right **9** Parotid Gland, Left **B** Parotid Duct, Right **C** Parotid Duct, Left **D** Sublingual Gland, Right **F** Sublingual Gland, Left **G** Submaxillary Gland, Right **H** Submaxillary Gland, Left **J** Minor Salivary Gland	**0** Open **3** Percutaneous	**Z** No Device	**Z** No Qualifier
M Pharynx **R** Epiglottis **S** Larynx **T** Vocal Cord, Right **V** Vocal Cord, Left	**0** Open **3** Percutaneous **4** Percutaneous Endoscopic **7** Via Natural or Artificial Opening **8** Via Natural or Artificial Opening Endoscopic	**Z** No Device	**Z** No Qualifier
W Upper Tooth **X** Lower Tooth	**0** Open **X** External	**Z** No Device	**0** Single **1** Multiple **2** All

Section **0** **Medical and Surgical**
Body System **C** **Mouth and Throat**
Operation **P** **Removal:** Taking out or off a device from a body part

Body Part (4th)	Approach (5th)	Device (6th)	Qualifier (7th)
A Salivary Gland	**0** Open **3** Percutaneous	**0** Drainage Device **C** Extraluminal Device **Y** Other Device	**Z** No Qualifier
A Salivary Gland	**7** Via Natural or Artificial Opening **8** Via Natural or Artificial Opening Endoscopic	**Y** Other Device	**Z** No Qualifier
S Larynx	**0** Open **3** Percutaneous **7** Via Natural or Artificial Opening **8** Via Natural or Artificial Opening Endoscopic	**0** Drainage Device **7** Autologous Tissue Substitute **D** Intraluminal Device **J** Synthetic Substitute **K** Nonautologous Tissue Substitute **Y** Other Device	**Z** No Qualifier
S Larynx	**X** External	**0** Drainage Device **7** Autologous Tissue Substitute **D** Intraluminal Device **J** Synthetic Substitute **K** Nonautologous Tissue Substitute	**Z** No Qualifier

Continued →

tion	0	**Medical and Surgical**
ly System	C	**Mouth and Throat**
eration	P	**Removal:** Taking out or off a device from a body part

Body Part (4th)	Approach (5th)	Device (6th)	Qualifier (7th)
Mouth and Throat	**0** Open **3** Percutaneous **7** Via Natural or Artificial Opening **8** Via Natural or Artificial Opening Endoscopic	**0** Drainage Device **1** Radioactive Element **7** Autologous Tissue Substitute **D** Intraluminal Device **J** Synthetic Substitute **K** Nonautologous Tissue Substitute **Y** Other Device	**Z** No Qualifier
Mouth and Throat	**X** External	**0** Drainage Device **1** Radioactive Element **7** Autologous Tissue Substitute **D** Intraluminal Device **J** Synthetic Substitute **K** Nonautologous Tissue Substitute	**Z** No Qualifier

tion	0	**Medical and Surgical**
dy System	C	**Mouth and Throat**
eration	Q	**Repair:** Restoring, to the extent possible, a body part to its normal anatomic structure and function

Body Part (4th)	Approach (5th)	Device (6th)	Qualifier (7th)
Upper Lip Lower Lip Hard Palate Soft Palate Buccal Mucosa Upper Gingiva Lower Gingiva Tongue Uvula Tonsils Adenoids	**0** Open **3** Percutaneous **X** External	**Z** No Device	**Z** No Qualifier
Parotid Gland, Right Parotid Gland, Left Parotid Duct, Right Parotid Duct, Left Sublingual Gland, Right Sublingual Gland, Left Submaxillary Gland, Right Submaxillary Gland, Left Minor Salivary Gland	**0** Open **3** Percutaneous	**Z** No Device	**Z** No Qualifier
M Pharynx Epiglottis Larynx Vocal Cord, Right Vocal Cord, Left	**0** Open **3** Percutaneous **4** Percutaneous Endoscopic **7** Via Natural or Artificial Opening **8** Via Natural or Artificial Opening Endoscopic	**Z** No Device	**Z** No Qualifier
W Upper Tooth **X** Lower Tooth	**0** Open **X** External	**Z** No Device	**0** Single **1** Multiple **2** All

Section 0 **Medical and Surgical**
Body System C **Mouth and Throat**
Operation R **Replacement:** Putting in or on biological or synthetic material that physically takes the place and/or function of all or a portion of a body part

Body Part (4th)	Approach (5th)	Device (6th)	Qualifier (7th)
0 Upper Lip **1** Lower Lip **2** Hard Palate **3** Soft Palate **4** Buccal Mucosa **5** Upper Gingiva **6** Lower Gingiva **7** Tongue **N** Uvula	**0** Open **3** Percutaneous **X** External	**7** Autologous Tissue Substitute **J** Synthetic Substitute **K** Nonautologous Tissue Substitute	**Z** No Qualifier
B Parotid Duct, Right **C** Parotid Duct, Left	**0** Open **3** Percutaneous	**7** Autologous Tissue Substitute **J** Synthetic Substitute **K** Nonautologous Tissue Substitute	**Z** No Qualifier
M Pharynx **R** Epiglottis **S** Larynx **T** Vocal Cord, Right **V** Vocal Cord, Left	**0** Open **7** Via Natural or Artificial Opening **8** Via Natural or Artificial Opening Endoscopic	**7** Autologous Tissue Substitute **J** Synthetic Substitute **K** Nonautologous Tissue Substitute	**Z** No Qualifier
W Upper Tooth **X** Lower Tooth	**0** Open **X** External	**7** Autologous Tissue Substitute **J** Synthetic Substitute **K** Nonautologous Tissue Substitute	**0** Single **1** Multiple **2** All

Section 0 **Medical and Surgical**
Body System C **Mouth and Throat**
Operation S **Reposition:** Moving to its normal location, or other suitable location, all or a portion of a body part

Body Part (4th)	Approach (5th)	Device (6th)	Qualifier (7th)
0 Upper Lip **1** Lower Lip **2** Hard Palate **3** Soft Palate **7** Tongue **N** Uvula	**0** Open **X** External	**Z** No Device	**Z** No Qualifier
B Parotid Duct, Right **C** Parotid Duct, Left	**0** Open **3** Percutaneous	**Z** No Device	**Z** No Qualifier
R Epiglottis **T** Vocal Cord, Right **V** Vocal Cord, Left	**0** Open **7** Via Natural or Artificial Opening **8** Via Natural or Artificial Opening Endoscopic	**Z** No Device	**Z** No Qualifier
W Upper Tooth **X** Lower Tooth	**0** Open **X** External	**5** External Fixation Device **Z** No Device	**0** Single **1** Multiple **2** All

tion 0 **Medical and Surgical**
dy System C **Mouth and Throat**
eration T **Resection:** Cutting out or off, without replacement, all of a body part

Body Part (4th)	Approach (5th)	Device (6th)	Qualifier (7th)
Upper Lip Lower Lip Hard Palate Soft Palate Tongue Uvula Tonsils Adenoids	**0** Open **X** External	**Z** No Device	**Z** No Qualifier
Parotid Gland, Right Parotid Gland, Left Parotid Duct, Right Parotid Duct, Left Sublingual Gland, Right Sublingual Gland, Left Submaxillary Gland, Right Submaxillary Gland, Left Minor Salivary Gland	**0** Open	**Z** No Device	**Z** No Qualifier
Pharynx Epiglottis Larynx Vocal Cord, Right Vocal Cord, Left	**0** Open **4** Percutaneous Endoscopic **7** Via Natural or Artificial Opening **8** Via Natural or Artificial Opening Endoscopic	**Z** No Device	**Z** No Qualifier
Upper Tooth Lower Tooth	**0** Open	**Z** No Device	**0** Single **1** Multiple **2** All

ction 0 **Medical and Surgical**
dy System C **Mouth and Throat**
eration U **Supplement:** Putting in or on biological or synthetic material that physically reinforces and/or augments the function of a portion of a body part

Body Part (4th)	Approach (5th)	Device (6th)	Qualifier (7th)
Upper Lip Lower Lip Hard Palate Soft Palate Buccal Mucosa Upper Gingiva Lower Gingiva Tongue Uvula	**0** Open **3** Percutaneous **X** External	**7** Autologous Tissue Substitute **J** Synthetic Substitute **K** Nonautologous Tissue Substitute	**Z** No Qualifier
Pharynx Epiglottis Larynx Vocal Cord, Right Vocal Cord, Left	**0** Open **7** Via Natural or Artificial Opening **8** Via Natural or Artificial Opening Endoscopic	**7** Autologous Tissue Substitute **J** Synthetic Substitute **K** Nonautologous Tissue Substitute	**Z** No Qualifier

Section 0 **Medical and Surgical**
Body System C **Mouth and Throat**
Operation V **Restriction:** Partially closing an orifice or the lumen of a tubular body part

Body Part (4th)	Approach (5th)	Device (6th)	Qualifier (7th)
B Parotid Duct, Right **C** Parotid Duct, Left	**0** Open **3** Percutaneous	**C** Extraluminal Device **D** Intraluminal Device **Z** No Device	**Z** No Qualifier
B Parotid Duct, Right **C** Parotid Duct, Left	**7** Via Natural or Artificial Opening **8** Via Natural or Artificial Opening Endoscopic	**D** Intraluminal Device **Z** No Device	**Z** No Qualifier

Section 0 **Medical and Surgical**
Body System C **Mouth and Throat**
Operation W **Revision:** Correcting, to the extent possible, a portion of a malfunctioning device or the position of a displaced device

Body Part (4th)	Approach (5th)	Device (6th)	Qualifier (7th)
A Salivary Gland	**0** Open **3** Percutaneous	**0** Drainage Device **C** Extraluminal Device **Y** Other Device	**Z** No Qualifier
A Salivary Gland	**7** Via Natural or Artificial Opening **8** Via Natural or Artificial Opening Endoscopic	**Y** Other Device	**Z** No Qualifier
A Salivary Gland	**X** External	**0** Drainage Device **C** Extraluminal Device	**Z** No Qualifier
S Larynx	**0** Open **3** Percutaneous **7** Via Natural or Artificial Opening **8** Via Natural or Artificial Opening Endoscopic	**0** Drainage Device **7** Autologous Tissue Substitute **D** Intraluminal Device **J** Synthetic Substitute **K** Nonautologous Tissue Substitute **Y** Other Device	**Z** No Qualifier
S Larynx	**X** External	**0** Drainage Device **7** Autologous Tissue Substitute **D** Intraluminal Device **J** Synthetic Substitute **K** Nonautologous Tissue Substitute	**Z** No Qualifier
Y Mouth and Throat	**0** Open **3** Percutaneous **7** Via Natural or Artificial Opening **8** Via Natural or Artificial Opening Endoscopic	**0** Drainage Device **1** Radioactive Element **7** Autologous Tissue Substitute **D** Intraluminal Device **J** Synthetic Substitute **K** Nonautologous Tissue Substitute **Y** Other Device	**Z** No Qualifier
Y Mouth and Throat	**X** External	**0** Drainage Device **1** Radioactive Element **7** Autologous Tissue Substitute **D** Intraluminal Device **J** Synthetic Substitute **K** Nonautologous Tissue Substitute	**Z** No Qualifier

ction **0** **Medical and Surgical**
dy System **C** **Mouth and Throat**
eration **X** **Transfer:** Moving, without taking out, all or a portion of a body part to another location to take over the function of all or a portion of a body part

Body Part (4th)	Approach (5th)	Device (6th)	Qualifier (7th)
0 Upper Lip 1 Lower Lip 3 Soft Palate 4 Buccal Mucosa 5 Upper Gingiva 6 Lower Gingiva 7 Tongue	**0** Open **X** External	**Z** No Device	**Z** No Qualifier

HA Coding Clinic

CB80ZZ Excision of Right Parotid Gland, Open Approach—AHA CC: 3Q, 2014, 21-22
CBM8ZX Excision of Pharynx, Via Natural or Artificial Opening Endoscopic, Diagnostic—AHA CC: 2Q, 2016, 20
CBM8ZZ Excision of Pharynx, Via Natural or Artificial Opening Endoscopic—AHA CC: 3Q, 2016, 28-29
CCH3ZZ Extirpation of Matter from Left Submaxillary Gland, Percutaneous Approach—AHA CC: 2Q, 2016, 20
CQ50ZZ Repair Upper Gingiva, Open Approach—AHA CC: 1Q, 2017, 20-21
CR3XJZ Replacement of Soft Palate with Synthetic Substitute, External Approach—AHA CC: 3Q, 2014, 25
CR4XKZ Replacement of Buccal Mucosa with Nonautologous Tissue Substitute, External Approach—AHA CC: 2Q, 2014, 5-6
CSR8ZZ Reposition Epiglottis, Via Natural or Artificial Opening Endoscopic—AHA CC: 3Q, 2016, 28-29
CT90ZZ Resection of Left Parotid Gland, Open Approach—AHA CC: 2Q, 2016, 12-14
CTW0Z1 Resection of Upper Tooth, Multiple, Open Approach—AHA CC: 3Q, 2014, 23-24
CTX0Z1 Resection of Lower Tooth, Multiple, Open Approach—AHA CC: 3Q, 2014, 23-24

Upper Gastrointestinal System

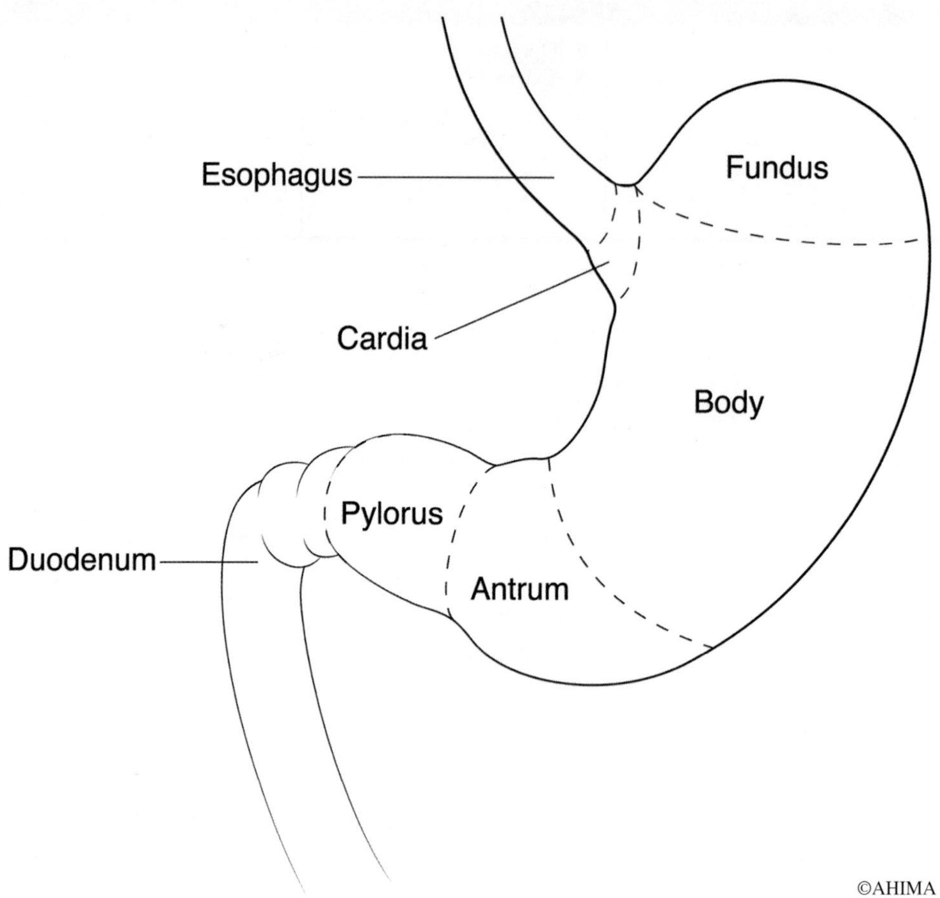

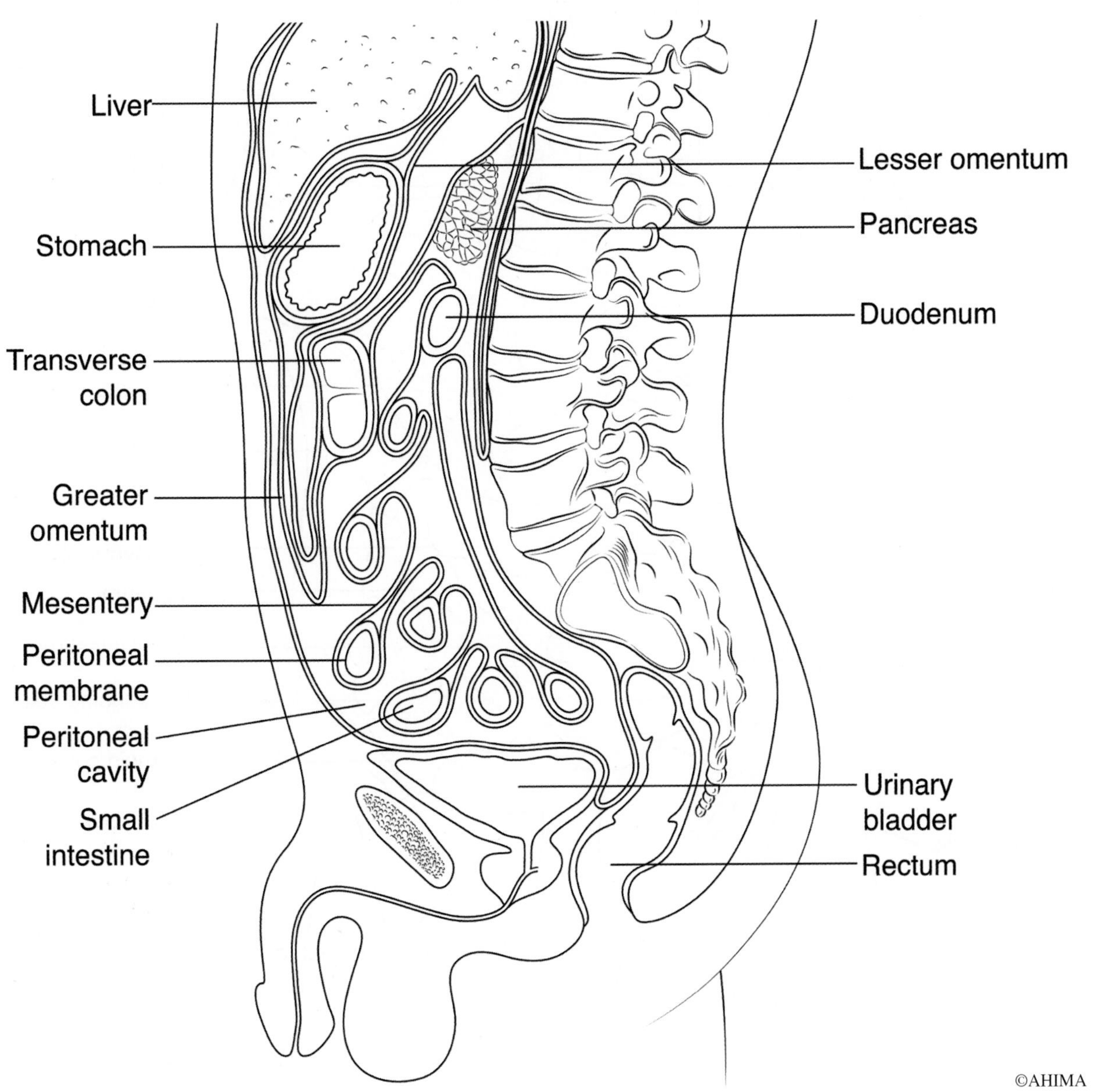
Liver
Stomach
Transverse colon
Greater omentum
Mesentery
Peritoneal membrane
Peritoneal cavity
Small intestine
Lesser omentum
Pancreas
Duodenum
Urinary bladder
Rectum

Gastrointestinal System

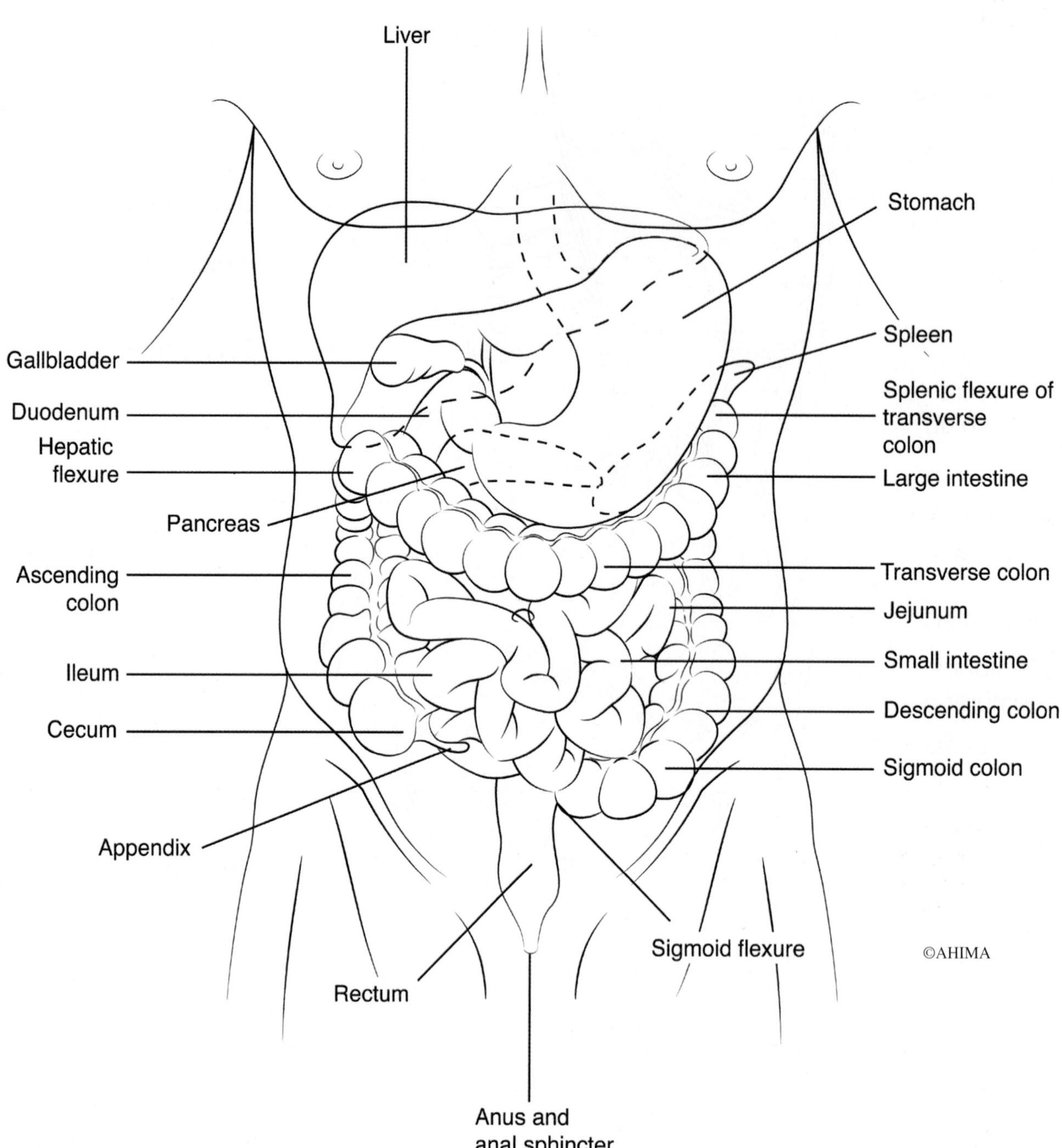

Large Intestine Structure of Colon

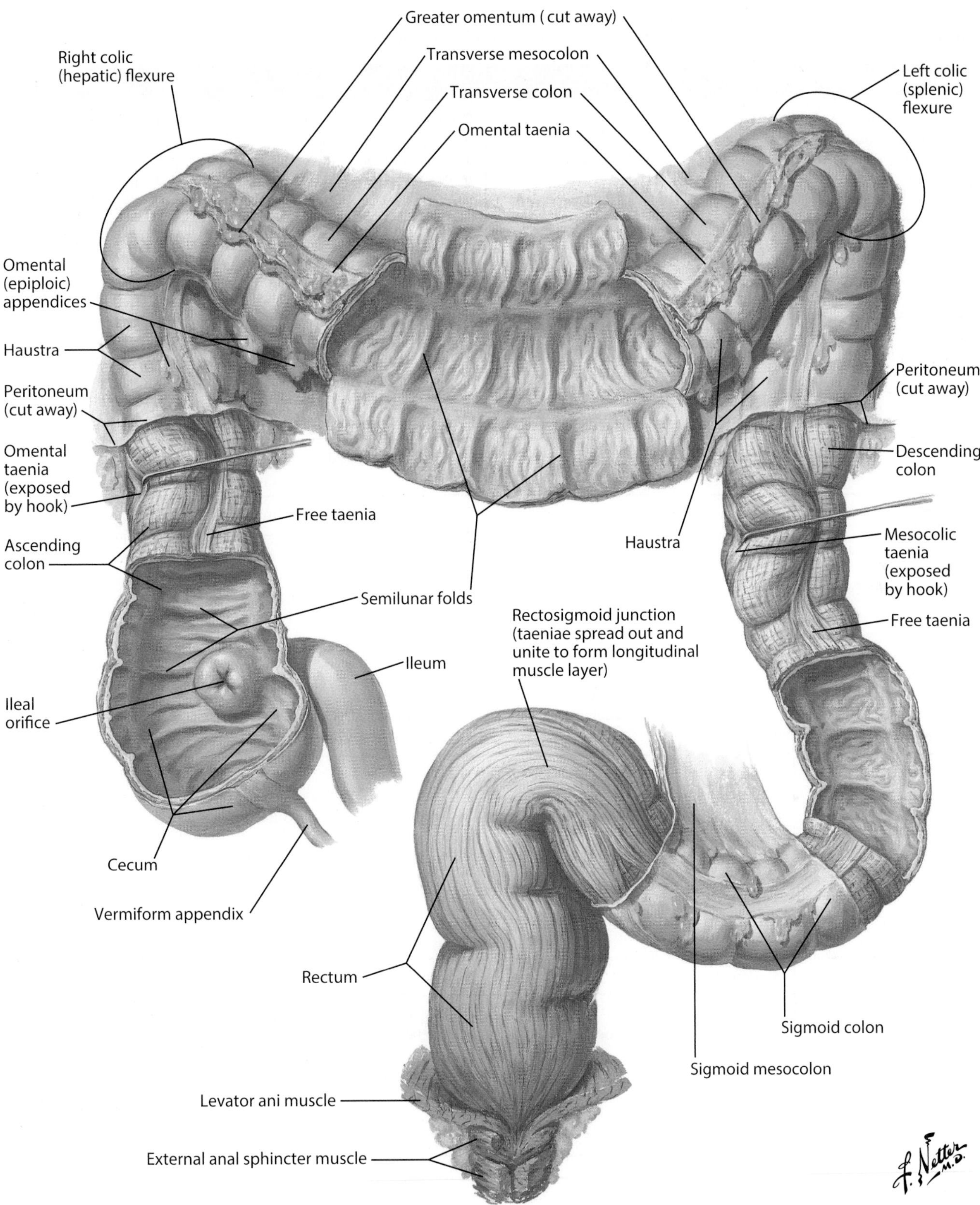

Gastrointestinal System Tables 0D1–0DY

Section 0 **Medical and Surgical**
Body System D **Gastrointestinal System**
Operation 1 **Bypass:** Altering the route of passage of the contents of a tubular body part

Body Part (4th)	Approach (5th)	Device (6th)	Qualifier (7th)
1 Esophagus, Upper **2** Esophagus, Middle **3** Esophagus, Lower **5** Esophagus	**0** Open **4** Percutaneous Endoscopic **8** Via Natural or Artificial Opening Endoscopic	**7** Autologous Tissue Substitute **J** Synthetic Substitute **K** Nonautologous Tissue Substitute **Z** No Device	**4** Cutaneous **6** Stomach **9** Duodenum **A** Jejunum **B** Ileum
1 Esophagus, Upper **2** Esophagus, Middle **3** Esophagus, Lower **5** Esophagus	**3** Percutaneous	**J** Synthetic Substitute	**4** Cutaneous
6 Stomach **9** Duodenum	**0** Open **4** Percutaneous Endoscopic **8** Via Natural or Artificial Opening Endoscopic	**7** Autologous Tissue Substitute **J** Synthetic Substitute **K** Nonautologous Tissue Substitute **Z** No Device	**4** Cutaneous **9** Duodenum **A** Jejunum **B** Ileum **L** Transverse Colon
6 Stomach **9** Duodenum	**3** Percutaneous	**J** Synthetic Substitute	**4** Cutaneous
A Jejunum	**0** Open **4** Percutaneous Endoscopic **8** Via Natural or Artificial Opening Endoscopic	**7** Autologous Tissue Substitute **J** Synthetic Substitute **K** Nonautologous Tissue Substitute **Z** No Device	**4** Cutaneous **A** Jejunum **B** Ileum **H** Cecum **K** Ascending Colon **L** Transverse Colon **M** Descending Colon **N** Sigmoid Colon **P** Rectum **Q** Anus
A Jejunum	**3** Percutaneous	**J** Synthetic Substitute	**4** Cutaneous
B Ileum	**0** Open **4** Percutaneous Endoscopic **8** Via Natural or Artificial Opening Endoscopic	**7** Autologous Tissue Substitute **J** Synthetic Substitute **K** Nonautologous Tissue Substitute **Z** No Device	**4** Cutaneous **B** Ileum **H** Cecum **K** Ascending Colon **L** Transverse Colon **M** Descending Colon **N** Sigmoid Colon **P** Rectum **Q** Anus
B Ileum	**3** Percutaneous	**J** Synthetic Substitute	**4** Cutaneous
H Cecum	**0** Open **4** Percutaneous Endoscopic **8** Via Natural or Artificial Opening Endoscopic	**7** Autologous Tissue Substitute **J** Synthetic Substitute **K** Nonautologous Tissue Substitute **Z** No Device	**4** Cutaneous **H** Cecum **K** Ascending Colon **L** Transverse Colon **M** Descending Colon **N** Sigmoid Colon **P** Rectum
H Cecum	**3** Percutaneous	**J** Synthetic Substitute	**4** Cutaneous
K Ascending Colon	**0** Open **4** Percutaneous Endoscopic **8** Via Natural or Artificial Opening Endoscopic	**7** Autologous Tissue Substitute **J** Synthetic Substitute **K** Nonautologous Tissue Substitute **Z** No Device	**4** Cutaneous **K** Ascending Colon **L** Transverse Colon **M** Descending Colon **N** Sigmoid Colon **P** Rectum
K Ascending Colon	**3** Percutaneous	**J** Synthetic Substitute	**4** Cutaneous

Continued →

0D1 Continued

Section 0 **Medical and Surgical**
Body System D **Gastrointestinal System**
Operation 1 **Bypass:** Altering the route of passage of the contents of a tubular body part

Body Part (4th)	Approach (5th)	Device (6th)	Qualifier (7th)
L Transverse Colon	**0** Open **4** Percutaneous Endoscopic **8** Via Natural or Artificial Opening Endoscopic	**7** Autologous Tissue Substitute **J** Synthetic Substitute **K** Nonautologous Tissue Substitute **Z** No Device	**4** Cutaneous **L** Transverse Colon **M** Descending Colon **N** Sigmoid Colon **P** Rectum
L Transverse Colon	**3** Percutaneous	**J** Synthetic Substitute	**4** Cutaneous
M Descending Colon	**0** Open **4** Percutaneous Endoscopic **8** Via Natural or Artificial Opening Endoscopic	**7** Autologous Tissue Substitute **J** Synthetic Substitute **K** Nonautologous Tissue Substitute **Z** No Device	**4** Cutaneous **M** Descending Colon **N** Sigmoid Colon **P** Rectum
M Descending Colon	**3** Percutaneous	**J** Synthetic Substitute	**4** Cutaneous
N Sigmoid Colon	**0** Open **4** Percutaneous Endoscopic **8** Via Natural or Artificial Opening Endoscopic	**7** Autologous Tissue Substitute **J** Synthetic Substitute **K** Nonautologous Tissue Substitute **Z** No Device	**4** Cutaneous **N** Sigmoid Colon **P** Rectum
N Sigmoid Colon	**3** Percutaneous	**J** Synthetic Substitute	**4** Cutaneous

Section 0 **Medical and Surgical**
Body System D **Gastrointestinal System**
Operation 2 **Change:** Taking out or off a device from a body part and putting back an identical or similar device in or on the same body part without cutting or puncturing the skin or a mucous membrane

Body Part (4th)	Approach (5th)	Device (6th)	Qualifier (7th)
0 Upper Intestinal Tract **D** Lower Intestinal Tract	**X** External	**0** Drainage Device **U** Feeding Device **Y** Other Device	**Z** No Qualifier
U Omentum **V** Mesentery **W** Peritoneum	**X** External	**0** Drainage Device **Y** Other Device	**Z** No Qualifier

Section 0 **Medical and Surgical**
Body System D **Gastrointestinal System**
Operation 5 **Destruction:** Physical eradication of all or a portion of a body part by the direct use of energy, force, or a destructive age

Body Part (4th)	Approach (5th)	Device (6th)	Qualifier (7th)
1 Esophagus, Upper **2** Esophagus, Middle **3** Esophagus, Lower **4** Esophagogastric Junction **5** Esophagus **6** Stomach **7** Stomach, Pylorus **8** Small Intestine **9** Duodenum **A** Jejunum **B** Ileum **C** Ileocecal Valve **E** Large Intestine **F** Large Intestine, Right **G** Large Intestine, Left **H** Cecum **J** Appendix **K** Ascending Colon **L** Transverse Colon **M** Descending Colon **N** Sigmoid Colon **P** Rectum	**0** Open **3** Percutaneous **4** Percutaneous Endoscopic **7** Via Natural or Artificial Opening **8** Via Natural or Artificial Opening Endoscopic	**Z** No Device	**Z** No Qualifier
Q Anus	**0** Open **3** Percutaneous **4** Percutaneous Endoscopic **7** Via Natural or Artificial Opening **8** Via Natural or Artificial Opening Endoscopic **X** External	**Z** No Device	**Z** No Qualifier
R Anal Sphincter **U** Omentum **V** Mesentery **W** Peritoneum	**0** Open **3** Percutaneous **4** Percutaneous Endoscopic	**Z** No Device	**Z** No Qualifier

Section 0 **Medical and Surgical**
Body System D **Gastrointestinal System**
Operation 7 **Dilation:** Expanding an orifice or the lumen of a tubular body part

Body Part (4th)	Approach (5th)	Device (6th)	Qualifier (7th)
1 Esophagus, Upper **2** Esophagus, Middle **3** Esophagus, Lower **4** Esophagogastric Junction **5** Esophagus **6** Stomach **7** Stomach, Pylorus **8** Small Intestine **9** Duodenum **A** Jejunum **B** Ileum **C** Ileocecal Valve **E** Large Intestine **F** Large Intestine, Right **G** Large Intestine, Left **H** Cecum **K** Ascending Colon **L** Transverse Colon **M** Descending Colon **N** Sigmoid Colon **P** Rectum **Q** Anus	**0** Open **3** Percutaneous **4** Percutaneous Endoscopic **7** Via Natural or Artificial Opening **8** Via Natural or Artificial Opening Endoscopic	**D** Intraluminal Device **Z** No Device	**Z** No Qualifier

Section **0** **Medical and Surgical**
Body System **D** **Gastrointestinal System**
Operation **8** **Division:** Cutting into a body part, without draining fluids and/or gases from the body part, in order to separate or transect a body part

Body Part (4th)	Approach (5th)	Device (6th)	Qualifier (7th)
4 Esophagogastric Junction **7** Stomach, Pylorus	**0** Open **3** Percutaneous **4** Percutaneous Endoscopic **7** Via Natural or Artificial Opening **8** Via Natural or Artificial Opening Endoscopic	**Z** No Device	**Z** No Qualifier
R Anal Sphincter	**0** Open **3** Percutaneous	**Z** No Device	**Z** No Qualifier

Section **0** **Medical and Surgical**
Body System **D** **Gastrointestinal System**
Operation **9** **Drainage:** Taking or letting out fluids and/or gases from a body part

Body Part (4th)	Approach (5th)	Device (6th)	Qualifier (7th)
1 Esophagus, Upper **2** Esophagus, Middle **3** Esophagus, Lower **4** Esophagogastric Junction **5** Esophagus **6** Stomach **7** Stomach, Pylorus **8** Small Intestine **9** Duodenum **A** Jejunum **B** Ileum **C** Ileocecal Valve **E** Large Intestine **F** Large Intestine, Right **G** Large Intestine, Left **H** Cecum **J** Appendix **K** Ascending Colon **L** Transverse Colon **M** Descending Colon **N** Sigmoid Colon **P** Rectum	**0** Open **3** Percutaneous **4** Percutaneous Endoscopic **7** Via Natural or Artificial Opening **8** Via Natural or Artificial Opening Endoscopic	**0** Drainage Device	**Z** No Qualifier
1 Esophagus, Upper **2** Esophagus, Middle **3** Esophagus, Lower **4** Esophagogastric Junction **5** Esophagus **6** Stomach **7** Stomach, Pylorus **8** Small Intestine **9** Duodenum **A** Jejunum **B** Ileum **C** Ileocecal Valve **E** Large Intestine **F** Large Intestine, Right **G** Large Intestine, Left **H** Cecum **J** Appendix **K** Ascending Colon **L** Transverse Colon **M** Descending Colon **N** Sigmoid Colon **P** Rectum	**0** Open **3** Percutaneous **4** Percutaneous Endoscopic **7** Via Natural or Artificial Opening **8** Via Natural or Artificial Opening Endoscopic	**Z** No Device	**X** Diagnostic **Z** No Qualifier

Continued →

0D9 Continued

Section 0 **Medical and Surgical**
Body System D **Gastrointestinal System**
Operation 9 **Drainage:** Taking or letting out fluids and/or gases from a body part

Body Part (4th)	Approach (5th)	Device (6th)	Qualifier (7th)
Q Anus	**0** Open **3** Percutaneous **4** Percutaneous Endoscopic **7** Via Natural or Artificial Opening **8** Via Natural or Artificial Opening Endoscopic **X** External	**0** Drainage Device	**Z** No Qualifier
Q Anus	**0** Open **3** Percutaneous **4** Percutaneous Endoscopic **7** Via Natural or Artificial Opening **8** Via Natural or Artificial Opening Endoscopic **X** External	**Z** No Device	**X** Diagnostic **Z** No Qualifier
R Anal Sphincter **U** Omentum **V** Mesentery **W** Peritoneum	**0** Open **3** Percutaneous **4** Percutaneous Endoscopic	**0** Drainage Device	**Z** No Qualifier
R Anal Sphincter **U** Omentum **V** Mesentery **W** Peritoneum	**0** Open **3** Percutaneous **4** Percutaneous Endoscopic	**Z** No Device	**X** Diagnostic **Z** No Qualifier

Section 0 **Medical and Surgical**
Body System D **Gastrointestinal System**
Operation B **Excision:** Cutting out or off, without replacement, a portion of a body part

Body Part (4th)	Approach (5th)	Device (6th)	Qualifier (7th)
1 Esophagus, Upper **2** Esophagus, Middle **3** Esophagus, Lower **4** Esophagogastric Junction **5** Esophagus **7** Stomach, Pylorus **8** Small Intestine **9** Duodenum **A** Jejunum **B** Ileum **C** Ileocecal Valve **E** Large Intestine **F** Large Intestine, Right **H** Cecum **J** Appendix **K** Ascending Colon **P** Rectum	**0** Open **3** Percutaneous **4** Percutaneous Endoscopic **7** Via Natural or Artificial Opening **8** Via Natural or Artificial Opening Endoscopic	**Z** No Device	**X** Diagnostic **Z** No Qualifier
6 Stomach	**0** Open **3** Percutaneous **4** Percutaneous Endoscopic **7** Via Natural or Artificial Opening **8** Via Natural or Artificial Opening Endoscopic	**Z** No Device	**3** Vertical **X** Diagnostic **Z** No Qualifier
G Large Intestine, Left **L** Transverse Colon **M** Descending Colon **N** Sigmoid Colon	**0** Open **3** Percutaneous **4** Percutaneous Endoscopic **7** Via Natural or Artificial Opening **8** Via Natural or Artificial Opening Endoscopic	**Z** No Device	**X** Diagnostic **Z** No Qualifier

Continued →

ction	**0**	**Medical and Surgical**
dy System	**D**	**Gastrointestinal System**
eration	**B**	**Excision:** Cutting out or off, without replacement, a portion of a body part

Body Part (4th)	Approach (5th)	Device (6th)	Qualifier (7th)
G Large Intestine, Left L Transverse Colon M Descending Colon N Sigmoid Colon	**F** Via Natural or Artificial Opening With Percutaneous Endoscopic Assistance	**Z** No Device	**Z** No Qualifier
Q Anus	**0** Open **3** Percutaneous **4** Percutaneous Endoscopic **7** Via Natural or Artificial Opening **8** Via Natural or Artificial Opening Endoscopic **X** External	**Z** No Device	**X** Diagnostic **Z** No Qualifier
R Anal Sphincter U Omentum V Mesentery W Peritoneum	**0** Open **3** Percutaneous **4** Percutaneous Endoscopic	**Z** No Device	**X** Diagnostic **Z** No Qualifier

ction	**0**	**Medical and Surgical**
dy System	**D**	**Gastrointestinal System**
eration	**C**	**Extirpation:** Taking or cutting out solid matter from a body part

Body Part (4th)	Approach (5th)	Device (6th)	Qualifier (7th)
1 Esophagus, Upper 2 Esophagus, Middle 3 Esophagus, Lower 4 Esophagogastric Junction 5 Esophagus 6 Stomach 7 Stomach, Pylorus 8 Small Intestine 9 Duodenum A Jejunum B Ileum C Ileocecal Valve E Large Intestine F Large Intestine, Right G Large Intestine, Left H Cecum J Appendix K Ascending Colon L Transverse Colon M Descending Colon N Sigmoid Colon P Rectum	**0** Open **3** Percutaneous **4** Percutaneous Endoscopic **7** Via Natural or Artificial Opening **8** Via Natural or Artificial Opening Endoscopic	**Z** No Device	**Z** No Qualifier
Q Anus	**0** Open **3** Percutaneous **4** Percutaneous Endoscopic **7** Via Natural or Artificial Opening **8** Via Natural or Artificial Opening Endoscopic **X** External	**Z** No Device	**Z** No Qualifier
R Anal Sphincter U Omentum V Mesentery W Peritoneum	**0** Open **3** Percutaneous **4** Percutaneous Endoscopic	**Z** No Device	**Z** No Qualifier

Section 0 **Medical and Surgical**
Body System D **Gastrointestinal System**
Operation D **Extraction:** Pulling or stripping out or off all or a portion of a body part by the use of force

Body Part (4th)	Approach (5th)	Device (6th)	Qualifier (7th)
1 Esophagus, Upper **2** Esophagus, Middle **3** Esophagus, Lower **4** Esophagogastric Junction **5** Esophagus **6** Stomach **7** Stomach, Pylorus **8** Small Intestine **9** Duodenum **A** Jejunum **B** Ileum **C** Ileocecal Valve **E** Large Intestine **F** Large Intestine, Right **G** Large Intestine, Left **H** Cecum **J** Appendix **K** Ascending Colon **L** Transverse Colon **M** Descending Colon **N** Sigmoid Colon **P** Rectum	**3** Percutaneous **4** Percutaneous Endoscopic **8** Via Natural or Artificial Opening Endoscopic	**Z** No Device	**X** Diagnostic
Q Anus	**3** Percutaneous **4** Percutaneous Endoscopic **8** Via Natural or Artificial Opening Endoscopic **X** External	**Z** No Device	**X** Diagnostic

Section 0 **Medical and Surgical**
Body System D **Gastrointestinal System**
Operation F **Fragmentation:** Breaking solid matter in a body part into pieces

Body Part (4th)	Approach (5th)	Device (6th)	Qualifier (7th)
5 Esophagus **6** Stomach **8** Small Intestine **9** Duodenum **A** Jejunum **B** Ileum **E** Large Intestine **F** Large Intestine, Right **G** Large Intestine, Left **H** Cecum **J** Appendix **K** Ascending Colon **L** Transverse Colon **M** Descending Colon **N** Sigmoid Colon **P** Rectum **Q** Anus	**0** Open **3** Percutaneous **4** Percutaneous Endoscopic **7** Via Natural or Artificial Opening **8** Via Natural or Artificial Opening Endoscopic **X** External	**Z** No Device	**Z** No Qualifier

tion 0 **Medical and Surgical**
dy System D **Gastrointestinal System**
eration H **Insertion:** Putting in a nonbiological appliance that monitors, assists, performs, or prevents a physiological function but does not physically take the place of a body part

Body Part (4th)	Approach (5th)	Device (6th)	Qualifier (7th)
Upper Intestinal Tract Lower Intestinal Tract	**0** Open **3** Percutaneous **4** Percutaneous Endoscopic **7** Via Natural or Artificial Opening **8** Via Natural or Artificial Opening Endoscopic	**Y** Other Device	**Z** No Qualifier
Esophagus	**0** Open **3** Percutaneous **4** Percutaneous Endoscopic	**1** Radioactive Element **2** Monitoring Device **3** Infusion Device **D** Intraluminal Device **U** Feeding Device **Y** Other Device	**Z** No Qualifier
Esophagus	**7** Via Natural or Artificial Opening **8** Via Natural or Artificial Opening Endoscopic	**1** Radioactive Element **2** Monitoring Device **3** Infusion Device **B** Intraluminal Device, Airway **D** Intraluminal Device **U** Feeding Device **Y** Other Device	**Z** No Qualifier
Stomach	**0** Open **3** Percutaneous **4** Percutaneous Endoscopic	**2** Monitoring Device **3** Infusion Device **D** Intraluminal Device **M** Stimulator Lead **U** Feeding Device **Y** Other Device	**Z** No Qualifier
Stomach	**7** Via Natural or Artificial Opening **8** Via Natural or Artificial Opening Endoscopic	**2** Monitoring Device **3** Infusion Device **D** Intraluminal Device **U** Feeding Device **Y** Other Device	**Z** No Qualifier
Small Intestine Duodenum Jejunum Ileum	**0** Open **3** Percutaneous **4** Percutaneous Endoscopic **7** Via Natural or Artificial Opening **8** Via Natural or Artificial Opening Endoscopic	**2** Monitoring Device **3** Infusion Device **D** Intraluminal Device **U** Feeding Device	**Z** No Qualifier
Large Intestine	**0** Open **3** Percutaneous **4** Percutaneous Endoscopic **7** Via Natural or Artificial Opening **8** Via Natural or Artificial Opening Endoscopic	**D** Intraluminal Device	**Z** No Qualifier
Rectum	**0** Open **3** Percutaneous **4** Percutaneous Endoscopic **7** Via Natural or Artificial Opening **8** Via Natural or Artificial Opening Endoscopic	**1** Radioactive Element **D** Intraluminal Device	**Z** No Qualifier
Anus	**0** Open **3** Percutaneous **4** Percutaneous Endoscopic	**D** Intraluminal Device **L** Artificial Sphincter	**Z** No Qualifier
Anus	**7** Via Natural or Artificial Opening **8** Via Natural or Artificial Opening Endoscopic	**D** Intraluminal Device	**Z** No Qualifier
Anal Sphincter	**0** Open **3** Percutaneous **4** Percutaneous Endoscopic	**M** Stimulator Lead	**Z** No Qualifier

Section 0 **Medical and Surgical**
Body System D **Gastrointestinal System**
Operation J **Inspection:** Visually and/or manually exploring a body part

Body Part (4th)	Approach (5th)	Device (6th)	Qualifier (7th)
0 Upper Intestinal Tract **6** Stomach **D** Lower Intestinal Tract	**0** Open **3** Percutaneous **4** Percutaneous Endoscopic **7** Via Natural or Artificial Opening **8** Via Natural or Artificial Opening Endoscopic **X** External	**Z** No Device	**Z** No Qualifier
U Omentum **V** Mesentery **W** Peritoneum	**0** Open **3** Percutaneous **4** Percutaneous Endoscopic **X** External	**Z** No Device	**Z** No Qualifier

Section 0 **Medical and Surgical**
Body System D **Gastrointestinal System**
Operation L **Occlusion:** Completely closing an orifice or the lumen of a tubular body part

Body Part (4th)	Approach (5th)	Device (6th)	Qualifier (7th)
1 Esophagus, Upper **2** Esophagus, Middle **3** Esophagus, Lower **4** Esophagogastric Junction **5** Esophagus **6** Stomach **7** Stomach, Pylorus **8** Small Intestine **9** Duodenum **A** Jejunum **B** Ileum **C** Ileocecal Valve **E** Large Intestine **F** Large Intestine, Right **G** Large Intestine, Left **H** Cecum **K** Ascending Colon **L** Transverse Colon **M** Descending Colon **N** Sigmoid Colon **P** Rectum	**0** Open **3** Percutaneous **4** Percutaneous Endoscopic	**C** Extraluminal Device **D** Intraluminal Device **Z** No Device	**Z** No Qualifier
1 Esophagus, Upper **2** Esophagus, Middle **3** Esophagus, Lower **4** Esophagogastric Junction **5** Esophagus **6** Stomach **7** Stomach, Pylorus **8** Small Intestine **9** Duodenum **A** Jejunum **B** Ileum **C** Ileocecal Valve **E** Large Intestine **F** Large Intestine, Right **G** Large Intestine, Left **H** Cecum **K** Ascending Colon **L** Transverse Colon **M** Descending Colon **N** Sigmoid Colon **P** Rectum	**7** Via Natural or Artificial Opening **8** Via Natural or Artificial Opening Endoscopic	**D** Intraluminal Device **Z** No Device	**Z** No Qualifier

Continued →

tion	0	**Medical and Surgical**
ly System	D	**Gastrointestinal System**
eration	L	**Occlusion:** Completely closing an orifice or the lumen of a tubular body part

Body Part (4th)	Approach (5th)	Device (6th)	Qualifier (7th)
Anus	**0** Open **3** Percutaneous **4** Percutaneous Endoscopic **X** External	**C** Extraluminal Device **D** Intraluminal Device **Z** No Device	**Z** No Qualifier
Anus	**7** Via Natural or Artificial Opening **8** Via Natural or Artificial Opening Endoscopic	**D** Intraluminal Device **Z** No Device	**Z** No Qualifier

tion	0	**Medical and Surgical**
ly System	D	**Gastrointestinal System**
eration	M	**Reattachment:** Putting back in or on all or a portion of a separated body part to its normal location or other suitable location

Body Part (4th)	Approach (5th)	Device (6th)	Qualifier (7th)
Esophagus Stomach Small Intestine Duodenum Jejunum Ileum Large Intestine Large Intestine, Right Large Intestine, Left Cecum Ascending Colon Transverse Colon Descending Colon Sigmoid Colon Rectum	**0** Open **4** Percutaneous Endoscopic	**Z** No Device	**Z** No Qualifier

tion	0	**Medical and Surgical**
dy System	D	**Gastrointestinal System**
eration	N	**Release:** Freeing a body part from an abnormal physical constraint by cutting or by the use of force

Body Part (4th)	Approach (5th)	Device (6th)	Qualifier (7th)
Esophagus, Upper Esophagus, Middle Esophagus, Lower Esophagogastric Junction Esophagus Stomach Stomach, Pylorus Small Intestine Duodenum Jejunum Ileum Ileocecal Valve Large Intestine Large Intestine, Right Large Intestine, Left Cecum Appendix Ascending Colon Transverse Colon Descending Colon Sigmoid Colon Rectum	**0** Open **3** Percutaneous **4** Percutaneous Endoscopic **7** Via Natural or Artificial Opening **8** Via Natural or Artificial Opening Endoscopic	**Z** No Device	**Z** No Qualifier

Continued →

Section 0 **Medical and Surgical**
Body System D **Gastrointestinal System**
Operation N **Release:** Freeing a body part from an abnormal physical constraint by cutting or by the use of force

Body Part (4th)	Approach (5th)	Device (6th)	Qualifier (7th)
Q Anus	**0** Open **3** Percutaneous **4** Percutaneous Endoscopic **7** Via Natural or Artificial Opening **8** Via Natural or Artificial Opening Endoscopic **X** External	**Z** No Device	**Z** No Qualifier
R Anal Sphincter **U** Omentum **V** Mesentery **W** Peritoneum	**0** Open **3** Percutaneous **4** Percutaneous Endoscopic	**Z** No Device	**Z** No Qualifier

Section 0 **Medical and Surgical**
Body System D **Gastrointestinal System**
Operation P **Removal:** Taking out or off a device from a body part

Body Part (4th)	Approach (5th)	Device (6th)	Qualifier (7th
0 Upper Intestinal Tract **D** Lower Intestinal Tract	**0** Open **3** Percutaneous **4** Percutaneous Endoscopic **7** Via Natural or Artificial Opening **8** Via Natural or Artificial Opening Endoscopic	**0** Drainage Device **2** Monitoring Device **3** Infusion Device **7** Autologous Tissue Substitute **C** Extraluminal Device **D** Intraluminal Device **J** Synthetic Substitute **K** Nonautologous Tissue Substitute **U** Feeding Device **Y** Other Device	**Z** No Qualifier
0 Upper Intestinal Tract **D** Lower Intestinal Tract	**X** External	**0** Drainage Device **2** Monitoring Device **3** Infusion Device **D** Intraluminal Device **U** Feeding Device	**Z** No Qualifier
5 Esophagus	**0** Open **3** Percutaneous **4** Percutaneous Endoscopic	**1** Radioactive Element **2** Monitoring Device **3** Infusion Device **U** Feeding Device **Y** Other Device	**Z** No Qualifier
5 Esophagus	**7** Via Natural or Artificial Opening **8** Via Natural or Artificial Opening Endoscopic	**1** Radioactive Element **D** Intraluminal Device **Y** Other Device	**Z** No Qualifier
5 Esophagus	**X** External	**1** Radioactive Element **2** Monitoring Device **3** Infusion Device **D** Intraluminal Device **U** Feeding Device	**Z** No Qualifier

Continued →

tion 0 **Medical and Surgical**
dy System D **Gastrointestinal System**
eration P **Removal:** Taking out or off a device from a body part

Body Part (4th)	Approach (5th)	Device (6th)	Qualifier (7th)
Stomach	**0** Open **3** Percutaneous **4** Percutaneous Endoscopic	**0** Drainage Device **2** Monitoring Device **3** Infusion Device **7** Autologous Tissue Substitute **C** Extraluminal Device **D** Intraluminal Device **J** Synthetic Substitute **K** Nonautologous Tissue Substitute **M** Stimulator Lead **U** Feeding Device **Y** Other Device	**Z** No Qualifier
Stomach	**7** Via Natural or Artificial Opening **8** Via Natural or Artificial Opening Endoscopic	**0** Drainage Device **2** Monitoring Device **3** Infusion Device **7** Autologous Tissue Substitute **C** Extraluminal Device **D** Intraluminal Device **J** Synthetic Substitute **K** Nonautologous Tissue Substitute **U** Feeding Device **Y** Other Device	**Z** No Qualifier
Stomach	**X** External	**0** Drainage Device **2** Monitoring Device **3** Infusion Device **D** Intraluminal Device **U** Feeding Device	**Z** No Qualifier
Rectum	**0** Open **3** Percutaneous **4** Percutaneous Endoscopic **7** Via Natural or Artificial Opening **8** Via Natural or Artificial Opening Endoscopic **X** External	**1** Radioactive Element	**Z** No Qualifier
Q Anus	**0** Open **3** Percutaneous **4** Percutaneous Endoscopic **7** Via Natural or Artificial Opening **8** Via Natural or Artificial Opening Endoscopic	**L** Artificial Sphincter	**Z** No Qualifier
R Anal Sphincter	**0** Open **3** Percutaneous **4** Percutaneous Endoscopic	**M** Stimulator Lead	**Z** No Qualifier
U Omentum V Mesentery W Peritoneum	**0** Open **3** Percutaneous **4** Percutaneous Endoscopic	**0** Drainage Device **1** Radioactive Element **7** Autologous Tissue Substitute **J** Synthetic Substitute **K** Nonautologous Tissue Substitute	**Z** No Qualifier

Section **0** **Medical and Surgical**
Body System **D** **Gastrointestinal System**
Operation **Q** **Repair:** Restoring, to the extent possible, a body part to its normal anatomic structure and function

Body Part (4th)	Approach (5th)	Device (6th)	Qualifier (7th)
1 Esophagus, Upper **2** Esophagus, Middle **3** Esophagus, Lower **4** Esophagogastric Junction **5** Esophagus **6** Stomach **7** Stomach, Pylorus **8** Small Intestine **9** Duodenum **A** Jejunum **B** Ileum **C** Ileocecal Valve **E** Large Intestine **F** Large Intestine, Right **G** Large Intestine, Left **H** Cecum **J** Appendix **K** Ascending Colon **L** Transverse Colon **M** Descending Colon **N** Sigmoid Colon **P** Rectum	**0** Open **3** Percutaneous **4** Percutaneous Endoscopic **7** Via Natural or Artificial Opening **8** Via Natural or Artificial Opening Endoscopic	**Z** No Device	**Z** No Qualifier
Q Anus	**0** Open **3** Percutaneous **4** Percutaneous Endoscopic **7** Via Natural or Artificial Opening **8** Via Natural or Artificial Opening Endoscopic **X** External	**Z** No Device	**Z** No Qualifier
R Anal Sphincter **U** Omentum **V** Mesentery **W** Peritoneum	**0** Open **3** Percutaneous **4** Percutaneous Endoscopic	**Z** No Device	**Z** No Qualifier

Section **0** **Medical and Surgical**
Body System **D** **Gastrointestinal System**
Operation **R** **Replacement:** Putting in or on biological or synthetic material that physically takes the place and/or function of all or a portion of a body part

Body Part (4th)	Approach (5th)	Device (6th)	Qualifier (7th)
5 Esophagus	**0** Open **4** Percutaneous Endoscopic **7** Via Natural or Artificial Opening **8** Via Natural or Artificial Opening Endoscopic	**7** Autologous Tissue Substitute **J** Synthetic Substitute **K** Nonautologous Tissue Substitute	**Z** No Qualifier
R Anal Sphincter **U** Omentum **V** Mesentery **W** Peritoneum	**0** Open **4** Percutaneous Endoscopic	**7** Autologous Tissue Substitute **J** Synthetic Substitute **K** Nonautologous Tissue Substitute	**Z** No Qualifier

tion	0	**Medical and Surgical**
dy System	D	**Gastrointestinal System**
eration	S	**Reposition:** Moving to its normal location, or other suitable location, all or a portion of a body part

Body Part (4th)	Approach (5th)	Device (6th)	Qualifier (7th)
Esophagus Stomach Duodenum Jejunum Ileum Cecum Ascending Colon Transverse Colon Descending Colon Sigmoid Colon Rectum Anus	**0** Open **4** Percutaneous Endoscopic **7** Via Natural or Artificial Opening **8** Via Natural or Artificial Opening Endoscopic **X** External	**Z** No Device	**Z** No Qualifier
Small Intestine Large Intestine	**0** Open **4** Percutaneous Endoscopic **7** Via Natural or Artificial Opening **8** Via Natural or Artificial Opening Endoscopic	**Z** No Device	**Z** No Qualifier

tion	0	**Medical and Surgical**
dy System	D	**Gastrointestinal System**
eration	T	**Resection:** Cutting out or off, without replacement, all of a body part

Body Part (4th)	Approach (5th)	Device (6th)	Qualifier (7th)
Esophagus, Upper Esophagus, Middle Esophagus, Lower Esophagogastric Junction Esophagus Stomach Stomach, Pylorus Small Intestine Duodenum Jejunum Ileum Ileocecal Valve Large Intestine Large Intestine, Right Cecum Appendix Ascending Colon Rectum Anus	**0** Open **4** Percutaneous Endoscopic **7** Via Natural or Artificial Opening **8** Via Natural or Artificial Opening Endoscopic	**Z** No Device	**Z** No Qualifier
G Large Intestine, Left Transverse Colon M Descending Colon N Sigmoid Colon	**0** Open **4** Percutaneous Endoscopic **7** Via Natural or Artificial Opening **8** Via Natural or Artificial Opening Endoscopic **F** Via Natural or Artificial Opening With Percutaneous Endoscopic Assistance	**Z** No Device	**Z** No Qualifier
R Anal Sphincter J Omentum	**0** Open **4** Percutaneous Endoscopic	**Z** No Device	**Z** No Qualifier

Section 0 **Medical and Surgical**
Body System D **Gastrointestinal System**
Operation U **Supplement:** Putting in or on biological or synthetic material that physically reinforces and/or augments the function of a portion of a body part

Body Part (4th)	Approach (5th)	Device (6th)	Qualifier (7th)
1 Esophagus, Upper **2** Esophagus, Middle **3** Esophagus, Lower **4** Esophagogastric Junction **5** Esophagus **6** Stomach **7** Stomach, Pylorus **8** Small Intestine **9** Duodenum **A** Jejunum **B** Ileum **C** Ileocecal Valve **E** Large Intestine **F** Large Intestine, Right **G** Large Intestine, Left **H** Cecum **K** Ascending Colon **L** Transverse Colon **M** Descending Colon **N** Sigmoid Colon **P** Rectum	**0** Open **4** Percutaneous Endoscopic **7** Via Natural or Artificial Opening **8** Via Natural or Artificial Opening Endoscopic	**7** Autologous Tissue Substitute **J** Synthetic Substitute **K** Nonautologous Tissue Substitute	**Z** No Qualifier
Q Anus	**0** Open **4** Percutaneous Endoscopic **7** Via Natural or Artificial Opening **8** Via Natural or Artificial Opening Endoscopic **X** External	**7** Autologous Tissue Substitute **J** Synthetic Substitute **K** Nonautologous Tissue Substitute	**Z** No Qualifier
R Anal Sphincter **U** Omentum **V** Mesentery **W** Peritoneum	**0** Open **4** Percutaneous Endoscopic	**7** Autologous Tissue Substitute **J** Synthetic Substitute **K** Nonautologous Tissue Substitute	**Z** No Qualifier

Section 0 **Medical and Surgical**
Body System D **Gastrointestinal System**
Operation V **Restriction:** Partially closing an orifice or the lumen of a tubular body part

Body Part (4th)	Approach (5th)	Device (6th)	Qualifier (7th)
1 Esophagus, Upper **2** Esophagus, Middle **3** Esophagus, Lower **4** Esophagogastric Junction **5** Esophagus **6** Stomach **7** Stomach, Pylorus **8** Small Intestine **9** Duodenum **A** Jejunum **B** Ileum **C** Ileocecal Valve **E** Large Intestine **F** Large Intestine, Right **G** Large Intestine, Left **H** Cecum **K** Ascending Colon **L** Transverse Colon **M** Descending Colon **N** Sigmoid Colon **P** Rectum	**0** Open **3** Percutaneous **4** Percutaneous Endoscopic	**C** Extraluminal Device **D** Intraluminal Device **Z** No Device	**Z** No Qualifier

Continued →

tion **0** **Medical and Surgical**
dy System **D** **Gastrointestinal System**
eration **V** **Restriction:** Partially closing an orifice or the lumen of a tubular body part

Body Part (4th)	Approach (5th)	Device (6th)	Qualifier (7th)
Esophagus, Upper Esophagus, Middle Esophagus, Lower Esophagogastric Junction Esophagus Stomach Stomach, Pylorus Small Intestine Duodenum Jejunum Ileum Ileocecal Valve Large Intestine Large Intestine, Right Large Intestine, Left Cecum Ascending Colon Transverse Colon Descending Colon Sigmoid Colon Rectum	**7** Via Natural or Artificial Opening **8** Via Natural or Artificial Opening Endoscopic	**D** Intraluminal Device **Z** No Device	**Z** No Qualifier
Anus	**0** Open **3** Percutaneous **4** Percutaneous Endoscopic **X** External	**C** Extraluminal Device **D** Intraluminal Device **Z** No Device	**Z** No Qualifier
Anus	**7** Via Natural or Artificial Opening **8** Via Natural or Artificial Opening Endoscopic	**D** Intraluminal Device **Z** No Device	**Z** No Qualifier

ction **0** **Medical and Surgical**
dy System **D** **Gastrointestinal System**
eration **W** **Revision:** Correcting, to the extent possible, a portion of a malfunctioning device or the position of a displaced device

Body Part (4th)	Approach (5th)	Device (6th)	Qualifier (7th)
Upper Intestinal Tract Lower Intestinal Tract	**0** Open **3** Percutaneous **4** Percutaneous Endoscopic **7** Via Natural or Artificial Opening **8** Via Natural or Artificial Opening Endoscopic	**0** Drainage Device **2** Monitoring Device **3** Infusion Device **7** Autologous Tissue Substitute **C** Extraluminal Device **D** Intraluminal Device **J** Synthetic Substitute **K** Nonautologous Tissue Substitute **U** Feeding Device **Y** Other Device	**Z** No Qualifier
Upper Intestinal Tract **D** Lower Intestinal Tract	**X** External	**0** Drainage Device **2** Monitoring Device **3** Infusion Device **7** Autologous Tissue Substitute **C** Extraluminal Device **D** Intraluminal Device **J** Synthetic Substitute **K** Nonautologous Tissue Substitute **U** Feeding Device	**Z** No Qualifier

Continued →

Section	**0**	**Medical and Surgical**	***0DW Contin...***
Body System	**D**	**Gastrointestinal System**	
Operation	**W**	**Revision:** Correcting, to the extent possible, a portion of a malfunctioning device or the position of a displaced device	

Body Part (4th)	Approach (5th)	Device (6th)	Qualifier (7th)
5 Esophagus	**0** Open **3** Percutaneous **4** Percutaneous Endoscopic	**Y** Other Device	**Z** No Qualifier
5 Esophagus	**7** Via Natural or Artificial Opening **8** Via Natural or Artificial Opening Endoscopic	**D** Intraluminal Device **Y** Other Device	**Z** No Qualifier
5 Esophagus	**X** External	**D** Intraluminal Device	**Z** No Qualifier
6 Stomach	**0** Open **3** Percutaneous **4** Percutaneous Endoscopic	**0** Drainage Device **2** Monitoring Device **3** Infusion Device **7** Autologous Tissue Substitute **C** Extraluminal Device **D** Intraluminal Device **J** Synthetic Substitute **K** Nonautologous Tissue Substitute **M** Stimulator Lead **U** Feeding Device **Y** Other Device	**Z** No Qualifier
6 Stomach	**7** Via Natural or Artificial Opening **8** Via Natural or Artificial Opening Endoscopic	**0** Drainage Device **2** Monitoring Device **3** Infusion Device **7** Autologous Tissue Substitute **C** Extraluminal Device **D** Intraluminal Device **J** Synthetic Substitute **K** Nonautologous Tissue Substitute **U** Feeding Device **Y** Other Device	**Z** No Qualifier
6 Stomach	**X** External	**0** Drainage Device **2** Monitoring Device **3** Infusion Device **7** Autologous Tissue Substitute **C** Extraluminal Device **D** Intraluminal Device **J** Synthetic Substitute **K** Nonautologous Tissue Substitute **U** Feeding Device	**Z** No Qualifier
8 Small Intestine **E** Large Intestine	**0** Open **4** Percutaneous Endoscopic **7** Via Natural or Artificial Opening **8** Via Natural or Artificial Opening Endoscopic	**7** Autologous Tissue Substitute **J** Synthetic Substitute **K** Nonautologous Tissue Substitute	**Z** No Qualifier
Q Anus	**0** Open **3** Percutaneous **4** Percutaneous Endoscopic **7** Via Natural or Artificial Opening **8** Via Natural or Artificial Opening Endoscopic	**L** Artificial Sphincter	**Z** No Qualifier
R Anal Sphincter	**0** Open **3** Percutaneous **4** Percutaneous Endoscopic	**M** Stimulator Lead	**Z** No Qualifier
U Omentum **V** Mesentery **W** Peritoneum	**0** Open **3** Percutaneous **4** Percutaneous Endoscopic	**0** Drainage Device **7** Autologous Tissue Substitute **J** Synthetic Substitute **K** Nonautologous Tissue Substitute	**Z** No Qualifier

ction 0 **Medical and Surgical**
dy System D **Gastrointestinal System**
eration X **Transfer:** Moving, without taking out, all or a portion of a body part to another location to take over the function of all or a portion of a body part

Body Part (4th)	Approach (5th)	Device (6th)	Qualifier (7th)
Stomach Small Intestine Large Intestine	**0** Open **4** Percutaneous Endoscopic	**Z** No Device	**5** Esophagus

ction 0 **Medical and Surgical**
dy System D **Gastrointestinal System**
eration Y **Transplantation:** Putting in or on all or a portion of a living body part taken from another individual or animal to physically take the place and/or function of all or a portion of a similar body part

Body Part (4th)	Approach (5th)	Device (6th)	Qualifier (7th)
Esophagus Stomach Small Intestine Large Intestine	**0** Open	**Z** No Device	**0** Allogeneic **1** Syngeneic **2** Zooplastic

HA Coding Clinic

D160ZA Bypass Stomach to Jejunum, Open Approach— AHA CC: 2Q, 2017, 17-18
D194ZB Bypass Duodenum to Ileum, Percutaneous Endoscopic Approach—AHA CC: 2Q, 2016, 31
D1N0Z4 Bypass Sigmoid Colon to Cutaneous, Open Approach—AHA CC: 4Q, 2014, 41-42
D5W0ZZ Destruction of Peritoneum, Open Approach—AHA CC: 1Q, 2017, 34-35
D768ZZ Dilation of Stomach, Via Natural or Artificial Opening Endoscopic—AHA CC: 4Q, 2014, 40
D7A8ZZ Dilation of Jejunum, Via Natural or Artificial Opening Endoscopic—AHA CC: 4Q, 2014, 40
D844ZZ Division of Esophagogastric Junction, Percutaneous Endoscopic Approach—AHA CC: 3Q, 2017, 22-23
D874ZZ Division of Stomach, Pylorus, Percutaneous Endoscopic Approach—AHA CC: 3Q, 2017, 23-24
D9670Z Drainage of Stomach with Drainage Device, Via Natural or Artificial Opening—AHA CC: 2Q, 2015, 29
DB28ZX Excision of Middle Esophagus, Via Natural or Artificial Opening Endoscopic, Diagnostic—AHA CC: 1Q, 2016, 24-25
DB60ZZ Excision of Stomach, Open Approach—AHA CC: 2Q, 2017, 17-18
DB64Z3 Excision of Stomach, Percutaneous Endoscopic Approach, Vertical—AHA CC: 2Q, 2016, 31
DB90ZZ Excision of Duodenum, Open Approach—AHA CC: 3Q, 2014, 32-33
DBB0ZZ Excision of Ileum, Open Approach—AHA CC: 3Q, 2014, 28-29; 3Q, 2016, 5-6
DBK8ZZ Excision of Ascending Colon, Via Natural or Artificial Opening Endoscopic—AHA CC: 1Q, 2017, 16
DBN0ZZ Excision of Sigmoid Colon, Open Approach—AHA CC: 4Q, 2014, 40-41
DBP7ZZ Excision of Rectum, Via Natural or Artificial Opening—AHA CC: 1Q, 2016, 22
DD68ZX Extraction of Stomach, Via Natural or Artificial Opening Endoscopic, Diagnostic—AHA CC: 4Q, 2017, 42
DH63UZ Insertion of Feeding Device into Stomach, Percutaneous Approach—AHA CC: 4Q, 2013, 117
DH67UZ Insertion of Feeding Device into Stomach, Via Natural or Artificial Opening—AHA CC: 3Q, 2016, 26-27
DJ07ZZ Inspection of Upper Intestinal Tract, Via Natural or Artificial Opening—AHA CC: 2Q, 2016, 20-21
DJ08ZZ Inspection of Upper Intestinal Tract, Via Natural or Artificial Opening Endoscopic—AHA CC: 3Q, 2015, 24-25
DJD8ZZ Inspection of Lower Intestinal Tract, Via Natural or Artificial Opening Endoscopic—AHA CC: 2Q, 2017, 15-16
DN50ZZ Release Esophagus, Open Approach—AHA CC: 3Q, 2015, 15-16
DN80ZZ Release Small Intestine, Open Approach—AHA CC: 4Q, 2017, 49-50
DNW0ZZ Release Peritoneum, Open Approach—AHA CC: 1Q, 2017, 35
DQ98ZZ Repair Duodenum, Via Natural or Artificial Opening Endoscopic—AHA CC: 4Q, 2014, 20
DQP0ZZ Repair Rectum, Open Approach—AHA CC: 1Q, 2016, 7-8
DQR0ZZ Repair Anal Sphincter, Open Approach—AHA CC: 1Q, 2016, 7-8
DQV4ZZ Repair Mesentery, Percutaneous Endoscopic Approach— AHA CC: 1Q, 2018, 11-12

0DS80ZZ Reposition Small Intestine, Open Approach—AHA CC: 4Q, 2017, 49-50

0DSB7ZZ Reposition Ileum, Via Natural or Artificial Opening—AHA CC: 3Q, 2017, 9-10

0DSE0ZZ Reposition Large Intestine, Open Approach—AHA CC: 4Q, 2017, 49-50

0DSK7ZZ Reposition Ascending Colon, Via Natural or Artificial Opening—AHA CC: 3Q, 2017, 9-10

0DSM4ZZ Reposition Descending Colon, Percutaneous Endoscopic Approach—AHA CC: 3Q, 2016, 5-6

0DSP0ZZ Reposition Rectum, Open Approach—AHA CC: 3Q, 2017, 17-18

0DTF0ZZ Resection of Right Large Intestine, Open Approach—AHA CC: 3Q, 2014, 6-7; 4Q, 2014, 42-43

0DTH0ZZ Resection of Cecum, Open Approach—AHA CC: 3Q, 2014, 6

0DTJ0ZZ Resection of Appendix, Open Approach—AHA CC: 4Q, 2017, 49-50

0DTP0ZZ Resection of Rectum, Open Approach—AHA CC: 4Q, 2014, 40-41

0DTQ0ZZ Resection of Anus, Open Approach—AHA CC: 4Q, 2014, 40-41

0DV40ZZ Restriction of Esophagogastric Junction, Open Approach—AHA CC: 2Q, 2016, 22-23

0DV44ZZ Restriction of Esophagogastric Junction, Percutaneous Endoscopic Approach—AHA CC: 3Q, 2014, 28; 3Q, 2017, 22-23

0DW63CZ Revision of Extraluminal Device in Stomach, Percutaneous Approach—AHA CC: 1Q, 2018, 20

0DX60Z5 Transfer Stomach to Esophagus, Open Approach—AHA CC: 2Q, 2016, 22-23; 2Q, 2017, 18

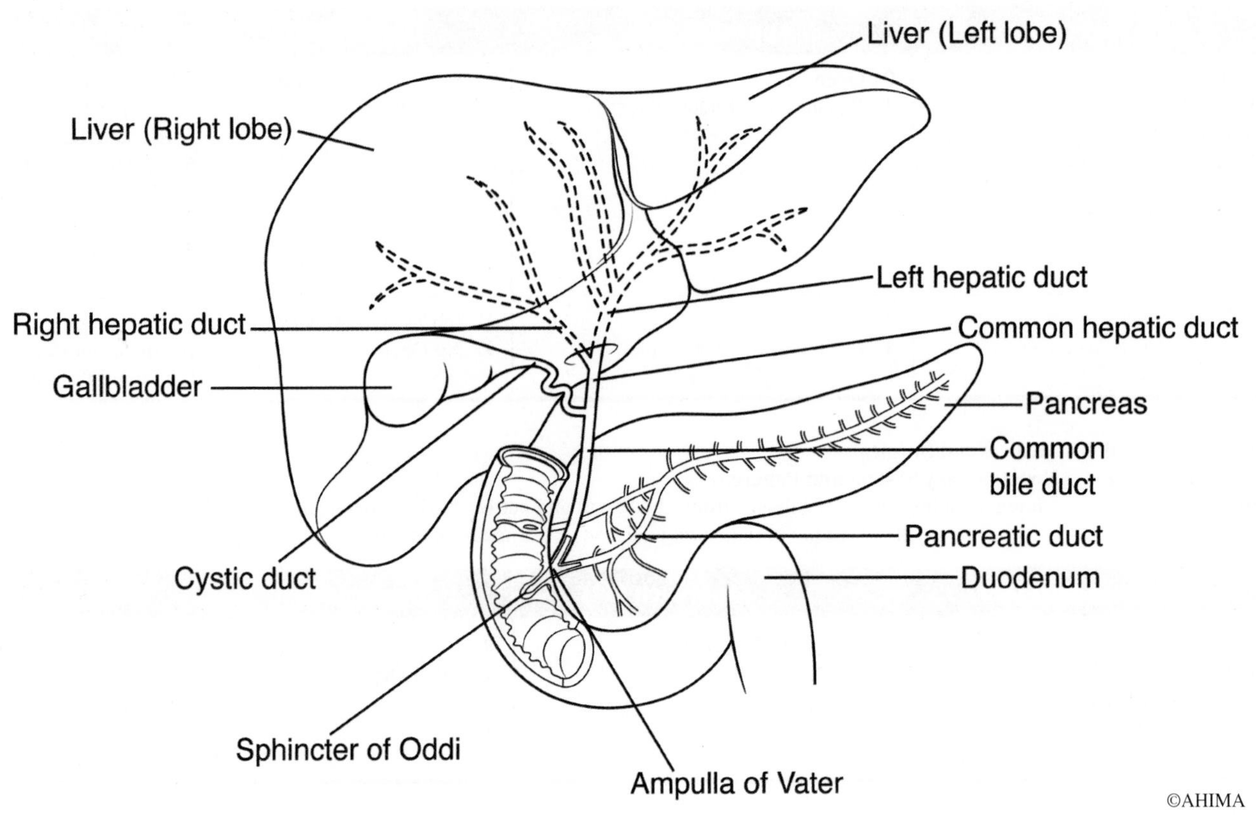
Hepatobiliary System and Pancreas
Liver (Left lobe)
Liver (Right lobe)
Left hepatic duct
Right hepatic duct
Common hepatic duct
Gallbladder
Pancreas
Common bile duct
Pancreatic duct
Cystic duct
Duodenum
Sphincter of Oddi
Ampulla of Vater
©AHIMA

Hepatobiliary System and Pancreas Tables 0F1–0FY

Section **0** **Medical and Surgical**
Body System **F** **Hepatobiliary System and Pancreas**
Operation **1** **Bypass:** Altering the route of passage of the contents of a tubular body part

Body Part (4th)	Approach (5th)	Device (6th)	Qualifier (7th)
4 Gallbladder **5** Hepatic Duct, Right **6** Hepatic Duct, Left **7** Hepatic Duct, Common **8** Cystic Duct **9** Common Bile Duct	**0** Open **4** Percutaneous Endoscopic	**D** Intraluminal Device **Z** No Device	**3** Duodenum **4** Stomach **5** Hepatic Duct, Right **6** Hepatic Duct, Left **7** Hepatic Duct, Caudate **8** Cystic Duct **9** Common Bile Duct **B** Small Intestine
D Pancreatic Duct **F** Pancreatic Duct, Accessory **G** Pancreas	**0** Open **4** Percutaneous Endoscopic	**D** Intraluminal Device **Z** No Device	**3** Duodenum **B** Small Intestine **C** Large Intestine

Section **0** **Medical and Surgical**
Body System **F** **Hepatobiliary System and Pancreas**
Operation **2** **Change:** Taking out or off a device from a body part and putting back an identical or similar device in or on the same bc part without cutting or puncturing the skin or a mucous membrane

Body Part (4th)	Approach (5th)	Device (6th)	Qualifier (7th)
0 Liver **4** Gallbladder **B** Hepatobiliary Duct **D** Pancreatic Duct **G** Pancreas	**X** External	**0** Drainage Device **Y** Other Device	**Z** No Qualifier

Section **0** **Medical and Surgical**
Body System **F** **Hepatobiliary System and Pancreas**
Operation **5** **Destruction:** Physical eradication of all or a portion of a body part by the direct use of energy, force, or a destructive age

Body Part (4th)	Approach (5th)	Device (6th)	Qualifier (7th)
0 Liver **1** Liver, Right Lobe **2** Liver, Left Lobe	**0** Open **3** Percutaneous **4** Percutaneous Endoscopic	**Z** No Device	**F** Irreversible Electroporation **Z** No Qualifier
4 Gallbladder	**0** Open **3** Percutaneous **4** Percutaneous Endoscopic **8** Via Natural or Artificial Opening Endoscopic	**Z** No Device	**Z** No Qualifier
5 Hepatic Duct, Right **6** Hepatic Duct, Left **7** Hepatic Duct, Common **8** Cystic Duct **9** Common Bile Duct **C** Ampulla of Vater **D** Pancreatic Duct **F** Pancreatic Duct, Accessory	**0** Open **3** Percutaneous **4** Percutaneous Endoscopic **7** Via Natural or Artificial Opening **8** Via Natural or Artificial Opening Endoscopic	**Z** No Device	**Z** No Qualifier
G Pancreas	**0** Open **3** Percutaneous **4** Percutaneous Endoscopic	**Z** No Device	**F** Irreversible Electroporation **Z** No Qualifier
G Pancreas	**8** Via Natural or Artificial Opening Endoscopic	**Z** No Device	**Z** No Qualifier

tion	**0**	**Medical and Surgical**
ly System	**F**	**Hepatobiliary System and Pancreas**
eration	**7**	**Dilation:** Expanding an orifice or the lumen of a tubular body part

Body Part (4th)	Approach (5th)	Device (6th)	Qualifier (7th)
Hepatic Duct, Right Hepatic Duct, Left Hepatic Duct, Common Cystic Duct Common Bile Duct Ampulla of Vater Pancreatic Duct Pancreatic Duct, Accessory	**0** Open **3** Percutaneous **4** Percutaneous Endoscopic **7** Via Natural or Artificial Opening **8** Via Natural or Artificial Opening Endoscopic	**D** Intraluminal Device **Z** No Device	**Z** No Qualifier

tion	**0**	**Medical and Surgical**
dy System	**F**	**Hepatobiliary System and Pancreas**
eration	**8**	**Division:** Cutting into a body part, without draining fluids and/or gases from the body part, in order to separate or transect a body part

Body Part (4th)	Approach (5th)	Device (6th)	Qualifier (7th)
Pancreas	**0** Open **3** Percutaneous **4** Percutaneous Endoscopic	**Z** No Device	**Z** No Qualifier

tion	**0**	**Medical and Surgical**
dy System	**F**	**Hepatobiliary System and Pancreas**
eration	**9**	**Drainage:** Taking or letting out fluids and/or gases from a body part

Body Part (4th)	Approach (5th)	Device (6th)	Qualifier (7th)
Liver Liver, Right Lobe Liver, Left Lobe	**0** Open **3** Percutaneous **4** Percutaneous Endoscopic	**0** Drainage Device	**Z** No Qualifier
Liver Liver, Right Lobe Liver, Left Lobe	**0** Open **3** Percutaneous **4** Percutaneous Endoscopic	**Z** No Device	**X** Diagnostic **Z** No Qualifier
Gallbladder Pancreas	**0** Open **3** Percutaneous **4** Percutaneous Endoscopic **8** Via Natural or Artificial Opening Endoscopic	**0** Drainage Device	**Z** No Qualifier
Gallbladder Pancreas	**0** Open **3** Percutaneous **4** Percutaneous Endoscopic **8** Via Natural or Artificial Opening Endoscopic	**Z** No Device	**X** Diagnostic **Z** No Qualifier
Hepatic Duct, Right Hepatic Duct, Left Hepatic Duct, Common Cystic Duct Common Bile Duct Ampulla of Vater Pancreatic Duct Pancreatic Duct, Accessory	**0** Open **3** Percutaneous **4** Percutaneous Endoscopic **7** Via Natural or Artificial Opening **8** Via Natural or Artificial Opening Endoscopic	**0** Drainage Device	**Z** No Qualifier
Hepatic Duct, Right Hepatic Duct, Left Hepatic Duct, Common Cystic Duct Common Bile Duct Ampulla of Vater Pancreatic Duct Pancreatic Duct, Accessory	**0** Open **3** Percutaneous **4** Percutaneous Endoscopic **7** Via Natural or Artificial Opening **8** Via Natural or Artificial Opening Endoscopic	**Z** No Device	**X** Diagnostic **Z** No Qualifier

Section 0 **Medical and Surgical**
Body System F **Hepatobiliary System and Pancreas**
Operation B **Excision:** Cutting out or off, without replacement, a portion of a body part

Body Part (4th)	Approach (5th)	Device (6th)	Qualifier (7th)
0 Liver **1** Liver, Right Lobe **2** Liver, Left Lobe	**0** Open **3** Percutaneous **4** Percutaneous Endoscopic	**Z** No Device	**X** Diagnostic **Z** No Qualifier
4 Gallbladder **G** Pancreas	**0** Open **3** Percutaneous **4** Percutaneous Endoscopic **8** Via Natural or Artificial Opening Endoscopic	**Z** No Device	**X** Diagnostic **Z** No Qualifier
5 Hepatic Duct, Right **6** Hepatic Duct, Left **7** Hepatic Duct, Common **8** Cystic Duct **9** Common Bile Duct **C** Ampulla of Vater **D** Pancreatic Duct **F** Pancreatic Duct, Accessory	**0** Open **3** Percutaneous **4** Percutaneous Endoscopic **7** Via Natural or Artificial Opening **8** Via Natural or Artificial Opening Endoscopic	**Z** No Device	**X** Diagnostic **Z** No Qualifier

Section 0 **Medical and Surgical**
Body System F **Hepatobiliary System and Pancreas**
Operation C **Extirpation:** Taking or cutting out solid matter from a body part

Body Part (4th)	Approach (5th)	Device (6th)	Qualifier (7th)
0 Liver **1** Liver, Right Lobe **2** Liver, Left Lobe	**0** Open **3** Percutaneous **4** Percutaneous Endoscopic	**Z** No Device	**Z** No Qualifier
4 Gallbladder **G** Pancreas	**0** Open **3** Percutaneous **4** Percutaneous Endoscopic **8** Via Natural or Artificial Opening Endoscopic	**Z** No Device	**Z** No Qualifier
5 Hepatic Duct, Right **6** Hepatic Duct, Left **7** Hepatic Duct, Common **8** Cystic Duct **9** Common Bile Duct **C** Ampulla of Vater **D** Pancreatic Duct **F** Pancreatic Duct, Accessory	**0** Open **3** Percutaneous **4** Percutaneous Endoscopic **7** Via Natural or Artificial Opening **8** Via Natural or Artificial Opening Endoscopic	**Z** No Device	**Z** No Qualifier

Section 0 **Medical and Surgical**
Body System F **Hepatobiliary System and Pancreas**
Operation D **Extraction:** Pulling or stripping out or off all or a portion of a body part by the use of force

Body Part (4th)	Approach (5th)	Device (6th)	Qualifier (7th)
0 Liver **1** Liver, Right Lobe **2** Liver, Left Lobe	**3** Percutaneous **4** Percutaneous Endoscopic	**Z** No Device	**X** Diagnostic
4 Gallbladder **5** Hepatic Duct, Right **6** Hepatic Duct, Left **7** Hepatic Duct, Common **8** Cystic Duct **9** Common Bile Duct **C** Ampulla of Vater **D** Pancreatic Duct **F** Pancreatic Duct, Accessory **G** Pancreas	**3** Percutaneous **4** Percutaneous Endoscopic **8** Via Natural or Artificial Opening Endoscopic	**Z** No Device	**X** Diagnostic

tion	**0**	**Medical and Surgical**
dy System	**F**	**Hepatobiliary System and Pancreas**
eration	**F**	**Fragmentation:** Breaking solid matter in a body part into pieces

Body Part (4th)	Approach (5th)	Device (6th)	Qualifier (7th)
Gallbladder Hepatic Duct, Right Hepatic Duct, Left Hepatic Duct, Common Cystic Duct Common Bile Duct Ampulla of Vater Pancreatic Duct Pancreatic Duct, Accessory	**0** Open **3** Percutaneous **4** Percutaneous Endoscopic **7** Via Natural or Artificial Opening **8** Via Natural or Artificial Opening Endoscopic **X** External	**Z** No Device	**Z** No Qualifier

tion	**0**	**Medical and Surgical**
dy System	**F**	**Hepatobiliary System and Pancreas**
eration	**H**	**Insertion:** Putting in a nonbiological appliance that monitors, assists, performs, or prevents a physiological function but does not physically take the place of a body part

Body Part (4th)	Approach (5th)	Device (6th)	Qualifier (7th)
Liver Gallbladder Pancreas	**0** Open **3** Percutaneous **4** Percutaneous Endoscopic	**2** Monitoring Device **3** Infusion Device **Y** Other Device	**Z** No Qualifier
Liver, Right Lobe Liver, Left Lobe	**0** Open **3** Percutaneous **4** Percutaneous Endoscopic	**2** Monitoring Device **3** Infusion Device	**Z** No Qualifier
Hepatobiliary Duct Pancreatic Duct	**0** Open **3** Percutaneous **4** Percutaneous Endoscopic **7** Via Natural or Artificial Opening **8** Via Natural or Artificial Opening Endoscopic	**1** Radioactive Element **2** Monitoring Device **3** Infusion Device **D** Intraluminal Device **Y** Other Device	**Z** No Qualifier

ction	**0**	**Medical and Surgical**
dy System	**F**	**Hepatobiliary System and Pancreas**
eration	**J**	**Inspection:** Visually and/or manually exploring a body part

Body Part (4th)	Approach (5th)	Device (6th)	Qualifier (7th)
Liver	**0** Open **3** Percutaneous **4** Percutaneous Endoscopic **X** External	**Z** No Device	**Z** No Qualifier
Gallbladder Pancreas	**0** Open **3** Percutaneous **4** Percutaneous Endoscopic **8** Via Natural or Artificial Opening Endoscopic **X** External	**Z** No Device	**Z** No Qualifier
B Hepatobiliary Duct **D** Pancreatic Duct	**0** Open **3** Percutaneous **4** Percutaneous Endoscopic **7** Via Natural or Artificial Opening **8** Via Natural or Artificial Opening Endoscopic	**Z** No Device	**Z** No Qualifier

Section 0 **Medical and Surgical**
Body System F **Hepatobiliary System and Pancreas**
Operation L **Occlusion:** Completely closing an orifice or the lumen of a tubular body part

Body Part (4th)	Approach (5th)	Device (6th)	Qualifier (7th)
5 Hepatic Duct, Right **6** Hepatic Duct, Left **7** Hepatic Duct, Common **8** Cystic Duct **9** Common Bile Duct **C** Ampulla of Vater **D** Pancreatic Duct **F** Pancreatic Duct, Accessory	**0** Open **3** Percutaneous **4** Percutaneous Endoscopic	**C** Extraluminal Device **D** Intraluminal Device **Z** No Device	**Z** No Qualifier
5 Hepatic Duct, Right **6** Hepatic Duct, Left **7** Hepatic Duct, Common **8** Cystic Duct **9** Common Bile Duct **C** Ampulla of Vater **D** Pancreatic Duct **F** Pancreatic Duct, Accessory	**7** Via Natural or Artificial Opening **8** Via Natural or Artificial Opening Endoscopic	**D** Intraluminal Device **Z** No Device	**Z** No Qualifier

Section 0 **Medical and Surgical**
Body System F **Hepatobiliary System and Pancreas**
Operation M **Reattachment:** Putting back in or on all or a portion of a separated body part to its normal location or other suitable location

Body Part (4th)	Approach (5th)	Device (6th)	Qualifier (7th)
0 Liver **1** Liver, Right Lobe **2** Liver, Left Lobe **4** Gallbladder **5** Hepatic Duct, Right **6** Hepatic Duct, Left **7** Hepatic Duct, Common **8** Cystic Duct **9** Common Bile Duct **C** Ampulla of Vater **D** Pancreatic Duct **F** Pancreatic Duct, Accessory **G** Pancreas	**0** Open **4** Percutaneous Endoscopic	**Z** No Device	**Z** No Qualifier

Section 0 **Medical and Surgical**
Body System F **Hepatobiliary System and Pancreas**
Operation N **Release:** Freeing a body part from an abnormal physical constraint by cutting or by the use of force

Body Part (4th)	Approach (5th)	Device (6th)	Qualifier (7th)
0 Liver **1** Liver, Right Lobe **2** Liver, Left Lobe	**0** Open **3** Percutaneous **4** Percutaneous Endoscopic	**Z** No Device	**Z** No Qualifier
4 Gallbladder **G** Pancreas	**0** Open **3** Percutaneous **4** Percutaneous Endoscopic **8** Via Natural or Artificial Opening Endoscopic	**Z** No Device	**Z** No Qualifier
5 Hepatic Duct, Right **6** Hepatic Duct, Left **7** Hepatic Duct, Common **8** Cystic Duct **9** Common Bile Duct **C** Ampulla of Vater **D** Pancreatic Duct **F** Pancreatic Duct, Accessory	**0** Open **3** Percutaneous **4** Percutaneous Endoscopic **7** Via Natural or Artificial Opening **8** Via Natural or Artificial Opening Endoscopic	**Z** No Device	**Z** No Qualifier

tion	**0**	**Medical and Surgical**
dy System	**F**	**Hepatobiliary System and Pancreas**
eration	**P**	**Removal:** Taking out or off a device from a body part

Body Part (4th)	Approach (5th)	Device (6th)	Qualifier (7th)
Liver	**0** Open **3** Percutaneous **4** Percutaneous Endoscopic	**0** Drainage Device **2** Monitoring Device **3** Infusion Device **Y** Other Device	**Z** No Qualifier
Liver	**X** External	**0** Drainage Device **2** Monitoring Device **3** Infusion Device	**Z** No Qualifier
4 Gallbladder **G** Pancreas	**0** Open **3** Percutaneous **4** Percutaneous Endoscopic **X** External	**0** Drainage Device **2** Monitoring Device **3** Infusion Device **D** Intraluminal Device **Y** Other Device	**Z** No Qualifier
4 Gallbladder **G** Pancreas	**X** External	**0** Drainage Device **2** Monitoring Device **3** Infusion Device **D** Intraluminal Device	**Z** No Qualifier
B Hepatobiliary Duct **D** Pancreatic Duct	**0** Open **3** Percutaneous **4** Percutaneous Endoscopic **7** Via Natural or Artificial Opening **8** Via Natural or Artificial Opening Endoscopic	**0** Drainage Device **1** Radioactive Element **2** Monitoring Device **3** Infusion Device **7** Autologous Tissue Substitute **C** Extraluminal Device **D** Intraluminal Device **J** Synthetic Substitute **K** Nonautologous Tissue Substitute **Y** Other Device	**Z** No Qualifier
B Hepatobiliary Duct **D** Pancreatic Duct	**X** External	**0** Drainage Device **1** Radioactive Element **2** Monitoring Device **3** Infusion Device **D** Intraluminal Device	**Z** No Qualifier

ction	**0**	**Medical and Surgical**
dy System	**F**	**Hepatobiliary System and Pancreas**
eration	**Q**	**Repair:** Restoring, to the extent possible, a body part to its normal anatomic structure and function

Body Part (4th)	Approach (5th)	Device (6th)	Qualifier (7th)
0 Liver **1** Liver, Right Lobe **2** Liver, Left Lobe	**0** Open **3** Percutaneous **4** Percutaneous Endoscopic	**Z** No Device	**Z** No Qualifier
4 Gallbladder **G** Pancreas	**0** Open **3** Percutaneous **4** Percutaneous Endoscopic **8** Via Natural or Artificial Opening Endoscopic	**Z** No Device	**Z** No Qualifier
5 Hepatic Duct, Right **6** Hepatic Duct, Left **7** Hepatic Duct, Common **8** Cystic Duct **9** Common Bile Duct **C** Ampulla of Vater **D** Pancreatic Duct **F** Pancreatic Duct, Accessory	**0** Open **3** Percutaneous **4** Percutaneous Endoscopic **7** Via Natural or Artificial Opening **8** Via Natural or Artificial Opening Endoscopic	**Z** No Device	**Z** No Qualifier

Section 0 **Medical and Surgical**
Body System F **Hepatobiliary System and Pancreas**
Operation R **Replacement:** Putting in or on biological or synthetic material that physically takes the place and/or function of all or a portion of a body part

Body Part (4th)	Approach (5th)	Device (6th)	Qualifier (7th)
5 Hepatic Duct, Right **6** Hepatic Duct, Left **7** Hepatic Duct, Common **8** Cystic Duct **9** Common Bile Duct **C** Ampulla of Vater **D** Pancreatic Duct **F** Pancreatic Duct, Accessory	**0** Open **4** Percutaneous Endoscopic **8** Via Natural or Artificial Opening Endoscopic	**7** Autologous Tissue Substitute **J** Synthetic Substitute **K** Nonautologous Tissue Substitute	**Z** No Qualifier

Section 0 **Medical and Surgical**
Body System F **Hepatobiliary System and Pancreas**
Operation S **Reposition:** Moving to its normal location, or other suitable location, all or a portion of a body part

Body Part (4th)	Approach (5th)	Device (6th)	Qualifier (7th)
0 Liver **4** Gallbladder **5** Hepatic Duct, Right **6** Hepatic Duct, Left **7** Hepatic Duct, Common **8** Cystic Duct **9** Common Bile Duct **C** Ampulla of Vater **D** Pancreatic Duct **F** Pancreatic Duct, Accessory **G** Pancreas	**0** Open **4** Percutaneous Endoscopic	**Z** No Device	**Z** No Qualifier

Section 0 **Medical and Surgical**
Body System F **Hepatobiliary System and Pancreas**
Operation T **Resection:** Cutting out or off, without replacement, all of a body part

Body Part (4th)	Approach (5th)	Device (6th)	Qualifier (7th)
0 Liver **1** Liver, Right Lobe **2** Liver, Left Lobe **4** Gallbladder **G** Pancreas	**0** Open **4** Percutaneous Endoscopic	**Z** No Device	**Z** No Qualifier
5 Hepatic Duct, Right **6** Hepatic Duct, Left **7** Hepatic Duct, Common **8** Cystic Duct **9** Common Bile Duct **C** Ampulla of Vater **D** Pancreatic Duct **F** Pancreatic Duct, Accessory	**0** Open **4** Percutaneous Endoscopic **7** Via Natural or Artificial Opening **8** Via Natural or Artificial Opening Endoscopic	**Z** No Device	**Z** No Qualifier

tion **0** **Medical and Surgical**
dy System **F** **Hepatobiliary System and Pancreas**
eration **U** **Supplement:** Putting in or on biological or synthetic material that physically reinforces and/or augments the function of a portion of a body part

Body Part (4th)	Approach (5th)	Device (6th)	Qualifier (7th)
Hepatic Duct, Right Hepatic Duct, Left Hepatic Duct, Common Cystic Duct Common Bile Duct Ampulla of Vater Pancreatic Duct Pancreatic Duct, Accessory	**0** Open **3** Percutaneous **4** Percutaneous Endoscopic **8** Via Natural or Artificial Opening Endoscopic	**7** Autologous Tissue Substitute **J** Synthetic Substitute **K** Nonautologous Tissue Substitute	**Z** No Qualifier

tion **0** **Medical and Surgical**
dy System **F** **Hepatobiliary System and Pancreas**
eration **V** **Restriction:** Partially closing an orifice or the lumen of a tubular body part

Body Part (4th)	Approach (5th)	Device (6th)	Qualifier (7th)
Hepatic Duct, Right Hepatic Duct, Left Hepatic Duct, Common Cystic Duct Common Bile Duct Ampulla of Vater Pancreatic Duct Pancreatic Duct, Accessory	**0** Open **3** Percutaneous **4** Percutaneous Endoscopic	**C** Extraluminal Device **D** Intraluminal Device **Z** No Device	**Z** No Qualifier
Hepatic Duct, Right Hepatic Duct, Left Hepatic Duct, Common Cystic Duct Common Bile Duct Ampulla of Vater Pancreatic Duct Pancreatic Duct, Accessory	**7** Via Natural or Artificial Opening **8** Via Natural or Artificial Opening Endoscopic	**D** Intraluminal Device **Z** No Device	**Z** No Qualifier

ction **0** **Medical and Surgical**
dy System **F** **Hepatobiliary System and Pancreas**
eration **W** **Revision:** Correcting, to the extent possible, a portion of a malfunctioning device or the position of a displaced device

Body Part (4th)	Approach (5th)	Device (6th)	Qualifier (7th)
Liver	**0** Open **3** Percutaneous **4** Percutaneous Endoscopic	**0** Drainage Device **2** Monitoring Device **3** Infusion Device **Y** Other Device	**Z** No Qualifier
Liver	**X** External	**0** Drainage Device **2** Monitoring Device **3** Infusion Device	**Z** No Qualifier
4 Gallbladder **G** Pancreas	**0** Open **3** Percutaneous **4** Percutaneous Endoscopic	**0** Drainage Device **2** Monitoring Device **3** Infusion Device **D** Intraluminal Device **Y** Other Device	**Z** No Qualifier
4 Gallbladder **G** Pancreas	**X** External	**0** Drainage Device **2** Monitoring Device **3** Infusion Device **D** Intraluminal Device	**Z** No Qualifier

Continued →

0FW Contin

Section 0 **Medical and Surgical**
Body System F **Hepatobiliary System and Pancreas**
Operation W **Revision:** Correcting, to the extent possible, a portion of a malfunctioning device or the position of a displaced device

Body Part (4th)	Approach (5th)	Device (6th)	Qualifier (7th)
B Hepatobiliary Duct **D** Pancreatic Duct	**0** Open **3** Percutaneous **4** Percutaneous Endoscopic **7** Via Natural or Artificial Opening **8** Via Natural or Artificial Opening Endoscopic	**0** Drainage Device **2** Monitoring Device **3** Infusion Device **7** Autologous Tissue Substitute **C** Extraluminal Device **D** Intraluminal Device **J** Synthetic Substitute **K** Nonautologous Tissue Substitute **Y** Other Device	**Z** No Qualifier
B Hepatobiliary Duct **D** Pancreatic Duct	**X** External	**0** Drainage Device **2** Monitoring Device **3** Infusion Device **7** Autologous Tissue Substitute **C** Extraluminal Device **D** Intraluminal Device **J** Synthetic Substitute **K** Nonautologous Tissue Substitute	**Z** No Qualifier

Section 0 **Medical and Surgical**
Body System F **Hepatobiliary System and Pancreas**
Operation Y **Transplantation:** Putting in or on all or a portion of a living body part taken from another individual or animal to physically take the place and/or function of all or a portion of a similar body part

Body Part (4th)	Approach (5th)	Device (6th)	Qualifier (7th)
0 Liver **G** Pancreas	**0** Open	**Z** No Device	**0** Allogeneic **1** Syngeneic **2** Zooplastic

AHA Coding Clinic

0F798DZ Dilation of Common Bile Duct with Intraluminal Device, Via Natural or Artificial Opening Endoscopic—AHA CC: 3Q, 20 15-16; 1Q, 2016, 25

0F7D8DZ Dilation of Pancreatic Duct with Intraluminal Device, Via Natural or Artificial Opening Endoscopic—AHA CC: 1Q, 2016, 3Q, 2016, 27-28

0F9630Z Drainage of Left Hepatic Duct with Drainage Device, Percutaneous Approach—AHA CC: 1Q, 2015, 32

0F9G40Z Drainage of Pancreas with Drainage Device, Percutaneous Endoscopic Approach AHA CC: 3Q, 2014, 15-16

0FB00ZX Excision of Liver, Open Approach, Diagnostic—AHA CC: 3Q, 2016, 41

0FB98ZX Excision of Common Bile Duct, Via Natural or Artificial Opening Endoscopic, Diagnostic—AHA CC: 1Q, 2016, 23-25

0FBD8ZX Excision of Pancreatic Duct, Via Natural or Artificial Opening Endoscopic, Diagnostic—AHA CC: 1Q, 2016, 25

0FBG0ZZ Excision of Pancreas, Open Approach—AHA CC: 3Q, 2014, 32-33

0FQ00ZZ Repair Liver, Open Approach—AHA CC: 4Q, 2013, 109-111

0FQ90ZZ Repair Common Bile Duct, Open Approach—AHA CC: 3Q, 2016, 27

0FT00ZZ Resection of Liver, Open Approach—AHA CC: 4Q, 2012, 99-101

0FY00Z0 Transplantation of Liver, Allogeneic, Open Approach—AHA CC: 4Q, 2012, 99-101; 3Q, 2014, 13-14

Endocrine System

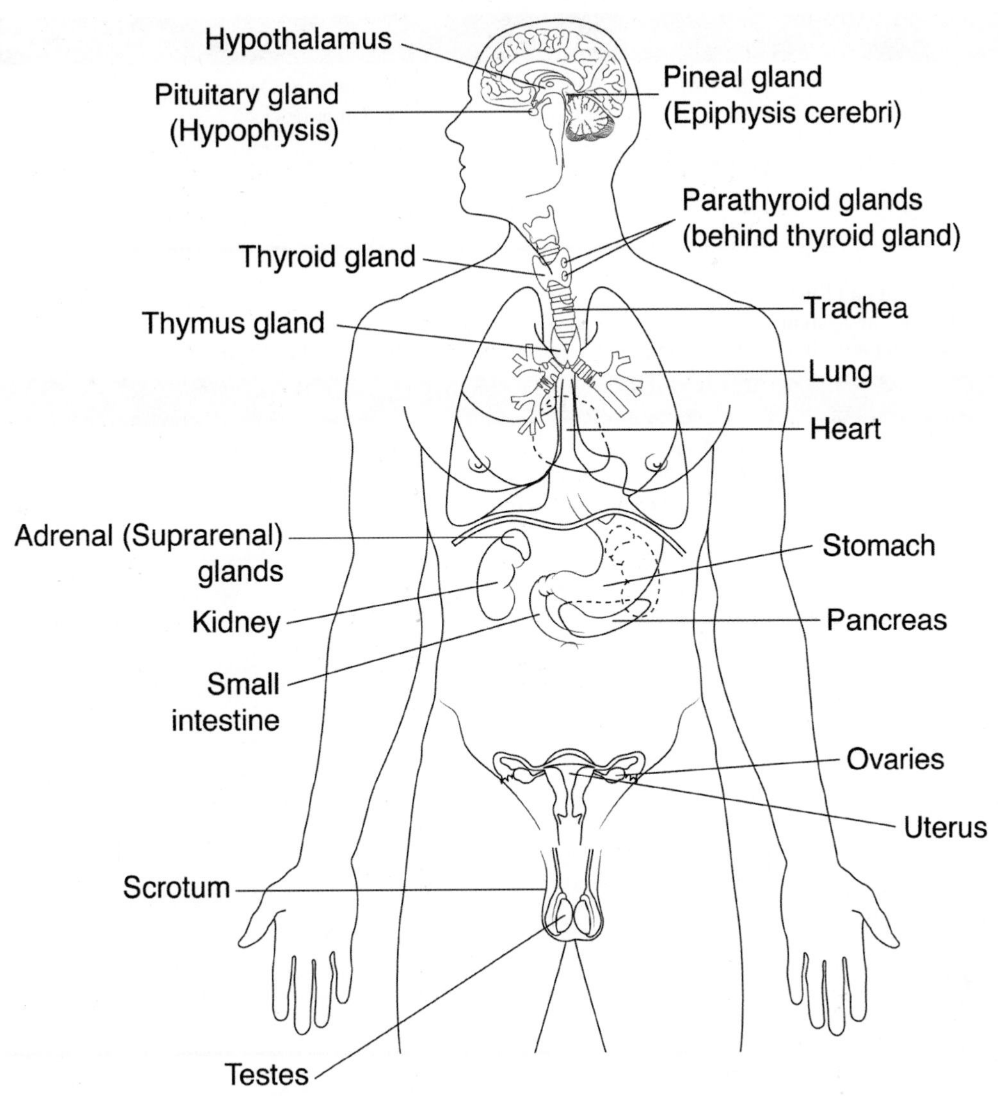

Endocrine System Tables 0G2–0GW

Section 0 **Medical and Surgical**
Body System G **Endocrine System**
Operation 2 **Change:** Taking out or off a device from a body part and putting back an identical or similar device in or on the same b part without cutting or puncturing the skin or a mucous membrane

Body Part (4th)	Approach (5th)	Device (6th)	Qualifier (7th)
0 Pituitary Gland **1** Pineal Body **5** Adrenal Gland **K** Thyroid Gland **R** Parathyroid Gland **S** Endocrine Gland	**X** External	**0** Drainage Device **Y** Other Device	**Z** No Qualifier

Section 0 **Medical and Surgical**
Body System G **Endocrine System**
Operation 5 **Destruction:** Physical eradication of all or a portion of a body part by the direct use of energy, force, or a destructive ag

Body Part (4th)	Approach (5th)	Device (6th)	Qualifier (7th)
0 Pituitary Gland **1** Pineal Body **2** Adrenal Gland, Left **3** Adrenal Gland, Right **4** Adrenal Glands, Bilateral **6** Carotid Body, Left **7** Carotid Body, Right **8** Carotid Bodies, Bilateral **9** Para-aortic Body **B** Coccygeal Glomus **C** Glomus Jugulare **D** Aortic Body **F** Paraganglion Extremity **G** Thyroid Gland Lobe, Left **H** Thyroid Gland Lobe, Right **K** Thyroid Gland **L** Superior Parathyroid Gland, Right **M** Superior Parathyroid Gland, Left **N** Inferior Parathyroid Gland, Right **P** Inferior Parathyroid Gland, Left **Q** Parathyroid Glands, Multiple **R** Parathyroid Gland	**0** Open **3** Percutaneous **4** Percutaneous Endoscopic	**Z** No Device	**Z** No Qualifier

Section 0 **Medical and Surgical**
Body System G **Endocrine System**
Operation 8 **Division:** Cutting into a body part, without draining fluids and/or gases from the body part, in order to separate or transe body part

Body Part (4th)	Approach (5th)	Device (6th)	Qualifier (7th)
0 Pituitary Gland **J** Thyroid Gland Isthmus	**0** Open **3** Percutaneous **4** Percutaneous Endoscopic	**Z** No Device	**Z** No Qualifier

Section 0 **Medical and Surgical**
Body System G **Endocrine System**
Operation 9 **Drainage:** Taking or letting out fluids and/or gases from a body part

Body Part (4th)	Approach (5th)	Device (6th)	Qualifier (7th)
0 Pituitary Gland **1** Pineal Body **2** Adrenal Gland, Left **3** Adrenal Gland, Right **4** Adrenal Glands, Bilateral **6** Carotid Body, Left **7** Carotid Body, Right **8** Carotid Bodies, Bilateral **9** Para-aortic Body **B** Coccygeal Glomus **C** Glomus Jugulare **D** Aortic Body **F** Paraganglion Extremity **G** Thyroid Gland Lobe, Left **H** Thyroid Gland Lobe, Right **K** Thyroid Gland **L** Superior Parathyroid Gland, Right **M** Superior Parathyroid Gland, Left **N** Inferior Parathyroid Gland, Right **P** Inferior Parathyroid Gland, Left **Q** Parathyroid Glands, Multiple **R** Parathyroid Gland	**0** Open **3** Percutaneous **4** Percutaneous Endoscopic	**0** Drainage Device	**Z** No Qualifier
0 Pituitary Gland **1** Pineal Body **2** Adrenal Gland, Left **3** Adrenal Gland, Right **4** Adrenal Glands, Bilateral **6** Carotid Body, Left **7** Carotid Body, Right **8** Carotid Bodies, Bilateral **9** Para-aortic Body **B** Coccygeal Glomus **C** Glomus Jugulare **D** Aortic Body **F** Paraganglion Extremity **G** Thyroid Gland Lobe, Left **H** Thyroid Gland Lobe, Right **K** Thyroid Gland **L** Superior Parathyroid Gland, Right **M** Superior Parathyroid Gland, Left **N** Inferior Parathyroid Gland, Right **P** Inferior Parathyroid Gland, Left **Q** Parathyroid Glands, Multiple **R** Parathyroid Gland	**0** Open **3** Percutaneous **4** Percutaneous Endoscopic	**Z** No Device	**X** Diagnostic **Z** No Qualifier

Section 0 **Medical and Surgical**
Body System G **Endocrine System**
Operation B **Excision:** Cutting out or off, without replacement, a portion of a body part

Body Part (4th)	Approach (5th)	Device (6th)	Qualifier (7th)
0 Pituitary Gland **1** Pineal Body **2** Adrenal Gland, Left **3** Adrenal Gland, Right **4** Adrenal Glands, Bilateral **6** Carotid Body, Left **7** Carotid Body, Right **8** Carotid Bodies, Bilateral **9** Para-aortic Body **B** Coccygeal Glomus **C** Glomus Jugulare **D** Aortic Body **F** Paraganglion Extremity **G** Thyroid Gland Lobe, Left **H** Thyroid Gland Lobe, Right **J** Thyroid Gland Isthmus **L** Superior Parathyroid Gland, Right **M** Superior Parathyroid Gland, Left **N** Inferior Parathyroid Gland, Right **P** Inferior Parathyroid Gland, Left **Q** Parathyroid Glands, Multiple **R** Parathyroid Gland	**0** Open **3** Percutaneous **4** Percutaneous Endoscopic	**Z** No Device	**X** Diagnostic **Z** No Qualifier

Section 0 **Medical and Surgical**
Body System G **Endocrine System**
Operation C **Extirpation:** Taking or cutting out solid matter from a body part

Body Part (4th)	Approach (5th)	Device (6th)	Qualifier (7th)
0 Pituitary Gland **1** Pineal Body **2** Adrenal Gland, Left **3** Adrenal Gland, Right **4** Adrenal Glands, Bilateral **6** Carotid Body, Left **7** Carotid Body, Right **8** Carotid Bodies, Bilateral **9** Para-aortic Body **B** Coccygeal Glomus **C** Glomus Jugulare **D** Aortic Body **F** Paraganglion Extremity **G** Thyroid Gland Lobe, Left **H** Thyroid Gland Lobe, Right **K** Thyroid Gland **L** Superior Parathyroid Gland, Right **M** Superior Parathyroid Gland, Left **N** Inferior Parathyroid Gland, Right **P** Inferior Parathyroid Gland, Left **Q** Parathyroid Glands, Multiple **R** Parathyroid Gland	**0** Open **3** Percutaneous **4** Percutaneous Endoscopic	**Z** No Device	**Z** No Qualifier

Section 0 **Medical and Surgical**
Body System G **Endocrine System**
Operation H **Insertion:** Putting in a nonbiological appliance that monitors, assists, performs, or prevents a physiological function but does not physically take the place of a body part

Body Part (4th)	Approach (5th)	Device (6th)	Qualifier (7th)
S Endocrine Gland	**0** Open **3** Percutaneous **4** Percutaneous Endoscopic	**2** Monitoring Device **3** Infusion Device **Y** Other Device	**Z** No Qualifier

ction	0	**Medical and Surgical**
dy System	G	**Endocrine System**
eration	J	**Inspection:** Visually and/or manually exploring a body part

Body Part (4th)	Approach (5th)	Device (6th)	Qualifier (7th)
Pituitary Gland Pineal Body Adrenal Gland K Thyroid Gland R Parathyroid Gland Endocrine Gland	0 Open 3 Percutaneous 4 Percutaneous Endoscopic	Z No Device	Z No Qualifier

ction	0	**Medical and Surgical**
dy System	G	**Endocrine System**
eration	M	**Reattachment:** Putting back in or on all or a portion of a separated body part to its normal location or other suitable location

Body Part (4th)	Approach (5th)	Device (6th)	Qualifier (7th)
2 Adrenal Gland, Left 3 Adrenal Gland, Right G Thyroid Gland Lobe, Left H Thyroid Gland Lobe, Right L Superior Parathyroid Gland, Right M Superior Parathyroid Gland, Left N Inferior Parathyroid Gland, Right P Inferior Parathyroid Gland, Left Q Parathyroid Glands, Multiple R Parathyroid Gland	0 Open 4 Percutaneous Endoscopic	Z No Device	Z No Qualifier

ction	0	**Medical and Surgical**
dy System	G	**Endocrine System**
eration	N	**Release:** Freeing a body part from an abnormal physical constraint by cutting or by the use of force

Body Part (4th)	Approach (5th)	Device (6th)	Qualifier (7th)
0 Pituitary Gland 1 Pineal Body 2 Adrenal Gland, Left 3 Adrenal Gland, Right 4 Adrenal Glands, Bilateral 6 Carotid Body, Left 7 Carotid Body, Right 8 Carotid Bodies, Bilateral 9 Para-aortic Body B Coccygeal Glomus C Glomus Jugulare D Aortic Body F Paraganglion Extremity G Thyroid Gland Lobe, Left H Thyroid Gland Lobe, Right K Thyroid Gland L Superior Parathyroid Gland, Right M Superior Parathyroid Gland, Left N Inferior Parathyroid Gland, Right P Inferior Parathyroid Gland, Left Q Parathyroid Glands, Multiple R Parathyroid Gland	0 Open 3 Percutaneous 4 Percutaneous Endoscopic	Z No Device	Z No Qualifier

Section 0 **Medical and Surgical**
Body System G **Endocrine System**
Operation P **Removal:** Taking out or off a device from a body part

Body Part (4th)	Approach (5th)	Device (6th)	Qualifier (7th)
0 Pituitary Gland **1** Pineal Body **5** Adrenal Gland **K** Thyroid Gland **R** Parathyroid Gland	**0** Open **3** Percutaneous **4** Percutaneous Endoscopic **X** External	**0** Drainage Device	**Z** No Qualifier
S Endocrine Gland	**0** Open **3** Percutaneous **4** Percutaneous Endoscopic	**0** Drainage Device **2** Monitoring Device **3** Infusion Device **Y** Other Device	**Z** No Qualifier
S Endocrine Gland	**X** External	**0** Drainage Device **2** Monitoring Device **3** Infusion Device	**Z** No Qualifier

Section 0 **Medical and Surgical**
Body System G **Endocrine System**
Operation Q **Repair:** Restoring, to the extent possible, a body part to its normal anatomic structure and function

Body Part (4th)	Approach (5th)	Device (6th)	Qualifier (7th)
0 Pituitary Gland **1** Pineal Body **2** Adrenal Gland, Left **3** Adrenal Gland, Right **4** Adrenal Glands, Bilateral **6** Carotid Body, Left **7** Carotid Body, Right **8** Carotid Bodies, Bilateral **9** Para-aortic Body **B** Coccygeal Glomus **C** Glomus Jugulare **D** Aortic Body **F** Paraganglion Extremity **G** Thyroid Gland Lobe, Left **H** Thyroid Gland Lobe, Right **J** Thyroid Gland Isthmus **K** Thyroid Gland **L** Superior Parathyroid Gland, Right **M** Superior Parathyroid Gland, Left **N** Inferior Parathyroid Gland, Right **P** Inferior Parathyroid Gland, Left **Q** Parathyroid Glands, Multiple **R** Parathyroid Gland	**0** Open **3** Percutaneous **4** Percutaneous Endoscopic	**Z** No Device	**Z** No Qualifier

Section 0 **Medical and Surgical**
Body System G **Endocrine System**
Operation S **Reposition:** Moving to its normal location, or other suitable location, all or a portion of a body part

Body Part (4th)	Approach (5th)	Device (6th)	Qualifier (7th)
2 Adrenal Gland, Left **3** Adrenal Gland, Right **G** Thyroid Gland Lobe, Left **H** Thyroid Gland Lobe, Right **L** Superior Parathyroid Gland, Right **M** Superior Parathyroid Gland, Left **N** Inferior Parathyroid Gland, Right **P** Inferior Parathyroid Gland, Left **Q** Parathyroid Glands, Multiple **R** Parathyroid Gland	**0** Open **4** Percutaneous Endoscopic	**Z** No Device	**Z** No Qualifier

ction **0** **Medical and Surgical**
dy System **G** **Endocrine System**
eration **T** **Resection:** Cutting out or off, without replacement, all of a body part

Body Part (4th)	Approach (5th)	Device (6th)	Qualifier (7th)
0 Pituitary Gland 1 Pineal Body 2 Adrenal Gland, Left 3 Adrenal Gland, Right 4 Adrenal Glands, Bilateral 6 Carotid Body, Left 7 Carotid Body, Right 8 Carotid Bodies, Bilateral 9 Para-aortic Body B Coccygeal Glomus C Glomus Jugulare D Aortic Body F Paraganglion Extremity G Thyroid Gland Lobe, Left H Thyroid Gland Lobe, Right J Thyroid Gland Isthmus K Thyroid Gland L Superior Parathyroid Gland, Right M Superior Parathyroid Gland, Left N Inferior Parathyroid Gland, Right P Inferior Parathyroid Gland, Left Q Parathyroid Glands, Multiple R Parathyroid Gland	**0** Open **4** Percutaneous Endoscopic	**Z** No Device	**Z** No Qualifier

ction **0** **Medical and Surgical**
dy System **G** **Endocrine System**
eration **W** **Revision:** Correcting, to the extent possible, a portion of a malfunctioning device or the position of a displaced device

Body Part (4th)	Approach (5th)	Device (6th)	Qualifier (7th)
0 Pituitary Gland 1 Pineal Body 5 Adrenal Gland K Thyroid Gland R Parathyroid Gland	**0** Open **3** Percutaneous **4** Percutaneous Endoscopic **X** External	**0** Drainage Device	**Z** No Qualifier
S Endocrine Gland	**0** Open **3** Percutaneous **4** Percutaneous Endoscopic	**0** Drainage Device **2** Monitoring Device **3** Infusion Device **Y** Other Device	**Z** No Qualifier
S Endocrine Gland	**X** External	**0** Drainage Device **2** Monitoring Device **3** Infusion Device	**Z** No Qualifier

AHA Coding Clinic

0GB00ZZ Excision of Pituitary Gland, Open Approach—AHA CC: 3Q, 2014, 22-23
0GBG0ZZ Excision of Left Thyroid Gland Lobe, Open Approach—AHA CC: 2Q, 2017, 20
0GBH0ZZ Excision of Right Thyroid Gland Lobe, Open Approach—AHA CC: 2Q, 2017, 20

Skin and Subcutaneous Tissue

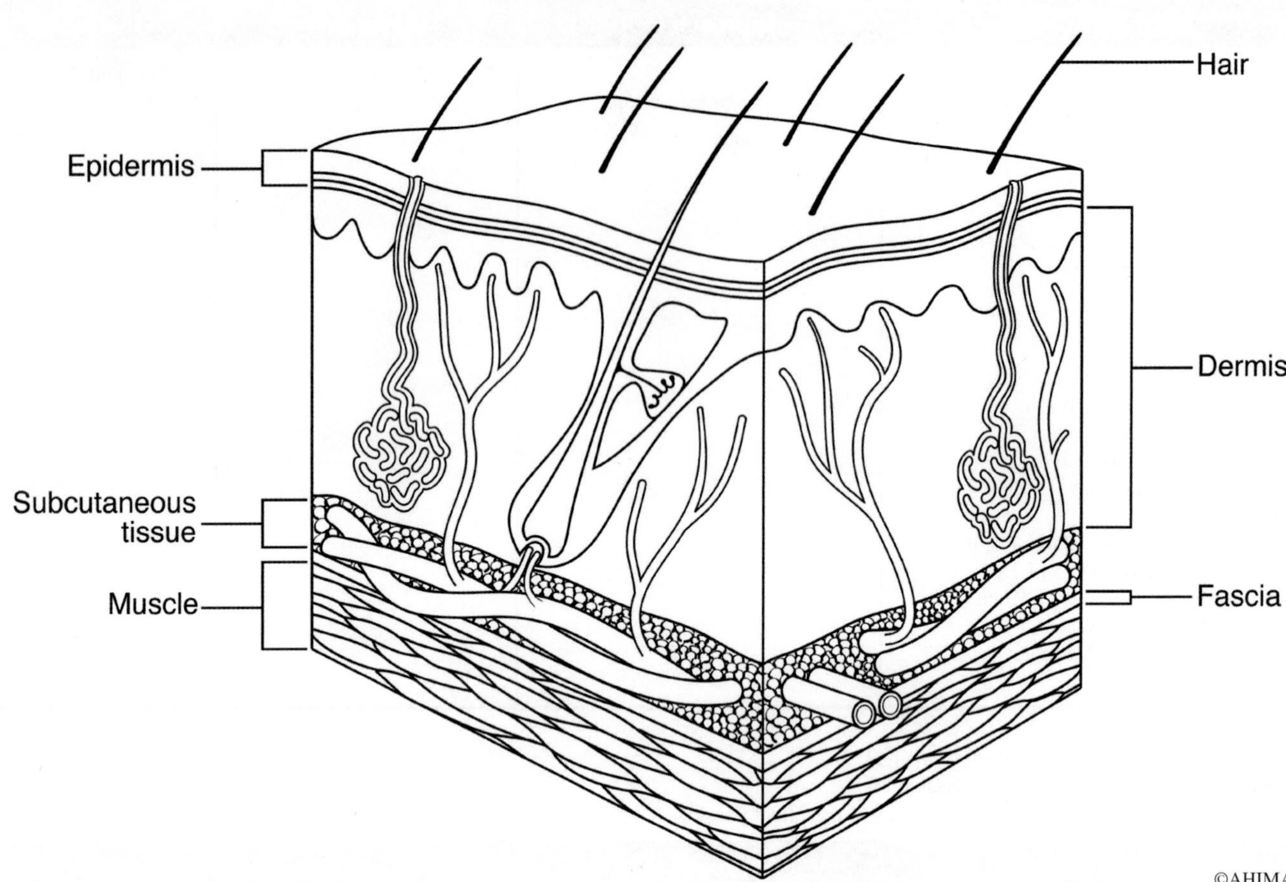

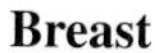

Breast

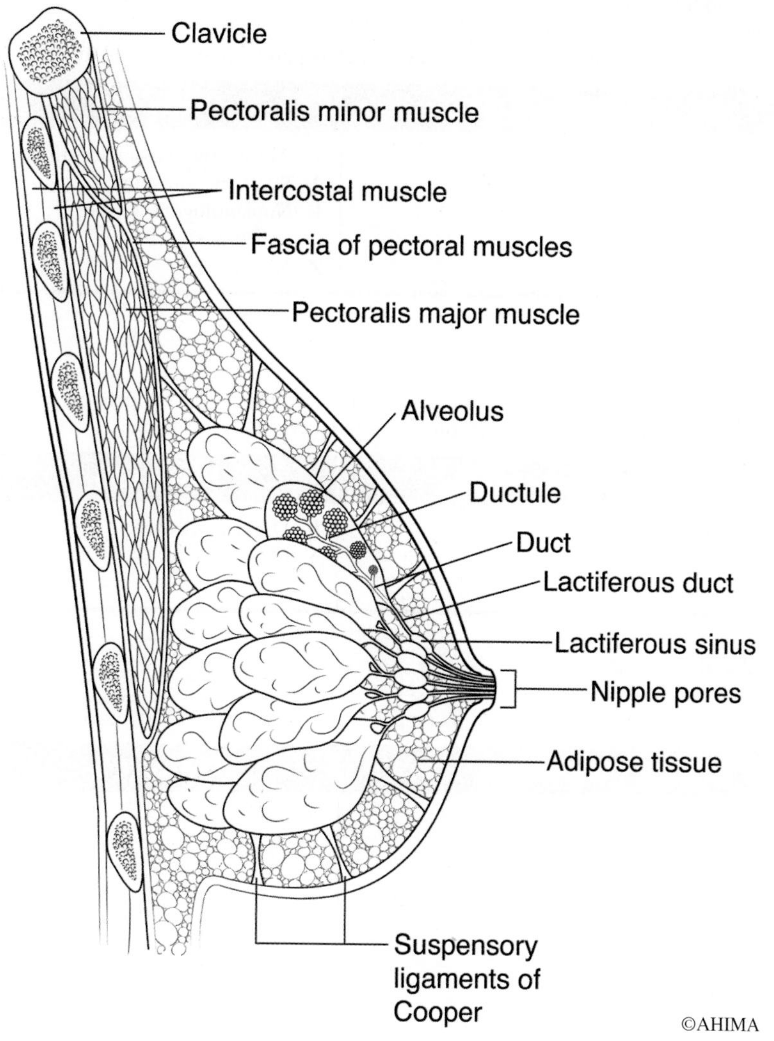

Nail Bed

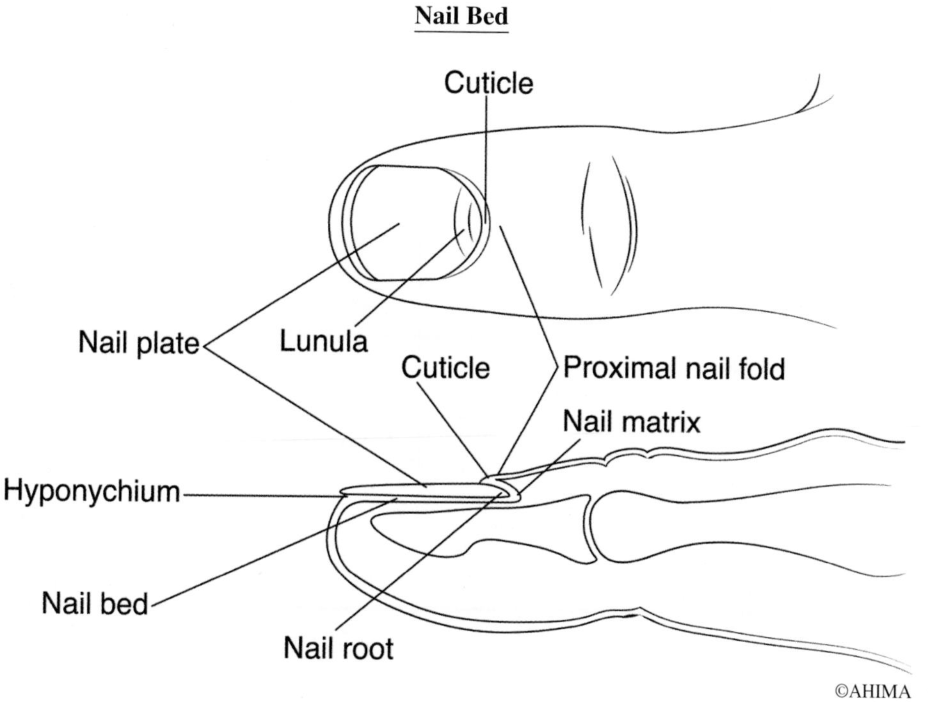

Skin and Breast Tables 0H0–0HX

Section 0 **Medical and Surgical**
Body System H **Skin and Breast**
Operation 0 **Alteration:** Modifying the anatomic structure of a body part without affecting the function of the body part

Body Part (4th)	Approach (5th)	Device (6th)	Qualifier (7th)
T Breast, Right **U** Breast, Left **V** Breast, Bilateral	**0** Open **3** Percutaneous **X** External	**7** Autologous Tissue Substitute **J** Synthetic Substitute **K** Nonautologous Tissue Substitute **Z** No Device	**Z** No Qualifier

Section 0 **Medical and Surgical**
Body System H **Skin and Breast**
Operation 2 **Change:** Taking out or off a device from a body part and putting back an identical or similar device in or on the same bo part without cutting or puncturing the skin or a mucous membrane

Body Part (4th)	Approach (5th)	Device (6th)	Qualifier (7th)
P Skin **T** Breast, Right **U** Breast, Left	**X** External	**0** Drainage Device **Y** Other Device	**Z** No Qualifier

Section 0 **Medical and Surgical**
Body System H **Skin and Breast**
Operation 5 **Destruction:** Physical eradication of all or a portion of a body part by the direct use of energy, force, or a destructive age

Body Part (4th)	Approach (5th)	Device (6th)	Qualifier (7th)
0 Skin, Scalp **1** Skin, Face **2** Skin, Right Ear **3** Skin, Left Ear **4** Skin, Neck **5** Skin, Chest **6** Skin, Back **7** Skin, Abdomen **8** Skin, Buttock **9** Skin, Perineum **A** Skin, Inguinal **B** Skin, Right Upper Arm **C** Skin, Left Upper Arm **D** Skin, Right Lower Arm **E** Skin, Left Lower Arm **F** Skin, Right Hand **G** Skin, Left Hand **H** Skin, Right Upper Leg **J** Skin, Left Upper Leg **K** Skin, Right Lower Leg **L** Skin, Left Lower Leg **M** Skin, Right Foot **N** Skin, Left Foot	**X** External	**Z** No Device	**D** Multiple **Z** No Qualifier
Q Finger Nail **R** Toe Nail	**X** External	**Z** No Device	**Z** No Qualifier
T Breast, Right **U** Breast, Left **V** Breast, Bilateral **W** Nipple, Right **X** Nipple, Left	**0** Open **3** Percutaneous **7** Via Natural or Artificial Opening **8** Via Natural or Artificial Opening Endoscopic **X** External	**Z** No Device	**Z** No Qualifier

ction 0 **Medical and Surgical**
dy System H **Skin and Breast**
eration 8 **Division:** Cutting into a body part, without draining fluids and/or gases from the body part, in order to separate or transect a body part

Body Part (4th)	Approach (5th)	Device (6th)	Qualifier (7th)
0 Skin, Scalp	X External	Z No Device	Z No Qualifier
1 Skin, Face			
2 Skin, Right Ear			
3 Skin, Left Ear			
4 Skin, Neck			
5 Skin, Chest			
6 Skin, Back			
7 Skin, Abdomen			
8 Skin, Buttock			
9 Skin, Perineum			
A Skin, Inguinal			
B Skin, Right Upper Arm			
C Skin, Left Upper Arm			
D Skin, Right Lower Arm			
E Skin, Left Lower Arm			
F Skin, Right Hand			
G Skin, Left Hand			
H Skin, Right Upper Leg			
J Skin, Left Upper Leg			
K Skin, Right Lower Leg			
L Skin, Left Lower Leg			
M Skin, Right Foot			
N Skin, Left Foot			

ction 0 **Medical and Surgical**
dy System H **Skin and Breast**
peration 9 **Drainage:** Taking or letting out fluids and/or gases from a body part

Body Part (4th)	Approach (5th)	Device (6th)	Qualifier (7th)
0 Skin, Scalp	X External	0 Drainage Device	Z No Qualifier
1 Skin, Face			
2 Skin, Right Ear			
3 Skin, Left Ear			
4 Skin, Neck			
5 Skin, Chest			
6 Skin, Back			
7 Skin, Abdomen			
8 Skin, Buttock			
9 Skin, Perineum			
A Skin, Inguinal			
B Skin, Right Upper Arm			
C Skin, Left Upper Arm			
D Skin, Right Lower Arm			
E Skin, Left Lower Arm			
F Skin, Right Hand			
G Skin, Left Hand			
H Skin, Right Upper Leg			
J Skin, Left Upper Leg			
K Skin, Right Lower Leg			
L Skin, Left Lower Leg			
M Skin, Right Foot			
N Skin, Left Foot			
Q Finger Nail			
R Toe Nail			

Continued →

Section **0** **Medical and Surgical**
Body System **H** **Skin and Breast**
Operation **9** **Drainage:** Taking or letting out fluids and/or gases from a body part

0H9 Contin

Body Part (4th)	Approach (5th)	Device (6th)	Qualifier (7th)
0 Skin, Scalp **1** Skin, Face **2** Skin, Right Ear **3** Skin, Left Ear **4** Skin, Neck **5** Skin, Chest **6** Skin, Back **7** Skin, Abdomen **8** Skin, Buttock **9** Skin, Perineum **A** Skin, Inguinal **B** Skin, Right Upper Arm **C** Skin, Left Upper Arm **D** Skin, Right Lower Arm **E** Skin, Left Lower Arm **F** Skin, Right Hand **G** Skin, Left Hand **H** Skin, Right Upper Leg **J** Skin, Left Upper Leg **K** Skin, Right Lower Leg **L** Skin, Left Lower Leg **M** Skin, Right Foot **N** Skin, Left Foot **Q** Finger Nail **R** Toe Nail	**X** External	**Z** No Device	**X** Diagnostic **Z** No Qualifier
T Breast, Right **U** Breast, Left **V** Breast, Bilateral **W** Nipple, Right **X** Nipple, Left	**0** Open **3** Percutaneous **7** Via Natural or Artificial Opening **8** Via Natural or Artificial Opening Endoscopic **X** External	**0** Drainage Device	**Z** No Qualifier
T Breast, Right **U** Breast, Left **V** Breast, Bilateral **W** Nipple, Right **X** Nipple, Left	**0** Open **3** Percutaneous **7** Via Natural or Artificial Opening **8** Via Natural or Artificial Opening Endoscopic **X** External	**Z** No Device	**X** Diagnostic **Z** No Qualifier

tion **0** **Medical and Surgical**
dy System **H** **Skin and Breast**
eration **B** **Excision:** Cutting out or off, without replacement, a portion of a body part

Body Part (4th)	Approach (5th)	Device (6th)	Qualifier (7th)
Skin, Scalp Skin, Face Skin, Right Ear Skin, Left Ear Skin, Neck Skin, Chest Skin, Back Skin, Abdomen Skin, Buttock Skin, Perineum Skin, Inguinal Skin, Right Upper Arm Skin, Left Upper Arm Skin, Right Lower Arm Skin, Left Lower Arm Skin, Right Hand Skin, Left Hand Skin, Right Upper Leg Skin, Left Upper Leg Skin, Right Lower Leg Skin, Left Lower Leg Skin, Right Foot Skin, Left Foot Finger Nail Toe Nail	**X** External	**Z** No Device	**X** Diagnostic **Z** No Qualifier
Breast, Right Breast, Left Breast, Bilateral Nipple, Right Nipple, Left Supernumerary Breast	**0** Open **3** Percutaneous **7** Via Natural or Artificial Opening **8** Via Natural or Artificial Opening Endoscopic **X** External	**Z** No Device	**X** Diagnostic **Z** No Qualifier

Section **0** **Medical and Surgical**
Body System **H** **Skin and Breast**
Operation **C** **Extirpation:** Taking or cutting out solid matter from a body part

Body Part (4th)	Approach (5th)	Device (6th)	Qualifier (7th)
0 Skin, Scalp **1** Skin, Face **2** Skin, Right Ear **3** Skin, Left Ear **4** Skin, Neck **5** Skin, Chest **6** Skin, Back **7** Skin, Abdomen **8** Skin, Buttock **9** Skin, Perineum **A** Skin, Inguinal **B** Skin, Right Upper Arm **C** Skin, Left Upper Arm **D** Skin, Right Lower Arm **E** Skin, Left Lower Arm **F** Skin, Right Hand **G** Skin, Left Hand **H** Skin, Right Upper Leg **J** Skin, Left Upper Leg **K** Skin, Right Lower Leg **L** Skin, Left Lower Leg **M** Skin, Right Foot **N** Skin, Left Foot **Q** Finger Nail **R** Toe Nail	**X** External	**Z** No Device	**Z** No Qualifier
T Breast, Right **U** Breast, Left **V** Breast, Bilateral **W** Nipple, Right **X** Nipple, Left	**0** Open **3** Percutaneous **7** Via Natural or Artificial Opening **8** Via Natural or Artificial Opening Endoscopic **X** External	**Z** No Device	**Z** No Qualifier

tion **0** **Medical and Surgical**
dy System **H** **Skin and Breast**
eration **D** **Extraction:** Pulling or stripping out or off all or a portion of a body part by the use of force

Body Part (4th)	Approach (5th)	Device (6th)	Qualifier (7th)
Skin, Scalp Skin, Face Skin, Right Ear Skin, Left Ear Skin, Neck Skin, Chest Skin, Back Skin, Abdomen Skin, Buttock Skin, Perineum Skin, Inguinal Skin, Right Upper Arm Skin, Left Upper Arm Skin, Right Lower Arm Skin, Left Lower Arm Skin, Right Hand Skin, Left Hand Skin, Right Upper Leg Skin, Left Upper Leg Skin, Right Lower Leg Skin, Left Lower Leg Skin, Right Foot Skin, Left Foot Finger Nail Toe Nail Hair	**X** External	**Z** No Device	**Z** No Qualifier

ction **0** **Medical and Surgical**
dy System **H** **Skin and Breast**
eration **H** **Insertion:** Putting in a nonbiological appliance that monitors, assists, performs, or prevents a physiological function but does not physically take the place of a body part

Body Part (4th)	Approach (5th)	Device (6th)	Qualifier (7th)
Skin	**X** External	**Y** Other Device	**Z** No Qualifier
Breast, Right Breast, Left	**0** Open **3** Percutaneous **7** Via Natural or Artificial Opening **8** Via Natural or Artificial Opening Endoscopic	**1** Radioactive Element **N** Tissue Expander **Y** Other Device	**Z** No Qualifier
Breast, Right Breast, Left	**X** External	**1** Radioactive Element	**Z** No Qualifier
Breast, Bilateral **V** Nipple, Right Nipple, Left	**0** Open **3** Percutaneous **7** Via Natural or Artificial Opening **8** Via Natural or Artificial Opening Endoscopic	**1** Radioactive Element **N** Tissue Expander	**Z** No Qualifier
Breast, Bilateral **V** Nipple, Right Nipple, Left	**X** External	**1** Radioactive Element	**Z** No Qualifier

ction **0** **Medical and Surgical**
dy System **H** **Skin and Breast**
peration **J** **Inspection:** Visually and/or manually exploring a body part

Body Part (4th)	Approach (5th)	Device (6th)	Qualifier (7th)
Skin **Q** Finger Nail **R** Toe Nail	**X** External	**Z** No Device	**Z** No Qualifier
T Breast, Right **U** Breast, Left	**0** Open **3** Percutaneous **7** Via Natural or Artificial Opening **8** Via Natural or Artificial Opening Endoscopic **X** External	**Z** No Device	**Z** No Qualifier

Section 0 **Medical and Surgical**
Body System H **Skin and Breast**
Operation M **Reattachment:** Putting back in or on all or a portion of a separated body part to its normal location or other suitable location

Body Part (4th)	Approach (5th)	Device (6th)	Qualifier (7th)
0 Skin, Scalp **1** Skin, Face **2** Skin, Right Ear **3** Skin, Left Ear **4** Skin, Neck **5** Skin, Chest **6** Skin, Back **7** Skin, Abdomen **8** Skin, Buttock **9** Skin, Perineum **A** Skin, Inguinal **B** Skin, Right Upper Arm **C** Skin, Left Upper Arm **D** Skin, Right Lower Arm **E** Skin, Left Lower Arm **F** Skin, Right Hand **G** Skin, Left Hand **H** Skin, Right Upper Leg **J** Skin, Left Upper Leg **K** Skin, Right Lower Leg **L** Skin, Left Lower Leg **M** Skin, Right Foot **N** Skin, Left Foot **T** Breast, Right **U** Breast, Left **V** Breast, Bilateral **W** Nipple, Right **X** Nipple, Left	**X** External	**Z** No Device	**Z** No Qualifier

Section 0 **Medical and Surgical**
Body System H **Skin and Breast**
Operation N **Release:** Freeing a body part from an abnormal physical constraint by cutting or by the use of force

Body Part (4th)	Approach (5th)	Device (6th)	Qualifier (7th)
0 Skin, Scalp **1** Skin, Face **2** Skin, Right Ear **3** Skin, Left Ear **4** Skin, Neck **5** Skin, Chest **6** Skin, Back **7** Skin, Abdomen **8** Skin, Buttock **9** Skin, Perineum **A** Skin, Inguinal **B** Skin, Right Upper Arm **C** Skin, Left Upper Arm **D** Skin, Right Lower Arm **E** Skin, Left Lower Arm **F** Skin, Right Hand **G** Skin, Left Hand **H** Skin, Right Upper Leg **J** Skin, Left Upper Leg **K** Skin, Right Lower Leg **L** Skin, Left Lower Leg **M** Skin, Right Foot **N** Skin, Left Foot **Q** Finger Nail **R** Toe Nail	**X** External	**Z** No Device	**Z** No Qualifier

Continued →

ction 0 **Medical and Surgical**
ody System H **Skin and Breast**
peration N **Release:** Freeing a body part from an abnormal physical constraint by cutting or by the use of force

Body Part (4th)	Approach (5th)	Device (6th)	Qualifier (7th)
T Breast, Right U Breast, Left V Breast, Bilateral W Nipple, Right X Nipple, Left	0 Open 3 Percutaneous 7 Via Natural or Artificial Opening 8 Via Natural or Artificial Opening Endoscopic X External	Z No Device	Z No Qualifier

ction 0 **Medical and Surgical**
ody System H **Skin and Breast**
peration P **Removal:** Taking out or off a device from a body part

Body Part (4th)	Approach (5th)	Device (6th)	Qualifier (7th)
P Skin	X External	0 Drainage Device 7 Autologous Tissue Substitute J Synthetic Substitute K Nonautologous Tissue Substitute Y Other Device	Z No Qualifier
Q Finger Nail R Toe Nail	X External	0 Drainage Device 7 Autologous Tissue Substitute J Synthetic Substitute K Nonautologous Tissue Substitute	Z No Qualifier
S Hair	X External	7 Autologous Tissue Substitute J Synthetic Substitute K Nonautologous Tissue Substitute	Z No Qualifier
T Breast, Right U Breast, Left	0 Open 3 Percutaneous 7 Via Natural or Artificial Opening 8 Via Natural or Artificial Opening Endoscopic	0 Drainage Device 1 Radioactive Element 7 Autologous Tissue Substitute J Synthetic Substitute K Nonautologous Tissue Substitute N Tissue Expander Y Other Device	Z No Qualifier
T Breast, Right U Breast, Left	X External	0 Drainage Device 1 Radioactive Element 7 Autologous Tissue Substitute J Synthetic Substitute K Nonautologous Tissue Substitute	Z No Qualifier

Section 0 **Medical and Surgical**
Body System H **Skin and Breast**
Operation Q **Repair:** Restoring, to the extent possible, a body part to its normal anatomic structure and function

Body Part (4th)	Approach (5th)	Device (6th)	Qualifier (7th)
0 Skin, Scalp **1** Skin, Face **2** Skin, Right Ear **3** Skin, Left Ear **4** Skin, Neck **5** Skin, Chest **6** Skin, Back **7** Skin, Abdomen **8** Skin, Buttock **9** Skin, Perineum **A** Skin, Inguinal **B** Skin, Right Upper Arm **C** Skin, Left Upper Arm **D** Skin, Right Lower Arm **E** Skin, Left Lower Arm **F** Skin, Right Hand **G** Skin, Left Hand **H** Skin, Right Upper Leg **J** Skin, Left Upper Leg **K** Skin, Right Lower Leg **L** Skin, Left Lower Leg **M** Skin, Right Foot **N** Skin, Left Foot **Q** Finger Nail **R** Toe Nail	**X** External	**Z** No Device	**Z** No Qualifier
T Breast, Right **U** Breast, Left **V** Breast, Bilateral **W** Nipple, Right **X** Nipple, Left **Y** Supernumerary Breast	**0** Open **3** Percutaneous **7** Via Natural or Artificial Opening **8** Via Natural or Artificial Opening Endoscopic **X** External	**Z** No Device	**Z** No Qualifier

Section 0 **Medical and Surgical**
Body System H **Skin and Breast**
Operation R **Replacement:** Putting in or on biological or synthetic material that physically takes the place and/or function of all or a portion of a body part

Body Part (4th)	Approach (5th)	Device (6th)	Qualifier (7th)
0 Skin, Scalp **1** Skin, Face **2** Skin, Right Ear **3** Skin, Left Ear **4** Skin, Neck **5** Skin, Chest **6** Skin, Back **7** Skin, Abdomen **8** Skin, Buttock **9** Skin, Perineum **A** Skin, Inguinal **B** Skin, Right Upper Arm **C** Skin, Left Upper Arm **D** Skin, Right Lower Arm **E** Skin, Left Lower Arm **F** Skin, Right Hand **G** Skin, Left Hand **H** Skin, Right Upper Leg **J** Skin, Left Upper Leg **K** Skin, Right Lower Leg **L** Skin, Left Lower Leg **M** Skin, Right Foot **N** Skin, Left Foot	**X** External	**7** Autologous Tissue Substitute **K** Nonautologous Tissue Substitute	**3** Full Thickness **4** Partial Thickness

Continued →

tion 0 **Medical and Surgical**
dy System H **Skin and Breast**
eration R **Replacement:** Putting in or on biological or synthetic material that physically takes the place and/or function of all or a portion of a body part

Body Part (4th)	Approach (5th)	Device (6th)	Qualifier (7th)
Skin, Scalp Skin, Face Skin, Right Ear Skin, Left Ear Skin, Neck Skin, Chest Skin, Back Skin, Abdomen Skin, Buttock Skin, Perineum Skin, Inguinal Skin, Right Upper Arm Skin, Left Upper Arm Skin, Right Lower Arm Skin, Left Lower Arm Skin, Right Hand Skin, Left Hand Skin, Right Upper Leg Skin, Left Upper Leg Skin, Right Lower Leg Skin, Left Lower Leg Skin, Right Foot Skin, Left Foot	**X** External	**J** Synthetic Substitute	**3** Full Thickness **4** Partial Thickness **Z** No Qualifier
Finger Nail Toe Nail Hair	**X** External	**7** Autologous Tissue Substitute **J** Synthetic Substitute **K** Nonautologous Tissue Substitute	**Z** No Qualifier
Breast, Right Breast, Left Breast, Bilateral	**0** Open	**7** Autologous Tissue Substitute	**5** Latissimus Dorsi Myocutaneous Flap **6** Transverse Rectus Abdominis Myocutaneous Flap **7** Deep Inferior Epigastric Artery Perforator Flap **8** Superficial Inferior Epigastric Artery Flap **9** Gluteal Artery Perforator Flap **Z** No Qualifier
Breast, Right Breast, Left Breast, Bilateral	**0** Open	**J** Synthetic Substitute **K** Nonautologous Tissue Substitute	**Z** No Qualifier
Breast, Right Breast, Left Breast, Bilateral	**3** Percutaneous **X** External	**7** Autologous Tissue Substitute **J** Synthetic Substitute **K** Nonautologous Tissue Substitute	**Z** No Qualifier
W Nipple, Right **X** Nipple, Left	**0** Open **3** Percutaneous **X** External	**7** Autologous Tissue Substitute **J** Synthetic Substitute **K** Nonautologous Tissue Substitute	**Z** No Qualifier

ction 0 **Medical and Surgical**
dy System H **Skin and Breast**
eration S **Reposition:** Moving to its normal location, or other suitable location, all or a portion of a body part

Body Part (4th)	Approach (5th)	Device (6th)	Qualifier (7th)
Hair **W** Nipple, Right **X** Nipple, Left	**X** External	**Z** No Device	**Z** No Qualifier
T Breast, Right **U** Breast, Left **V** Breast, Bilateral	**0** Open	**Z** No Device	**Z** No Qualifier

Section 0 Medical and Surgical
Body System H Skin and Breast
Operation T **Resection:** Cutting out or off, without replacement, all of a body part

Body Part (4th)	Approach (5th)	Device (6th)	Qualifier (7th)
Q Finger Nail **R** Toe Nail **W** Nipple, Right **X** Nipple, Left	**X** External	**Z** No Device	**Z** No Qualifier
T Breast, Right **U** Breast, Left **V** Breast, Bilateral **Y** Supernumerary Breast	**0** Open	**Z** No Device	**Z** No Qualifier

Section 0 Medical and Surgical
Body System H Skin and Breast
Operation U **Supplement:** Putting in or on biological or synthetic material that physically reinforces and/or augments the function of a portion of a body part

Body Part (4th)	Approach (5th)	Device (6th)	Qualifier (7th)
T Breast, Right **U** Breast, Left **V** Breast, Bilateral **W** Nipple, Right **X** Nipple, Left	**0** Open **3** Percutaneous **7** Via Natural or Artificial Opening **8** Via Natural or Artificial Opening Endoscopic **X** External	**7** Autologous Tissue Substitute **J** Synthetic Substitute **K** Nonautologous Tissue Substitute	**Z** No Qualifier

Section 0 Medical and Surgical
Body System H Skin and Breast
Operation W **Revision:** Correcting, to the extent possible, a portion of a malfunctioning device or the position of a displaced device

Body Part (4th)	Approach (5th)	Device (6th)	Qualifier (7th)
P Skin	**X** External	**0** Drainage Device **7** Autologous Tissue Substitute **J** Synthetic Substitute **K** Nonautologous Tissue Substitute **Y** Other Device	**Z** No Qualifier
Q Finger Nail **R** Toe Nail	**X** External	**0** Drainage Device **7** Autologous Tissue Substitute **J** Synthetic Substitute **K** Nonautologous Tissue Substitute	**Z** No Qualifier
S Hair	**X** External	**7** Autologous Tissue Substitute **J** Synthetic Substitute **K** Nonautologous Tissue Substitute	**Z** No Qualifier
T Breast, Right **U** Breast, Left	**0** Open **3** Percutaneous **7** Via Natural or Artificial Opening **8** Via Natural or Artificial Opening Endoscopic	**0** Drainage Device **7** Autologous Tissue Substitute **J** Synthetic Substitute **K** Nonautologous Tissue Substitute **N** Tissue Expander **Y** Other Device	**Z** No Qualifier
T Breast, Right **U** Breast, Left	**X** External	**0** Drainage Device **7** Autologous Tissue Substitute **J** Synthetic Substitute **K** Nonautologous Tissue Substitute	**Z** No Qualifier

ction **0** **Medical and Surgical**
dy System **H** **Skin and Breast**
eration **X** **Transfer:** Moving, without taking out, all or a portion of a body part to another location to take over the function of all or a portion of a body part

Body Part (4th)	Approach (5th)	Device (6th)	Qualifier (7th)
0 Skin, Scalp 1 Skin, Face 2 Skin, Right Ear 3 Skin, Left Ear 4 Skin, Neck 5 Skin, Chest 6 Skin, Back 7 Skin, Abdomen 8 Skin, Buttock 9 Skin, Perineum A Skin, Inguinal B Skin, Right Upper Arm C Skin, Left Upper Arm D Skin, Right Lower Arm E Skin, Left Lower Arm F Skin, Right Hand G Skin, Left Hand H Skin, Right Upper Leg J Skin, Left Upper Leg K Skin, Right Lower Leg L Skin, Left Lower Leg M Skin, Right Foot N Skin, Left Foot	X External	Z No Device	Z No Qualifier

HA Coding Clinic

HB8XZZ Excision of Buttock Skin, External Approach—AHA CC: 3Q, 2015, 3

HBJXZZ Excision of Left Upper Leg Skin, External Approach—AHA CC: 3Q, 2016, 29-30

HBT0ZZ Excision of Right Breast, Open Approach—AHA CC: 1Q, 2018, 14-15

HD6XZZ Extraction of Back Skin, External Approach—AHA CC: 3Q, 2015, 5-6

HDHXZZ Extraction of Right Upper Leg Skin, External Approach—AHA CC: 3Q, 2015, 5; 1Q, 2016, 40

HHT0NZ Insertion of Tissue Expander into Right Breast, Open Approach—AHA CC: 4Q, 2017, 67

HHU0YZ Insertion of Other Device into Left Breast, Open Approach—AHA CC: 4Q, 2013, 107

HHV0NZ Insertion of Tissue Expander into Bilateral Breast, Open Approach—AHA CC: 2Q, 2014, 12

HPT07Z Removal of Autologous Tissue Substitute from Right Breast, Open Approach—AHA CC: 2Q, 2016, 27

HPU07Z Removal of Autologous Tissue Substitute from Left Breast, Open Approach—AHA CC: 2Q, 2016, 27

HQ9XZZ Repair Perineum Skin, External Approach—AHA CC: 1Q, 2016, 7

HQEXZZ Repair Left Lower Arm Skin, External Approach—AHA CC: 4Q, 2014, 31-32

HRMXK3 Replacement of Right Foot Skin with Nonautologous Tissue Substitute, Full Thickness, External Approach—AHA CC: 1Q, 2017, 35-36

HRNXK3 Replacement of Left Foot Skin with Nonautologous Tissue Substitute, Full Thickness, External Approach—AHA CC: 3Q, 2014, 14-15

HTT0ZZ Resection of Right Breast, Open Approach—AHA CC: 4Q, 2014, 34

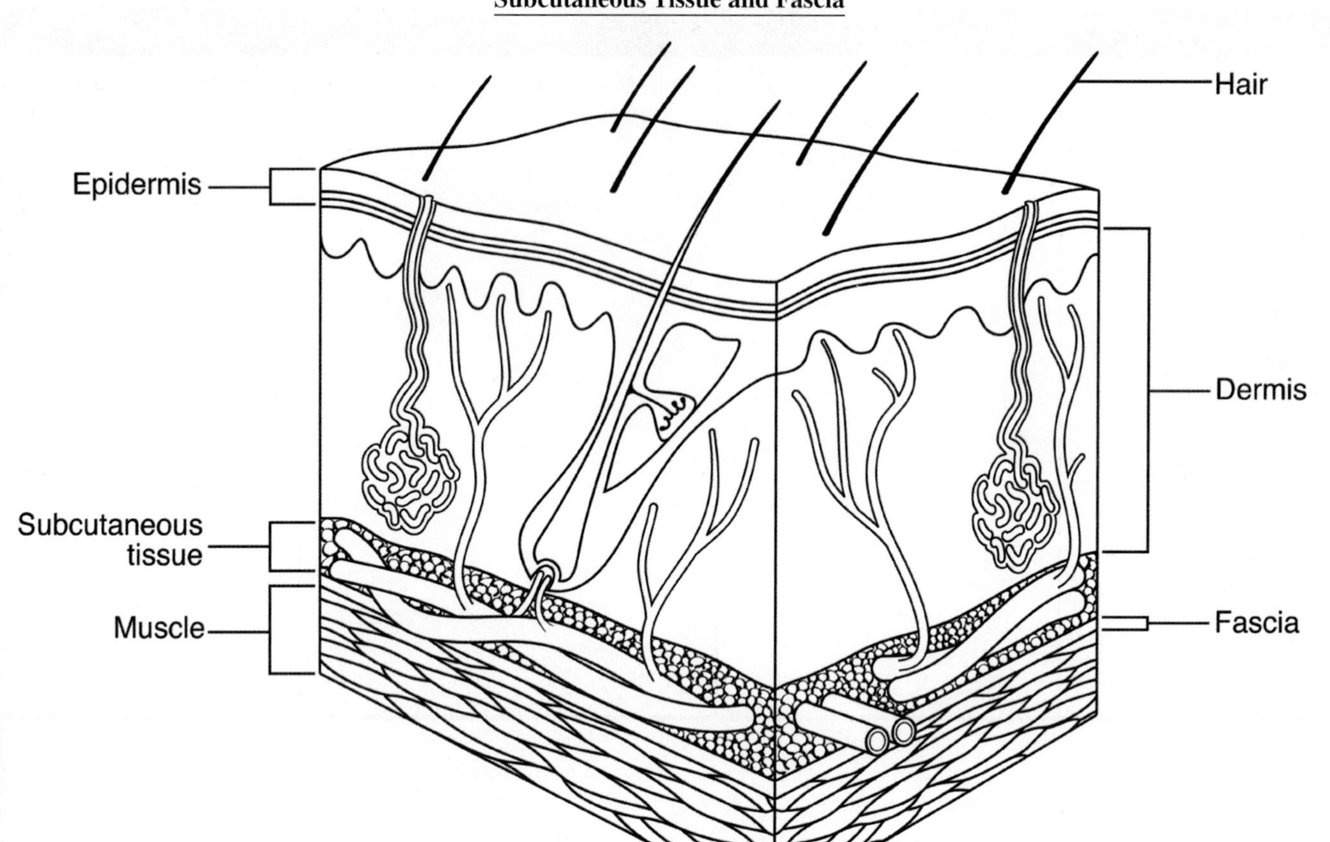
Subcutaneous Tissue and Fascia
Hair
Epidermis
Dermis
Subcutaneous tissue
Muscle
Fascia

Section 0 **Medical and Surgical**
Body System J **Subcutaneous Tissue and Fascia**
Operation 0 **Alteration:** Modifying the anatomic structure of a body part without affecting the function of the body part

Body Part (4th)	Approach (5th)	Device (6th)	Qualifier (7th)
1 Subcutaneous Tissue and Fascia, Face **4** Subcutaneous Tissue and Fascia, Right Neck **5** Subcutaneous Tissue and Fascia, Left Neck **6** Subcutaneous Tissue and Fascia, Chest **7** Subcutaneous Tissue and Fascia, Back **8** Subcutaneous Tissue and Fascia, Abdomen **9** Subcutaneous Tissue and Fascia, Buttock **D** Subcutaneous Tissue and Fascia, Right Upper Arm **F** Subcutaneous Tissue and Fascia, Left Upper Arm **G** Subcutaneous Tissue and Fascia, Right Lower Arm **H** Subcutaneous Tissue and Fascia, Left Lower Arm **L** Subcutaneous Tissue and Fascia, Right Upper Leg **M** Subcutaneous Tissue and Fascia, Left Upper Leg **N** Subcutaneous Tissue and Fascia, Right Lower Leg **P** Subcutaneous Tissue and Fascia, Left Lower Leg	**0** Open **3** Percutaneous	**Z** No Device	**Z** No Qualifier

Section 0 **Medical and Surgical**
Body System J **Subcutaneous Tissue and Fascia**
Operation 2 **Change:** Taking out or off a device from a body part and putting back an identical or similar device in or on the same body part without cutting or puncturing the skin or a mucous membrane

Body Part (4th)	Approach (5th)	Device (6th)	Qualifier (7th)
S Subcutaneous Tissue and Fascia, Head and Neck **T** Subcutaneous Tissue and Fascia, Trunk **V** Subcutaneous Tissue and Fascia, Upper Extremity **W** Subcutaneous Tissue and Fascia, Lower Extremity	**X** External	**0** Drainage Device **Y** Other Device	**Z** No Qualifier

Section 0 **Medical and Surgical**
Body System J **Subcutaneous Tissue and Fascia**
Operation 5 **Destruction:** Physical eradication of all or a portion of a body part by the direct use of energy, force, or a destructive agent

Body Part (4th)	Approach (5th)	Device (6th)	Qualifier (7th)
0 Subcutaneous Tissue and Fascia, Scalp **1** Subcutaneous Tissue and Fascia, Face **4** Subcutaneous Tissue and Fascia, Right Neck **5** Subcutaneous Tissue and Fascia, Left Neck **6** Subcutaneous Tissue and Fascia, Chest **7** Subcutaneous Tissue and Fascia, Back **8** Subcutaneous Tissue and Fascia, Abdomen **9** Subcutaneous Tissue and Fascia, Buttock **B** Subcutaneous Tissue and Fascia, Perineum **C** Subcutaneous Tissue and Fascia, Pelvic Region **D** Subcutaneous Tissue and Fascia, Right Upper Arm **F** Subcutaneous Tissue and Fascia, Left Upper Arm **G** Subcutaneous Tissue and Fascia, Right Lower Arm **H** Subcutaneous Tissue and Fascia, Left Lower Arm **J** Subcutaneous Tissue and Fascia, Right Hand **K** Subcutaneous Tissue and Fascia, Left Hand **L** Subcutaneous Tissue and Fascia, Right Upper Leg **M** Subcutaneous Tissue and Fascia, Left Upper Leg **N** Subcutaneous Tissue and Fascia, Right Lower Leg **P** Subcutaneous Tissue and Fascia, Left Lower Leg **Q** Subcutaneous Tissue and Fascia, Right Foot **R** Subcutaneous Tissue and Fascia, Left Foot	**0** Open **3** Percutaneous	**Z** No Device	**Z** No Qualifier

Section 0 **Medical and Surgical**
Body System J **Subcutaneous Tissue and Fascia**
Operation 8 **Division:** Cutting into a body part, without draining fluids and/or gases from the body part, in order to separate or transect a body part

Body Part (4th)	Approach (5th)	Device (6th)	Qualifier (7th)
0 Subcutaneous Tissue and Fascia, Scalp **1** Subcutaneous Tissue and Fascia, Face **4** Subcutaneous Tissue and Fascia, Right Neck **5** Subcutaneous Tissue and Fascia, Left Neck **6** Subcutaneous Tissue and Fascia, Chest **7** Subcutaneous Tissue and Fascia, Back **8** Subcutaneous Tissue and Fascia, Abdomen **9** Subcutaneous Tissue and Fascia, Buttock **B** Subcutaneous Tissue and Fascia, Perineum **C** Subcutaneous Tissue and Fascia, Pelvic Region **D** Subcutaneous Tissue and Fascia, Right Upper Arm **F** Subcutaneous Tissue and Fascia, Left Upper Arm **G** Subcutaneous Tissue and Fascia, Right Lower Arm **H** Subcutaneous Tissue and Fascia, Left Lower Arm **J** Subcutaneous Tissue and Fascia, Right Hand **K** Subcutaneous Tissue and Fascia, Left Hand **L** Subcutaneous Tissue and Fascia, Right Upper Leg **M** Subcutaneous Tissue and Fascia, Left Upper Leg **N** Subcutaneous Tissue and Fascia, Right Lower Leg **P** Subcutaneous Tissue and Fascia, Left Lower Leg **Q** Subcutaneous Tissue and Fascia, Right Foot **R** Subcutaneous Tissue and Fascia, Left Foot **S** Subcutaneous Tissue and Fascia, Head and Neck **T** Subcutaneous Tissue and Fascia, Trunk **V** Subcutaneous Tissue and Fascia, Upper Extremity **W** Subcutaneous Tissue and Fascia, Lower Extremity	**0** Open **3** Percutaneous	**Z** No Device	**Z** No Qualifier

Section 0 **Medical and Surgical**
Body System J **Subcutaneous Tissue and Fascia**
Operation 9 **Drainage:** Taking or letting out fluids and/or gases from a body part

Body Part (4th)	Approach (5th)	Device (6th)	Qualifier (7th)
0 Subcutaneous Tissue and Fascia, Scalp **1** Subcutaneous Tissue and Fascia, Face **4** Subcutaneous Tissue and Fascia, Right Neck **5** Subcutaneous Tissue and Fascia, Left Neck **6** Subcutaneous Tissue and Fascia, Chest **7** Subcutaneous Tissue and Fascia, Back **8** Subcutaneous Tissue and Fascia, Abdomen **9** Subcutaneous Tissue and Fascia, Buttock **B** Subcutaneous Tissue and Fascia, Perineum **C** Subcutaneous Tissue and Fascia, Pelvic Region **D** Subcutaneous Tissue and Fascia, Right Upper Arm **F** Subcutaneous Tissue and Fascia, Left Upper Arm **G** Subcutaneous Tissue and Fascia, Right Lower Arm **H** Subcutaneous Tissue and Fascia, Left Lower Arm **J** Subcutaneous Tissue and Fascia, Right Hand **K** Subcutaneous Tissue and Fascia, Left Hand **L** Subcutaneous Tissue and Fascia, Right Upper Leg **M** Subcutaneous Tissue and Fascia, Left Upper Leg **N** Subcutaneous Tissue and Fascia, Right Lower Leg **P** Subcutaneous Tissue and Fascia, Left Lower Leg **Q** Subcutaneous Tissue and Fascia, Right Foot **R** Subcutaneous Tissue and Fascia, Left Foot	**0** Open **3** Percutaneous	**0** Drainage Device	**Z** No Qualifier

Continued →

tion 0 **Medical and Surgical**
ly System J **Subcutaneous Tissue and Fascia**
eration 9 **Drainage:** Taking or letting out fluids and/or gases from a body part

Body Part (4th)	Approach (5th)	Device (6th)	Qualifier (7th)
Subcutaneous Tissue and Fascia, Scalp Subcutaneous Tissue and Fascia, Face Subcutaneous Tissue and Fascia, Right Neck Subcutaneous Tissue and Fascia, Left Neck Subcutaneous Tissue and Fascia, Chest Subcutaneous Tissue and Fascia, Back Subcutaneous Tissue and Fascia, Abdomen Subcutaneous Tissue and Fascia, Buttock Subcutaneous Tissue and Fascia, Perineum Subcutaneous Tissue and Fascia, Pelvic Region Subcutaneous Tissue and Fascia, Right Upper Arm Subcutaneous Tissue and Fascia, Left Upper Arm Subcutaneous Tissue and Fascia, Right Lower Arm Subcutaneous Tissue and Fascia, Left Lower Arm Subcutaneous Tissue and Fascia, Right Hand Subcutaneous Tissue and Fascia, Left Hand Subcutaneous Tissue and Fascia, Right Upper Leg Subcutaneous Tissue and Fascia, Left Upper Leg Subcutaneous Tissue and Fascia, Right Lower Leg Subcutaneous Tissue and Fascia, Left Lower Leg Subcutaneous Tissue and Fascia, Right Foot Subcutaneous Tissue and Fascia, Left Foot	**0** Open **3** Percutaneous	**Z** No Device	**X** Diagnostic **Z** No Qualifier

tion 0 **Medical and Surgical**
dy System J **Subcutaneous Tissue and Fascia**
eration B **Excision:** Cutting out or off, without replacement, a portion of a body part

Body Part (4th)	Approach (5th)	Device (6th)	Qualifier (7th)
Subcutaneous Tissue and Fascia, Scalp Subcutaneous Tissue and Fascia, Face Subcutaneous Tissue and Fascia, Right Neck Subcutaneous Tissue and Fascia, Left Neck Subcutaneous Tissue and Fascia, Chest Subcutaneous Tissue and Fascia, Back Subcutaneous Tissue and Fascia, Abdomen Subcutaneous Tissue and Fascia, Buttock Subcutaneous Tissue and Fascia, Perineum Subcutaneous Tissue and Fascia, Pelvic Region Subcutaneous Tissue and Fascia, Right Upper Arm Subcutaneous Tissue and Fascia, Left Upper Arm Subcutaneous Tissue and Fascia, Right Lower Arm Subcutaneous Tissue and Fascia, Left Lower Arm Subcutaneous Tissue and Fascia, Right Hand Subcutaneous Tissue and Fascia, Left Hand Subcutaneous Tissue and Fascia, Right Upper Leg Subcutaneous Tissue and Fascia, Left Upper Leg Subcutaneous Tissue and Fascia, Right Lower Leg Subcutaneous Tissue and Fascia, Left Lower Leg Subcutaneous Tissue and Fascia, Right Foot Subcutaneous Tissue and Fascia, Left Foot	**0** Open **3** Percutaneous	**Z** No Device	**X** Diagnostic **Z** No Qualifier

Section 0 **Medical and Surgical**
Body System J **Subcutaneous Tissue and Fascia**
Operation C **Extirpation:** Taking or cutting out solid matter from a body part

Body Part (4th)	Approach (5th)	Device (6th)	Qualifier (7th)
0 Subcutaneous Tissue and Fascia, Scalp **1** Subcutaneous Tissue and Fascia, Face **4** Subcutaneous Tissue and Fascia, Right Neck **5** Subcutaneous Tissue and Fascia, Left Neck **6** Subcutaneous Tissue and Fascia, Chest **7** Subcutaneous Tissue and Fascia, Back **8** Subcutaneous Tissue and Fascia, Abdomen **9** Subcutaneous Tissue and Fascia, Buttock **B** Subcutaneous Tissue and Fascia, Perineum **C** Subcutaneous Tissue and Fascia, Pelvic Region **D** Subcutaneous Tissue and Fascia, Right Upper Arm **F** Subcutaneous Tissue and Fascia, Left Upper Arm **G** Subcutaneous Tissue and Fascia, Right Lower Arm **H** Subcutaneous Tissue and Fascia, Left Lower Arm **J** Subcutaneous Tissue and Fascia, Right Hand **K** Subcutaneous Tissue and Fascia, Left Hand **L** Subcutaneous Tissue and Fascia, Right Upper Leg **M** Subcutaneous Tissue and Fascia, Left Upper Leg **N** Subcutaneous Tissue and Fascia, Right Lower Leg **P** Subcutaneous Tissue and Fascia, Left Lower Leg **Q** Subcutaneous Tissue and Fascia, Right Foot **R** Subcutaneous Tissue and Fascia, Left Foot	**0** Open **3** Percutaneous	**Z** No Device	**Z** No Qualifier

Section 0 **Medical and Surgical**
Body System J **Subcutaneous Tissue and Fascia**
Operation D **Extraction:** Pulling or stripping out or off all or a portion of a body part by the use of force

Body Part (4th)	Approach (5th)	Device (6th)	Qualifier (7th)
0 Subcutaneous Tissue and Fascia, Scalp **1** Subcutaneous Tissue and Fascia, Face **4** Subcutaneous Tissue and Fascia, Right Neck **5** Subcutaneous Tissue and Fascia, Left Neck **6** Subcutaneous Tissue and Fascia, Chest **7** Subcutaneous Tissue and Fascia, Back **8** Subcutaneous Tissue and Fascia, Abdomen **9** Subcutaneous Tissue and Fascia, Buttock **B** Subcutaneous Tissue and Fascia, Perineum **C** Subcutaneous Tissue and Fascia, Pelvic Region **D** Subcutaneous Tissue and Fascia, Right Upper Arm **F** Subcutaneous Tissue and Fascia, Left Upper Arm **G** Subcutaneous Tissue and Fascia, Right Lower Arm **H** Subcutaneous Tissue and Fascia, Left Lower Arm **J** Subcutaneous Tissue and Fascia, Right Hand **K** Subcutaneous Tissue and Fascia, Left Hand **L** Subcutaneous Tissue and Fascia, Right Upper Leg **M** Subcutaneous Tissue and Fascia, Left Upper Leg **N** Subcutaneous Tissue and Fascia, Right Lower Leg **P** Subcutaneous Tissue and Fascia, Left Lower Leg **Q** Subcutaneous Tissue and Fascia, Right Foot **R** Subcutaneous Tissue and Fascia, Left Foot	**0** Open **3** Percutaneous	**Z** No Device	**Z** No Qualifier

Section **0** **Medical and Surgical**
Body System **J** **Subcutaneous Tissue and Fascia**
Operation **H** **Insertion:** Putting in a nonbiological appliance that monitors, assists, performs, or prevents a physiological function but does not physically take the place of a body part

Body Part (4th)	Approach (5th)	Device (6th)	Qualifier (7th)
0 Subcutaneous Tissue and Fascia, Scalp **1** Subcutaneous Tissue and Fascia, Face **4** Subcutaneous Tissue and Fascia, Right Neck **5** Subcutaneous Tissue and Fascia, Left Neck **9** Subcutaneous Tissue and Fascia, Buttock **B** Subcutaneous Tissue and Fascia, Perineum **C** Subcutaneous Tissue and Fascia, Pelvic Region **J** Subcutaneous Tissue and Fascia, Right Hand **K** Subcutaneous Tissue and Fascia, Left Hand **Q** Subcutaneous Tissue and Fascia, Right Foot **R** Subcutaneous Tissue and Fascia, Left Foot	**0** Open **3** Percutaneous	**N** Tissue Expander	**Z** No Qualifier
6 Subcutaneous Tissue and Fascia, Chest **8** Subcutaneous Tissue and Fascia, Abdomen	**0** Open **3** Percutaneous	**0** Monitoring Device, Hemodynamic **2** Monitoring Device **4** Pacemaker, Single Chamber **5** Pacemaker, Single Chamber Rate Responsive **6** Pacemaker, Dual Chamber **7** Cardiac Resynchronization Pacemaker Pulse Generator **8** Defibrillator Generator **9** Cardiac Resynchronization Defibrillator Pulse Generator **A** Contractility Modulation Device **B** Stimulator Generator, Single Array **C** Stimulator Generator, Single Array Rechargeable **D** Stimulator Generator, Multiple Array **E** Stimulator Generator, Multiple Array Rechargeable **H** Contraceptive Device **M** Stimulator Generator **N** Tissue Expander **P** Cardiac Rhythm Related Device **V** Infusion Device, Pump **W** Vascular Access Device, Totally Implantable **X** Vascular Access Device, Tunneled	**Z** No Qualifier
7 Subcutaneous Tissue and Fascia, Back	**0** Open **3** Percutaneous	**B** Stimulator Generator, Single Array **C** Stimulator Generator, Single Array Rechargeable **D** Stimulator Generator, Multiple Array **E** Stimulator Generator, Multiple Array Rechargeable **M** Stimulator Generator **N** Tissue Expander **V** Infusion Device, Pump	**Z** No Qualifier
D Subcutaneous Tissue and Fascia, Right Upper Arm **F** Subcutaneous Tissue and Fascia, Left Upper Arm **G** Subcutaneous Tissue and Fascia, Right Lower Arm **H** Subcutaneous Tissue and Fascia, Left Lower Arm **L** Subcutaneous Tissue and Fascia, Right Upper Leg **M** Subcutaneous Tissue and Fascia, Left Upper Leg **N** Subcutaneous Tissue and Fascia, Right Lower Leg **P** Subcutaneous Tissue and Fascia, Left Lower Leg	**0** Open **3** Percutaneous	**H** Contraceptive Device **N** Tissue Expander **V** Infusion Device, Pump **W** Vascular Access Device, Totally Implantable **X** Vascular Access Device, Tunneled	**Z** No Qualifier
S Subcutaneous Tissue and Fascia, Head and Neck **V** Subcutaneous Tissue and Fascia, Upper Extremity **W** Subcutaneous Tissue and Fascia, Lower Extremity	**0** Open **3** Percutaneous	**1** Radioactive Element **3** Infusion Device **Y** Other Device	**Z** No Qualifier
T Subcutaneous Tissue and Fascia, Trunk	**0** Open **3** Percutaneous	**1** Radioactive Element **3** Infusion Device **V** Infusion Device, Pump **Y** Other Device	**Z** No Qualifier

Section 0 **Medical and Surgical**
Body System J **Subcutaneous Tissue and Fascia**
Operation J **Inspection:** Visually and/or manually exploring a body part

Body Part (4th)	Approach (5th)	Device (6th)	Qualifier (7th)
S Subcutaneous Tissue and Fascia, Head and Neck **T** Subcutaneous Tissue and Fascia, Trunk **V** Subcutaneous Tissue and Fascia, Upper Extremity **W** Subcutaneous Tissue and Fascia, Lower Extremity	**0** Open **3** Percutaneous **X** External	**Z** No Device	**Z** No Qualifier

Section 0 **Medical and Surgical**
Body System J **Subcutaneous Tissue and Fascia**
Operation N **Release:** Freeing a body part from an abnormal physical constraint by cutting or by the use of force

Body Part (4th)	Approach (5th)	Device (6th)	Qualifier (7th)
0 Subcutaneous Tissue and Fascia, Scalp **1** Subcutaneous Tissue and Fascia, Face **4** Subcutaneous Tissue and Fascia, Right Neck **5** Subcutaneous Tissue and Fascia, Left Neck **6** Subcutaneous Tissue and Fascia, Chest **7** Subcutaneous Tissue and Fascia, Back **8** Subcutaneous Tissue and Fascia, Abdomen **9** Subcutaneous Tissue and Fascia, Buttock **B** Subcutaneous Tissue and Fascia, Perineum **C** Subcutaneous Tissue and Fascia, Pelvic Region **D** Subcutaneous Tissue and Fascia, Right Upper Arm **F** Subcutaneous Tissue and Fascia, Left Upper Arm **G** Subcutaneous Tissue and Fascia, Right Lower Arm **H** Subcutaneous Tissue and Fascia, Left Lower Arm **J** Subcutaneous Tissue and Fascia, Right Hand **K** Subcutaneous Tissue and Fascia, Left Hand **L** Subcutaneous Tissue and Fascia, Right Upper Leg **M** Subcutaneous Tissue and Fascia, Left Upper Leg **N** Subcutaneous Tissue and Fascia, Right Lower Leg **P** Subcutaneous Tissue and Fascia, Left Lower Leg **Q** Subcutaneous Tissue and Fascia, Right Foot **R** Subcutaneous Tissue and Fascia, Left Foot	**0** Open **3** Percutaneous **X** External	**Z** No Device	**Z** No Qualifier

Section 0 **Medical and Surgical**
Body System J **Subcutaneous Tissue and Fascia**
Operation P **Removal:** Taking out or off a device from a body part

Body Part (4th)	Approach (5th)	Device (6th)	Qualifier (7th)
S Subcutaneous Tissue and Fascia, Head and Neck	**0** Open **3** Percutaneous	**0** Drainage Device **1** Radioactive Element **3** Infusion Device **7** Autologous Tissue Substitute **J** Synthetic Substitute **K** Nonautologous Tissue Substitute **N** Tissue Expander **Y** Other Device	**Z** No Qualifier
S Subcutaneous Tissue and Fascia, Head and Neck	**X** External	**0** Drainage Device **1** Radioactive Element **3** Infusion Device	**Z** No Qualifier

Continued→

ction	**0**	**Medical and Surgical**
dy System	**J**	**Subcutaneous Tissue and Fascia**
eration	**P**	**Removal:** Taking out or off a device from a body part

Body Part (4th)	Approach (5th)	Device (6th)	Qualifier (7th)
T Subcutaneous Tissue and Fascia, Trunk	**0** Open **3** Percutaneous	**0** Drainage Device **1** Radioactive Element **2** Monitoring Device **3** Infusion Device **7** Autologous Tissue Substitute **H** Contraceptive Device **J** Synthetic Substitute **K** Nonautologous Tissue Substitute **M** Stimulator Generator **N** Tissue Expander **P** Cardiac Rhythm Related Device **V** Infusion Device, Pump **W** Vascular Access Device, Totally Implantable **X** Vascular Access Device, Tunneled **Y** Other Device	**Z** No Qualifier
T Subcutaneous Tissue and Fascia, Trunk	**X** External	**0** Drainage Device **1** Radioactive Element **2** Monitoring Device **3** Infusion Device **H** Contraceptive Device **V** Infusion Device, Pump **X** Vascular Access Device, Tunneled	**Z** No Qualifier
V Subcutaneous Tissue and Fascia, Upper Extremity **W** Subcutaneous Tissue and Fascia, Lower Extremity	**0** Open **3** Percutaneous	**0** Drainage Device **1** Radioactive Element **3** Infusion Device **7** Autologous Tissue Substitute **H** Contraceptive Device **J** Synthetic Substitute **K** Nonautologous Tissue Substitute **N** Tissue Expander **V** Infusion Device, Pump **W** Vascular Access Device, Totally Implantable **X** Vascular Access Device, Tunneled **Y** Other Device	**Z** No Qualifier
V Subcutaneous Tissue and Fascia, Upper Extremity **W** Subcutaneous Tissue and Fascia, Lower Extremity	**X** External	**0** Drainage Device **1** Radioactive Element **3** Infusion Device **H** Contraceptive Device **V** Infusion Device, Pump **X** Vascular Access Device, Tunneled	**Z** No Qualifier

Section **0** **Medical and Surgical**
Body System **J** **Subcutaneous Tissue and Fascia**
Operation **Q** **Repair:** Restoring, to the extent possible, a body part to its normal anatomic structure and function

Body Part (4th)	Approach (5th)	Device (6th)	Qualifier (7th)
0 Subcutaneous Tissue and Fascia, Scalp **1** Subcutaneous Tissue and Fascia, Face **4** Subcutaneous Tissue and Fascia, Right Neck **5** Subcutaneous Tissue and Fascia, Left Neck **6** Subcutaneous Tissue and Fascia, Chest **7** Subcutaneous Tissue and Fascia, Back **8** Subcutaneous Tissue and Fascia, Abdomen **9** Subcutaneous Tissue and Fascia, Buttock **B** Subcutaneous Tissue and Fascia, Perineum **C** Subcutaneous Tissue and Fascia, Pelvic Region **D** Subcutaneous Tissue and Fascia, Right Upper Arm **F** Subcutaneous Tissue and Fascia, Left Upper Arm **G** Subcutaneous Tissue and Fascia, Right Lower Arm **H** Subcutaneous Tissue and Fascia, Left Lower Arm **J** Subcutaneous Tissue and Fascia, Right Hand **K** Subcutaneous Tissue and Fascia, Left Hand **L** Subcutaneous Tissue and Fascia, Right Upper Leg **M** Subcutaneous Tissue and Fascia, Left Upper Leg **N** Subcutaneous Tissue and Fascia, Right Lower Leg **P** Subcutaneous Tissue and Fascia, Left Lower Leg **Q** Subcutaneous Tissue and Fascia, Right Foot **R** Subcutaneous Tissue and Fascia, Left Foot	**0** Open **3** Percutaneous	**Z** No Device	**Z** No Qualifier

Section **0** **Medical and Surgical**
Body System **J** **Subcutaneous Tissue and Fascia**
Operation **R** **Replacement:** Putting in or on biological or synthetic material that physically takes the place and/or function of all or a portion of a body part

Body Part (4th)	Approach (5th)	Device (6th)	Qualifier (7th)
0 Subcutaneous Tissue and Fascia, Scalp **1** Subcutaneous Tissue and Fascia, Face **4** Subcutaneous Tissue and Fascia, Right Neck **5** Subcutaneous Tissue and Fascia, Left Neck **6** Subcutaneous Tissue and Fascia, Chest **7** Subcutaneous Tissue and Fascia, Back **8** Subcutaneous Tissue and Fascia, Abdomen **9** Subcutaneous Tissue and Fascia, Buttock **B** Subcutaneous Tissue and Fascia, Perineum **C** Subcutaneous Tissue and Fascia, Pelvic Region **D** Subcutaneous Tissue and Fascia, Right Upper Arm **F** Subcutaneous Tissue and Fascia, Left Upper Arm **G** Subcutaneous Tissue and Fascia, Right Lower Arm **H** Subcutaneous Tissue and Fascia, Left Lower Arm **J** Subcutaneous Tissue and Fascia, Right Hand **K** Subcutaneous Tissue and Fascia, Left Hand **L** Subcutaneous Tissue and Fascia, Right Upper Leg **M** Subcutaneous Tissue and Fascia, Left Upper Leg **N** Subcutaneous Tissue and Fascia, Right Lower Leg **P** Subcutaneous Tissue and Fascia, Left Lower Leg **Q** Subcutaneous Tissue and Fascia, Right Foot **R** Subcutaneous Tissue and Fascia, Left Foot	**0** Open **3** Percutaneous	**7** Autologous Tissue Substitute **J** Synthetic Substitute **K** Nonautologous Tissue Substitute	**Z** No Qualifier

tion	**0**	**Medical and Surgical**
dy System	**J**	**Subcutaneous Tissue and Fascia**
eration	**U**	**Supplement:** Putting in or on biological or synthetic material that physically reinforces and/or augments the function of a portion of a body part

Body Part (4th)	Approach (5th)	Device (6th)	Qualifier (7th)
Subcutaneous Tissue and Fascia, Scalp Subcutaneous Tissue and Fascia, Face Subcutaneous Tissue and Fascia, Right Neck Subcutaneous Tissue and Fascia, Left Neck Subcutaneous Tissue and Fascia, Chest Subcutaneous Tissue and Fascia, Back Subcutaneous Tissue and Fascia, Abdomen Subcutaneous Tissue and Fascia, Buttock B Subcutaneous Tissue and Fascia, Perineum C Subcutaneous Tissue and Fascia, Pelvic Region D Subcutaneous Tissue and Fascia, Right Upper Arm F Subcutaneous Tissue and Fascia, Left Upper Arm G Subcutaneous Tissue and Fascia, Right Lower Arm H Subcutaneous Tissue and Fascia, Left Lower Arm Subcutaneous Tissue and Fascia, Right Hand K Subcutaneous Tissue and Fascia, Left Hand L Subcutaneous Tissue and Fascia, Right Upper Leg M Subcutaneous Tissue and Fascia, Left Upper Leg N Subcutaneous Tissue and Fascia, Right Lower Leg P Subcutaneous Tissue and Fascia, Left Lower Leg Q Subcutaneous Tissue and Fascia, Right Foot R Subcutaneous Tissue and Fascia, Left Foot	**0** Open **3** Percutaneous	**7** Autologous Tissue Substitute **J** Synthetic Substitute **K** Nonautologous Tissue Substitute	**Z** No Qualifier

ction	**0**	**Medical and Surgical**
dy System	**J**	**Subcutaneous Tissue and Fascia**
eration	**W**	**Revision:** Correcting, to the extent possible, a portion of a malfunctioning device or the position of a displaced device

Body Part (4th)	Approach (5th)	Device (6th)	Qualifier (7th)
S Subcutaneous Tissue and Fascia, Head and Neck	**0** Open **3** Percutaneous	**0** Drainage Device **3** Infusion Device **7** Autologous Tissue Substitute **J** Synthetic Substitute **K** Nonautologous Tissue Substitute **N** Tissue Expander **Y** Other Device	**Z** No Qualifier
S Subcutaneous Tissue and Fascia, Head and Neck	**X** External	**0** Drainage Device **3** Infusion Device **7** Autologous Tissue Substitute **J** Synthetic Substitute **K** Nonautologous Tissue Substitute **N** Tissue Expander	**Z** No Qualifier
T Subcutaneous Tissue and Fascia, Trunk	**0** Open **3** Percutaneous	**0** Drainage Device **2** Monitoring Device **3** Infusion Device **7** Autologous Tissue Substitute **H** Contraceptive Device **J** Synthetic Substitute **K** Nonautologous Tissue Substitute **M** Stimulator Generator **N** Tissue Expander **P** Cardiac Rhythm Related Device **V** Infusion Device, Pump **W** Vascular Access Device, Totally Implantable **X** Vascular Access Device, Tunneled **Y** Other Device	**Z** No Qualifier

Continued →

Section 0 **Medical and Surgical**
Body System J **Subcutaneous Tissue and Fascia**
Operation W **Revision:** Correcting, to the extent possible, a portion of a malfunctioning device or the position of a displaced device

Body Part (4th)	Approach (5th)	Device (6th)	Qualifier (7th)
T Subcutaneous Tissue and Fascia, Trunk	**X** External	**0** Drainage Device **2** Monitoring Device **3** Infusion Device **7** Autologous Tissue Substitute **H** Contraceptive Device **J** Synthetic Substitute **K** Nonautologous Tissue Substitute **M** Stimulator Generator **N** Tissue Expander **P** Cardiac Rhythm Related Device **V** Infusion Device, Pump **W** Vascular Access Device, Totally Implantable **X** Vascular Access Device, Tunneled	**Z** No Qualifier
V Subcutaneous Tissue and Fascia, Upper Extremity **W** Subcutaneous Tissue and Fascia, Lower Extremity	**0** Open **3** Percutaneous	**0** Drainage Device **3** Infusion Device **7** Autologous Tissue Substitute **H** Contraceptive Device **J** Synthetic Substitute **K** Nonautologous Tissue Substitute **N** Tissue Expander **V** Infusion Device, Pump **W** Vascular Access Device, Totally Implantable **X** Vascular Access Device, Tunneled **Y** Other Device	**Z** No Qualifier
V Subcutaneous Tissue and Fascia, Upper Extremity **W** Subcutaneous Tissue and Fascia, Lower Extremity	**X** External	**0** Drainage Device **3** Infusion Device **7** Autologous Tissue Substitute **H** Contraceptive Device **J** Synthetic Substitute **K** Nonautologous Tissue Substitute **N** Tissue Expander **V** Infusion Device, Pump **W** Vascular Access Device, Totally Implantable **X** Vascular Access Device, Tunneled	**Z** No Qualifier

Section 0 **Medical and Surgical**
Body System J **Subcutaneous Tissue and Fascia**
Operation X **Transfer:** Moving, without taking out, all or a portion of a body part to another location to take over the function of all c portion of a body part

Body Part (4th)	Approach (5th)	Device (6th)	Qualifier (7th)
0 Subcutaneous Tissue and Fascia, Scalp **1** Subcutaneous Tissue and Fascia, Face **4** Subcutaneous Tissue and Fascia, Right Neck **5** Subcutaneous Tissue and Fascia, Left Neck **6** Subcutaneous Tissue and Fascia, Chest **7** Subcutaneous Tissue and Fascia, Back **8** Subcutaneous Tissue and Fascia, Abdomen **9** Subcutaneous Tissue and Fascia, Buttock **B** Subcutaneous Tissue and Fascia, Perineum **C** Subcutaneous Tissue and Fascia, Pelvic Region **D** Subcutaneous Tissue and Fascia, Right Upper Arm **F** Subcutaneous Tissue and Fascia, Left Upper Arm **G** Subcutaneous Tissue and Fascia, Right Lower Arm **H** Subcutaneous Tissue and Fascia, Left Lower Arm **J** Subcutaneous Tissue and Fascia, Right Hand **K** Subcutaneous Tissue and Fascia, Left Hand **L** Subcutaneous Tissue and Fascia, Right Upper Leg **M** Subcutaneous Tissue and Fascia, Left Upper Leg **N** Subcutaneous Tissue and Fascia, Right Lower Leg **P** Subcutaneous Tissue and Fascia, Left Lower Leg **Q** Subcutaneous Tissue and Fascia, Right Foot **R** Subcutaneous Tissue and Fascia, Left Foot	**0** Open **3** Percutaneous	**Z** No Device	**B** Skin and Subcutaneous Tissue **C** Skin, Subcutaneous Tissue and Fascia **Z** No Qualifier

HA Coding Clinic

J2TXYZ Change Other Device in Trunk Subcutaneous Tissue and Fascia, External Approach—AHA CC: 2Q, 2017, 26

J960ZZ Drainage of Chest Subcutaneous Tissue and Fascia, Open Approach—AHA CC: 3Q, 2015, 23-24

J9C0ZZ Drainage of Pelvic Region Subcutaneous Tissue and Fascia, Open Approach—AHA CC: 3Q, 2015, 23-24

J9D0ZZ Drainage of Right Upper Arm Subcutaneous Tissue and Fascia, Open Approach—AHA CC: 3Q, 2015, 23-24

J9F0ZZ Drainage of Left Upper Arm Subcutaneous Tissue and Fascia, Open Approach—AHA CC: 3Q, 2015, 23-24

J9L0ZZ Drainage of Right Upper Leg Subcutaneous Tissue and Fascia, Open Approach—AHA CC: 3Q, 2015, 23-24

J9M0ZZ Drainage of Left Upper Leg Subcutaneous Tissue and Fascia, Open Approach—AHA CC: 3Q, 2015, 23-24

JB70ZZ Excision of Back Subcutaneous Tissue and Fascia, Open Approach—AHA CC: 1Q, 2018, 7-8

JB80ZZ Excision of Abdomen Subcutaneous Tissue and Fascia, Open Approach—AHA CC: 3Q, 2014, 22-23; 4Q, 2014, 39-40

JB90ZZ Excision of Buttock Subcutaneous Tissue and Fascia, Open Approach—AHA CC: 3Q, 2015, 6-7

JBB0ZZ Excision of Perineum Subcutaneous Tissue and Fascia, Open Approach—AHA CC: 1Q, 2015, 29-30

JBH0ZZ Excision of Left Lower Arm Subcutaneous Tissue and Fascia, Open Approach—AHA CC: 2Q, 2015, 13

JC80ZZ Extirpation of Matter from Abdomen Subcutaneous Tissue and Fascia, Open Approach—AHA CC: 3Q, 2017, 22

JD70ZZ Extraction of Back Subcutaneous Tissue and Fascia, Open Approach—AHA CC: 3Q, 2016, 21

JDC0ZZ Extraction of Pelvic Region Subcutaneous Tissue and Fascia, Open Approach—AHA CC: 1Q, 2015, 23

JDL0ZZ Extraction of Right Upper Leg Subcutaneous Tissue and Fascia, Open Approach—AHA CC: 1Q, 2016, 40

JDN0ZZ Extraction of Right Lower Leg Subcutaneous Tissue and Fascia, Open Approach—AHA CC: 3Q, 2016, 20-21

JDR0ZZ Extraction of Left Foot Subcutaneous Tissue and Fascia, Open Approach—AHA CC: 3Q, 2016, 22

JH608Z Insertion of Defibrillator Generator into Chest Subcutaneous Tissue and Fascia, Open Approach—AHA CC: 4Q, 2012, 104-106

JH60MZ Insertion of Stimulator Generator into Chest Subcutaneous Tissue and Fascia, Open Approach—AHA CC: 4Q, 2016, 98-99

JH60PZ Insertion of Cardiac Rhythm Related Device into Chest Subcutaneous Tissue and Fascia, Open Approach—AHA CC: 4Q, 2012, 104-106

JH60WZ Insertion of Totally Implantable Vascular Access Device into Chest Subcutaneous Tissue and Fascia, Open Approach—AHA CC: 4Q, 2017, 63-64

JH60XZ Insertion of Tunneled Vascular Access Device into Chest Subcutaneous Tissue and Fascia, Open Approach—AHA CC: 2Q, 2015, 33-34

JH63VZ Insertion of Infusion Pump into Chest Subcutaneous Tissue and Fascia, Percutaneous Approach—AHA CC: 4Q, 2015, 14-15

JH63XZ Insertion of Tunneled Vascular Access Device into Chest Subcutaneous Tissue and Fascia, Percutaneous Approach—AHA CC: 2Q, 2015, 33-34; 4q, 2015, 30-32; 2Q, 2016, 15-16; 2Q, 2017, 24-26

JH80VZ Insertion of Infusion Pump into Abdomen Subcutaneous Tissue and Fascia, Open Approach—AHA CC: 3Q, 2014, 19-20

JH80WZ Insertion of Totally Implantable Vascular Access Device into Abdomen Subcutaneous Tissue and Fascia, Open Approach—AHA CC: 2Q, 2016, 14

JNL0ZZ Release Right Upper Leg Subcutaneous Tissue and Fascia, Open Approach—AHA CC: 3Q, 2017, 11-12

JNM0ZZ Release Left Upper Leg Subcutaneous Tissue and Fascia, Open Approach—AHA CC: 3Q, 2017, 11-12

JNN0ZZ Release Right Lower Leg Subcutaneous Tissue and Fascia, Open Approach—AHA CC: 3Q, 2017, 11-12

JNP0ZZ Release Left Lower Leg Subcutaneous Tissue and Fascia, Open Approach—AHA CC: 3Q, 2017, 11-12

JNQ0ZZ Release Right Foot Subcutaneous Tissue and Fascia, Open Approach—AHA CC: 3Q, 2017, 11-12

JNR0ZZ Release Left Foot Subcutaneous Tissue and Fascia, Open Approach—AHA CC: 3Q, 2017, 11-12

JPT0NZ Removal of Tissue Expander from Trunk Subcutaneous Tissue and Fascia, Open Approach—AHA CC: 4Q, 2013, 109-111

JPT0PZ Removal of Cardiac Rhythm Related Device from Trunk Subcutaneous Tissue and Fascia, Open Approach—AHA CC: 4Q, 2012, 104-106

JPT0VZ Removal of Infusion Pump from Trunk Subcutaneous Tissue and Fascia, Open Approach—AHA CC: 3Q, 2014, 19-20

JPT0XZ Removal of Tunneled Vascular Access Device from Trunk Subcutaneous Tissue and Fascia, Open Approach—AHA CC: 4Q, 2015, 31-32; 2Q, 2016, 15-16

JQC0ZZ Repair Pelvic Region Subcutaneous Tissue and Fascia, Open Approach—AHA CC: 4Q, 2014, 44-45; 3Q, 2017, 19

JR107Z Replacement of Face Subcutaneous Tissue and Fascia with Autologous Tissue Substitute, Open Approach—AHA CC: 2Q, 2015, 13

JU707Z Supplement of Back Subcutaneous Tissue and Fascia with Autologous Tissue Substitute, Open Approach—AHA CC: 1Q, 2018, 7-8

JUH0KZ Supplement of Left Lower Arm Subcutaneous Tissue and Fascia with Nonautologous Tissue Substitute, Open Approach—AHA CC: 2Q, 2018, 20

0JWS0JZ Revision of Synthetic Substitute in Head and Neck Subcutaneous Tissue and Fascia, Open Approach—AHA CC: 2Q, 2015, 9-

0JWT0JZ Revision of Synthetic Substitute in Trunk Subcutaneous Tissue and Fascia, Open Approach— AHA CC: 1Q, 2018, 8-9

0JWT0PZ Revision of Cardiac Rhythm Related Device in Trunk Subcutaneous Tissue and Fascia, Open Approach—AHA CC: 4Q, 201 104-106

0JWT33Z Revision of Infusion Device in Trunk Subcutaneous Tissue and Fascia, Percutaneous Approach—AHA CC: 4Q, 2015, 33

0JX00ZC Transfer Scalp Subcutaneous Tissue and Fascia with Skin, Subcutaneous Tissue and Fascia, Open Approach—AHA CC: 1 2018, 10

0JX60ZB Transfer Chest Subcutaneous Tissue and Fascia with Skin and Subcutaneous Tissue, Open Approach—AHA CC: 4Q, 201 109-111

0JX80ZB Transfer Abdomen Subcutaneous Tissue and Fascia with Skin and Subcutaneous Tissue, Open Approach—AHA CC: 4Q, 201 109-111

0JXN0ZC Transfer Right Lower Leg Subcutaneous Tissue and Fascia with Skin, Subcutaneous Tissue and Fascia, Open Approach—AH CC: 3Q, 2014, 18-19

Muscles

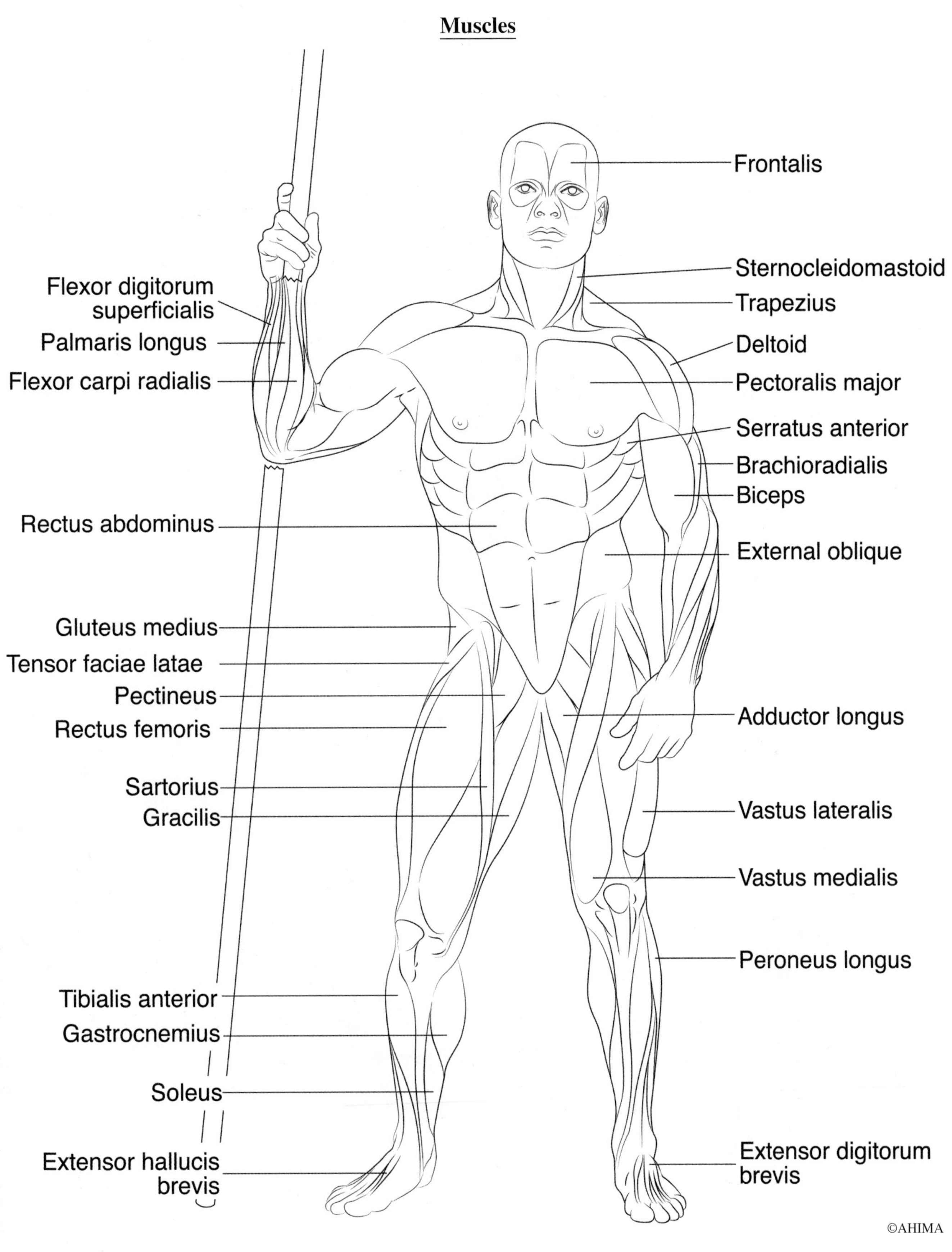
Frontalis
Sternocleidomastoid
Trapezius
Deltoid
Pectoralis major
Serratus anterior
Brachioradialis
Biceps
External oblique
Adductor longus
Vastus lateralis
Vastus medialis
Peroneus longus
Extensor digitorum brevis
Flexor digitorum superficialis
Palmaris longus
Flexor carpi radialis
Rectus abdominus
Gluteus medius
Tensor faciae latae
Pectineus
Rectus femoris
Sartorius
Gracilis
Tibialis anterior
Gastrocnemius
Soleus
Extensor hallucis brevis

Muscles of the Hand

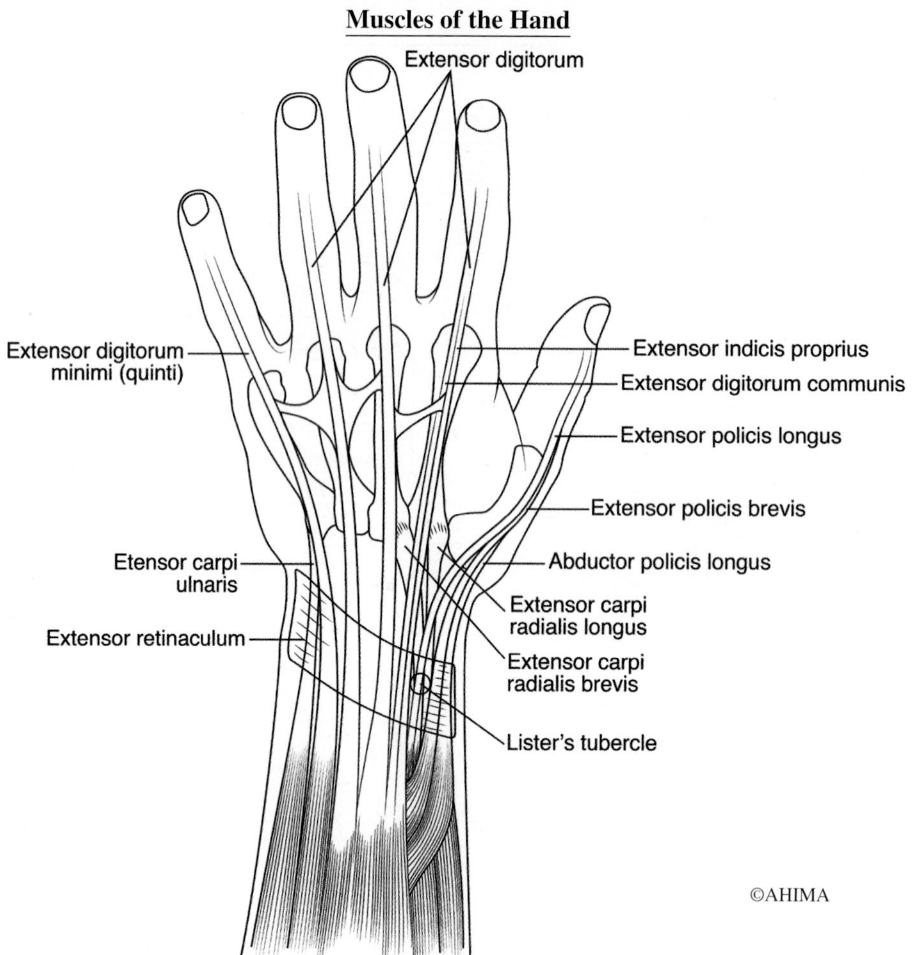

Muscles of the Foot

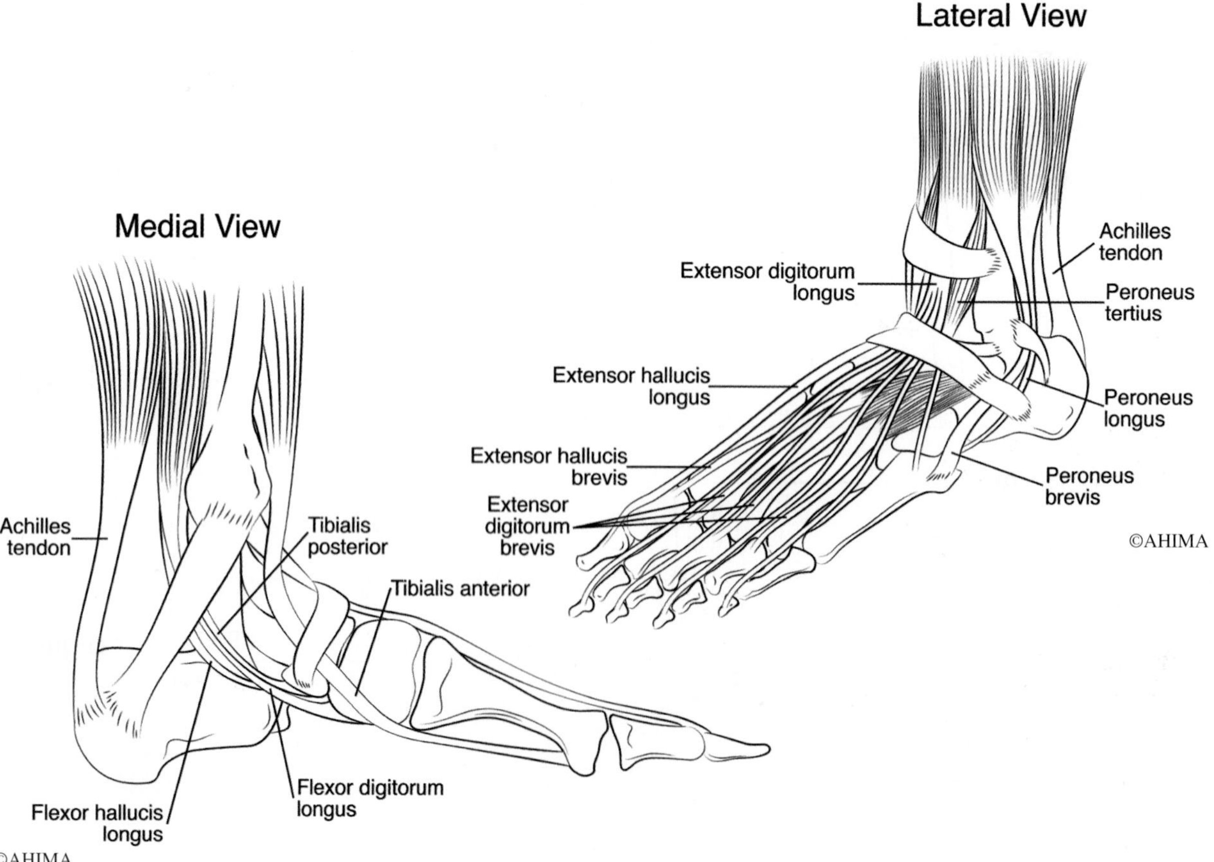

Section	0	**Medical and Surgical**
Body System	K	**Muscles**
Operation	2	**Change:** Taking out or off a device from a body part and putting back an identical or similar device in or on the same body part without cutting or puncturing the skin or a mucous membrane

Body Part (4th)	Approach (5th)	Device (6th)	Qualifier (7th)
X Upper Muscle Y Lower Muscle	X External	0 Drainage Device Y Other Device	Z No Qualifier

Section	0	**Medical and Surgical**
Body System	K	**Muscles**
Operation	5	**Destruction:** Physical eradication of all or a portion of a body part by the direct use of energy, force, or a destructive agent

Body Part (4th)	Approach (5th)	Device (6th)	Qualifier (7th)
0 Head Muscle 1 Facial Muscle 2 Neck Muscle, Right 3 Neck Muscle, Left 4 Tongue, Palate, Pharynx Muscle 5 Shoulder Muscle, Right 6 Shoulder Muscle, Left 7 Upper Arm Muscle, Right 8 Upper Arm Muscle, Left 9 Lower Arm and Wrist Muscle, Right B Lower Arm and Wrist Muscle, Left C Hand Muscle, Right D Hand Muscle, Left F Trunk Muscle, Right G Trunk Muscle, Left H Thorax Muscle, Right J Thorax Muscle, Left K Abdomen Muscle, Right L Abdomen Muscle, Left M Perineum Muscle N Hip Muscle, Right P Hip Muscle, Left Q Upper Leg Muscle, Right R Upper Leg Muscle, Left S Lower Leg Muscle, Right T Lower Leg Muscle, Left V Foot Muscle, Right W Foot Muscle, Left	0 Open 3 Percutaneous 4 Percutaneous Endoscopic	Z No Device	Z No Qualifier

Section 0 **Medical and Surgical**
Body System K **Muscles**
Operation 8 **Division:** Cutting into a body part, without draining fluids and/or gases from the body part, in order to separate or transec body part

Body Part (4th)	Approach (5th)	Device (6th)	Qualifier (7th)
0 Head Muscle **1** Facial Muscle **2** Neck Muscle, Right **3** Neck Muscle, Left **4** Tongue, Palate, Pharynx Muscle **5** Shoulder Muscle, Right **6** Shoulder Muscle, Left **7** Upper Arm Muscle, Right **8** Upper Arm Muscle, Left **9** Lower Arm and Wrist Muscle, Right **B** Lower Arm and Wrist Muscle, Left **C** Hand Muscle, Right **D** Hand Muscle, Left **F** Trunk Muscle, Right **G** Trunk Muscle, Left **H** Thorax Muscle, Right **J** Thorax Muscle, Left **K** Abdomen Muscle, Right **L** Abdomen Muscle, Left **M** Perineum Muscle **N** Hip Muscle, Right **P** Hip Muscle, Left **Q** Upper Leg Muscle, Right **R** Upper Leg Muscle, Left **S** Lower Leg Muscle, Right **T** Lower Leg Muscle, Left **V** Foot Muscle, Right **W** Foot Muscle, Left	**0** Open **3** Percutaneous **4** Percutaneous Endoscopic	**Z** No Device	**Z** No Qualifier

ction	**0**	**Medical and Surgical**
dy System	**K**	**Muscles**
eration	**9**	**Drainage:** Taking or letting out fluids and/or gases from a body part

Body Part (4th)	Approach (5th)	Device (6th)	Qualifier (7th)
0 Head Muscle **1** Facial Muscle **2** Neck Muscle, Right **3** Neck Muscle, Left **4** Tongue, Palate, Pharynx Muscle **5** Shoulder Muscle, Right **6** Shoulder Muscle, Left **7** Upper Arm Muscle, Right **8** Upper Arm Muscle, Left **9** Lower Arm and Wrist Muscle, Right **B** Lower Arm and Wrist Muscle, Left **C** Hand Muscle, Right **D** Hand Muscle, Left **F** Trunk Muscle, Right **G** Trunk Muscle, Left **H** Thorax Muscle, Right **J** Thorax Muscle, Left **K** Abdomen Muscle, Right **L** Abdomen Muscle, Left **M** Perineum Muscle **N** Hip Muscle, Right **P** Hip Muscle, Left **Q** Upper Leg Muscle, Right **R** Upper Leg Muscle, Left **S** Lower Leg Muscle, Right **T** Lower Leg Muscle, Left **V** Foot Muscle, Right **W** Foot Muscle, Left	**0** Open **3** Percutaneous **4** Percutaneous Endoscopic	**0** Drainage Device	**Z** No Qualifier
0 Head Muscle **1** Facial Muscle **2** Neck Muscle, Right **3** Neck Muscle, Left **4** Tongue, Palate, Pharynx Muscle **5** Shoulder Muscle, Right **6** Shoulder Muscle, Left **7** Upper Arm Muscle, Right **8** Upper Arm Muscle, Left **9** Lower Arm and Wrist Muscle, Right **B** Lower Arm and Wrist Muscle, Left **C** Hand Muscle, Right **D** Hand Muscle, Left **F** Trunk Muscle, Right **G** Trunk Muscle, Left **H** Thorax Muscle, Right **J** Thorax Muscle, Left **K** Abdomen Muscle, Right **L** Abdomen Muscle, Left **M** Perineum Muscle **N** Hip Muscle, Right **P** Hip Muscle, Left **Q** Upper Leg Muscle, Right **R** Upper Leg Muscle, Left **S** Lower Leg Muscle, Right **T** Lower Leg Muscle, Left **V** Foot Muscle, Right **W** Foot Muscle, Left	**0** Open **3** Percutaneous **4** Percutaneous Endoscopic	**Z** No Device	**X** Diagnostic **Z** No Qualifier

Section 0 **Medical and Surgical**
Body System K **Muscles**
Operation B **Excision:** Cutting out or off, without replacement, a portion of a body part

Body Part (4th)	Approach (5th)	Device (6th)	Qualifier (7th)
0 Head Muscle **1** Facial Muscle **2** Neck Muscle, Right **3** Neck Muscle, Left **4** Tongue, Palate, Pharynx Muscle **5** Shoulder Muscle, Right **6** Shoulder Muscle, Left **7** Upper Arm Muscle, Right **8** Upper Arm Muscle, Left **9** Lower Arm and Wrist Muscle, Right **B** Lower Arm and Wrist Muscle, Left **C** Hand Muscle, Right **D** Hand Muscle, Left **F** Trunk Muscle, Right **G** Trunk Muscle, Left **H** Thorax Muscle, Right **J** Thorax Muscle, Left **K** Abdomen Muscle, Right **L** Abdomen Muscle, Left **M** Perineum Muscle **N** Hip Muscle, Right **P** Hip Muscle, Left **Q** Upper Leg Muscle, Right **R** Upper Leg Muscle, Left **S** Lower Leg Muscle, Right **T** Lower Leg Muscle, Left **V** Foot Muscle, Right **W** Foot Muscle, Left	**0** Open **3** Percutaneous **4** Percutaneous Endoscopic	**Z** No Device	**X** Diagnostic **Z** No Qualifier

Section 0 **Medical and Surgical**
Body System K **Muscles**
Operation C **Extirpation:** Taking or cutting out solid matter from a body part

Body Part (4th)	Approach (5th)	Device (6th)	Qualifier (7th)
0 Head Muscle **1** Facial Muscle **2** Neck Muscle, Right **3** Neck Muscle, Left **4** Tongue, Palate, Pharynx Muscle **5** Shoulder Muscle, Right **6** Shoulder Muscle, Left **7** Upper Arm Muscle, Right **8** Upper Arm Muscle, Left **9** Lower Arm and Wrist Muscle, Right **B** Lower Arm and Wrist Muscle, Left **C** Hand Muscle, Right **D** Hand Muscle, Left **F** Trunk Muscle, Right **G** Trunk Muscle, Left **H** Thorax Muscle, Right **J** Thorax Muscle, Left **K** Abdomen Muscle, Right **L** Abdomen Muscle, Left **M** Perineum Muscle **N** Hip Muscle, Right **P** Hip Muscle, Left **Q** Upper Leg Muscle, Right **R** Upper Leg Muscle, Left **S** Lower Leg Muscle, Right **T** Lower Leg Muscle, Left **V** Foot Muscle, Right **W** Foot Muscle, Left	**0** Open **3** Percutaneous **4** Percutaneous Endoscopic	**Z** No Device	**Z** No Qualifier

on **0** **Medical and Surgical**
System **K** **Muscles**
ation **D** **Extirpation:** Pulling or stripping out or off all or a portion of a body part by the use of force

Body Part (4th)	Approach (5th)	Device (6th)	Qualifier (7th)
Head Muscle Facial Muscle Neck Muscle, Right Neck Muscle, Left Tongue, Palate, Pharynx Muscle Shoulder Muscle, Right Shoulder Muscle, Left Upper Arm Muscle, Right Upper Arm Muscle, Left Lower Arm and Wrist Muscle, Right Lower Arm and Wrist Muscle, Left Hand Muscle, Right Hand Muscle, Left Trunk Muscle, Right Trunk Muscle, Left Thorax Muscle, Right Thorax Muscle, Left Abdomen Muscle, Right Abdomen Muscle, Left Perineum Hip Muscle, Right Hip Muscle, Left Upper Leg Muscle, Right Upper Leg Muscle, Left Lower Leg Muscle, Right Lower Leg Muscle, Left Foot Muscle, Right Foot Muscle, Left	**0** Open	**Z** No Device	**Z** No Qualifier

ion **0** **Medical and Surgical**
System **K** **Muscles**
ration **H** **Insertion:** Putting in a nonbiological appliance that monitors, assists, performs, or prevents a physiological function but does not physically take the place of a body part

Body Part (4th)	Approach (5th)	Device (6th)	Qualifier (7th)
Upper Muscle Lower Muscle	**0** Open **3** Percutaneous **4** Percutaneous Endoscopic	**M** Stimulator Lead **Y** Other Device	**Z** No Qualifier

ion **0** **Medical and Surgical**
y System **K** **Muscles**
ration **J** **Inspection:** Visually and/or manually exploring a body part

Body Part (4th)	Approach (5th)	Device (6th)	Qualifier (7th)
Upper Muscle Lower Muscle	**0** Open **3** Percutaneous **4** Percutaneous Endoscopic **X** External	**Z** No Device	**Z** No Qualifier

Section 0 **Medical and Surgical**
Body System K **Muscles**
Operation M **Reattachment:** Putting back in or on all or a portion of a separated body part to its normal location or other suitable loc

Body Part (4th)	Approach (5th)	Device (6th)	Qualifier (7th)
0 Head Muscle **1** Facial Muscle **2** Neck Muscle, Right **3** Neck Muscle, Left **4** Tongue, Palate, Pharynx Muscle **5** Shoulder Muscle, Right **6** Shoulder Muscle, Left **7** Upper Arm Muscle, Right **8** Upper Arm Muscle, Left **9** Lower Arm and Wrist Muscle, Right **B** Lower Arm and Wrist Muscle, Left **C** Hand Muscle, Right **D** Hand Muscle, Left **F** Trunk Muscle, Right **G** Trunk Muscle, Left **H** Thorax Muscle, Right **J** Thorax Muscle, Left **K** Abdomen Muscle, Right **L** Abdomen Muscle, Left **M** Perineum Muscle **N** Hip Muscle, Right **P** Hip Muscle, Left **Q** Upper Leg Muscle, Right **R** Upper Leg Muscle, Left **S** Lower Leg Muscle, Right **T** Lower Leg Muscle, Left **V** Foot Muscle, Right **W** Foot Muscle, Left	**0** Open **4** Percutaneous Endoscopic	**Z** No Device	**Z** No Qualifier

Section 0 **Medical and Surgical**
Body System K **Muscles**
Operation N **Release:** Freeing a body part from an abnormal physical constraint by cutting or by the use of force

Body Part (4th)	Approach (5th)	Device (6th)	Qualifier (7th)
0 Head Muscle **1** Facial Muscle **2** Neck Muscle, Right **3** Neck Muscle, Left **4** Tongue, Palate, Pharynx Muscle **5** Shoulder Muscle, Right **6** Shoulder Muscle, Left **7** Upper Arm Muscle, Right **8** Upper Arm Muscle, Left **9** Lower Arm and Wrist Muscle, Right **B** Lower Arm and Wrist Muscle, Left **C** Hand Muscle, Right **D** Hand Muscle, Left **F** Trunk Muscle, Right **G** Trunk Muscle, Left **H** Thorax Muscle, Right **J** Thorax Muscle, Left **K** Abdomen Muscle, Right **L** Abdomen Muscle, Left **M** Perineum Muscle **N** Hip Muscle, Right **P** Hip Muscle, Left **Q** Upper Leg Muscle, Right **R** Upper Leg Muscle, Left **S** Lower Leg Muscle, Right **T** Lower Leg Muscle, Left **V** Foot Muscle, Right **W** Foot Muscle, Left	**0** Open **3** Percutaneous **4** Percutaneous Endoscopic **X** External	**Z** No Device	**Z** No Qualifier

tion 0 **Medical and Surgical**
dy System K **Muscles**
eration P **Removal:** Taking out or off a device from a body part

Body Part (4th)	Approach (5th)	Device (6th)	Qualifier (7th)
X Upper Muscle Y Lower Muscle	**0** Open **3** Percutaneous **4** Percutaneous Endoscopic	**0** Drainage Device **7** Autologous Tissue Substitute **J** Synthetic Substitute **K** Nonautologous Tissue Substitute **M** Stimulator Lead **Y** Other Device	**Z** No Qualifier
X Upper Muscle Y Lower Muscle	**X** External	**0** Drainage Device **M** Stimulator Lead	**Z** No Qualifier

ction 0 **Medical and Surgical**
dy System K **Muscles**
eration Q **Repair:** Restoring, to the extent possible, a body part to its normal anatomic structure and function

Body Part (4th)	Approach (5th)	Device (6th)	Qualifier (7th)
0 Head Muscle 1 Facial Muscle 2 Neck Muscle, Right 3 Neck Muscle, Left 4 Tongue, Palate, Pharynx Muscle 5 Shoulder Muscle, Right 6 Shoulder Muscle, Left 7 Upper Arm Muscle, Right 8 Upper Arm Muscle, Left 9 Lower Arm and Wrist Muscle, Right B Lower Arm and Wrist Muscle, Left C Hand Muscle, Right D Hand Muscle, Left F Trunk Muscle, Right G Trunk Muscle, Left H Thorax Muscle, Right J Thorax Muscle, Left K Abdomen Muscle, Right L Abdomen Muscle, Left M Perineum Muscle N Hip Muscle, Right P Hip Muscle, Left Q Upper Leg Muscle, Right R Upper Leg Muscle, Left S Lower Leg Muscle, Right T Lower Leg Muscle, Left V Foot Muscle, Right W Foot Muscle, Left	**0** Open **3** Percutaneous **4** Percutaneous Endoscopic	**Z** No Device	**Z** No Qualifier

Section 0 **Medical and Surgical**
Body System K **Muscles**
Operation R **Replacement:** Putting in or on biological or synthetic material that physically takes the place and/or function of all or a portion of a body part

Body Part (4th)	Approach (5th)	Device (6th)	Qualifier (7th)
0 Head Muscle **1** Facial Muscle **2** Neck Muscle, Right **3** Neck Muscle, Left **4** Tongue, Palate, Pharynx Muscle **5** Shoulder Muscle, Right **6** Shoulder Muscle, Left **7** Upper Arm Muscle, Right **8** Upper Arm Muscle, Left **9** Lower Arm and Wrist Muscle, Right **B** Lower Arm and Wrist Muscle, Left **C** Hand Muscle, Right **D** Hand Muscle, Left **F** Trunk Muscle, Right **G** Trunk Muscle, Left **H** Thorax Muscle, Right **J** Thorax Muscle, Left **K** Abdomen Muscle, Right **L** Abdomen Muscle, Left **M** Perineum **N** Hip Muscle, Right **P** Hip Muscle, Left **Q** Upper Leg Muscle, Right **R** Upper Leg Muscle, Left **S** Lower Leg Muscle, Right **T** Lower Leg Muscle, Left **V** Foot Muscle, Right **W** Foot Muscle, Left	**0** Open **4** Percutaneous Endoscopic	**7** Autologous Tissue Substitute **J** Synthetic Substitute **K** Nonautologous Tissue Substitute	**Z** No Qualifier

Section 0 **Medical and Surgical**
Body System K **Muscles**
Operation S **Reposition:** Moving to its normal location, or other suitable location, all or a portion of a body part

Body Part (4th)	Approach (5th)	Device (6th)	Qualifier (7th)
0 Head Muscle **1** Facial Muscle **2** Neck Muscle, Right **3** Neck Muscle, Left **4** Tongue, Palate, Pharynx Muscle **5** Shoulder Muscle, Right **6** Shoulder Muscle, Left **7** Upper Arm Muscle, Right **8** Upper Arm Muscle, Left **9** Lower Arm and Wrist Muscle, Right **B** Lower Arm and Wrist Muscle, Left **C** Hand Muscle, Right **D** Hand Muscle, Left **F** Trunk Muscle, Right **G** Trunk Muscle, Left **H** Thorax Muscle, Right **J** Thorax Muscle, Left **K** Abdomen Muscle, Right **L** Abdomen Muscle, Left **M** Perineum Muscle **N** Hip Muscle, Right **P** Hip Muscle, Left **Q** Upper Leg Muscle, Right **R** Upper Leg Muscle, Left **S** Lower Leg Muscle, Right **T** Lower Leg Muscle, Left **V** Foot Muscle, Right **W** Foot Muscle, Left	**0** Open **4** Percutaneous Endoscopic	**Z** No Device	**Z** No Qualifier

tion	**0**	**Medical and Surgical**
dy System	**K**	**Muscles**
eration	**T**	**Resection:** Cutting out or off, without replacement, all of a body part

Body Part (4th)	Approach (5th)	Device (6th)	Qualifier (7th)
0 Head Muscle **1** Facial Muscle **2** Neck Muscle, Right **3** Neck Muscle, Left **4** Tongue, Palate, Pharynx Muscle **5** Shoulder Muscle, Right **6** Shoulder Muscle, Left **7** Upper Arm Muscle, Right **8** Upper Arm Muscle, Left **9** Lower Arm and Wrist Muscle, Right **B** Lower Arm and Wrist Muscle, Left **C** Hand Muscle, Right **D** Hand Muscle, Left **F** Trunk Muscle, Right **G** Trunk Muscle, Left **H** Thorax Muscle, Right **J** Thorax Muscle, Left **K** Abdomen Muscle, Right **L** Abdomen Muscle, Left **M** Perineum Muscle **N** Hip Muscle, Right **P** Hip Muscle, Left **Q** Upper Leg Muscle, Right **R** Upper Leg Muscle, Left **S** Lower Leg Muscle, Right **T** Lower Leg Muscle, Left **V** Foot Muscle, Right **W** Foot Muscle, Left	**0** Open **4** Percutaneous Endoscopic	**Z** No Device	**Z** No Qualifier

ction	**0**	**Medical and Surgical**
dy System	**K**	**Muscles**
eration	**U**	**Supplement:** Putting in or on biological or synthetic material that physically reinforces and/or augments the function of a portion of a body part

Body Part (4th)	Approach (5th)	Device (6th)	Qualifier (7th)
0 Head Muscle **1** Facial Muscle **2** Neck Muscle, Right **3** Neck Muscle, Left **4** Tongue, Palate, Pharynx Muscle **5** Shoulder Muscle, Right **6** Shoulder Muscle, Left **7** Upper Arm Muscle, Right **8** Upper Arm Muscle, Left **9** Lower Arm and Wrist Muscle, Right **B** Lower Arm and Wrist Muscle, Left **C** Hand Muscle, Right **D** Hand Muscle, Left **F** Trunk Muscle, Right **G** Trunk Muscle, Left **H** Thorax Muscle, Right **J** Thorax Muscle, Left **K** Abdomen Muscle, Right **L** Abdomen Muscle, Left **M** Perineum Muscle **N** Hip Muscle, Right **P** Hip Muscle, Left **Q** Upper Leg Muscle, Right **R** Upper Leg Muscle, Left **S** Lower Leg Muscle, Right **T** Lower Leg Muscle, Left **V** Foot Muscle, Right **W** Foot Muscle, Left	**0** Open **4** Percutaneous Endoscopic	**7** Autologous Tissue Substitute **J** Synthetic Substitute **K** Nonautologous Tissue Substitute	**Z** No Qualifier

Section 0 **Medical and Surgical**
Body System K **Muscles**
Operation W **Revision:** Correcting, to the extent possible, a portion of a malfunctioning device or the position of a displaced device

Body Part (4th)	Approach (5th)	Device (6th)	Qualifier (7th)
X Upper Muscle **Y** Lower Muscle	**0** Open **3** Percutaneous **4** Percutaneous Endoscopic	**0** Drainage Device **7** Autologous Tissue Substitute **J** Synthetic Substitute **K** Nonautologous Tissue Substitute **M** Stimulator Lead **Y** Other Device	**Z** No Qualifier
X Upper Muscle **Y** Lower Muscle	**X** External	**0** Drainage Device **7** Autologous Tissue Substitute **J** Synthetic Substitute **K** Nonautologous Tissue Substitute **M** Stimulator Lead	**Z** No Qualifier

Section 0 **Medical and Surgical**
Body System K **Muscles**
Operation X **Transfer:** Moving, without taking out, all or a portion of a body part to another location to take over the function of all or a portion of a body part

Body Part (4th)	Approach (5th)	Device (6th)	Qualifier (7th)
0 Head Muscle **1** Facial Muscle **2** Neck Muscle, Right **3** Neck Muscle, Left **4** Tongue, Palate, Pharynx Muscle **5** Shoulder Muscle, Right **6** Shoulder Muscle, Left **7** Upper Arm Muscle, Right **8** Upper Arm Muscle, Left **9** Lower Arm and Wrist Muscle, Right **B** Lower Arm and Wrist Muscle, Left **C** Hand Muscle, Right **D** Hand Muscle, Left **H** Thorax Muscle, Right **J** Thorax Muscle, Left **M** Perineum Muscle **N** Hip Muscle, Right **P** Hip Muscle, Left **Q** Upper Leg Muscle, Right **R** Upper Leg Muscle, Left **S** Lower Leg Muscle, Right **T** Lower Leg Muscle, Left **V** Foot Muscle, Right **W** Foot Muscle, Left	**0** Open **4** Percutaneous Endoscopic	**Z** No Device	**0** Skin **1** Subcutaneous Tissue **2** Skin and Subcutaneous Tissue **Z** No Qualifier
F Trunk Muscle, Right **G** Trunk Muscle, Left	**0** Open **4** Percutaneous Endoscopic	**Z** No Device	**0** Skin **1** Subcutaneous Tissue **2** Skin and Subcutaneous Tissue **5** Latissimus Dorsi Myocutaneous Flap **7** Deep Inferior Epigastric Artery Perforator Flap **8** Superficial Inferior Epigastric Artery Flap **9** Gluteal Artery Perforator Flap **Z** No Qualifier
K Abdomen Muscle, Right **L** Abdomen Muscle, Left	**0** Open **4** Percutaneous Endoscopic	**Z** No Device	**0** Skin **1** Subcutaneous Tissue **2** Skin and Subcutaneous Tissue **6** Transverse Rectus Abdominis Myocutaneous Flap **Z** No Qualifier

HA Coding Clinic

KBN0ZZ Excision of Right Hip Muscle, Open Approach—AHA CC: 3Q, 2016, 20
KBP0ZZ Excision of Left Hip Muscle, Open Approach—AHA CC: 3Q, 2016, 20
KDS0ZZ Extraction of Right Lower Leg Muscle, Open Approach—AHA CC: 4Q, 2017, 42
KN84ZZ Release Left Upper Arm Muscle, Percutaneous Endoscopic Approach—AHA CC: 2Q, 2015, 22-23
KNK0ZZ Release Right Abdomen Muscle, Open Approach—AHA CC: 4Q, 2014, 39-40
KNL0ZZ Release Left Abdomen Muscle, Open Approach—AHA CC: 4Q, 2014, 39-40
KNT0ZZ Release Left Lower Leg Muscle, Open Approach—AHA CC: 2Q, 2017, 12-14
KNV0ZZ Release Right Foot Muscle, Open Approach—AHA CC: 2Q, 2017, 12-14
KQM0ZZ Repair Perineum Muscle, Open Approach—AHA CC: 4Q, 2013, 120; 1Q, 2016, 7; 2Q, 2016, 34-35
KT30ZZ Resection of Left Neck Muscle, Open Approach—AHA CC: 2Q, 2016, 12-14
KTM0ZZ Resection of Perineum Muscle, Open Approach—AHA CC: 4Q, 2014, 40-41; 1Q, 2015, 38
KX10Z2 Transfer Facial Muscle with Skin and Subcutaneous Tissue, Open Approach—AHA CC: 3Q, 2015, 33
KX40Z2 Transfer Tongue, Palate, Pharynx Muscle with Skin and Subcutaneous Tissue, Open Approach—AHA CC: 2Q, 2015, 26
KXF0Z2 Transfer Right Trunk Muscle with Skin and Subcutaneous Tissue, Open Approach—AHA CC: 2Q, 2014, 12
KXF0Z5 Transfer Right Trunk Muscle, Latissimus Dorsi Myocutaneous Flap, Open Approach—AHA CC: 4Q, 2017, 67
KXK0Z6 Transfer Right Abdomen Muscle, Transverse Rectus Abdominis Myocutaneous Flap, Open Approach—AHA CC: 4Q, 2014, 41
KXL0Z6 Transfer Left Abdomen Muscle, Transverse Rectus Abdominis Myocutaneous Flap, Open Approach—AHA CC: 2Q, 2014, 10-11
KXQ0ZZ Transfer Right Upper Leg Muscle, Open Approach—AHA CC: 3Q, 2016, 30-31
KXR0ZZ Transfer Left Upper Leg Muscle, Open Approach—AHA CC: 3Q, 2016, 30-31

Shoulder Tendons and Ligaments

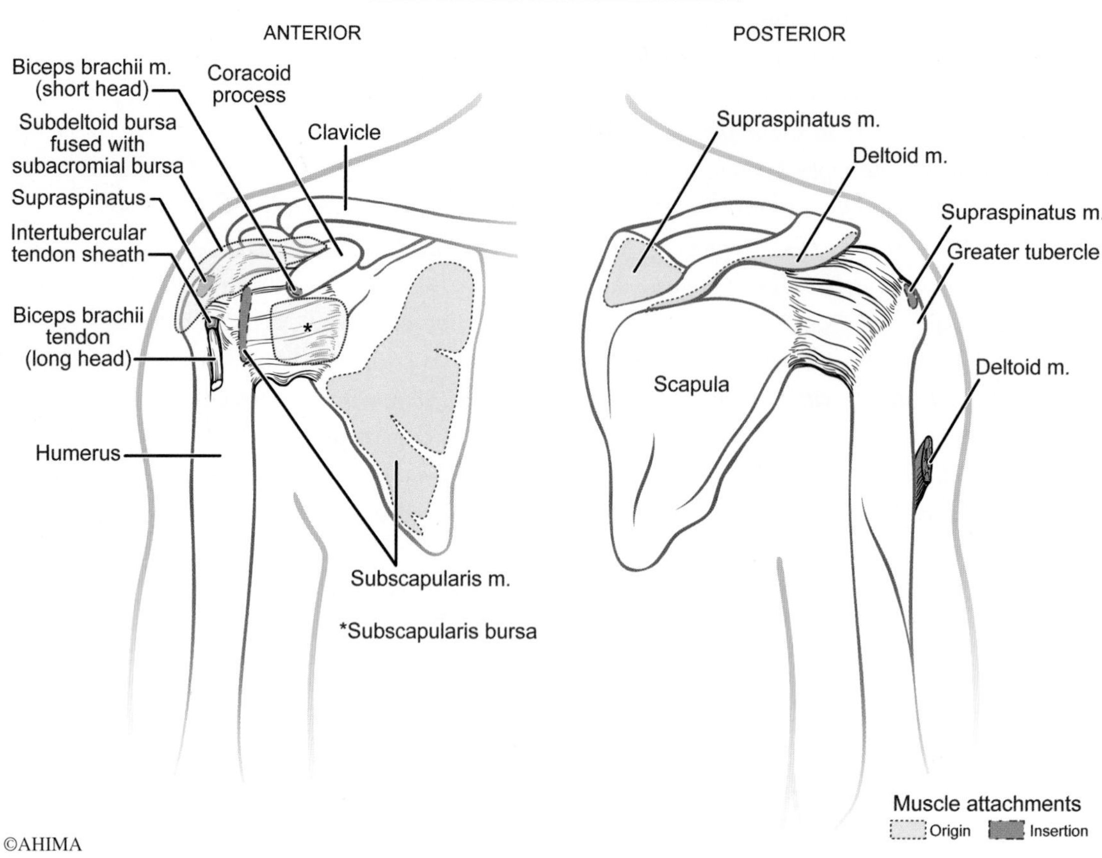

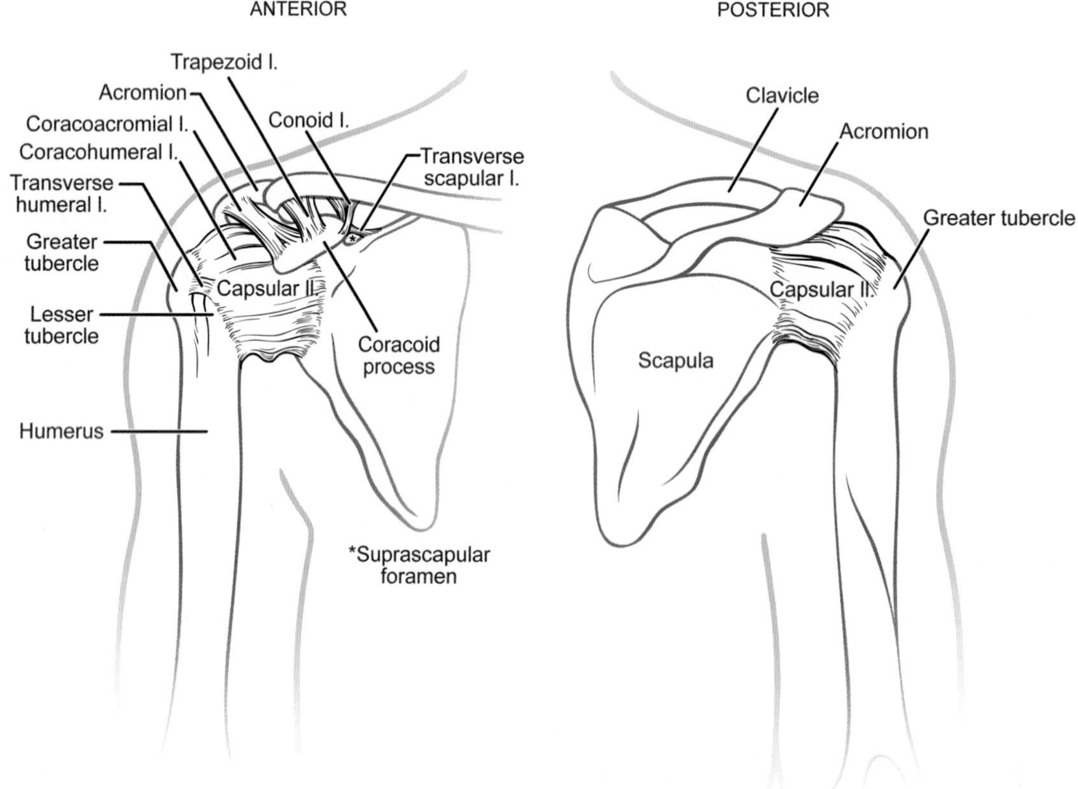

Hip Tendons and Ligaments

ANTERIOR
POSTERIOR
Anterior sacroiliac l.
Iliopectinea bursa
Pubofemoral l.
Iliofemoral l.
Greater trochanter
Lesser trochanter
Intertrochanteric line
*
**
*
Posterior sacroiliac ll.
**Sacrospinous l.
Iliotibial band
Acetabular labrum
Iliofemoral l.
Ischiofemoral l.
Greater trochanter
Zona orbicularis
Protrusion of synovial membrane
Lesser trochanter
*Sacrotuberous l.

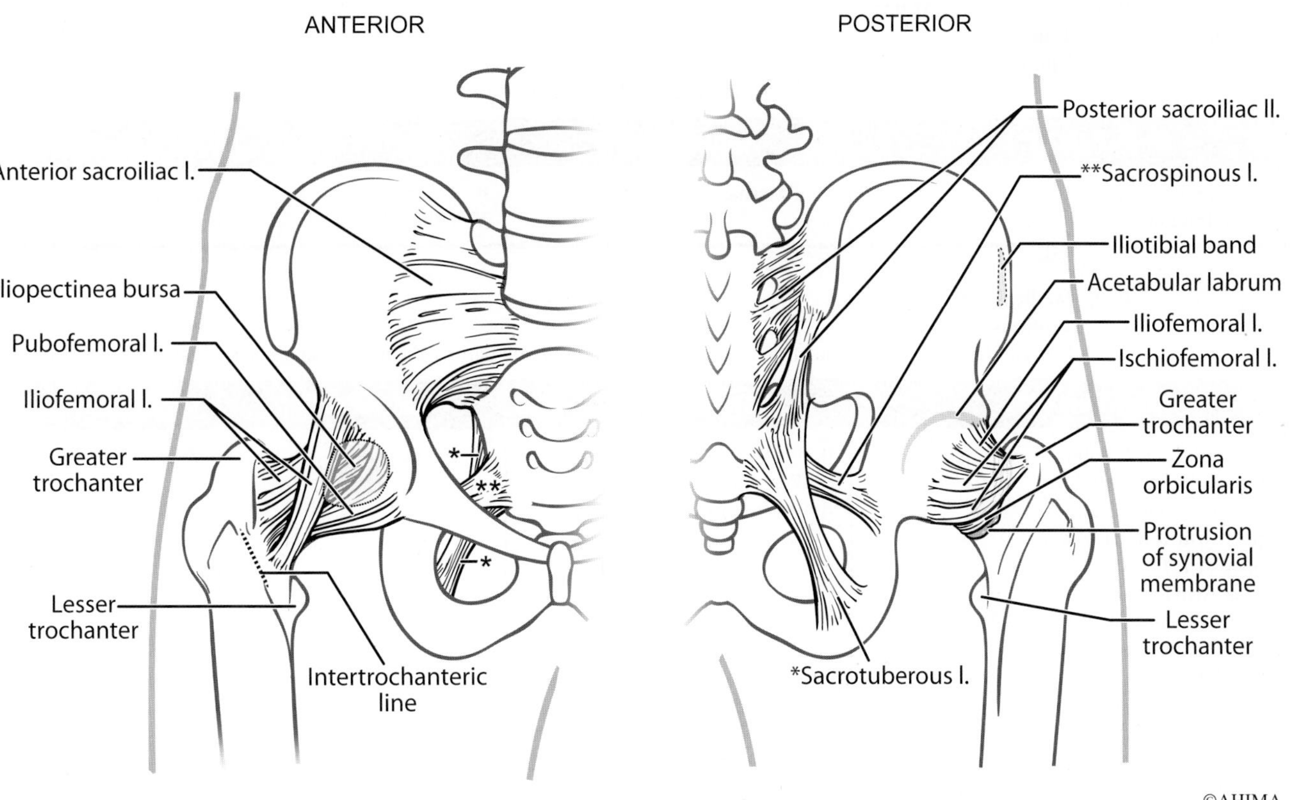

Knee Tendons and Ligaments

ANTERIOR
POSTERIOR
Femur
Patella
Lat. condyle of femur
Ant. cruciate l.
Fibular collateral l.
Lat. meniscus
Lat. condyle of tibia
Head of fibula
Tibia
Post. cruciate l.
Med. condyle of femur
Tibial collateral l.
Med. meniscus
Med. condyle of tibia
Transverse l. of knee
Tibial tuberosity
Femur
Post. meniscofemoral l.
Ant. cruciate l.
Lat. condyle of femur
Fibular collateral l.
Popliteus tendon
Lat. meniscus
Head of fibula
Post. cruciate l.
Tibia

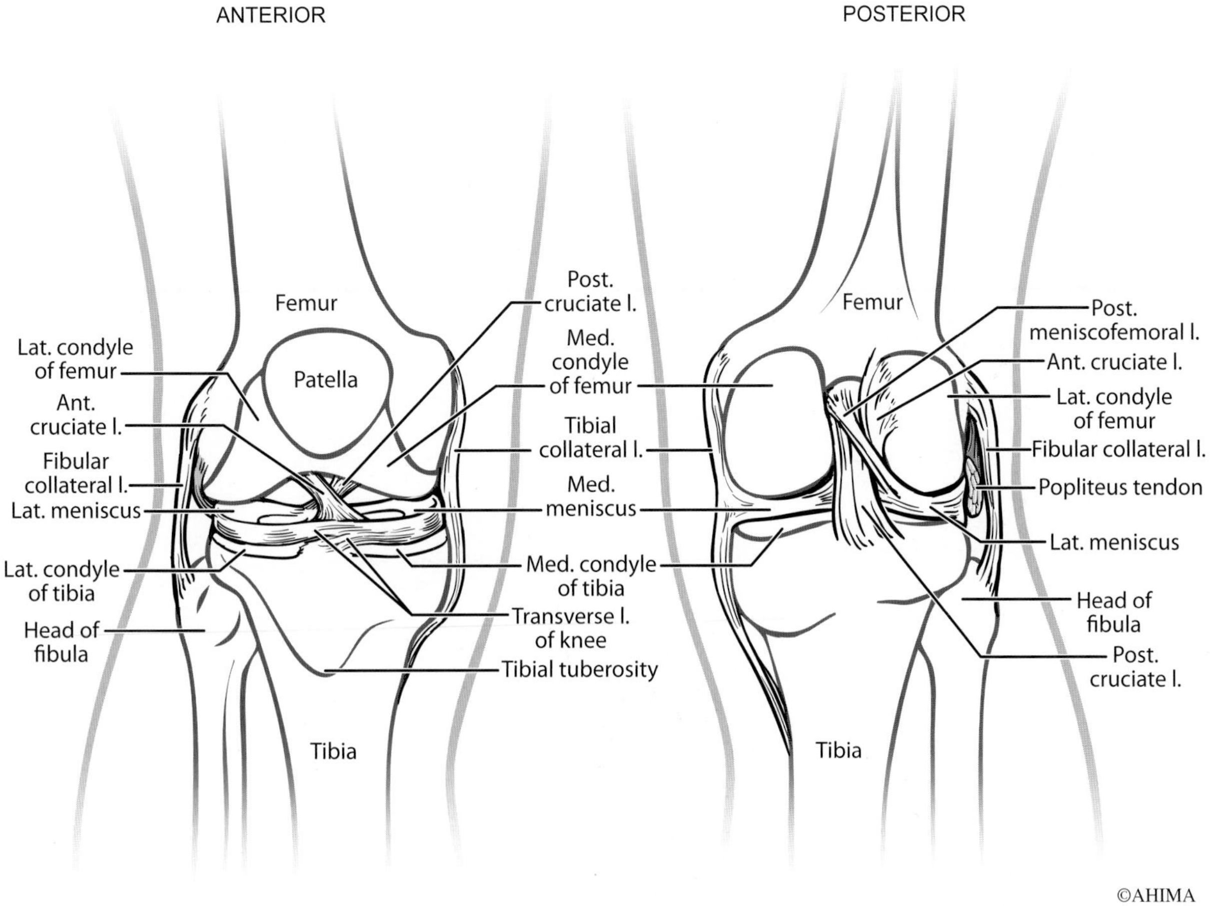

Tendons Tables 0L2–0LX

Section 0 **Medical and Surgical**
Body System L **Tendons**
Operation 2 **Change:** Taking out or off a device from a body part and putting back an identical or similar device in or on the same bo part without cutting or puncturing the skin or a mucous membrane

Body Part (4th)	Approach (5th)	Device (6th)	Qualifier (7th)
X Upper Tendon **Y** Lower Tendon	**X** External	**0** Drainage Device **Y** Other Device	**Z** No Qualifier

Section 0 **Medical and Surgical**
Body System L **Tendons**
Operation 5 **Destruction:** Physical eradication of all or a portion of a body part by the direct use of energy, force, or a destructive age

Body Part (4th)	Approach (5th)	Device (6th)	Qualifier (7th)
0 Head and Neck Tendon **1** Shoulder Tendon, Right **2** Shoulder Tendon, Left **3** Upper Arm Tendon, Right **4** Upper Arm Tendon, Left **5** Lower Arm and Wrist Tendon, Right **6** Lower Arm and Wrist Tendon, Left **7** Hand Tendon, Right **8** Hand Tendon, Left **9** Trunk Tendon, Right **B** Trunk Tendon, Left **C** Thorax Tendon, Right **D** Thorax Tendon, Left **F** Abdomen Tendon, Right **G** Abdomen Tendon, Left **H** Perineum Tendon **J** Hip Tendon, Right **K** Hip Tendon, Left **L** Upper Leg Tendon, Right **M** Upper Leg Tendon, Left **N** Lower Leg Tendon, Right **P** Lower Leg Tendon, Left **Q** Knee Tendon, Right **R** Knee Tendon, Left **S** Ankle Tendon, Right **T** Ankle Tendon, Left **V** Foot Tendon, Right **W** Foot Tendon, Left	**0** Open **3** Percutaneous **4** Percutaneous Endoscopic	**Z** No Device	**Z** No Qualifier

ction 0 **Medical and Surgical**
dy System L **Tendons**
eration 8 **Division:** Cutting into a body part, without draining fluids and/or gases from the body part, in order to separate or transect a body part

Body Part (4th)	Approach (5th)	Device (6th)	Qualifier (7th)
0 Head and Neck Tendon	**0** Open	**Z** No Device	**Z** No Qualifier
Shoulder Tendon, Right	**3** Percutaneous		
2 Shoulder Tendon, Left	**4** Percutaneous Endoscopic		
3 Upper Arm Tendon, Right			
4 Upper Arm Tendon, Left			
5 Lower Arm and Wrist Tendon, Right			
6 Lower Arm and Wrist Tendon, Left			
7 Hand Tendon, Right			
8 Hand Tendon, Left			
9 Trunk Tendon, Right			
B Trunk Tendon, Left			
C Thorax Tendon, Right			
D Thorax Tendon, Left			
F Abdomen Tendon, Right			
G Abdomen Tendon, Left			
H Perineum Tendon			
J Hip Tendon, Right			
K Hip Tendon, Left			
L Upper Leg Tendon, Right			
M Upper Leg Tendon, Left			
N Lower Leg Tendon, Right			
P Lower Leg Tendon, Left			
Q Knee Tendon, Right			
R Knee Tendon, Left			
S Ankle Tendon, Right			
T Ankle Tendon, Left			
V Foot Tendon, Right			
W Foot Tendon, Left			

ction 0 **Medical and Surgical**
dy System L **Tendons**
peration 9 **Drainage:** Taking or letting out fluids and/or gases from a body part

Body Part (4th)	Approach (5th)	Device (6th)	Qualifier (7th)
0 Head and Neck Tendon	**0** Open	**0** Drainage Device	**Z** No Qualifier
1 Shoulder Tendon, Right	**3** Percutaneous		
2 Shoulder Tendon, Left	**4** Percutaneous Endoscopic		
3 Upper Arm Tendon, Right			
4 Upper Arm Tendon, Left			
5 Lower Arm and Wrist Tendon, Right			
6 Lower Arm and Wrist Tendon, Left			
7 Hand Tendon, Right			
8 Hand Tendon, Left			
9 Trunk Tendon, Right			
B Trunk Tendon, Left			
C Thorax Tendon, Right			
D Thorax Tendon, Left			
F Abdomen Tendon, Right			
G Abdomen Tendon, Left			
H Perineum Tendon			
J Hip Tendon, Right			
K Hip Tendon, Left			
L Upper Leg Tendon, Right			
M Upper Leg Tendon, Left			
N Lower Leg Tendon, Right			
P Lower Leg Tendon, Left			
Q Knee Tendon, Right			
R Knee Tendon, Left			
S Ankle Tendon, Right			
T Ankle Tendon, Left			
V Foot Tendon, Right			
W Foot Tendon, Left			

Continued →

Section 0 **Medical and Surgical**
Body System L **Tendons**
Operation 9 **Drainage:** Taking or letting out fluids and/or gases from a body part

Body Part (4th)	Approach (5th)	Device (6th)	Qualifier (7th)
0 Head and Neck Tendon **1** Shoulder Tendon, Right **2** Shoulder Tendon, Left **3** Upper Arm Tendon, Right **4** Upper Arm Tendon, Left **5** Lower Arm and Wrist Tendon, Right **6** Lower Arm and Wrist Tendon, Left **7** Hand Tendon, Right **8** Hand Tendon, Left **9** Trunk Tendon, Right **B** Trunk Tendon, Left **C** Thorax Tendon, Right **D** Thorax Tendon, Left **F** Abdomen Tendon, Right **G** Abdomen Tendon, Left **H** Perineum Tendon **J** Hip Tendon, Right **K** Hip Tendon, Left **L** Upper Leg Tendon, Right **M** Upper Leg Tendon, Left **N** Lower Leg Tendon, Right **P** Lower Leg Tendon, Left **Q** Knee Tendon, Right **R** Knee Tendon, Left **S** Ankle Tendon, Right **T** Ankle Tendon, Left **V** Foot Tendon, Right **W** Foot Tendon, Left	**0** Open **3** Percutaneous **4** Percutaneous Endoscopic	**Z** No Device	**X** Diagnostic **Z** No Qualifier

Section 0 **Medical and Surgical**
Body System L **Tendons**
Operation B **Excision:** Cutting out or off, without replacement, a portion of a body part

Body Part (4th)	Approach (5th)	Device (6th)	Qualifier (7th)
0 Head and Neck Tendon **1** Shoulder Tendon, Right **2** Shoulder Tendon, Left **3** Upper Arm Tendon, Right **4** Upper Arm Tendon, Left **5** Lower Arm and Wrist Tendon, Right **6** Lower Arm and Wrist Tendon, Left **7** Hand Tendon, Right **8** Hand Tendon, Left **9** Trunk Tendon, Right **B** Trunk Tendon, Left **C** Thorax Tendon, Right **D** Thorax Tendon, Left **F** Abdomen Tendon, Right **G** Abdomen Tendon, Left **H** Perineum Tendon **J** Hip Tendon, Right **K** Hip Tendon, Left **L** Upper Leg Tendon, Right **M** Upper Leg Tendon, Left **N** Lower Leg Tendon, Right **P** Lower Leg Tendon, Left **Q** Knee Tendon, Right **R** Knee Tendon, Left **S** Ankle Tendon, Right **T** Ankle Tendon, Left **V** Foot Tendon, Right **W** Foot Tendon, Left	**0** Open **3** Percutaneous **4** Percutaneous Endoscopic	**Z** No Device	**X** Diagnostic **Z** No Qualifier

tion	**0**	**Medical and Surgical**
dy System	**L**	**Tendons**
eration	**C**	**Extirpation:** Taking or cutting out solid matter from a body part

Body Part (4th)	Approach (5th)	Device (6th)	Qualifier (7th)
Head and Neck Tendon Shoulder Tendon, Right Shoulder Tendon, Left Upper Arm Tendon, Right Upper Arm Tendon, Left Lower Arm and Wrist Tendon, Right Lower Arm and Wrist Tendon, Left Hand Tendon, Right Hand Tendon, Left Trunk Tendon, Right B Trunk Tendon, Left C Thorax Tendon, Right D Thorax Tendon, Left F Abdomen Tendon, Right G Abdomen Tendon, Left H Perineum Tendon Hip Tendon, Right K Hip Tendon, Left L Upper Leg Tendon, Right M Upper Leg Tendon, Left N Lower Leg Tendon, Right P Lower Leg Tendon, Left Q Knee Tendon, Right R Knee Tendon, Left S Ankle Tendon, Right T Ankle Tendon, Left V Foot Tendon, Right W Foot Tendon, Left	**0** Open **3** Percutaneous **4** Percutaneous Endoscopic	**Z** No Device	**Z** No Qualifier

ction	**0**	**Medical and Surgical**
dy System	**L**	**Tendons**
eration	**D**	**Extraction:** Pulling or stripping out or off all or a portion of a body part by the use of force

Body Part (4th)	Approach (5th)	Device (6th)	Qualifier (7th)
0 Head and Neck Tendon 1 Shoulder Tendon, Right 2 Shoulder Tendon, Left 3 Upper Arm Tendon, Right 4 Upper Arm Tendon, Left 5 Lower Arm and Wrist Tendon, Right 6 Lower Arm and Wrist Tendon, Left 7 Hand Tendon, Right 8 Hand Tendon, Left 9 Trunk Tendon, Right B Trunk Tendon, Left C Thorax Tendon, Right D Thorax Tendon, Left F Abdomen Tendon, Right G Abdomen Tendon, Left H Perineum Tendon J Hip Tendon, Right K Hip Tendon, Left L Upper Leg Tendon, Right M Upper Leg Tendon, Left N Lower Leg Tendon, Right P Lower Leg Tendon, Left Q Knee Tendon, Right R Knee Tendon, Left S Ankle Tendon, Right T Ankle Tendon, Left V Foot Tendon, Right W Foot Tendon, Left	**0** Open	**Z** No Device	**Z** No Qualifier

Section 0 **Medical and Surgical**
Body System L **Tendons**
Operation H **Inspection:** Putting in a nonbiological appliance that monitors, assists, performs, or prevents a physiological function b does not physically take the place of a body part

Body Part (4th)	Approach (5th)	Device (6th)	Qualifier (7th)
X Upper Tendon **Y** Lower Tendon	**0** Open **3** Percutaneous **4** Percutaneous Endoscopic	**Y** Other Device	**Z** No Qualifier

Section 0 **Medical and Surgical**
Body System L **Tendons**
Operation J **Inspection:** Visually and/or manually exploring a body part

Body Part (4th)	Approach (5th)	Device (6th)	Qualifier (7th)
X Upper Tendon **Y** Lower Tendon	**0** Open **3** Percutaneous **4** Percutaneous Endoscopic **X** External	**Z** No Device	**Z** No Qualifier

Section 0 **Medical and Surgical**
Body System L **Tendons**
Operation M **Reattachment:** Putting back in or on all or a portion of a separated body part to its normal location or other suitable locati

Body Part (4th)	Approach (5th)	Device (6th)	Qualifier (7th)
0 Head and Neck Tendon **1** Shoulder Tendon, Right **2** Shoulder Tendon, Left **3** Upper Arm Tendon, Right **4** Upper Arm Tendon, Left **5** Lower Arm and Wrist Tendon, Right **6** Lower Arm and Wrist Tendon, Left **7** Hand Tendon, Right **8** Hand Tendon, Left **9** Trunk Tendon, Right **B** Trunk Tendon, Left **C** Thorax Tendon, Right **D** Thorax Tendon, Left **F** Abdomen Tendon, Right **G** Abdomen Tendon, Left **H** Perineum Tendon **J** Hip Tendon, Right **K** Hip Tendon, Left **L** Upper Leg Tendon, Right **M** Upper Leg Tendon, Left **N** Lower Leg Tendon, Right **P** Lower Leg Tendon, Left **Q** Knee Tendon, Right **R** Knee Tendon, Left **S** Ankle Tendon, Right **T** Ankle Tendon, Left **V** Foot Tendon, Right **W** Foot Tendon, Left	**0** Open **4** Percutaneous Endoscopic	**Z** No Device	**Z** No Qualifier

ction	**0**	**Medical and Surgical**
dy System	**L**	**Tendons**
eration	**N**	**Release:** Freeing a body part from an abnormal physical constraint by cutting or by the use of force

Body Part (4th)	Approach (5th)	Device (6th)	Qualifier (7th)
0 Head and Neck Tendon **1** Shoulder Tendon, Right **2** Shoulder Tendon, Left **3** Upper Arm Tendon, Right **4** Upper Arm Tendon, Left **5** Lower Arm and Wrist Tendon, Right **6** Lower Arm and Wrist Tendon, Left **7** Hand Tendon, Right **8** Hand Tendon, Left **9** Trunk Tendon, Right **B** Trunk Tendon, Left **C** Thorax Tendon, Right **D** Thorax Tendon, Left **F** Abdomen Tendon, Right **G** Abdomen Tendon, Left **H** Perineum Tendon **J** Hip Tendon, Right **K** Hip Tendon, Left **L** Upper Leg Tendon, Right **M** Upper Leg Tendon, Left **N** Lower Leg Tendon, Right **P** Lower Leg Tendon, Left **Q** Knee Tendon, Right **R** Knee Tendon, Left **S** Ankle Tendon, Right **T** Ankle Tendon, Left **V** Foot Tendon, Right **W** Foot Tendon, Left	**0** Open **3** Percutaneous **4** Percutaneous Endoscopic **X** External	**Z** No Device	**Z** No Qualifier

ction	**0**	**Medical and Surgical**
dy System	**L**	**Tendons**
peration	**P**	**Removal:** Taking out or off a device from a body part

Body Part (4th)	Approach (5th)	Device (6th)	Qualifier (7th)
X Upper Tendon **Y** Lower Tendon	**0** Open **3** Percutaneous **4** Percutaneous Endoscopic	**0** Drainage Device **7** Autologous Tissue Substitute **J** Synthetic Substitute **K** Nonautologous Tissue Substitute **Y** Other Device	**Z** No Qualifier
X Upper Tendon **Y** Lower Tendon	**X** External	**0** Drainage Device	**Z** No Qualifier

Section 0 **Medical and Surgical**
Body System L **Tendons**
Operation Q **Repair:** Restoring, to the extent possible, a body part to its normal anatomic structure and function

Body Part (4th)	Approach (5th)	Device (6th)	Qualifier (7th)
0 Head and Neck Tendon **1** Shoulder Tendon, Right **2** Shoulder Tendon, Left **3** Upper Arm Tendon, Right **4** Upper Arm Tendon, Left **5** Lower Arm and Wrist Tendon, Right **6** Lower Arm and Wrist Tendon, Left **7** Hand Tendon, Right **8** Hand Tendon, Left **9** Trunk Tendon, Right **B** Trunk Tendon, Left **C** Thorax Tendon, Right **D** Thorax Tendon, Left **F** Abdomen Tendon, Right **G** Abdomen Tendon, Left **H** Perineum Tendon **J** Hip Tendon, Right **K** Hip Tendon, Left **L** Upper Leg Tendon, Right **M** Upper Leg Tendon, Left **N** Lower Leg Tendon, Right **P** Lower Leg Tendon, Left **Q** Knee Tendon, Right **R** Knee Tendon, Left **S** Ankle Tendon, Right **T** Ankle Tendon, Left **V** Foot Tendon, Right **W** Foot Tendon, Left	**0** Open **3** Percutaneous **4** Percutaneous Endoscopic	**Z** No Device	**Z** No Qualifier

Section 0 **Medical and Surgical**
Body System L **Tendons**
Operation R **Replacement:** Putting in or on biological or synthetic material that physically takes the place and/or function of all or a portion of a body part

Body Part (4th)	Approach (5th)	Device (6th)	Qualifier (7th)
0 Head and Neck Tendon **1** Shoulder Tendon, Right **2** Shoulder Tendon, Left **3** Upper Arm Tendon, Right **4** Upper Arm Tendon, Left **5** Lower Arm and Wrist Tendon, Right **6** Lower Arm and Wrist Tendon, Left **7** Hand Tendon, Right **8** Hand Tendon, Left **9** Trunk Tendon, Right **B** Trunk Tendon, Left **C** Thorax Tendon, Right **D** Thorax Tendon, Left **F** Abdomen Tendon, Right **G** Abdomen Tendon, Left **H** Perineum Tendon **J** Hip Tendon, Right **K** Hip Tendon, Left **L** Upper Leg Tendon, Right **M** Upper Leg Tendon, Left **N** Lower Leg Tendon, Right **P** Lower Leg Tendon, Left **Q** Knee Tendon, Right **R** Knee Tendon, Left **S** Ankle Tendon, Right **T** Ankle Tendon, Left **V** Foot Tendon, Right **W** Foot Tendon, Left	**0** Open **4** Percutaneous Endoscopic	**7** Autologous Tissue Substitute **J** Synthetic Substitute **K** Nonautologous Tissue Substitute	**Z** No Qualifier

tion **0 Medical and Surgical**
dy System **L Tendons**
eration **S Reposition:** Moving to its normal location, or other suitable location, all or a portion of a body part

Body Part (4th)	Approach (5th)	Device (6th)	Qualifier (7th)
0 Head and Neck Tendon 1 Shoulder Tendon, Right 2 Shoulder Tendon, Left 3 Upper Arm Tendon, Right 4 Upper Arm Tendon, Left 5 Lower Arm and Wrist Tendon, Right 6 Lower Arm and Wrist Tendon, Left 7 Hand Tendon, Right 8 Hand Tendon, Left 9 Trunk Tendon, Right B Trunk Tendon, Left C Thorax Tendon, Right D Thorax Tendon, Left F Abdomen Tendon, Right G Abdomen Tendon, Left H Perineum Tendon J Hip Tendon, Right K Hip Tendon, Left L Upper Leg Tendon, Right M Upper Leg Tendon, Left N Lower Leg Tendon, Right P Lower Leg Tendon, Left Q Knee Tendon, Right R Knee Tendon, Left S Ankle Tendon, Right T Ankle Tendon, Left V Foot Tendon, Right W Foot Tendon, Left	**0** Open **4** Percutaneous Endoscopic	**Z** No Device	**Z** No Qualifier

ction **0 Medical and Surgical**
dy System **L Tendons**
eration **T Resection:** Cutting out or off, without replacement, all of a body part

Body Part (4th)	Approach (5th)	Device (6th)	Qualifier (7th)
0 Head and Neck Tendon 1 Shoulder Tendon, Right 2 Shoulder Tendon, Left 3 Upper Arm Tendon, Right 4 Upper Arm Tendon, Left 5 Lower Arm and Wrist Tendon, Right 6 Lower Arm and Wrist Tendon, Left 7 Hand Tendon, Right 8 Hand Tendon, Left 9 Trunk Tendon, Right B Trunk Tendon, Left C Thorax Tendon, Right D Thorax Tendon, Left F Abdomen Tendon, Right G Abdomen Tendon, Left H Perineum Tendon J Hip Tendon, Right K Hip Tendon, Left L Upper Leg Tendon, Right M Upper Leg Tendon, Left N Lower Leg Tendon, Right P Lower Leg Tendon, Left Q Knee Tendon, Right R Knee Tendon, Left S Ankle Tendon, Right T Ankle Tendon, Left V Foot Tendon, Right W Foot Tendon, Left	**0** Open **4** Percutaneous Endoscopic	**Z** No Device	**Z** No Qualifier

Section 0 **Medical and Surgical**
Body System L **Tendons**
Operation U **Supplement:** Putting in or on biological or synthetic material that physically reinforces and/or augments the function of a portion of a body part

Body Part (4th)	Approach (5th)	Device (6th)	Qualifier (7th)
0 Head and Neck Tendon **1** Shoulder Tendon, Right **2** Shoulder Tendon, Left **3** Upper Arm Tendon, Right **4** Upper Arm Tendon, Left **5** Lower Arm and Wrist Tendon, Right **6** Lower Arm and Wrist Tendon, Left **7** Hand Tendon, Right **8** Hand Tendon, Left **9** Trunk Tendon, Right **B** Trunk Tendon, Left **C** Thorax Tendon, Right **D** Thorax Tendon, Left **F** Abdomen Tendon, Right **G** Abdomen Tendon, Left **H** Perineum Tendon **J** Hip Tendon, Right **K** Hip Tendon, Left **L** Upper Leg Tendon, Right **M** Upper Leg Tendon, Left **N** Lower Leg Tendon, Right **P** Lower Leg Tendon, Left **Q** Knee Tendon, Right **R** Knee Tendon, Left **S** Ankle Tendon, Right **T** Ankle Tendon, Left **V** Foot Tendon, Right **W** Foot Tendon, Left	**0** Open **4** Percutaneous Endoscopic	**7** Autologous Tissue Substitute **J** Synthetic Substitute **K** Nonautologous Tissue Substitute	**Z** No Qualifier

Section 0 **Medical and Surgical**
Body System L **Tendons**
Operation W **Revision:** Correcting, to the extent possible, a portion of a malfunctioning device or the position of a displaced device

Body Part (4th)	Approach (5th)	Device (6th)	Qualifier (7th)
X Upper Tendon **Y** Lower Tendon	**0** Open **3** Percutaneous **4** Percutaneous Endoscopic	**0** Drainage Device **7** Autologous Tissue Substitute **J** Synthetic Substitute **K** Nonautologous Tissue Substitute **Y** Other Device	**Z** No Qualifier
X Upper Tendon **Y** Lower Tendon	**X** External	**0** Drainage Device **7** Autologous Tissue Substitute **J** Synthetic Substitute **K** Nonautologous Tissue Substitute	**Z** No Qualifier

ection **0** **Medical and Surgical**
ody System **L** **Tendons**
peration **X** **Transfer:** Moving, without taking out, all or a portion of a body part to another location to take over the function of all or a portion of a body part

Body Part (4th)	Approach (5th)	Device (6th)	Qualifier (7th)
0 Head and Neck Tendon **1** Shoulder Tendon, Right **2** Shoulder Tendon, Left **3** Upper Arm Tendon, Right **4** Upper Arm Tendon, Left **5** Lower Arm and Wrist Tendon, Right **6** Lower Arm and Wrist Tendon, Left **7** Hand Tendon, Right **8** Hand Tendon, Left **9** Trunk Tendon, Right **B** Trunk Tendon, Left **C** Thorax Tendon, Right **D** Thorax Tendon, Left **F** Abdomen Tendon, Right **G** Abdomen Tendon, Left **H** Perineum Tendon **J** Hip Tendon, Right **K** Hip Tendon, Left **L** Upper Leg Tendon, Right **M** Upper Leg Tendon, Left **N** Lower Leg Tendon, Right **P** Lower Leg Tendon, Left **Q** Knee Tendon, Right **R** Knee Tendon, Left **S** Ankle Tendon, Right **T** Ankle Tendon, Left **V** Foot Tendon, Right **W** Foot Tendon, Left	**0** Open **4** Percutaneous Endoscopic	**Z** No Device	**Z** No Qualifier

HA Coding Clinic

L8J0ZZ Division of Right Hip Tendon, Open Approach—AHA CC: 3Q, 2016, 30-31
LB60ZZ Excision of Left Lower Arm and Wrist Tendon, Open Approach—AHA CC: 3Q, 2015, 26-27
LBL0ZZ Excision of Right Upper Leg Tendon, Open Approach—AHA CC: 2Q, 2017, 21-22
LBP0ZZ Excision of Left Lower Leg Tendon, Open Approach—AHA CC: 3Q, 2014, 18-19
LBT0ZZ Excision of Left Ankle Tendon, Open Approach—AHA CC: 3Q, 2014, 14-15
LQ14ZZ Repair Right Shoulder Tendon, Percutaneous Endoscopic Approach—AHA CC: 3Q, 2013, 20-22; 3Q, 2016, 32-33
LS30ZZ Reposition Right Upper Arm Tendon, Open Approach—AHA CC: 3Q, 2016, 32-33
LS40ZZ Reposition Left Upper Arm Tendon, Open Approach—AHA CC: 3Q, 2015, 14-15
LUM0KZ Supplement Left Upper Leg Tendon with Nonautologous Tissue Substitute, Open Approach—AHA CC: 2Q, 2015, 11
LUQ0KZ Supplement Right Knee Tendon with Nonautologous Tissue Substitute, Open Approach—AHA CC: 2Q, 2015, 11

Bursa of the Knee

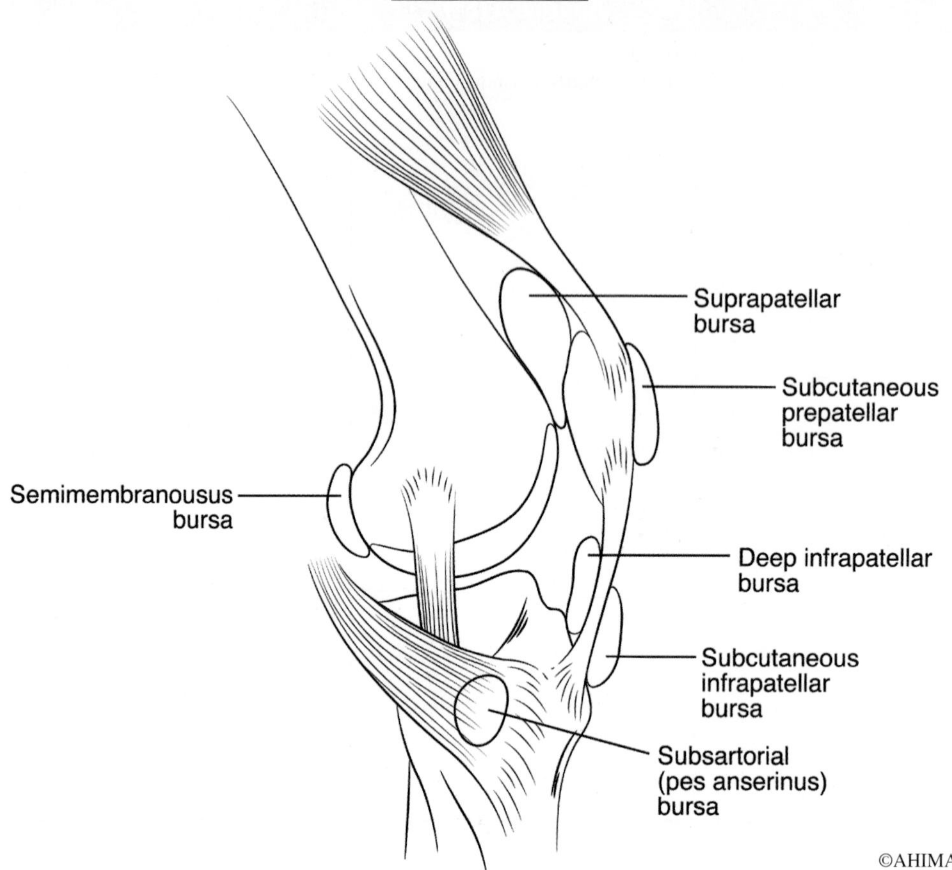

Ligaments of the Knee

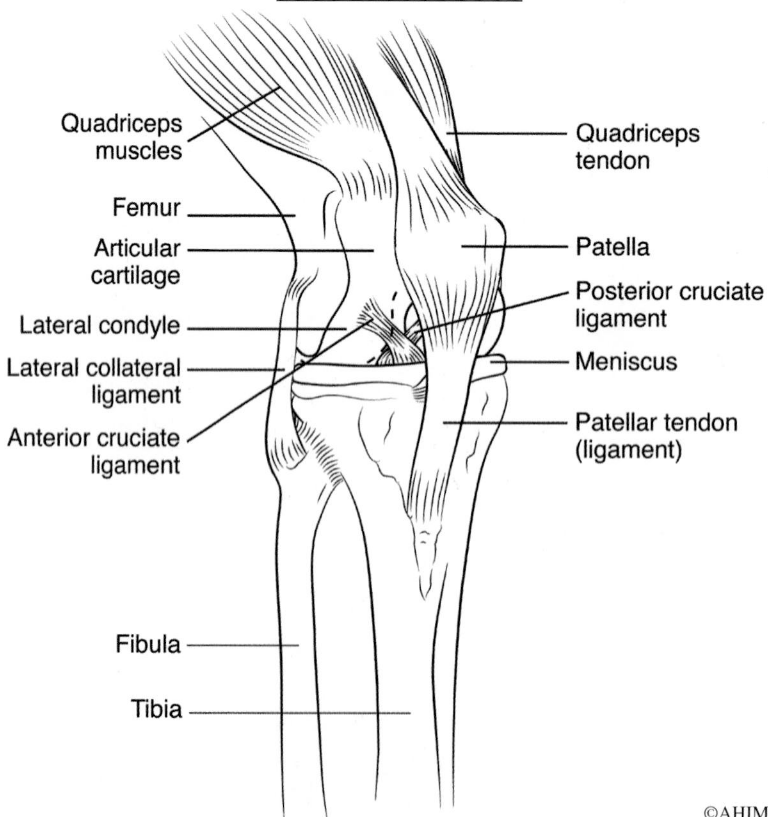

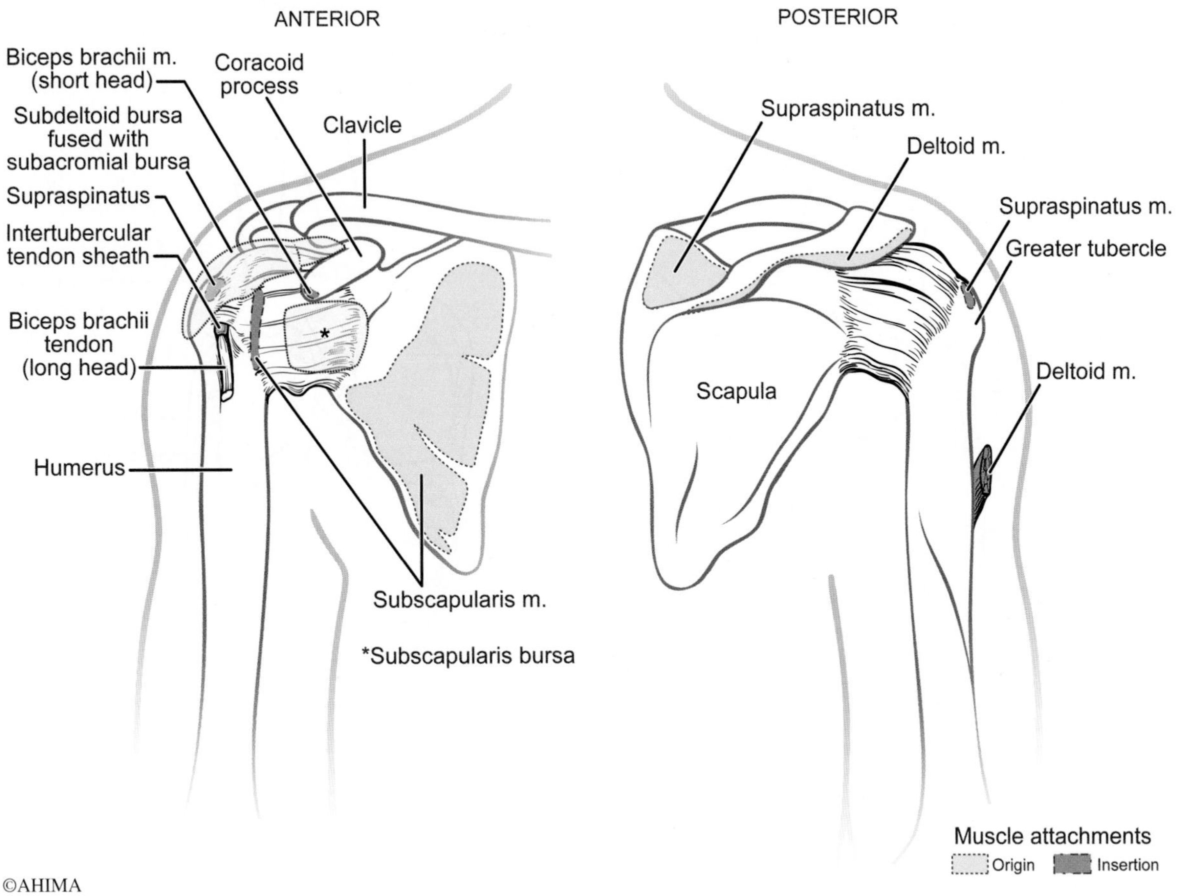

Shoulder Tendons and Ligaments

ANTERIOR

POSTERIOR

Biceps brachii m. (short head)

Coracoid process

Clavicle

Subdeltoid bursa fused with subacromial bursa

Supraspinatus

Intertubercular tendon sheath

Biceps brachii tendon (long head)

Humerus

Subscapularis m.

*Subscapularis bursa

Supraspinatus m.

Deltoid m.

Supraspinatus m.

Greater tubercle

Scapula

Deltoid m.

Muscle attachments

Origin Insertion

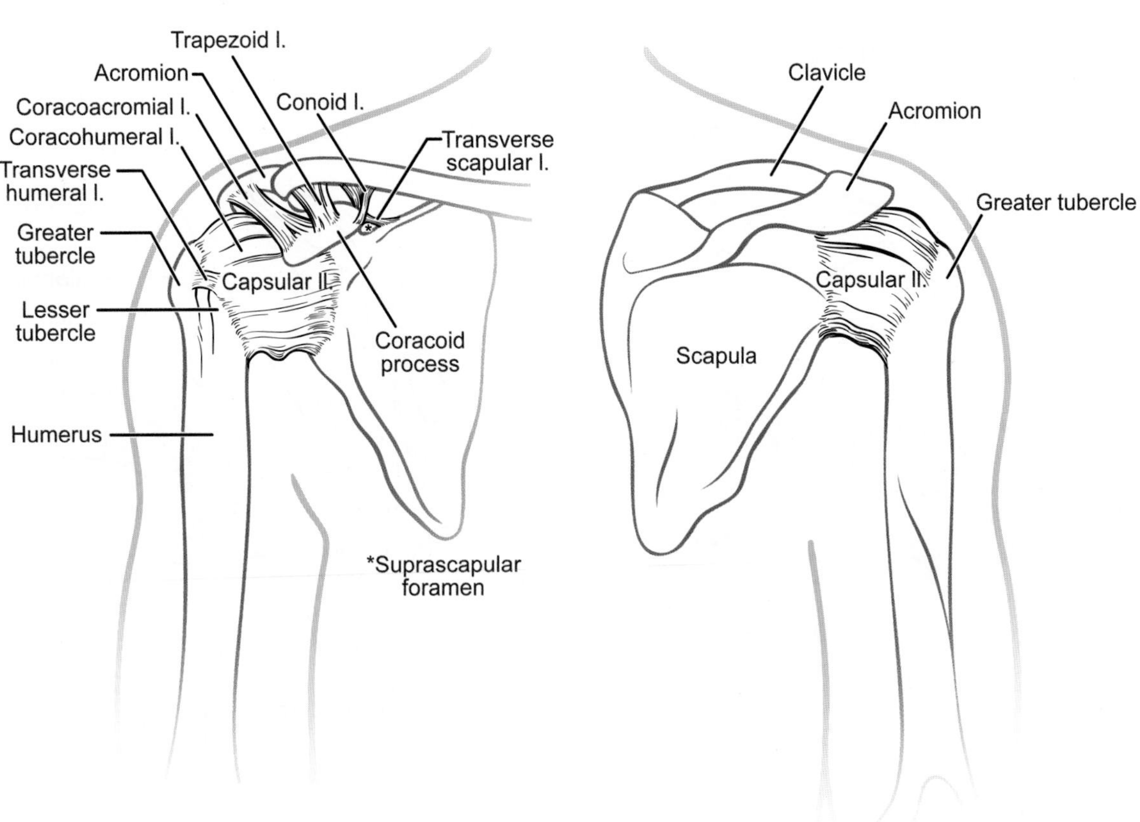

Knee Tendons and Ligaments

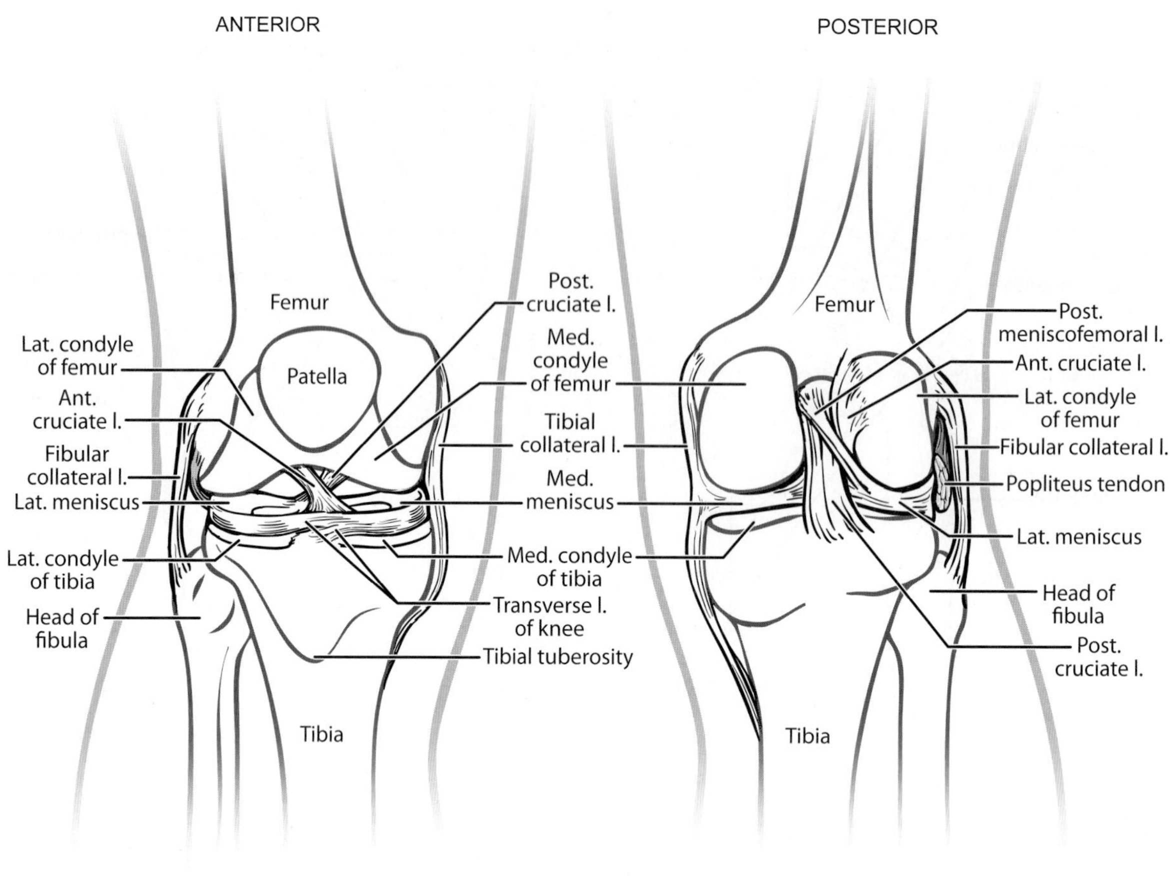

Hip Tendons and Ligaments

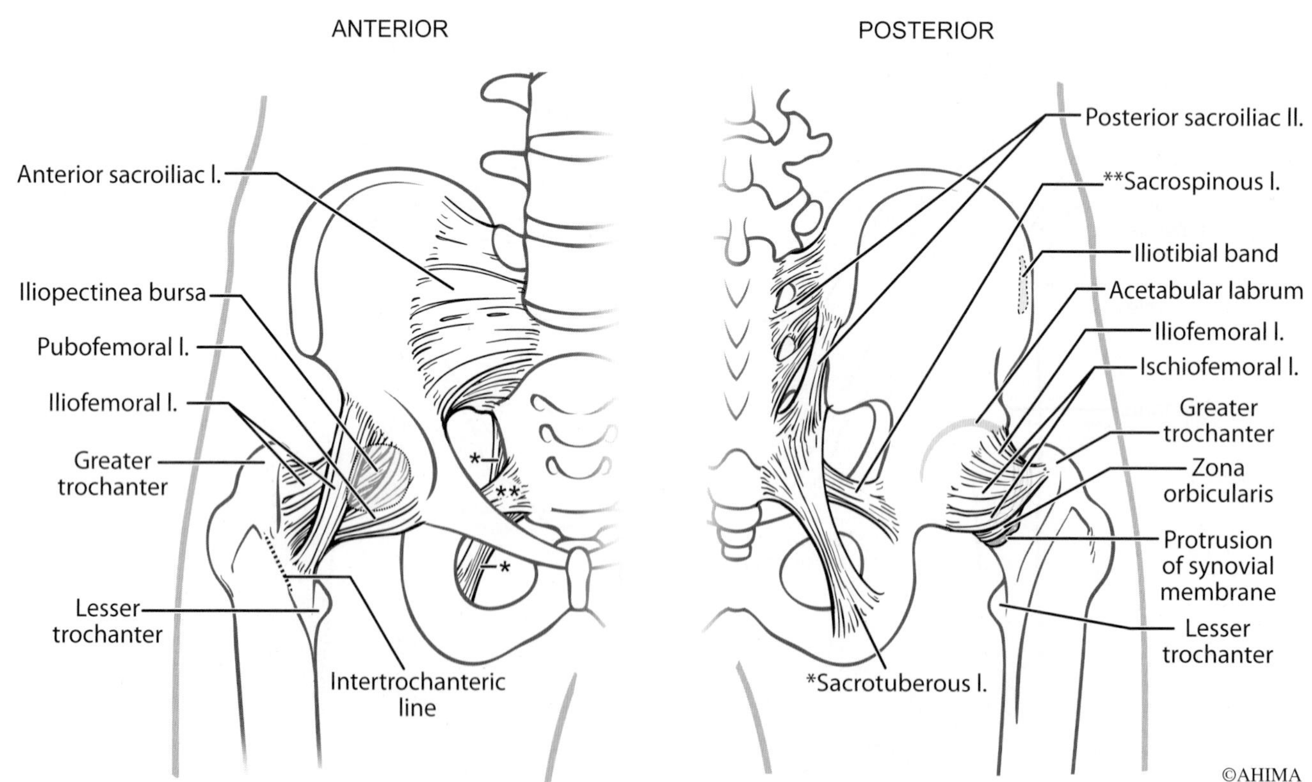

ction	**0**	**Medical and Surgical**
dy System	**M**	**Bursae and Ligaments**
eration	**2**	**Change:** Taking out or off a device from a body part and putting back an identical or similar device in or on the same body part without cutting or puncturing the skin or a mucous membrane

Body Part (4th)	Approach (5th)	Device (6th)	Qualifier (7th)
X Upper Bursa and Ligament Y Lower Bursa and Ligament	**X** External	**0** Drainage Device **Y** Other Device	**Z** No Qualifier

ction	**0**	**Medical and Surgical**
dy System	**M**	**Bursae and Ligaments**
eration	**5**	**Destruction:** Physical eradication of all or a portion of a body part by the direct use of energy, force, or a destructive agent

Body Part (4th)	Approach (5th)	Device (6th)	Qualifier (7th)
0 Head and Neck Bursa and Ligament **1** Shoulder Bursa and Ligament, Right **2** Shoulder Bursa and Ligament, Left **3** Elbow Bursa and Ligament, Right **4** Elbow Bursa and Ligament, Left **5** Wrist Bursa and Ligament, Right **6** Wrist Bursa and Ligament, Left **7** Hand Bursa and Ligament, Right **8** Hand Bursa and Ligament, Left **9** Upper Extremity Bursa and Ligament, Right **B** Upper Extremity Bursa and Ligament, Left **C** Upper Spine Bursa and Ligament, Right **D** Lower Spine Bursa and Ligament, Left **F** Sternum Bursa and Ligament, Right **G** Rib(s) Bursa and Ligament, Left **H** Abdomen Bursa and Ligament, Right **J** Abdomen Bursa and Ligament, Left **K** Perineum Bursa and Ligament **L** Hip Bursa and Ligament, Right **M** Hip Bursa and Ligament, Left **N** Knee Bursa and Ligament, Right **P** Knee Bursa and Ligament, Left **Q** Ankle Bursa and Ligament, Right **R** Ankle Bursa and Ligament, Left **S** Foot Bursa and Ligament, Right **T** Foot Bursa and Ligament, Left **V** Lower Extremity Bursa and Ligament, Right **W** Lower Extremity Bursa and Ligament, Left	**0** Open **3** Percutaneous **4** Percutaneous Endoscopic	**Z** No Device	**Z** No Qualifier

Section 0 **Medical and Surgical**
Body System M **Bursae and Ligaments**
Operation 8 **Division:** Cutting into a body part, without draining fluids and/or gases from the body part, in order to separate or transect a body part

Body Part (4th)	Approach (5th)	Device (6th)	Qualifier (7th)
0 Head and Neck Bursa and Ligament	**0** Open	**Z** No Device	**Z** No Qualifier
1 Shoulder Bursa and Ligament, Right	**3** Percutaneous		
2 Shoulder Bursa and Ligament, Left	**4** Percutaneous Endoscopic		
3 Elbow Bursa and Ligament, Right			
4 Elbow Bursa and Ligament, Left			
5 Wrist Bursa and Ligament, Right			
6 Wrist Bursa and Ligament, Left			
7 Hand Bursa and Ligament, Right			
8 Hand Bursa and Ligament, Left			
9 Upper Extremity Bursa and Ligament, Right			
B Upper Extremity Bursa and Ligament, Left			
C Upper Spine Bursa and Ligament, Right			
D Lower Spine Bursa and Ligament, Left			
F Sternum Bursa and Ligament, Right			
G Rib(s) Bursa and Ligament, Left			
H Abdomen Bursa and Ligament, Right			
J Abdomen Bursa and Ligament, Left			
K Perineum Bursa and Ligament			
L Hip Bursa and Ligament, Right			
M Hip Bursa and Ligament, Left			
N Knee Bursa and Ligament, Right			
P Knee Bursa and Ligament, Left			
Q Ankle Bursa and Ligament, Right			
R Ankle Bursa and Ligament, Left			
S Foot Bursa and Ligament, Right			
T Foot Bursa and Ligament, Left			
V Lower Extremity Bursa and Ligament, Right			
W Lower Extremity Bursa and Ligament, Left			

Section 0 **Medical and Surgical**
Body System M **Bursae and Ligaments**
Operation 9 **Drainage:** Taking or letting out fluids and/or gases from a body part

Body Part (4th)	Approach (5th)	Device (6th)	Qualifier (7th)
0 Head and Neck Bursa and Ligament	**0** Open	**0** Drainage Device	**Z** No Qualifier
1 Shoulder Bursa and Ligament, Right	**3** Percutaneous		
2 Shoulder Bursa and Ligament, Left	**4** Percutaneous Endoscopic		
3 Elbow Bursa and Ligament, Right			
4 Elbow Bursa and Ligament, Left			
5 Wrist Bursa and Ligament, Right			
6 Wrist Bursa and Ligament, Left			
7 Hand Bursa and Ligament, Right			
8 Hand Bursa and Ligament, Left			
9 Upper Extremity Bursa and Ligament, Right			
B Upper Extremity Bursa and Ligament, Left			
C Upper Spine Bursa and Ligament, Right			
D Lower Spine Bursa and Ligament, Left			
F Sternum Bursa and Ligament, Right			
G Rib(s) Bursa and Ligament, Left			
H Abdomen Bursa and Ligament, Right			
J Abdomen Bursa and Ligament, Left			
K Perineum Bursa and Ligament			
L Hip Bursa and Ligament, Right			
M Hip Bursa and Ligament, Left			
N Knee Bursa and Ligament, Right			
P Knee Bursa and Ligament, Left			
Q Ankle Bursa and Ligament, Right			
R Ankle Bursa and Ligament, Left			
S Foot Bursa and Ligament, Right			
T Foot Bursa and Ligament, Left			
V Lower Extremity Bursa and Ligament, Right			
W Lower Extremity Bursa and Ligament, Left			

Continued →

tion	**0**	**Medical and Surgical**
dy System	**M**	**Bursae and Ligaments**
eration	**9**	**Drainage:** Taking or letting out fluids and/or gases from a body part

Body Part (4th)	Approach (5th)	Device (6th)	Qualifier (7th)
Head and Neck Bursa and Ligament Shoulder Bursa and Ligament, Right Shoulder Bursa and Ligament, Left Elbow Bursa and Ligament, Right Elbow Bursa and Ligament, Left Wrist Bursa and Ligament, Right Wrist Bursa and Ligament, Left Hand Bursa and Ligament, Right Hand Bursa and Ligament, Left Upper Extremity Bursa and Ligament, Right B Upper Extremity Bursa and Ligament, Left C Upper Spine Bursa and Ligament, Right D Lower Spine Bursa and Ligament, Left F Sternum Bursa and Ligament, Right G Rib(s) Bursa and Ligament, Left H Abdomen Bursa and Ligament, Right Abdomen Bursa and Ligament, Left K Perineum Bursa and Ligament L Hip Bursa and Ligament, Right M Hip Bursa and Ligament, Left N Knee Bursa and Ligament, Right P Knee Bursa and Ligament, Left Q Ankle Bursa and Ligament, Right R Ankle Bursa and Ligament, Left S Foot Bursa and Ligament, Right T Foot Bursa and Ligament, Left V Lower Extremity Bursa and Ligament, Right W Lower Extremity Bursa and Ligament, Left	**0** Open **3** Percutaneous **4** Percutaneous Endoscopic	**Z** No Device	**X** Diagnostic **Z** No Qualifier

ction	**0**	**Medical and Surgical**
dy System	**M**	**Bursae and Ligaments**
eration	**B**	**Excision:** Cutting out or off, without replacement, a portion of a body part

Body Part (4th)	Approach (5th)	Device (6th)	Qualifier (7th)
0 Head and Neck Bursa and Ligament 1 Shoulder Bursa and Ligament, Right 2 Shoulder Bursa and Ligament, Left 3 Elbow Bursa and Ligament, Right 4 Elbow Bursa and Ligament, Left 5 Wrist Bursa and Ligament, Right 6 Wrist Bursa and Ligament, Left 7 Hand Bursa and Ligament, Right 8 Hand Bursa and Ligament, Left 9 Upper Extremity Bursa and Ligament, Right B Upper Extremity Bursa and Ligament, Left C Upper Spine Bursa and Ligament, Right D Lower Spine Bursa and Ligament, Left F Sternum Bursa and Ligament, Right G Rib(s) Bursa and Ligament, Left H Abdomen Bursa and Ligament, Right J Abdomen Bursa and Ligament, Left K Perineum Bursa and Ligament L Hip Bursa and Ligament, Right M Hip Bursa and Ligament, Left N Knee Bursa and Ligament, Right P Knee Bursa and Ligament, Left Q Ankle Bursa and Ligament, Right R Ankle Bursa and Ligament, Left S Foot Bursa and Ligament, Right T Foot Bursa and Ligament, Left V Lower Extremity Bursa and Ligament, Right W Lower Extremity Bursa and Ligament, Left	**0** Open **3** Percutaneous **4** Percutaneous Endoscopic	**Z** No Device	**X** Diagnostic **Z** No Qualifier

Section **0** **Medical and Surgical**
Body System **M** **Bursae and Ligaments**
Operation **C** **Extirpation:** Taking or cutting out solid matter from a body part

Body Part (4th)	Approach (5th)	Device (6th)	Qualifier (7th)
0 Head and Neck Bursa and Ligament	**0** Open	**Z** No Device	**Z** No Qualifier
1 Shoulder Bursa and Ligament, Right	**3** Percutaneous		
2 Shoulder Bursa and Ligament, Left	**4** Percutaneous Endoscopic		
3 Elbow Bursa and Ligament, Right			
4 Elbow Bursa and Ligament, Left			
5 Wrist Bursa and Ligament, Right			
6 Wrist Bursa and Ligament, Left			
7 Hand Bursa and Ligament, Right			
8 Hand Bursa and Ligament, Left			
9 Upper Extremity Bursa and Ligament, Right			
B Upper Extremity Bursa and Ligament, Left			
C Upper Spine Bursa and Ligament, Right			
D Trunk Bursa and Ligament, Left			
F Sternum Bursa and Ligament, Right			
G Rib(s) Bursa and Ligament, Left			
H Abdomen Bursa and Ligament, Right			
J Abdomen Bursa and Ligament, Left			
K Perineum Bursa and Ligament			
L Hip Bursa and Ligament, Right			
M Hip Bursa and Ligament, Left			
N Knee Bursa and Ligament, Right			
P Knee Bursa and Ligament, Left			
Q Ankle Bursa and Ligament, Right			
R Ankle Bursa and Ligament, Left			
S Foot Bursa and Ligament, Right			
T Foot Bursa and Ligament, Left			
V Lower Extremity Bursa and Ligament, Right			
W Lower Extremity Bursa and Ligament, Left			

Section **0** **Medical and Surgical**
Body System **M** **Bursae and Ligaments**
Operation **D** **Extraction:** Pulling or stripping out or off all or a portion of a body part by the use of force

Body Part (4th)	Approach (5th)	Device (6th)	Qualifier (7th)
0 Head and Neck Bursa and Ligament	**0** Open	**Z** No Device	**Z** No Qualifier
1 Shoulder Bursa and Ligament, Right	**3** Percutaneous		
2 Shoulder Bursa and Ligament, Left	**4** Percutaneous Endoscopic		
3 Elbow Bursa and Ligament, Right			
4 Elbow Bursa and Ligament, Left			
5 Wrist Bursa and Ligament, Right			
6 Wrist Bursa and Ligament, Left			
7 Hand Bursa and Ligament, Right			
8 Hand Bursa and Ligament, Left			
9 Upper Extremity Bursa and Ligament, Right			
B Upper Extremity Bursa and Ligament, Left			
C Upper Spine Bursa and Ligament, Right			
D Lower Spine Bursa and Ligament, Left			
F Sternum Bursa and Ligament, Right			
G Rib(s) Bursa and Ligament, Left			
H Abdomen Bursa and Ligament, Right			
J Abdomen Bursa and Ligament, Left			
K Perineum Bursa and Ligament			
L Hip Bursa and Ligament, Right			
M Hip Bursa and Ligament, Left			
N Knee Bursa and Ligament, Right			
P Knee Bursa and Ligament, Left			
Q Ankle Bursa and Ligament, Right			
R Ankle Bursa and Ligament, Left			
S Foot Bursa and Ligament, Right			
T Foot Bursa and Ligament, Left			
V Lower Extremity Bursa and Ligament, Right			
W Lower Extremity Bursa and Ligament, Left			

ction 0 **Medical and Surgical**
dy System M **Bursae and Ligaments**
eration H **Insertion:** Putting in a nonbiological appliance that monitors, assists, performs, or prevents a physiological function but does not physically take the place of a body part

Body Part (4th)	Approach (5th)	Device (6th)	Qualifier (7th)
X Upper Bursa and Ligament Y Lower Bursa and Ligament	0 Open 3 Percutaneous 4 Percutaneous Endoscopic	Y Other Device	Z No Qualifier

ction 0 **Medical and Surgical**
dy System M **Bursae and Ligaments**
eration J **Inspection:** Visually and/or manually exploring a body part

Body Part (4th)	Approach (5th)	Device (6th)	Qualifier (7th)
X Upper Bursa and Ligament Y Lower Bursa and Ligament	0 Open 3 Percutaneous 4 Percutaneous Endoscopic X External	Z No Device	Z No Qualifier

ction 0 **Medical and Surgical**
dy System M **Bursae and Ligaments**
eration M **Reattachment:** Putting back in or on all or a portion of a separated body part to its normal location or other suitable location

Body Part (4th)	Approach (5th)	Device (6th)	Qualifier (7th)
0 Head and Neck Bursa and Ligament 1 Shoulder Bursa and Ligament, Right 2 Shoulder Bursa and Ligament, Left 3 Elbow Bursa and Ligament, Right 4 Elbow Bursa and Ligament, Left 5 Wrist Bursa and Ligament, Right 6 Wrist Bursa and Ligament, Left 7 Hand Bursa and Ligament, Right 8 Hand Bursa and Ligament, Left 9 Upper Extremity Bursa and Ligament, Right B Upper Extremity Bursa and Ligament, Left C Upper Spine Bursa and Ligament, Right D Lower Spine Bursa and Ligament, Left F Sternum Bursa and Ligament, Right G Rib(s) Bursa and Ligament, Left H Abdomen Bursa and Ligament, Right J Abdomen Bursa and Ligament, Left K Perineum Bursa and Ligament L Hip Bursa and Ligament, Right M Hip Bursa and Ligament, Left N Knee Bursa and Ligament, Right P Knee Bursa and Ligament, Left Q Ankle Bursa and Ligament, Right R Ankle Bursa and Ligament, Left S Foot Bursa and Ligament, Right T Foot Bursa and Ligament, Left V Lower Extremity Bursa and Ligament, Right W Lower Extremity Bursa and Ligament, Left	0 Open 4 Percutaneous Endoscopic	Z No Device	Z No Qualifier

Section 0 **Medical and Surgical**
Body System M **Bursae and Ligaments**
Operation N **Release:** Freeing a body part from an abnormal physical constraint by cutting or by the use of force

Body Part (4th)	Approach (5th)	Device (6th)	Qualifier (7th)
0 Head and Neck Bursa and Ligament **1** Shoulder Bursa and Ligament, Right **2** Shoulder Bursa and Ligament, Left **3** Elbow Bursa and Ligament, Right **4** Elbow Bursa and Ligament, Left **5** Wrist Bursa and Ligament, Right **6** Wrist Bursa and Ligament, Left **7** Hand Bursa and Ligament, Right **8** Hand Bursa and Ligament, Left **9** Upper Extremity Bursa and Ligament, Right **B** Upper Extremity Bursa and Ligament, Left **C** Upper Spine Bursa and Ligament, Right **D** Lower Spine Bursa and Ligament, Left **F** Sternum Bursa and Ligament, Right **G** Rib(s) Bursa and Ligament, Left **H** Abdomen Bursa and Ligament, Right **J** Abdomen Bursa and Ligament, Left **K** Perineum Bursa and Ligament **L** Hip Bursa and Ligament, Right **M** Hip Bursa and Ligament, Left **N** Knee Bursa and Ligament, Right **P** Knee Bursa and Ligament, Left **Q** Ankle Bursa and Ligament, Right **R** Ankle Bursa and Ligament, Left **S** Foot Bursa and Ligament, Right **T** Foot Bursa and Ligament, Left **V** Lower Extremity Bursa and Ligament, Right **W** Lower Extremity Bursa and Ligament, Left	**0** Open **3** Percutaneous **4** Percutaneous Endoscopic **X** External	**Z** No Device	**Z** No Qualifier

Section 0 **Medical and Surgical**
Body System M **Bursae and Ligaments**
Operation P **Removal:** Taking out or off a device from a body part

Body Part (4th)	Approach (5th)	Device (6th)	Qualifier (7th)
X Upper Bursa and Ligament **Y** Lower Bursa and Ligament	**0** Open **3** Percutaneous **4** Percutaneous Endoscopic	**0** Drainage Device **7** Autologous Tissue Substitute **J** Synthetic Substitute **K** Nonautologous Tissue Substitute **Y** Other Device	**Z** No Qualifier
X Upper Bursa and Ligament **Y** Lower Bursa and Ligament	**X** External	**0** Drainage Device	**Z** No Qualifier

tion	0	Medical and Surgical
dy System	M	Bursae and Ligaments
eration	Q	**Repair:** Restoring, to the extent possible, a body part to its normal anatomic structure and function

Body Part (4th)	Approach (5th)	Device (6th)	Qualifier (7th)
Head and Neck Bursa and Ligament Shoulder Bursa and Ligament, Right Shoulder Bursa and Ligament, Left Elbow Bursa and Ligament, Right Elbow Bursa and Ligament, Left Wrist Bursa and Ligament, Right Wrist Bursa and Ligament, Left Hand Bursa and Ligament, Right Hand Bursa and Ligament, Left Upper Extremity Bursa and Ligament, Right Upper Extremity Bursa and Ligament, Left Upper Spine Bursa and Ligament, Right Lower Spine Bursa and Ligament, Left Sternum Bursa and Ligament, Right Rib(s) Bursa and Ligament, Left Abdomen Bursa and Ligament, Right Abdomen Bursa and Ligament, Left Perineum Bursa and Ligament Hip Bursa and Ligament, Right Hip Bursa and Ligament, Left Knee Bursa and Ligament, Right Knee Bursa and Ligament, Left Ankle Bursa and Ligament, Right Ankle Bursa and Ligament, Left Foot Bursa and Ligament, Right Foot Bursa and Ligament, Left Lower Extremity Bursa and Ligament, Right Lower Extremity Bursa and Ligament, Left	**0** Open **3** Percutaneous **4** Percutaneous Endoscopic	**Z** No Device	**Z** No Qualifier

ction	0	Medical and Surgical
dy System	M	Bursae and Ligaments
eration	R	**Replacement:** Putting in or on biological or synthetic material that physically takes the place and/or function of all or a portion of a body part

Body Part (4th)	Approach (5th)	Device (6th)	Qualifier (7th)
Head and Neck Bursa and Ligament Shoulder Bursa and Ligament, Right Shoulder Bursa and Ligament, Left Elbow Bursa and Ligament, Right Elbow Bursa and Ligament, Left Wrist Bursa and Ligament, Right Wrist Bursa and Ligament, Left Hand Bursa and Ligament, Right Hand Bursa and Ligament, Left Upper Extremity Bursa and Ligament, Right Upper Extremity Bursa and Ligament, Left Upper Spine Bursa and Ligament Lower Spine Bursa and Ligament Sternum Bursa and Ligament Rib(s) Bursa and Ligament Abdomen Bursa and Ligament, Right Abdomen Bursa and Ligament, Left Perineum Bursa and Ligament Hip Bursa and Ligament, Right Hip Bursa and Ligament, Left Knee Bursa and Ligament, Right Knee Bursa and Ligament, Left Ankle Bursa and Ligament, Right Ankle Bursa and Ligament, Left Foot Bursa and Ligament, Right Foot Bursa and Ligament, Left Lower Extremity Bursa and Ligament, Right Lower Extremity Bursa and Ligament, Left	**0** Open **4** Percutaneous Endoscopic	**7** Autologous Tissue Substitute **J** Synthetic Substitute **K** Nonautologous Tissue Substitute	**Z** No Qualifier

Section 0 **Medical and Surgical**
Body System M **Bursae and Ligaments**
Operation S **Reposition:** Moving to its normal location, or other suitable location, all or a portion of a body part

Body Part (4th)	Approach (5th)	Device (6th)	Qualifier (7th)
0 Head and Neck Bursa and Ligament **1** Shoulder Bursa and Ligament, Right **2** Shoulder Bursa and Ligament, Left **3** Elbow Bursa and Ligament, Right **4** Elbow Bursa and Ligament, Left **5** Wrist Bursa and Ligament, Right **6** Wrist Bursa and Ligament, Left **7** Hand Bursa and Ligament, Right **8** Hand Bursa and Ligament, Left **9** Upper Extremity Bursa and Ligament, Right **B** Upper Extremity Bursa and Ligament, Left **C** Upper Spine Bursa and Ligament, Right **D** Lower Spine Bursa and Ligament, Left **F** Sternum Bursa and Ligament, Right **G** Rib(s) Bursa and Ligament, Left **H** Abdomen Bursa and Ligament, Right **J** Abdomen Bursa and Ligament, Left **K** Perineum Bursa and Ligament **L** Hip Bursa and Ligament, Right **M** Hip Bursa and Ligament, Left **N** Knee Bursa and Ligament, Right **P** Knee Bursa and Ligament, Left **Q** Ankle Bursa and Ligament, Right **R** Ankle Bursa and Ligament, Left **S** Foot Bursa and Ligament, Right **T** Foot Bursa and Ligament, Left **V** Lower Extremity Bursa and Ligament, Right **W** Lower Extremity Bursa and Ligament, Left	**0** Open **4** Percutaneous Endoscopic	**Z** No Device	**Z** No Qualifier

Section 0 **Medical and Surgical**
Body System M **Bursae and Ligaments**
Operation T **Resection:** Cutting out or off, without replacement, all of a body part

Body Part (4th)	Approach (5th)	Device (6th)	Qualifier (7th)
0 Head and Neck Bursa and Ligament **1** Shoulder Bursa and Ligament, Right **2** Shoulder Bursa and Ligament, Left **3** Elbow Bursa and Ligament, Right **4** Elbow Bursa and Ligament, Left **5** Wrist Bursa and Ligament, Right **6** Wrist Bursa and Ligament, Left **7** Hand Bursa and Ligament, Right **8** Hand Bursa and Ligament, Left **9** Upper Extremity Bursa and Ligament, Right **B** Upper Extremity Bursa and Ligament, Left **C** Upper Spine Bursa and Ligament, Right **D** Lower Spine Bursa and Ligament, Left **F** Sternum Bursa and Ligament, Right **G** Rib(s) Bursa and Ligament, Left **H** Abdomen Bursa and Ligament, Right **J** Abdomen Bursa and Ligament, Left **K** Perineum Bursa and Ligament **L** Hip Bursa and Ligament, Right **M** Hip Bursa and Ligament, Left **N** Knee Bursa and Ligament, Right **P** Knee Bursa and Ligament, Left **Q** Ankle Bursa and Ligament, Right **R** Ankle Bursa and Ligament, Left **S** Foot Bursa and Ligament, Right **T** Foot Bursa and Ligament, Left **V** Lower Extremity Bursa and Ligament, Right **W** Lower Extremity Bursa and Ligament, Left	**0** Open **4** Percutaneous Endoscopic	**Z** No Device	**Z** No Qualifier

ction **0 Medical and Surgical**
dy System **M Bursae and Ligaments**
eration **U Supplement:** Putting in or on biological or synthetic material that physically reinforces and/or augments the function of a portion of a body part

Body Part (4th)	Approach (5th)	Device (6th)	Qualifier (7th)
0 Head and Neck Bursa and Ligament 1 Shoulder Bursa and Ligament, Right 2 Shoulder Bursa and Ligament, Left 3 Elbow Bursa and Ligament, Right 4 Elbow Bursa and Ligament, Left 5 Wrist Bursa and Ligament, Right 6 Wrist Bursa and Ligament, Left 7 Hand Bursa and Ligament, Right 8 Hand Bursa and Ligament, Left 9 Upper Extremity Bursa and Ligament, Right B Upper Extremity Bursa and Ligament, Left C Upper Spine Bursa and Ligament, Right D Lower Spine Bursa and Ligament, Left F Sternum Bursa and Ligament, Right G Rib(s) Bursa and Ligament, Left H Abdomen Bursa and Ligament, Right J Abdomen Bursa and Ligament, Left K Perineum Bursa and Ligament L Hip Bursa and Ligament, Right M Hip Bursa and Ligament, Left N Knee Bursa and Ligament, Right P Knee Bursa and Ligament, Left Q Ankle Bursa and Ligament, Right R Ankle Bursa and Ligament, Left S Foot Bursa and Ligament, Right T Foot Bursa and Ligament, Left V Lower Extremity Bursa and Ligament, Right W Lower Extremity Bursa and Ligament, Left	**0** Open **4** Percutaneous Endoscopic	**7** Autologous Tissue Substitute **J** Synthetic Substitute **K** Nonautologous Tissue Substitute	**Z** No Qualifier

ction **0 Medical and Surgical**
dy System **M Bursae and Ligaments**
eration **W Revision:** Correcting, to the extent possible, a portion of a malfunctioning device or the position of a displaced device

Body Part (4th)	Approach (5th)	Device (6th)	Qualifier (7th)
X Upper Bursa and Ligament Y Lower Bursa and Ligament	**0** Open **3** Percutaneous **4** Percutaneous Endoscopic	**0** Drainage Device **7** Autologous Tissue Substitute **J** Synthetic Substitute **K** Nonautologous Tissue Substitute **Y** Other Device	**Z** No Qualifier
X Upper Bursa and Ligament Y Lower Bursa and Ligament	**X** External	**0** Drainage Device **7** Autologous Tissue Substitute **J** Synthetic Substitute **K** Nonautologous Tissue Substitute	**Z** No Qualifier

Section 0 **Medical and Surgical**
Body System M **Bursae and Ligaments**
Operation X **Transfer:** Moving, without taking out, all or a portion of a body part to another location to take over the function of all c portion of a body part

Body Part (4th)	Approach (5th)	Device (6th)	Qualifier (7th)
0 Head and Neck Bursa and Ligament **1** Shoulder Bursa and Ligament, Right **2** Shoulder Bursa and Ligament, Left **3** Elbow Bursa and Ligament, Right **4** Elbow Bursa and Ligament, Left **5** Wrist Bursa and Ligament, Right **6** Wrist Bursa and Ligament, Left **7** Hand Bursa and Ligament, Right **8** Hand Bursa and Ligament, Left **9** Upper Extremity Bursa and Ligament, Right **B** Upper Extremity Bursa and Ligament, Left **C** Upper Spine Bursa and Ligament, Right **D** Lower Spine Bursa and Ligament, Left **F** Sternum Bursa and Ligament, Right **G** Rib(s) Bursa and Ligament, Left **H** Abdomen Bursa and Ligament, Right **J** Abdomen Bursa and Ligament, Left **K** Perineum Bursa and Ligament **L** Hip Bursa and Ligament, Right **M** Hip Bursa and Ligament, Left **N** Knee Bursa and Ligament, Right **P** Knee Bursa and Ligament, Left **Q** Ankle Bursa and Ligament, Right **R** Ankle Bursa and Ligament, Left **S** Foot Bursa and Ligament, Right **T** Foot Bursa and Ligament, Left **V** Lower Extremity Bursa and Ligament, Right **W** Lower Extremity Bursa and Ligament, Left	**0** Open **4** Percutaneous Endoscopic	**Z** No Device	**Z** No Qualifier

AHA Coding Clinic

0MM14ZZ Reattachment of Right Shoulder Bursa and Ligament, Percutaneous Endoscopic Approach—AHA CC: 3Q, 2013, 20-22

0MQ00ZZ Repair Head and Neck Bursa and Ligament, Open Approach—AHA CC: 3Q, 2014, 9

0MUN47Z Supplement Right Knee Bursa and Ligament with Autologous Tissue Substitute, Percutaneous Endoscopic Approach—AI CC: 2Q, 2017, 21-22

Head and Facial Bones

Temporal bone
Temporal fossa
External acoustic meatus
Styloid process
Mastoid process
Stylomandibular ligament
Stylohyoid ligament
Angle of mandible
Sphenoid bone
Zygomatic arch
Mandibular notch
Ramus of mandible
Mandible
Hyoid bone
Epiglottis
Thyroid cartilage
Trachea
1st rib

©AHIMA

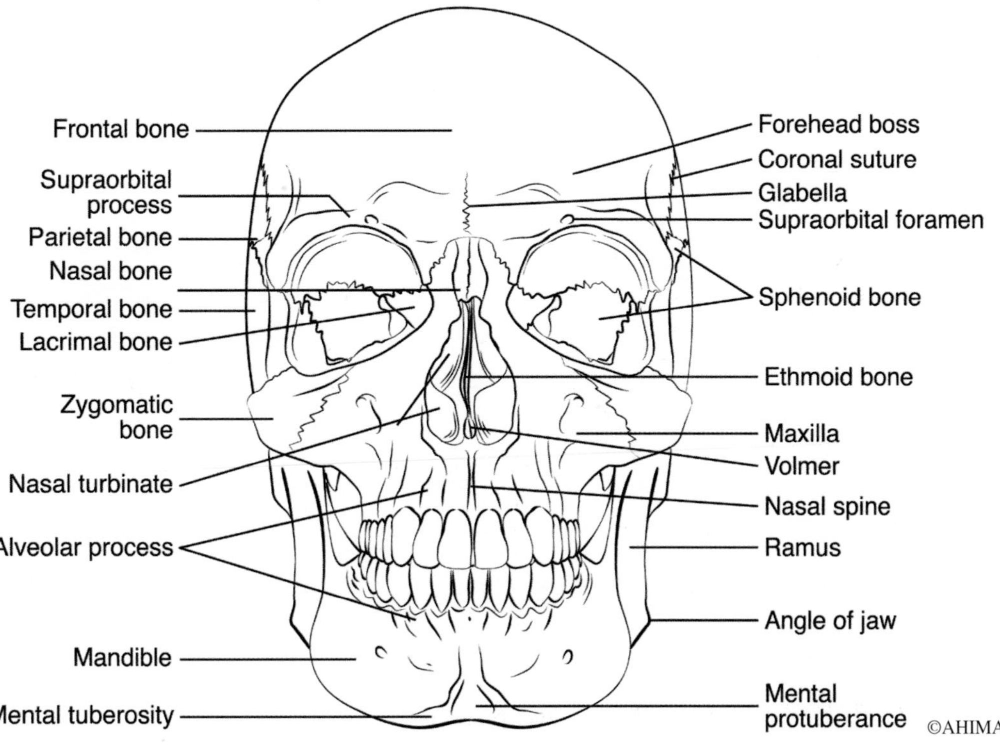

Head and Facial Bones Tables 0N2–0NW

Section 0 **Medical and Surgical**
Body System N **Head and Facial Bones**
Operation 2 **Change:** Taking out or off a device from a body part and putting back an identical or similar device in or on the same bo
part without cutting or puncturing the skin or a mucous membrane

Body Part (4th)	Approach (5th)	Device (6th)	Qualifier (7th)
0 Skull **B** Nasal Bone **W** Facial Bone	**X** External	**0** Drainage Device **Y** Other Device	**Z** No Qualifier

Section 0 **Medical and Surgical**
Body System N **Head and Facial Bones**
Operation 5 **Destruction:** Physical eradication of all or a portion of a body part by the direct use of energy, force, or a destructive age

Body Part (4th)	Approach (5th)	Device (6th)	Qualifier (7th)
0 Skull **1** Frontal Bone **3** Parietal Bone, Right **4** Parietal Bone, Left **5** Temporal Bone, Right **6** Temporal Bone, Left **7** Occipital Bone **B** Nasal Bone **C** Sphenoid Bone **F** Ethmoid Bone, Right **G** Ethmoid Bone, Left **H** Lacrimal Bone, Right **J** Lacrimal Bone, Left **K** Palatine Bone, Right **L** Palatine Bone, Left **M** Zygomatic Bone, Right **N** Zygomatic Bone, Left **P** Orbit, Right **Q** Orbit, Left **R** Maxilla **T** Mandible, Right **V** Mandible, Left **X** Hyoid Bone	**0** Open **3** Percutaneous **4** Percutaneous Endoscopic	**Z** No Device	**Z** No Qualifier

ction 0 **Medical and Surgical**
dy System N **Head and Facial Bones**
eration 8 **Division:** Cutting into a body part, without draining fluids and/or gases from the body part, in order to separate or transect a body part

Body Part (4th)	Approach (5th)	Device (6th)	Qualifier (7th)
0 Skull	**0** Open	**Z** No Device	**Z** No Qualifier
Frontal Bone	**3** Percutaneous		
3 Parietal Bone, Right	**4** Percutaneous Endoscopic		
4 Parietal Bone, Left			
5 Temporal Bone, Right			
6 Temporal Bone, Left			
7 Occipital Bone			
B Nasal Bone			
C Sphenoid Bone			
F Ethmoid Bone, Right			
G Ethmoid Bone, Left			
H Lacrimal Bone, Right			
J Lacrimal Bone, Left			
K Palatine Bone, Right			
L Palatine Bone, Left			
M Zygomatic Bone, Right			
N Zygomatic Bone, Left			
P Orbit, Right			
Q Orbit, Left			
R Maxilla			
T Mandible, Right			
V Mandible, Left			
X Hyoid Bone			

ction 0 **Medical and Surgical**
dy System N **Head and Facial Bones**
eration 9 **Drainage:** Taking or letting out fluids and/or gases from a body part

Body Part (4th)	Approach (5th)	Device (6th)	Qualifier (7th)
0 Skull	**0** Open	**0** Drainage Device	**Z** No Qualifier
1 Frontal Bone	**3** Percutaneous		
3 Parietal Bone, Right	**4** Percutaneous Endoscopic		
4 Parietal Bone, Left			
5 Temporal Bone, Right			
6 Temporal Bone, Left			
7 Occipital Bone			
B Nasal Bone			
C Sphenoid Bone			
F Ethmoid Bone, Right			
G Ethmoid Bone, Left			
H Lacrimal Bone, Right			
J Lacrimal Bone, Left			
K Palatine Bone, Right			
L Palatine Bone, Left			
M Zygomatic Bone, Right			
N Zygomatic Bone, Left			
P Orbit, Right			
Q Orbit, Left			
R Maxilla			
T Mandible, Right			
V Mandible, Left			
X Hyoid Bone			

Continued →

Section 0 **Medical and Surgical**
Body System N **Head and Facial Bones**
Operation 9 **Drainage:** Taking or letting out fluids and/or gases from a body part

Body Part (4th)	Approach (5th)	Device (6th)	Qualifier (7th)
0 Skull **1** Frontal Bone **3** Parietal Bone, Right **4** Parietal Bone, Left **5** Temporal Bone, Right **6** Temporal Bone, Left **7** Occipital Bone **B** Nasal Bone **C** Sphenoid Bone **F** Ethmoid Bone, Right **G** Ethmoid Bone, Left **H** Lacrimal Bone, Right **J** Lacrimal Bone, Left **K** Palatine Bone, Right **L** Palatine Bone, Left **M** Zygomatic Bone, Right **N** Zygomatic Bone, Left **P** Orbit, Right **Q** Orbit, Left **R** Maxilla **T** Mandible, Right **V** Mandible, Left **X** Hyoid Bone	**0** Open **3** Percutaneous **4** Percutaneous Endoscopic	**Z** No Device	**X** Diagnostic **Z** No Qualifier

Section 0 **Medical and Surgical**
Body System N **Head and Facial Bones**
Operation B **Excision:** Cutting out or off, without replacement, a portion of a body part

Body Part (4th)	Approach (5th)	Device (6th)	Qualifier (7th)
0 Skull **1** Frontal Bone **3** Parietal Bone, Right **4** Parietal Bone, Left **5** Temporal Bone, Right **6** Temporal Bone, Left **7** Occipital Bone **B** Nasal Bone **C** Sphenoid Bone **F** Ethmoid Bone, Right **G** Ethmoid Bone, Left **H** Lacrimal Bone, Right **J** Lacrimal Bone, Left **K** Palatine Bone, Right **L** Palatine Bone, Left **M** Zygomatic Bone, Right **N** Zygomatic Bone, Left **P** Orbit, Right **Q** Orbit, Left **R** Maxilla **T** Mandible, Right **V** Mandible, Left **X** Hyoid Bone	**0** Open **3** Percutaneous **4** Percutaneous Endoscopic	**Z** No Device	**X** Diagnostic **Z** No Qualifier

tion	0	**Medical and Surgical**
dy System	N	**Head and Facial Bones**
eration	C	**Extirpation: Taking or cutting out solid matter from a body part**

Body Part (4th)	Approach (5th)	Device (6th)	Qualifier (7th)
Frontal Bone	**0** Open	**Z** No Device	**Z** No Qualifier
Parietal Bone, Right	**3** Percutaneous		
Parietal Bone, Left	**4** Percutaneous Endoscopic		
Temporal Bone, Right			
Temporal Bone, Left			
Occipital Bone			
B Nasal Bone			
C Sphenoid Bone			
F Ethmoid Bone, Right			
G Ethmoid Bone, Left			
H Lacrimal Bone, Right			
Lacrimal Bone, Left			
K Palatine Bone, Right			
L Palatine Bone, Left			
M Zygomatic Bone, Right			
N Zygomatic Bone, Left			
P Orbit, Right			
Q Orbit, Left			
R Maxilla			
T Mandible, Right			
V Mandible, Left			
X Hyoid Bone			

ction	0	**Medical and Surgical**
dy System	N	**Head and Facial Bones**
eration	D	**Extraction:** Pulling or stripping out or off all or a portion of a body part by the use of force

Body Part (4th)	Approach (5th)	Device (6th)	Qualifier (7th)
0 Skull	**0** Open	**Z** No Device	**Z** No Qualifier
1 Frontal Bone			
3 Parietal Bone, Right			
4 Parietal Bone, Left			
5 Temporal Bone, Right			
6 Temporal Bone, Left			
7 Occipital Bone			
B Nasal Bone			
C Sphenoid Bone			
F Ethmoid Bone, Right			
G Ethmoid Bone, Left			
H Lacrimal Bone, Right			
J Lacrimal Bone, Left			
K Palatine Bone, Right			
L Palatine Bone, Left			
M Zygomatic Bone, Right			
N Zygomatic Bone, Left			
P Orbit, Right			
Q Orbit, Left			
R Maxilla			
T Mandible, Right			
V Mandible, Left			
X Hyoid Bone			

Section 0 **Medical and Surgical**
Body System N **Head and Facial Bones**
Operation H **Insertion:** Putting in a nonbiological appliance that monitors, assists, performs, or prevents a physiological function but does not physically take the place of a body part

Body Part (4th)	Approach (5th)	Device (6th)	Qualifier (7th)
0 Skull	**0** Open	**4** Internal Fixation Device **5** External Fixation Device **M** Bone Growth Stimulator **N** Neurostimulator Generator	**Z** No Qualifier
0 Skull	**3** Percutaneous **4** Percutaneous Endoscopic	**4** Internal Fixation Device **5** External Fixation Device **M** Bone Growth Stimulator	**Z** No Qualifier
1 Frontal Bone **3** Parietal Bone, Right **4** Parietal Bone, Left **7** Occipital Bone **C** Sphenoid Bone **F** Ethmoid Bone, Right **G** Ethmoid Bone, Left **H** Lacrimal Bone, Right **J** Lacrimal Bone, Left **K** Palatine Bone, Right **L** Palatine Bone, Left **M** Zygomatic Bone, Right **N** Zygomatic Bone, Left **P** Orbit, Right **Q** Orbit, Left **X** Hyoid Bone	**0** Open **3** Percutaneous **4** Percutaneous Endoscopic	**4** Internal Fixation Device	**Z** No Qualifier
5 Temporal Bone, Right **6** Temporal Bone, Left	**0** Open **3** Percutaneous **4** Percutaneous Endoscopic	**4** Internal Fixation Device **S** Hearing Device	**Z** No Qualifier
B Nasal Bone	**0** Open **3** Percutaneous **4** Percutaneous Endoscopic	**4** Internal Fixation Device **M** Bone Growth Stimulator	**Z** No Qualifier
R Maxilla **T** Mandible, Right **V** Mandible, Left	**0** Open **3** Percutaneous **4** Percutaneous Endoscopic	**4** Internal Fixation Device **5** External Fixation Device	**Z** No Qualifier
W Facial Bone	**0** Open **3** Percutaneous **4** Percutaneous Endoscopic	**M** Bone Growth Stimulator	**Z** No Qualifier

Section 0 **Medical and Surgical**
Body System N **Head and Facial Bones**
Operation J **Inspection:** Visually and/or manually exploring a body part

Body Part (4th)	Approach (5th)	Device (6th)	Qualifier (7th)
0 Skull **B** Nasal Bone **W** Facial Bone	**0** Open **3** Percutaneous **4** Percutaneous Endoscopic **X** External	**Z** No Device	**Z** No Qualifier

tion	0	**Medical and Surgical**
ly System	N	**Head and Facial Bones**
eration	N	**Release:** Freeing a body part from an abnormal physical constraint by cutting or by the use of force

Body Part (4th)	Approach (5th)	Device (6th)	Qualifier (7th)
Frontal Bone Parietal Bone, Right Parietal Bone, Left Temporal Bone, Right Temporal Bone, Left Occipital Bone Nasal Bone Sphenoid Bone Ethmoid Bone, Right Ethmoid Bone, Left Lacrimal Bone, Right Lacrimal Bone, Left Palatine Bone, Right Palatine Bone, Left Zygomatic Bone, Right Zygomatic Bone, Left Orbit, Right Orbit, Left Maxilla Mandible, Right Mandible, Left Hyoid Bone	**0** Open **3** Percutaneous **4** Percutaneous Endoscopic	**Z** No Device	**Z** No Qualifier

tion	0	**Medical and Surgical**
dy System	N	**Head and Facial Bones**
eration	P	**Removal:** Taking out or off a device from a body part

Body Part (4th)	Approach (5th)	Device (6th)	Qualifier (7th)
Skull	**0** Open	**0** Drainage Device **4** Internal Fixation Device **5** External Fixation Device **7** Autologous Tissue Substitute **J** Synthetic Substitute **K** Nonautologous Tissue Substitute **M** Bone Growth Stimulator **N** Neurostimulator Generator **S** Hearing Device	**Z** No Qualifier
Skull	**3** Percutaneous **4** Percutaneous Endoscopic	**0** Drainage Device **4** Internal Fixation Device **5** External Fixation Device **7** Autologous Tissue Substitute **J** Synthetic Substitute **K** Nonautologous Tissue Substitute **M** Bone Growth Stimulator **S** Hearing Device	**Z** No Qualifier
Skull	**X** External	**0** Drainage Device **4** Internal Fixation Device **5** External Fixation Device **M** Bone Growth Stimulator **S** Hearing Device	**Z** No Qualifier
B Nasal Bone **W** Facial Bone	**0** Open **3** Percutaneous **4** Percutaneous Endoscopic	**0** Drainage Device **4** Internal Fixation Device **7** Autologous Tissue Substitute **J** Synthetic Substitute **K** Nonautologous Tissue Substitute **M** Bone Growth Stimulator	**Z** No Qualifier
B Nasal Bone **W** Facial Bone	**X** External	**0** Drainage Device **4** Internal Fixation Device **M** Bone Growth Stimulator	**Z** No Qualifier

Section 0 **Medical and Surgical**
Body System N **Head and Facial Bones**
Operation Q **Repair:** Restoring, to the extent possible, a body part to its normal anatomic structure and function

Body Part (4th)	Approach (5th)	Device (6th)	Qualifier (7th)
0 Skull **1** Frontal Bone **3** Parietal Bone, Right **4** Parietal Bone, Left **5** Temporal Bone, Right **6** Temporal Bone, Left **7** Occipital Bone **B** Nasal Bone **C** Sphenoid Bone **F** Ethmoid Bone, Right **G** Ethmoid Bone, Left **H** Lacrimal Bone, Right **J** Lacrimal Bone, Left **K** Palatine Bone, Right **L** Palatine Bone, Left **M** Zygomatic Bone, Right **N** Zygomatic Bone, Left **P** Orbit, Right **Q** Orbit, Left **R** Maxilla **T** Mandible, Right **V** Mandible, Left **X** Hyoid Bone	**0** Open **3** Percutaneous **4** Percutaneous Endoscopic **X** External	**Z** No Device	**Z** No Qualifier

Section 0 **Medical and Surgical**
Body System N **Head and Facial Bones**
Operation R **Replacement:** Putting in or on biological or synthetic material that physically takes the place and/or function of all or a portion of a body part

Body Part (4th)	Approach (5th)	Device (6th)	Qualifier (7th)
0 Skull **1** Frontal Bone **3** Parietal Bone, Right **4** Parietal Bone, Left **5** Temporal Bone, Right **6** Temporal Bone, Left **7** Occipital Bone **B** Nasal Bone **C** Sphenoid Bone **F** Ethmoid Bone, Right **G** Ethmoid Bone, Left **H** Lacrimal Bone, Right **J** Lacrimal Bone, Left **K** Palatine Bone, Right **L** Palatine Bone, Left **M** Zygomatic Bone, Right **N** Zygomatic Bone, Left **P** Orbit, Right **Q** Orbit, Left **R** Maxilla **T** Mandible, Right **V** Mandible, Left **X** Hyoid Bone	**0** Open **3** Percutaneous **4** Percutaneous Endoscopic	**7** Autologous Tissue Substitute **J** Synthetic Substitute **K** Nonautologous Tissue Substitute	**Z** No Qualifier

ction **0** **Medical and Surgical**
dy System **N** **Head and Facial Bones**
peration **S** **Reposition:** Moving to its normal location, or other suitable location, all or a portion of a body part

Body Part (4th)	Approach (5th)	Device (6th)	Qualifier (7th)
0 Skull **R** Maxilla **T** Mandible, Right **V** Mandible, Left	**0** Open **3** Percutaneous **4** Percutaneous Endoscopic	**4** Internal Fixation Device **5** External Fixation Device **Z** No Device	**Z** No Qualifier
0 Skull **R** Maxilla **T** Mandible, Right **V** Mandible, Left	**X** External	**Z** No Device	**Z** No Qualifier
1 Frontal Bone **3** Parietal Bone, Right **4** Parietal Bone, Left **5** Temporal Bone, Right **6** Temporal Bone, Left **7** Occipital Bone **B** Nasal Bone **C** Sphenoid Bone **F** Ethmoid Bone, Right **G** Ethmoid Bone, Left **H** Lacrimal Bone, Right **J** Lacrimal Bone, Left **K** Palatine Bone, Right **L** Palatine Bone, Left **M** Zygomatic Bone, Right **N** Zygomatic Bone, Left **P** Orbit, Right **Q** Orbit, Left **X** Hyoid Bone	**0** Open **3** Percutaneous **4** Percutaneous Endoscopic	**4** Internal Fixation Device **Z** No Device	**Z** No Qualifier
1 Frontal Bone **3** Parietal Bone, Right **4** Parietal Bone, Left **5** Temporal Bone, Right **6** Temporal Bone, Left **7** Occipital Bone **B** Nasal Bone **C** Sphenoid Bone **F** Ethmoid Bone, Right **G** Ethmoid Bone, Left **H** Lacrimal Bone, Right **J** Lacrimal Bone, Left **K** Palatine Bone, Right **L** Palatine Bone, Left **M** Zygomatic Bone, Right **N** Zygomatic Bone, Left **P** Orbit, Right **Q** Orbit, Left **X** Hyoid Bone	**X** External	**Z** No Device	**Z** No Qualifier

Section 0 **Medical and Surgical**
Body System N **Head and Facial Bones**
Operation T **Resection:** Cutting out or off, without replacement, all of a body part

Body Part (4th)	Approach (5th)	Device (6th)	Qualifier (7th)
1 Frontal Bone **3** Parietal Bone, Right **4** Parietal Bone, Left **5** Temporal Bone, Right **6** Temporal Bone, Left **7** Occipital Bone **B** Nasal Bone **C** Sphenoid Bone **F** Ethmoid Bone, Right **G** Ethmoid Bone, Left **H** Lacrimal Bone, Right **J** Lacrimal Bone, Left **K** Palatine Bone, Right **L** Palatine Bone, Left **M** Zygomatic Bone, Right **N** Zygomatic Bone, Left **P** Orbit, Right **Q** Orbit, Left **R** Maxilla **T** Mandible, Right **V** Mandible, Left **X** Hyoid Bone	**0** Open	**Z** No Device	**Z** No Qualifier

Section 0 **Medical and Surgical**
Body System N **Head and Facial Bones**
Operation U **Supplement:** Putting in or on biological or synthetic material that physically reinforces and/or augments the function of a portion of a body part

Body Part (4th)	Approach (5th)	Device (6th)	Qualifier (7th)
0 Skull **1** Frontal Bone **3** Parietal Bone, Right **4** Parietal Bone, Left **5** Temporal Bone, Right **6** Temporal Bone, Left **7** Occipital Bone **B** Nasal Bone **C** Sphenoid Bone **F** Ethmoid Bone, Right **G** Ethmoid Bone, Left **H** Lacrimal Bone, Right **J** Lacrimal Bone, Left **K** Palatine Bone, Right **L** Palatine Bone, Left **M** Zygomatic Bone, Right **N** Zygomatic Bone, Left **P** Orbit, Right **Q** Orbit, Left **R** Maxilla **T** Mandible, Right **V** Mandible, Left **X** Hyoid Bone	**0** Open **3** Percutaneous **4** Percutaneous Endoscopic	**7** Autologous Tissue Substitute **J** Synthetic Substitute **K** Nonautologous Tissue Substitute	**Z** No Qualifier

:tion 0 **Medical and Surgical**
dy System N **Head and Facial Bones**
eration W **Revision:** Correcting, to the extent possible, a portion of a malfunctioning device or the position of a displaced device

Body Part (4th)	Approach (5th)	Device (6th)	Qualifier (7th)
Skull	**0** Open	**0** Drainage Device **4** Internal Fixation Device **5** External Fixation Device **7** Autologous Tissue Substitute **J** Synthetic Substitute **K** Nonautologous Tissue Substitute **M** Bone Growth Stimulator **N** Neurostimulator Generator **S** Hearing Device	**Z** No Qualifier
Skull	**3** Percutaneous **4** Percutaneous Endoscopic **X** External	**0** Drainage Device **4** Internal Fixation Device **5** External Fixation Device **7** Autologous Tissue Substitute **J** Synthetic Substitute **K** Nonautologous Tissue Substitute **M** Bone Growth Stimulator **S** Hearing Device	**Z** No Qualifier
B Nasal Bone **W** Facial Bone	**0** Open **3** Percutaneous **4** Percutaneous Endoscopic **X** External	**0** Drainage Device **4** Internal Fixation Device **7** Autologous Tissue Substitute **J** Synthetic Substitute **K** Nonautologous Tissue Substitute **M** Bone Growth Stimulator	**Z** No Qualifier

HA Coding Clinic

NBB0ZZ Excision of Nasal Bone, Open Approach—AHA CC: 1Q, 2017, 20-21
NBQ0ZZ Excision of Left Orbit, Open Approach—AHA CC: 2Q, 2015, 12-1
NH004Z Insertion of Internal Fixation Device into Skull, Open Approach—AHA CC: 3Q, 2015, 13-14
NP004Z Removal of Internal Fixation Device from Skull, Open Approach—AHA CC: 3Q, 2015, 13-14
NR00JZ Replacement of Skull with Synthetic Substitute, Open Approach—AHA CC: 3Q, 2014, 7-8
NR70JZ Replacement of Occipital Bone with Synthetic Substitute, Open Approach—AHA CC: 3Q, 2017, 17
NRV07Z Replacement of Left Mandible with Autologous Tissue Substitute, Open Approach—AHA CC: 1Q, 2017, 23-24
NRV0JZ Replacement of Left Mandible with Synthetic Substitute, Open Approach—AHA CC: 1Q, 2017, 23-24
NS004Z Reposition Skull with Internal Fixation Device, Open Approach—AHA CC: 3Q, 2017, 22
NS005Z Reposition Skull with External Fixation Device, Open Approach—AHA CC: 3Q, 2013, 24-25
NS00ZZ Reposition Skull, Open Approach—AHA CC: 3Q, 2015, 17-18; 2Q, 2016, 30
NS104Z Reposition Frontal Bone with Internal Fixation Device, Open Approach—AHA CC: 3Q, 2013, 25
NS504Z Reposition Right Temporal Bone with Internal Fixation Device, Open Approach—AHA CC: 3Q, 2015, 27-28
NSR04Z Reposition Maxilla with Internal Fixation Device, Open Approach—AHA CC: 3Q, 2014, 23-24
NSR0ZZ Reposition Maxilla, Open Approach—AHA CC: 1Q, 2017, 20-21
NU00JZ Supplement Skull with Synthetic Substitute, Open Approach—AHA CC: 3Q, 2013, 24-25
NUR07Z Supplement Maxilla with Autologous Tissue Substitute, Open Approach—AHA CC: 3Q, 2016, 29-30

Bones - Front and Back Views

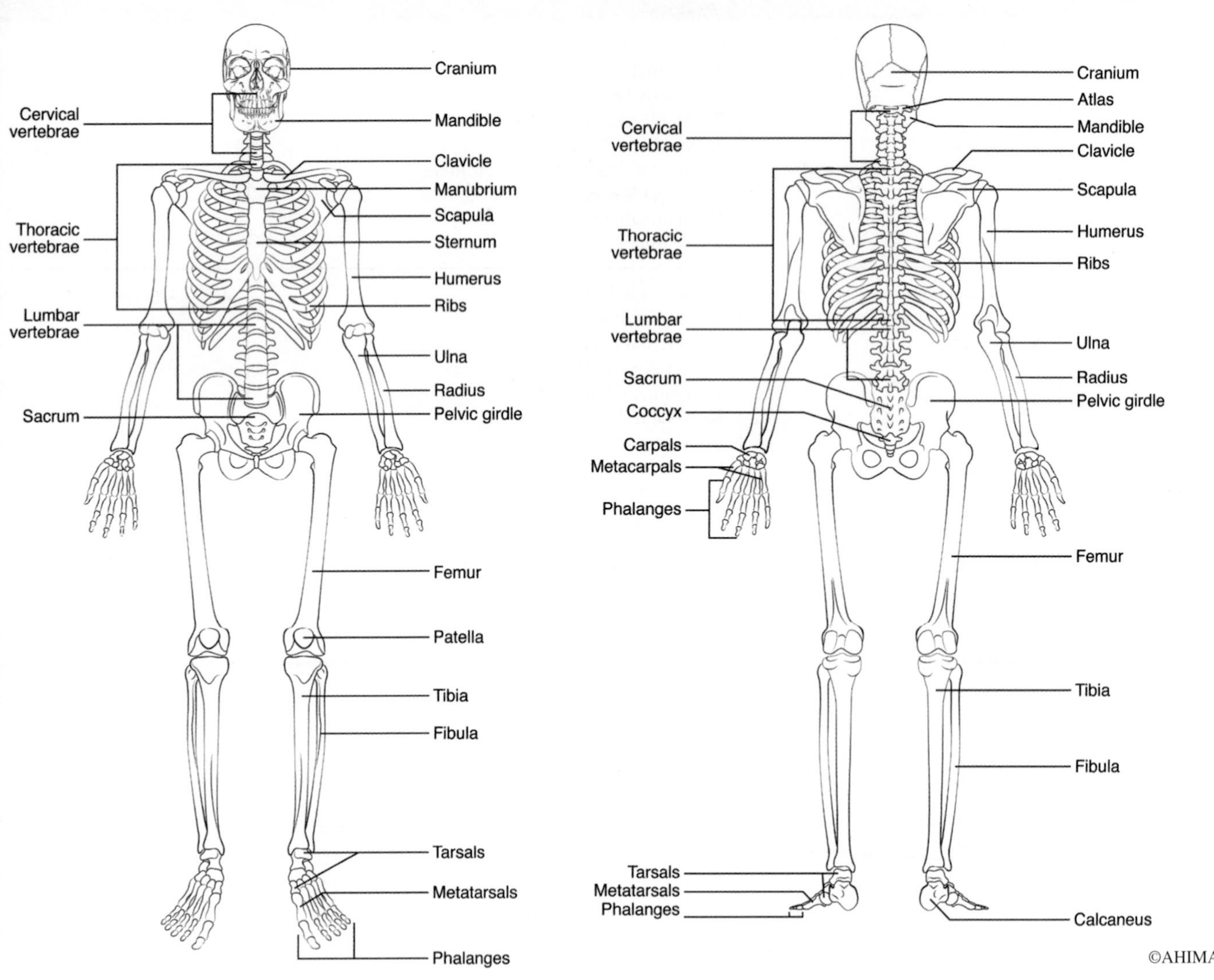

Vertebrae

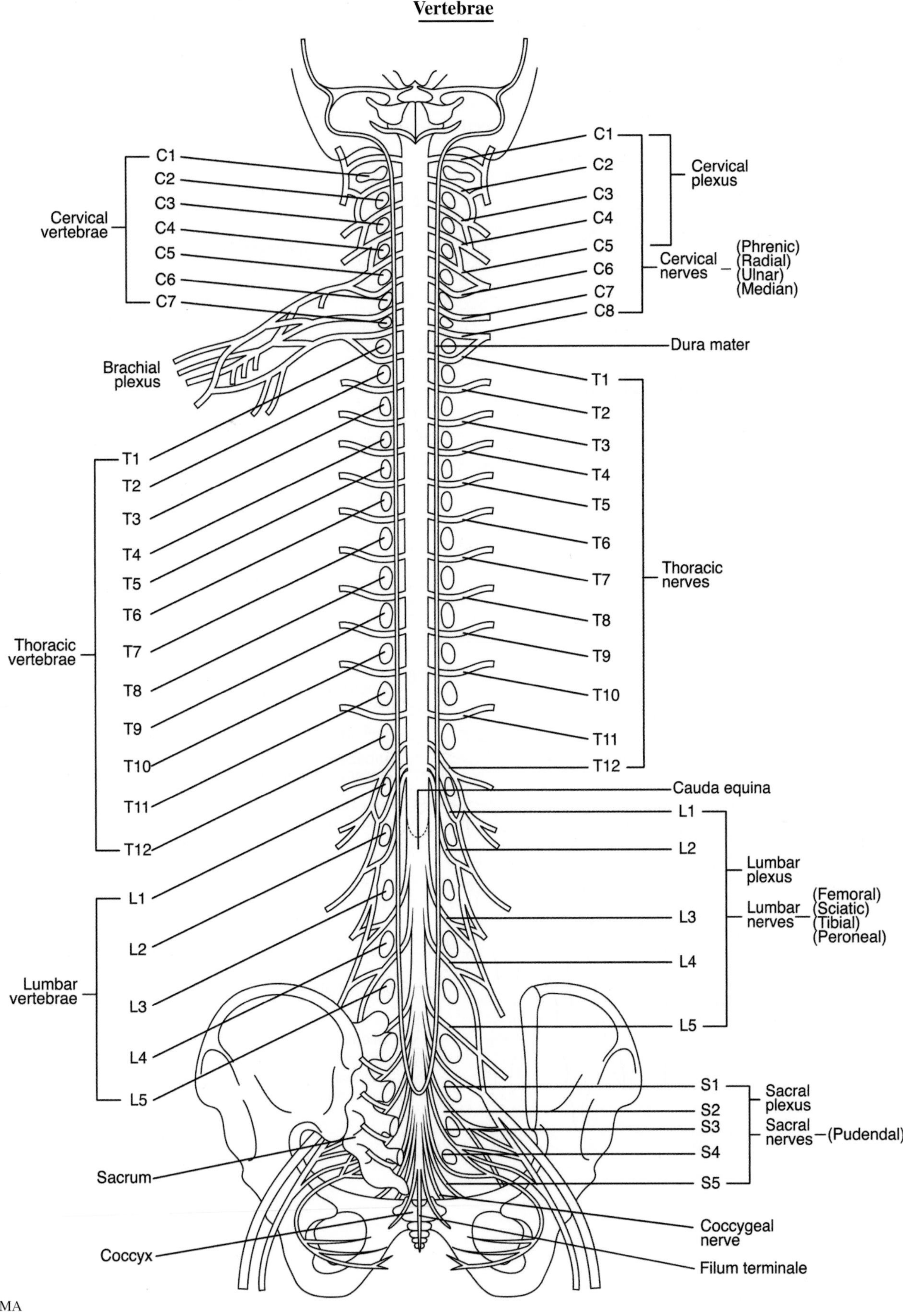

AHIMA

Cross-section Spine

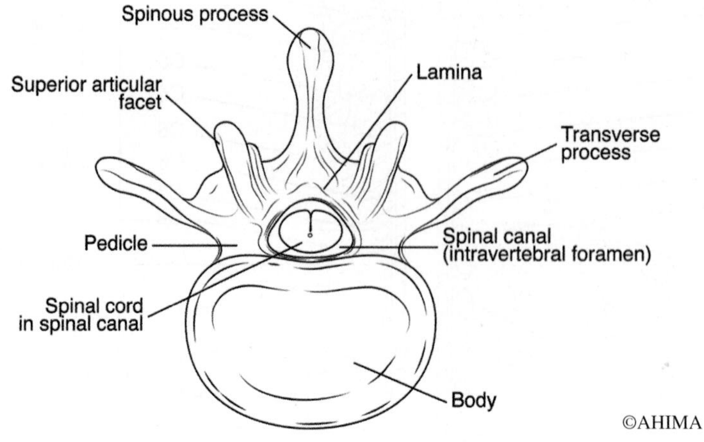

Hand Bones

Ulna
Radius
Lunate (semilunar)
Scaphoid (navicular)
Carpals
Triangular (triquetrum)
Capitate
Carpals
Trapezoid (lesser multangular)
Pisiform
Hamate (unciform)
Trapezium (greater multangular)
1
Metacarpals
5
4
3
2
Phalanges
Proimal phalanx
Middle phalanx
Distal phalanx

©AHIMA

pper Bones Tables 0P2–0PW

ection 0 **Medical and Surgical**
ody System P **Upper Bones**
peration 2 **Change:** Taking out or off a device from a body part and putting back an identical or similar device in or on the same body part without cutting or puncturing the skin or a mucous membrane

Body Part (4th)	Approach (5th)	Device (6th)	Qualifier (7th)
Y Upper Bone	X External	0 Drainage Device Y Other Device	Z No Qualifier

ection 0 **Medical and Surgical**
ody System P **Upper Bones**
peration 5 **Destruction:** Physical eradication of all or a portion of a body part by the direct use of energy, force, or a destructive agent

Body Part (4th)	Approach (5th)	Device (6th)	Qualifier (7th)
0 Sternum 1 Ribs, 1 to 2 2 Ribs, 3 or More 3 Cervical Vertebra 4 Thoracic Vertebra 5 Scapula, Right 6 Scapula, Left 7 Glenoid Cavity, Right 8 Glenoid Cavity, Left 9 Clavicle, Right B Clavicle, Left C Humeral Head, Right D Humeral Head, Left F Humeral Shaft, Right G Humeral Shaft, Left H Radius, Right J Radius, Left K Ulna, Right L Ulna, Left M Carpal, Right N Carpal, Left P Metacarpal, Right Q Metacarpal, Left R Thumb Phalanx, Right S Thumb Phalanx, Left T Finger Phalanx, Right V Finger Phalanx, Left	0 Open 3 Percutaneous 4 Percutaneous Endoscopic	Z No Device	Z No Qualifier

Section 0 **Medical and Surgical**
Body System P **Upper Bones**
Operation 8 **Division:** Cutting into a body part, without draining fluids and/or gases from the body part, in order to separate or transec body part

Body Part (4th)	Approach (5th)	Device (6th)	Qualifier (7th)
0 Sternum **1** Ribs, 1 to 2 **2** Ribs, 3 or More **3** Cervical Vertebra **4** Thoracic Vertebra **5** Scapula, Right **6** Scapula, Left **7** Glenoid Cavity, Right **8** Glenoid Cavity, Left **9** Clavicle, Right **B** Clavicle, Left **C** Humeral Head, Right **D** Humeral Head, Left **F** Humeral Shaft, Right **G** Humeral Shaft, Left **H** Radius, Right **J** Radius, Left **K** Ulna, Right **L** Ulna, Left **M** Carpal, Right **N** Carpal, Left **P** Metacarpal, Right **Q** Metacarpal, Left **R** Thumb Phalanx, Right **S** Thumb Phalanx, Left **T** Finger Phalanx, Right **V** Finger Phalanx, Left	**0** Open **3** Percutaneous **4** Percutaneous Endoscopic	**Z** No Device	**Z** No Qualifier

Section 0 **Medical and Surgical**
Body System P **Upper Bones**
Operation 9 **Drainage:** Taking or letting out fluids and/or gases from a body part

Body Part (4th)	Approach (5th)	Device (6th)	Qualifier (7th)
0 Sternum **1** Ribs, 1 to 2 **2** Ribs, 3 or More **3** Cervical Vertebra **4** Thoracic Vertebra **5** Scapula, Right **6** Scapula, Left **7** Glenoid Cavity, Right **8** Glenoid Cavity, Left **9** Clavicle, Right **B** Clavicle, Left **C** Humeral Head, Right **D** Humeral Head, Left **F** Humeral Shaft, Right **G** Humeral Shaft, Left **H** Radius, Right **J** Radius, Left **K** Ulna, Right **L** Ulna, Left **M** Carpal, Right **N** Carpal, Left **P** Metacarpal, Right **Q** Metacarpal, Left **R** Thumb Phalanx, Right **S** Thumb Phalanx, Left **T** Finger Phalanx, Right **V** Finger Phalanx, Left	**0** Open **3** Percutaneous **4** Percutaneous Endoscopic	**0** Drainage Device	**Z** No Qualifier

Continued →

0P9 Continued

tion	**0**	**Medical and Surgical**
dy System	**P**	**Upper Bones**
eration	**9**	**Drainage:** Taking or letting out fluids and/or gases from a body part

Body Part (4th)	Approach (5th)	Device (6th)	Qualifier (7th)
Sternum Ribs, 1 to 2 Ribs, 3 or More Cervical Vertebra Thoracic Vertebra Scapula, Right Scapula, Left Glenoid Cavity, Right Glenoid Cavity, Left Clavicle, Right Clavicle, Left Humeral Head, Right Humeral Head, Left Humeral Shaft, Right Humeral Shaft, Left Radius, Right Radius, Left Ulna, Right Ulna, Left Carpal, Right Carpal, Left Metacarpal, Right Metacarpal, Left Thumb Phalanx, Right Thumb Phalanx, Left Finger Phalanx, Right Finger Phalanx, Left	**0** Open **3** Percutaneous **4** Percutaneous Endoscopic	**Z** No Device	**X** Diagnostic **Z** No Qualifier

tion	**0**	**Medical and Surgical**
dy System	**P**	**Upper Bones**
eration	**B**	**Excision:** Cutting out or off, without replacement, a portion of a body part

Body Part (4th)	Approach (5th)	Device (6th)	Qualifier (7th)
Sternum Ribs, 1 to 2 Ribs, 3 or More Cervical Vertebra Thoracic Vertebra Scapula, Right Scapula, Left Glenoid Cavity, Right Glenoid Cavity, Left Clavicle, Right Clavicle, Left Humeral Head, Right Humeral Head, Left Humeral Shaft, Right Humeral Shaft, Left Radius, Right Radius, Left Ulna, Right Ulna, Left Carpal, Right Carpal, Left Metacarpal, Right Metacarpal, Left Thumb Phalanx, Right Thumb Phalanx, Left Finger Phalanx, Right Finger Phalanx, Left	**0** Open **3** Percutaneous **4** Percutaneous Endoscopic	**Z** No Device	**X** Diagnostic **Z** No Qualifier

Section 0 **Medical and Surgical**
Body System P **Upper Bones**
Operation C **Extirpation:** Taking or cutting out solid matter from a body part

Body Part (4th)	Approach (5th)	Device (6th)	Qualifier (7th)
0 Sternum **1** Ribs, 1 to 2 **2** Ribs, 3 or More **3** Cervical Vertebra **4** Thoracic Vertebra **5** Scapula, Right **6** Scapula, Left **7** Glenoid Cavity, Right **8** Glenoid Cavity, Left **9** Clavicle, Right **B** Clavicle, Left **C** Humeral Head, Right **D** Humeral Head, Left **F** Humeral Shaft, Right **G** Humeral Shaft, Left **H** Radius, Right **J** Radius, Left **K** Ulna, Right **L** Ulna, Left **M** Carpal, Right **N** Carpal, Left **P** Metacarpal, Right **Q** Metacarpal, Left **R** Thumb Phalanx, Right **S** Thumb Phalanx, Left **T** Finger Phalanx, Right **V** Finger Phalanx, Left	**0** Open **3** Percutaneous **4** Percutaneous Endoscopic	**Z** No Device	**Z** No Qualifier

Section 0 **Medical and Surgical**
Body System P **Upper Bones**
Operation D **Extraction:** Pulling or stripping out or off all or a portion of a body part by the use of force

Body Part (4th)	Approach (5th)	Device (6th)	Qualifier (7th)
0 Sternum **1** Ribs, 1 to 2 **2** Ribs, 3 or More **3** Cervical Vertebra **4** Thoracic Vertebra **5** Scapula, Right **6** Scapula, Left **7** Glenoid Cavity, Right **8** Glenoid Cavity, Left **9** Clavical, Right **B** Clavical, Left **C** Humeral Head, Right **D** Humeral Head, Left **F** Humeral Shaft, Right **G** Humeral Shaft, Left **H** Radius, Right **J** Radius, Left **K** Ulna, Right **L** Ulna, Left **M** Carpal, Right **N** Carpal, Left **P** Metacarpal, Right **Q** Metacarpal, Left **R** Thumb Phalanx, Right **S** Thumb Phalanx, Left **T** Finger Phalanx, Right **V** Finger Phalanx, Left	**0** Open	**Z** No Device	**Z** No Qualifier

ction	**0**	**Medical and Surgical**
dy System	**P**	**Upper Bones**
eration	**H**	**Insertion:** Putting in a nonbiological appliance that monitors, assists, performs, or prevents a physiological function but does not physically take the place of a body part

Body Part (4th)	Approach (5th)	Device (6th)	Qualifier (7th)
0 Sternum	**0** Open **3** Percutaneous **4** Percutaneous Endoscopic	**0** Internal Fixation Device, Rigid Plate **4** Internal Fixation Device	**Z** No Qualifier
1 Ribs, 1 to 2 2 Ribs, 3 or More 3 Cervical Vertebra 4 Thoracic Vertebra 5 Scapula, Right 6 Scapula, Left 7 Glenoid Cavity, Right 8 Glenoid Cavity, Left 9 Clavicle, Right B Clavicle, Left	**0** Open **3** Percutaneous **4** Percutaneous Endoscopic	**4** Internal Fixation Device	**Z** No Qualifier
C Humeral Head, Right D Humeral Head, Left F Humeral Shaft, Right G Humeral Shaft, Left H Radius, Right J Radius, Left K Ulna, Right L Ulna, Left	**0** Open **3** Percutaneous **4** Percutaneous Endoscopic	**4** Internal Fixation Device **5** External Fixation Device **6** Internal Fixation Device, Intramedullary **8** External Fixation Device, Limb Lengthening **B** External Fixation Device, Monoplanar **C** External Fixation Device, Ring **D** External Fixation Device, Hybrid	**Z** No Qualifier
M Carpal, Right N Carpal, Left P Metacarpal, Right Q Metacarpal, Left R Thumb Phalanx, Right S Thumb Phalanx, Left T Finger Phalanx, Right V Finger Phalanx, Left	**0** Open **3** Percutaneous **4** Percutaneous Endoscopic	**4** Internal Fixation Device **5** External Fixation Device	**Z** No Qualifier
Y Upper Bone	**0** Open **3** Percutaneous **4** Percutaneous Endoscopic	**M** Bone Growth Stimulator	**Z** No Qualifier

ction	**0**	**Medical and Surgical**
dy System	**P**	**Upper Bones**
eration	**J**	**Inspection:** Visually and/or manually exploring a body part

Body Part (4th)	Approach (5th)	Device (6th)	Qualifier (7th)
Y Upper Bone	**0** Open **3** Percutaneous **4** Percutaneous Endoscopic **X** External	**Z** No Device	**Z** No Qualifier

Section 0 **Medical and Surgical**
Body System P **Upper Bones**
Operation N **Release:** Freeing a body part from an abnormal physical constraint by cutting or by the use of force

Body Part (4th)	Approach (5th)	Device (6th)	Qualifier (7th)
0 Sternum **1** Ribs, 1 to 2 **2** Ribs, 3 or More **3** Cervical Vertebra **4** Thoracic Vertebra **5** Scapula, Right **6** Scapula, Left **7** Glenoid Cavity, Right **8** Glenoid Cavity, Left **9** Clavicle, Right **B** Clavicle, Left **C** Humeral Head, Right **D** Humeral Head, Left **F** Humeral Shaft, Right **G** Humeral Shaft, Left **H** Radius, Right **J** Radius, Left **K** Ulna, Right **L** Ulna, Left **M** Carpal, Right **N** Carpal, Left **P** Metacarpal, Right **Q** Metacarpal, Left **R** Thumb Phalanx, Right **S** Thumb Phalanx, Left **T** Finger Phalanx, Right **V** Finger Phalanx, Left	**0** Open **3** Percutaneous **4** Percutaneous Endoscopic	**Z** No Device	**Z** No Qualifier

Section 0 **Medical and Surgical**
Body System P **Upper Bones**
Operation P **Removal:** Taking out or off a device from a body part

Body Part (4th)	Approach (5th)	Device (6th)	Qualifier (7th)
0 Sternum **1** Ribs, 1 to 2 **2** Ribs, 3 or More **3** Cervical Vertebra **4** Thoracic Vertebra **5** Scapula, Right **6** Scapula, Left **7** Glenoid Cavity, Right **8** Glenoid Cavity, Left **9** Clavicle, Right **B** Clavicle, Left	**0** Open **3** Percutaneous **4** Percutaneous Endoscopic	**4** Internal Fixation Device **7** Autologous Tissue Substitute **J** Synthetic Substitute **K** Nonautologous Tissue Substitute	**Z** No Qualifier
0 Sternum **1** Ribs, 1 to 2 **2** Ribs, 3 or More **3** Cervical Vertebra **4** Thoracic Vertebra **5** Scapula, Right **6** Scapula, Left **7** Glenoid Cavity, Right **8** Glenoid Cavity, Left **9** Clavicle, Right **B** Clavicle, Left	**X** External	**4** Internal Fixation Device	**Z** No Qualifier

Continued →

Section 0 **Medical and Surgical**
Body System P **Upper Bones**
Operation P **Removal:** Taking out or off a device from a body part

Body Part (4th)	Approach (5th)	Device (6th)	Qualifier (7th)
C Humeral Head, Right **D** Humeral Head, Left **F** Humeral Shaft, Right **G** Humeral Shaft, Left **H** Radius, Right **J** Radius, Left **K** Ulna, Right **L** Ulna, Left **M** Carpal, Right **N** Carpal, Left **P** Metacarpal, Right **Q** Metacarpal, Left **R** Thumb Phalanx, Right **S** Thumb Phalanx, Left **T** Finger Phalanx, Right **V** Finger Phalanx, Left	**0** Open **3** Percutaneous **4** Percutaneous Endoscopic	**4** Internal Fixation Device **5** External Fixation Device **7** Autologous Tissue Substitute **J** Synthetic Substitute **K** Nonautologous Tissue Substitute	**Z** No Qualifier
C Humeral Head, Right **D** Humeral Head, Left **F** Humeral Shaft, Right **G** Humeral Shaft, Left **H** Radius, Right **J** Radius, Left **K** Ulna, Right **L** Ulna, Left **M** Carpal, Right **N** Carpal, Left **P** Metacarpal, Right **Q** Metacarpal, Left **R** Thumb Phalanx, Right **S** Thumb Phalanx, Left **T** Finger Phalanx, Right **V** Finger Phalanx, Left	**X** External	**4** Internal Fixation Device **5** External Fixation Device	**Z** No Qualifier
Y Upper Bone	**0** Open **3** Percutaneous **4** Percutaneous Endoscopic **X** External	**0** Drainage Device **M** Bone Growth Stimulator	**Z** No Qualifier

Section 0 **Medical and Surgical**
Body System P **Upper Bones**
Operation Q **Repair:** Restoring, to the extent possible, a body part to its normal anatomic structure and function

Body Part (4th)	Approach (5th)	Device (6th)	Qualifier (7th)
0 Sternum **1** Ribs, 1 to 2 **2** Ribs, 3 or More **3** Cervical Vertebra **4** Thoracic Vertebra **5** Scapula, Right **6** Scapula, Left **7** Glenoid Cavity, Right **8** Glenoid Cavity, Left **9** Clavicle, Right **B** Clavicle, Left **C** Humeral Head, Right **D** Humeral Head, Left **F** Humeral Shaft, Right **G** Humeral Shaft, Left **H** Radius, Right **J** Radius, Left **K** Ulna, Right **L** Ulna, Left **M** Carpal, Right **N** Carpal, Left **P** Metacarpal, Right **Q** Metacarpal, Left **R** Thumb Phalanx, Right **S** Thumb Phalanx, Left **T** Finger Phalanx, Right **V** Finger Phalanx, Left	**0** Open **3** Percutaneous **4** Percutaneous Endoscopic **X** External	**Z** No Device	**Z** No Qualifier

Section 0 **Medical and Surgical**
Body System P **Upper Bones**
Operation R **Replacement:** Putting in or on biological or synthetic material that physically takes the place and/or function of all or a portion of a body part

Body Part (4th)	Approach (5th)	Device (6th)	Qualifier (7th)
0 Sternum **1** Ribs, 1 to 2 **2** Ribs, 3 or More **3** Cervical Vertebra **4** Thoracic Vertebra **5** Scapula, Right **6** Scapula, Left **7** Glenoid Cavity, Right **8** Glenoid Cavity, Left **9** Clavicle, Right **B** Clavicle, Left **C** Humeral Head, Right **D** Humeral Head, Left **F** Humeral Shaft, Right **G** Humeral Shaft, Left **H** Radius, Right **J** Radius, Left **K** Ulna, Right **L** Ulna, Left **M** Carpal, Right **N** Carpal, Left **P** Metacarpal, Right **Q** Metacarpal, Left **R** Thumb Phalanx, Right **S** Thumb Phalanx, Left **T** Finger Phalanx, Right **V** Finger Phalanx, Left	**0** Open **3** Percutaneous **4** Percutaneous Endoscopic	**7** Autologous Tissue Substitute **J** Synthetic Substitute **K** Nonautologous Tissue Substitute	**Z** No Qualifier

ection 0 Medical and Surgical
ody System P Upper Bones
peration S Reposition: Moving to its normal location, or other suitable location, all or a portion of a body part

Body Part (4th)	Approach (5th)	Device (6th)	Qualifier (7th)
0 Sternum	0 Open 3 Percutaneous 4 Percutaneous Endoscopic	0 Internal Fixation Device, Rigid Plate 4 Internal Fixation Device Z No Device	Z No Qualifier
0 Sternum	X External	Z No Device	Z No Qualifier
1 Ribs, 1 to 2 2 Ribs, 3 or More 3 Cervical Vertebra 4 Thoracic Vertebra 5 Scapula, Right 6 Scapula, Left 7 Glenoid Cavity, Right 8 Glenoid Cavity, Left 9 Clavicle, Right B Clavicle, Left	0 Open 3 Percutaneous 4 Percutaneous Endoscopic	4 Internal Fixation Device Z No Device	Z No Qualifier
1 Ribs, 1 to 2 2 Ribs, 3 or More 3 Cervical Vertebra 4 Thoracic Vertebra 5 Scapula, Right 6 Scapula, Left 7 Glenoid Cavity, Right 8 Glenoid Cavity, Left 9 Clavicle, Right B Clavicle, Left	X External	Z No Device	Z No Qualifier
C Humeral Head, Right D Humeral Head, Left F Humeral Shaft, Right G Humeral Shaft, Left H Radius, Right J Radius, Left K Ulna, Right L Ulna, Left	0 Open 3 Percutaneous 4 Percutaneous Endoscopic	4 Internal Fixation Device 5 External Fixation Device 6 Internal Fixation Device, Intramedullary B External Fixation Device, Monoplanar C External Fixation Device, Ring D External Fixation Device, Hybrid Z No Device	Z No Qualifier
C Humeral Head, Right D Humeral Head, Left F Humeral Shaft, Right G Humeral Shaft, Left H Radius, Right J Radius, Left K Ulna, Right L Ulna, Left	X External	Z No Device	Z No Qualifier
M Carpal, Right N Carpal, Left P Metacarpal, Right Q Metacarpal, Left R Thumb Phalanx, Right S Thumb Phalanx, Left T Finger Phalanx, Right V Finger Phalanx, Left	0 Open 3 Percutaneous 4 Percutaneous Endoscopic	4 Internal Fixation Device 5 External Fixation Device Z No Device	Z No Qualifier
M Carpal, Right N Carpal, Left P Metacarpal, Right Q Metacarpal, Left R Thumb Phalanx, Right S Thumb Phalanx, Left T Finger Phalanx, Right V Finger Phalanx, Left	X External	Z No Device	Z No Qualifier

Section 0 **Medical and Surgical**
Body System P **Upper Bones**
Operation T **Resection:** Cutting out or off, without replacement, all of a body part

Body Part (4th)	Approach (5th)	Device (6th)	Qualifier (7th)
0 Sternum **1** Ribs, 1 to 2 **2** Ribs, 3 or More **5** Scapula, Right **6** Scapula, Left **7** Glenoid Cavity, Right **8** Glenoid Cavity, Left **9** Clavicle, Right **B** Clavicle, Left **C** Humeral Head, Right **D** Humeral Head, Left **F** Humeral Shaft, Right **G** Humeral Shaft, Left **H** Radius, Right **J** Radius, Left **K** Ulna, Right **L** Ulna, Left **M** Carpal, Right **N** Carpal, Left **P** Metacarpal, Right **Q** Metacarpal, Left **R** Thumb Phalanx, Right **S** Thumb Phalanx, Left **T** Finger Phalanx, Right **V** Finger Phalanx, Left	**0** Open	**Z** No Device	**Z** No Qualifier

Section 0 **Medical and Surgical**
Body System P **Upper Bones**
Operation U **Supplement:** Putting in or on biological or synthetic material that physically reinforces and/or augments the function of a portion of a body part

Body Part (4th)	Approach (5th)	Device (6th)	Qualifier (7th)
0 Sternum **1** Ribs, 1 to 2 **2** Ribs, 3 or More **3** Cervical Vertebra **4** Thoracic Vertebra **5** Scapula, Right **6** Scapula, Left **7** Glenoid Cavity, Right **8** Glenoid Cavity, Left **9** Clavicle, Right **B** Clavicle, Left **C** Humeral Head, Right **D** Humeral Head, Left **F** Humeral Shaft, Right **G** Humeral Shaft, Left **H** Radius, Right **J** Radius, Left **K** Ulna, Right **L** Ulna, Left **M** Carpal, Right **N** Carpal, Left **P** Metacarpal, Right **Q** Metacarpal, Left **R** Thumb Phalanx, Right **S** Thumb Phalanx, Left **T** Finger Phalanx, Right **V** Finger Phalanx, Left	**0** Open **3** Percutaneous **4** Percutaneous Endoscopic	**7** Autologous Tissue Substitute **J** Synthetic Substitute **K** Nonautologous Tissue Substitute	**Z** No Qualifier

ction 0 **Medical and Surgical**
dy System P **Upper Bones**
eration W **Revision:** Correcting, to the extent possible, a portion of a malfunctioning device or the position of a displaced device

Body Part (4th)	Approach (5th)	Device (6th)	Qualifier (7th)
0 Sternum 1 Ribs, 1 to 2 2 Ribs, 3 or More 3 Cervical Vertebra 4 Thoracic Vertebra 5 Scapula, Right 6 Scapula, Left 7 Glenoid Cavity, Right 8 Glenoid Cavity, Left 9 Clavicle, Right B Clavicle, Left	**0** Open **3** Percutaneous **4** Percutaneous Endoscopic **X** External	**4** Internal Fixation Device **7** Autologous Tissue Substitute **J** Synthetic Substitute **K** Nonautologous Tissue Substitute	**Z** No Qualifier
C Humeral Head, Right D Humeral Head, Left F Humeral Shaft, Right G Humeral Shaft, Left H Radius, Right J Radius, Left K Ulna, Right L Ulna, Left M Carpal, Right N Carpal, Left P Metacarpal, Right Q Metacarpal, Left R Thumb Phalanx, Right S Thumb Phalanx, Left T Finger Phalanx, Right V Finger Phalanx, Left	**0** Open **3** Percutaneous **4** Percutaneous Endoscopic **X** External	**4** Internal Fixation Device **5** External Fixation Device **7** Autologous Tissue Substitute **J** Synthetic Substitute **K** Nonautologous Tissue Substitute	**Z** No Qualifier
Y Upper Bone	**0** Open **3** Percutaneous **4** Percutaneous Endoscopic **X** External	**0** Drainage Device **M** Bone Growth Stimulator	**Z** No Qualifier

HA Coding Clinic

PB10ZZ Excision of 1 to 2 Ribs, Open Approach—AHA CC: 4Q, 2012, 101-102; 4Q, 2013, 109-111
PB20ZZ Excision of 3 or More Ribs, Open Approach—AHA CC: 4Q, 2013, 109-111
PB54ZZ Excision of Right Scapula, Percutaneous Endoscopic Approach—AHA CC: 3Q, 2013, 20-22
PH404Z Insertion of Internal Fixation Device into Thoracic Vertebra, Open Approach—AHA CC: 4Q, 2014, 28-29
PP404Z Removal of Internal Fixation Device from Thoracic Vertebra, Open Approach—AHA CC: 4Q, 2014, 28-29
PS00ZZ Reposition Sternum, Open Approach—AHA CC: 4Q, 2015, 34
PS204Z Reposition 3 or More Ribs with Internal Fixation Device, Open Approach—AHA CC: 4Q, 2014, 26; 4Q, 2017, 53
PS3XZZ Reposition Cervical Vertebra, External Approach—AHA CC: 2Q, 2015, 35
PS4XZZ Reposition Thoracic Vertebra, External Approach—AHA CC: 1Q, 2016, 21
PSJ04Z Reposition Left Radius with Internal Fixation Device, Open Approach—AHA CC: 3Q, 2014, 33-34; 4Q, 2014, 32-33
PSL04Z Reposition Left Ulna with Internal Fixation Device, Open Approach—AHA CC: 4Q, 2014, 32-33
PTN0ZZ Resection of Left Carpal, Open Approach—AHA CC: 3Q, 2015, 26-27
PU00JZ Supplement Sternum with Synthetic Substitute, Open Approach—AHA CC: 4Q, 2013, 109-111
PU30KZ Supplement Cervical Vertebra with Nonautologous Tissue Substitute, Open Approach—AHA CC: 2Q, 2015, 20-21
PW104Z Revision of Internal Fixation Device in 1 to 2 Ribs, Open Approach—AHA CC: 4Q, 2014, 26-27
PW204Z Revision of Internal Fixation Device in 3 or More Ribs, Open Approach—AHA CC: 4Q, 2014, 26-27
PW404Z Revision of Internal Fixation Device in Thoracic Vertebra, Open Approach—AHA CC: 4Q, 2014, 27-28

Bones - Front and Back Views

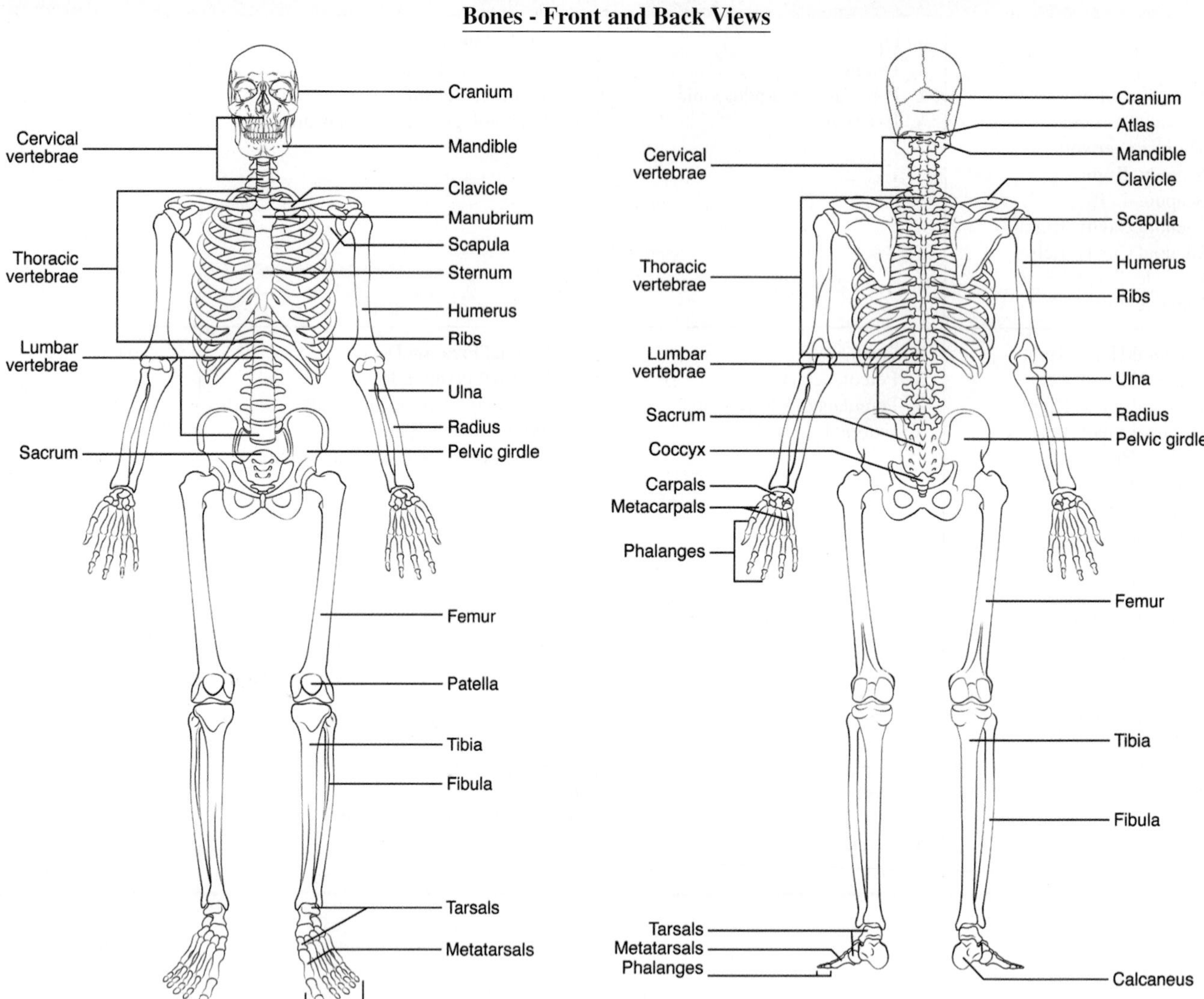

Vertebrae

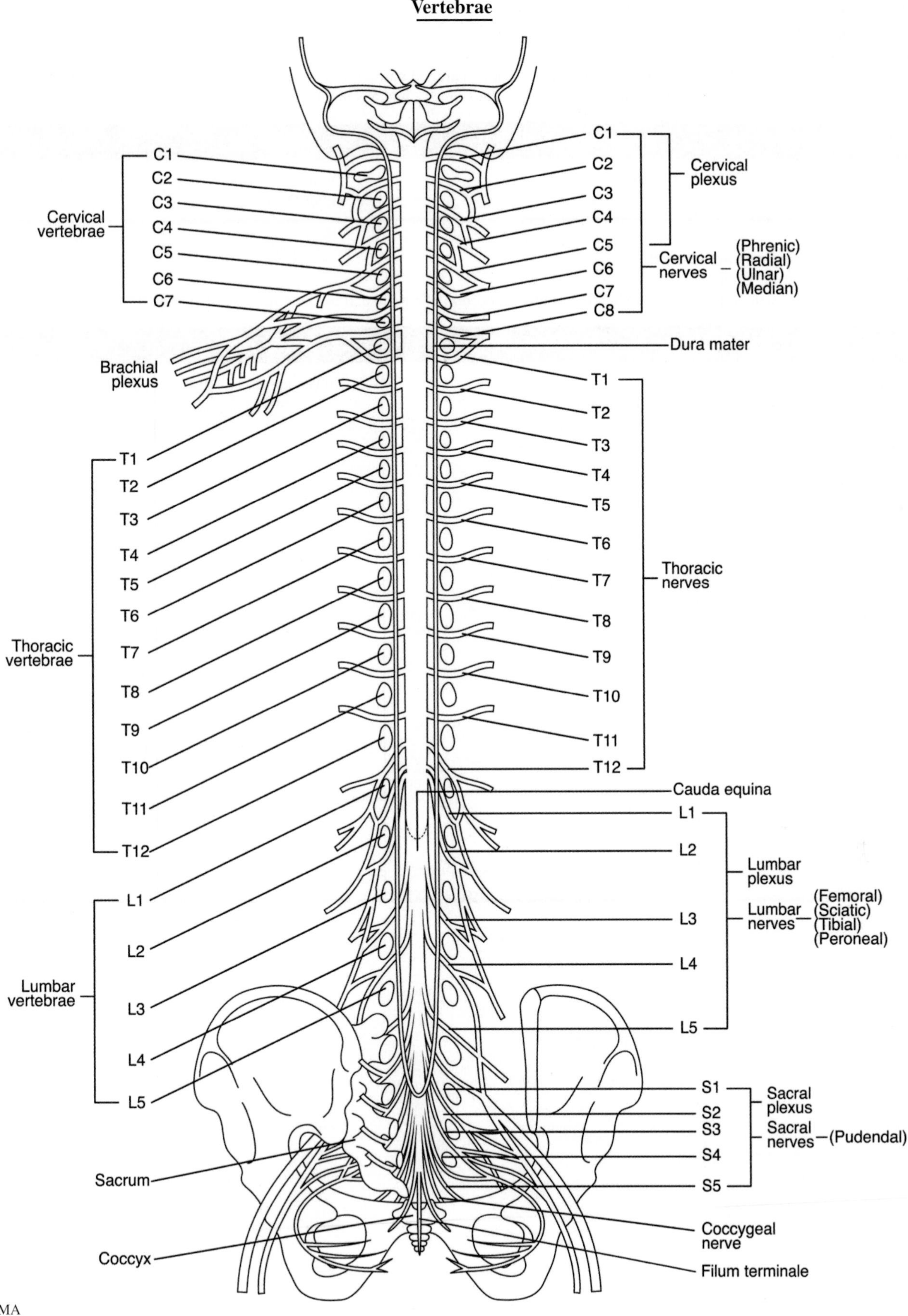

AHIMA

Lower Bones Tables 0Q2–0QW

Section 0 **Medical and Surgical**
Body System Q **Lower Bones**
Operation 2 **Change:** Taking out or off a device from a body part and putting back an identical or similar device in or on the same bo part without cutting or puncturing the skin or a mucous membrane

Body Part (4th)	Approach (5th)	Device (6th)	Qualifier (7th)
Y Lower Bone	**X** External	**0** Drainage Device **Y** Other Device	**Z** No Qualifier

Section 0 **Medical and Surgical**
Body System Q **Lower Bones**
Operation 5 **Destruction:** Physical eradication of all or a portion of a body part by the direct use of energy, force, or a destructive age

Body Part (4th)	Approach (5th)	Device (6th)	Qualifier (7th)
0 Lumbar Vertebra **1** Sacrum **2** Pelvic Bone, Right **3** Pelvic Bone, Left **4** Acetabulum, Right **5** Acetabulum, Left **6** Upper Femur, Right **7** Upper Femur, Left **8** Femoral Shaft, Right **9** Femoral Shaft, Left **B** Lower Femur, Right **C** Lower Femur, Left **D** Patella, Right **F** Patella, Left **G** Tibia, Right **H** Tibia, Left **J** Fibula, Right **K** Fibula, Left **L** Tarsal, Right **M** Tarsal, Left **N** Metatarsal, Right **P** Metatarsal, Left **Q** Toe Phalanx, Right **R** Toe Phalanx, Left **S** Coccyx	**0** Open **3** Percutaneous **4** Percutaneous Endoscopic	**Z** No Device	**Z** No Qualifier

ction 0 **Medical and Surgical**
dy System Q **Lower Bones**
eration 8 **Division:** Cutting into a body part, without draining fluids and/or gases from the body part, in order to separate or transect a body part

Body Part (4th)	Approach (5th)	Device (6th)	Qualifier (7th)
0 Lumbar Vertebra 1 Sacrum 2 Pelvic Bone, Right 3 Pelvic Bone, Left 4 Acetabulum, Right 5 Acetabulum, Left 6 Upper Femur, Right 7 Upper Femur, Left 8 Femoral Shaft, Right 9 Femoral Shaft, Left B Lower Femur, Right C Lower Femur, Left D Patella, Right F Patella, Left G Tibia, Right H Tibia, Left J Fibula, Right K Fibula, Left L Tarsal, Right M Tarsal, Left N Metatarsal, Right P Metatarsal, Left Q Toe Phalanx, Right R Toe Phalanx, Left S Coccyx	0 Open 3 Percutaneous 4 Percutaneous Endoscopic	Z No Device	Z No Qualifier

ction 0 **Medical and Surgical**
ody System Q **Lower Bones**
peration 9 **Drainage:** Taking or letting out fluids and/or gases from a body part

Body Part (4th)	Approach (5th)	Device (6th)	Qualifier (7th)
0 Lumbar Vertebra 1 Sacrum 2 Pelvic Bone, Right 3 Pelvic Bone, Left 4 Acetabulum, Right 5 Acetabulum, Left 6 Upper Femur, Right 7 Upper Femur, Left 8 Femoral Shaft, Right 9 Femoral Shaft, Left B Lower Femur, Right C Lower Femur, Left D Patella, Right F Patella, Left G Tibia, Right H Tibia, Left J Fibula, Right K Fibula, Left L Tarsal, Right M Tarsal, Left N Metatarsal, Right P Metatarsal, Left Q Toe Phalanx, Right R Toe Phalanx, Left S Coccyx	0 Open 3 Percutaneous 4 Percutaneous Endoscopic	0 Drainage Device	Z No Qualifier

Continued →

Section 0 **Medical and Surgical**
Body System Q **Lower Bones**
Operation 9 **Drainage:** Taking or letting out fluids and/or gases from a body part

Body Part (4th)	Approach (5th)	Device (6th)	Qualifier (7th)
0 Lumbar Vertebra **1** Sacrum **2** Pelvic Bone, Right **3** Pelvic Bone, Left **4** Acetabulum, Right **5** Acetabulum, Left **6** Upper Femur, Right **7** Upper Femur, Left **8** Femoral Shaft, Right **9** Femoral Shaft, Left **B** Lower Femur, Right **C** Lower Femur, Left **D** Patella, Right **F** Patella, Left **G** Tibia, Right **H** Tibia, Left **J** Fibula, Right **K** Fibula, Left **L** Tarsal, Right **M** Tarsal, Left **N** Metatarsal, Right **P** Metatarsal, Left **Q** Toe Phalanx, Right **R** Toe Phalanx, Left **S** Coccyx	**0** Open **3** Percutaneous **4** Percutaneous Endoscopic	**Z** No Device	**X** Diagnostic **Z** No Qualifier

Section 0 **Medical and Surgical**
Body System Q **Lower Bones**
Operation B **Excision:** Cutting out or off, without replacement, a portion of a body part

Body Part (4th)	Approach (5th)	Device (6th)	Qualifier (7th)
0 Lumbar Vertebra **1** Sacrum **2** Pelvic Bone, Right **3** Pelvic Bone, Left **4** Acetabulum, Right **5** Acetabulum, Left **6** Upper Femur, Right **7** Upper Femur, Left **8** Femoral Shaft, Right **9** Femoral Shaft, Left **B** Lower Femur, Right **C** Lower Femur, Left **D** Patella, Right **F** Patella, Left **G** Tibia, Right **H** Tibia, Left **J** Fibula, Right **K** Fibula, Left **L** Tarsal, Right **M** Tarsal, Left **N** Metatarsal, Right **P** Metatarsal, Left **Q** Toe Phalanx, Right **R** Toe Phalanx, Left **S** Coccyx	**0** Open **3** Percutaneous **4** Percutaneous Endoscopic	**Z** No Device	**X** Diagnostic **Z** No Qualifier

ction 0 **Medical and Surgical**
dy System Q **Lower Bones**
eration C **Extirpation:** Taking or cutting out solid matter from a body part

Body Part (4th)	Approach (5th)	Device (6th)	Qualifier (7th)
0 Lumbar Vertebra 1 Sacrum 2 Pelvic Bone, Right 3 Pelvic Bone, Left 4 Acetabulum, Right 5 Acetabulum, Left 6 Upper Femur, Right 7 Upper Femur, Left 8 Femoral Shaft, Right 9 Femoral Shaft, Left B Lower Femur, Right C Lower Femur, Left D Patella, Right F Patella, Left G Tibia, Right H Tibia, Left J Fibula, Right K Fibula, Left L Tarsal, Right M Tarsal, Left N Metatarsal, Right P Metatarsal, Left Q Toe Phalanx, Right R Toe Phalanx, Left S Coccyx	**0** Open **3** Percutaneous **4** Percutaneous Endoscopic	**Z** No Device	**Z** No Qualifier

ction 0 **Medical and Surgical**
dy System Q **Lower Bones**
peration D **Extraction:** Pulling or stripping out or off all or a portion of a body part by the use of force

Body Part (4th)	Approach (5th)	Device (6th)	Qualifier (7th)
0 Lumbar Vertebra 1 Sacrum 2 Pelvic Bone, Right 3 Pelvic Bone, Left 4 Acetabulum, Right 5 Acetabulum, Left 6 Upper Femur, Right 7 Upper Femur, Left 8 Femoral Shaft, Right 9 Femoral Shaft, Left B Lower Femur, Right C Lower Femur, Left D Patella, Right F Patella, Left G Tibia, Right H Tibia, Left J Fibula, Right K Fibula, Left L Tarsal, Right M Tarsal, Left N Metatarsal, Right P Metatarsal, Left Q Toe Phalanx, Right R Toe Phalanx, Left S Coccyx	**0** Open	**Z** No Device	**Z** No Qualifier

Section **0** **Medical and Surgical**
Body System **Q** **Lower Bones**
Operation **H** **Insertion:** Putting in a nonbiological appliance that monitors, assists, performs, or prevents a physiological function but does not physically take the place of a body part

Body Part (4th)	Approach (5th)	Device (6th)	Qualifier (7th)
0 Lumbar Vertebra **1** Sacrum **2** Pelvic Bone, Right **3** Pelvic Bone, Left **4** Acetabulum, Right **5** Acetabulum, Left **D** Patella, Right **F** Patella, Left **L** Tarsal, Right **M** Tarsal, Left **N** Metatarsal, Right **P** Metatarsal, Left **Q** Toe Phalanx, Right **R** Toe Phalanx, Left **S** Coccyx	**0** Open **3** Percutaneous **4** Percutaneous Endoscopic	**4** Internal Fixation Device **5** External Fixation Device	**Z** No Qualifier
6 Upper Femur, Right **7** Upper Femur, Left **8** Femoral Shaft, Right **9** Femoral Shaft, Left **B** Lower Femur, Right **C** Lower Femur, Left **G** Tibia, Right **H** Tibia, Left **J** Fibula, Right **K** Fibula, Left	**0** Open **3** Percutaneous **4** Percutaneous Endoscopic	**4** Internal Fixation Device **5** External Fixation Device **6** Internal Fixation Device, Intramedullary **8** External Fixation Device, Limb Lengthening **B** External Fixation Device, Monoplanar **C** External Fixation Device, Ring **D** External Fixation Device, Hybrid	**Z** No Qualifier
Y Lower Bone	**0** Open **3** Percutaneous **4** Percutaneous Endoscopic	**M** Bone Growth Stimulator	**Z** No Qualifier

Section **0** **Medical and Surgical**
Body System **Q** **Lower Bones**
Operation **J** **Inspection:** Visually and/or manually exploring a body part

Body Part (4th)	Approach (5th)	Device (6th)	Qualifier (7th)
Y Lower Bone	**0** Open **3** Percutaneous **4** Percutaneous Endoscopic **X** External	**Z** No Device	**Z** No Qualifier

ction 0 **Medical and Surgical**
dy System Q **Lower Bones**
eration N **Release:** Freeing a body part from an abnormal physical constraint by cutting or by the use of force

Body Part (4th)	Approach (5th)	Device (6th)	Qualifier (7th)
0 Lumbar Vertebra 1 Sacrum 2 Pelvic Bone, Right 3 Pelvic Bone, Left 4 Acetabulum, Right 5 Acetabulum, Left 6 Upper Femur, Right 7 Upper Femur, Left 8 Femoral Shaft, Right 9 Femoral Shaft, Left B Lower Femur, Right C Lower Femur, Left D Patella, Right F Patella, Left G Tibia, Right H Tibia, Left J Fibula, Right K Fibula, Left L Tarsal, Right M Tarsal, Left N Metatarsal, Right P Metatarsal, Left Q Toe Phalanx, Right R Toe Phalanx, Left S Coccyx	**0** Open **3** Percutaneous **4** Percutaneous Endoscopic	**Z** No Device	**Z** No Qualifier

ction 0 **Medical and Surgical**
dy System Q **Lower Bones**
eration P **Removal:** Taking out or off a device from a body part

Body Part (4th)	Approach (5th)	Device (6th)	Qualifier (7th)
0 Lumbar Vertebra 1 Sacrum 4 Acetabulum, Right 5 Acetabulum, Left S Coccyx	**0** Open **3** Percutaneous **4** Percutaneous Endoscopic	**4** Internal Fixation Device **7** Autologous Tissue Substitute **J** Synthetic Substitute **K** Nonautologous Tissue Substitute	**Z** No Qualifier
0 Lumbar Vertebra 1 Sacrum 4 Acetabulum, Right 5 Acetabulum, Left S Coccyx	**X** External	**4** Internal Fixation Device	**Z** No Qualifier

Continued →

Section 0 **Medical and Surgical**
Body System Q **Lower Bones**
Operation P **Removal:** Taking out or off a device from a body part

Body Part (4th)	Approach (5th)	Device (6th)	Qualifier (7th)
2 Pelvic Bone, Right **3** Pelvic Bone, Left **6** Upper Femur, Right **7** Upper Femur, Left **8** Femoral Shaft, Right **9** Femoral Shaft, Left **B** Lower Femur, Right **C** Lower Femur, Left **D** Patella, Right **F** Patella, Left **G** Tibia, Right **H** Tibia, Left **J** Fibula, Right **K** Fibula, Left **L** Tarsal, Right **M** Tarsal, Left **N** Metatarsal, Right **P** Metatarsal, Left **Q** Toe Phalanx, Right **R** Toe Phalanx, Left	**0** Open **3** Percutaneous **4** Percutaneous Endoscopic	**4** Internal Fixation Device **5** External Fixation Device **7** Autologous Tissue Substitute **J** Synthetic Substitute **K** Nonautologous Tissue Substitute	**Z** No Qualifier
2 Pelvic Bone, Right **3** Pelvic Bone, Left **6** Upper Femur, Right **7** Upper Femur, Left **8** Femoral Shaft, Right **9** Femoral Shaft, Left **B** Lower Femur, Right **C** Lower Femur, Left **D** Patella, Right **F** Patella, Left **G** Tibia, Right **H** Tibia, Left **J** Fibula, Right **K** Fibula, Left **L** Tarsal, Right **M** Tarsal, Left **N** Metatarsal, Right **P** Metatarsal, Left **Q** Toe Phalanx, Right **R** Toe Phalanx, Left	**X** External	**4** Internal Fixation Device **5** External Fixation Device	**Z** No Qualifier
Y Lower Bone	**0** Open **3** Percutaneous **4** Percutaneous Endoscopic **X** External	**0** Drainage Device **M** Bone Growth Stimulator	**Z** No Qualifier

ction 0 Medical and Surgical
dy System Q Lower Bones
peration Q **Repair:** Restoring, to the extent possible, a body part to its normal anatomic structure and function

Body Part (4th)	Approach (5th)	Device (6th)	Qualifier (7th)
0 Lumbar Vertebra 1 Sacrum 2 Pelvic Bone, Right 3 Pelvic Bone, Left 4 Acetabulum, Right 5 Acetabulum, Left 6 Upper Femur, Right 7 Upper Femur, Left 8 Femoral Shaft, Right 9 Femoral Shaft, Left B Lower Femur, Right C Lower Femur, Left D Patella, Right F Patella, Left G Tibia, Right H Tibia, Left J Fibula, Right K Fibula, Left L Tarsal, Right M Tarsal, Left N Metatarsal, Right P Metatarsal, Left Q Toe Phalanx, Right R Toe Phalanx, Left S Coccyx	0 Open 3 Percutaneous 4 Percutaneous Endoscopic X External	Z No Device	Z No Qualifier

ction 0 Medical and Surgical
dy System Q Lower Bones
peration R **Replacement:** Putting in or on biological or synthetic material that physically takes the place and/or function of all or a portion of a body part

Body Part (4th)	Approach (5th)	Device (6th)	Qualifier (7th)
0 Lumbar Vertebra 1 Sacrum 2 Pelvic Bone, Right 3 Pelvic Bone, Left 4 Acetabulum, Right 5 Acetabulum, Left 6 Upper Femur, Right 7 Upper Femur, Left 8 Femoral Shaft, Right 9 Femoral Shaft, Left B Lower Femur, Right C Lower Femur, Left D Patella, Right F Patella, Left G Tibia, Right H Tibia, Left J Fibula, Right K Fibula, Left L Tarsal, Right M Tarsal, Left N Metatarsal, Right P Metatarsal, Left Q Toe Phalanx, Right R Toe Phalanx, Left S Coccyx	0 Open 3 Percutaneous 4 Percutaneous Endoscopic	7 Autologous Tissue Substitute J Synthetic Substitute K Nonautologous Tissue Substitute	Z No Qualifier

Section 0 **Medical and Surgical**
Body System Q **Lower Bones**
Operation S **Reposition:** Moving to its normal location, or other suitable location, all or a portion of a body part

Body Part (4th)	Approach (5th)	Device (6th)	Qualifier (7th)
0 Lumbar Vertebra **1** Sacrum **4** Acetabulum, Right **5** Acetabulum, Left **S** Coccyx	**0** Open **3** Percutaneous **4** Percutaneous Endoscopic	**4** Internal Fixation Device **Z** No Device	**Z** No Qualifier
0 Lumbar Vertebra **1** Sacrum **4** Acetabulum, Right **5** Acetabulum, Left **S** Coccyx	**X** External	**Z** No Device	**Z** No Qualifier
2 Pelvic Bone, Right **3** Pelvic Bone, Left **D** Patella, Right **F** Patella, Left **L** Tarsal, Right **M** Tarsal, Left **Q** Toe Phalanx, Right **R** Toe Phalanx, Left	**0** Open **3** Percutaneous **4** Percutaneous Endoscopic	**4** Internal Fixation Device **5** External Fixation Device **Z** No Device	**Z** No Qualifier
2 Pelvic Bone, Right **3** Pelvic Bone, Left **D** Patella, Right **F** Patella, Left **L** Tarsal, Right **M** Tarsal, Left **Q** Toe Phalanx, Right **R** Toe Phalanx, Left	**X** External	**Z** No Device	**Z** No Qualifier
6 Upper Femur, Right **7** Upper Femur, Left **8** Femoral Shaft, Right **9** Femoral Shaft, Left **B** Lower Femur, Right **C** Lower Femur, Left **G** Tibia, Right **H** Tibia, Left **J** Fibula, Right **K** Fibula, Left	**0** Open **3** Percutaneous **4** Percutaneous Endoscopic	**4** Internal Fixation Device **5** External Fixation Device **6** Internal Fixation Device, Intramedullary **B** External Fixation Device, Monoplanar **C** External Fixation Device, Ring **D** External Fixation Device, Hybrid **Z** No Device	**Z** No Qualifier
6 Upper Femur, Right **7** Upper Femur, Left **8** Femoral Shaft, Right **9** Femoral Shaft, Left **B** Lower Femur, Right **C** Lower Femur, Left **G** Tibia, Right **H** Tibia, Left **J** Fibula, Right **K** Fibula, Left	**X** External	**Z** No Device	**Z** No Qualifier
N Metatarsal, Right **P** Metatarsal, Left	**0** Open **3** Percutaneous **4** Percutaneous Endoscopic	**4** Internal Fixation Device **5** External Fixation Device **Z** No Device	**2** Sesamoid Bone(s) 1st Toe **Z** No Qualifier
N Metatarsal, Right **P** Metatarsal, Left	**X** External	**Z** No Device	**2** Sesamoid Bone(s) 1st Toe **Z** No Qualifier

tion	**0**	**Medical and Surgical**
dy System	**Q**	**Lower Bones**
eration	**T**	**Resection:** Cutting out or off, without replacement, all of a body part

Body Part (4th)	Approach (5th)	Device (6th)	Qualifier (7th)
Pelvic Bone, Right Pelvic Bone, Left Acetabulum, Right Acetabulum, Left Upper Femur, Right Upper Femur, Left Femoral Shaft, Right Femoral Shaft, Left B Lower Femur, Right C Lower Femur, Left D Patella, Right Patella, Left G Tibia, Right H Tibia, Left Fibula, Right K Fibula, Left L Tarsal, Right M Tarsal, Left N Metatarsal, Right P Metatarsal, Left Q Toe Phalanx, Right R Toe Phalanx, Left Coccyx	**0** Open	**Z** No Device	**Z** No Qualifier

tion	**0**	**Medical and Surgical**
dy System	**Q**	**Lower Bones**
eration	**U**	**Supplement:** Putting in or on biological or synthetic material that physically reinforces and/or augments the function of a portion of a body part

Body Part (4th)	Approach (5th)	Device (6th)	Qualifier (7th)
Lumbar Vertebra Sacrum Pelvic Bone, Right Pelvic Bone, Left Acetabulum, Right Acetabulum, Left Upper Femur, Right Upper Femur, Left Femoral Shaft, Right Femoral Shaft, Left B Lower Femur, Right C Lower Femur, Left D Patella, Right Patella, Left G Tibia, Right H Tibia, Left Fibula, Right K Fibula, Left L Tarsal, Right M Tarsal, Left N Metatarsal, Right P Metatarsal, Left Q Toe Phalanx, Right R Toe Phalanx, Left S Coccyx	**0** Open **3** Percutaneous **4** Percutaneous Endoscopic	**7** Autologous Tissue Substitute **J** Synthetic Substitute **K** Nonautologous Tissue Substitute	**Z** No Qualifier

Section 0 **Medical and Surgical**
Body System Q **Lower Bones**
Operation W **Revision:** Correcting, to the extent possible, a portion of a malfunctioning device or the position of a displaced device

Body Part (4th)	Approach (5th)	Device (6th)	Qualifier (7th)
0 Lumbar Vertebra **1** Sacrum **4** Acetabulum, Right **5** Acetabulum, Left **S** Coccyx	**0** Open **3** Percutaneous **4** Percutaneous Endoscopic **X** External	**4** Internal Fixation Device **7** Autologous Tissue Substitute **J** Synthetic Substitute **K** Nonautologous Tissue Substitute	**Z** No Qualifier
2 Pelvic Bone, Right **3** Pelvic Bone, Left **6** Upper Femur, Right **7** Upper Femur, Left **8** Femoral Shaft, Right **9** Femoral Shaft, Left **B** Lower Femur, Right **C** Lower Femur, Left **D** Patella, Right **F** Patella, Left **G** Tibia, Right **H** Tibia, Left **J** Fibula, Right **K** Fibula, Left **L** Tarsal, Right **M** Tarsal, Left **N** Metatarsal, Right **P** Metatarsal, Left **Q** Toe Phalanx, Right **R** Toe Phalanx, Left	**0** Open **3** Percutaneous **4** Percutaneous Endoscopic **X** External	**4** Internal Fixation Device **5** External Fixation Device **7** Autologous Tissue Substitute **J** Synthetic Substitute **K** Nonautologous Tissue Substitute	**Z** No Qualifier
Y Lower Bone	**0** Open **3** Percutaneous **4** Percutaneous Endoscopic **X** External	**0** Drainage Device **M** Bone Growth Stimulator	**Z** No Qualifier

AHA Coding Clinic

0Q830ZZ Division of Left Pelvic Bone, Open Approach—AHA CC: 2Q, 2016, 32
0QB20ZZ Excision of Right Pelvic Bone, Open Approach—AHA CC: 2Q, 2014, 6-7
0QB74ZZ Excision of Left Upper Femur, Percutaneous Endoscopic Approach—AHA CC: 4Q, 2014, 25-26
0QBJ0ZZ Excision of Right Fibula, Open Approach—AHA CC: 1Q, 2017, 23-24
0QBK0ZZ Excision of Left Fibula, Open Approach—AHA CC: 2Q, 2013, 39-40
0QH204Z Insertion of Internal Fixation Device into Right Pelvic Bone, Open Approach—AHA CC: 1Q, 2017, 21-22
0QH304Z Insertion of Internal Fixation Device into Left Pelvic Bone, Open Approach—AHA CC: 1Q, 2017, 21-22
0QHG04Z Insertion of Internal Fixation Device into Right Tibia, Open Approach—AHA CC: 3Q, 2016, 34-35
0QHJ04Z Insertion of Internal Fixation Device into Right Fibula, Open Approach—AHA CC: 3Q, 2016, 34-35
0QP004Z Removal of Internal Fixation Device from Lumbar Vertebra, Open Approach—AHA CC: 4Q, 2017, 75
0QPG04Z Removal of Internal Fixation Device from Right Tibia, Open Approach—AHA CC: 2Q, 2015, 6-7
0QQ10ZZ Repair Sacrum, Open Approach—AHA CC: 3Q, 2014, 24
0QQ20ZZ Repair Right Pelvic Bone, Open Approach—AHA CC: 1Q, 2018, 15
0QQ30ZZ Repair Left Pelvic Bone, Open Approach—AHA CC: 1Q, 2018, 15
0QS504Z Reposition Left Acetabulum with Internal Fixation Device, Open Approach—AHA CC: 2Q, 2016, 32; 1Q, 2018, 25
0QSC04Z Reposition Left Lower Femur with Internal Fixation Device, Open Approach—AHA CC: 4Q, 2014, 31
0QSF04Z Reposition Left Patella with Internal Fixation Device, Open Approach—AHA CC: 3Q, 2016, 34-35
0QSH04Z Reposition Left Tibia with Internal Fixation Device, Open Approach—AHA CC: 4Q, 2014, 30-31; 3Q, 2016, 34-35
0QSK0ZZ Reposition Left Fibula, Open Approach—AHA CC: 3Q, 2016, 34-35
0QSL04Z Reposition Right Tarsal with Internal Fixation Device, Open Approach—AHA CC: 1Q, 2018, 13
0QSM04Z Reposition Left Tarsal with Internal Fixation Device, Open Approach—AHA CC: 1Q, 2018, 13
0QT60ZZ Resection of Right Upper Femur, Open Approach—AHA CC: 3Q, 2016, 30-31

T70ZZ Resection of Left Upper Femur, Open Approach—AHA CC: 3Q, 2015, 26; 3Q, 2016, 30-31
TC0ZZ Resection of Left Lower Femur, Open Approach—AHA CC: 4Q, 2014, 30-31
U03JZ Supplement Lumbar Vertebra with Synthetic Substitute, Percutaneous Approach—AHA CC: 2Q, 2014, 12-13
U20JZ Supplement Right Pelvic Bone with Synthetic Substitute, Open Approach—AHA CC: 2Q, 2013, 35-36
U50JZ Supplement Left Acetabulum with Synthetic Substitute, Open Approach—AHA CC: 3Q, 2015, 18-19
UC0KZ Supplement Left Lower Femur with—Nonautologous Tissue Substitute, Open Approach—AHA CC: 4Q, 2014, 31
W034Z Revision of Internal Fixation Device in Lumbar Vertebra, Percutaneous Approach—AHA CC: 4Q, 2017, 75

Intervertebral Joint

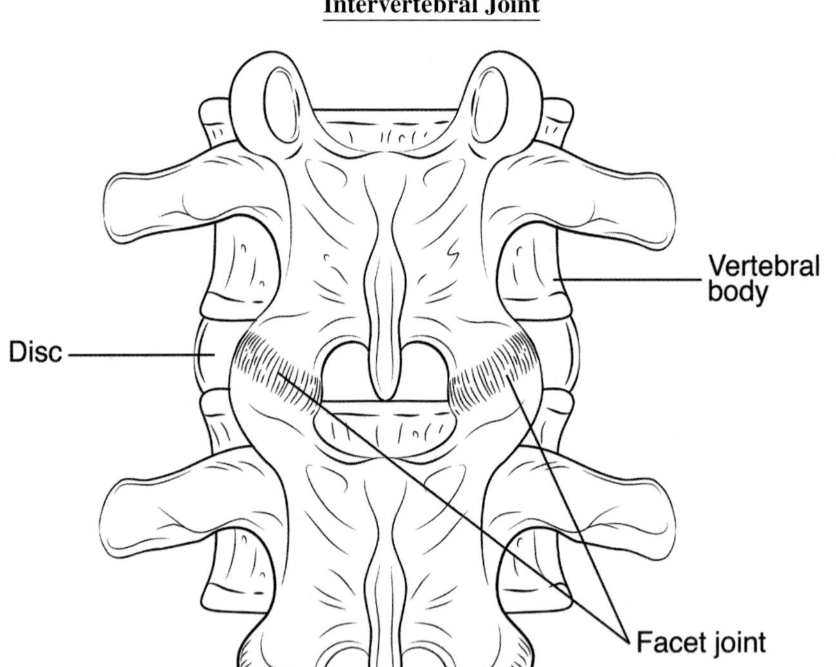

Shoulder

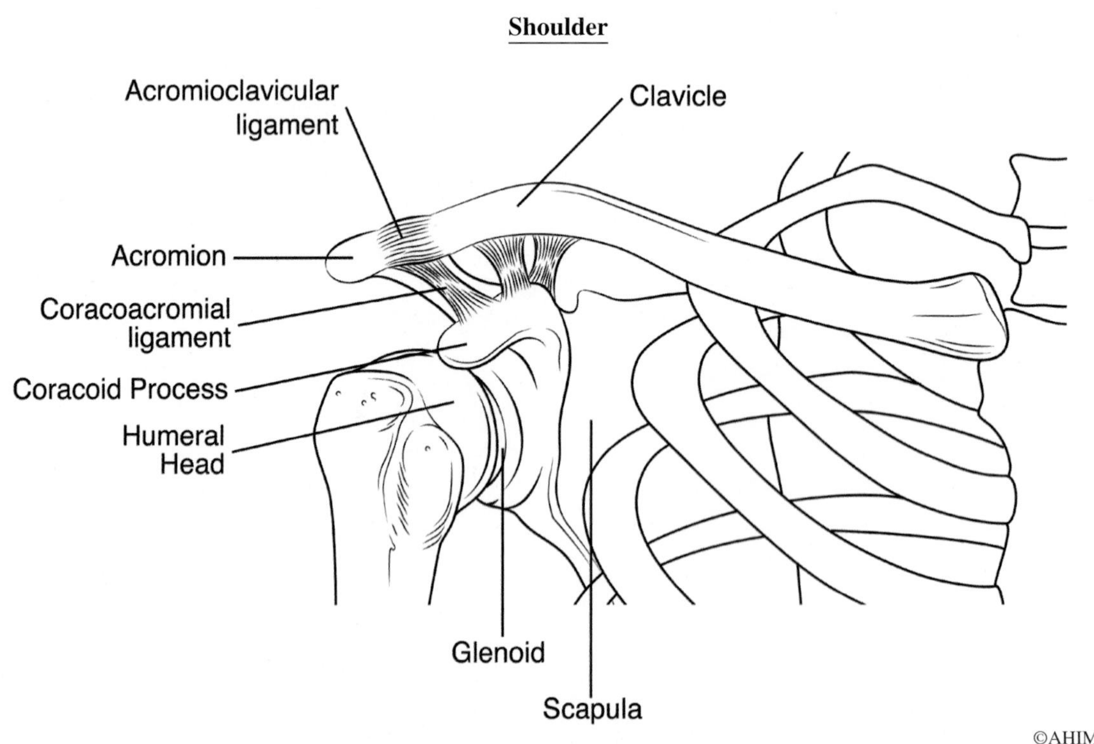

Anterior Interbody Fusion by Dowel Graft

Cervical Spine Injury: Anterior Interbody Fusion by Dowel Graft (Cloward)

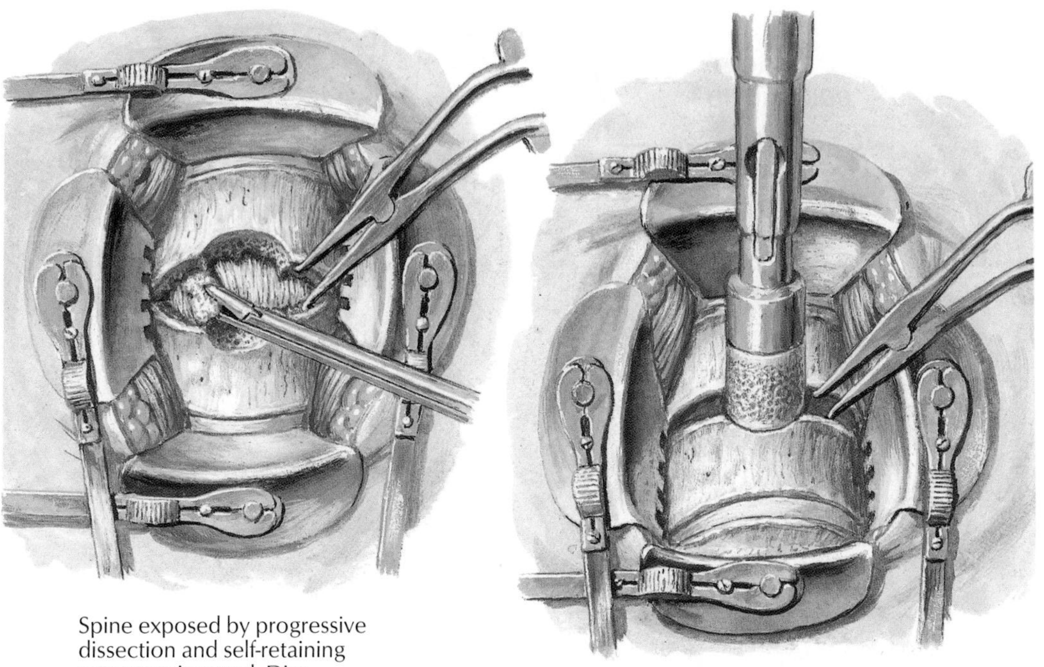

Spine exposed by progressive dissection and self-retaining retractors inserted. Disc, osteophytes and bone fragments removed under direct vision

Dowel bone graft obtained from ilium or bone bank is cut 2 mm wider and 2 mm shorter than drill hole. It is impacted after hole is widened with vertebra spreader

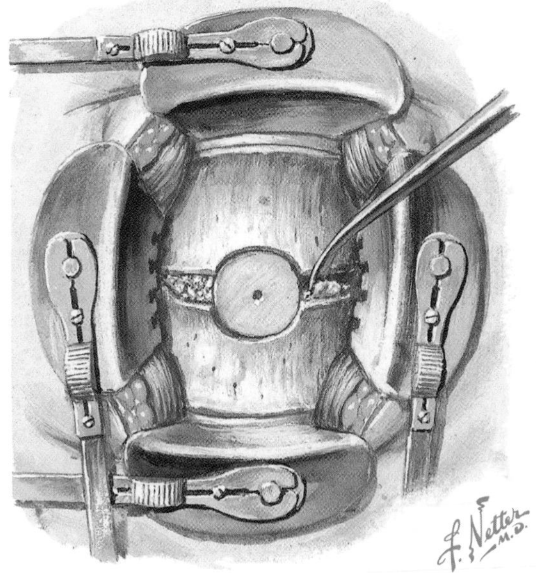

Dowel recessed 2 mm below anterior margin of drill hole. When spreader is removed, graft is locked securely in place. Cortical end plates lateral to dowel are perforated and interspace packed with bone dust removed from drill

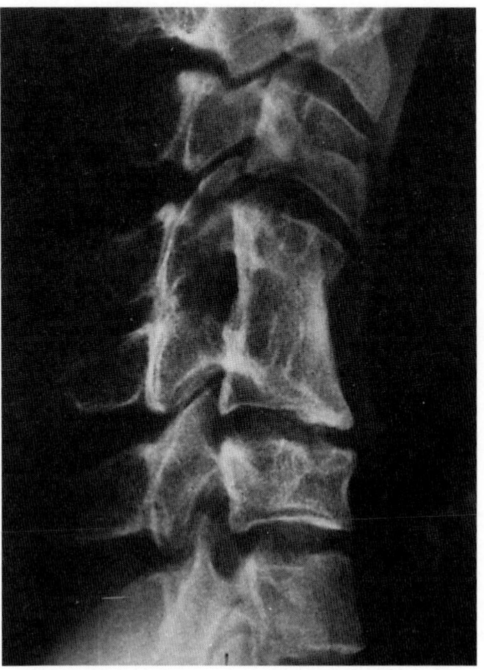

Follow-up x-ray film. Dowel graft fusion of C5-6 with good union

Elbow

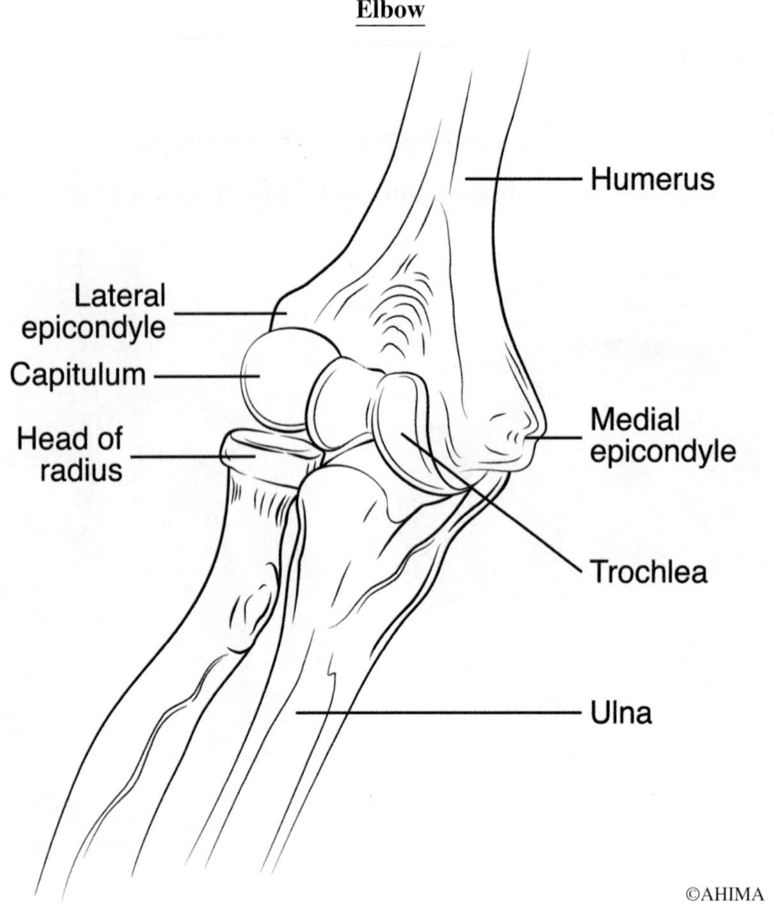
Humerus
Lateral epicondyle
Capitulum
Head of radius
Medial epicondyle
Trochlea
Ulna
©AHIMA

Wrist

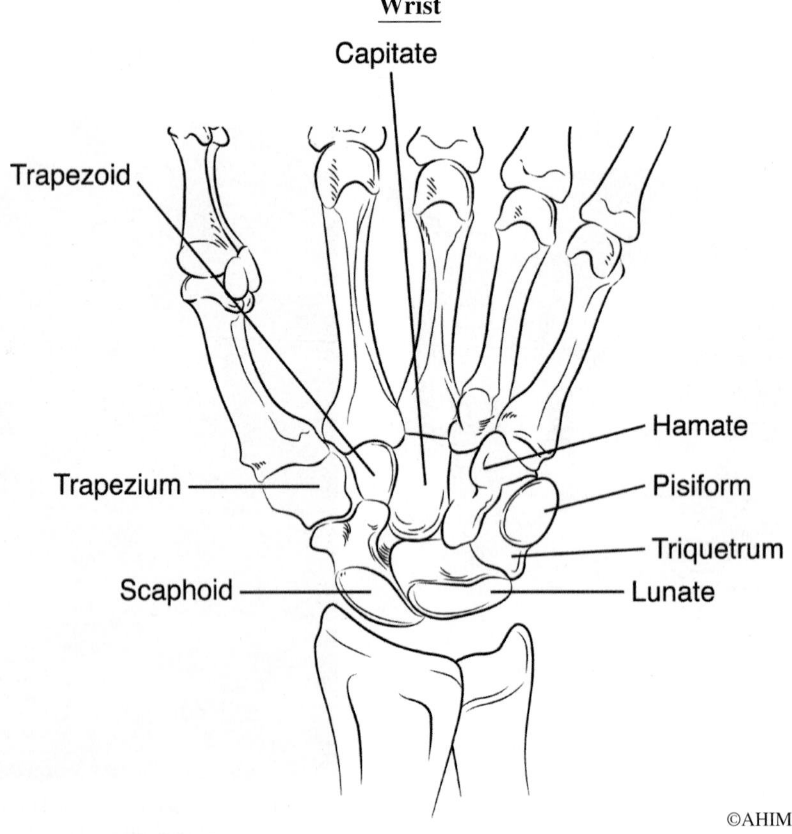
Capitate
Trapezoid
Hamate
Trapezium
Pisiform
Triquetrum
Scaphoid
Lunate
©AHIMA

tion	0	**Medical and Surgical**
dy System	R	**Upper Joints**
eration	2	**Change:** Taking out or off a device from a body part and putting back an identical or similar device in or on the same body part without cutting or puncturing the skin or a mucous membrane

Body Part (4th)	Approach (5th)	Device (6th)	Qualifier (7th)
Y Upper Joint	**X** External	**0** Drainage Device **Y** Other Device	**Z** No Qualifier

tion	0	**Medical and Surgical**
dy System	R	**Upper Joints**
eration	5	**Destruction:** Physical eradication of all or a portion of a body part by the direct use of energy, force, or a destructive agent

Body Part (4th)	Approach (5th)	Device (6th)	Qualifier (7th)
0 Occipital-cervical Joint **1** Cervical Vertebral Joint **3** Cervical Vertebral Disc **4** Cervicothoracic Vertebral Joint **5** Cervicothoracic Vertebral Disc **6** Thoracic Vertebral Joint **9** Thoracic Vertebral Disc **A** Thoracolumbar Vertebral Joint **B** Thoracolumbar Vertebral Disc **C** Temporomandibular Joint, Right **D** Temporomandibular Joint, Left **E** Sternoclavicular Joint, Right **F** Sternoclavicular Joint, Left **G** Acromioclavicular Joint, Right **H** Acromioclavicular Joint, Left **J** Shoulder Joint, Right **K** Shoulder Joint, Left **L** Elbow Joint, Right **M** Elbow Joint, Left **N** Wrist Joint, Right **P** Wrist Joint, Left **Q** Carpal Joint, Right **R** Carpal Joint, Left **S** Carpometacarpal Joint, Right **T** Carpometacarpal Joint, Left **U** Metacarpophalangeal Joint, Right **V** Metacarpophalangeal Joint, Left **W** Finger Phalangeal Joint, Right **X** Finger Phalangeal Joint, Left	**0** Open **3** Percutaneous **4** Percutaneous Endoscopic	**Z** No Device	**Z** No Qualifier

Section 0 **Medical and Surgical**
Body System R **Upper Joints**
Operation 9 **Drainage:** Taking or letting out fluids and/or gases from a body part

Body Part (4th)	Approach (5th)	Device (6th)	Qualifier (7th)
0 Occipital-cervical Joint **1** Cervical Vertebral Joint **3** Cervical Vertebral Disc **4** Cervicothoracic Vertebral Joint **5** Cervicothoracic Vertebral Disc **6** Thoracic Vertebral Joint **9** Thoracic Vertebral Disc **A** Thoracolumbar Vertebral Joint **B** Thoracolumbar Vertebral Disc **C** Temporomandibular Joint, Right **D** Temporomandibular Joint, Left **E** Sternoclavicular Joint, Right **F** Sternoclavicular Joint, Left **G** Acromioclavicular Joint, Right **H** Acromioclavicular Joint, Left **J** Shoulder Joint, Right **K** Shoulder Joint, Left **L** Elbow Joint, Right **M** Elbow Joint, Left **N** Wrist Joint, Right **P** Wrist Joint, Left **Q** Carpal Joint, Right **R** Carpal Joint, Left **S** Carpometacarpal Joint, Right **T** Carpometacarpal Joint, Left **U** Metacarpophalangeal Joint, Right **V** Metacarpophalangeal Joint, Left **W** Finger Phalangeal Joint, Right **X** Finger Phalangeal Joint, Left	**0** Open **3** Percutaneous **4** Percutaneous Endoscopic	**0** Drainage Device	**Z** No Qualifier
0 Occipital-cervical Joint **1** Cervical Vertebral Joint **3** Cervical Vertebral Disc **4** Cervicothoracic Vertebral Joint **5** Cervicothoracic Vertebral Disc **6** Thoracic Vertebral Joint **9** Thoracic Vertebral Disc **A** Thoracolumbar Vertebral Joint **B** Thoracolumbar Vertebral Disc **C** Temporomandibular Joint, Right **D** Temporomandibular Joint, Left **E** Sternoclavicular Joint, Right **F** Sternoclavicular Joint, Left **G** Acromioclavicular Joint, Right **H** Acromioclavicular Joint, Left **J** Shoulder Joint, Right **K** Shoulder Joint, Left **L** Elbow Joint, Right **M** Elbow Joint, Left **N** Wrist Joint, Right **P** Wrist Joint, Left **Q** Carpal Joint, Right **R** Carpal Joint, Left **S** Carpometacarpal Joint, Right **T** Carpometacarpal Joint, Left **U** Metacarpophalangeal Joint, Right **V** Metacarpophalangeal Joint, Left **W** Finger Phalangeal Joint, Right **X** Finger Phalangeal Joint, Left	**0** Open **3** Percutaneous **4** Percutaneous Endoscopic	**Z** No Device	**X** Diagnostic **Z** No Qualifier

ction 0 **Medical and Surgical**
dy System R **Upper Joints**
peration B **Excision:** Cutting out or off, without replacement, a portion of a body part

Body Part (4th)	Approach (5th)	Device (6th)	Qualifier (7th)
0 Occipital-cervical Joint **1** Cervical Vertebral Joint **3** Cervical Vertebral Disc **4** Cervicothoracic Vertebral Joint **5** Cervicothoracic Vertebral Disc **6** Thoracic Vertebral Joint **9** Thoracic Vertebral Disc **A** Thoracolumbar Vertebral Joint **B** Thoracolumbar Vertebral Disc **C** Temporomandibular Joint, Right **D** Temporomandibular Joint, Left **E** Sternoclavicular Joint, Right **F** Sternoclavicular Joint, Left **G** Acromioclavicular Joint, Right **H** Acromioclavicular Joint, Left **J** Shoulder Joint, Right **K** Shoulder Joint, Left **L** Elbow Joint, Right **M** Elbow Joint, Left **N** Wrist Joint, Right **P** Wrist Joint, Left **Q** Carpal Joint, Right **R** Carpal Joint, Left **S** Carpometacarpal Joint, Right **T** Carpometacarpal Joint, Left **U** Metacarpophalangeal Joint, Right **V** Metacarpophalangeal Joint, Left **W** Finger Phalangeal Joint, Right **X** Finger Phalangeal Joint, Left	**0** Open **3** Percutaneous **4** Percutaneous Endoscopic	**Z** No Device	**X** Diagnostic **Z** No Qualifier

Section 0 **Medical and Surgical**
Body System R **Upper Joints**
Operation C **Extirpation:** Taking or cutting out solid matter from a body part

Body Part (4th)	Approach (5th)	Device (6th)	Qualifier (7th)
0 Occipital-cervical Joint **1** Cervical Vertebral Joint **3** Cervical Vertebral Disc **4** Cervicothoracic Vertebral Joint **5** Cervicothoracic Vertebral Disc **6** Thoracic Vertebral Joint **9** Thoracic Vertebral Disc **A** Thoracolumbar Vertebral Joint **B** Thoracolumbar Vertebral Disc **C** Temporomandibular Joint, Right **D** Temporomandibular Joint, Left **E** Sternoclavicular Joint, Right **F** Sternoclavicular Joint, Left **G** Acromioclavicular Joint, Right **H** Acromioclavicular Joint, Left **J** Shoulder Joint, Right **K** Shoulder Joint, Left **L** Elbow Joint, Right **M** Elbow Joint, Left **N** Wrist Joint, Right **P** Wrist Joint, Left **Q** Carpal Joint, Right **R** Carpal Joint, Left **S** Carpometacarpal Joint, Right **T** Carpometacarpal Joint, Left **U** Metacarpophalangeal Joint, Right **V** Metacarpophalangeal Joint, Left **W** Finger Phalangeal Joint, Right **X** Finger Phalangeal Joint, Left	**0** Open **3** Percutaneous **4** Percutaneous Endoscopic	**Z** No Device	**Z** No Qualifier

Section 0 **Medical and Surgical**
Body System R **Upper Joints**
Operation G **Fusion:** Joining together portions of an articular body part rendering the articular body part immobile

Body Part (4th)	Approach (5th)	Device (6th)	Qualifier (7th)
0 Occipital-cervical Joint **1** Cervical Vertebral Joint **2** Cervical Vertebral Joints, 2 or more **4** Cervicothoracic Vertebral Joint **6** Thoracic Vertebral Joint **7** Thoracic Vertebral Joints, 2 to 7 **8** Thoracic Vertebral Joints, 8 or more **A** Thoracolumbar Vertebral Joint	**0** Open **3** Percutaneous **4** Percutaneous Endoscopic	**7** Autologous Tissue Substitute **J** Synthetic Substitute **K** Nonautologous Tissue Substitute	**0** Anterior Approach, Anterior Column **1** Posterior Approach, Posterior Column **J** Posterior Approach, Anterior Column
0 Occipital-cervical Joint **1** Cervical Vertebral Joint **2** Cervical Vertebral Joints, 2 or more **4** Cervicothoracic Vertebral Joint **6** Thoracic Vertebral Joint **7** Thoracic Vertebral Joints, 2 to 7 **8** Thoracic Vertebral Joints, 8 or more **A** Thoracolumbar Vertebral Joint	**0** Open **3** Percutaneous **4** Percutaneous Endoscopic	**A** Interbody Fusion Device	**0** Anterior Approach, Anterior Column **J** Posterior Approach, Anterior Column
C Temporomandibular Joint, Right **D** Temporomandibular Joint, Left **E** Sternoclavicular Joint, Right **F** Sternoclavicular Joint, Left **G** Acromioclavicular Joint, Right **H** Acromioclavicular Joint, Left **J** Shoulder Joint, Right **K** Shoulder Joint, Left	**0** Open **3** Percutaneous **4** Percutaneous Endoscopic	**4** Internal Fixation Device **7** Autologous Tissue Substitute **J** Synthetic Substitute **K** Nonautologous Tissue Substitute	**Z** No Qualifier

Continued →

ction 0 **Medical and Surgical**
dy System R **Upper Joints**
peration G **Fusion:** Joining together portions of an articular body part rendering the articular body part immobile

Body Part (4th)	Approach (5th)	Device (6th)	Qualifier (7th)
L Elbow Joint, Right **M** Elbow Joint, Left **N** Wrist Joint, Right **P** Wrist Joint, Left **Q** Carpal Joint, Right **R** Carpal Joint, Left **S** Carpometacarpal Joint, Right **T** Carpometacarpal Joint, Left **U** Metacarpophalangeal Joint, Right **V** Metacarpophalangeal Joint, Left **W** Finger Phalangeal Joint, Right **X** Finger Phalangeal Joint, Left	**0** Open **3** Percutaneous **4** Percutaneous Endoscopic	**4** Internal Fixation Device **5** External Fixation Device **7** Autologous Tissue Substitute **J** Synthetic Substitute **K** Nonautologous Tissue Substitute	**Z** No Qualifier

ction 0 **Medical and Surgical**
dy System R **Upper Joints**
peration H **Insertion:** Putting in a nonbiological appliance that monitors, assists, performs, or prevents a physiological function but does not physically take the place of a body part

Body Part (4th)	Approach (5th)	Device (6th)	Qualifier (7th)
0 Occipital-cervical Joint **1** Cervical Vertebral Joint **4** Cervicothoracic Vertebral Joint **6** Thoracic Vertebral Joint **A** Thoracolumbar Vertebral Joint	**0** Open **3** Percutaneous **4** Percutaneous Endoscopic	**3** Infusion Device **4** Internal Fixation Device **8** Spacer **B** Spinal Stabilization Device, Interspinous Process **C** Spinal Stabilization Device, Pedicle-Based **D** Spinal Stabilization Device, Facet Replacement	**Z** No Qualifier
3 Cervical Vertebral Disc **5** Cervicothoracic Vertebral Disc **9** Thoracic Vertebral Disc **B** Thoracolumbar Vertebral Disc	**0** Open **3** Percutaneous **4** Percutaneous Endoscopic	**3** Infusion Device	**Z** No Qualifier
C Temporomandibular Joint, Right **D** Temporomandibular Joint, Left **E** Sternoclavicular Joint, Right **F** Sternoclavicular Joint, Left **G** Acromioclavicular Joint, Right **H** Acromioclavicular Joint, Left **J** Shoulder Joint, Right **K** Shoulder Joint, Left	**0** Open **3** Percutaneous **4** Percutaneous Endoscopic	**3** Infusion Device **4** Internal Fixation Device **8** Spacer	**Z** No Qualifier
L Elbow Joint, Right **M** Elbow Joint, Left **N** Wrist Joint, Right **P** Wrist Joint, Left **Q** Carpal Joint, Right **R** Carpal Joint, Left **S** Carpometacarpal Joint, Right **T** Carpometacarpal Joint, Left **U** Metacarpophalangeal Joint, Right **V** Metacarpophalangeal Joint, Left **W** Finger Phalangeal Joint, Right **X** Finger Phalangeal Joint, Left	**0** Open **3** Percutaneous **4** Percutaneous Endoscopic	**3** Infusion Device **4** Internal Fixation Device **5** External Fixation Device **8** Spacer	**Z** No Qualifier

Section 0 **Medical and Surgical**
Body System R **Upper Joints**
Operation J **Inspection:** Visually and/or manually exploring a body part

Body Part (4th)	Approach (5th)	Device (6th)	Qualifier (7th)
0 Occipital-cervical Joint **1** Cervical Vertebral Joint **3** Cervical Vertebral Disc **4** Cervicothoracic Vertebral Joint **5** Cervicothoracic Vertebral Disc **6** Thoracic Vertebral Joint **9** Thoracic Vertebral Disc **A** Thoracolumbar Vertebral Joint **B** Thoracolumbar Vertebral Disc **C** Temporomandibular Joint, Right **D** Temporomandibular Joint, Left **E** Sternoclavicular Joint, Right **F** Sternoclavicular Joint, Left **G** Acromioclavicular Joint, Right **H** Acromioclavicular Joint, Left **J** Shoulder Joint, Right **K** Shoulder Joint, Left **L** Elbow Joint, Right **M** Elbow Joint, Left **N** Wrist Joint, Right **P** Wrist Joint, Left **Q** Carpal Joint, Right **R** Carpal Joint, Left **S** Carpometacarpal Joint, Right **T** Carpometacarpal Joint, Left **U** Metacarpophalangeal Joint, Right **V** Metacarpophalangeal Joint, Left **W** Finger Phalangeal Joint, Right **X** Finger Phalangeal Joint, Left	**0** Open **3** Percutaneous **4** Percutaneous Endoscopic **X** External	**Z** No Device	**Z** No Qualifier

Section 0 **Medical and Surgical**
Body System R **Upper Joints**
Operation N **Release:** Freeing a body part from an abnormal physical constraint by cutting or by the use of force

Body Part (4th)	Approach (5th)	Device (6th)	Qualifier (7th)
0 Occipital-cervical Joint **1** Cervical Vertebral Joint **3** Cervical Vertebral Disc **4** Cervicothoracic Vertebral Joint **5** Cervicothoracic Vertebral Disc **6** Thoracic Vertebral Joint **9** Thoracic Vertebral Disc **A** Thoracolumbar Vertebral Joint **B** Thoracolumbar Vertebral Disc **C** Temporomandibular Joint, Right **D** Temporomandibular Joint, Left **E** Sternoclavicular Joint, Right **F** Sternoclavicular Joint, Left **G** Acromioclavicular Joint, Right **H** Acromioclavicular Joint, Left **J** Shoulder Joint, Right **K** Shoulder Joint, Left **L** Elbow Joint, Right **M** Elbow Joint, Left **N** Wrist Joint, Right **P** Wrist Joint, Left **Q** Carpal Joint, Right **R** Carpal Joint, Left **S** Carpometacarpal Joint, Right **T** Carpometacarpal Joint, Left **U** Metacarpophalangeal Joint, Right **V** Metacarpophalangeal Joint, Left **W** Finger Phalangeal Joint, Right **X** Finger Phalangeal Joint, Left	**0** Open **3** Percutaneous **4** Percutaneous Endoscopic **X** External	**Z** No Device	**Z** No Qualifier

tion 0 **Medical and Surgical**
dy System R **Upper Joints**
eration P **Removal:** Taking out or off a device from a body part

Body Part (4th)	Approach (5th)	Device (6th)	Qualifier (7th)
Occipital-cervical Joint Cervical Vertebral Joint Cervicothoracic Vertebral Joint Thoracic Vertebral Joint Thoracolumbar Vertebral Joint	**0** Open **3** Percutaneous **4** Percutaneous Endoscopic	**0** Drainage Device **3** Infusion Device **4** Internal Fixation Device **7** Autologous Tissue Substitute **8** Spacer **A** Interbody Fusion Device **J** Synthetic Substitute **K** Nonautologous Tissue Substitute	**Z** No Qualifier
Occipital-cervical Joint Cervical Vertebral Joint Cervicothoracic Vertebral Joint Thoracic Vertebral Joint Thoracolumbar Vertebral Joint	**X** External	**0** Drainage Device **3** Infusion Device **4** Internal Fixation Device	**Z** No Qualifier
Cervical Vertebral Disc Cervicothoracic Vertebral Disc Thoracic Vertebral Disc Thoracolumbar Vertebral Disc	**0** Open **3** Percutaneous **4** Percutaneous Endoscopic	**0** Drainage Device **3** Infusion Device **7** Autologous Tissue Substitute **J** Synthetic Substitute **K** Nonautologous Tissue Substitute	**Z** No Qualifier
Cervical Vertebral Disc Cervicothoracic Vertebral Disc Thoracic Vertebral Disc Thoracolumbar Vertebral Disc	**X** External	**0** Drainage Device **3** Infusion Device	**Z** No Qualifier
Temporomandibular Joint, Right Temporomandibular Joint, Left Sternoclavicular Joint, Right Sternoclavicular Joint, Left Acromioclavicular Joint, Right Acromioclavicular Joint, Left Shoulder Joint, Right Shoulder Joint, Left	**0** Open **3** Percutaneous **4** Percutaneous Endoscopic	**0** Drainage Device **3** Infusion Device **4** Internal Fixation Device **7** Autologous Tissue Substitute **8** Spacer **J** Synthetic Substitute **K** Nonautologous Tissue Substitute	**Z** No Qualifier
Temporomandibular Joint, Right Temporomandibular Joint, Left Sternoclavicular Joint, Right Sternoclavicular Joint, Left Acromioclavicular Joint, Right Acromioclavicular Joint, Left Shoulder Joint, Right Shoulder Joint, Left	**X** External	**0** Drainage Device **3** Infusion Device **4** Internal Fixation Device	**Z** No Qualifier
Elbow Joint, Right **M** Elbow Joint, Left Wrist Joint, Right Wrist Joint, Left **Q** Carpal Joint, Right **R** Carpal Joint, Left Carpometacarpal Joint, Right Carpometacarpal Joint, Left Metacarpophalangeal Joint, Right Metacarpophalangeal Joint, Left **W** Finger Phalangeal Joint, Right **X** Finger Phalangeal Joint, Left	**0** Open **3** Percutaneous **4** Percutaneous Endoscopic	**0** Drainage Device **3** Infusion Device **4** Internal Fixation Device **5** External Fixation Device **7** Autologous Tissue Substitute **8** Spacer **J** Synthetic Substitute **K** Nonautologous Tissue Substitute	**Z** No Qualifier

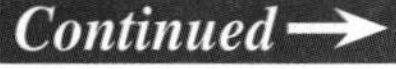
Continued →

Section 0 Medical and Surgical
Body System R Upper Joints
Operation P **Removal:** Taking out or off a device from a body part

0RP Continu

Body Part (4th)	Approach (5th)	Device (6th)	Qualifier (7th)
L Elbow Joint, Right **M** Elbow Joint, Left **N** Wrist Joint, Right **P** Wrist Joint, Left **Q** Carpal Joint, Right **R** Carpal Joint, Left **S** Carpometacarpal Joint, Right **T** Carpometacarpal Joint, Left **U** Metacarpophalangeal Joint, Right **V** Metacarpophalangeal Joint, Left **W** Finger Phalangeal Joint, Right **X** Finger Phalangeal Joint, Left	**X** External	**0** Drainage Device **3** Infusion Device **4** Internal Fixation Device **5** External Fixation Device	**Z** No Qualifier

Section 0 Medical and Surgical
Body System R Upper Joints
Operation Q **Repair:** Restoring, to the extent possible, a body part to its normal anatomic structure and function

Body Part (4th)	Approach (5th)	Device (6th)	Qualifier (7th)
0 Occipital-cervical Joint **1** Cervical Vertebral Joint **3** Cervical Vertebral Disc **4** Cervicothoracic Vertebral Joint **5** Cervicothoracic Vertebral Disc **6** Thoracic Vertebral Joint **9** Thoracic Vertebral Disc **A** Thoracolumbar Vertebral Joint **B** Thoracolumbar Vertebral Disc **C** Temporomandibular Joint, Right **D** Temporomandibular Joint, Left **E** Sternoclavicular Joint, Right **F** Sternoclavicular Joint, Left **G** Acromioclavicular Joint, Right **H** Acromioclavicular Joint, Left **J** Shoulder Joint, Right **K** Shoulder Joint, Left **L** Elbow Joint, Right **M** Elbow Joint, Left **N** Wrist Joint, Right **P** Wrist Joint, Left **Q** Carpal Joint, Right **R** Carpal Joint, Left **S** Carpometacarpal Joint, Right **T** Carpometacarpal Joint, Left **U** Metacarpophalangeal Joint, Right **V** Metacarpophalangeal Joint, Left **W** Finger Phalangeal Joint, Right **X** Finger Phalangeal Joint, Left	**0** Open **3** Percutaneous **4** Percutaneous Endoscopic **X** External	**Z** No Device	**Z** No Qualifier

ction	0	**Medical and Surgical**
dy System	R	**Upper Joints**
peration	R	**Replacement:** Putting in or on biological or synthetic material that physically takes the place and/or function of all or a portion of a body part

Body Part (4th)	Approach (5th)	Device (6th)	Qualifier (7th)
0 Occipital-cervical Joint **1** Cervical Vertebral Joint **3** Cervical Vertebral Disc **4** Cervicothoracic Vertebral Joint **5** Cervicothoracic Vertebral Disc **6** Thoracic Vertebral Joint **9** Thoracic Vertebral Disc **A** Thoracolumbar Vertebral Joint **B** Thoracolumbar Vertebral Disc **C** Temporomandibular Joint, Right **D** Temporomandibular Joint, Left **E** Sternoclavicular Joint, Right **F** Sternoclavicular Joint, Left **G** Acromioclavicular Joint, Right **H** Acromioclavicular Joint, Left **L** Elbow Joint, Right **M** Elbow Joint, Left **N** Wrist Joint, Right **P** Wrist Joint, Left **Q** Carpal Joint, Right **R** Carpal Joint, Left **S** Carpometacarpal Joint, Right **T** Carpometacarpal Joint, Left **U** Metacarpophalangeal Joint, Right **V** Metacarpophalangeal Joint, Left **W** Finger Phalangeal Joint, Right **X** Finger Phalangeal Joint, Left	**0** Open	**7** Autologous Tissue Substitute **J** Synthetic Substitute **K** Nonautologous Tissue Substitute	**Z** No Qualifier
J Shoulder Joint, Right **K** Shoulder Joint, Left	**0** Open	**0** Synthetic Substitute, Reverse Ball and Socket **7** Autologous Tissue Substitute **K** Nonautologous Tissue Substitute	**Z** No Qualifier
J Shoulder Joint, Right **K** Shoulder Joint, Left	**0** Open	**J** Synthetic Substitute	**6** Humeral Surface **7** Glenoid Surface **Z** No Qualifier

ection	0	**Medical and Surgical**
ody System	R	**Upper Joints**
peration	S	**Reposition:** Moving to its normal location, or other suitable location, all or a portion of a body part

Body Part (4th)	Approach (5th)	Device (6th)	Qualifier (7th)
0 Occipital-cervical Joint **1** Cervical Vertebral Joint **4** Cervicothoracic Vertebral Joint **6** Thoracic Vertebral Joint **A** Thoracolumbar Vertebral Joint **C** Temporomandibular Joint, Right **D** Temporomandibular Joint, Left **E** Sternoclavicular Joint, Right **F** Sternoclavicular Joint, Left **G** Acromioclavicular Joint, Right **H** Acromioclavicular Joint, Left **J** Shoulder Joint, Right **K** Shoulder Joint, Left	**0** Open **3** Percutaneous **4** Percutaneous Endoscopic **X** External	**4** Internal Fixation Device **Z** No Device	**Z** No Qualifier

Continued →

0RS Continu

Section 0 **Medical and Surgical**
Body System R **Upper Joints**
Operation S **Reposition:** Moving to its normal location, or other suitable location, all or a portion of a body part

Body Part (4th)	Approach (5th)	Device (6th)	Qualifier (7th)
L Elbow Joint, Right **M** Elbow Joint, Left **N** Wrist Joint, Right **P** Wrist Joint, Left **Q** Carpal Joint, Right **R** Carpal Joint, Left **S** Carpometacarpal Joint, Right **T** Carpometacarpal Joint, Left **U** Metacarpophalangeal Joint, Right **V** Metacarpophalangeal Joint, Left **W** Finger Phalangeal Joint, Right **X** Finger Phalangeal Joint, Left	**0** Open **3** Percutaneous **4** Percutaneous Endoscopic **X** External	**4** Internal Fixation Device **5** External Fixation Device **Z** No Device	**Z** No Qualifier

Section 0 **Medical and Surgical**
Body System R **Upper Joints**
Operation T **Resection:** Cutting out or off, without replacement, all of a body part

Body Part (4th)	Approach (5th)	Device (6th)	Qualifier (7th)
3 Cervical Vertebral Disc **4** Cervicothoracic Vertebral Joint **5** Cervicothoracic Vertebral Disc **9** Thoracic Vertebral Disc **B** Thoracolumbar Vertebral Disc **C** Temporomandibular Joint, Right **D** Temporomandibular Joint, Left **E** Sternoclavicular Joint, Right **F** Sternoclavicular Joint, Left **G** Acromioclavicular Joint, Right **H** Acromioclavicular Joint, Left **J** Shoulder Joint, Right **K** Shoulder Joint, Left **L** Elbow Joint, Right **M** Elbow Joint, Left **N** Wrist Joint, Right **P** Wrist Joint, Left **Q** Carpal Joint, Right **R** Carpal Joint, Left **S** Carpometacarpal Joint, Right **T** Carpometacarpal Joint, Left **U** Metacarpophalangeal Joint, Right **V** Metacarpophalangeal Joint, Left **W** Finger Phalangeal Joint, Right **X** Finger Phalangeal Joint, Left	**0** Open	**Z** No Device	**Z** No Qualifier

tion **0** **Medical and Surgical**
dy System **R** **Upper Joints**
eration **U** **Supplement:** Putting in or on biological or synthetic material that physically reinforces and/or augments the function of a portion of a body part

Body Part (4th)	Approach (5th)	Device (6th)	Qualifier (7th)
Occipital-cervical Joint Cervical Vertebral Joint Cervical Vertebral Disc Cervicothoracic Vertebral Joint Cervicothoracic Vertebral Disc Thoracic Vertebral Joint Thoracic Vertebral Disc Thoracolumbar Vertebral Joint Thoracolumbar Vertebral Disc Temporomandibular Joint, Right Temporomandibular Joint, Left Sternoclavicular Joint, Right Sternoclavicular Joint, Left Acromioclavicular Joint, Right Acromioclavicular Joint, Left Shoulder Joint, Right Shoulder Joint, Left Elbow Joint, Right Elbow Joint, Left Wrist Joint, Right Wrist Joint, Left Carpal Joint, Right Carpal Joint, Left Carpometacarpal Joint, Right Carpometacarpal Joint, Left Metacarpophalangeal Joint, Right Metacarpophalangeal Joint, Left V Finger Phalangeal Joint, Right Finger Phalangeal Joint, Left	**0** Open **3** Percutaneous **4** Percutaneous Endoscopic	**7** Autologous Tissue Substitute **J** Synthetic Substitute **K** Nonautologous Tissue Substitute	**Z** No Qualifier

tion **0** **Medical and Surgical**
dy System **R** **Upper Joints**
eration **W** **Revision:** Correcting, to the extent possible, a portion of a malfunctioning device or the position of a displaced device

Body Part (4th)	Approach (5th)	Device (6th)	Qualifier (7th)
Occipital-cervical Joint Cervical Vertebral Joint Cervicothoracic Vertebral Joint Thoracic Vertebral Joint Thoracolumbar Vertebral Joint	**0** Open **3** Percutaneous **4** Percutaneous Endoscopic **X** External	**0** Drainage Device **3** Infusion Device **4** Internal Fixation Device **7** Autologous Tissue Substitute **8** Spacer **A** Interbody Fusion Device **J** Synthetic Substitute **K** Nonautologous Tissue Substitute	**Z** No Qualifier
Cervical Vertebral Disc Cervicothoracic Vertebral Disc Thoracic Vertebral Disc Thoracolumbar Vertebral Disc	**0** Open **3** Percutaneous **4** Percutaneous Endoscopic **X** External	**0** Drainage Device **3** Infusion Device **7** Autologous Tissue Substitute **J** Synthetic Substitute **K** Nonautologous Tissue Substitute	**Z** No Qualifier
Temporomandibular Joint, Right Temporomandibular Joint, Left Sternoclavicular Joint, Right Sternoclavicular Joint, Left Acromioclavicular Joint, Right Acromioclavicular Joint, Left Shoulder Joint, Right Shoulder Joint, Left	**0** Open **3** Percutaneous **4** Percutaneous Endoscopic **X** External	**0** Drainage Device **3** Infusion Device **4** Internal Fixation Device **7** Autologous Tissue Substitute **8** Spacer **J** Synthetic Substitute **K** Nonautologous Tissue Substitute	**Z** No Qualifier

Continued →

Section **0** **Medical and Surgical**
Body System **R** **Upper Joints**
Operation **W** **Revision:** Correcting, to the extent possible, a portion of a malfunctioning device or the position of a displaced device

0RW Contin.

Body Part (4th)	Approach (5th)	Device (6th)	Qualifier (7t
L Elbow Joint, Right **M** Elbow Joint, Left **N** Wrist Joint, Right **P** Wrist Joint, Left **Q** Carpal Joint, Right **R** Carpal Joint, Left **S** Carpometacarpal Joint, Right **T** Carpometacarpal Joint, Left **U** Metacarpophalangeal Joint, Right **V** Metacarpophalangeal Joint, Left **W** Finger Phalangeal Joint, Right **X** Finger Phalangeal Joint, Left	**0** Open **3** Percutaneous **4** Percutaneous Endoscopic **X** External	**0** Drainage Device **3** Infusion Device **4** Internal Fixation Device **5** External Fixation Device **7** Autologous Tissue Substitute **8** Spacer **J** Synthetic Substitute **K** Nonautologous Tissue Substitute	**Z** No Qualifie

AHA Coding Clinic

0RG40A0 Fusion of Cervicothoracic Vertebral Joint with Interbody Fusion Device, Anterior Approach, Anterior Column, O Approach—AHA CC: 1Q, 2013, 29-30; 2Q, 2014, 7-8

0RG7071 Fusion of 2 to 7 Thoracic Vertebral Joints with Autologous Tissue Substitute, Posterior Approach, Posterior Column, O Approach—AHA CC: 1Q, 2013, 21-23

0RGA071 Fusion of Thoracolumbar Vertebral Joint with Autologous Tissue Substitute, Posterior Approach, Posterior Column, O Approach—AHA CC: 1Q, 2013, 21-23

0RGW04Z Fusion of Right Finger Phalangeal Joint with Internal Fixation Device, Open Approach—AHA CC: 4Q, 2017, 62

0RH104Z Insertion of Internal Fixation Device into Cervical Vertebral Joint, Open Approach—AHA CC: 2Q, 2017, 23-24

0RHJ04Z Insertion of Internal Fixation Device into Right Shoulder Joint, Open Approach—AHA CC: 3Q, 2016, 32-33

0RNJ4ZZ Release Right Shoulder Joint, Percutaneous Endoscopic Approach—AHA CC: 3Q, 2016, 32-33

0RNK4ZZ Release Left Shoulder Joint, Percutaneous Endoscopic Approach—AHA CC: 2Q, 2015, 22-23

0RQJ4ZZ Repair Right Shoulder Joint, Percutaneous Endoscopic Approach—AHA CC: 1Q, 2016, 30-31

0RRJ00Z Replacement of Right Shoulder Joint with Reverse Ball and Socket Synthetic Substitute, Open Approach—AHA CC: 2015, 27

0RRK0J6 Replacement of Left Shoulder Joint with Synthetic Substitute, Humeral Surface, Open Approach—AHA CC: 3Q, 2015, 14-1

0RS1XZZ Reposition Cervical Vertebral Joint, External Approach—AHA CC: 2Q, 2015, 35

0RSPXZZ Reposition Left Wrist Joint, External Approach—AHA CC: 4Q, 2014, 32-33

0RSR04Z Reposition Left Carpal Joint with Internal Fixation Device, Open Approach—AHA CC: 3Q, 2014, 33-34

0RT50ZZ Resection of Cervicothoracic Vertebral Disc, Open Approach—AHA CC: 2Q, 2014, 7-8

0RUT07Z Supplement Left Carpometacarpal Joint with Autologous Tissue Substitute, Open Approach—AHA CC: 3Q, 2015, 26-27

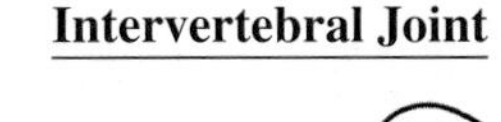

Intervertebral Joint

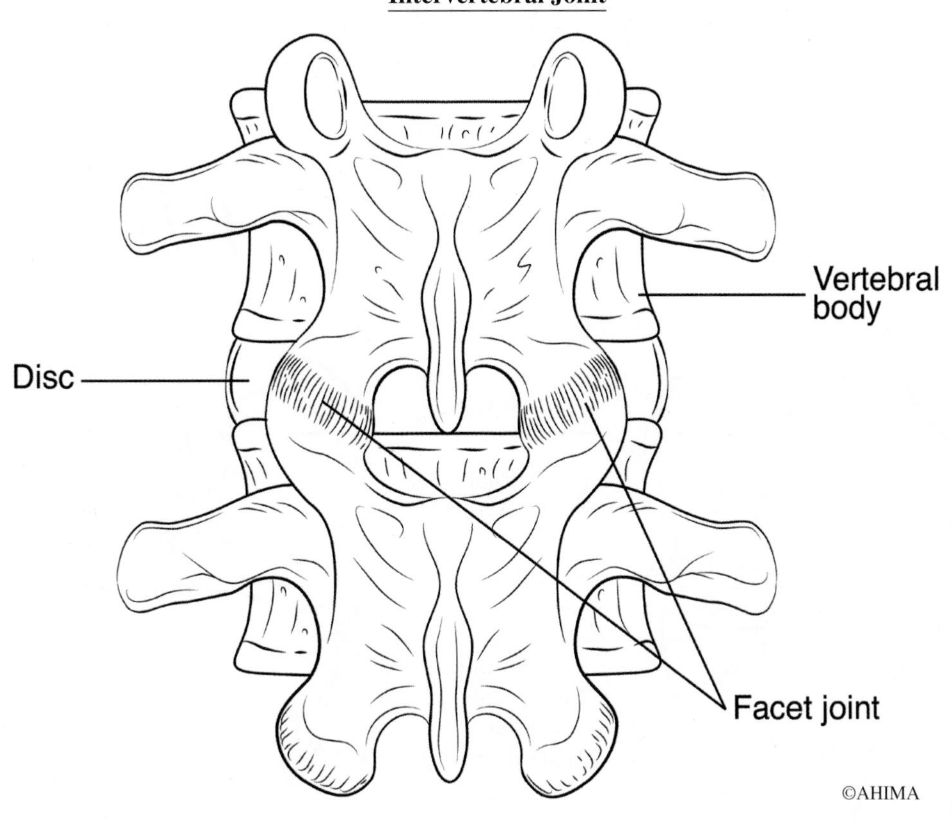

©AHIMA

Hip

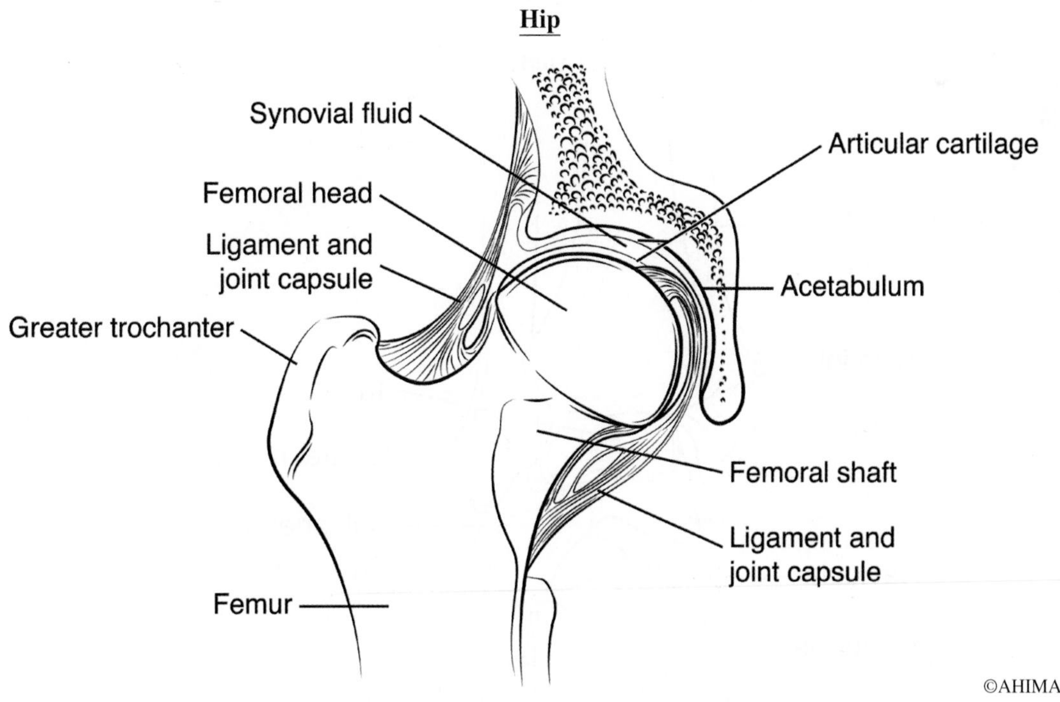

©AHIMA

Knee Joint

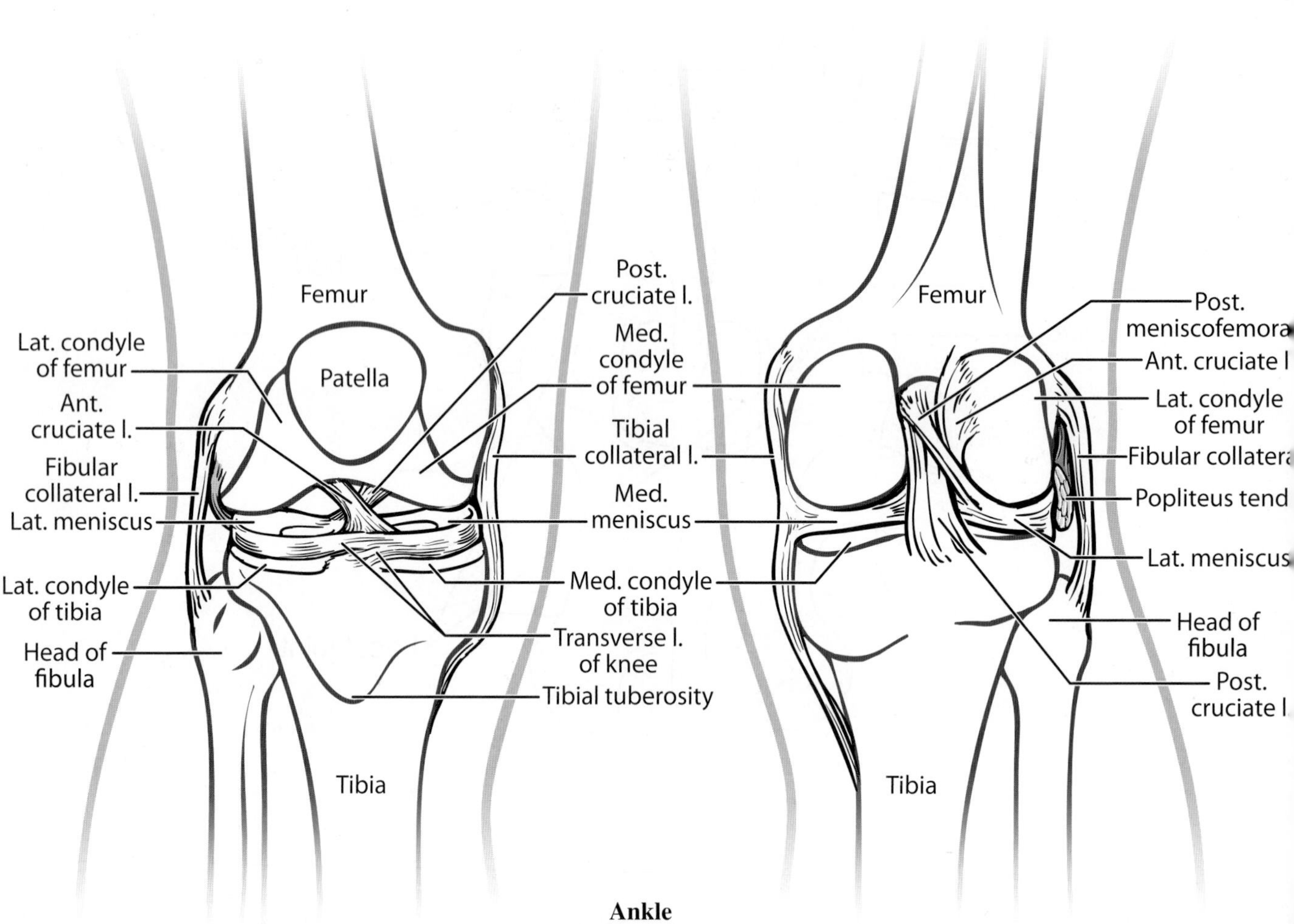
ANTERIOR
POSTERIOR
Femur
Patella
Lat. condyle of femur
Ant. cruciate l.
Fibular collateral l.
Lat. meniscus
Lat. condyle of tibia
Head of fibula
Post. cruciate l.
Med. condyle of femur
Tibial collateral l.
Med. meniscus
Med. condyle of tibia
Transverse l. of knee
Tibial tuberosity
Tibia
Femur
Post. meniscofemora
Ant. cruciate l
Lat. condyle of femur
Fibular collatera
Popliteus tend
Lat. meniscus
Head of fibula
Post. cruciate l
Tibia

Ankle

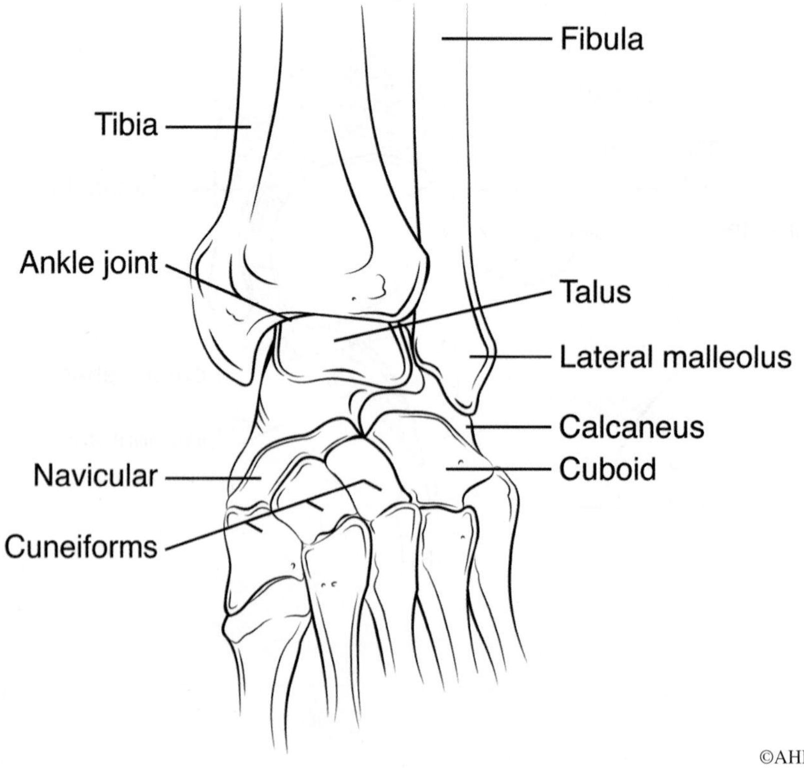
Fibula
Tibia
Ankle joint
Talus
Lateral malleolus
Calcaneus
Cuboid
Navicular
Cuneiforms

Total Knee Replacement Technique: Steps 1-5

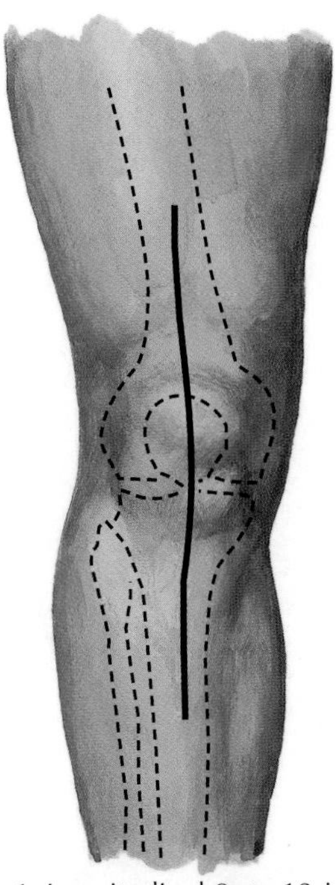

1. Longitudinal 8- to 12-in. skin incision is centered on patella.

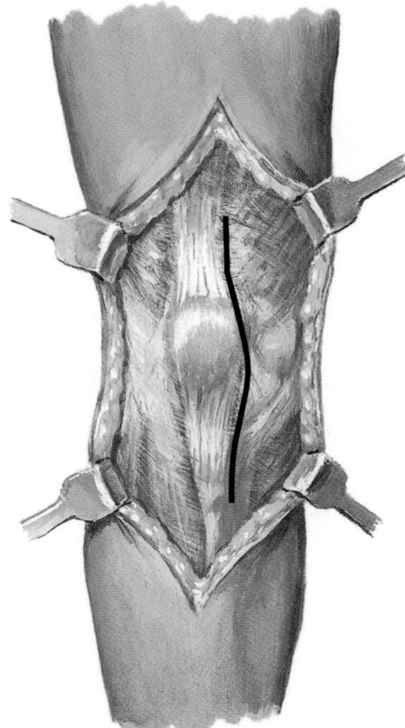

2. Capsular incision skirts medial margin of patella and courses distally through periosteum medial to tibial tuberosity.

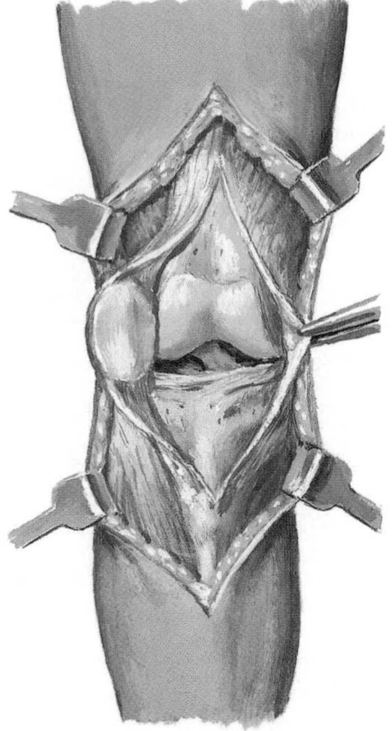

3. Patella is reflected laterally by raising patellar ligament in continuity with periosteum.

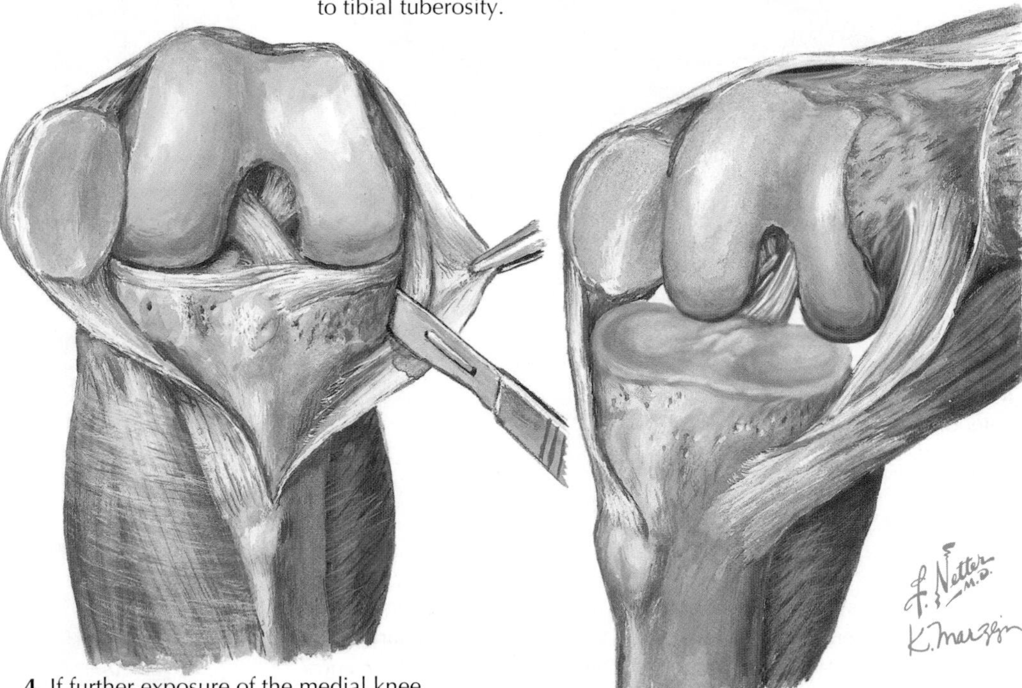

4. If further exposure of the medial knee is needed, a flap can be raised by elevating the deep medial collateral ligament and pes anserinus subperiosteally, aided by external rotation of the tibia.

5. The anterior cruciate ligament and both menisci are excised, and the tibia is subluxated anteriorly.

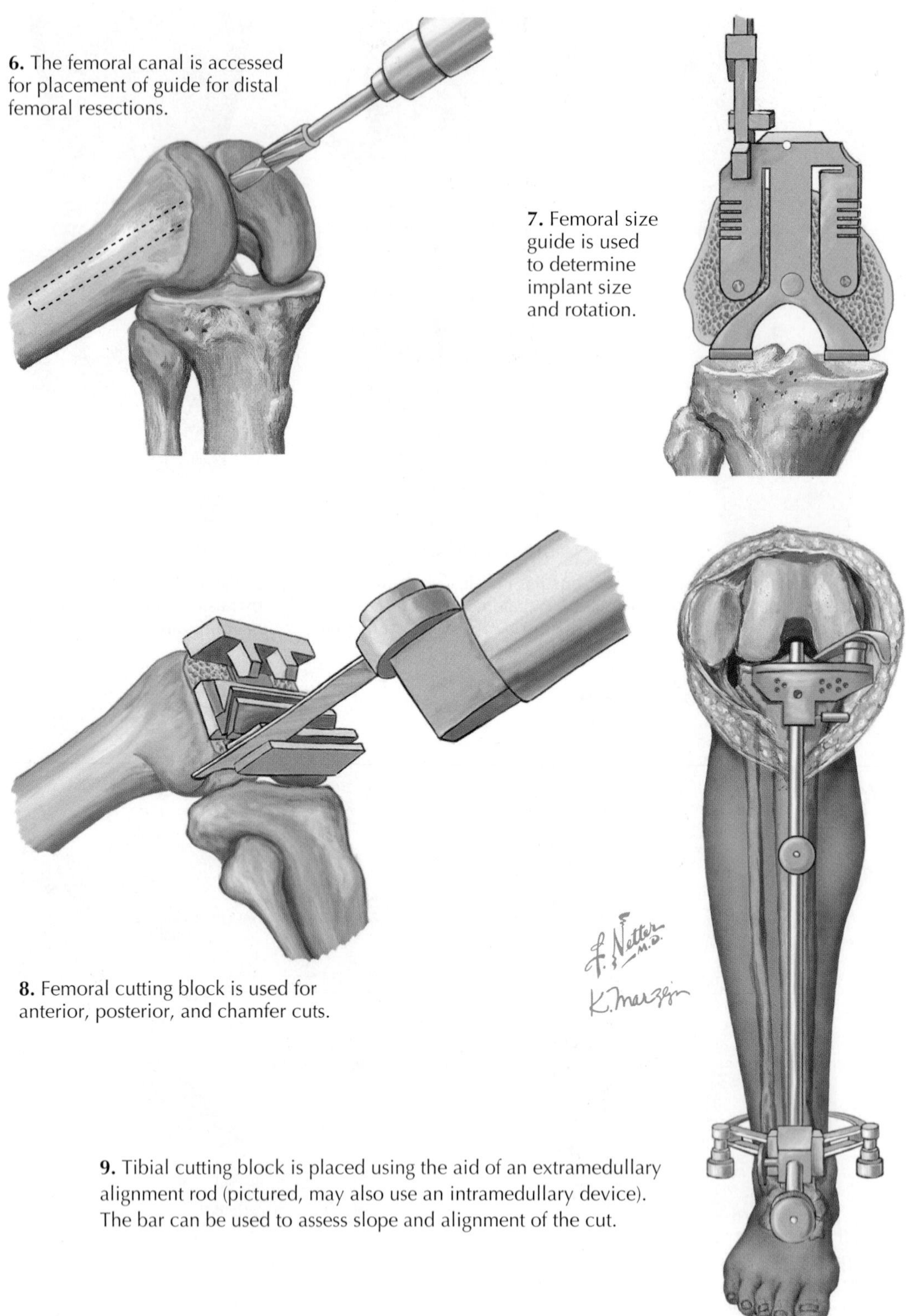

6. The femoral canal is accessed for placement of guide for distal femoral resections.

7. Femoral size guide is used to determine implant size and rotation.

8. Femoral cutting block is used for anterior, posterior, and chamfer cuts.

9. Tibial cutting block is placed using the aid of an extramedullary alignment rod (pictured, may also use an intramedullary device). The bar can be used to assess slope and alignment of the cut.

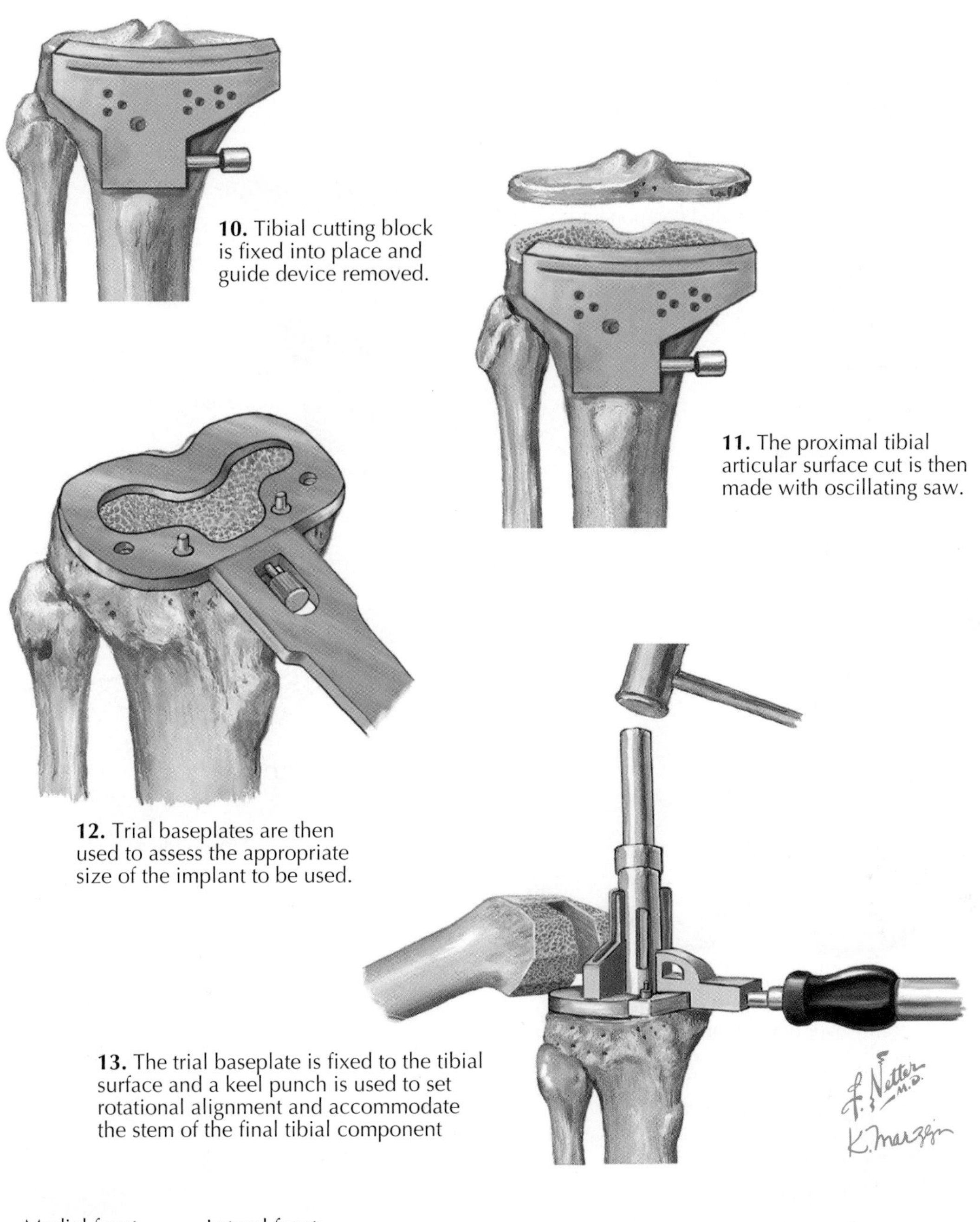

14. Articular surface of patella resected to leave flat surface. Equal amounts to be removed from medial and lateral facets, but at least 1 cm of bone must be left to ensure adequate strength. Using a patella drill template, three holes are drilled into the surface to accommodate the final patellar component, which is cemented in place.

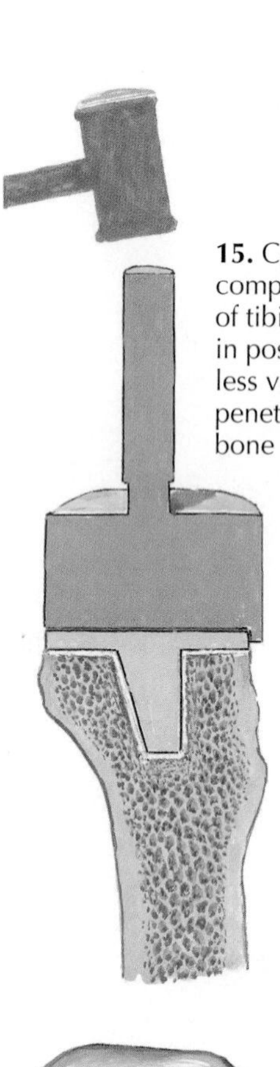

15. Cement is applied to tibial component and cut surfaces of tibia, and component is placed in position. Cement is somewhat less viscous to facilitate penetration into trabecular bone (sagittal section).

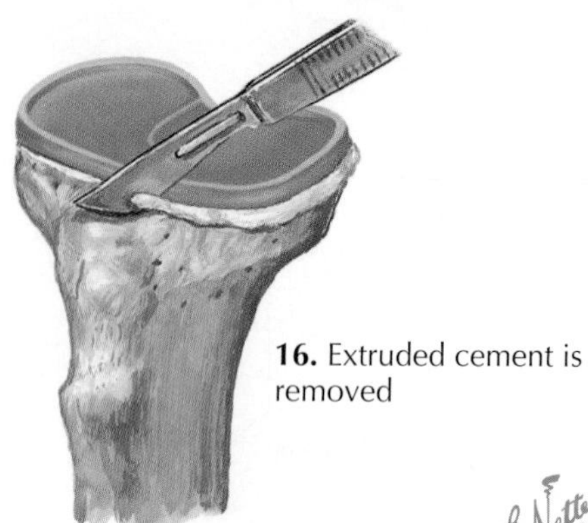

16. Extruded cement is removed

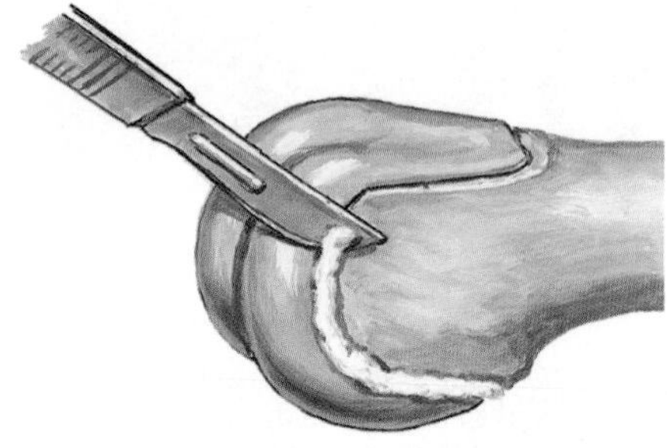

18. Extruded cement is removed

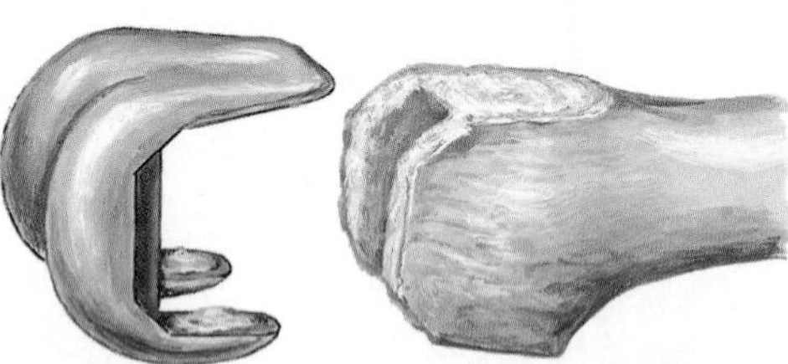

17. Cement is applied to posterior limb of femoral component and spread evenly over beveled ends of femur

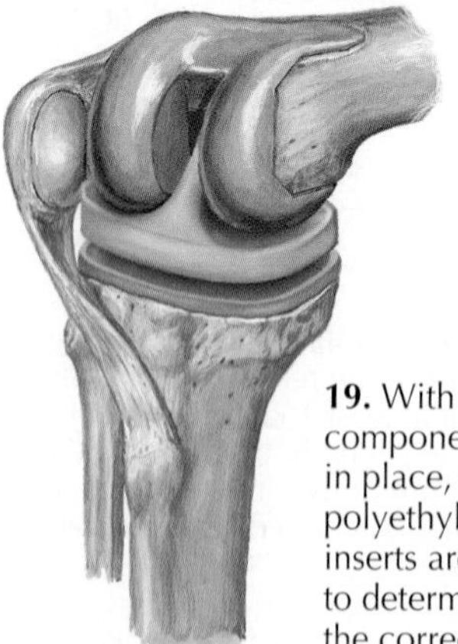

19. With all components in place, trial polyethylene inserts are used to determine the correct size.

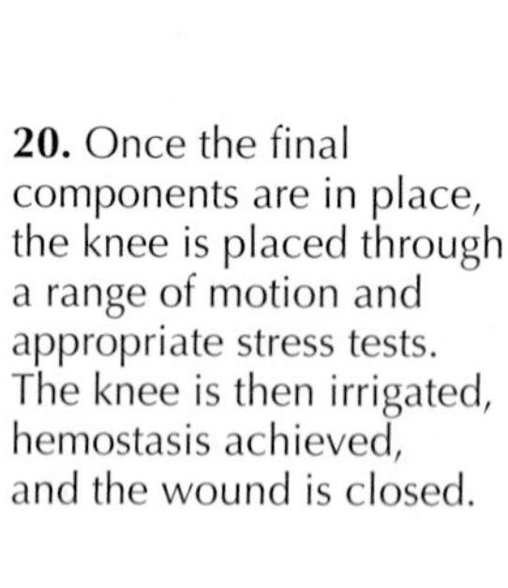

20. Once the final components are in place, the knee is placed through a range of motion and appropriate stress tests. The knee is then irrigated, hemostasis achieved, and the wound is closed.

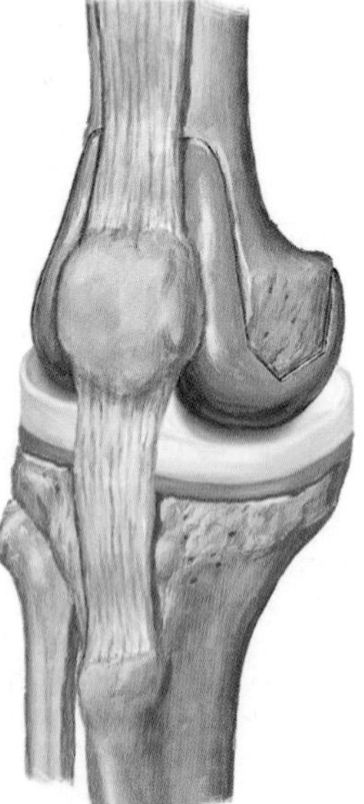

ction 0 **Medical and Surgical**
dy System S **Lower Joints**
peration 2 **Change:** Taking out or off a device from a body part and putting back an identical or similar device in or on the same body part without cutting or puncturing the skin or a mucous membrane

Body Part (4th)	Approach (5th)	Device (6th)	Qualifier (7th)
Y Lower Joint	X External	0 Drainage Device Y Other Device	Z No Qualifier

ction 0 **Medical and Surgical**
dy System S **Lower Joints**
peration 5 **Destruction:** Physical eradication of all or a portion of a body part by the direct use of energy, force, or a destructive agent

Body Part (4th)	Approach (5th)	Device (6th)	Qualifier (7th)
0 Lumbar Vertebral Joint 2 Lumbar Vertebral Disc 3 Lumbosacral Joint 4 Lumbosacral Disc 5 Sacrococcygeal Joint 6 Coccygeal Joint 7 Sacroiliac Joint, Right 8 Sacroiliac Joint, Left 9 Hip Joint, Right B Hip Joint, Left C Knee Joint, Right D Knee Joint, Left F Ankle Joint, Right G Ankle Joint, Left H Tarsal Joint, Right J Tarsal Joint, Left K Tarsometatarsal Joint, Right L Tarsometatarsal Joint, Left M Metatarsal-Phalangeal Joint, Right N Metatarsal-Phalangeal Joint, Left P Toe Phalangeal Joint, Right Q Toe Phalangeal Joint, Left	0 Open 3 Percutaneous 4 Percutaneous Endoscopic	Z No Device	Z No Qualifier

Section 0 **Medical and Surgical**
Body System S **Lower Joints**
Operation 9 **Drainage:** Taking or letting out fluids and/or gases from a body part

Body Part (4th)	Approach (5th)	Device (6th)	Qualifier (7th)
0 Lumbar Vertebral Joint **2** Lumbar Vertebral Disc **3** Lumbosacral Joint **4** Lumbosacral Disc **5** Sacrococcygeal Joint **6** Coccygeal Joint **7** Sacroiliac Joint, Right **8** Sacroiliac Joint, Left **9** Hip Joint, Right **B** Hip Joint, Left **C** Knee Joint, Right **D** Knee Joint, Left **F** Ankle Joint, Right **G** Ankle Joint, Left **H** Tarsal Joint, Right **J** Tarsal Joint, Left **K** Tarsometatarsal Joint, Right **L** Tarsometatarsal Joint, Left **M** Metatarsal-Phalangeal Joint, Right **N** Metatarsal-Phalangeal Joint, Left **P** Toe Phalangeal Joint, Right **Q** Toe Phalangeal Joint, Left	**0** Open **3** Percutaneous **4** Percutaneous Endoscopic	**0** Drainage Device	**Z** No Qualifier
0 Lumbar Vertebral Joint **2** Lumbar Vertebral Disc **3** Lumbosacral Joint **4** Lumbosacral Disc **5** Sacrococcygeal Joint **6** Coccygeal Joint **7** Sacroiliac Joint, Right **8** Sacroiliac Joint, Left **9** Hip Joint, Right **B** Hip Joint, Left **C** Knee Joint, Right **D** Knee Joint, Left **F** Ankle Joint, Right **G** Ankle Joint, Left **H** Tarsal Joint, Right **J** Tarsal Joint, Left **K** Tarsometatarsal Joint, Right **L** Tarsometatarsal Joint, Left **M** Metatarsal-Phalangeal Joint, Right **N** Metatarsal-Phalangeal Joint, Left **P** Toe Phalangeal Joint, Right **Q** Toe Phalangeal Joint, Left	**0** Open **3** Percutaneous **4** Percutaneous Endoscopic	**Z** No Device	**X** Diagnostic **Z** No Qualifier

Section 0 **Medical and Surgical**
Body System S **Lower Joints**
Operation B **Excision:** Cutting out or off, without replacement, a portion of a body part

Body Part (4th)	Approach (5th)	Device (6th)	Qualifier (7th)
0 Lumbar Vertebral Joint	**0** Open	**Z** No Device	**X** Diagnostic
2 Lumbar Vertebral Disc	**3** Percutaneous		**Z** No Qualifier
3 Lumbosacral Joint	**4** Percutaneous Endoscopic		
4 Lumbosacral Disc			
5 Sacrococcygeal Joint			
6 Coccygeal Joint			
7 Sacroiliac Joint, Right			
8 Sacroiliac Joint, Left			
9 Hip Joint, Right			
B Hip Joint, Left			
C Knee Joint, Right			
D Knee Joint, Left			
F Ankle Joint, Right			
G Ankle Joint, Left			
H Tarsal Joint, Right			
J Tarsal Joint, Left			
K Tarsometatarsal Joint, Right			
L Tarsometatarsal Joint, Left			
M Metatarsal-Phalangeal Joint, Right			
N Metatarsal-Phalangeal Joint, Left			
P Toe Phalangeal Joint, Right			
Q Toe Phalangeal Joint, Left			

Section 0 **Medical and Surgical**
Body System S **Lower Joints**
Operation C **Extirpation:** Taking or cutting out solid matter from a body part

Body Part (4th)	Approach (5th)	Device (6th)	Qualifier (7th)
0 Lumbar Vertebral Joint	**0** Open	**Z** No Device	**Z** No Qualifier
2 Lumbar Vertebral Disc	**3** Percutaneous		
3 Lumbosacral Joint	**4** Percutaneous Endoscopic		
4 Lumbosacral Disc			
5 Sacrococcygeal Joint			
6 Coccygeal Joint			
7 Sacroiliac Joint, Right			
8 Sacroiliac Joint, Left			
9 Hip Joint, Right			
B Hip Joint, Left			
C Knee Joint, Right			
D Knee Joint, Left			
F Ankle Joint, Right			
G Ankle Joint, Left			
H Tarsal Joint, Right			
J Tarsal Joint, Left			
K Tarsometatarsal Joint, Right			
L Tarsometatarsal Joint, Left			
M Metatarsal-Phalangeal Joint, Right			
N Metatarsal-Phalangeal Joint, Left			
P Toe Phalangeal Joint, Right			
Q Toe Phalangeal Joint, Left			

Section 0 **Medical and Surgical**
Body System S **Lower Joints**
Operation G **Fusion:** Joining together portions of an articular body part rendering the articular body part immobile

Body Part (4th)	Approach (5th)	Device (6th)	Qualifier (7th)
0 Lumbar Vertebral Joint **1** Lumbar Vertebral Joints, 2 or more **3** Lumbosacral Joint	**0** Open **3** Percutaneous **4** Percutaneous Endoscopic	**7** Autologous Tissue Substitute **J** Synthetic Substitute **K** Nonautologous Tissue Substitute	**0** Anterior Approach, Anterior Column **1** Posterior Approach, Posterior Column **J** Posterior Approach, Anterior Column
0 Lumbar Vertebral Joint **1** Lumbar Vertebral Joints, 2 or more **3** Lumbosacral Joint	**0** Open **3** Percutaneous **4** Percutaneous Endoscopic	**A** Interbody Fusion Device	**0** Anterior Approach, Anterior Column **J** Posterior Approach, Anterior Column
5 Sacrococcygeal Joint **6** Coccygeal Joint **7** Sacroiliac Joint, Right **8** Sacroiliac Joint, Left	**0** Open **3** Percutaneous **4** Percutaneous Endoscopic	**4** Internal Fixation Device **7** Autologous Tissue Substitute **J** Synthetic Substitute **K** Nonautologous Tissue Substitute	**Z** No Qualifier
9 Hip Joint, Right **B** Hip Joint, Left **C** Knee Joint, Right **D** Knee Joint, Left **F** Ankle Joint, Right **G** Ankle Joint, Left **H** Tarsal Joint, Right **J** Tarsal Joint, Left **K** Tarsometatarsal Joint, Right **L** Tarsometatarsal Joint, Left **M** Metatarsal-Phalangeal Joint, Right **N** Metatarsal-Phalangeal Joint, Left **P** Toe Phalangeal Joint, Right **Q** Toe Phalangeal Joint, Left	**0** Open **3** Percutaneous **4** Percutaneous Endoscopic	**4** Internal Fixation Device **5** External Fixation Device **7** Autologous Tissue Substitute **J** Synthetic Substitute **K** Nonautologous Tissue Substitute	**Z** No Qualifier

Section 0 **Medical and Surgical**
Body System S **Lower Joints**
Operation H **Insertion:** Putting in a nonbiological appliance that monitors, assists, performs, or prevents a physiological function but does not physically take the place of a body part

Body Part (4th)	Approach (5th)	Device (6th)	Qualifier (7th)
0 Lumbar Vertebral Joint **3** Lumbosacral Joint	**0** Open **3** Percutaneous **4** Percutaneous Endoscopic	**3** Infusion Device **4** Internal Fixation Device **8** Spacer **B** Spinal Stabilization Device, Interspinous Process **C** Spinal Stabilization Device, Pedicle-Based **D** Spinal Stabilization Device, Facet Replacement	**Z** No Qualifier
2 Lumbar Vertebral Disc **4** Lumbosacral Disc	**0** Open **3** Percutaneous **4** Percutaneous Endoscopic	**3** Infusion Device **8** Spacer	**Z** No Qualifier
5 Sacrococcygeal Joint **6** Coccygeal Joint **7** Sacroiliac Joint, Right **8** Sacroiliac Joint, Left	**0** Open **3** Percutaneous **4** Percutaneous Endoscopic	**3** Infusion Device **4** Internal Fixation Device **8** Spacer	**Z** No Qualifier

Continued →

tion	**0**	**Medical and Surgical**
dy System	**S**	**Lower Joints**
eration	**H**	**Insertion:** Putting in a nonbiological appliance that monitors, assists, performs, or prevents a physiological function but does not physically take the place of a body part

Body Part (4th)	Approach (5th)	Device (6th)	Qualifier (7th)
Hip Joint, Right Hip Joint, Left Knee Joint, Right Knee Joint, Left Ankle Joint, Right Ankle Joint, Left Tarsal Joint, Right Tarsal Joint, Left Tarsometatarsal Joint, Right Tarsometatarsal Joint, Left Metatarsal-Phalangeal Joint, Right Metatarsal-Phalangeal Joint, Left Toe Phalangeal Joint, Right Toe Phalangeal Joint, Left	**0** Open **3** Percutaneous **4** Percutaneous Endoscopic	**3** Infusion Device **4** Internal Fixation Device **5** External Fixation Device **8** Spacer	**Z** No Qualifier

tion	**0**	**Medical and Surgical**
dy System	**S**	**Lower Joints**
eration	**J**	**Inspection:** Visually and/or manually exploring a body part

Body Part (4th)	Approach (5th)	Device (6th)	Qualifier (7th)
Lumbar Vertebral Joint Lumbar Vertebral Disc Lumbosacral Joint Lumbosacral Disc Sacrococcygeal Joint Coccygeal Joint Sacroiliac Joint, Right Sacroiliac Joint, Left Hip Joint, Right Hip Joint, Left Knee Joint, Right Knee Joint, Left Ankle Joint, Right Ankle Joint, Left Tarsal Joint, Right Tarsal Joint, Left Tarsometatarsal Joint, Right Tarsometatarsal Joint, Left Metatarsal-Phalangeal Joint, Right Metatarsal-Phalangeal Joint, Left Toe Phalangeal Joint, Right Toe Phalangeal Joint, Left	**0** Open **3** Percutaneous **4** Percutaneous Endoscopic **X** External	**Z** No Device	**Z** No Qualifier

Section 0 **Medical and Surgical**
Body System S **Lower Joints**
Operation N **Release:** Freeing a body part from an abnormal physical constraint by cutting or by the use of force

Body Part (4th)	Approach (5th)	Device (6th)	Qualifier (7th)
0 Lumbar Vertebral Joint **2** Lumbar Vertebral Disc **3** Lumbosacral Joint **4** Lumbosacral Disc **5** Sacrococcygeal Joint **6** Coccygeal Joint **7** Sacroiliac Joint, Right **8** Sacroiliac Joint, Left **9** Hip Joint, Right **B** Hip Joint, Left **C** Knee Joint, Right **D** Knee Joint, Left **F** Ankle Joint, Right **G** Ankle Joint, Left **H** Tarsal Joint, Right **J** Tarsal Joint, Left **K** Tarsometatarsal Joint, Right **L** Tarsometatarsal Joint, Left **M** Metatarsal-Phalangeal Joint, Right **N** Metatarsal-Phalangeal Joint, Left **P** Toe Phalangeal Joint, Right **Q** Toe Phalangeal Joint, Left	**0** Open **3** Percutaneous **4** Percutaneous Endoscopic **X** External	**Z** No Device	**Z** No Qualifier

Section 0 **Medical and Surgical**
Body System S **Lower Joints**
Operation P **Removal:** Taking out or off a device from a body part

Body Part (4th)	Approach (5th)	Device (6th)	Qualifier (7th)
0 Lumbar Vertebral Joint **3** Lumbosacral Joint	**0** Open **3** Percutaneous **4** Percutaneous Endoscopic	**0** Drainage Device **3** Infusion Device **4** Internal Fixation Device **7** Autologous Tissue Substitute **8** Spacer **A** Interbody Fusion Device **J** Synthetic Substitute **K** Nonautologous Tissue Substitute	**Z** No Qualifier
0 Lumbar Vertebral Joint **3** Lumbosacral Joint	**X** External	**0** Drainage Device **3** Infusion Device **4** Internal Fixation Device	**Z** No Qualifier
2 Lumbar Vertebral Disc **4** Lumbosacral Disc	**0** Open **3** Percutaneous **4** Percutaneous Endoscopic	**0** Drainage Device **3** Infusion Device **7** Autologous Tissue Substitute **J** Synthetic Substitute **K** Nonautologous Tissue Substitute	**Z** No Qualifier
2 Lumbar Vertebral Disc **4** Lumbosacral Disc	**X** External	**0** Drainage Device **3** Infusion Device	**Z** No Qualifier
5 Sacrococcygeal Joint **6** Coccygeal Joint **7** Sacroiliac Joint, Right **8** Sacroiliac Joint, Left	**0** Open **3** Percutaneous **4** Percutaneous Endoscopic	**0** Drainage Device **3** Infusion Device **4** Internal Fixation Device **7** Autologous Tissue Substitute **8** Spacer **J** Synthetic Substitute **K** Nonautologous Tissue Substitute	**Z** No Qualifier

Continued →

ction 0 Medical and Surgical
dy System S Lower Joints
eration P Removal: Taking out or off a device from a body part

Body Part (4th)	Approach (5th)	Device (6th)	Qualifier (7th)
5 Sacrococcygeal Joint 6 Coccygeal Joint 7 Sacroiliac Joint, Right 8 Sacroiliac Joint, Left	X External	0 Drainage Device 3 Infusion Device 4 Internal Fixation Device	Z No Qualifier
9 Hip Joint, Right B Hip Joint, Left	0 Open	0 Drainage Device 3 Infusion Device 4 Internal Fixation Device 5 External Fixation Device 7 Autologous Tissue Substitute 8 Spacer 9 Liner B Resurfacing Device E Articulating Spacer J Synthetic Substitute K Nonautologous Tissue Substitute	Z No Qualifier
9 Hip Joint, Right B Hip Joint, Left	3 Percutaneous 4 Percutaneous Endoscopic	0 Drainage Device 3 Infusion Device 4 Internal Fixation Device 5 External Fixation Device 7 Autologous Tissue Substitute 8 Spacer J Synthetic Substitute K Nonautologous Tissue Substitute	Z No Qualifier
9 Hip Joint, Right B Hip Joint, Left	X External	0 Drainage Device 3 Infusion Device 4 Internal Fixation Device 5 External Fixation Device	Z No Qualifier
A Hip Joint, Acetabular Surface, Right E Hip Joint, Acetabular Surface, Left R Hip Joint, Femoral Surface, Right S Hip Joint, Femoral Surface, Left T Knee Joint, Femoral Surface, Right U Knee Joint, Femoral Surface, Left V Knee Joint, Tibial Surface, Right W Knee Joint, Tibial Surface, Left	0 Open 3 Percutaneous 4 Percutaneous Endoscopic	J Synthetic Substitute	Z No Qualifier
C Knee Joint, Right D Knee Joint, Left	0 Open	0 Drainage Device 3 Infusion Device 4 Internal Fixation Device 5 External Fixation Device 7 Autologous Tissue Substitute 8 Spacer 9 Liner E Articulating Spacer K Nonautologous Tissue Substitute L Synthetic Substitute, Unicondylar Medial M Synthetic Substitute, Unicondylar Lateral N Synthetic Substitute, Unicondylar Patellofemoral	Z No Qualifier
C Knee Joint, Right D Knee Joint, Left	0 Open	J Synthetic Substitute	C Patellar Surface Z No Qualifier

Continued →

Section **0** **Medical and Surgical**
Body System **S** **Lower Joints**
Operation **P** **Removal:** Taking out or off a device from a body part

0SP Continu

Body Part (4th)	Approach (5th)	Device (6th)	Qualifier (7th
C Knee Joint, Right **D** Knee Joint, Left	**3** Percutaneous **4** Percutaneous Endoscopic	**0** Drainage Device **3** Infusion Device **4** Internal Fixation Device **5** External Fixation Device **7** Autologous Tissue Substitute **8** Spacer **K** Nonautologous Tissue Substitute **L** Synthetic Substitute, Unicondylar Medial **M** Synthetic Substitute, Unicondylar Lateral **N** Synthetic Substitute, Unicondylar Patellofemoral	**Z** No Qualifier
C Knee Joint, Right **D** Knee Joint, Left	**3** Percutaneous **4** Percutaneous Endoscopic	**J** Synthetic Substitute	**C** Patellar Surface **Z** No Qualifier
C Knee Joint, Right **D** Knee Joint, Left	**X** External	**0** Drainage Device **3** Infusion Device **4** Internal Fixation Device **5** External Fixation Device	**Z** No Qualifier
F Ankle Joint, Right **G** Ankle Joint, Left **H** Tarsal Joint, Right **J** Tarsal Joint, Left **K** Tarsometatarsal Joint, Right **L** Tarsometatarsal Joint, Left **M** Metatarsal-Phalangeal Joint, Right **N** Metatarsal-Phalangeal Joint, Left **P** Toe Phalangeal Joint, Right **Q** Toe Phalangeal Joint, Left	**0** Open **3** Percutaneous **4** Percutaneous Endoscopic	**0** Drainage Device **3** Infusion Device **4** Internal Fixation Device **5** External Fixation Device **7** Autologous Tissue Substitute **8** Spacer **J** Synthetic Substitute **K** Nonautologous Tissue Substitute	**Z** No Qualifier
F Ankle Joint, Right **G** Ankle Joint, Left **H** Tarsal Joint, Right **J** Tarsal Joint, Left **K** Tarsometatarsal Joint, Right **L** Tarsometatarsal Joint, Left **M** Metatarsal-Phalangeal Joint, Right **N** Metatarsal-Phalangeal Joint, Left **P** Toe Phalangeal Joint, Right **Q** Toe Phalangeal Joint, Left	**X** External	**0** Drainage Device **3** Infusion Device **4** Internal Fixation Device **5** External Fixation Device	**Z** No Qualifier

Section 0 **Medical and Surgical**
Body System S **Lower Joints**
Operation Q **Repair:** Restoring, to the extent possible, a body part to its normal anatomic structure and function

Body Part (4th)	Approach (5th)	Device (6th)	Qualifier (7th)
0 Lumbar Vertebral Joint 2 Lumbar Vertebral Disc 3 Lumbosacral Joint 4 Lumbosacral Disc 5 Sacrococcygeal Joint 6 Coccygeal Joint 7 Sacroiliac Joint, Right 8 Sacroiliac Joint, Left 9 Hip Joint, Right B Hip Joint, Left C Knee Joint, Right D Knee Joint, Left F Ankle Joint, Right G Ankle Joint, Left H Tarsal Joint, Right J Tarsal Joint, Left K Tarsometatarsal Joint, Right L Tarsometatarsal Joint, Left M Metatarsal-Phalangeal Joint, Right N Metatarsal-Phalangeal Joint, Left P Toe Phalangeal Joint, Right Q Toe Phalangeal Joint, Left	0 Open 3 Percutaneous 4 Percutaneous Endoscopic X External	Z No Device	Z No Qualifier

Section 0 **Medical and Surgical**
Body System S **Lower Joints**
Operation R **Replacement:** Putting in or on biological or synthetic material that physically takes the place and/or function of all or a portion of a body part

Body Part (4th)	Approach (5th)	Device (6th)	Qualifier (7th)
0 Lumbar Vertebral Joint 2 Lumbar Vertebral Disc 3 Lumbosacral Joint 4 Lumbosacral Disc 5 Sacrococcygeal Joint 6 Coccygeal Joint 7 Sacroiliac Joint, Right 8 Sacroiliac Joint, Left H Tarsal Joint, Right J Tarsal Joint, Left K Tarsometatarsal Joint, Right L Tarsometatarsal Joint, Left M Metatarsal-Phalangeal Joint, Right N Metatarsal-Phalangeal Joint, Left P Toe Phalangeal Joint, Right Q Toe Phalangeal Joint, Left	0 Open	7 Autologous Tissue Substitute J Synthetic Substitute K Nonautologous Tissue Substitute	Z No Qualifier
9 Hip Joint, Right B Hip Joint, Left	0 Open	1 Synthetic Substitute, Metal 2 Synthetic Substitute, Metal on Polyethylene 3 Synthetic Substitute, Ceramic 4 Synthetic Substitute, Ceramic on Polyethylene 6 Synthetic Substitute, Oxidized Zirconium on Polyethylene J Synthetic Substitute	9 Cemented A Uncemented Z No Qualifier
9 Hip Joint, Right B Hip Joint, Left	0 Open	7 Autologous Tissue Substitute E Articulating Spacer K Nonautologous Tissue Substitute	Z No Qualifier
A Hip Joint, Acetabular Surface, Right E Hip Joint, Acetabular Surface, Left	0 Open	0 Synthetic Substitute, Polyethylene 1 Synthetic Substitute, Metal 3 Synthetic Substitute, Ceramic J Synthetic Substitute	9 Cemented A Uncemented Z No Qualifier

Continued →

Section 0 **Medical and Surgical**
Body System S **Lower Joints**
Operation R **Replacement:** Putting in or on biological or synthetic material that physically takes the place and/or function of all or a portion of a body part

Body Part (4th)	Approach (5th)	Device (6th)	Qualifier (7th)
A Hip Joint, Acetabular Surface, Right **E** Hip Joint, Acetabular Surface, Left	**0** Open	**7** Autologous Tissue Substitute **K** Nonautologous Tissue Substitute	**Z** No Qualifier
C Knee Joint, Right **D** Knee Joint, Left	**0** Open	**6** Synthetic Substitute, Oxidized Zirconium on Polyethylene **J** Synthetic Substitute **L** Synthetic Substitute, Unicondylar Medial **M** Synthetic Substitute, Unicondylar Lateral **N** Synthetic Substitute, Unicondylar Patellofemoral	**9** Cemented **A** Uncemented **Z** No Qualifier
C Knee Joint, Right **D** Knee Joint, Left	**0** Open	**7** Autologous Tissue Substitute **E** Articulating Spacer **K** Nonautologous Tissue Substitute	**Z** No Qualifier
F Ankle Joint, Right **G** Ankle Joint, Left **T** Knee Joint, Femoral Surface, Right **U** Knee Joint, Femoral Surface, Left **V** Knee Joint, Tibial Surface, Right **W** Knee Joint, Tibial Surface, Left	**0** Open	**7** Autologous Tissue Substitute **K** Nonautologous Tissue Substitute	**Z** No Qualifier
F Ankle Joint, Right **G** Ankle Joint, Left **T** Knee Joint, Femoral Surface, Right **U** Knee Joint, Femoral Surface, Left **V** Knee Joint, Tibial Surface, Right **W** Knee Joint, Tibial Surface, Left	**0** Open	**J** Synthetic Substitute	**9** Cemented **A** Uncemented **Z** No Qualifier
R Hip Joint, Femoral Surface, Right **S** Hip Joint, Femoral Surface, Left	**0** Open	**1** Synthetic Substitute, Metal **3** Synthetic Substitute, Ceramic **J** Synthetic Substitute	**9** Cemented **A** Uncemented **Z** No Qualifier
R Hip Joint, Femoral Surface, Right **S** Hip Joint, Femoral Surface, Left	**0** Open	**7** Autologous Tissue Substitute **K** Nonautologous Tissue Substitute	**Z** No Qualifier

Section 0 **Medical and Surgical**
Body System S **Lower Joints**
Operation S **Reposition:** Moving to its normal location, or other suitable location, all or a portion of a body part

Body Part (4th)	Approach (5th)	Device (6th)	Qualifier (7th)
0 Lumbar Vertebral Joint **3** Lumbosacral Joint **5** Sacrococcygeal Joint **6** Coccygeal Joint **7** Sacroiliac Joint, Right **8** Sacroiliac Joint, Left	**0** Open **3** Percutaneous **4** Percutaneous Endoscopic **X** External	**4** Internal Fixation Device **Z** No Device	**Z** No Qualifier
9 Hip Joint, Right **B** Hip Joint, Left **C** Knee Joint, Right **D** Knee Joint, Left **F** Ankle Joint, Right **G** Ankle Joint, Left **H** Tarsal Joint, Right **J** Tarsal Joint, Left **K** Tarsometatarsal Joint, Right **L** Tarsometatarsal Joint, Left **M** Metatarsal-Phalangeal Joint, Right **N** Metatarsal-Phalangeal Joint, Left **P** Toe Phalangeal Joint, Right **Q** Toe Phalangeal Joint, Left	**0** Open **3** Percutaneous **4** Percutaneous Endoscopic **X** External	**4** Internal Fixation Device **5** External Fixation Device **Z** No Device	**Z** No Qualifier

ection 0 Medical and Surgical
ody System S Lower Joints
peration T Resection: Cutting out or off, without replacement, all of a body part

Body Part (4th)	Approach (5th)	Device (6th)	Qualifier (7th)
2 Lumbar Vertebral Disc 4 Lumbosacral Disc 5 Sacrococcygeal Joint 6 Coccygeal Joint 7 Sacroiliac Joint, Right 8 Sacroiliac Joint, Left 9 Hip Joint, Right B Hip Joint, Left C Knee Joint, Right D Knee Joint, Left F Ankle Joint, Right G Ankle Joint, Left H Tarsal Joint, Right J Tarsal Joint, Left K Tarsometatarsal Joint, Right L Tarsometatarsal Joint, Left M Metatarsal-Phalangeal Joint, Right N Metatarsal-Phalangeal Joint, Left P Toe Phalangeal Joint, Right Q Toe Phalangeal Joint, Left	0 Open	Z No Device	Z No Qualifier

ection 0 Medical and Surgical
ody System S Lower Joints
peration U Supplement: Putting in or on biological or synthetic material that physically reinforces and/or augments the function of a portion of a body part

Body Part (4th)	Approach (5th)	Device (6th)	Qualifier (7th)
0 Lumbar Vertebral Joint 2 Lumbar Vertebral Disc 3 Lumbosacral Joint 4 Lumbosacral Disc 5 Sacrococcygeal Joint 6 Coccygeal Joint 7 Sacroiliac Joint, Right 8 Sacroiliac Joint, Left F Ankle Joint, Right G Ankle Joint, Left H Tarsal Joint, Right J Tarsal Joint, Left K Tarsometatarsal Joint, Right L Tarsometatarsal Joint, Left M Metatarsal-Phalangeal Joint, Right N Metatarsal-Phalangeal Joint, Left P Toe Phalangeal Joint, Right Q Toe Phalangeal Joint, Left	0 Open 3 Percutaneous 4 Percutaneous Endoscopic	7 Autologous Tissue Substitute J Synthetic Substitute K Nonautologous Tissue Substitute	Z No Qualifier
9 Hip Joint, Right B Hip Joint, Left	0 Open	7 Autologous Tissue Substitute 9 Liner B Resurfacing Device J Synthetic Substitute K Nonautologous Tissue Substitute	Z No Qualifier
9 Hip Joint, Right B Hip Joint, Left	3 Percutaneous 4 Percutaneous Endoscopic	7 Autologous Tissue Substitute J Synthetic Substitute K Nonautologous Tissue Substitute	Z No Qualifier
A Hip Joint, Acetabular Surface, Right E Hip Joint, Acetabular Surface, Left R Hip Joint, Femoral Surface, Right S Hip Joint, Femoral Surface, Left	0 Open	9 Liner B Resurfacing Device	Z No Qualifier

Continued →

0SU Continu

Section 0 **Medical and Surgical**
Body System S **Lower Joints**
Operation U **Supplement:** Putting in or on biological or synthetic material that physically reinforces and/or augments the function of a portion of a body part

Body Part (4th)	Approach (5th)	Device (6th)	Qualifier (7th)
C Knee Joint, Right **D** Knee Joint, Left	**0** Open	**7** Autologous Tissue Substitute **J** Synthetic Substitute **K** Nonautologous Tissue Substitute	**Z** No Qualifier
C Knee Joint, Right **D** Knee Joint, Left	**0** Open	**9** Liner	**C** Patellar Surface **Z** No Qualifier
C Knee Joint, Right **D** Knee Joint, Left	**3** Percutaneous **4** Percutaneous Endoscopic	**7** Autologous Tissue Substitute **J** Synthetic Substitute **K** Nonautologous Tissue Substitute	**Z** No Qualifier
T Knee Joint, Femoral Surface, Right **U** Knee Joint, Femoral Surface, Left **V** Knee Joint, Tibial Surface, Right **W** Knee Joint, Tibial Surface, Left	**0** Open	**9** Liner	**Z** No Qualifier

Section 0 **Medical and Surgical**
Body System S **Lower Joints**
Operation W **Revision:** Correcting, to the extent possible, a portion of a malfunctioning device or the position of a displaced device

Body Part (4th)	Approach (5th)	Device (6th)	Qualifier (7th)
0 Lumbar Vertebral Joint **3** Lumbosacral Joint	**0** Open **3** Percutaneous **4** Percutaneous Endoscopic **X** External	**0** Drainage Device **3** Infusion Device **4** Internal Fixation Device **7** Autologous Tissue Substitute **8** Spacer **A** Interbody Fusion Device **J** Synthetic Substitute **K** Nonautologous Tissue Substitute	**Z** No Qualifier
2 Lumbar Vertebral Disc **4** Lumbosacral Disc	**0** Open **3** Percutaneous **4** Percutaneous Endoscopic **X** External	**0** Drainage Device **3** Infusion Device **7** Autologous Tissue Substitute **J** Synthetic Substitute **K** Nonautologous Tissue Substitute	**Z** No Qualifier
5 Sacrococcygeal Joint **6** Coccygeal Joint **7** Sacroiliac Joint, Right **8** Sacroiliac Joint, Left	**0** Open **3** Percutaneous **4** Percutaneous Endoscopic **X** External	**0** Drainage Device **3** Infusion Device **4** Internal Fixation Device **7** Autologous Tissue Substitute **8** Spacer **J** Synthetic Substitute **K** Nonautologous Tissue Substitute	**Z** No Qualifier
9 Hip Joint, Right **B** Hip Joint, Left	**0** Open	**0** Drainage Device **3** Infusion Device **4** Internal Fixation Device **5** External Fixation Device **7** Autologous Tissue Substitute **8** Spacer **9** Liner **B** Resurfacing Device **J** Synthetic Substitute **K** Nonautologous Tissue Substitute	**Z** No Qualifier

Continued →

ction	0	**Medical and Surgical**
dy System	S	**Lower Joints**
eration	W	**Revision:** Correcting, to the extent possible, a portion of a malfunctioning device or the position of a displaced device

Body Part (4th)	Approach (5th)	Device (6th)	Qualifier (7th)
9 Hip Joint, Right B Hip Joint, Left	3 Percutaneous 4 Percutaneous Endoscopic X External	0 Drainage Device 3 Infusion Device 4 Internal Fixation Device 5 External Fixation Device 7 Autologous Tissue Substitute 8 Spacer J Synthetic Substitute K Nonautologous Tissue Substitute	Z No Qualifier
A Hip Joint, Acetabular Surface, Right E Hip Joint, Acetabular Surface, Left R Hip Joint, Femoral Surface, Right S Hip Joint, Femoral Surface, Left T Knee Joint, Femoral Surface, Right U Knee Joint, Femoral Surface, Left V Knee Joint, Tibial Surface, Right W Knee Joint, Tibial Surface, Left	0 Open 3 Percutaneous 4 Percutaneous Endoscopic X External	J Synthetic Substitute	Z No Qualifier
C Knee Joint, Right D Knee Joint, Left	0 Open	0 Drainage Device 3 Infusion Device 4 Internal Fixation Device 5 External Fixation Device 7 Autologous Tissue Substitute 8 Spacer 9 Liner K Nonautologous Tissue Substitute	Z No Qualifier
C Knee Joint, Right D Knee Joint, Left	0 Open	J Synthetic Substitute	C Patellar Surface Z No Qualifier
C Knee Joint, Right D Knee Joint, Left	3 Percutaneous 4 Percutaneous Endoscopic X External	0 Drainage Device 3 Infusion Device 4 Internal Fixation Device 5 External Fixation Device 7 Autologous Tissue Substitute 8 Spacer K Nonautologous Tissue Substitute	Z No Qualifier
C Knee Joint, Right E Knee Joint, Left	3 Percutaneous 4 Percutaneous Endoscopic X External	J Synthetic Substitute	C Patellar Surface Z No Qualifier
F Ankle Joint, Right G Ankle Joint, Left H Tarsal Joint, Right J Tarsal Joint, Left K Tarsometatarsal Joint, Right L Tarsometatarsal Joint, Left M Metatarsal-Phalangeal Joint, Right N Metatarsal-Phalangeal Joint, Left P Toe Phalangeal Joint, Right Q Toe Phalangeal Joint, Left	0 Open 3 Percutaneous 4 Percutaneous Endoscopic X External	0 Drainage Device 3 Infusion Device 4 Internal Fixation Device 5 External Fixation Device 7 Autologous Tissue Substitute 8 Spacer J Synthetic Substitute K Nonautologous Tissue Substitute	Z No Qualifier

AHA Coding Clinic

0S9D4ZZ Drainage of Left Knee Joint, Percutaneous Endoscopic Approach— AHA CC: 2Q, 2018, 17

0SB20ZZ Excision of Lumbar Vertebral Disc, Open Approach—AHA CC: 2Q, 2014, 6-7; 2Q, 2016, 16; 4Q, 2017, 76-77

0SB40ZZ Excision of Lumbosacral Disc, Open Approach—AHA CC: 4Q, 2017, 76-77

0SBD4ZZ Excision of Left Knee Joint, Percutaneous Endoscopic Approach—AHA CC: 1Q, 2015, 34

0SG0071 Fusion of Lumbar Vertebral Joint with Autologous Tissue Substitute, Posterior Approach, Posterior Column, Open Approach AHA CC: 1Q, 2013, 21-23; 3Q, 2013, 25-26

0SG00AJ Fusion of Lumbar Vertebral Joint with Interbody Fusion Device, Posterior Approach, Anterior Column, Open Approach—AH CC: 3Q, 2013, 25-26

0SG107J Fusion of 2 or more Lumbar Vertebral Joints with Autologous Tissue Substitute, Posterior Approach, Anterior Column, Op Approach—AHA CC: 3Q, 2014, 36

0SGG04Z Fusion of Left Ankle Joint with Internal Fixation Device, Open Approach—AHA CC: 2Q, 2013, 39-40

0SGG07Z Fusion of Left Ankle Joint with Autologous Tissue Substitute, Open Approach—AHA CC: 2Q, 2013, 39-40

0SJG3ZZ Inspection of Left Ankle Joint, Percutaneous Approach—AHA CC: 1Q, 2017, 50

0SP909Z Removal of Liner from Right Hip Joint, Open Approach—AHA CC: 2Q, 2015, 19-20; 4Q, 2016, 111-112

0SP90JZ Removal of Synthetic Substitute from Right Hip Joint, Open Approach—AHA CC: 2Q, 2015, 19-20

0SPC0JZ Removal of Synthetic Substitute from Right Knee Joint, Open Approach—AHA CC: 2Q, 2015, 18-19

0SPF0JZ Removal of Synthetic Substitute from Right Ankle Joint, Open Approach—AHA CC: 4Q, 2017, 107-108

0SPG04Z Removal of Internal Fixation Device from Left Ankle Joint, Open Approach—AHA CC: 2Q, 2013, 39-40

0SPR0JZ Removal of Synthetic Substitute from Right Hip Joint, Femoral Surface, Open Approach—AHA CC: 4Q, 2016, 111-112

0SPW0JZ Removal of Synthetic Substitute from Left Knee Joint, Tibial Surface, Open Approach—AHA CC: 2Q, 2018, 16-17

0SQB4ZZ Repair Left Hip Joint, Percutaneous Endoscopic Approach—AHA CC: 4Q, 2014, 25-26

0SRB06Z Replacement of Left Hip Joint with Oxidized Zirconium on Polyethylene Synthetic Substitute, Open Approach—AHA CC: 4 2017, 39

0SRB0J9 Replacement of Left Hip Joint with Synthetic Substitute, Cemented, Open Approach—AHA CC: 3Q, 2015, 18-19

0SRC0J9 Replacement of Right Knee Joint with Synthetic Substitute, Cemented, Open Approach—AHA CC: 2Q, 2015, 18-19

0SRD0JZ Replacement of Left Knee Joint with Synthetic Substitute, Open Approach—AHA CC: 4Q, 2016, 109-110

0SRD0LZ Replacement of Left Knee Joint with Unicondylar Synthetic Substitute, Open Approach—AHA CC: 4Q, 2016, 110

0SRF0JA Replacement of Right Ankle Joint with Synthetic Substitute, Uncemented, Open Approach—AHA CC: 4Q, 2017, 107-108

0SRR03A Replacement of Right Hip Joint, Femoral Surface with Ceramic Synthetic Substitute, Uncemented, Open Approach—AHA C 2Q, 2015, 19-20

0SRR0J9 Replacement of Right Hip Joint, Femoral Surface with Synthetic Substitute, Cemented, Open Approach—AHA CC: 4Q, 201 111-112

0SRW0JZ Replacement of Left Knee Joint, Tibial Surface with Synthetic Substitute, Open Approach—AHA CC: 2Q, 2018, 16-17

0SSB04Z Reposition Left Hip Joint with Internal Fixation Device, Open Approach—AHA CC: 2Q, 2016, 32

0STD0ZZ Resection of Left Knee Joint, Open Approach—AHA CC: 4Q, 2014, 30-31

0STM0ZZ Resection of Right Metatarsal-Phalangeal Joint, Open Approach—AHA CC: 1Q, 2016, 20-21

0SUA09Z Supplement Right Hip Joint, Acetabular Surface with Liner, Open Approach—AHA CC: 2Q, 2015, 19-20; 4Q, 2016, 111-11

0SWF0JZ Revision of Synthetic Substitute in Right Ankle Joint, Open Approach—AHA CC: 4Q, 2017, 107-108

0SWW0JZ Revision of Synthetic Substitute in Left Knee Joint, Tibial Surface, Open Approach—AHA CC: 4Q, 2016, 112

Urinary System

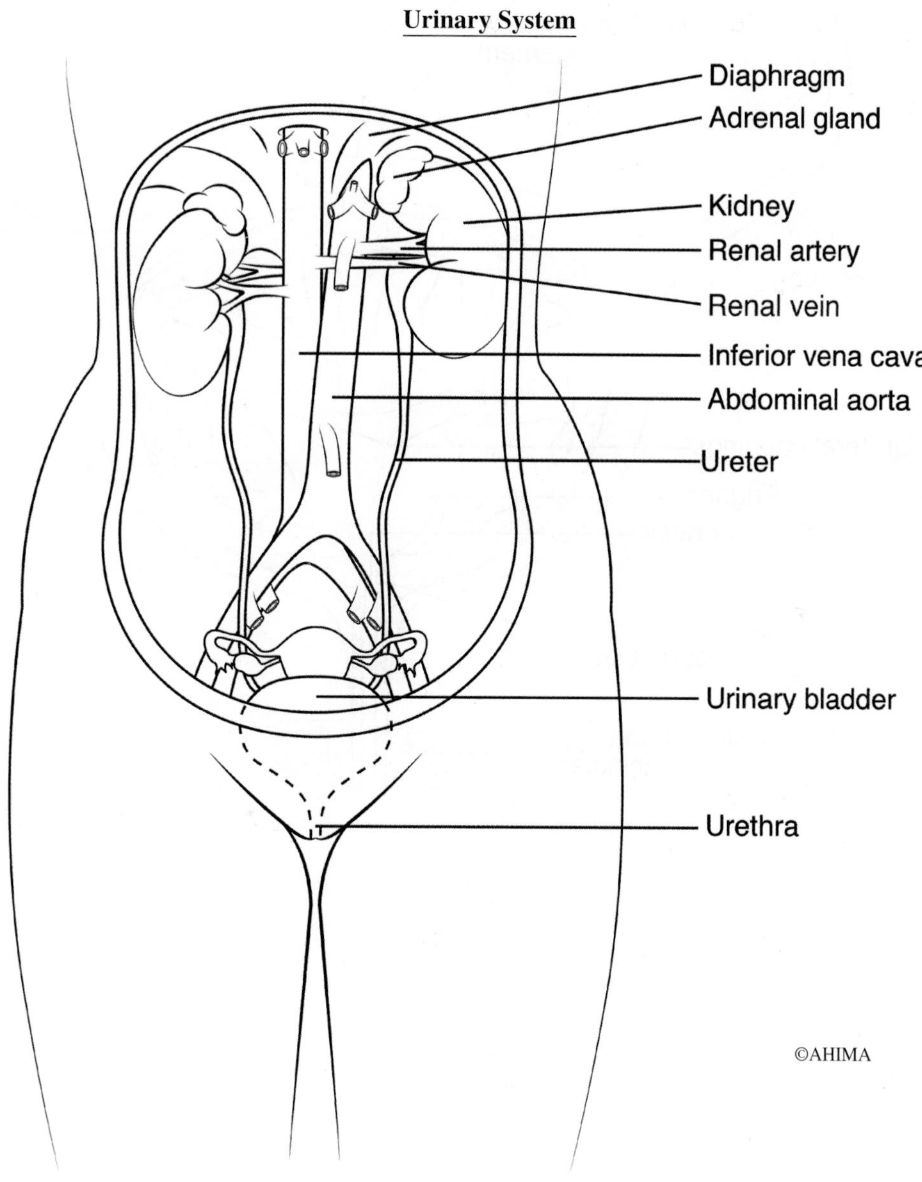

Lower Urinary Tract

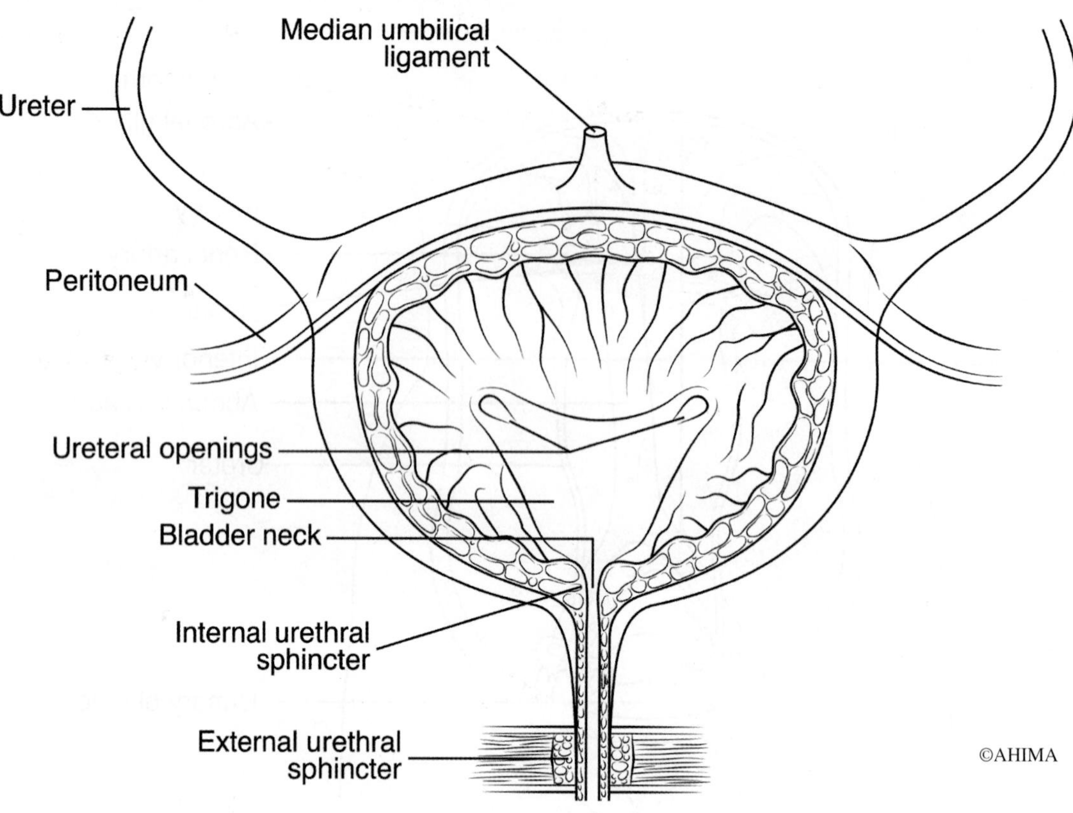

Kidney

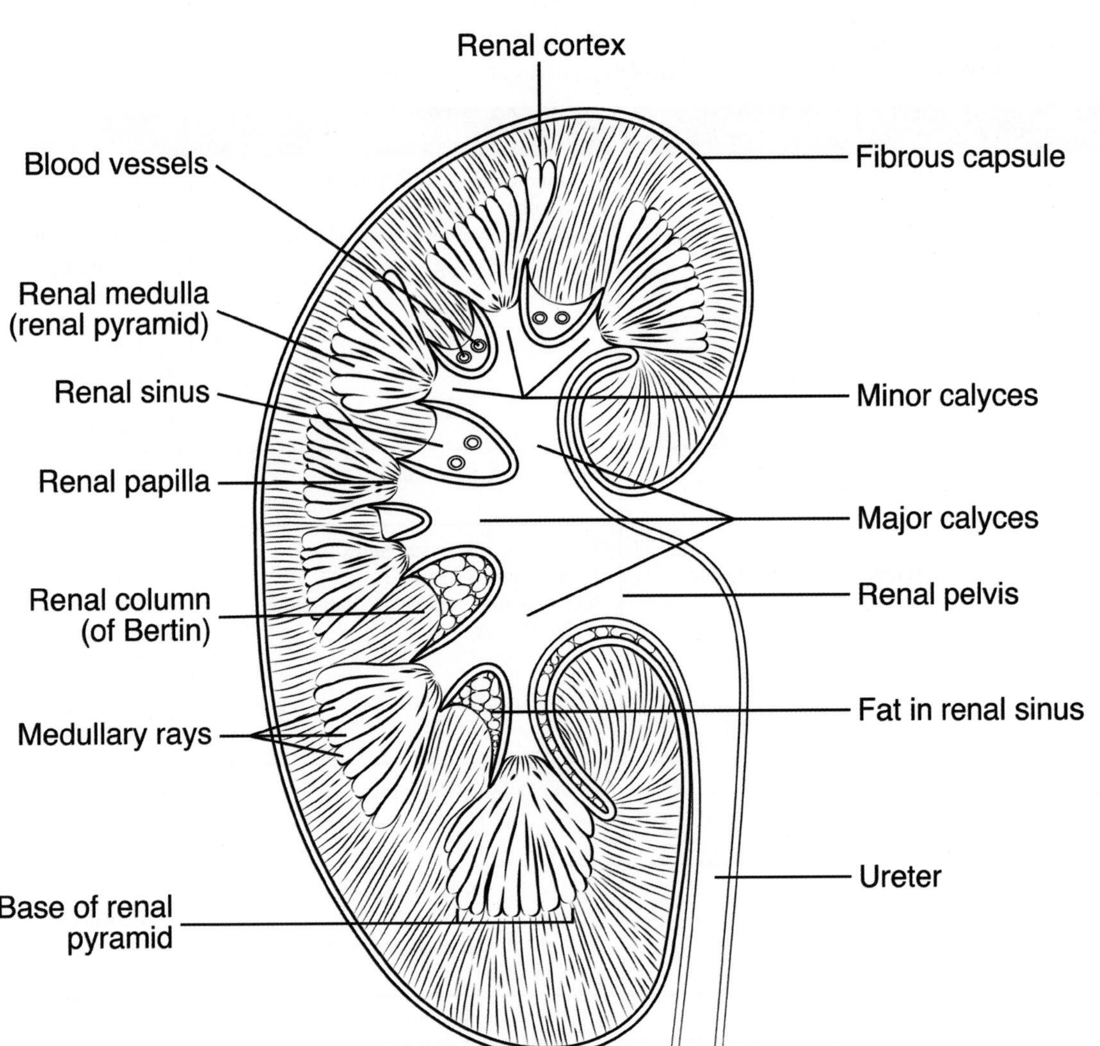

Renal cortex
Blood vessels
Fibrous capsule
Renal medulla (renal pyramid)
Renal sinus
Minor calyces
Renal papilla
Major calyces
Renal column (of Bertin)
Renal pelvis
Fat in renal sinus
Medullary rays
Ureter
Base of renal pyramid

Urinary System Tables 0T1–0TY

Section	**0**	**Medical and Surgical**
Body System	**T**	**Urinary System**
Operation	**1**	**Bypass:** Altering the route of passage of the contents of a tubular body part

Body Part (4th)	Approach (5th)	Device (6th)	Qualifier (7th)
3 Kidney Pelvis, Right **4** Kidney Pelvis, Left	**0** Open **4** Percutaneous Endoscopic	**7** Autologous Tissue Substitute **J** Synthetic Substitute **K** Nonautologous Tissue Substitute **Z** No Device	**3** Kidney Pelvis, Right **4** Kidney Pelvis, Left **6** Ureter, Right **7** Ureter, Left **8** Colon **9** Colocutaneous **A** Ileum **B** Bladder **C** Ileocutaneous **D** Cutaneous
3 Kidney Pelvis, Right **4** Kidney Pelvis, Left	**3** Percutaneous	**J** Synthetic Substitute	**D** Cutaneous
6 Ureter, Right **7** Ureter, Left **8** Ureters, Bilateral	**0** Open **4** Percutaneous Endoscopic	**7** Autologous Tissue Substitute **J** Synthetic Substitute **K** Nonautologous Tissue Substitute **Z** No Device	**6** Ureter, Right **7** Ureter, Left **8** Colon **9** Colocutaneous **A** Ileum **B** Bladder **C** Ileocutaneous **D** Cutaneous
6 Ureter, Right **7** Ureter, Left **8** Ureters, Bilateral	**3** Percutaneous	**J** Synthetic Substitute	**D** Cutaneous
B Bladder	**0** Open **4** Percutaneous Endoscopic	**7** Autologous Tissue Substitute **J** Synthetic Substitute **K** Nonautologous Tissue Substitute **Z** No Device	**9** Colocutaneous **C** Ileocutaneous **D** Cutaneous
B Bladder	**3** Percutaneous	**J** Synthetic Substitute	**D** Cutaneous

Section	**0**	**Medical and Surgical**
Body System	**T**	**Urinary System**
Operation	**2**	**Change:** Taking out or off a device from a body part and putting back an identical or similar device in or on the same body part without cutting or puncturing the skin or a mucous membrane

Body Part (4th)	Approach (5th)	Device (6th)	Qualifier (7th)
5 Kidney **9** Ureter **B** Bladder **D** Urethra	**X** External	**0** Drainage Device **Y** Other Device	**Z** No Qualifier

Section	**0**	**Medical and Surgical**
Body System	**T**	**Urinary System**
Operation	**5**	**Destruction:** Physical eradication of all or a portion of a body part by the direct use of energy, force, or a destructive agent

Body Part (4th)	Approach (5th)	Device (6th)	Qualifier (7th)
0 Kidney, Right **1** Kidney, Left **3** Kidney Pelvis, Right **4** Kidney Pelvis, Left **6** Ureter, Right **7** Ureter, Left **B** Bladder **C** Bladder Neck	**0** Open **3** Percutaneous **4** Percutaneous Endoscopic **7** Via Natural or Artificial Opening **8** Via Natural or Artificial Opening Endoscopic	**Z** No Device	**Z** No Qualifier

Continued →

ion 0 **Medical and Surgical**
y System T **Urinary System**
ration 5 **Destruction:** Physical eradication of all or a portion of a body part by the direct use of energy, force, or a destructive agent

Body Part (4th)	Approach (5th)	Device (6th)	Qualifier (7th)
Urethra	0 Open 3 Percutaneous 4 Percutaneous Endoscopic 7 Via Natural or Artificial Opening 8 Via Natural or Artificial Opening Endoscopic X External	Z No Device	Z No Qualifier

tion 0 **Medical and Surgical**
y System T **Urinary System**
ration 7 **Dilation:** Expanding an orifice or the lumen of a tubular body part

Body Part (4th)	Approach (5th)	Device (6th)	Qualifier (7th)
Kidney Pelvis, Right Kidney Pelvis, Left Ureter, Right Ureter, Left Ureters, Bilateral Bladder Bladder Neck Urethra	0 Open 3 Percutaneous 4 Percutaneous Endoscopic 7 Via Natural or Artificial Opening 8 Via Natural or Artificial Opening Endoscopic	D Intraluminal Device Z No Device	Z No Qualifier

tion 0 **Medical and Surgical**
y System T **Urinary System**
eration 8 **Division:** Cutting into a body part, without draining fluids and/or gases from the body part, in order to separate or transect a body part

Body Part (4th)	Approach (5th)	Device (6th)	Qualifier (7th)
Kidneys, Bilateral Bladder Neck	0 Open 3 Percutaneous 4 Percutaneous Endoscopic	Z No Device	Z No Qualifier

tion 0 **Medical and Surgical**
ly System T **Urinary System**
eration 9 **Drainage:** Taking or letting out fluids and/or gases from a body part

Body Part (4th)	Approach (5th)	Device (6th)	Qualifier (7th)
Kidney, Right Kidney, Left Kidney Pelvis, Right Kidney Pelvis, Left Ureter, Right Ureter, Left Ureters, Bilateral Bladder Bladder Neck	0 Open 3 Percutaneous 4 Percutaneous Endoscopic 7 Via Natural or Artificial Opening 8 Via Natural or Artificial Opening Endoscopic	0 Drainage Device	Z No Qualifier
Kidney, Right Kidney, Left Kidney Pelvis, Right Kidney Pelvis, Left Ureter, Right Ureter, Left Ureters, Bilateral Bladder Bladder Neck	0 Open 3 Percutaneous 4 Percutaneous Endoscopic 7 Via Natural or Artificial Opening 8 Via Natural or Artificial Opening Endoscopic	Z No Device	X Diagnostic Z No Qualifier

Continued →

Section 0 **Medical and Surgical**
Body System T **Urinary System**
Operation 9 **Drainage:** Taking or letting out fluids and/or gases from a body part

Body Part (4th)	Approach (5th)	Device (6th)	Qualifier (7th)
D Urethra	**0** Open **3** Percutaneous **4** Percutaneous Endoscopic **7** Via Natural or Artificial Opening **8** Via Natural or Artificial Opening Endoscopic **X** External	**0** Drainage Device	**Z** No Qualifier
D Urethra	**0** Open **3** Percutaneous **4** Percutaneous Endoscopic **7** Via Natural or Artificial Opening **8** Via Natural or Artificial Opening Endoscopic **X** External	**Z** No Device	**X** Diagnostic **Z** No Qualifier

Section 0 **Medical and Surgical**
Body System T **Urinary System**
Operation B **Excision:** Cutting out or off, without replacement, a portion of a body part

Body Part (4th)	Approach (5th)	Device (6th)	Qualifier (7th)
0 Kidney, Right **1** Kidney, Left **3** Kidney Pelvis, Right **4** Kidney Pelvis, Left **6** Ureter, Right **7** Ureter, Left **B** Bladder **C** Bladder Neck	**0** Open **3** Percutaneous **4** Percutaneous Endoscopic **7** Via Natural or Artificial Opening **8** Via Natural or Artificial Opening Endoscopic	**Z** No Device	**X** Diagnostic **Z** No Qualifier
D Urethra	**0** Open **3** Percutaneous **4** Percutaneous Endoscopic **7** Via Natural or Artificial Opening **8** Via Natural or Artificial Opening Endoscopic **X** External	**Z** No Device	**X** Diagnostic **Z** No Qualifier

Section 0 **Medical and Surgical**
Body System T **Urinary System**
Operation C **Extirpation:** Taking or cutting out solid matter from a body part

Body Part (4th)	Approach (5th)	Device (6th)	Qualifier (7th)
0 Kidney, Right **1** Kidney, Left **3** Kidney Pelvis, Right **4** Kidney Pelvis, Left **6** Ureter, Right **7** Ureter, Left **B** Bladder **C** Bladder Neck	**0** Open **3** Percutaneous **4** Percutaneous Endoscopic **7** Via Natural or Artificial Opening **8** Via Natural or Artificial Opening Endoscopic	**Z** No Device	**Z** No Qualifier
D Urethra	**0** Open **3** Percutaneous **4** Percutaneous Endoscopic **7** Via Natural or Artificial Opening **8** Via Natural or Artificial Opening Endoscopic **X** External	**Z** No Device	**Z** No Qualifier

tion 0 **Medical and Surgical**
ly System T **Urinary System**
eration D **Extraction:** Pulling or stripping out or off all or a portion of a body part by the use of force

Body Part (4th)	Approach (5th)	Device (6th)	Qualifier (7th)
Kidney, Right Kidney, Left	0 Open 3 Percutaneous 4 Percutaneous Endoscopic	Z No Device	Z No Qualifier

tion 0 **Medical and Surgical**
ly System T **Urinary System**
eration F **Fragmentation:** Breaking solid matter in a body part into pieces

Body Part (4th)	Approach (5th)	Device (6th)	Qualifier (7th)
Kidney Pelvis, Right Kidney Pelvis, Left Ureter, Right Ureter, Left B Bladder C Bladder Neck D Urethra	0 Open 3 Percutaneous 4 Percutaneous Endoscopic 7 Via Natural or Artificial Opening 8 Via Natural or Artificial Opening Endoscopic X External	Z No Device	Z No Qualifier

tion 0 **Medical and Surgical**
dy System T **Urinary System**
eration H **Insertion:** Putting in a nonbiological appliance that monitors, assists, performs, or prevents a physiological function but does not physically take the place of a body part

Body Part (4th)	Approach (5th)	Device (6th)	Qualifier (7th)
Kidney	0 Open 3 Percutaneous 4 Percutaneous Endoscopic 7 Via Natural or Artificial Opening 8 Via Natural or Artificial Opening Endoscopic	2 Monitoring Device 3 Infusion Device Y Other Device	Z No Qualifier
Ureter	0 Open 3 Percutaneous 4 Percutaneous Endoscopic 7 Via Natural or Artificial Opening 8 Via Natural or Artificial Opening Endoscopic	2 Monitoring Device 3 Infusion Device M Stimulator Lead Y Other Device	Z No Qualifier
B Bladder	0 Open 3 Percutaneous 4 Percutaneous Endoscopic 7 Via Natural or Artificial Opening 8 Via Natural or Artificial Opening Endoscopic	2 Monitoring Device 3 Infusion Device L Artificial Sphincter M Stimulator Lead Y Other Device	Z No Qualifier
C Bladder Neck	0 Open 3 Percutaneous 4 Percutaneous Endoscopic 7 Via Natural or Artificial Opening 8 Via Natural or Artificial Opening Endoscopic	L Artificial Sphincter	Z No Qualifier
D Urethra	0 Open 3 Percutaneous 4 Percutaneous Endoscopic 7 Via Natural or Artificial Opening 8 Via Natural or Artificial Opening Endoscopic	2 Monitoring Device 3 Infusion Device L Artificial Sphincter Y Other Device	Z No Qualifier
D Urethra	X External	2 Monitoring Device 3 Infusion Device L Artificial Sphincter	Z No Qualifier

Section 0 **Medical and Surgical**
Body System T **Urinary System**
Operation J **Inspection:** Visually and/or manually exploring a body part

Body Part (4th)	Approach (5th)	Device (6th)	Qualifier (7th)
5 Kidney **9** Ureter **B** Bladder **D** Urethra	**0** Open **3** Percutaneous **4** Percutaneous Endoscopic **7** Via Natural or Artificial Opening **8** Via Natural or Artificial Opening Endoscopic **X** External	**Z** No Device	**Z** No Qualifier

Section 0 **Medical and Surgical**
Body System T **Urinary System**
Operation L **Occlusion:** Completely closing an orifice or the lumen of a tubular body part

Body Part (4th)	Approach (5th)	Device (6th)	Qualifier (7th)
3 Kidney Pelvis, Right **4** Kidney Pelvis, Left **6** Ureter, Right **7** Ureter, Left **B** Bladder **C** Bladder Neck	**0** Open **3** Percutaneous **4** Percutaneous Endoscopic	**C** Extraluminal Device **D** Intraluminal Device **Z** No Device	**Z** No Qualifier
3 Kidney Pelvis, Right **4** Kidney Pelvis, Left **6** Ureter, Right **7** Ureter, Left **B** Bladder **C** Bladder Neck	**7** Via Natural or Artificial Opening **8** Via Natural or Artificial Opening Endoscopic	**D** Intraluminal Device **Z** No Device	**Z** No Qualifier
D Urethra	**0** Open **3** Percutaneous **4** Percutaneous Endoscopic **X** External	**C** Extraluminal Device **D** Intraluminal Device **Z** No Device	**Z** No Qualifier
D Urethra	**7** Via Natural or Artificial Opening **8** Via Natural or Artificial Opening Endoscopic	**D** Intraluminal Device **Z** No Device	**Z** No Qualifier

Section 0 **Medical and Surgical**
Body System T **Urinary System**
Operation M **Reattachment:** Putting back in or on all or a portion of a separated body part to its normal location or other suitable location

Body Part (4th)	Approach (5th)	Device (6th)	Qualifier (7th)
0 Kidney, Right **1** Kidney, Left **2** Kidneys, Bilateral **3** Kidney Pelvis, Right **4** Kidney Pelvis, Left **6** Ureter, Right **7** Ureter, Left **8** Ureters, Bilateral **B** Bladder **C** Bladder Neck **D** Urethra	**0** Open **4** Percutaneous Endoscopic	**Z** No Device	**Z** No Qualifier

ection **0** **Medical and Surgical**
ody System **T** **Urinary System**
peration **N** **Release:** Freeing a body part from an abnormal physical constraint by cutting or by the use of force

Body Part (4th)	Approach (5th)	Device (6th)	Qualifier (7th)
0 Kidney, Right **1** Kidney, Left **3** Kidney Pelvis, Right **4** Kidney Pelvis, Left **6** Ureter, Right **7** Ureter, Left **B** Bladder **C** Bladder Neck	**0** Open **3** Percutaneous **4** Percutaneous Endoscopic **7** Via Natural or Artificial Opening **8** Via Natural or Artificial Opening Endoscopic	**Z** No Device	**Z** No Qualifier
D Urethra	**0** Open **3** Percutaneous **4** Percutaneous Endoscopic **7** Via Natural or Artificial Opening **8** Via Natural or Artificial Opening Endoscopic **X** External	**Z** No Device	**Z** No Qualifier

ection **0** **Medical and Surgical**
ody System **T** **Urinary System**
peration **P** **Removal:** Taking out or off a device from a body part

Body Part (4th)	Approach (5th)	Device (6th)	Qualifier (7th)
5 Kidney	**0** Open **3** Percutaneous **4** Percutaneous Endoscopic **7** Via Natural or Artificial Opening **8** Via Natural or Artificial Opening Endoscopic	**0** Drainage Device **2** Monitoring Device **3** Infusion Device **7** Autologous Tissue Substitute **C** Extraluminal Device **D** Intraluminal Device **J** Synthetic Substitute **K** Nonautologous Tissue Substitute **Y** Other Device	**Z** No Qualifier
5 Kidney	**X** External	**0** Drainage Device **2** Monitoring Device **3** Infusion Device **D** Intraluminal Device	**Z** No Qualifier
9 Ureter	**0** Open **3** Percutaneous **4** Percutaneous Endoscopic **7** Via Natural or Artificial Opening **8** Via Natural or Artificial Opening Endoscopic	**0** Drainage Device **2** Monitoring Device **3** Infusion Device **7** Autologous Tissue Substitute **C** Extraluminal Device **D** Intraluminal Device **J** Synthetic Substitute **K** Nonautologous Tissue Substitute **M** Stimulator Lead **Y** Other Device	**Z** No Qualifier
9 Ureter	**X** External	**0** Drainage Device **2** Monitoring Device **3** Infusion Device **D** Intraluminal Device **M** Stimulator Lead	**Z** No Qualifier

Continued →

Section 0 **Medical and Surgical**
Body System T **Urinary System**
Operation P **Removal:** Taking out or off a device from a body part

Body Part (4th)	Approach (5th)	Device (6th)	Qualifier (7th)
B Bladder	**0** Open **3** Percutaneous **4** Percutaneous Endoscopic **7** Via Natural or Artificial Opening **8** Via Natural or Artificial Opening Endoscopic	**0** Drainage Device **2** Monitoring Device **3** Infusion Device **7** Autologous Tissue Substitute **C** Extraluminal Device **D** Intraluminal Device **J** Synthetic Substitute **K** Nonautologous Tissue Substitute **L** Artificial Sphincter **M** Stimulator Lead **Y** Other Device	**Z** No Qualifier
B Bladder	**X** External	**0** Drainage Device **2** Monitoring Device **3** Infusion Device **D** Intraluminal Device **L** Artificial Sphincter **M** Stimulator Lead	**Z** No Qualifier
D Urethra	**0** Open **3** Percutaneous **4** Percutaneous Endoscopic **7** Via Natural or Artificial Opening **8** Via Natural or Artificial Opening Endoscopic	**0** Drainage Device **2** Monitoring Device **3** Infusion Device **7** Autologous Tissue Substitute **C** Extraluminal Device **D** Intraluminal Device **J** Synthetic Substitute **K** Nonautologous Tissue Substitute **L** Artificial Sphincter **Y** Other Device	**Z** No Qualifier
D Urethra	**X** External	**0** Drainage Device **2** Monitoring Device **3** Infusion Device **D** Intraluminal Device **L** Artificial Sphincter	**Z** No Qualifier

Section 0 **Medical and Surgical**
Body System T **Urinary System**
Operation Q **Repair:** Restoring, to the extent possible, a body part to its normal anatomic structure and function

Body Part (4th)	Approach (5th)	Device (6th)	Qualifier (7th)
0 Kidney, Right **1** Kidney, Left **3** Kidney Pelvis, Right **4** Kidney Pelvis, Left **6** Ureter, Right **7** Ureter, Left **B** Bladder **C** Bladder Neck	**0** Open **3** Percutaneous **4** Percutaneous Endoscopic **7** Via Natural or Artificial Opening **8** Via Natural or Artificial Opening Endoscopic	**Z** No Device	**Z** No Qualifier
D Urethra	**0** Open **3** Percutaneous **4** Percutaneous Endoscopic **7** Via Natural or Artificial Opening **8** Via Natural or Artificial Opening Endoscopic **X** External	**Z** No Device	**Z** No Qualifier

ction	0	**Medical and Surgical**
dy System	T	**Urinary System**
eration	R	**Replacement:** Putting in or on biological or synthetic material that physically takes the place and/or function of all or a portion of a body part

Body Part (4th)	Approach (5th)	Device (6th)	Qualifier (7th)
3 Kidney Pelvis, Right 4 Kidney Pelvis, Left 6 Ureter, Right 7 Ureter, Left B Bladder C Bladder Neck	**0** Open **4** Percutaneous Endoscopic **7** Via Natural or Artificial Opening **8** Via Natural or Artificial Opening Endoscopic	**7** Autologous Tissue Substitute **J** Synthetic Substitute **K** Nonautologous Tissue Substitute	**Z** No Qualifier
D Urethra	**0** Open **4** Percutaneous Endoscopic **7** Via Natural or Artificial Opening **8** Via Natural or Artificial Opening Endoscopic **X** External	**7** Autologous Tissue Substitute **J** Synthetic Substitute **K** Nonautologous Tissue Substitute	**Z** No Qualifier

ction	0	**Medical and Surgical**
dy System	T	**Urinary System**
eration	S	**Reposition:** Moving to its normal location, or other suitable location, all or a portion of a body part

Body Part (4th)	Approach (5th)	Device (6th)	Qualifier (7th)
0 Kidney, Right 1 Kidney, Left 2 Kidneys, Bilateral 3 Kidney Pelvis, Right 4 Kidney Pelvis, Left 6 Ureter, Right 7 Ureter, Left 8 Ureters, Bilateral B Bladder C Bladder Neck D Urethra	**0** Open **4** Percutaneous Endoscopic	**Z** No Device	**Z** No Qualifier

ction	0	**Medical and Surgical**
dy System	T	**Urinary System**
eration	T	**Resection:** Cutting out or off, without replacement, all of a body part

Body Part (4th)	Approach (5th)	Device (6th)	Qualifier (7th)
0 Kidney, Right 1 Kidney, Left 2 Kidneys, Bilateral	**0** Open **4** Percutaneous Endoscopic	**Z** No Device	**Z** No Qualifier
3 Kidney Pelvis, Right 4 Kidney Pelvis, Left 6 Ureter, Right 7 Ureter, Left B Bladder C Bladder Neck D Urethra	**0** Open **4** Percutaneous Endoscopic **7** Via Natural or Artificial Opening **8** Via Natural or Artificial Opening Endoscopic	**Z** No Device	**Z** No Qualifier

Section 0 **Medical and Surgical**
Body System T **Urinary System**
Operation U **Supplement:** Putting in or on biological or synthetic material that physically reinforces and/or augments the function of portion of a body part

Body Part (4th)	Approach (5th)	Device (6th)	Qualifier (7th)
3 Kidney Pelvis, Right **4** Kidney Pelvis, Left **6** Ureter, Right **7** Ureter, Left **B** Bladder **C** Bladder Neck	**0** Open **4** Percutaneous Endoscopic **7** Via Natural or Artificial Opening **8** Via Natural or Artificial Opening Endoscopic	**7** Autologous Tissue Substitute **J** Synthetic Substitute **K** Nonautologous Tissue Substitute	**Z** No Qualifier
D Urethra	**0** Open **4** Percutaneous Endoscopic **7** Via Natural or Artificial Opening **8** Via Natural or Artificial Opening Endoscopic **X** External	**7** Autologous Tissue Substitute **J** Synthetic Substitute **K** Nonautologous Tissue Substitute	**Z** No Qualifier

Section 0 **Medical and Surgical**
Body System T **Urinary System**
Operation V **Restriction:** Partially closing an orifice or the lumen of a tubular body part

Body Part (4th)	Approach (5th)	Device (6th)	Qualifier (7th)
3 Kidney Pelvis, Right **4** Kidney Pelvis, Left **6** Ureter, Right **7** Ureter, Left **B** Bladder **C** Bladder Neck	**0** Open **3** Percutaneous **4** Percutaneous Endoscopic	**C** Extraluminal Device **D** Intraluminal Device **Z** No Device	**Z** No Qualifier
3 Kidney Pelvis, Right **4** Kidney Pelvis, Left **6** Ureter, Right **7** Ureter, Left **B** Bladder **C** Bladder Neck	**7** Via Natural or Artificial Opening **8** Via Natural or Artificial Opening Endoscopic	**D** Intraluminal Device **Z** No Device	**Z** No Qualifier
D Urethra	**0** Open **3** Percutaneous **4** Percutaneous Endoscopic	**C** Extraluminal Device **D** Intraluminal Device **Z** No Device	**Z** No Qualifier
D Urethra	**7** Via Natural or Artificial Opening **8** Via Natural or Artificial Opening Endoscopic	**D** Intraluminal Device **Z** No Device	**Z** No Qualifier
D Urethra	**X** External	**Z** No Device	**Z** No Qualifier

Section 0 **Medical and Surgical**
Body System T **Urinary System**
Operation W **Revision:** Correcting, to the extent possible, a portion of a malfunctioning device or the position of a displaced device

Body Part (4th)	Approach (5th)	Device (6th)	Qualifier (7th)
5 Kidney	**0** Open **3** Percutaneous **4** Percutaneous Endoscopic **7** Via Natural or Artificial Opening **8** Via Natural or Artificial Opening Endoscopic	**0** Drainage Device **2** Monitoring Device **3** Infusion Device **7** Autologous Tissue Substitute **C** Extraluminal Device **D** Intraluminal Device **J** Synthetic Substitute **K** Nonautologous Tissue Substitute **Y** Other Device	**Z** No Qualifier

Continued →

Body Part (4th)	Approach (5th)	Device (6th)	Qualifier (7th)
5 Kidney	X External	0 Drainage Device 2 Monitoring Device 3 Infusion Device 7 Autologous Tissue Substitute C Extraluminal Device D Intraluminal Device J Synthetic Substitute K Nonautologous Tissue Substitute	Z No Qualifier
9 Ureter	0 Open 3 Percutaneous 4 Percutaneous Endoscopic 7 Via Natural or Artificial Opening 8 Via Natural or Artificial Opening Endoscopic	0 Drainage Device 2 Monitoring Device 3 Infusion Device 7 Autologous Tissue Substitute C Extraluminal Device D Intraluminal Device J Synthetic Substitute K Nonautologous Tissue Substitute M Stimulator Lead Y Other Device	Z No Qualifier
9 Ureter	X External	0 Drainage Device 2 Monitoring Device 3 Infusion Device 7 Autologous Tissue Substitute C Extraluminal Device D Intraluminal Device J Synthetic Substitute K Nonautologous Tissue Substitute M Stimulator Lead	Z No Qualifier
B Bladder	0 Open 3 Percutaneous 4 Percutaneous Endoscopic 7 Via Natural or Artificial Opening 8 Via Natural or Artificial Opening Endoscopic	0 Drainage Device 2 Monitoring Device 3 Infusion Device 7 Autologous Tissue Substitute C Extraluminal Device D Intraluminal Device J Synthetic Substitute K Nonautologous Tissue Substitute L Artificial Sphincter M Stimulator Lead Y Other Device	Z No Qualifier
B Bladder	X External	0 Drainage Device 2 Monitoring Device 3 Infusion Device 7 Autologous Tissue Substitute C Extraluminal Device D Intraluminal Device J Synthetic Substitute K Nonautologous Tissue Substitute L Artificial Sphincter M Stimulator Lead	Z No Qualifier
D Urethra	0 Open 3 Percutaneous 4 Percutaneous Endoscopic 7 Via Natural or Artificial Opening 8 Via Natural or Artificial Opening Endoscopic	0 Drainage Device 2 Monitoring Device 3 Infusion Device 7 Autologous Tissue Substitute C Extraluminal Device D Intraluminal Device J Synthetic Substitute K Nonautologous Tissue Substitute L Artificial Sphincter Y Other Device	Z No Qualifier

Continued →

0TW Continued

Section 0 **Medical and Surgical**
Body System T **Urinary System**
Operation W **Revision:** Correcting, to the extent possible, a portion of a malfunctioning device or the position of a displaced device

Body Part (4th)	Approach (5th)	Device (6th)	Qualifier (7th)
D Urethra	**X** External	**0** Drainage Device **2** Monitoring Device **3** Infusion Device **7** Autologous Tissue Substitute **C** Extraluminal Device **D** Intraluminal Device **J** Synthetic Substitute **K** Nonautologous Tissue Substitute **L** Artificial Sphincter	**Z** No Qualifier

Section 0 **Medical and Surgical**
Body System T **Urinary System**
Operation Y **Transplantation:** Putting in or on all or a portion of a living body part taken from another individual or animal to physically take the place and/or function of all or a portion of a similar body part

Body Part (4th)	Approach (5th)	Device (6th)	Qualifier (7th)
0 Kidney, Right **1** Kidney, Left	**0** Open	**Z** No Device	**0** Allogeneic **1** Syngeneic **2** Zooplastic

AHA Coding Clinic

0T170ZB Bypass Left Ureter to Bladder, Open Approach—AHA CC: 3Q, 2015, 34-35
0T180ZC Bypass Bilateral Ureters to Ileocutaneous, Open Approach—AHA CC: 3Q, 2017, 20-21
0T1B0Z9 Bypass Bladder to Colocutaneous, Open Approach—AHA CC: 3Q, 2017, 21-22
0T768DZ Dilation of Right Ureter with Intraluminal Device, Via Natural or Artificial Opening Endoscopic—AHA CC: 2Q, 2016, 27-28; 4Q, 2017, 111
0T778DZ Dilation of Left Ureter with Intraluminal Device, Via Natural or Artificial Opening Endoscopic—AHA CC: 2Q, 2015, 8-9
0T7D8DZ Dilation of Urethra with Intraluminal Device, Via Natural or Artificial Opening Endoscopic—AHA CC: 4Q, 2013, 123
0T9680Z Drainage of Right Ureter with Drainage Device, Via Natural or Artificial Opening Endoscopic—AHA CC: 3Q, 2017, 19-20
0TBB8ZX Excision of Bladder, Via Natural or Artificial Opening Endoscopic, Diagnostic—AHA CC: 1Q, 2016, 19
0TBB8ZZ Excision of Bladder, Via Natural or Artificial Opening Endoscopic—AHA CC: 2Q, 2014, 8
0TBD8ZZ Excision of Urethra, Via Natural or Artificial Opening Endoscopic—AHA CC: 3Q, 2015, 34
0TC18ZZ Extirpation of Matter from Left Kidney, Via Natural or Artificial Opening Endoscopic—AHA CC: 2Q, 2015, 8-9
0TC48ZZ Extirpation of Matter from Left Kidney Pelvis, Via Natural or Artificial Opening Endoscopic—AHA CC: 2Q, 2015, 7-8
0TC68ZZ Extirpation of Matter from Right Ureter, Via Natural or Artificial Opening Endoscopic—AHA CC: 4Q, 2013, 122-123
0TC78ZZ Extirpation of Matter from Left Ureter, Via Natural or Artificial Opening Endoscopic—AHA CC: 2Q, 2015, 8-9
0TCB8ZZ Extirpation of Matter from Bladder, Via Natural or Artificial Opening Endoscopic—AHA CC: 2Q, 2015, 8-9; 3Q, 2016, 23-2
0TF3XZZ Fragmentation in Right Kidney Pelvis, External Approach—AHA CC: 4Q, 2013, 122
0TP98DZ Removal of Intraluminal Device from Ureter, Via Natural or Artificial Opening Endoscopic—AHA CC: 2Q, 2016, 27-28
0TQD0ZZ Repair Urethra, Open Approach—AHA CC: 1Q, 2017, 37-38
0TRB07Z Replacement of Bladder with Autologous Tissue Substitute, Open Approach—AHA CC: 3Q, 2017, 20-21
0TS60ZZ Reposition Right Ureter, Open Approach—AHA CC: 1Q, 2017, 36-37
0TSD0ZZ Reposition Urethra, Open Approach—AHA CC: 1Q, 2016, 15-16
0TT10ZZ Resection of Left Kidney, Open Approach—AHA CC: 3Q, 2014, 16
0TT70ZZ Resection of Left Ureter, Open Approach—AHA CC: 3Q, 2014, 16
0TUB07Z Supplement Bladder with Autologous Tissue Substitute, Open Approach—AHA CC: 3Q, 2017, 21-22
0TV68ZZ Restriction of Right Ureter, Via Natural or Artificial Opening Endoscopic—AHA CC: 2Q, 2015, 11-12
0TV78ZZ Restriction of Left Ureter, Via Natural or Artificial Opening Endoscopic—AHA CC: 2Q, 2015, 11-12

Female Reproductive System

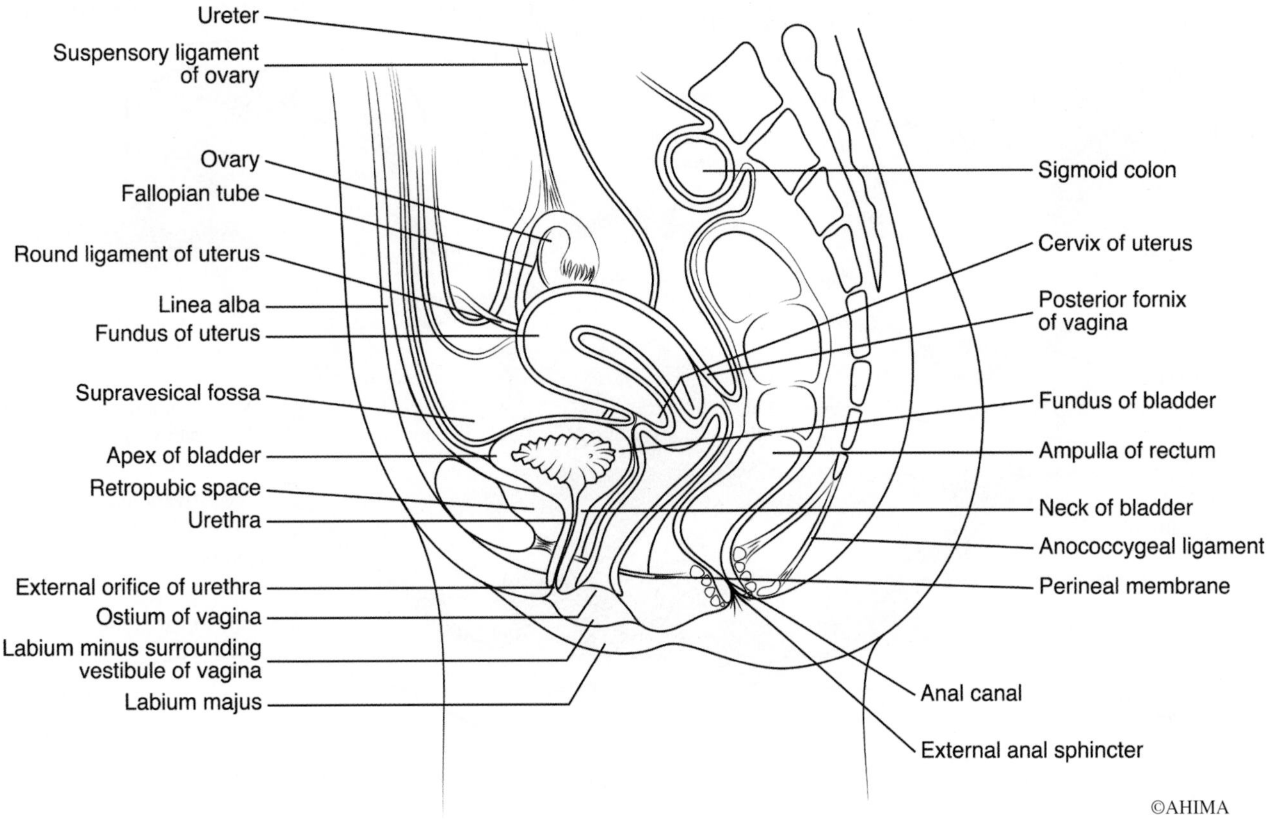

Ureter
Suspensory ligament of ovary
Ovary
Fallopian tube
Round ligament of uterus
Linea alba
Fundus of uterus
Supravesical fossa
Apex of bladder
Retropubic space
Urethra
External orifice of urethra
Ostium of vagina
Labium minus surrounding vestibule of vagina
Labium majus
Sigmoid colon
Cervix of uterus
Posterior fornix of vagina
Fundus of bladder
Ampulla of rectum
Neck of bladder
Anococcygeal ligament
Perineal membrane
Anal canal
External anal sphincter

Urethral opening (meatus)
Labium majus
Vaginal opening
Opening of greater vestibular (Bartholin's gland)
Vestibular fossa
Clitoris
Labium minus
Openings of paraurethral (Skene's) ducts
Vestibule
Hymen
Labium
Anus

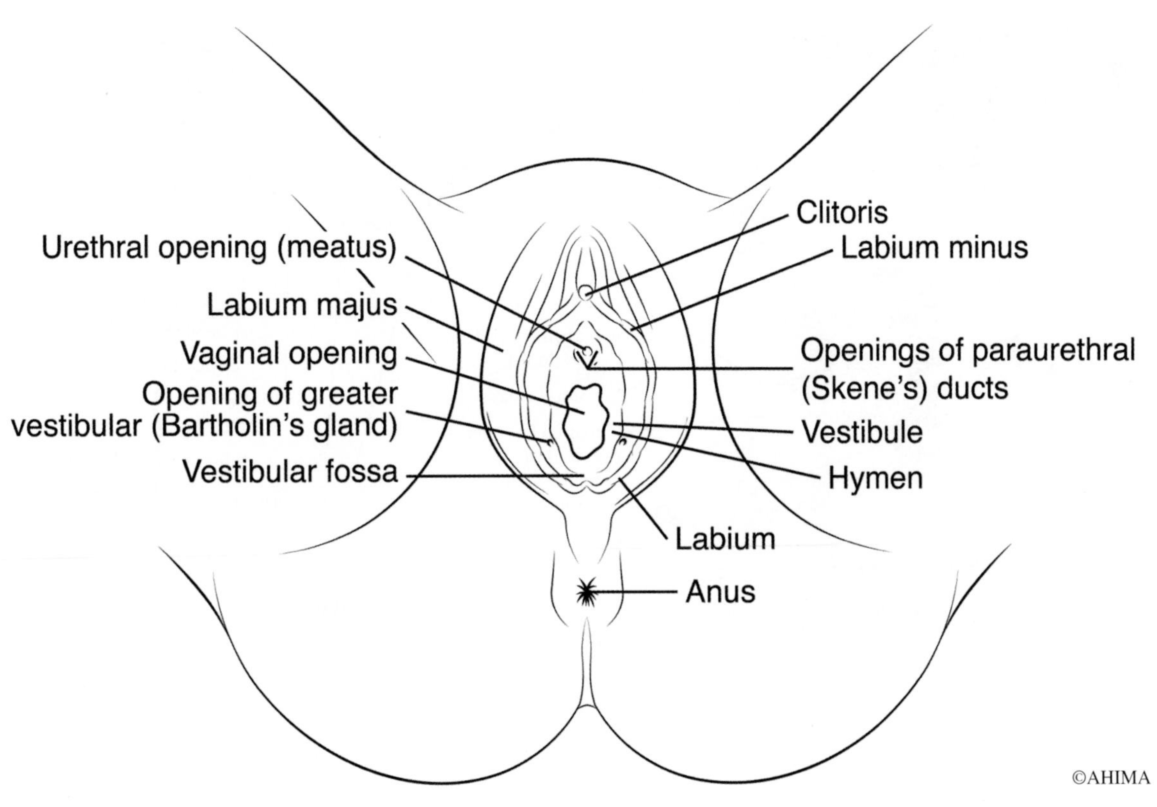

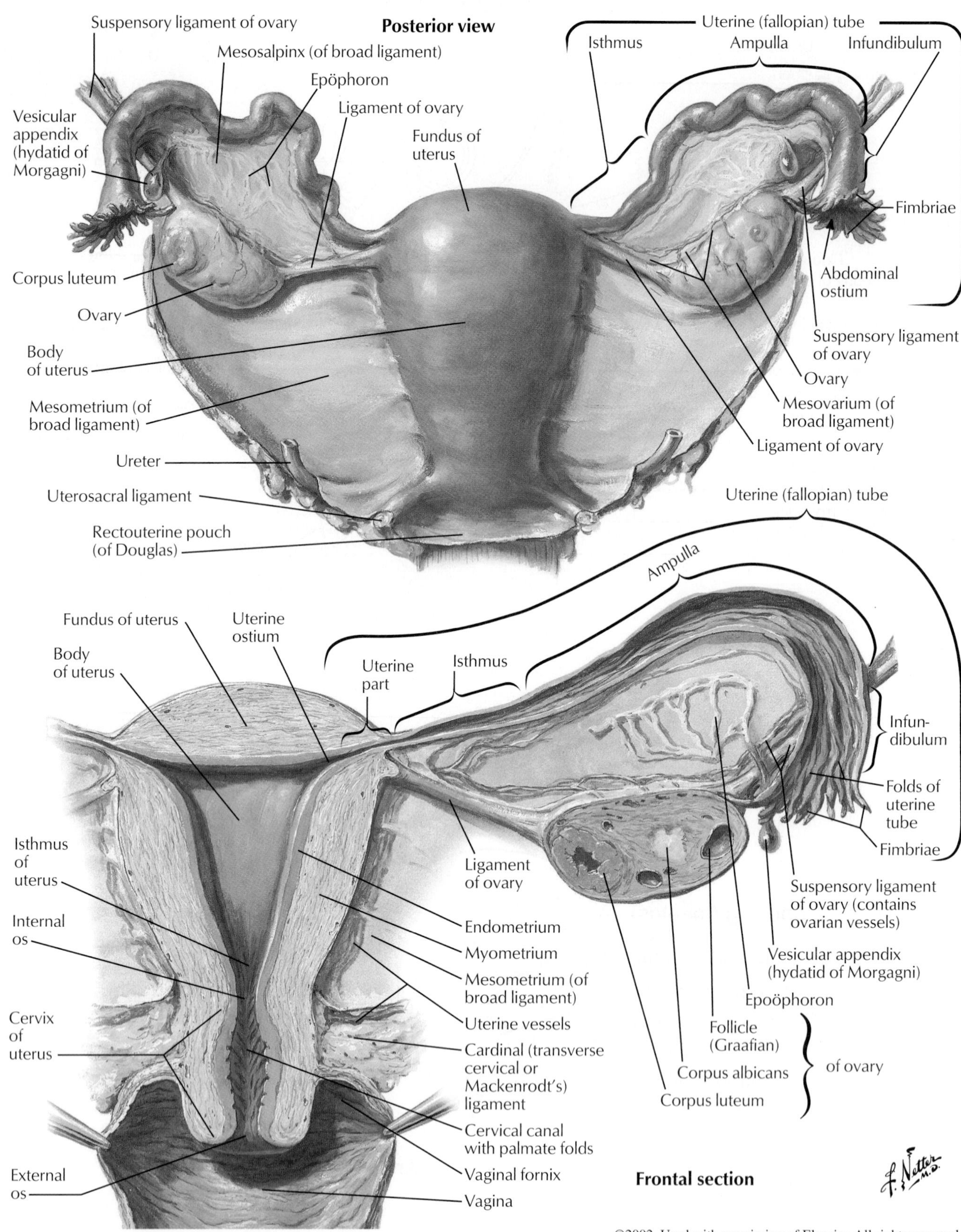
Posterior view
Suspensory ligament of ovary
Mesosalpinx (of broad ligament)
Epöphoron
Ligament of ovary
Fundus of uterus
Vesicular appendix (hydatid of Morgagni)
Corpus luteum
Ovary
Body of uterus
Mesometrium (of broad ligament)
Ureter
Uterosacral ligament
Rectouterine pouch (of Douglas)
Uterine (fallopian) tube
Isthmus
Ampulla
Infundibulum
Fimbriae
Abdominal ostium
Suspensory ligament of ovary
Ovary
Mesovarium (of broad ligament)
Ligament of ovary
Uterine (fallopian) tube
Ampulla
Fundus of uterus
Uterine ostium
Body of uterus
Uterine part
Isthmus
Infun-dibulum
Folds of uterine tube
Fimbriae
Ligament of ovary
Isthmus of uterus
Internal os
Endometrium
Myometrium
Mesometrium (of broad ligament)
Uterine vessels
Cardinal (transverse cervical or Mackenrodt's) ligament
Cervical canal with palmate folds
Vaginal fornix
Vagina
Cervix of uterus
External os
Suspensory ligament of ovary (contains ovarian vessels)
Vesicular appendix (hydatid of Morgagni)
Epoöphoron
Follicle (Graafian)
Corpus albicans
Corpus luteum
of ovary
Frontal section
F. Netter M.D.

nale Reproductive System Tables 0U1–0UY

tion **0** **Medical and Surgical**
ly System **U** **Female Reproductive System**
eration **1** **Bypass:** Altering the route of passage of the contents of a tubular body part

Body Part (4th)	Approach (5th)	Device (6th)	Qualifier (7th)
Fallopian Tube, Right Fallopian Tube, Left	**0** Open **4** Percutaneous Endoscopic	**7** Autologous Tissue Substitute **J** Synthetic Substitute **K** Nonautologous Tissue Substitute **Z** No Device	**5** Fallopian Tube, Right **6** Fallopian Tube, Left **9** Uterus

tion **0** **Medical and Surgical**
ly System **U** **Female Reproductive System**
eration **2** **Change:** Taking out or off a device from a body part and putting back an identical or similar device in or on the same body part without cutting or puncturing the skin or a mucous membrane

Body Part (4th)	Approach (5th)	Device (6th)	Qualifier (7th)
Ovary Fallopian Tube Vulva	**X** External	**0** Drainage Device **Y** Other Device	**Z** No Qualifier
Uterus and Cervix	**X** External	**0** Drainage Device **H** Contraceptive Device **Y** Other Device	**Z** No Qualifier
Vagina and Cul-de-sac	**X** External	**0** Drainage Device **G** Intraluminal Device, Pessary **Y** Other Device	**Z** No Qualifier

tion **0** **Medical and Surgical**
dy System **U** **Female Reproductive System**
eration **5** **Destruction:** Physical eradication of all or a portion of a body part by the direct use of energy, force, or a destructive agent

Body Part (4th)	Approach (5th)	Device (6th)	Qualifier (7th)
Ovary, Right Ovary, Left Ovaries, Bilateral Uterine Supporting Structure	**0** Open **3** Percutaneous **4** Percutaneous Endoscopic **8** Via Natural or Artificial Opening Endoscopic	**Z** No Device	**Z** No Qualifier
Fallopian Tube, Right Fallopian Tube, Left Fallopian Tubes, Bilateral Uterus Endometrium Cervix Cul-de-sac	**0** Open **3** Percutaneous **4** Percutaneous Endoscopic **7** Via Natural or Artificial Opening **8** Via Natural or Artificial Opening Endoscopic	**Z** No Device	**Z** No Qualifier
Vagina Hymen	**0** Open **3** Percutaneous **4** Percutaneous Endoscopic **7** Via Natural or Artificial Opening **8** Via Natural or Artificial Opening Endoscopic **X** External	**Z** No Device	**Z** No Qualifier
Clitoris Vestibular Gland M Vulva	**0** Open **X** External	**Z** No Device	**Z** No Qualifier

Section 0 **Medical and Surgical**
Body System U **Female Reproductive System**
Operation 7 **Dilation:** Expanding an orifice or the lumen of a tubular body part

Body Part (4th)	Approach (5th)	Device (6th)	Qualifier (7t
5 Fallopian Tube, Right **6** Fallopian Tube, Left **7** Fallopian Tubes, Bilateral **9** Uterus **C** Cervix **G** Vagina	**0** Open **3** Percutaneous **4** Percutaneous Endoscopic **7** Via Natural or Artificial Opening **8** Via Natural or Artificial Opening Endoscopic	**D** Intraluminal Device **Z** No Device	**Z** No Qualifie
K Hymen	**0** Open **3** Percutaneous **4** Percutaneous Endoscopic **7** Via Natural or Artificial Opening **8** Via Natural or Artificial Opening Endoscopic **X** External	**D** Intraluminal Device **Z** No Device	**Z** No Qualifie

Section 0 **Medical and Surgical**
Body System U **Female Reproductive System**
Operation 8 **Division:** Cutting into a body part, without draining fluids and/or gases from the body part, in order to separate or trans body part

Body Part (4th)	Approach (5th)	Device (6th)	Qualifier (7t
0 Ovary, Right **1** Ovary, Left **2** Ovaries, Bilateral **4** Uterine Supporting Structure	**0** Open **3** Percutaneous **4** Percutaneous Endoscopic	**Z** No Device	**Z** No Qualifier
K Hymen	**7** Via Natural or Artificial Opening **8** Via Natural or Artificial Opening Endoscopic **X** External	**Z** No Device	**Z** No Qualifier

Section 0 **Medical and Surgical**
Body System U **Female Reproductive System**
Operation 9 **Drainage:** Taking or letting out fluids and/or gases from a body part

Body Part (4th)	Approach (5th)	Device (6th)	Qualifier (7th
0 Ovary, Right **1** Ovary, Left **2** Ovaries, Bilateral	**0** Open **3** Percutaneous **4** Percutaneous Endoscopic **8** Via Natural or Artificial Opening Endoscopic	**0** Drainage Device	**Z** No Qualifier
0 Ovary, Right **1** Ovary, Left **2** Ovaries, Bilateral	**0** Open **3** Percutaneous **4** Percutaneous Endoscopic **8** Via Natural or Artificial Opening Endoscopic	**Z** No Device	**X** Diagnostic **Z** No Qualifier
0 Ovary, Right **1** Ovary, Left **2** Ovaries, Bilateral	**X** External	**Z** No Device	**Z** No Qualifier
4 Uterine Supporting Structure	**0** Open **3** Percutaneous **4** Percutaneous Endoscopic **8** Via Natural or Artificial Opening Endoscopic	**0** Drainage Device	**Z** No Qualifier
4 Uterine Supporting Structure	**0** Open **3** Percutaneous **4** Percutaneous Endoscopic **8** Via Natural or Artificial Opening Endoscopic	**Z** No Device	**X** Diagnostic **Z** No Qualifier

Continued

tion 0 **Medical and Surgical**
ly System U **Female Reproductive System**
eration 9 **Drainage:** Taking or letting out fluids and/or gases from a body part

Body Part (4th)	Approach (5th)	Device (6th)	Qualifier (7th)
Fallopian Tube, Right Fallopian Tube, Left Fallopian Tubes, Bilateral Uterus Cervix Cul-de-sac	**0** Open **3** Percutaneous **4** Percutaneous Endoscopic **7** Via Natural or Artificial Opening **8** Via Natural or Artificial Opening Endoscopic	**0** Drainage Device	**Z** No Qualifier
Fallopian Tube, Right Fallopian Tube, Left Fallopian Tubes, Bilateral Uterus Cervix Cul-de-sac	**0** Open **3** Percutaneous **4** Percutaneous Endoscopic **7** Via Natural or Artificial Opening **8** Via Natural or Artificial Opening Endoscopic	**Z** No Device	**X** Diagnostic **Z** No Qualifier
Vagina Hymen	**0** Open **3** Percutaneous **4** Percutaneous Endoscopic **7** Via Natural or Artificial Opening **8** Via Natural or Artificial Opening Endoscopic **X** External	**0** Drainage Device	**Z** No Qualifier
Vagina Hymen	**0** Open **3** Percutaneous **4** Percutaneous Endoscopic **7** Via Natural or Artificial Opening **8** Via Natural or Artificial Opening Endoscopic **X** External	**Z** No Device	**X** Diagnostic **Z** No Qualifier
Clitoris Vestibular Gland M Vulva	**0** Open **X** External	**0** Drainage Device	**Z** No Qualifier
Clitoris Vestibular Gland M Vulva	**0** Open **X** External	**Z** No Device	**X** Diagnostic **Z** No Qualifier

ction 0 **Medical and Surgical**
dy System U **Female Reproductive System**
eration B **Excision:** Cutting out or off, without replacement, a portion of a body part

Body Part (4th)	Approach (5th)	Device (6th)	Qualifier (7th)
Ovary, Right Ovary, Left Ovaries, Bilateral Uterine Supporting Structure Fallopian Tube, Right Fallopian Tube, Left Fallopian Tubes, Bilateral Uterus Cervix Cul-de-sac	**0** Open **3** Percutaneous **4** Percutaneous Endoscopic **7** Via Natural or Artificial Opening **8** Via Natural or Artificial Opening Endoscopic	**Z** No Device	**X** Diagnostic **Z** No Qualifier

Continued →

Section 0 **Medical and Surgical**
Body System U **Female Reproductive System**
Operation B **Excision:** Cutting out or off, without replacement, a portion of a body part

Body Part (4th)	Approach (5th)	Device (6th)	Qualifier (7th)
G Vagina **K** Hymen	**0** Open **3** Percutaneous **4** Percutaneous Endoscopic **7** Via Natural or Artificial Opening **8** Via Natural or Artificial Opening Endoscopic **X** External	**Z** No Device	**X** Diagnostic **Z** No Qualifier
J Clitoris **L** Vestibular Gland **M** Vulva	**0** Open **X** External	**Z** No Device	**X** Diagnostic **Z** No Qualifier

Section 0 **Medical and Surgical**
Body System U **Female Reproductive System**
Operation C **Extirpation:** Taking or cutting out solid matter from a body part

Body Part (4th)	Approach (5th)	Device (6th)	Qualifier (7th)
0 Ovary, Right **1** Ovary, Left **2** Ovaries, Bilateral **4** Uterine Supporting Structure	**0** Open **3** Percutaneous **4** Percutaneous Endoscopic **8** Via Natural or Artificial Opening Endoscopic	**Z** No Device	**Z** No Qualifier
5 Fallopian Tube, Right **6** Fallopian Tube, Left **7** Fallopian Tubes, Bilateral **9** Uterus **B** Endometrium **C** Cervix **F** Cul-de-sac	**0** Open **3** Percutaneous **4** Percutaneous Endoscopic **7** Via Natural or Artificial Opening **8** Via Natural or Artificial Opening Endoscopic	**Z** No Device	**Z** No Qualifier
G Vagina **K** Hymen	**0** Open **3** Percutaneous **4** Percutaneous Endoscopic **7** Via Natural or Artificial Opening **8** Via Natural or Artificial Opening Endoscopic **X** External	**Z** No Device	**Z** No Qualifier
J Clitoris **L** Vestibular Gland **M** Vulva	**0** Open **X** External	**Z** No Device	**Z** No Qualifier

Section 0 **Medical and Surgical**
Body System U **Female Reproductive System**
Operation D **Extraction:** Pulling or stripping out or off all or a portion of a body part by the use of force

Body Part (4th)	Approach (5th)	Device (6th)	Qualifier (7th)
B Endometrium	**7** Via Natural or Artificial Opening **8** Via Natural or Artificial Opening Endoscopic	**Z** No Device	**X** Diagnostic **Z** No Qualifier
N Ova	**0** Open **3** Percutaneous **4** Percutaneous Endoscopic	**Z** No Device	**Z** No Qualifier

tion	**0**	**Medical and Surgical**
dy System	**U**	**Female Reproductive System**
eration	**F**	**Fragmentation:** Breaking solid matter in a body part into pieces

Body Part (4th)	Approach (5th)	Device (6th)	Qualifier (7th)
Fallopian Tube, Right Fallopian Tube, Left Fallopian Tubes, Bilateral Uterus	**0** Open **3** Percutaneous **4** Percutaneous Endoscopic **7** Via Natural or Artificial Opening **8** Via Natural or Artificial Opening Endoscopic **X** External	**Z** No Device	**Z** No Qualifier

tion	**0**	**Medical and Surgical**
dy System	**U**	**Female Reproductive System**
eration	**H**	**Insertion:** Putting in a nonbiological appliance that monitors, assists, performs, or prevents a physiological function but does not physically take the place of a body part

Body Part (4th)	Approach (5th)	Device (6th)	Qualifier (7th)
Ovary	**0** Open **3** Percutaneous **4** Percutaneous Endoscopic	**3** Infusion Device **Y** Other Device	**Z** No Qualifier
Ovary	**7** Via Natural or Artificial Opening **8** Via Natural or Artificial Opening Endoscopic	**Y** Other Device	**Z** No Qualifier
Fallopian Tube Uterus and Cervix Vagina and Cul-de-sac	**0** Open **3** Percutaneous **4** Percutaneous Endoscopic **7** Via Natural or Artificial Opening **8** Via Natural or Artificial Opening Endoscopic	**3** Infusion Device **Y** Other Device	**Z** No Qualifier
Uterus	**0** Open **7** Via Natural or Artificial Opening **8** Via Natural or Artificial Opening Endoscopic	**H** Contraceptive Device	**Z** No Qualifier
C Cervix	**0** Open **3** Percutaneous **4** Percutaneous Endoscopic	**1** Radioactive Element	**Z** No Qualifier
C Cervix	**7** Via Natural or Artificial Opening **8** Via Natural or Artificial Opening Endoscopic	**1** Radioactive Element **H** Contraceptive Device	**Z** No Qualifier
Cul-de-sac	**7** Via Natural or Artificial Opening **8** Via Natural or Artificial Opening Endoscopic	**G** Intraluminal Device, Pessary	**Z** No Qualifier
G Vagina	**0** Open **3** Percutaneous **4** Percutaneous Endoscopic **X** External	**1** Radioactive Element	**Z** No Qualifier
G Vagina	**7** Via Natural or Artificial Opening **8** Via Natural or Artificial Opening Endoscopic	**1** Radioactive Element **G** Intraluminal Device, Pessary	**Z** No Qualifier

ction	**0**	**Medical and Surgical**
dy System	**U**	**Female Reproductive System**
eration	**J**	**Inspection:** Visually and/or manually exploring a body part

Body Part (4th)	Approach (5th)	Device (6th)	Qualifier (7th)
3 Ovary	**0** Open **3** Percutaneous **4** Percutaneous Endoscopic **8** Via Natural or Artificial Opening Endoscopic **X** External	**Z** No Device	**Z** No Qualifier

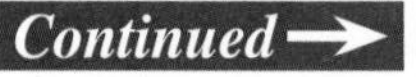
Continued →

0UJ Contin...

Section 0 **Medical and Surgical**
Body System U **Female Reproductive System**
Operation J **Inspection:** Visually and/or manually exploring a body part

Body Part (4th)	Approach (5th)	Device (6th)	Qualifier (7th)
8 Fallopian Tube **D** Uterus and Cervix **H** Vagina and Cul-de-sac	**0** Open **3** Percutaneous **4** Percutaneous Endoscopic **7** Via Natural or Artificial Opening **8** Via Natural or Artificial Opening Endoscopic **X** External	**Z** No Device	**Z** No Qualifier
M Vulva	**0** Open **X** External	**Z** No Device	**Z** No Qualifier

Section 0 **Medical and Surgical**
Body System U **Female Reproductive System**
Operation L **Occlusion:** Completely closing an orifice or the lumen of a tubular body part

Body Part (4th)	Approach (5th)	Device (6th)	Qualifier (7th)
5 Fallopian Tube, Right **6** Fallopian Tube, Left **7** Fallopian Tubes, Bilateral	**0** Open **3** Percutaneous **4** Percutaneous Endoscopic	**C** Extraluminal Device **D** Intraluminal Device **Z** No Device	**Z** No Qualifier
5 Fallopian Tube, Right **6** Fallopian Tube, Left **7** Fallopian Tubes, Bilateral	**7** Via Natural or Artificial Opening **8** Via Natural or Artificial Opening Endoscopic	**D** Intraluminal Device **Z** No Device	**Z** No Qualifier
F Cul-de-sac **G** Vagina	**7** Via Natural or Artificial Opening **8** Via Natural or Artificial Opening Endoscopic	**D** Intraluminal Device **Z** No Device	**Z** No Qualifier

Section 0 **Medical and Surgical**
Body System U **Female Reproductive System**
Operation M **Reattachment:** Putting back in or on all or a portion of a separated body part to its normal location or other suitable location

Body Part (4th)	Approach (5th)	Device (6th)	Qualifier (7th)
0 Ovary, Right **1** Ovary, Left **2** Ovaries, Bilateral **4** Uterine Supporting Structure **5** Fallopian Tube, Right **6** Fallopian Tube, Left **7** Fallopian Tubes, Bilateral **9** Uterus **C** Cervix **F** Cul-de-sac **G** Vagina	**0** Open **4** Percutaneous Endoscopic	**Z** No Device	**Z** No Qualifier
J Clitoris **M** Vulva	**X** External	**Z** No Device	**Z** No Qualifier
K Hymen	**0** Open **4** Percutaneous Endoscopic **X** External	**Z** No Device	**Z** No Qualifier

tion 0 **Medical and Surgical**
dy System U **Female Reproductive System**
eration N **Release:** Freeing a body part from an abnormal physical constraint by cutting or by the use of force

Body Part (4th)	Approach (5th)	Device (6th)	Qualifier (7th)
Ovary, Right Ovary, Left Ovaries, Bilateral Uterine Supporting Structure	**0** Open **3** Percutaneous **4** Percutaneous Endoscopic **8** Via Natural or Artificial Opening Endoscopic	**Z** No Device	**Z** No Qualifier
Fallopian Tube, Right Fallopian Tube, Left Fallopian Tubes, Bilateral Uterus Cervix Cul-de-sac	**0** Open **3** Percutaneous **4** Percutaneous Endoscopic **7** Via Natural or Artificial Opening **8** Via Natural or Artificial Opening Endoscopic	**Z** No Device	**Z** No Qualifier
Vagina Hymen	**0** Open **3** Percutaneous **4** Percutaneous Endoscopic **7** Via Natural or Artificial Opening **8** Via Natural or Artificial Opening Endoscopic **X** External	**Z** No Device	**Z** No Qualifier
Clitoris Vestibular Gland Vulva	**0** Open **X** External	**Z** No Device	**Z** No Qualifier

tion 0 **Medical and Surgical**
dy System U **Female Reproductive System**
eration P **Removal:** Taking out or off a device from a body part

Body Part (4th)	Approach (5th)	Device (6th)	Qualifier (7th)
Ovary	**0** Open **3** Percutaneous **4** Percutaneous Endoscopic	**0** Drainage Device **3** Infusion Device **Y** Other Device	**Z** No Qualifier
Ovary	**7** Via Natural or Artificial Opening **8** Via Natural or Artificial Opening Endoscopic	**Y** Other Device	**Z** No Qualifier
Ovary	**X** External	**0** Drainage Device **3** Infusion Device	**Z** No Qualifier
Fallopian Tube	**0** Open **3** Percutaneous **4** Percutaneous Endoscopic **7** Via Natural or Artificial Opening **8** Via Natural or Artificial Opening Endoscopic	**0** Drainage Device **3** Infusion Device **7** Autologous Tissue Substitute **C** Extraluminal Device **D** Intraluminal Device **J** Synthetic Substitute **K** Nonautologous Tissue Substitute **Y** Other Device	**Z** No Qualifier
Fallopian Tube	**X** External	**0** Drainage Device **3** Infusion Device **D** Intraluminal Device	**Z** No Qualifier
Uterus and Cervix	**0** Open **3** Percutaneous **4** Percutaneous Endoscopic **7** Via Natural or Artificial Opening **8** Via Natural or Artificial Opening Endoscopic	**0** Drainage Device **1** Radioactive Element **3** Infusion Device **7** Autologous Tissue Substitute **C** Extraluminal Device **D** Intraluminal Device **H** Contraceptive Device **J** Synthetic Substitute **K** Nonautologous Tissue Substitute **Y** Other Device	**Z** No Qualifier

Continued →

Section	0	Medical and Surgical
Body System	U	Female Reproductive System
Operation	P	**Removal:** Taking out or off a device from a body part

Body Part (4th)	Approach (5th)	Device (6th)	Qualifier (7th)
D Uterus and Cervix	**X** External	**0** Drainage Device **3** Infusion Device **D** Intraluminal Device **H** Contraceptive Device	**Z** No Qualifier
H Vagina and Cul-de-sac	**0** Open **3** Percutaneous **4** Percutaneous Endoscopic **7** Via Natural or Artificial Opening **8** Via Natural or Artificial Opening Endoscopic	**0** Drainage Device **1** Radioactive Element **3** Infusion Device **7** Autologous Tissue Substitute **D** Intraluminal Device **J** Synthetic Substitute **K** Nonautologous Tissue Substitute **Y** Other Device	**Z** No Qualifier
H Vagina and Cul-de-sac	**X** External	**0** Drainage Device **1** Radioactive Element **3** Infusion Device **D** Intraluminal Device	**Z** No Qualifier
M Vulva	**0** Open	**0** Drainage Device **7** Autologous Tissue Substitute **J** Synthetic Substitute **K** Nonautologous Tissue Substitute	**Z** No Qualifier
M Vulva	**X** External	**0** Drainage Device	**Z** No Qualifier

Section	0	Medical and Surgical
Body System	U	Female Reproductive System
Operation	Q	**Repair:** Restoring, to the extent possible, a body part to its normal anatomic structure and function

Body Part (4th)	Approach (5th)	Device (6th)	Qualifier (7th)
0 Ovary, Right **1** Ovary, Left **2** Ovaries, Bilateral **4** Uterine Supporting Structure	**0** Open **3** Percutaneous **4** Percutaneous Endoscopic **8** Via Natural or Artificial Opening Endoscopic	**Z** No Device	**Z** No Qualifier
5 Fallopian Tube, Right **6** Fallopian Tube, Left **7** Fallopian Tubes, Bilateral **9** Uterus **C** Cervix **F** Cul-de-sac	**0** Open **3** Percutaneous **4** Percutaneous Endoscopic **7** Via Natural or Artificial Opening **8** Via Natural or Artificial Opening Endoscopic	**Z** No Device	**Z** No Qualifier
G Vagina **K** Hymen	**0** Open **3** Percutaneous **4** Percutaneous Endoscopic **7** Via Natural or Artificial Opening **8** Via Natural or Artificial Opening Endoscopic **X** External	**Z** No Device	**Z** No Qualifier
J Clitoris **L** Vestibular Gland **M** Vulva	**0** Open **X** External	**Z** No Device	**Z** No Qualifier

Section 0 **Medical and Surgical**
Body System U **Female Reproductive System**
Operation S **Reposition:** Moving to its normal location, or other suitable location, all or a portion of a body part

Body Part (4th)	Approach (5th)	Device (6th)	Qualifier (7th)
0 Ovary, Right **1** Ovary, Left **2** Ovaries, Bilateral **4** Uterine Supporting Structure **5** Fallopian Tube, Right **6** Fallopian Tube, Left **7** Fallopian Tubes, Bilateral **C** Cervix **F** Cul-de-sac	**0** Open **4** Percutaneous Endoscopic **8** Via Natural or Artificial Opening Endoscopic	**Z** No Device	**Z** No Qualifier
9 Uterus **G** Vagina	**0** Open **4** Percutaneous Endoscopic **7** Via Natural or Artificial Opening **8** Via Natural or Artificial Opening Endoscopic **X** External	**Z** No Device	**Z** No Qualifier

Section 0 **Medical and Surgical**
Body System U **Female Reproductive System**
Operation T **Resection:** Cutting out or off, without replacement, all of a body part

Body Part (4th)	Approach (5th)	Device (6th)	Qualifier (7th)
0 Ovary, Right **1** Ovary, Left **2** Ovaries, Bilateral **5** Fallopian Tube, Right **6** Fallopian Tube, Left **7** Fallopian Tubes, Bilateral	**0** Open **4** Percutaneous Endoscopic **7** Via Natural or Artificial Opening **8** Via Natural or Artificial Opening Endoscopic **F** Via Natural or Artificial Opening With Percutaneous Endoscopic Assistance	**Z** No Device	**Z** No Qualifier
4 Uterine Supporting Structure **C** Cervix **F** Cul-de-sac **G** Vagina	**0** Open **4** Percutaneous Endoscopic **7** Via Natural or Artificial Opening **8** Via Natural or Artificial Opening Endoscopic	**Z** No Device	**Z** No Qualifier
9 Uterus	**0** Open **4** Percutaneous Endoscopic **7** Via Natural or Artificial Opening **8** Via Natural or Artificial Opening Endoscopic **F** Via Natural or Artificial Opening with Percutaneous Endoscopic Assistance	**Z** No Device	**L** Supracervical **Z** No Qualifier
J Clitoris **L** Vestibular Gland **M** Vulva	**0** Open **X** External	**Z** No Device	**Z** No Qualifier
K Hymen	**0** Open **4** Percutaneous Endoscopic **7** Via Natural or Artificial Opening **8** Via Natural or Artificial Opening Endoscopic **X** External	**Z** No Device	**Z** No Qualifier

Section 0 **Medical and Surgical**
Body System U **Female Reproductive System**
Operation U **Supplement:** Putting in or on biological or synthetic material that physically reinforces and/or augments the function of a portion of a body part

Body Part (4th)	Approach (5th)	Device (6th)	Qualifier (7th)
4 Uterine Supporting Structure	**0** Open **4** Percutaneous Endoscopic	**7** Autologous Tissue Substitute **J** Synthetic Substitute **K** Nonautologous Tissue Substitute	**Z** No Qualifier
5 Fallopian Tube, Right **6** Fallopian Tube, Left **7** Fallopian Tubes, Bilateral **F** Cul-de-sac	**0** Open **4** Percutaneous Endoscopic **7** Via Natural or Artificial Opening **8** Via Natural or Artificial Opening Endoscopic	**7** Autologous Tissue Substitute **J** Synthetic Substitute **K** Nonautologous Tissue Substitute	**Z** No Qualifier
G Vagina **K** Hymen	**0** Open **4** Percutaneous Endoscopic **7** Via Natural or Artificial Opening **8** Via Natural or Artificial Opening Endoscopic **X** External	**7** Autologous Tissue Substitute **J** Synthetic Substitute **K** Nonautologous Tissue Substitute	**Z** No Qualifier
J Clitoris **M** Vulva	**0** Open **X** External	**7** Autologous Tissue Substitute **J** Synthetic Substitute **K** Nonautologous Tissue Substitute	**Z** No Qualifier

Section 0 **Medical and Surgical**
Body System U **Female Reproductive System**
Operation V **Restriction:** Partially closing an orifice or the lumen of a tubular body part

Body Part (4th)	Approach (5th)	Device (6th)	Qualifier (7th)
C Cervix	**0** Open **3** Percutaneous **4** Percutaneous Endoscopic	**C** Extraluminal Device **D** Intraluminal Device **Z** No Device	**Z** No Qualifier
C Cervix	**7** Via Natural or Artificial Opening **8** Via Natural or Artificial Opening Endoscopic	**D** Intraluminal Device **Z** No Device	**Z** No Qualifier

Section 0 **Medical and Surgical**
Body System U **Female Reproductive System**
Operation W **Revision:** Correcting, to the extent possible, a portion of a malfunctioning device or the position of a displaced device

Body Part (4th)	Approach (5th)	Device (6th)	Qualifier (7th)
3 Ovary	**0** Open **3** Percutaneous **4** Percutaneous Endoscopic	**0** Drainage Device **3** Infusion Device **Y** Other Device	**Z** No Qualifier
3 Ovary	**7** Via Natural or Artificial Opening **8** Via Natural or Artificial Opening Endoscopic	**Y** Other Device	**Z** No Qualifier
3 Ovary	**X** External	**0** Drainage Device **3** Infusion Device	**Z** No Qualifier
8 Fallopian Tube	**0** Open **3** Percutaneous **4** Percutaneous Endoscopic **7** Via Natural or Artificial Opening **8** Via Natural or Artificial Opening Endoscopic **X** External	**0** Drainage Device **3** Infusion Device **7** Autologous Tissue Substitute **C** Extraluminal Device **D** Intraluminal Device **J** Synthetic Substitute **K** Nonautologous Tissue Substitute **Y** Other Device	**Z** No Qualifier

Continued →

ection 0 Medical and Surgical
ody System U Female Reproductive System
peration W Revision: Correcting, to the extent possible, a portion of a malfunctioning device or the position of a displaced device

Body Part (4th)	Approach (5th)	Device (6th)	Qualifier (7th)
8 Fallopian Tube	X External	0 Drainage Device 3 Infusion Device 7 Autologous Tissue Substitute C Extraluminal Device D Intraluminal Device J Synthetic Substitute K Nonautologous Tissue Substitute	Z No Qualifier
D Uterus and Cervix	0 Open 3 Percutaneous 4 Percutaneous Endoscopic 7 Via Natural or Artificial Opening 8 Via Natural or Artificial Opening Endoscopic	0 Drainage Device 1 Radioactive Element 3 Infusion Device 7 Autologous Tissue Substitute C Extraluminal Device D Intraluminal Device H Contraceptive Device J Synthetic Substitute K Nonautologous Tissue Substitute Y Other Device	Z No Qualifier
D Uterus and Cervix	X External	0 Drainage Device 3 Infusion Device 7 Autologous Tissue Substitute C Extraluminal Device D Intraluminal Device H Contraceptive Device J Synthetic Substitute K Nonautologous Tissue Substitute	Z No Qualifier
H Vagina and Cul-de-sac	0 Open 3 Percutaneous 4 Percutaneous Endoscopic 7 Via Natural or Artificial Opening 8 Via Natural or Artificial Opening Endoscopic	0 Drainage Device 1 Radioactive Element 3 Infusion Device 7 Autologous Tissue Substitute D Intraluminal Device J Synthetic Substitute K Nonautologous Tissue Substitute Y Other Device	Z No Qualifier
H Vagina and Cul-de-sac	X External	0 Drainage Device 3 Infusion Device 7 Autologous Tissue Substitute D Intraluminal Device J Synthetic Substitute K Nonautologous Tissue Substitute	Z No Qualifier
M Vulva	0 Open X External	0 Drainage Device 7 Autologous Tissue Substitute J Synthetic Substitute K Nonautologous Tissue Substitute	Z No Qualifier

ection 0 Medical and Surgical
ody System U Female Reproductive System
peration Y

ransplantation: Putting in or on all or a portion of a living body part taken from another individual or animal to physically take the place and/or function of all or a portion of a similar body part

Body Part (4th)	Approach (5th)	Device (6th)	Qualifier (7th)
0 Ovary, Right 1 Ovary, Left 9 Uterus	0 Open	Z No Device	0 Allogeneic 1 Syngeneic 2 Zooplastic

AHA Coding Clinic

0U9G7ZZ Drainage of Vagina, Via Natural or Artificial Opening—AHA CC: 4Q, 2016, 58-59
0UB64ZZ Excision of Left Fallopian Tube, Percutaneous Endoscopic Approach—AHA CC: 3Q, 2015, 31-32
0UB70ZZ Excision of Bilateral Fallopian Tubes, Open Approach—AHA CC: 3Q, 2015, 31
0UB90ZZ Excision of Uterus, Open Approach—AHA CC: 4Q, 2014, 16
0UBMXZZ Excision of Vulva, External Approach—AHA CC: 3Q, 2014, 12
0UC97ZZ Extirpation of Matter from Uterus, Via Natural or Artificial Opening—AHA CC: 2Q, 2013, 38
0UCC7ZZ Extirpation of Matter from Cervix, Via Natural or Artificial Opening—AHA CC: 3Q, 2015, 30
0UCC8ZZ Extirpation of Matter from Cervix, Via Natural or Artificial Opening Endoscopic—AHA CC: 3Q, 2015, 30-31
0UH97HZ Insertion of Contraceptive Device into Uterus, Via Natural or Artificial Opening—AHA CC: 2Q, 2013, 34
0UHD7YZ Insertion of Other Device into Uterus and Cervix, Via Natural or Artificial Opening—AHA CC: 4Q, 2017, 104; 1Q, 2018,
0UJD4ZZ Inspection of Uterus and Cervix, Percutaneous Endoscopic Approach—AHA CC: 1Q, 2015, 33-34
0UQJXZZ Repair Clitoris, External Approach—AHA CC: 4Q, 2013, 120-121
0UQMXZZ Repair Vulva, External Approach—AHA CC: 4Q, 2014, 18-19
0US9XZZ Reposition Uterus, External Approach—AHA CC: 1Q, 2016, 9
0UT00ZZ Resection of Right Ovary, Open Approach—AHA CC: 1Q, 2013, 24
0UT20ZZ Resection of Bilateral Ovaries, Open Approach—AHA CC: 1Q, 2015, 33-34
0UT70ZZ Resection of Bilateral Fallopian Tubes, Open Approach—AHA CC: 1Q, 2015, 33-34
0UT90ZZ Resection of Uterus, Open Approach—AHA CC: 3Q, 2013, 28; 1Q, 2015, 33-34; 4Q, 2017, 68
0UT97ZL Resection of Uterus, Supracervical, Via Natural or Artificial Opening—AHA CC: 4Q, 2017, 68
0UTC0ZZ Resection of Cervix, Open Approach—AHA CC: 3Q, 2013, 28; 1Q, 2015, 33-34
0UVC7ZZ Restriction of Cervix, Via Natural or Artificial Opening—AHA CC: 3Q, 2015, 30

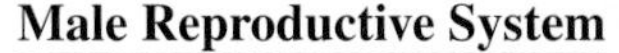

Male Reproductive System

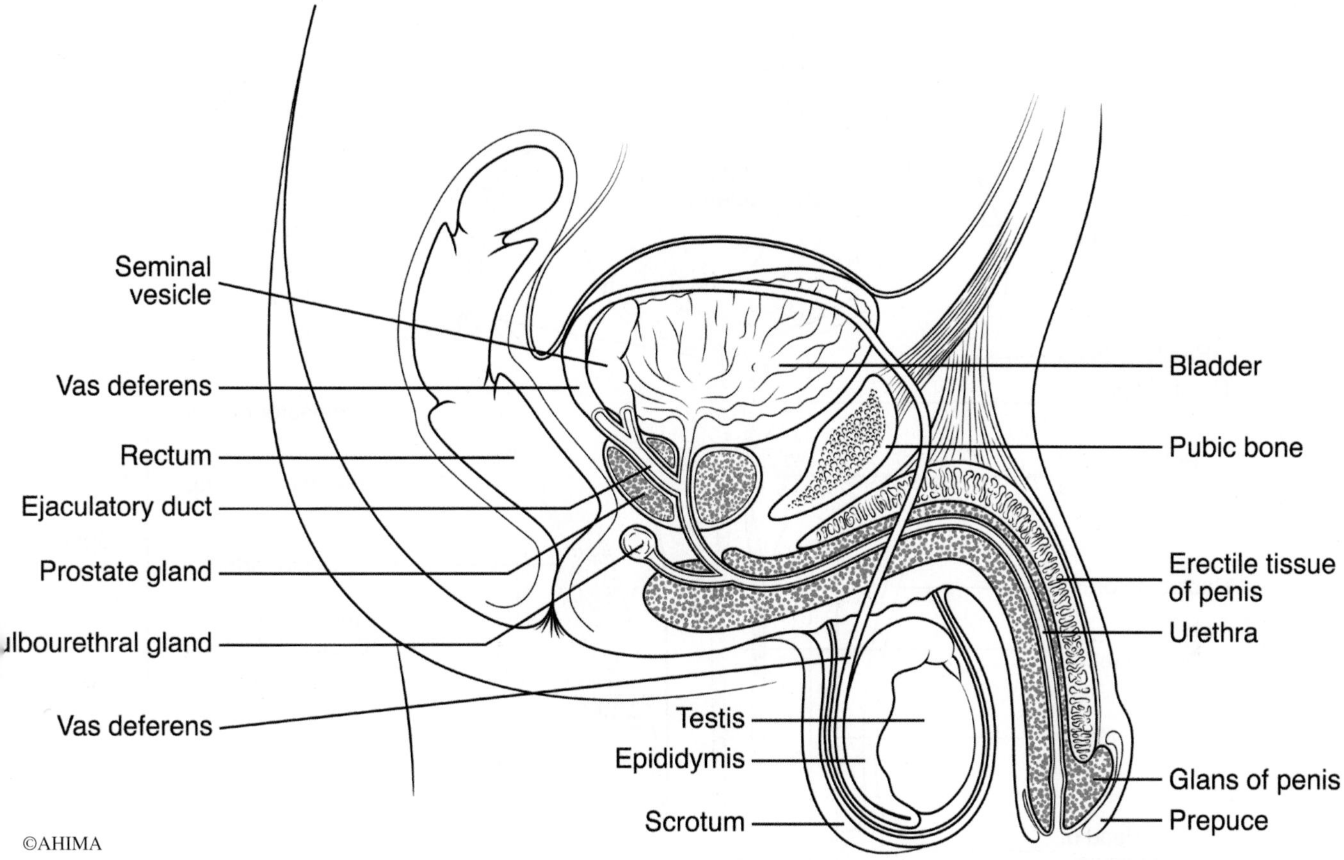

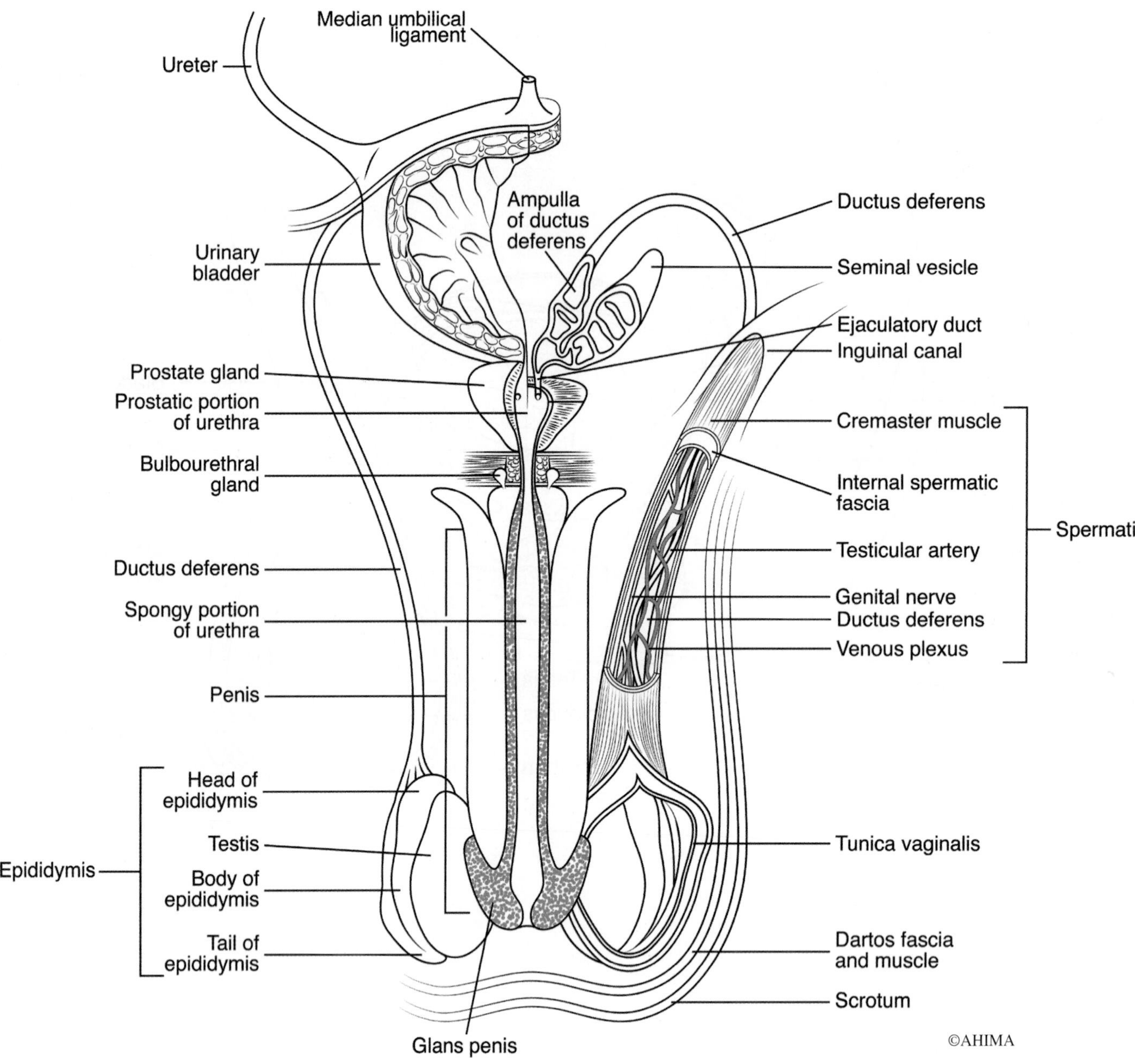
Median umbilical ligament
Ureter
Ampulla of ductus deferens
Ductus deferens
Seminal vesicle
Urinary bladder
Ejaculatory duct
Inguinal canal
Prostate gland
Prostatic portion of urethra
Cremaster muscle
Bulbourethral gland
Internal spermatic fascia
Spermatic
Testicular artery
Ductus deferens
Genital nerve
Spongy portion of urethra
Ductus deferens
Venous plexus
Penis
Head of epididymis
Testis
Tunica vaginalis
Epididymis
Body of epididymis
Tail of epididymis
Dartos fascia and muscle
Scrotum
Glans penis
©AHIMA

ction	**0**	**Medical and Surgical**
ody System	**V**	**Male Reproductive System**
peration	**1**	**Bypass:** Altering the route of passage of the contents of a tubular body part

Body Part (4th)	Approach (5th)	Device (6th)	Qualifier (7th)
N Vas Deferens, Right **P** Vas Deferens, Left **Q** Vas Deferens, Bilateral	**0** Open **4** Percutaneous Endoscopic	**7** Autologous Tissue Substitute **J** Synthetic Substitute **K** Nonautologous Tissue Substitute **Z** No Device	**J** Epididymis, Right **K** Epididymis, Left **N** Vas Deferens, Right **P** Vas Deferens, Left

ection	**0**	**Medical and Surgical**
ody System	**V**	**Male Reproductive System**
peration	**2**	**Change:** Taking out or off a device from a body part and putting back an identical or similar device in or on the same body part without cutting or puncturing the skin or a mucous membrane

Body Part (4th)	Approach (5th)	Device (6th)	Qualifier (7th)
4 Prostate and Seminal Vesicles **8** Scrotum and Tunica Vaginalis **D** Testis **M** Epididymis and Spermatic Cord **R** Vas Deferens **S** Penis	**X** External	**0** Drainage Device **Y** Other Device	**Z** No Qualifier

ection	**0**	**Medical and Surgical**
ody System	**V**	**Male Reproductive System**
peration	**5**	**Destruction:** Physical eradication of all or a portion of a body part by the direct use of energy, force, or a destructive agent

Body Part (4th)	Approach (5th)	Device (6th)	Qualifier (7th)
0 Prostate	**0** Open **3** Percutaneous **4** Percutaneous Endoscopic **7** Via Natural or Artificial Opening **8** Via Natural or Artificial Opening Endoscopic	**Z** No Device	**Z** No Qualifier
1 Seminal Vesicle, Right **2** Seminal Vesicle, Left **3** Seminal Vesicles, Bilateral **6** Tunica Vaginalis, Right **7** Tunica Vaginalis, Left **9** Testis, Right **B** Testis, Left **C** Testes, Bilateral	**0** Open **3** Percutaneous **4** Percutaneous Endoscopic	**Z** No Device	**Z** No Qualifier
5 Scrotum **S** Penis **T** Prepuce	**0** Open **3** Percutaneous **4** Percutaneous Endoscopic **X** External	**Z** No Device	**Z** No Qualifier
F Spermatic Cord, Right **G** Spermatic Cord, Left **H** Spermatic Cords, Bilateral **J** Epididymis, Right **K** Epididymis, Left **L** Epididymis, Bilateral **N** Vas Deferens, Right **P** Vas Deferens, Left **Q** Vas Deferens, Bilateral	**0** Open **3** Percutaneous **4** Percutaneous Endoscopic **8** Via Natural or Artificial Opening Endoscopic	**Z** No Device	**Z** No Qualifier

Section 0 **Medical and Surgical**
Body System V **Male Reproductive System**
Operation 7 **Dilation:** Expanding an orifice or the lumen of a tubular body part

Body Part (4th)	Approach (5th)	Device (6th)	Qualifier (7th)
N Vas Deferens, Right **P** Vas Deferens, Left **Q** Vas Deferens, Bilateral	**0** Open **3** Percutaneous **4** Percutaneous Endoscopic	**D** Intraluminal Device **Z** No Device	**Z** No Qualifier

Section 0 **Medical and Surgical**
Body System V **Male Reproductive System**
Operation 9 **Drainage:** Taking or letting out fluids and/or gases from a body part

Body Part (4th)	Approach (5th)	Device (6th)	Qualifier (7th)
0 Prostate	**0** Open **3** Percutaneous **4** Percutaneous Endoscopic **7** Via Natural or Artificial Opening **8** Via Natural or Artificial Opening Endoscopic	**0** Drainage Device	**Z** No Qualifier
0 Prostate	**0** Open **3** Percutaneous **4** Percutaneous Endoscopic **7** Via Natural or Artificial Opening **8** Via Natural or Artificial Opening Endoscopic	**Z** No Device	**X** Diagnostic **Z** No Qualifier
1 Seminal Vesicle, Right **2** Seminal Vesicle, Left **3** Seminal Vesicles, Bilateral **6** Tunica Vaginalis, Right **7** Tunica Vaginalis, Left **9** Testis, Right **B** Testis, Left **C** Testes, Bilateral **F** Spermatic Cord, Right **G** Spermatic Cord, Left **H** Spermatic Cords, Bilateral **J** Epididymis, Right **K** Epididymis, Left **L** Epididymis, Bilateral **N** Vas Deferens, Right **P** Vas Deferens, Left **Q** Vas Deferens, Bilateral	**0** Open **3** Percutaneous **4** Percutaneous Endoscopic	**0** Drainage Device	**Z** No Qualifier
1 Seminal Vesicle, Right **2** Seminal Vesicle, Left **3** Seminal Vesicles, Bilateral **6** Tunica Vaginalis, Right **7** Tunica Vaginalis, Left **9** Testis, Right **B** Testis, Left **C** Testes, Bilateral **F** Spermatic Cord, Right **G** Spermatic Cord, Left **H** Spermatic Cords, Bilateral **J** Epididymis, Right **K** Epididymis, Left **L** Epididymis, Bilateral **N** Vas Deferens, Right **P** Vas Deferens, Left **Q** Vas Deferens, Bilateral	**0** Open **3** Percutaneous **4** Percutaneous Endoscopic	**Z** No Device	**X** Diagnostic **Z** No Qualifier
5 Scrotum **S** Penis **T** Prepuce	**0** Open **3** Percutaneous **4** Percutaneous Endoscopic **X** External	**0** Drainage Device	**Z** No Qualifier

Continued →

tion	**0**	**Medical and Surgical**
dy System	**V**	**Male Reproductive System**
eration	**9**	**Drainage:** Taking or letting out fluids and/or gases from a body part

Body Part (4th)	Approach (5th)	Device (6th)	Qualifier (7th)
Scrotum Penis Prepuce	**0** Open **3** Percutaneous **4** Percutaneous Endoscopic **X** External	**Z** No Device	**X** Diagnostic **Z** No Qualifier

tion	**0**	**Medical and Surgical**
dy System	**V**	**Male Reproductive System**
eration	**B**	**Excision:** Cutting out or off, without replacement, a portion of a body part

Body Part (4th)	Approach (5th)	Device (6th)	Qualifier (7th)
Prostate	**0** Open **3** Percutaneous **4** Percutaneous Endoscopic **7** Via Natural or Artificial Opening **8** Via Natural or Artificial Opening Endoscopic	**Z** No Device	**X** Diagnostic **Z** No Qualifier
Seminal Vesicle, Right Seminal Vesicle, Left Seminal Vesicles, Bilateral Tunica Vaginalis, Right Tunica Vaginalis, Left Testis, Right Testis, Left Testes, Bilateral	**0** Open **3** Percutaneous **4** Percutaneous Endoscopic	**Z** No Device	**X** Diagnostic **Z** No Qualifier
Scrotum Penis Prepuce	**0** Open **3** Percutaneous **4** Percutaneous Endoscopic **X** External	**Z** No Device	**X** Diagnostic **Z** No Qualifier
Spermatic Cord, Right Spermatic Cord, Left Spermatic Cords, Bilateral Epididymis, Right Epididymis, Left Epididymis, Bilateral Vas Deferens, Right Vas Deferens, Left Vas Deferens, Bilateral	**0** Open **3** Percutaneous **4** Percutaneous Endoscopic **8** Via Natural or Artificial Opening Endoscopic	**Z** No Device	**X** Diagnostic **Z** No Qualifier

ction	**0**	**Medical and Surgical**
dy System	**V**	**Male Reproductive System**
eration	**C**	**Extirpation:** Taking or cutting out solid matter from a body part

Body Part (4th)	Approach (5th)	Device (6th)	Qualifier (7th)
Prostate	**0** Open **3** Percutaneous **4** Percutaneous Endoscopic **7** Via Natural or Artificial Opening **8** Via Natural or Artificial Opening Endoscopic	**Z** No Device	**Z** No Qualifier

Continued →

0VC Continued

Section 0 **Medical and Surgical**
Body System V **Male Reproductive System**
Operation C **Extirpation:** Taking or cutting out solid matter from a body part

Body Part (4th)	Approach (5th)	Device (6th)	Qualifier (7th)
1 Seminal Vesicle, Right **2** Seminal Vesicle, Left **3** Seminal Vesicles, Bilateral **6** Tunica Vaginalis, Right **7** Tunica Vaginalis, Left **9** Testis, Right **B** Testis, Left **C** Testes, Bilateral **F** Spermatic Cord, Right **G** Spermatic Cord, Left **H** Spermatic Cords, Bilateral **J** Epididymis, Right **K** Epididymis, Left **L** Epididymis, Bilateral **N** Vas Deferens, Right **P** Vas Deferens, Left **Q** Vas Deferens, Bilateral	**0** Open **3** Percutaneous **4** Percutaneous Endoscopic	**Z** No Device	**Z** No Qualifier
5 Scrotum **S** Penis **T** Prepuce	**0** Open **3** Percutaneous **4** Percutaneous Endoscopic **X** External	**Z** No Device	**Z** No Qualifier

Section 0 **Medical and Surgical**
Body System V **Male Reproductive System**
Operation H **Insertion:** Putting in a nonbiological appliance that monitors, assists, performs, or prevents a physiological function but does not physically take the place of a body part

Body Part (4th)	Approach (5th)	Device (6th)	Qualifier (7th)
0 Prostate	**0** Open **3** Percutaneous **4** Percutaneous Endoscopic **7** Via Natural or Artificial Opening **8** Via Natural or Artificial Opening Endoscopic	**1** Radioactive Element	**Z** No Qualifier
4 Prostate and Seminal Vesicles **8** Scrotum and Tunica Vaginalis **D** Testis **M** Epididymis and Spermatic Cord **R** Vas Deferens	**0** Open **3** Percutaneous **4** Percutaneous Endoscopic **7** Via Natural or Artificial Opening **8** Via Natural or Artificial Opening Endoscopic	**3** Infusion Device **Y** Other Device	**Z** No Qualifier
S Penis	**0** Open **3** Percutaneous **4** Percutaneous Endoscopic	**3** Infusion Device **Y** Other Device	**Z** No Qualifier
S Penis	**7** Via Natural or Artificial Opening **8** Via Natural or Artificial Opening Endoscopic	**Y** Other Device	**Z** No Qualifier
S Penis	**X** External	**3** Infusion Device	**Z** No Qualifier

tion	0	**Medical and Surgical**
ly System	V	**Male Reproductive System**
eration	J	**Inspection:** Visually and/or manually exploring a body part

Body Part (4th)	Approach (5th)	Device (6th)	Qualifier (7th)
Prostate and Seminal Vesicles Scrotum and Tunica Vaginalis Testis I Epididymis and Spermatic Cord Vas Deferens Penis	**0** Open **3** Percutaneous **4** Percutaneous Endoscopic **X** External	**Z** No Device	**Z** No Qualifier

tion	0	**Medical and Surgical**
dy System	V	**Male Reproductive System**
eration	L	**Occlusion:** Completely closing an orifice or the lumen of a tubular body part

Body Part (4th)	Approach (5th)	Device (6th)	Qualifier (7th)
Spermatic Cord, Right Spermatic Cord, Left Spermatic Cords, Bilateral Vas Deferens, Right Vas Deferens, Left Vas Deferens, Bilateral	**0** Open **3** Percutaneous **4** Percutaneous Endoscopic **8** Via Natural or Artificial Opening Endoscopic	**C** Extraluminal Device **D** Intraluminal Device **Z** No Device	**Z** No Qualifier

tion	0	**Medical and Surgical**
dy System	V	**Male Reproductive System**
eration	M	**Reattachment:** Putting back in or on all or a portion of a separated body part to its normal location or other suitable location

Body Part (4th)	Approach (5th)	Device (6th)	Qualifier (7th)
Scrotum Penis	**X** External	**Z** No Device	**Z** No Qualifier
Tunica Vaginalis, Right Tunica Vaginalis, Left Testis, Right B Testis, Left C Testes, Bilateral Spermatic Cord, Right Spermatic Cord, Left I Spermatic Cords, Bilateral	**0** Open **4** Percutaneous Endoscopic	**Z** No Device	**Z** No Qualifier

ction	0	**Medical and Surgical**
dy System	V	**Male Reproductive System**
eration	N	**Release:** Freeing a body part from an abnormal physical constraint by cutting or by the use of force

Body Part (4th)	Approach (5th)	Device (6th)	Qualifier (7th)
Prostate	**0** Open **3** Percutaneous **4** Percutaneous Endoscopic **7** Via Natural or Artificial Opening **8** Via Natural or Artificial Opening Endoscopic	**Z** No Device	**Z** No Qualifier
Seminal Vesicle, Right 2 Seminal Vesicle, Left 3 Seminal Vesicles, Bilateral 6 Tunica Vaginalis, Right 7 Tunica Vaginalis, Left 9 Testis, Right B Testis, Left C Testes, Bilateral	**0** Open **3** Percutaneous **4** Percutaneous Endoscopic	**Z** No Device	**Z** No Qualifier

Continued →

0VN Continued

Section 0 **Medical and Surgical**
Body System V **Male Reproductive System**
Operation N **Release:** Freeing a body part from an abnormal physical constraint by cutting or by the use of force

Body Part (4th)	Approach (5th)	Device (6th)	Qualifier (7th)
5 Scrotum **S** Penis **T** Prepuce	**0** Open **3** Percutaneous **4** Percutaneous Endoscopic **X** External	**Z** No Device	**Z** No Qualifier
F Spermatic Cord, Right **G** Spermatic Cord, Left **H** Spermatic Cords, Bilateral **J** Epididymis, Right **K** Epididymis, Left **L** Epididymis, Bilateral **N** Vas Deferens, Right **P** Vas Deferens, Left **Q** Vas Deferens, Bilateral	**0** Open **3** Percutaneous **4** Percutaneous Endoscopic **8** Via Natural or Artificial Opening Endoscopic	**Z** No Device	**Z** No Qualifier

Section 0 **Medical and Surgical**
Body System V **Male Reproductive System**
Operation P **Removal:** Taking out or off a device from a body part

Body Part (4th)	Approach (5th)	Device (6th)	Qualifier (7th)
4 Prostate and Seminal Vesicles	**0** Open **3** Percutaneous **4** Percutaneous Endoscopic **7** Via Natural or Artificial Opening **8** Via Natural or Artificial Opening Endoscopic	**0** Drainage Device **1** Radioactive Element **3** Infusion Device **7** Autologous Tissue Substitute **J** Synthetic Substitute **K** Nonautologous Tissue Substitute **Y** Other Device	**Z** No Qualifier
4 Prostate and Seminal Vesicles	**X** External	**0** Drainage Device **1** Radioactive Element **3** Infusion Device	**Z** No Qualifier
8 Scrotum and Tunica Vaginalis **D** Testis **S** Penis	**0** Open **3** Percutaneous **4** Percutaneous Endoscopic **7** Via Natural or Artificial Opening **8** Via Natural or Artificial Opening Endoscopic	**0** Drainage Device **3** Infusion Device **7** Autologous Tissue Substitute **J** Synthetic Substitute **K** Nonautologous Tissue Substitute **Y** Other Device	**Z** No Qualifier
8 Scrotum and Tunica Vaginalis **D** Testis **S** Penis	**X** External	**0** Drainage Device **3** Infusion Device	**Z** No Qualifier
M Epididymis and Spermatic Cord	**0** Open **3** Percutaneous **4** Percutaneous Endoscopic **7** Via Natural or Artificial Opening **8** Via Natural or Artificial Opening Endoscopic	**0** Drainage Device **3** Infusion Device **7** Autologous Tissue Substitute **C** Extraluminal Device **J** Synthetic Substitute **K** Nonautologous Tissue Substitute **Y** Other Device	**Z** No Qualifier
M Epididymis and Spermatic Cord	**X** External	**0** Drainage Device **3** Infusion Device	**Z** No Qualifier

Continued →

tion 0 **Medical and Surgical**
ly System V **Male Reproductive System**
eration P **Removal:** Taking out or off a device from a body part

Body Part (4th)	Approach (5th)	Device (6th)	Qualifier (7th)
Vas Deferens	**0** Open **3** Percutaneous **4** Percutaneous Endoscopic **7** Via Natural or Artificial Opening **8** Via Natural or Artificial Opening Endoscopic	**0** Drainage Device **3** Infusion Device **7** Autologous Tissue Substitute **C** Extraluminal Device **D** Intraluminal Device **J** Synthetic Substitute **K** Nonautologous Tissue Substitute **Y** Other Device	**Z** No Qualifier
Vas Deferens	**X** External	**0** Drainage Device **3** Infusion Device **D** Intraluminal Device	**Z** No Qualifier

tion 0 **Medical and Surgical**
dy System V **Male Reproductive System**
eration Q **Repair:** Restoring, to the extent possible, a body part to its normal anatomic structure and function

Body Part (4th)	Approach (5th)	Device (6th)	Qualifier (7th)
Prostate	**0** Open **3** Percutaneous **4** Percutaneous Endoscopic **7** Via Natural or Artificial Opening **8** Via Natural or Artificial Opening Endoscopic	**Z** No Device	**Z** No Qualifier
Seminal Vesicle, Right Seminal Vesicle, Left Seminal Vesicles, Bilateral Tunica Vaginalis, Right Tunica Vaginalis, Left Testis, Right Testis, Left Testes, Bilateral	**0** Open **3** Percutaneous **4** Percutaneous Endoscopic	**Z** No Device	**Z** No Qualifier
Scrotum Penis Prepuce	**0** Open **3** Percutaneous **4** Percutaneous Endoscopic **X** External	**Z** No Device	**Z** No Qualifier
Spermatic Cord, Right **G** Spermatic Cord, Left **H** Spermatic Cords, Bilateral Epididymis, Right **K** Epididymis, Left **L** Epididymis, Bilateral **N** Vas Deferens, Right **P** Vas Deferens, Left **Q** Vas Deferens, Bilateral	**0** Open **3** Percutaneous **4** Percutaneous Endoscopic **8** Via Natural or Artificial Opening Endoscopic	**Z** No Device	**Z** No Qualifier

ction 0 **Medical and Surgical**
dy System V **Male Reproductive System**
peration R **Replacement:** Putting in or on biological or synthetic material that physically takes the place and/or function of all or a portion of a body part

Body Part (4th)	Approach (5th)	Device (6th)	Qualifier (7th)
9 Testis, Right **B** Testis, Left **C** Testes, Bilateral	**0** Open	**J** Synthetic Substitute	**Z** No Qualifier

Section 0 **Medical and Surgical**
Body System V **Male Reproductive System**
Operation S **Reposition:** Moving to its normal location, or other suitable location, all or a portion of a body part

Body Part (4th)	Approach (5th)	Device (6th)	Qualifier (7th)
9 Testis, Right **B** Testis, Left **C** Testes, Bilateral **F** Spermatic Cord, Right **G** Spermatic Cord, Left **H** Spermatic Cords, Bilateral	**0** Open **3** Percutaneous **4** Percutaneous Endoscopic **8** Via Natural or Artificial Opening Endoscopic	**Z** No Device	**Z** No Qualifier

Section 0 **Medical and Surgical**
Body System V **Male Reproductive System**
Operation T **Resection:** Cutting out or off, without replacement, all of a body part

Body Part (4th)	Approach (5th)	Device (6th)	Qualifier (7th)
0 Prostate	**0** Open **4** Percutaneous Endoscopic **7** Via Natural or Artificial Opening **8** Via Natural or Artificial Opening Endoscopic	**Z** No Device	**Z** No Qualifier
1 Seminal Vesicle, Right **2** Seminal Vesicle, Left **3** Seminal Vesicles, Bilateral **6** Tunica Vaginalis, Right **7** Tunica Vaginalis, Left **9** Testis, Right **B** Testis, Left **C** Testes, Bilateral **F** Spermatic Cord, Right **G** Spermatic Cord, Left **H** Spermatic Cords, Bilateral **J** Epididymis, Right **K** Epididymis, Left **L** Epididymis, Bilateral **N** Vas Deferens, Right **P** Vas Deferens, Left **Q** Vas Deferens, Bilateral	**0** Open **4** Percutaneous Endoscopic	**Z** No Device	**Z** No Qualifier
5 Scrotum **S** Penis **T** Prepuce	**0** Open **4** Percutaneous Endoscopic **X** External	**Z** No Device	**Z** No Qualifier

Section 0 **Medical and Surgical**
Body System V **Male Reproductive System**
Operation U **Supplement:** Putting in or on biological or synthetic material that physically reinforces and/or augments the function of portion of a body part

Body Part (4th)	Approach (5th)	Device (6th)	Qualifier (7th)
1 Seminal Vesicle, Right **2** Seminal Vesicle, Left **3** Seminal Vesicles, Bilateral **6** Tunica Vaginalis, Right **7** Tunica Vaginalis, Left **F** Spermatic Cord, Right **G** Spermatic Cord, Left **H** Spermatic Cords, Bilateral **J** Epididymis, Right **K** Epididymis, Left **L** Epididymis, Bilateral **N** Vas Deferens, Right **P** Vas Deferens, Left **Q** Vas Deferens, Bilateral	**0** Open **4** Percutaneous Endoscopic **8** Via Natural or Artificial Opening Endoscopic	**7** Autologous Tissue Substitute **J** Synthetic Substitute **K** Nonautologous Tissue Substitute	**Z** No Qualifier

Continued →

ion	**0**	**Medical and Surgical**
y System	**V**	**Male Reproductive System**
ration	**U**	**Supplement:** Putting in or on biological or synthetic material that physically reinforces and/or augments the function of a portion of a body part

Body Part (4th)	Approach (5th)	Device (6th)	Qualifier (7th)
Scrotum Penis Prepuce	**0** Open **4** Percutaneous Endoscopic **X** External	**7** Autologous Tissue Substitute **J** Synthetic Substitute **K** Nonautologous Tissue Substitute	**Z** No Qualifier
Testis, Right Testis, Left Testes, Bilateral	**0** Open	**7** Autologous Tissue Substitute **J** Synthetic Substitute **K** Nonautologous Tissue Substitute	**Z** No Qualifier

tion	**0**	**Medical and Surgical**
y System	**V**	**Male Reproductive System**
eration	**W**	**Revision:** Correcting, to the extent possible, a portion of a malfunctioning device or the position of a displaced device

Body Part (4th)	Approach (5th)	Device (6th)	Qualifier (7th)
Prostate and Seminal Vesicles Scrotum and Tunica Vaginalis Testis Penis	**0** Open **3** Percutaneous **4** Percutaneous Endoscopic **7** Via Natural or Artificial Opening **8** Via Natural or Artificial Opening Endoscopic	**0** Drainage Device **3** Infusion Device **7** Autologous Tissue Substitute **J** Synthetic Substitute **K** Nonautologous Tissue Substitute **Y** Other Device	**Z** No Qualifier
Prostate and Seminal Vesicles Scrotum and Tunica Vaginalis Testis Penis	**X** External	**0** Drainage Device **3** Infusion Device **7** Autologous Tissue Substitute **J** Synthetic Substitute **K** Nonautologous Tissue Substitute	**Z** No Qualifier
Epididymis and Spermatic Cord	**0** Open **3** Percutaneous **4** Percutaneous Endoscopic **7** Via Natural or Artificial Opening **8** Via Natural or Artificial Opening Endoscopic	**0** Drainage Device **3** Infusion Device **7** Autologous Tissue Substitute **C** Extraluminal Device **J** Synthetic Substitute **K** Nonautologous Tissue Substitute **Y** Other Device	**Z** No Qualifier
Epididymis and Spermatic Cord	**X** External	**0** Drainage Device **3** Infusion Device **7** Autologous Tissue Substitute **C** Extraluminal Device **J** Synthetic Substitute **K** Nonautologous Tissue Substitute	**Z** No Qualifier
Vas Deferens	**0** Open **3** Percutaneous **4** Percutaneous Endoscopic **7** Via Natural or Artificial Opening **8** Via Natural or Artificial Opening Endoscopic	**0** Drainage Device **3** Infusion Device **7** Autologous Tissue Substitute **C** Extraluminal Device **D** Intraluminal Device **J** Synthetic Substitute **K** Nonautologous Tissue Substitute **Y** Other Device	**Z** No Qualifier
Vas Deferens	**X** External	**0** Drainage Device **3** Infusion Device **7** Autologous Tissue Substitute **C** Extraluminal Device **C** Intraluminal Device **J** Synthetic Substitute **K** Nonautologous Tissue Substitute	**Z** No Qualifier

Section **0** **Medical and Surgical**
Body System **V** **Male Reproductive System**
Operation **X** **Transfer:** Moving, without taking out, all or a portion of a body part to another location to take over the function of all portion of a body part

Body Part (4th)	Approach (5th)	Device (6th)	Qualifier (7th)
T Prepuce	**0** Open **X** External	**Z** No Device	**D** Urethra **S** Penis

AHA Coding Clinic

0VBQ4ZZ Excision of Bilateral Vas Deferens, Percutaneous Endoscopic Approach—AHA CC: 4Q, 2014, 33-34; 1Q, 2016, 23
0VPS0JZ Removal of Synthetic Substitute from Penis, Open Approach—AHA CC: 2Q, 2016, 28-29
0VT04ZZ Resection of Prostate, Percutaneous Endoscopic Approach— AHA CC: 4Q, 2014, 33-34
0VT34ZZ Resection of Bilateral Seminal Vesicles, Percutaneous Endoscopic Approach—AHA CC: 4Q, 2014, 33-34
0VUS0JZ Supplement Penis with Synthetic Substitute, Open Approach—AHA CC: 3Q, 2015, 25; 2Q, 2016, 28-29

Body Cavities

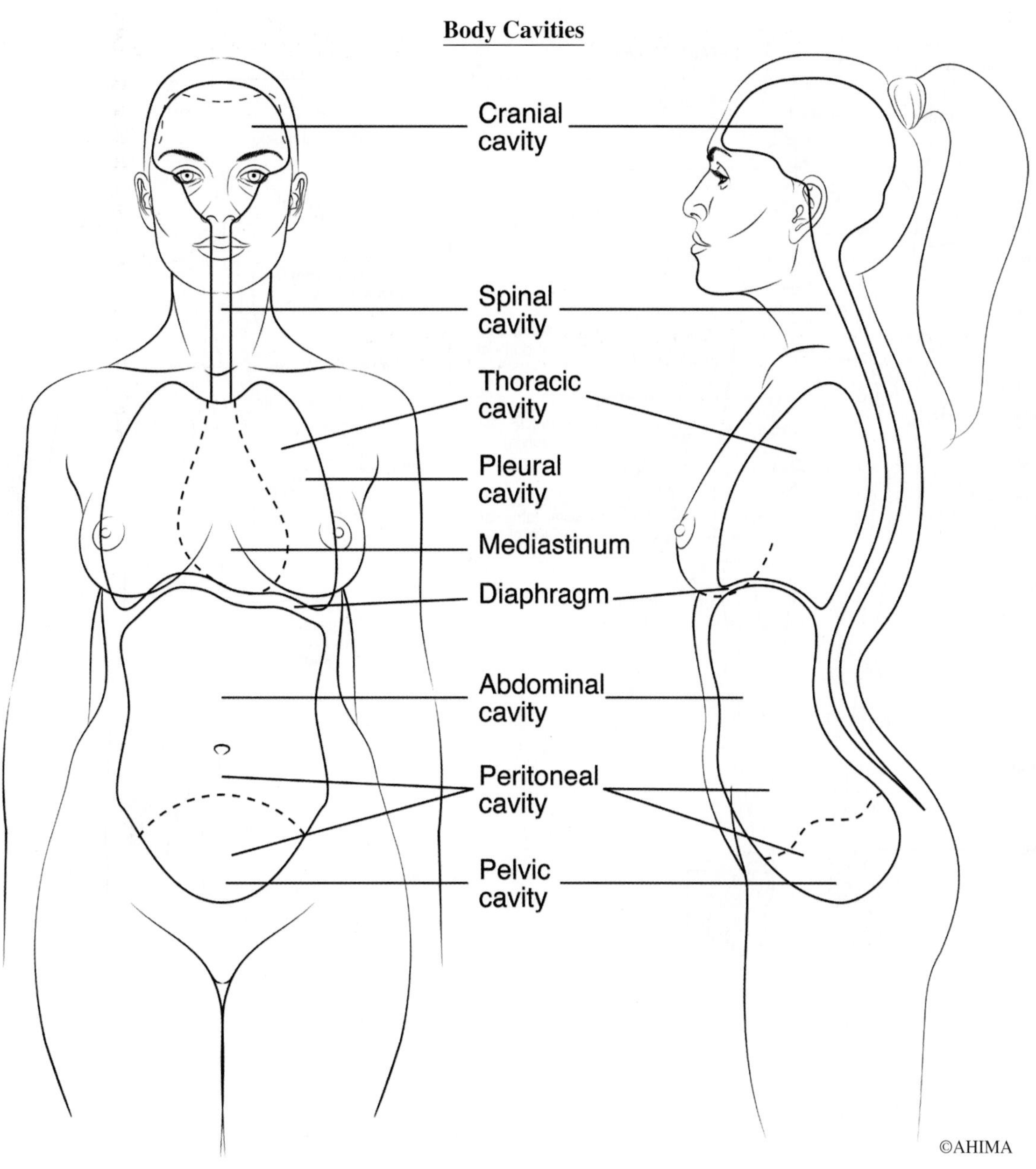

Body Areas

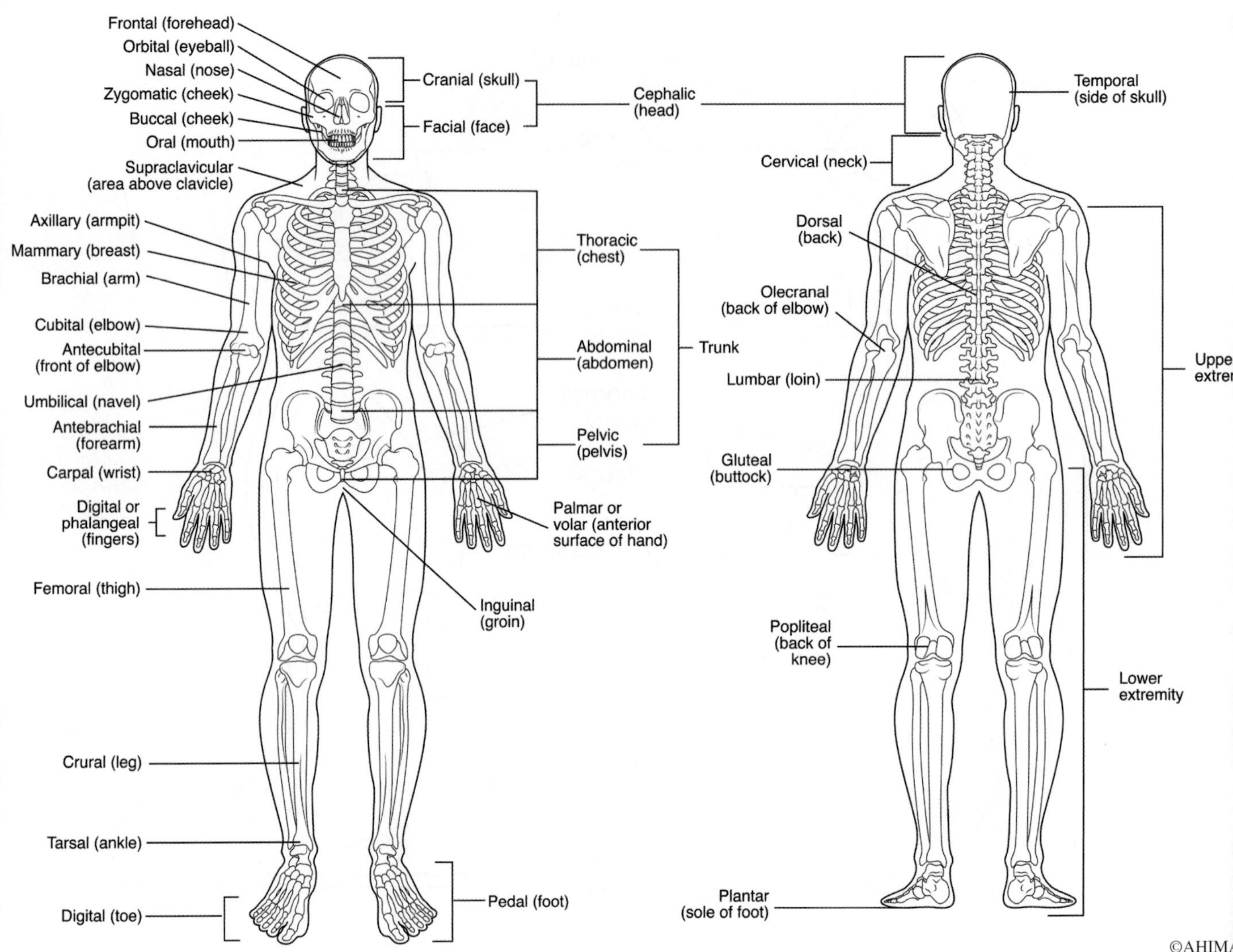

Frontal (forehead)
Orbital (eyeball)
Nasal (nose)
Zygomatic (cheek)
Buccal (cheek)
Oral (mouth)
Supraclavicular (area above clavicle)
Axillary (armpit)
Mammary (breast)
Brachial (arm)
Cubital (elbow)
Antecubital (front of elbow)
Umbilical (navel)
Antebrachial (forearm)
Carpal (wrist)
Digital or phalangeal (fingers)
Femoral (thigh)
Crural (leg)
Tarsal (ankle)
Digital (toe)
Cranial (skull)
Facial (face)
Cephalic (head)
Thoracic (chest)
Abdominal (abdomen)
Trunk
Pelvic (pelvis)
Palmar or volar (anterior surface of hand)
Inguinal (groin)
Pedal (foot)
Temporal (side of skull)
Cervical (neck)
Dorsal (back)
Olecranal (back of elbow)
Lumbar (loin)
Gluteal (buttock)
Popliteal (back of knee)
Plantar (sole of foot)
Lower extremity

Peritoneum of Posterior Abdominal Wall

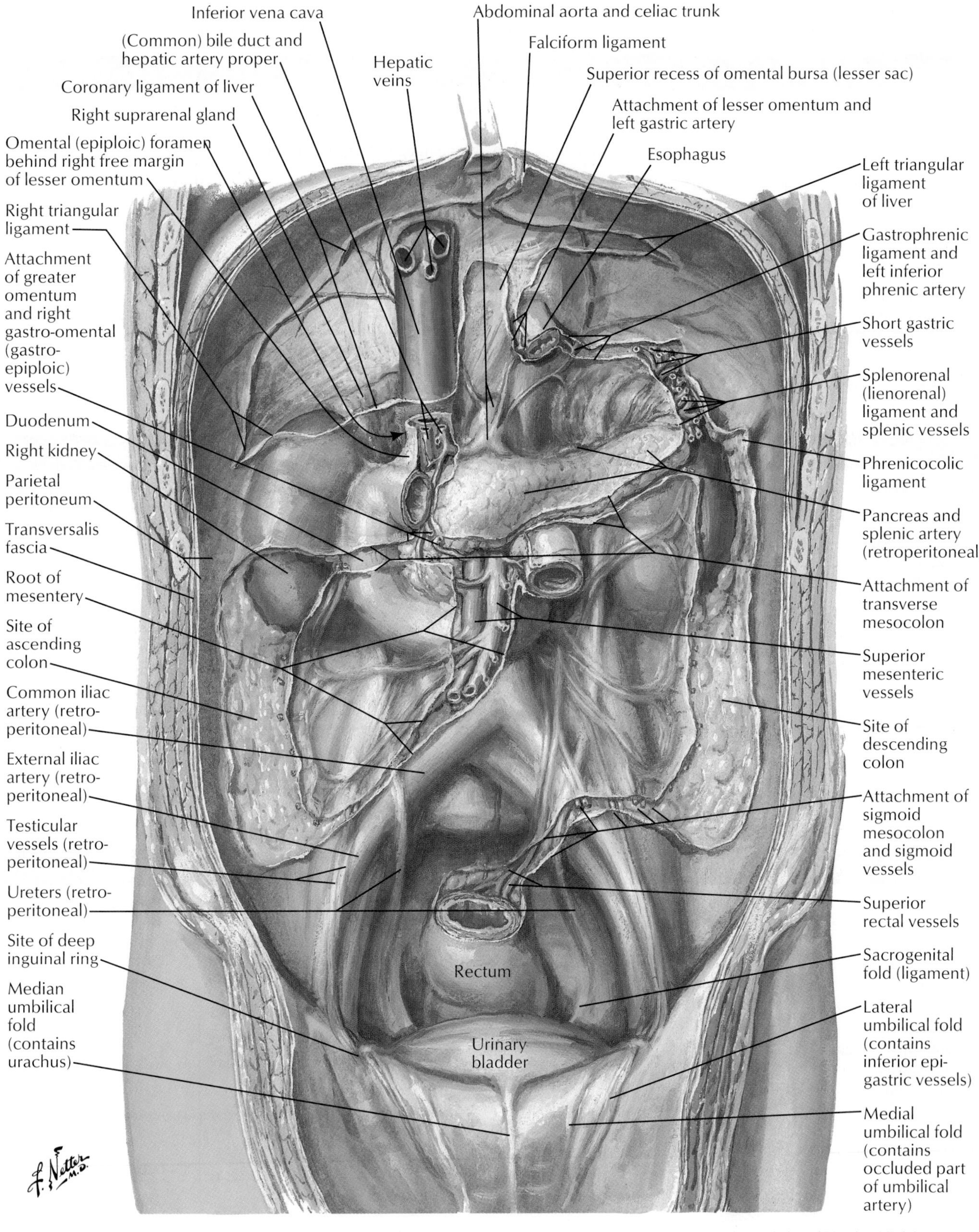

Anatomical Regions, General Tables 0W0–0WY

Section 0 **Medical and Surgical**
Body System W **Anatomical Regions, General**
Operation 0 **Alteration:** Modifying the anatomic structure of a body part without affecting the function of the body part

Body Part (4th)	Approach (5th)	Device (6th)	Qualifier (7th)
0 Head **2** Face **4** Upper Jaw **5** Lower Jaw **6** Neck **8** Chest Wall **F** Abdominal Wall **K** Upper Back **L** Lower Back **M** Perineum, Male **N** Perineum, Female	**0** Open **3** Percutaneous **4** Percutaneous Endoscopic	**7** Autologous Tissue Substitute **J** Synthetic Substitute **K** Nonautologous Tissue Substitute **Z** No Device	**Z** No Qualifier

Section 0 **Medical and Surgical**
Body System W **Anatomical Regions, General**
Operation 1 **Bypass:** Altering the route of passage of the contents of a tubular body part

Body Part (4th)	Approach (5th)	Device (6th)	Qualifier (7th)
1 Cranial Cavity	**0** Open	**J** Synthetic Substitute	**9** Pleural Cavity, Right **B** Pleural Cavity, Left **G** Peritoneal Cavity **J** Pelvic Cavity
9 Pleural Cavity, Right **B** Pleural Cavity, Left **G** Peritoneal Cavity **J** Pelvic Cavity	**0** Open **3** Percutaneous **4** Percutaneous Endoscopic	**J** Synthetic Substitute	**4** Cutaneous **9** Pleural Cavity, Right **B** Pleural Cavity, Left **G** Peritoneal Cavity **J** Pelvic Cavity **W** Upper Vein **Y** Lower Vein

Section 0 **Medical and Surgical**
Body System W **Anatomical Regions, General**
Operation 2 **Change:** Taking out or off a device from a body part and putting back an identical or similar device in or on the same body part without cutting or puncturing the skin or a mucous membrane

Body Part (4th)	Approach (5th)	Device (6th)	Qualifier (7th)
0 Head **1** Cranial Cavity **2** Face **4** Upper Jaw **5** Lower Jaw **6** Neck **8** Chest Wall **9** Pleural Cavity, Right **B** Pleural Cavity, Left **C** Mediastinum **D** Pericardial Cavity **F** Abdominal Wall **G** Peritoneal Cavity **H** Retroperitoneum **J** Pelvic Cavity **K** Upper Back **L** Lower Back **M** Perineum, Male **N** Perineum, Female	**X** External	**0** Drainage Device **Y** Other Device	**Z** No Qualifier

Section 0 Medical and Surgical
Body System W Anatomical Regions, General
Operation 3 **Control:** Stopping, or attempting to stop, postprocedural or other acute bleeding

Body Part (4th)	Approach (5th)	Device (6th)	Qualifier (7th)
0 Head **1** Cranial Cavity **2** Face **4** Upper Jaw **5** Lower Jaw **6** Neck **8** Chest Wall **9** Pleural Cavity, Right **B** Pleural Cavity, Left **C** Mediastinum **D** Pericardial Cavity **F** Abdominal Wall **G** Peritoneal Cavity **H** Retroperitoneum **J** Pelvic Cavity **K** Upper Back **L** Lower Back **M** Perineum, Male **N** Perineum, Female	**0** Open **3** Percutaneous **4** Percutaneous Endoscopic	**Z** No Device	**Z** No Qualifier
3 Oral Cavity and Throat	**0** Open **3** Percutaneous **4** Percutaneous Endoscopic **7** Via Natural or Artificial Opening **8** Via Natural or Artificial Opening Endoscopic **X** External	**Z** No Device	**Z** No Qualifier
P Gastrointestinal Tract **Q** Respiratory Tract **R** Genitourinary Tract	**0** Open **3** Percutaneous **4** Percutaneous Endoscopic **7** Via Natural or Artificial Opening **8** Via Natural or Artificial Opening Endoscopic	**Z** No Device	**Z** No Qualifier

Section 0 Medical and Surgical
Body System W Anatomical Regions, General
Operation 4 **Creation:** Putting in or on biological or synthetic material to form a new body part that to the extent possible replicates the anatomic structure or function of an absent body part

Body Part (4th)	Approach (5th)	Device (6th)	Qualifier (7th)
M Perineum, Male	**0** Open	**7** Autologous Tissue Substitute **J** Synthetic Substitute **K** Nonautologous Tissue Substitute	**0** Vagina
N Perineum, Female	**0** Open	**7** Autologous Tissue Substitute **J** Synthetic Substitute **K** Nonautologous Tissue Substitute	**1** Penis

Section 0 Medical and Surgical
Body System W Anatomical Regions, General
Operation 8 **Division:** Cutting into a body part, without draining fluids and/or gases from the body part, in order to separate or transect a body part

Body Part (4th)	Approach (5th)	Device (6th)	Qualifier (7th)
N Perineum, Female	**X** External	**Z** No Device	**Z** No Qualifier

Section 0 **Medical and Surgical**
Body System W **Anatomical Regions, General**
Operation 9 **Drainage:** Taking or letting out fluids and/or gases from a body part

Body Part (4th)	Approach (5th)	Device (6th)	Qualifier (7th)
0 Head **1** Cranial Cavity **2** Face **3** Oral Cavity and Throat **4** Upper Jaw **5** Lower Jaw **6** Neck **8** Chest Wall **9** Pleural Cavity, Right **B** Pleural Cavity, Left **C** Mediastinum **D** Pericardial Cavity **F** Abdominal Wall **G** Peritoneal Cavity **H** Retroperitoneum **J** Pelvic Cavity **K** Upper Back **L** Lower Back **M** Perineum, Male **N** Perineum, Female	**0** Open **3** Percutaneous **4** Percutaneous Endoscopic	**0** Drainage Device	**Z** No Qualifier
0 Head **1** Cranial Cavity **2** Face **3** Oral Cavity and Throat **4** Upper Jaw **5** Lower Jaw **6** Neck **8** Chest Wall **9** Pleural Cavity, Right **B** Pleural Cavity, Left **C** Mediastinum **D** Pericardial Cavity **F** Abdominal Wall **G** Peritoneal Cavity **H** Retroperitoneum **J** Pelvic Cavity **K** Upper Back **L** Lower Back **M** Perineum, Male **N** Perineum, Female	**0** Open **3** Percutaneous **4** Percutaneous Endoscopic	**Z** No Device	**X** Diagnostic **Z** No Qualifier

Section 0 **Medical and Surgical**
Body System W **Anatomical Regions, General**
Operation B **Excision:** Cutting out or off, without replacement, a portion of a body part

Body Part (4th)	Approach (5th)	Device (6th)	Qualifier (7th)
0 Head **2** Face **3** Oral Cavity and Throat **4** Upper Jaw **5** Lower Jaw **8** Chest Wall **K** Upper Back **L** Lower Back **M** Perineum, Male **N** Perineum, Female	**0** Open **3** Percutaneous **4** Percutaneous Endoscopic **X** External	**Z** No Device	**X** Diagnostic **Z** No Qualifier

Continued →

ection 0 **Medical and Surgical**
ody System W **Anatomical Regions, General**
peration B **Excision:** Cutting out or off, without replacement, a portion of a body part

Body Part (4th)	Approach (5th)	Device (6th)	Qualifier (7th)
6 Neck **F** Abdominal Wall	**0** Open **3** Percutaneous **4** Percutaneous Endoscopic	**Z** No Device	**X** Diagnostic **Z** No Qualifier
6 Neck **F** Abdominal Wall	**X** External	**Z** No Device	**2** Stoma **X** Diagnostic **Z** No Qualifier
C Mediastinum **H** Retroperitoneum	**0** Open **3** Percutaneous **4** Percutaneous Endoscopic	**Z** No Device	**X** Diagnostic **Z** No Qualifier

ection 0 **Medical and Surgical**
ody System W **Anatomical Regions, General**
peration C **Extirpation:** Taking or cutting out solid matter from a body part

Body Part (4th)	Approach (5th)	Device (6th)	Qualifier (7th)
1 Cranial Cavity **3** Oral Cavity and Throat **9** Pleural Cavity, Right **B** Pleural Cavity, Left **C** Mediastinum **D** Pericardial Cavity **G** Peritoneal Cavity **H** Retroperitoneum **J** Pelvic Cavity	**0** Open **3** Percutaneous **4** Percutaneous Endoscopic **X** External	**Z** No Device	**Z** No Qualifier
P Gastrointestinal Tract **Q** Respiratory Tract **R** Genitourinary Tract	**0** Open **3** Percutaneous **4** Percutaneous Endoscopic **7** Via Natural or Artificial Opening **8** Via Natural or Artificial Opening Endoscopic **X** External	**Z** No Device	**Z** No Qualifier

ection 0 **Medical and Surgical**
ody System W **Anatomical Regions, General**
peration F **Fragmentation:** Breaking solid matter in a body part into pieces

Body Part (4th)	Approach (5th)	Device (6th)	Qualifier (7th)
1 Cranial Cavity **3** Oral Cavity and Throat **9** Pleural Cavity, Right **B** Pleural Cavity, Left **C** Mediastinum **D** Pericardial Cavity **G** Peritoneal Cavity **J** Pelvic Cavity	**0** Open **3** Percutaneous **4** Percutaneous Endoscopic **X** External	**Z** No Device	**Z** No Qualifier
P Gastrointestinal Tract **Q** Respiratory Tract **R** Genitourinary Tract	**0** Open **3** Percutaneous **4** Percutaneous Endoscopic **7** Via Natural or Artificial Opening **8** Via Natural or Artificial Opening Endoscopic **X** External	**Z** No Device	**Z** No Qualifier

Section 0 **Medical and Surgical**
Body System W **Anatomical Regions, General**
Operation H **Insertion:** Putting in a nonbiological appliance that monitors, assists, performs, or prevents a physiological function but does not physically take the place of a body part

Body Part (4th)	Approach (5th)	Device (6th)	Qualifier (7th)
0 Head **1** Cranial Cavity **2** Face **3** Oral Cavity and Throat **4** Upper Jaw **5** Lower Jaw **6** Neck **8** Chest Wall **9** Pleural Cavity, Right **B** Pleural Cavity, Left **C** Mediastinum **D** Pericardial Cavity **F** Abdominal Wall **G** Peritoneal Cavity **H** Retroperitoneum **J** Pelvic Cavity **K** Upper Back **L** Lower Back **M** Perineum, Male **N** Perineum, Female	**0** Open **3** Percutaneous **4** Percutaneous Endoscopic	**1** Radioactive Element **3** Infusion Device **Y** Other Device	**Z** No Qualifier
P Gastrointestinal Tract **Q** Respiratory Tract **R** Genitourinary Tract	**0** Open **3** Percutaneous **4** Percutaneous Endoscopic **7** Via Natural or Artificial Opening **8** Via Natural or Artificial Opening Endoscopic	**1** Radioactive Element **3** Infusion Device **Y** Other Device	**Z** No Qualifier

Section 0 **Medical and Surgical**
Body System W **Anatomical Regions, General**
Operation J **Inspection:** Visually and/or manually exploring a body part

Body Part (4th)	Approach (5th)	Device (6th)	Qualifier (7th)
0 Head **2** Face **3** Oral Cavity and Throat **4** Upper Jaw **5** Lower Jaw **6** Neck **8** Chest Wall **F** Abdominal Wall **K** Upper Back **L** Lower Back **M** Perineum, Male **N** Perineum, Female	**0** Open **3** Percutaneous **4** Percutaneous Endoscopic **X** External	**Z** No Device	**Z** No Qualifier
1 Cranial Cavity **9** Pleural Cavity, Right **B** Pleural Cavity, Left **C** Mediastinum **D** Pericardial Cavity **G** Peritoneal Cavity **H** Retroperitoneum **J** Pelvic Cavity	**0** Open **3** Percutaneous **4** Percutaneous Endoscopic	**Z** No Device	**Z** No Qualifier
P Gastrointestinal Tract **Q** Respiratory Tract **R** Genitourinary Tract	**0** Open **3** Percutaneous **4** Percutaneous Endoscopic **7** Via Natural or Artificial Opening **8** Via Natural or Artificial Opening Endoscopic	**Z** No Device	**Z** No Qualifier

Section	**0**	**Medical and Surgical**
Body System	**W**	**Anatomical Regions, General**
Operation	**M**	**Reattachment:** Putting back in or on all or a portion of a separated body part to its normal location or other suitable location

Body Part (4th)	Approach (5th)	Device (6th)	Qualifier (7th)
2 Face 4 Upper Jaw 5 Lower Jaw 6 Neck 8 Chest Wall F Abdominal Wall K Upper Back L Lower Back M Perineum, Male N Perineum, Female	**0** Open	**Z** No Device	**Z** No Qualifier

Section	**0**	**Medical and Surgical**
Body System	**W**	**Anatomical Regions, General**
Operation	**P**	**Removal:** Taking out or off a device from a body part

Body Part (4th)	Approach (5th)	Device (6th)	Qualifier (7th)
0 Head 2 Face 4 Upper Jaw 5 Lower Jaw 6 Neck 8 Chest Wall C Mediastinum F Abdominal Wall K Upper Back L Lower Back M Perineum, Male N Perineum, Female	**0** Open **3** Percutaneous **4** Percutaneous Endoscopic **X** External	**0** Drainage Device **1** Radioactive Element **3** Infusion Device **7** Autologous Tissue Substitute **J** Synthetic Substitute **K** Nonautologous Tissue Substitute **Y** Other Device	**Z** No Qualifier
1 Cranial Cavity 9 Pleural Cavity, Right B Pleural Cavity, Left G Peritoneal Cavity J Pelvic Cavity	**0** Open **3** Percutaneous **4** Percutaneous Endoscopic	**0** Drainage Device **1** Radioactive Element **3** Infusion Device **J** Synthetic Substitute **Y** Other Device	**Z** No Qualifier
1 Cranial Cavity 9 Pleural Cavity, Right B Pleural Cavity, Left G Peritoneal Cavity J Pelvic Cavity	**X** External	**0** Drainage Device **1** Radioactive Element **3** Infusion Device	**Z** No Qualifier
D Pericardial Cavity H Retroperitoneum	**0** Open **3** Percutaneous **4** Percutaneous Endoscopic	**0** Drainage Device **1** Radioactive Element **3** Infusion Device **Y** Other Device	**Z** No Qualifier
D Pericardial Cavity H Retroperitoneum	**X** External	**0** Drainage Device **1** Radioactive Element **3** Infusion Device	**Z** No Qualifier
P Gastrointestinal Tract Q Respiratory Tract R Genitourinary Tract	**0** Open **3** Percutaneous **4** Percutaneous Endoscopic **7** Via Natural or Artificial Opening **8** Via Natural or Artificial Opening Endoscopic **X** External	**1** Radioactive Element **3** Infusion Device **Y** Other Device	**Z** No Qualifier

Section 0 **Medical and Surgical**
Body System W **Anatomical Regions, General**
Operation Q **Repair:** Restoring, to the extent possible, a body part to its normal anatomic structure and function

Body Part (4th)	Approach (5th)	Device (6th)	Qualifier (7th)
0 Head **2** Face **3** Oral Cavity and Throat **4** Upper Jaw **5** Lower Jaw **8** Chest Wall **K** Upper Back **L** Lower Back **M** Perineum, Male **N** Perineum, Female	**0** Open **3** Percutaneous **4** Percutaneous Endoscopic **X** External	**Z** No Device	**Z** No Qualifier
6 Neck **F** Abdominal Wall	**0** Open **3** Percutaneous **4** Percutaneous Endoscopic	**Z** No Device	**Z** No Qualifier
6 Neck **F** Abdominal Wall	**X** External	**Z** No Device	**2** Stoma **Z** No Qualifier
C Mediastinum	**0** Open **3** Percutaneous **4** Percutaneous Endoscopic	**Z** No Device	**Z** No Qualifier

Section 0 **Medical and Surgical**
Body System W **Anatomical Regions, General**
Operation U **Supplement:** Putting in or on biological or synthetic material that physically reinforces and/or augments the function of portion of a body part

Body Part (4th)	Approach (5th)	Device (6th)	Qualifier (7th)
0 Head **2** Face **4** Upper Jaw **5** Lower Jaw **6** Neck **8** Chest Wall **C** Mediastinum **F** Abdominal Wall **K** Upper Back **L** Lower Back **M** Perineum, Male **N** Perineum, Female	**0** Open **4** Percutaneous Endoscopic	**7** Autologous Tissue Substitute **J** Synthetic Substitute **K** Nonautologous Tissue Substitute	**Z** No Qualifier

Section 0 **Medical and Surgical**
Body System W **Anatomical Regions, General**
Operation W **Revision:** Correcting, to the extent possible, a portion of a malfunctioning device or the position of a displaced device

Body Part (4th)	Approach (5th)	Device (6th)	Qualifier (7th)
0 Head **2** Face **4** Upper Jaw **5** Lower Jaw **6** Neck **8** Chest Wall **C** Mediastinum **F** Abdominal Wall **K** Upper Back **L** Lower Back **M** Perineum, Male **N** Perineum, Female	**0** Open **3** Percutaneous **4** Percutaneous Endoscopic **X** External	**0** Drainage Device **1** Radioactive Element **3** Infusion Device **7** Autologous Tissue Substitute **J** Synthetic Substitute **K** Nonautologous Tissue Substitute **Y** Other Device	**Z** No Qualifier

Continued →

ction 0 Medical and Surgical
dy System W Anatomical Regions, General
eration W Revision: Correcting, to the extent possible, a portion of a malfunctioning device or the position of a displaced device

Body Part (4th)	Approach (5th)	Device (6th)	Qualifier (7th)
Cranial Cavity Pleural Cavity, Right **B** Pleural Cavity, Left **G** Peritoneal Cavity Pelvic Cavity	**0** Open **3** Percutaneous **4** Percutaneous Endoscopic **X** External	**0** Drainage Device **1** Radioactive Element **3** Infusion Device **J** Synthetic Substitute **Y** Other Device	**Z** No Qualifier
D Pericardial Cavity **H** Retroperitoneum	**0** Open **3** Percutaneous **4** Percutaneous Endoscopic **X** External	**0** Drainage Device **1** Radioactive Element **3** Infusion Device **Y** Other Device	**Z** No Qualifier
P Gastrointestinal Tract **Q** Respiratory Tract **R** Genitourinary Tract	**0** Open **3** Percutaneous **4** Percutaneous Endoscopic **7** Via Natural or Artificial Opening **8** Via Natural or Artificial Opening Endoscopic **X** External	**1** Radioactive Element **3** Infusion Device **Y** Other Device	**Z** No Qualifier

ction 0 Medical and Surgical
dy System W Anatomical Regions, General
eration Y Transplantation: Putting in or on all or a portion of a living body part taken from another individual or animal to physically take the place and/or function of all or a portion of a similar body part

Body Part (4th)	Approach (5th)	Device (6th)	Qualifier (7th)
2 Face	**0** Open	**Z** No Device	**0** Allogeneic **1** Syngeneic

HA Coding Clinic

W020ZZ Alteration of Face, Open Approach—AHA CC: 1Q, 2015, 31

W1G3J4 Bypass Peritoneal Cavity to Cutaneous with Synthetic Substitute, Percutaneous Approach—AHA CC: 4Q, 2013, 126-127

W1G4J4 Bypass Peritoneal Cavity to Cutaneous with Synthetic Substitute, Percutaneous Endoscopic Approach—AHA CC: 2Q, 2015, 36

W3F0ZZ Control Bleeding in Abdominal Wall, Open Approach—AHA CC: 4Q, 2016, 100-101

W3P8ZZ Control Bleeding in Gastrointestinal Tract, Via Natural or Artificial Opening Endoscopic—AHA CC: 4Q, 2016, 99-100; 4Q, 2017, 105; 1Q, 2018, 19

W3Q7ZZ Control Bleeding in Respiratory Tract, Via Natural or Artificial Opening—AHA CC: 4Q, 2017, 106

W3Q8ZZ Control Bleeding in Respiratory Tract, Via Natural or Artificial Opening Endoscopic—AHA CC: 1Q, 2018, 19-20

W3R7ZZ Control Bleeding in Genitourinary Tract, Via Natural or Artificial Opening—AHA CC: 4Q, 2014, 44

W930ZZ Drainage of Oral Cavity and Throat, Open Approach—AHA CC: 2Q, 2017, 16-17

W9G3ZZ Drainage of Peritoneal Cavity, Percutaneous Approach—AHA CC: 3Q, 2017, 12-13

WBF4ZZ Excision of Abdominal Wall, Percutaneous Endoscopic Approach—AHA CC: 1Q, 2016, 21-22

WBNXZZ Excision of Female Perineum, External Approach—AHA CC: 4Q, 2013, 119-120

WC30ZZ Extirpation of Matter from Oral Cavity and Throat, Open Approach—AHA CC: 2Q, 2017, 16

WHG33Z Insertion of Infusion Device into Peritoneal Cavity, Percutaneous Approach—AHA CC: 2Q, 2015, 36; 2Q, 2016, 14

WJG4ZZ Inspection of Peritoneal Cavity, Percutaneous Endoscopic Approach—AHA CC: 2Q, 2013, 36-37

WJJ4ZZ Inspection of Pelvic Cavity, Percutaneous Endoscopic Approach—AHA CC: 4Q, 2016, 58-59

WQF0ZZ Repair Abdominal Wall, Open Approach—AHA CC: 4Q, 2014, 38-39; 3Q, 2014, 28-29; 3Q, 2016, 6; 3Q, 2017, 8-9

WU80JZ Supplement Chest Wall with Synthetic Substitute, Open Approach—AHA CC: 4Q, 2012, 101-102

WUF07Z Supplement Abdominal Wall with Autologous Tissue Substitute, Open Approach—AHA CC: 3Q, 2016, 40-41

WUF0JZ Supplement Abdominal Wall with Synthetic Substitute, Open Approach—AHA CC: 4Q, 2014, 39-40; 3Q, 2017, 8

WWG4JZ Revision of Synthetic Substitute in Peritoneal Cavity, Percutaneous Endoscopic Approach—AHA CC: 2Q, 2015, 9-10

Anatomical Regions, Upper Extremities

Anatomical Regions, Upper Extremities Tables 0X0–0XY

Section 0 **Medical and Surgical**
Body System X **Anatomical Regions, Upper Extremities**
Operation 0 **Alteration:** Modifying the anatomic structure of a body part without affecting the function of the body part

Body Part (4th)	Approach (5th)	Device (6th)	Qualifier (7th)
2 Shoulder Region, Right **3** Shoulder Region, Left **4** Axilla, Right **5** Axilla, Left **6** Upper Extremity, Right **7** Upper Extremity, Left **8** Upper Arm, Right **9** Upper Arm, Left **B** Elbow Region, Right **C** Elbow Region, Left **D** Lower Arm, Right **F** Lower Arm, Left **G** Wrist Region, Right **H** Wrist Region, Left	**0** Open **3** Percutaneous **4** Percutaneous Endoscopic	**7** Autologous Tissue Substitute **J** Synthetic Substitute **K** Nonautologous Tissue Substitute **Z** No Device	**Z** No Qualifier

Section 0 **Medical and Surgical**
Body System X **Anatomical Regions, Upper Extremities**
Operation 2 **Change:** Taking out or off a device from a body part and putting back an identical or similar device in or on the same bo part without cutting or puncturing the skin or a mucous membrane

Body Part (4th)	Approach (5th)	Device (6th)	Qualifier (7th)
6 Upper Extremity, Right **7** Upper Extremity, Left	**X** External	**0** Drainage Device **Y** Other Device	**Z** No Qualifier

Section 0 **Medical and Surgical**
Body System X **Anatomical Regions, Upper Extremities**
Operation 3 **Control:** Stopping, or attempting to stop, postprocedural or other acute bleeding

Body Part (4th)	Approach (5th)	Device (6th)	Qualifier (7th)
2 Shoulder Region, Right **3** Shoulder Region, Left **4** Axilla, Right **5** Axilla, Left **6** Upper Extremity, Right **7** Upper Extremity, Left **8** Upper Arm, Right **9** Upper Arm, Left **B** Elbow Region, Right **C** Elbow Region, Left **D** Lower Arm, Right **F** Lower Arm, Left **G** Wrist Region, Right **H** Wrist Region, Left **J** Hand, Right **K** Hand, Left	**0** Open **3** Percutaneous **4** Percutaneous Endoscopic	**Z** No Device	**Z** No Qualifier

tion	0	**Medical and Surgical**
dy System	X	**Anatomical Regions, Upper Extremities**
eration	6	**Detachment:** Cutting off all or a portion of the upper or lower extremities

Body Part (4th)	Approach (5th)	Device (6th)	Qualifier (7th)
Forequarter, Right Forequarter, Left Shoulder Region, Right Shoulder Region, Left Elbow Region, Right Elbow Region, Left	**0** Open	**Z** No Device	**Z** No Qualifier
Upper Arm, Right Upper Arm, Left Lower Arm, Right Lower Arm, Left	**0** Open	**Z** No Device	**1** High **2** Mid **3** Low
Hand, Right **K** Hand, Left	**0** Open	**Z** No Device	**0** Complete **4** Complete 1st Ray **5** Complete 2nd Ray **6** Complete 3rd Ray **7** Complete 4th Ray **8** Complete 5th Ray **9** Partial 1st Ray **B** Partial 2nd Ray **C** Partial 3rd Ray **D** Partial 4th Ray **F** Partial 5th Ray
L Thumb, Right **M** Thumb, Left **N** Index Finger, Right **P** Index Finger, Left **Q** Middle Finger, Right **R** Middle Finger, Left **S** Ring Finger, Right **T** Ring Finger, Left **V** Little Finger, Right **W** Little Finger, Left	**0** Open	**Z** No Device	**0** Complete **1** High **2** Mid **3** Low

ction	0	**Medical and Surgical**
dy System	X	**Anatomical Regions, Upper Extremities**
peration	9	**Drainage:** Taking or letting out fluids and/or gases from a body part

Body Part (4th)	Approach (5th)	Device (6th)	Qualifier (7th)
2 Shoulder Region, Right **3** Shoulder Region, Left **4** Axilla, Right **5** Axilla, Left **6** Upper Extremity, Right **7** Upper Extremity, Left **8** Upper Arm, Right **9** Upper Arm, Left **B** Elbow Region, Right **C** Elbow Region, Left **D** Lower Arm, Right **F** Lower Arm, Left **G** Wrist Region, Right **H** Wrist Region, Left **J** Hand, Right **K** Hand, Left	**0** Open **3** Percutaneous **4** Percutaneous Endoscopic	**0** Drainage Device	**Z** No Qualifier

Continued →

Section	**0**	**Medical and Surgical**
Body System	**X**	**Anatomical Regions, Upper Extremities**
Operation	**9**	**Drainage:** Taking or letting out fluids and/or gases from a body part

Body Part (4th)	Approach (5th)	Device (6th)	Qualifier (7th)
2 Shoulder Region, Right **3** Shoulder Region, Left **4** Axilla, Right **5** Axilla, Left **6** Upper Extremity, Right **7** Upper Extremity, Left **8** Upper Arm, Right **9** Upper Arm, Left **B** Elbow Region, Right **C** Elbow Region, Left **D** Lower Arm, Right **F** Lower Arm, Left **G** Wrist Region, Right **H** Wrist Region, Left **J** Hand, Right **K** Hand, Left	**0** Open **3** Percutaneous **4** Percutaneous Endoscopic	**Z** No Device	**X** Diagnostic **Z** No Qualifier

Section	**0**	**Medical and Surgical**
Body System	**X**	**Anatomical Regions, Upper Extremities**
Operation	**B**	**Excision:** Cutting out or off, without replacement, a portion of a body part

Body Part (4th)	Approach (5th)	Device (6th)	Qualifier (7th)
2 Shoulder Region, Right **3** Shoulder Region, Left **4** Axilla, Right **5** Axilla, Left **6** Upper Extremity, Right **7** Upper Extremity, Left **8** Upper Arm, Right **9** Upper Arm, Left **B** Elbow Region, Right **C** Elbow Region, Left **D** Lower Arm, Right **F** Lower Arm, Left **G** Wrist Region, Right **H** Wrist Region, Left **J** Hand, Right **K** Hand, Left	**0** Open **3** Percutaneous **4** Percutaneous Endoscopic	**Z** No Device	**X** Diagnostic **Z** No Qualifier

Section	**0**	**Medical and Surgical**
Body System	**X**	**Anatomical Regions, Upper Extremities**
Operation	**H**	**Insertion:** Putting in a nonbiological appliance that monitors, assists, performs, or prevents a physiological function but does not physically take the place of a body part

Body Part (4th)	Approach (5th)	Device (6th)	Qualifier (7th)
2 Shoulder Region, Right **3** Shoulder Region, Left **4** Axilla, Right **5** Axilla, Left **6** Upper Extremity, Right **7** Upper Extremity, Left **8** Upper Arm, Right **9** Upper Arm, Left **B** Elbow Region, Right **C** Elbow Region, Left **D** Lower Arm, Right **F** Lower Arm, Left **G** Wrist Region, Right **H** Wrist Region, Left **J** Hand, Right **K** Hand, Left	**0** Open **3** Percutaneous **4** Percutaneous Endoscopic	**1** Radioactive Element **3** Infusion Device **Y** Other Device	**Z** No Qualifier

tion **0 Medical and Surgical**
ly System **X Anatomical Regions, Upper Extremities**
eration **J Inspection:** Visually and/or manually exploring a body part

Body Part (4th)	Approach (5th)	Device (6th)	Qualifier (7th)
Shoulder Region, Right Shoulder Region, Left Axilla, Right Axilla, Left Upper Extremity, Right Upper Extremity, Left Upper Arm, Right Upper Arm, Left Elbow Region, Right Elbow Region, Left Lower Arm, Right Lower Arm, Left Wrist Region, Right Wrist Region, Left Hand, Right Hand, Left	**0** Open **3** Percutaneous **4** Percutaneous Endoscopic **X** External	**Z** No Device	**Z** No Qualifier

tion **0 Medical and Surgical**
dy System **X Anatomical Regions, Upper Extremities**
eration **M Reattachment:** Putting back in or on all or a portion of a separated body part to its normal location or other suitable location

Body Part (4th)	Approach (5th)	Device (6th)	Qualifier (7th)
Forequarter, Right Forequarter, Left Shoulder Region, Right Shoulder Region, Left Axilla, Right Axilla, Left Upper Extremity, Right Upper Extremity, Left Upper Arm, Right Upper Arm, Left Elbow Region, Right Elbow Region, Left Lower Arm, Right Lower Arm, Left Wrist Region, Right H Wrist Region, Left Hand, Right K Hand, Left L Thumb, Right M Thumb, Left N Index Finger, Right P Index Finger, Left Q Middle Finger, Right R Middle Finger, Left S Ring Finger, Right T Ring Finger, Left V Little Finger, Right W Little Finger, Left	**0** Open	**Z** No Device	**Z** No Qualifier

Section 0 **Medical and Surgical**
Body System X **Anatomical Regions, Upper Extremities**
Operation P **Removal:** Taking out or off a device from a body part

Body Part (4th)	Approach (5th)	Device (6th)	Qualifier (7th)
6 Upper Extremity, Right **7** Upper Extremity, Left	**0** Open **3** Percutaneous **4** Percutaneous Endoscopic **X** External	**0** Drainage Device **1** Radioactive Element **3** Infusion Device **7** Autologous Tissue Substitute **J** Synthetic Substitute **K** Nonautologous Tissue Substitute **Y** Other Device	**Z** No Qualifier

Section 0 **Medical and Surgical**
Body System X **Anatomical Regions, Upper Extremities**
Operation Q **Repair:** Restoring, to the extent possible, a body part to its normal anatomic structure and function

Body Part (4th)	Approach (5th)	Device (6th)	Qualifier (7th)
2 Shoulder Region, Right **3** Shoulder Region, Left **4** Axilla, Right **5** Axilla, Left **6** Upper Extremity, Right **7** Upper Extremity, Left **8** Upper Arm, Right **9** Upper Arm, Left **B** Elbow Region, Right **C** Elbow Region, Left **D** Lower Arm, Right **F** Lower Arm, Left **G** Wrist Region, Right **H** Wrist Region, Left **J** Hand, Right **K** Hand, Left **L** Thumb, Right **M** Thumb, Left **N** Index Finger, Right **P** Index Finger, Left **Q** Middle Finger, Right **R** Middle Finger, Left **S** Ring Finger, Right **T** Ring Finger, Left **V** Little Finger, Right **W** Little Finger, Left	**0** Open **3** Percutaneous **4** Percutaneous Endoscopic **X** External	**Z** No Device	**Z** No Qualifier

Section 0 **Medical and Surgical**
Body System X **Anatomical Regions, Upper Extremities**
Operation R **Replacement:** Putting in or on biological or synthetic material that physically takes the place and/or function of all or a portion of a body part

Body Part (4th)	Approach (5th)	Device (6th)	Qualifier (7th)
L Thumb, Right **M** Thumb, Left	**0** Open **4** Percutaneous Endoscopic	**7** Autologous Tissue Substitute	**N** Toe, Right **P** Toe, Left

tion **0** **Medical and Surgical**
dy System **X** **Anatomical Regions, Upper Extremities**
eration **U** **Supplement:** Putting in or on biological or synthetic material that physically reinforces and/or augments the function of a portion of a body part

Body Part (4th)	Approach (5th)	Device (6th)	Qualifier (7th)
Shoulder Region, Right Shoulder Region, Left Axilla, Right Axilla, Left Upper Extremity, Right Upper Extremity, Left Upper Arm, Right Upper Arm, Left Elbow Region, Right Elbow Region, Left Lower Arm, Right Lower Arm, Left Wrist Region, Right Wrist Region, Left Hand, Right Hand, Left Thumb, Right Thumb, Left Index Finger, Right Index Finger, Left Middle Finger, Right Middle Finger, Left Ring Finger, Right Ring Finger, Left Little Finger, Right V Little Finger, Left	**0** Open **4** Percutaneous Endoscopic	**7** Autologous Tissue Substitute **J** Synthetic Substitute **K** Nonautologous Tissue Substitute	**Z** No Qualifier

ction **0** **Medical and Surgical**
dy System **X** **Anatomical Regions, Upper Extremities**
eration **W** **Revision:** Correcting, to the extent possible, a portion of a malfunctioning device or the position of a displaced device

Body Part (4th)	Approach (5th)	Device (6th)	Qualifier (7th)
Upper Extremity, Right Upper Extremity, Left	**0** Open **3** Percutaneous **4** Percutaneous Endoscopic **X** External	**0** Drainage Device **3** Infusion Device **7** Autologous Tissue Substitute **J** Synthetic Substitute **K** Nonautologous Tissue Substitute **Y** Other Device	**Z** No Qualifier

ction **0** **Medical and Surgical**
dy System **X** **Anatomical Regions, Upper Extremities**
eration **X** **Transfer:** Moving, without taking out, all or a portion of a body part to another location to take over the function of all or a portion of a body part

Body Part (4th)	Approach (5th)	Device (6th)	Qualifier (7th)
Index Finger, Right	**0** Open	**Z** No Device	**L** Thumb, Right
Index Finger, Left	**0** Open	**Z** No Device	**M** Thumb, Left

ction **0** **Medical and Surgical**
dy System **X** **Anatomical Regions, Upper Extremities**
eration **Y** **Transplantation:** Putting in or on all or a portion of a living body part taken from another individual or animal to physically take the place and/or function of all or a portion of a similar body part

Body Part (4th)	Approach (5th)	Device (6th)	Qualifier (7th)
Hand, Right Hand, Left	**0** Open	**Z** No Device	**0** Allogeneic **1** Syngeneic

AHA Coding Clinic

0X370ZZ Control Bleeding in Left Upper Extremity, Open Approach—AHA CC: 1Q, 2015, 35

0X6M0Z3 Detachment at Left Thumb, Low, Open Approach—AHA CC: 3Q, 2016, 33-34; 1Q, 2017, 52

0X6T0Z3 Detachment at Left Ring Finger, Low, Open Approach—AHA CC: 3Q, 2016, 33-34; 1Q, 2017, 52

0X6V0Z0 Detachment at Right Little Finger, Complete, Open Approach—AHA CC: 2Q, 2017, 18-19

0X6W0Z3 Detachment at Left Little Finger, Low, Open Approach—AHA CC: 3Q, 2016, 33-34; 1Q, 2017, 52

0XH90YZ Insertion of Other Device into Left Upper Arm, Open Approach—AHA CC: 2Q, 2017, 20-21

0XP70YZ Removal of Other Device from Left Upper Extremity, Open Approach—AHA CC: 2Q, 2017, 20-21

natomical Regions, Lower Extremities 0Y0–0YW

tion	0	**Medical and Surgical**
dy System	Y	**Anatomical Regions, Lower Extremities**
eration	0	**Alteration:** Modifying the anatomic structure of a body part without affecting the function of the body part

Body Part (4th)	Approach (5th)	Device (6th)	Qualifier (7th)
Buttock, Right Buttock, Left Lower Extremity, Right Lower Extremity, Left Upper Leg, Right Upper Leg, Left Knee Region, Right Knee Region, Left Lower Leg, Right Lower Leg, Left Ankle Region, Right Ankle Region, Left	0 Open 3 Percutaneous 4 Percutaneous Endoscopic	7 Autologous Tissue Substitute J Synthetic Substitute K Nonautologous Tissue Substitute Z No Device	Z No Qualifier

tion	0	**Medical and Surgical**
dy System	Y	**Anatomical Regions, Lower Extremities**
eration	2	**Change:** Taking out or off a device from a body part and putting back an identical or similar device in or on the same body part without cutting or puncturing the skin or a mucous membrane

Body Part (4th)	Approach (5th)	Device (6th)	Qualifier (7th)
Lower Extremity, Right Lower Extremity, Left	X External	0 Drainage Device Y Other Device	Z No Qualifier

tion	0	**Medical and Surgical**
dy System	Y	**Anatomical Regions, Lower Extremities**
eration	3	**Control:** Stopping, or attempting to stop, postprocedural or other acute bleeding

Body Part (4th)	Approach (5th)	Device (6th)	Qualifier (7th)
Buttock, Right Buttock, Left Inguinal Region, Right Inguinal Region, Left Femoral Region, Right Femoral Region, Left Lower Extremity, Right Lower Extremity, Left Upper Leg, Right Upper Leg, Left Knee Region, Right Knee Region, Left Lower Leg, Right Lower Leg, Left Ankle Region, Right Ankle Region, Left Foot, Right Foot, Left	0 Open 3 Percutaneous 4 Percutaneous Endoscopic	Z No Device	Z No Qualifier

Section 0 **Medical and Surgical**
Body System Y **Anatomical Regions, Lower Extremities**
Operation 6 **Detachment:** Cutting off all or a portion of the upper or lower extremities

Body Part (4th)	Approach (5th)	Device (6th)	Qualifier (7th)
2 Hindquarter, Right **3** Hindquarter, Left **4** Hindquarter, Bilateral **7** Femoral Region, Right **8** Femoral Region, Left **F** Knee Region, Right **G** Knee Region, Left	**0** Open	**Z** No Device	**Z** No Qualifier
C Upper Leg, Right **D** Upper Leg, Left **H** Lower Leg, Right **J** Lower Leg, Left	**0** Open	**Z** No Device	**1** High **2** Mid **3** Low
M Foot, Right **N** Foot, Left	**0** Open	**Z** No Device	**0** Complete **4** Complete 1st Ray **5** Complete 2nd Ray **6** Complete 3rd Ray **7** Complete 4th Ray **8** Complete 5th Ray **9** Partial 1st Ray **B** Partial 2nd Ray **C** Partial 3rd Ray **D** Partial 4th Ray **F** Partial 5th Ray
P 1st Toe, Right **Q** 1st Toe, Left **R** 2nd Toe, Right **S** 2nd Toe, Left **T** 3rd Toe, Right **U** 3rd Toe, Left **V** 4th Toe, Right **W** 4th Toe, Left **X** 5th Toe, Right **Y** 5th Toe, Left	**0** Open	**Z** No Device	**0** Complete **1** High **2** Mid **3** Low

Section 0 **Medical and Surgical**
Body System Y **Anatomical Regions, Lower Extremities**
Operation 9 **Drainage:** Taking or letting out fluids and/or gases from a body part

Body Part (4th)	Approach (5th)	Device (6th)	Qualifier (7th)
0 Buttock, Right **1** Buttock, Left **5** Inguinal Region, Right **6** Inguinal Region, Left **7** Femoral Region, Right **8** Femoral Region, Left **9** Lower Extremity, Right **B** Lower Extremity, Left **C** Upper Leg, Right **D** Upper Leg, Left **F** Knee Region, Right **G** Knee Region, Left **H** Lower Leg, Right **J** Lower Leg, Left **K** Ankle Region, Right **L** Ankle Region, Left **M** Foot, Right **N** Foot, Left	**0** Open **3** Percutaneous **4** Percutaneous Endoscopic	**0** Drainage Device	**Z** No Qualifier

Continued →

tion 0 **Medical and Surgical**
dy System Y **Anatomical Regions, Lower Extremities**
eration 9 **Drainage:** Taking or letting out fluids and/or gases from a body part

Body Part (4th)	Approach (5th)	Device (6th)	Qualifier (7th)
Buttock, Right Buttock, Left Inguinal Region, Right Inguinal Region, Left Femoral Region, Right Femoral Region, Left Lower Extremity, Right Lower Extremity, Left Upper Leg, Right Upper Leg, Left Knee Region, Right Knee Region, Left Lower Leg, Right Lower Leg, Left Ankle Region, Right Ankle Region, Left Foot, Right Foot, Left	**0** Open **3** Percutaneous **4** Percutaneous Endoscopic	**Z** No Device	**X** Diagnostic **Z** No Qualifier

ction 0 **Medical and Surgical**
dy System Y **Anatomical Regions, Lower Extremities**
eration B **Excision:** Cutting out or off, without replacement, a portion of a body part

Body Part (4th)	Approach (5th)	Device (6th)	Qualifier (7th)
Buttock, Right Buttock, Left Inguinal Region, Right Inguinal Region, Left Femoral Region, Right Femoral Region, Left Lower Extremity, Right B Lower Extremity, Left C Upper Leg, Right D Upper Leg, Left F Knee Region, Right G Knee Region, Left H Lower Leg, Right J Lower Leg, Left K Ankle Region, Right L Ankle Region, Left M Foot, Right N Foot, Left	**0** Open **3** Percutaneous **4** Percutaneous Endoscopic	**Z** No Device	**X** Diagnostic **Z** No Qualifier

Section **0** **Medical and Surgical**
Body System **Y** **Anatomical Regions, Lower Extremities**
Operation **H** **Insertion:** Putting in a nonbiological appliance that monitors, assists, performs, or prevents a physiological function but does not physically take the place of a body part

Body Part (4th)	Approach (5th)	Device (6th)	Qualifier (7th)
0 Buttock, Right **1** Buttock, Left **5** Inguinal Region, Right **6** Inguinal Region, Left **7** Femoral Region, Right **8** Femoral Region, Left **9** Lower Extremity, Right **B** Lower Extremity, Left **C** Upper Leg, Right **D** Upper Leg, Left **F** Knee Region, Right **G** Knee Region, Left **H** Lower Leg, Right **J** Lower Leg, Left **K** Ankle Region, Right **L** Ankle Region, Left **M** Foot, Right **N** Foot, Left	**0** Open **3** Percutaneous **4** Percutaneous Endoscopic	**1** Radioactive Element **3** Infusion Device **Y** Other Device	**Z** No Qualifier

Section **0** **Medical and Surgical**
Body System **Y** **Anatomical Regions, Lower Extremities**
Operation **J** **Inspection:** Visually and/or manually exploring a body part

Body Part (4th)	Approach (5th)	Device (6th)	Qualifier (7th)
0 Buttock, Right **1** Buttock, Left **5** Inguinal Region, Right **6** Inguinal Region, Left **7** Femoral Region, Right **8** Femoral Region, Left **9** Lower Extremity, Right **A** Inguinal Region, Bilateral **B** Lower Extremity, Left **C** Upper Leg, Right **D** Upper Leg, Left **E** Femoral Region, Bilateral **F** Knee Region, Right **G** Knee Region, Left **H** Lower Leg, Right **J** Lower Leg, Left **K** Ankle Region, Right **L** Ankle Region, Left **M** Foot, Right **N** Foot, Left	**0** Open **3** Percutaneous **4** Percutaneous Endoscopic **X** External	**Z** No Device	**Z** No Qualifier

ction | **0** | **Medical and Surgical**
dy System | **Y** | **Anatomical Regions, Lower Extremities**
eration | **M** | **Reattachment:** Putting back in or on all or a portion of a separated body part to its normal location or other suitable location

Body Part (4th)	Approach (5th)	Device (6th)	Qualifier (7th)
0 Buttock, Right	**0** Open	**Z** No Device	**Z** No Qualifier
1 Buttock, Left			
2 Hindquarter, Right			
3 Hindquarter, Left			
4 Hindquarter, Bilateral			
5 Inguinal Region, Right			
6 Inguinal Region, Left			
7 Femoral Region, Right			
8 Femoral Region, Left			
9 Lower Extremity, Right			
B Lower Extremity, Left			
C Upper Leg, Right			
D Upper Leg, Left			
F Knee Region, Right			
G Knee Region, Left			
H Lower Leg, Right			
J Lower Leg, Left			
K Ankle Region, Right			
L Ankle Region, Left			
M Foot, Right			
N Foot, Left			
P 1st Toe, Right			
Q 1st Toe, Left			
R 2nd Toe, Right			
S 2nd Toe, Left			
T 3rd Toe, Right			
U 3rd Toe, Left			
V 4th Toe, Right			
W 4th Toe, Left			
X 5th Toe, Right			
Y 5th Toe, Left			

ction | **0** | **Medical and Surgical**
ody System | **Y** | **Anatomical Regions, Lower Extremities**
peration | **P** | **Removal:** Taking out or off a device from a body part

Body Part (4th)	Approach (5th)	Device (6th)	Qualifier (7th)
9 Lower Extremity, Right	**0** Open	**0** Drainage Device	**Z** No Qualifier
B Lower Extremity, Left	**3** Percutaneous	**1** Radioactive Element	
	4 Percutaneous Endoscopic	**3** Infusion Device	
	X External	**7** Autologous Tissue Substitute	
		J Synthetic Substitute	
		K Nonautologous Tissue Substitute	
		Y Other Device	

Section 0 **Medical and Surgical**
Body System Y **Anatomical Regions, Lower Extremities**
Operation Q **Repair:** Restoring, to the extent possible, a body part to its normal anatomic structure and function

Body Part (4th)	Approach (5th)	Device (6th)	Qualifier (7th)
0 Buttock, Right **1** Buttock, Left **5** Inguinal Region, Right **6** Inguinal Region, Left **7** Femoral Region, Right **8** Femoral Region, Left **9** Lower Extremity, Right **A** Inguinal Region, Bilateral **B** Lower Extremity, Left **C** Upper Leg, Right **D** Upper Leg, Left **E** Femoral Region, Bilateral **F** Knee Region, Right **G** Knee Region, Left **H** Lower Leg, Right **J** Lower Leg, Left **K** Ankle Region, Right **L** Ankle Region, Left **M** Foot, Right **N** Foot, Left **P** 1st Toe, Right **Q** 1st Toe, Left **R** 2nd Toe, Right **S** 2nd Toe, Left **T** 3rd Toe, Right **U** 3rd Toe, Left **V** 4th Toe, Right **W** 4th Toe, Left **X** 5th Toe, Right **Y** 5th Toe, Left	**0** Open **3** Percutaneous **4** Percutaneous Endoscopic **X** External	**Z** No Device	**Z** No Qualifier

Section 0 **Medical and Surgical**
Body System Y **Anatomical Regions, Lower Extremities**
Operation U **Supplement:** Putting in or on biological or synthetic material that physically reinforces and/or augments the function of a portion of a body part

Body Part (4th)	Approach (5th)	Device (6th)	Qualifier (7th)
0 Buttock, Right **1** Buttock, Left **5** Inguinal Region, Right **6** Inguinal Region, Left **7** Femoral Region, Right **8** Femoral Region, Left **9** Lower Extremity, Right **A** Inguinal Region, Bilateral **B** Lower Extremity, Left **C** Upper Leg, Right **D** Upper Leg, Left **E** Femoral Region, Bilateral **F** Knee Region, Right **G** Knee Region, Left **H** Lower Leg, Right **J** Lower Leg, Left **K** Ankle Region, Right **L** Ankle Region, Left **M** Foot, Right **N** Foot, Left **P** 1st Toe, Right **Q** 1st Toe, Left **R** 2nd Toe, Right **S** 2nd Toe, Left **T** 3rd Toe, Right **U** 3rd Toe, Left **V** 4th Toe, Right **W** 4th Toe, Left **X** 5th Toe, Right **Y** 5th Toe, Left	**0** Open **4** Percutaneous Endoscopic	**7** Autologous Tissue Substitute **J** Synthetic Substitute **K** Nonautologous Tissue Substitute	**Z** No Qualifier

Section 0 **Medical and Surgical**
Body System Y **Anatomical Regions, Lower Extremities**
Operation W **Revision:** Correcting, to the extent possible, a portion of a malfunctioning device or the position of a displaced device

Body Part (4th)	Approach (5th)	Device (6th)	Qualifier (7th)
9 Lower Extremity, Right **B** Lower Extremity, Left	**0** Open **3** Percutaneous **4** Percutaneous Endoscopic **X** External	**0** Drainage Device **3** Infusion Device **7** Autologous Tissue Substitute **J** Synthetic Substitute **K** Nonautologous Tissue Substitute **Y** Other Device	**Z** No Qualifier

AHA Coding Clinic

0Y6N0Z0 Detachment at Left Foot, Complete, Open Approach—AHA CC: 1Q, 2015, 28; 1Q, 2017, 22-23
0Y6P0Z3 Detachment at Right 1st Toe, Low, Open Approach—AHA CC: 2Q, 2015, 28-29
0Y6Q0Z3 Detachment at Left 1st Toe, Low, Open Approach—AHA CC: 2Q, 2015, 28-29
0Y950ZZ Drainage of Right Inguinal Region, Open Approach—AHA CC: 1Q, 2015, 23
0Y980ZZ Drainage of Left Femoral Region, Open Approach—AHA CC: 1Q, 2015, 22

Obstetrics Section (102–10Y)

Within each section of ICD-10-PCS the characters have different meanings. The seven character meanings for the Obstetrics section a illustrated here through the procedure example of *Manually-assisted delivery*.

Section	Body System	Root Operation	Body Part	Approach	Device	Qualifier
Obstetrics	Pregnancy	Delivery	Products of Conception	External	None	None
1	0	E	0	X	Z	Z

Section (Character 1)

All Obstetric procedure codes have a first character value of 1.

Body System (Character 2)

The alphanumeric character for the body system is placed in the second position. The body system applicable to the Obstetrics section Pregnancy and has a character value of 0.

Root Operations (Character 3)

The alphanumeric character value for root operations is placed in the third position. Listed below are the root operations applicable to t Obstetrics section with their associated meaning.

Character Value	Root Operation	Root Operation Definition
2	Change	Taking out or off a device from a body part and putting back an identical or similar device in or on the same body part without cutting or puncturing the skin or a mucous membrane
9	Drainage	Taking or letting out fluids and/or gases from a body part
A	Abortion	Artificially terminating a pregnancy
D	Extraction	Pulling or stripping out or off all or a portion of a body part by the use of force
E	Delivery	Assisting the passage of the products of conception from the genital canal
H	Insertion	Putting in a nonbiological appliance that monitors, assists, performs, or prevents a physiological function but does not physically take the place of a body part
J	Inspection	Visually and/or manually exploring a body part
P	Removal	Taking out or off a device from a body part, region or orifice
Q	Repair	Restoring, to the extent possible, a body part to its normal anatomic structure and function
S	Reposition	Moving to its normal location, or other suitable location, all or a portion of a body part
T	Resection	Cutting out or off, without replacement, all of a body part
Y	Transplantation	Putting in or on all or a portion of a living body part taken from another individual or animal to physically take the place and/or function of all or a portion of a similar body part

Body Part (Character 4)

For each body system the applicable body part character values will be available for procedure code construction. An example of a bo part is Products of Conception.

Approach (Character 5)

The approach is the technique used to reach the procedure site. The following are the approach character values for the Obstetrics secti with the associated definitions.

Character Value	Approach	Approach Definition
0	Open	Cutting through the skin or mucous membrane and any other body layers necessary to expose the site of the procedure
3	Percutaneous	Entry, by puncture or minor incision, of instrumentation through the skin or mucous membrane and any other body layers necessary to reach the site of the procedure

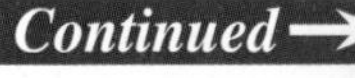

Character Value	Approach	Approach Definition
4	Percutaneous Endoscopic	Entry, by puncture or minor incision, of instrumentation through the skin or mucous membrane and any other body layers necessary to reach and visualize the site of the procedure
7	Via Natural or Artificial Opening	Entry of instrumentation through a natural or artificial external opening to reach the site of the procedure
8	Via Natural or Artificial Opening Endoscopic	Entry of instrumentation through a natural or artificial external opening to reach and visualize the site of the procedure
X	External	Procedures performed directly on the skin or mucous membrane and procedures performed indirectly by the application of external force through the skin or mucous membrane

evice (Character 6)

epending on the procedure performed there may or may not be a device used. There are two types of devices included in the Obstetrics ction: monitoring electrode and other device. When a device is not utilized during the procedure, the placeholder Z is the character value at should be reported.

ualifier (Character 7)

e qualifier represents an additional attribute for the procedure when applicable. For example, drainage procedures in this section include veral qualifiers including fetal cerebrospinal fluid that is reported with the character value of A. If there is no qualifier for a procedure, e placeholder Z is the character valve that should be reported.

bstetric Section Guidelines (section 1)

. Obstetrics Section

roducts of Conception

1. Procedures performed on the products of conception are coded to the Obstetrics section. Procedures performed on the pregnant female her than the products of conception are coded to the appropriate root operation in the Medical and Surgical section.

xample: Amniocentesis is coded to the products of conception body part in the Obstetrics section. Repair of obstetric urethral laceration coded to the urethra body part in the Medical and Surgical section.

rocedures following delivery or abortion

2. Procedures performed following a delivery or abortion for curettage of the endometrium or evacuation of retained products of nception are all coded in the Obstetrics section, to the root operation Extraction and the body part Products of Conception, Retained. iagnostic or therapeutic dilation and curettage performed during times other than the postpartum or post-abortion period are all coded in e Medical and Surgical section, to the root operation Extraction and the body part Endometrium.

oding Guidelines References

he table below links ICD-10-PCS coding guidelines to Obstetrics section body system tables. The guidelines identified in the table are ovided in order to remind users to reference the coding guidelines prior to code reporting. It is imperative to review the ICD-10-PCS oding guidelines to ensure the procedure code being reported is accurate and complete.

able References

Table	Root Operation	Coding Guideline(s)
102	Change	C1
10D	Extraction	C2

Obstetrics Section Tables

Obstetrics Tables 102–10Y

Section 1 **Obstetrics**
Body System 0 **Pregnancy**
Operation 2 **Change:** Taking out or off a device from a body part and putting back an identical or similar device in or on the same bo part without cutting or puncturing the skin or a mucous membrane

Body Part (4th)	Approach (5th)	Device (6th)	Qualifier (7th)
0 Products of Conception	**7** Via Natural or Artificial Opening	**3** Monitoring Electrode **Y** Other Device	**Z** No Qualifier

Section 1 **Obstetrics**
Body System 0 **Pregnancy**
Operation 9 **Drainage:** Taking or letting out fluids and/or gases from a body part

Body Part (4th)	Approach (5th)	Device (6th)	Qualifier (7th)
0 Products of Conception	**0** Open **3** Percutaneous **4** Percutaneous Endoscopic **7** Via Natural or Artificial Opening **8** Via Natural or Artificial Opening Endoscopic	**Z** No Device	**9** Fetal Blood **A** Fetal Cerebrospinal Fluid **B** Fetal Fluid, Other **C** Amniotic Fluid, Therapeutic **D** Fluid, Other **U** Amniotic Fluid, Diagnostic

Section 1 **Obstetrics**
Body System 0 **Pregnancy**
Operation A **Abortion:** Artificially terminating a pregnancy

Body Part (4th)	Approach (5th)	Device (6th)	Qualifier (7th)
0 Products of Conception	**0** Open **3** Percutaneous **4** Percutaneous Endoscopic **8** Via Natural or Artificial Opening Endoscopic	**Z** No Device	**Z** No Qualifier
0 Products of Conception	**7** Via Natural or Artificial Opening	**Z** No Device	**6** Vacuum **W** Laminaria **X** Abortifacient **Z** No Qualifier

Section 1 **Obstetrics**
Body System 0 **Pregnancy**
Operation D **Extraction:** Pulling or stripping out or off all or a portion of a body part by the use of force

Body Part (4th)	Approach (5th)	Device (6th)	Qualifier (7th)
0 Products of Conception	**0** Open	**Z** No Device	**0** High **1** Low **2** Extraperitoneal
0 Products of Conception	**7** Via Natural or Artificial Opening	**Z** No Device	**3** Low Forceps **4** Mid Forceps **5** High Forceps **6** Vacuum **7** Internal Version **8** Other

Continued →

ection **1 Obstetrics**
ody System **0 Pregnancy**
peration **D Extraction:** Pulling or stripping out or off all or a portion of a body part by the use of force

Body Part (4th)	Approach (5th)	Device (6th)	Qualifier (7th)
1 Products of Conception, Retained	**7** Via Natural or Artificial Opening **8** Via Natural or Artificial Opening Endoscopic	**Z** No Device	**9** Manual **Z** No Qualifier
2 Products of Conception, Ectopic	**7** Via Natural or Artificial Opening **8** Via Natural or Artificial Opening Endoscopic	**Z** No Device	**Z** No Qualifier

ection **1 Obstetrics**
ody System **0 Pregnancy**
peration **E Delivery:** Assisting the passage of the products of conception from the genital canal

Body Part (4th)	Approach (5th)	Device (6th)	Qualifier (7th)
0 Products of Conception	**X** External	**Z** No Device	**Z** No Qualifier

ection **1 Obstetrics**
ody System **0 Pregnancy**
peration **H Insertion:** Putting in a nonbiological appliance that monitors, assists, performs, or prevents a physiological function but does not physically take the place of a body part

Body Part (4th)	Approach (5th)	Device (6th)	Qualifier (7th)
0 Products of Conception	**0** Open **7** Via Natural or Artificial Opening	**3** Monitoring Electrode **Y** Other Device	**Z** No Qualifier

ection **1 Obstetrics**
ody System **0 Pregnancy**
peration **J Inspection:** Visually and/or manually exploring a body part

Body Part (4th)	Approach (5th)	Device (6th)	Qualifier (7th)
0 Products of Conception **1** Products of Conception, Retained **2** Products of Conception, Ectopic	**0** Open **3** Percutaneous **4** Percutaneous Endoscopic **7** Via Natural or Artificial Opening **8** Via Natural or Artificial Opening Endoscopic **X** External	**Z** No Device	**Z** No Qualifier

ection **1 Obstetrics**
ody System **0 Pregnancy**
peration **P Removal:** Taking out or off a device from a body part, region or orifice

Body Part (4th)	Approach (5th)	Device (6th)	Qualifier (7th)
0 Products of Conception	**0** Open **7** Via Natural or Artificial Opening	**3** Monitoring Electrode **Y** Other Device	**Z** No Qualifier

Section 1 **Obstetrics**
Body System 0 **Pregnancy**
Operation Q **Repair:** Restoring, to the extent possible, a body part to its normal anatomic structure and function

Body Part (4th)	Approach (5th)	Device (6th)	Qualifier (7th)
0 Products of Conception	**0** Open **3** Percutaneous **4** Percutaneous Endoscopic **7** Via Natural or Artificial Opening **8** Via Natural or Artificial Opening Endoscopic	**Y** Other Device **Z** No Device	**E** Nervous System **F** Cardiovascular System **G** Lymphatics and Hemic **H** Eye **J** Ear, Nose and Sinus **K** Respiratory System **L** Mouth and Throat **M** Gastrointestinal System **N** Hepatobiliary and Pancreas **P** Endocrine System **Q** Skin **R** Musculoskeletal System **S** Urinary System **T** Female Reproductive System **V** Male Reproductive System **Y** Other Body System

Section 1 **Obstetrics**
Body System 0 **Pregnancy**
Operation S **Reposition:** Moving to its normal location, or other suitable location, all or a portion of a body part

Body Part (4th)	Approach (5th)	Device (6th)	Qualifier (7th)
0 Products of Conception	**7** Via Natural or Artificial Opening **X** External	**Z** No Device	**Z** No Qualifier
2 Products of Conception, Ectopic	**0** Open **3** Percutaneous **4** Percutaneous Endoscopic **7** Via Natural or Artificial Opening **8** Via Natural or Artificial Opening Endoscopic	**Z** No Device	**Z** No Qualifier

Section 1 **Obstetrics**
Body System 0 **Pregnancy**
Operation T **Resection:** Cutting out or off, without replacement, all of a body part

Body Part (4th)	Approach (5th)	Device (6th)	Qualifier (7th)
2 Products of Conception, Ectopic	**0** Open **3** Percutaneous **4** Percutaneous Endoscopic **7** Via Natural or Artificial Opening **8** Via Natural or Artificial Opening Endoscopic	**Z** No Device	**Z** No Qualifier

ction 1 **Obstetrics**
dy System 0 **Pregnancy**
peration Y **Transplantation:** Putting in or on all or a portion of a living body part taken from another individual or animal to physically take the place and/or function of all or a portion of a similar body part

Body Part (4th)	Approach (5th)	Device (6th)	Qualifier (7th)
0 Products of Conception	3 Percutaneous 4 Percutaneous Endoscopic 7 Via Natural or Artificial Opening	Z No Device	E Nervous System F Cardiovascular System G Lymphatics and Hemic H Eye J Ear, Nose and Sinus K Respiratory System L Mouth and Throat M Gastrointestinal System N Hepatobiliary and Pancreas P Endocrine System Q Skin R Musculoskeletal System S Urinary System T Female Reproductive System V Male Reproductive System Y Other Body System

HA Coding Clinic

)904ZC Drainage of Amniotic Fluid, Therapeutic from Products of Conception, Percutaneous Endoscopic Approach—AHA CC: 3Q, 2014, 12-13

)907ZC Drainage of Amniotic Fluid, Therapeutic from Products of Conception, Via Natural or Artificial Opening—AHA CC: 2Q, 2014, 9-10

)D00Z0 Extraction of Products of Conception, High, Open Approach— AHA CC: 2Q, 2018, 17-18

)D07Z3 Extraction of Products of Conception, Low Forceps, Via Natural or Artificial Opening—AHA CC: 1Q, 2016, 9-10

)D07Z6 Extraction of Products of Conception, Vacuum, Via Natural or Artificial Opening—AHA CC: 4Q, 2014, 43

)E0XZZ Delivery of Products of Conception, External Approach—AHA CC: 2Q, 2014, 9-10; 4Q, 2014, 17-18; 2Q, 2016, 34-35; 3Q, 2017, 5

)H07YZ Insertion of Other Device into Products of Conception, Via Natural or Artificial Opening—AHA CC: 2Q, 2013, 36

)Q04ZY Repair Other Body System in Products of Conception, Percutaneous Endoscopic Approach—AHA CC: 3Q, 2014, 12-13

)T24ZZ Resection of Products of Conception, Ectopic, Percutaneous Endoscopic Approach—AHA CC: 3Q, 2015, 32

Placement Section (2W0–2Y5)

Within each section of ICD-10-PCS the characters have different meanings. The seven character meanings for the Placement section illustrated below through the procedure example of *Placement of pressure dressing on abdominal wall.*

Section	Body System	Root Operation	Body Region	Approach	Device	Qualifier
Placement	Anatomical Regions	Compression	Abdominal Wall	External	Pressure Dressing	None
2	W	1	3	X	6	Z

Section (Character 1)

All Placement procedure codes have a first character value of 2.

Body System (Character 2)

The alphanumeric character for the body system is placed in the second position. There are two character values applicable for Placement section. The character value of W is reported for anatomical regions. The character value Y is reported for anatomical orific

Root Operations (Character 3)

The alphanumeric character value for root operations is placed in the third position. The following are the root operations applicable the Placement section with their associated meaning.

Character Value	Root Operation	Root Operation Definition
0	Change	Taking out or off a device from a body part and putting back an identical or similar device in or on the same body part without cutting or puncturing the skin or a mucous membrane
1	Compression	Putting pressure on a body region
2	Dressing	Putting material on a body region for protection
3	Immobilization	Limiting or preventing motion of a body region
4	Packing	Putting material in a body region or orifice
5	Removal	Taking out or off a device from a body part
6	Traction	Exerting a pulling force on a body region in a distal direction

Body Region (Character 4)

For each body system the applicable body part character values will be available for procedure code construction. An example of a bo region is Chest Wall.

Approach (Character 5)

The only approach technique utilized for the Placement section is External approach and is reported with the character value of X.

Character Value	Approach	Approach Definition
X	External	Procedures performed directly on the skin or mucous membrane and procedures performed indirectly by the application of external force through the skin or mucous membrane

Device (Character 6)

Depending on the procedure performed there may or may not be a device used. There are several types of devices included in t Placement section. Here is a sample list of the devices included in this section:

- Cast
- Packing material
- Pressure dressing
- Traction apparatus

en a device is not utilized during the procedure, the placeholder Z is the character value that should be reported.

alifier (Character 7)

e qualifier represents an additional attribute for the procedure when applicable. Currently, there are no qualifiers in the Placement tion; therefore, the placeholder character value of Z should be reported.

ding Guideline References

fore reporting Change and Removal procedures in this section users should review coding guideline B6.1c.

acement Section Tables

acement Tables 2W0–2Y5

tion 2 **Placement**
dy System W **Anatomical Regions**
eration 0 **Change:** Taking out or off a device from a body part and putting back an identical or similar device in or on the same body part without cutting or puncturing the skin or a mucous membrane

Body Region (4th)	Approach (5th)	Device (6th)	Qualifier (7th)
0 Head 2 Neck 3 Abdominal Wall 4 Chest Wall 5 Back 6 Inguinal Region, Right 7 Inguinal Region, Left 8 Upper Extremity, Right 9 Upper Extremity, Left A Upper Arm, Right B Upper Arm, Left C Lower Arm, Right D Lower Arm, Left E Hand, Right F Hand, Left G Thumb, Right H Thumb, Left J Finger, Right K Finger, Left L Lower Extremity, Right M Lower Extremity, Left N Upper Leg, Right P Upper Leg, Left Q Lower Leg, Right R Lower Leg, Left S Foot, Right T Foot, Left U Toe, Right V Toe, Left	**X** External	**0** Traction Apparatus **1** Splint **2** Cast **3** Brace **4** Bandage **5** Packing Material **6** Pressure Dressing **7** Intermittent Pressure Device **Y** Other Device	**Z** No Qualifier
1 Face	**X** External	**0** Traction Apparatus **1** Splint **2** Cast **3** Brace **4** Bandage **5** Packing Material **6** Pressure Dressing **7** Intermittent Pressure Device **9** Wire **Y** Other Device	**Z** No Qualifier

Section 2 **Placement**
Body System W **Anatomical Regions**
Operation 1 **Compression:** Putting pressure on a body region

Body Region (4th)	Approach (5th)	Device (6th)	Qualifier (7th)
0 Head **1** Face **2** Neck **3** Abdominal Wall **4** Chest Wall **5** Back **6** Inguinal Region, Right **7** Inguinal Region, Left **8** Upper Extremity, Right **9** Upper Extremity, Left **A** Upper Arm, Right **B** Upper Arm, Left **C** Lower Arm, Right **D** Lower Arm, Left **E** Hand, Right **F** Hand, Left **G** Thumb, Right **H** Thumb, Left **J** Finger, Right **K** Finger, Left **L** Lower Extremity, Right **M** Lower Extremity, Left **N** Upper Leg, Right **P** Upper Leg, Left **Q** Lower Leg, Right **R** Lower Leg, Left **S** Foot, Right **T** Foot, Left **U** Toe, Right **V** Toe, Left	**X** External	**6** Pressure Dressing **7** Intermittent Pressure Device	**Z** No Qualifier

tion	**2**	**Placement**
dy System	**W**	**Anatomical Regions**
eration	**2**	**Dressing:** Putting material on a body region for protection

Body Region (4th)	Approach (5th)	Device (6th)	Qualifier (7th)
Head Face Neck Abdominal Wall Chest Wall Back Inguinal Region, Right Inguinal Region, Left Upper Extremity, Right Upper Extremity, Left Upper Arm, Right Upper Arm, Left Lower Arm, Right Lower Arm, Left Hand, Right Hand, Left Thumb, Right Thumb, Left Finger, Right Finger, Left Lower Extremity, Right Lower Extremity, Left Upper Leg, Right Upper Leg, Left Lower Leg, Right Lower Leg, Left Foot, Right Foot, Left Toe, Right Toe, Left	**X** External	**4** Bandage	**Z** No Qualifier

Section 2 **Placement**
Body System W **Anatomical Regions**
Operation 3 **Immobilization:** Limiting or preventing motion of a body region

Body Region (4th)	Approach (5th)	Device (6th)	Qualifier (7th)
0 Head **2** Neck **3** Abdominal Wall **4** Chest Wall **5** Back **6** Inguinal Region, Right **7** Inguinal Region, Left **8** Upper Extremity, Right **9** Upper Extremity, Left **A** Upper Arm, Right **B** Upper Arm, Left **C** Lower Arm, Right **D** Lower Arm, Left **E** Hand, Right **F** Hand, Left **G** Thumb, Right **H** Thumb, Left **J** Finger, Right **K** Finger, Left **L** Lower Extremity, Right **M** Lower Extremity, Left **N** Upper Leg, Right **P** Upper Leg, Left **Q** Lower Leg, Right **R** Lower Leg, Left **S** Foot, Right **T** Foot, Left **U** Toe, Right **V** Toe, Left	**X** External	**1** Splint **2** Cast **3** Brace **Y** Other Device	**Z** No Qualifier
1 Face	**X** External	**1** Splint **2** Cast **3** Brace **9** Wire **Y** Other Device	**Z** No Qualifier

tion	2	**Placement**
ly System	W	**Anatomical Regions**
eration	4	**Packing:** Putting material in a body region or orifice

Body Region (4th)	Approach (5th)	Device (6th)	Qualifier (7th)
Head Face Neck Abdominal Wall Chest Wall Back Inguinal Region, Right Inguinal Region, Left Upper Extremity, Right Upper Extremity, Left Upper Arm, Right Upper Arm, Left Lower Arm, Right Lower Arm, Left Hand, Right Hand, Left Thumb, Right Thumb, Left Finger, Right Finger, Left Lower Extremity, Right M Lower Extremity, Left Upper Leg, Right Upper Leg, Left Lower Leg, Right Lower Leg, Left Foot, Right Foot, Left Toe, Right Toe, Left	**X** External	**5** Packing Material	**Z** No Qualifier

Section 2 **Placement**
Body System W **Anatomical Regions**
Operation 5 **Removal:** Taking out or off a device from a body part

Body Region (4th)	Approach (5th)	Device (6th)	Qualifier (7th)
0 Head **2** Neck **3** Abdominal Wall **4** Chest Wall **5** Back **6** Inguinal Region, Right **7** Inguinal Region, Left **8** Upper Extremity, Right **9** Upper Extremity, Left **A** Upper Arm, Right **B** Upper Arm, Left **C** Lower Arm, Right **D** Lower Arm, Left **E** Hand, Right **F** Hand, Left **G** Thumb, Right **H** Thumb, Left **J** Finger, Right **K** Finger, Left **L** Lower Extremity, Right **M** Lower Extremity, Left **N** Upper Leg, Right **P** Upper Leg, Left **Q** Lower Leg, Right **R** Lower Leg, Left **S** Foot, Right **T** Foot, Left **U** Toe, Right **V** Toe, Left	**X** External	**0** Traction Apparatus **1** Splint **2** Cast **3** Brace **4** Bandage **5** Packing Material **6** Pressure Dressing **7** Intermittent Pressure Device **Y** Other Device	**Z** No Qualifier
1 Face	**X** External	**0** Traction Apparatus **1** Splint **2** Cast **3** Brace **4** Bandage **5** Packing Material **6** Pressure Dressing **7** Intermittent Pressure Device **9** Wire **Y** Other Device	**Z** No Qualifier

ction	2	Placement
dy System	W	Anatomical Regions
eration	6	**Traction:** Exerting a pulling force on a body region in a distal direction

Body Region (4th)	Approach (5th)	Device (6th)	Qualifier (7th)
0 Head 1 Face 2 Neck 3 Abdominal Wall 4 Chest Wall 5 Back 6 Inguinal Region, Right 7 Inguinal Region, Left 8 Upper Extremity, Right 9 Upper Extremity, Left A Upper Arm, Right B Upper Arm, Left C Lower Arm, Right D Lower Arm, Left E Hand, Right F Hand, Left G Thumb, Right H Thumb, Left J Finger, Right K Finger, Left L Lower Extremity, Right M Lower Extremity, Left N Upper Leg, Right P Upper Leg, Left Q Lower Leg, Right R Lower Leg, Left S Foot, Right T Foot, Left U Toe, Right V Toe, Left	X External	0 Traction Apparatus Z No Device	Z No Qualifier

ction	2	Placement
dy System	Y	Anatomical Orifices
peration	0	**Change:** Taking out or off a device from a body part and putting back an identical or similar device in or on the same body part without cutting or puncturing the skin or a mucous membrane

Body Region (4th)	Approach (5th)	Device (6th)	Qualifier (7th)
0 Mouth and Pharynx 1 Nasal 2 Ear 3 Anorectal 4 Female Genital Tract 5 Urethra	X External	5 Packing Material	Z No Qualifier

ction	2	Placement
ody System	Y	Anatomical Orifices
peration	4	**Packing:** Putting material in a body region or orifice

Body Region (4th)	Approach (5th)	Device (6th)	Qualifier (7th)
0 Mouth and Pharynx 1 Nasal 2 Ear 3 Anorectal 4 Female Genital Tract 5 Urethra	X External	5 Packing Material	Z No Qualifier

Section 2 **Placement**
Body System Y **Anatomical Orifices**
Operation 5 **Removal:** Taking out or off a device from a body part

Body Region (4th)	Approach (5th)	Device (6th)	Qualifier (7th)
0 Mouth and Pharynx **1** Nasal **2** Ear **3** Anorectal **4** Female Genital Tract **5** Urethra	**X** External	**5** Packing Material	**Z** No Qualifier

AHA Coding Clinic

2W60X0Z Traction of Head using Traction Apparatus - AHA CC: 2Q, 2013, 39; 2Q, 2015, 35

2W62X0Z Traction of Neck using Traction Apparatus - AHA CC: 2Q, 2015, 35

2Y41X5Z Packing of Nasal Region using Packing Material—AHA CC: 4Q, 2017, 106

ithin each section of ICD-10-PCS, the characters have different meanings. The seven character meanings for the Administration section e illustrated here through the procedure example of *Nerve block injection to median nerve*.

Section	Body System	Root Operation	Body System/ Region	Approach	Substance	Qualifier
Administration	Physiological System and Anatomical Region	Introduction	Peripheral Nerves and Plexi	Percutaneous	Regional Anesthetic	None
3	E	0	T	3	C	Z

ection (Character 1)

ll Administration procedure codes have a first character value of 3.

ody System (Character 2)

ne alphanumeric character for the body system is placed in the second position. There are three character values applicable for the dministration section.

Character Value	Character Value Description
0	Circulatory
C	Indwelling Device
E	Physiological System and Anatomical Region

oot Operations (Character 3)

he alphanumeric character value for root operations is placed in the third position. Listed here are the root operations applicable to the dministration section with their associated meaning.

Character Value	Root Operation	Root Operation Definition
0	Introduction	Putting in or on a therapeutic, diagnostic, nutritional, physiological, or prophylactic substance except blood or blood products
1	Irrigation	Putting in or on a cleansing substance
2	Transfusion	Putting in blood or blood products

ody System/Region (Character 4)

or each body system the applicable body part character values will be available for procedure code construction. An example of a body egion is upper GI.

pproach (Character 5)

he approach is the technique used to reach the procedure site. Listed here are the approach character values for the Administration with ne associated definitions.

Character Value	Approach	Approach Definition
0	Open	Cutting through the skin or mucous membrane and any other body layers necessary to expose the site of the procedure
3	Percutaneous	Entry, by puncture or minor incision, of instrumentation through the skin or mucous membrane and any other body layers necessary to reach the site of the procedure
4	Percutaneous Endoscopic	Entry, by puncture or minor incision, of instrumentation through the skin or mucous membrane and any other body layers necessary to reach and visualize the site of the procedure
7	Via Natural or Artificial Opening	Entry of instrumentation through a natural or artificial external opening to reach the site of the procedure
8	Via Natural or Artificial Opening Endoscopic	Entry of instrumentation through a natural or artificial external opening to reach and visualize the site of the procedure
X	External	Procedures performed directly on the skin or mucous membrane and procedures performed indirectly by the application of external force through the skin or mucous membrane

Substance (Character 6)

In the Administration section a substance is always utilized. The substance is reported in the sixth character position by the type substance utilized. The following is a sample list of the substances included in this section:

- Anti-inflammatory
- Antineoplastic
- Bone marrow
- Platelet inhibitor
- Whole blood

Qualifier (Character 7)

The qualifier represents an additional attribute for the procedure when applicable. There are several qualifiers included in the Administrati section. For example, transfusion procedures in this section include qualifiers including Autologous and Nonautologous that are reported with character values of 0 and 1, respectively. If there is no qualifier for a procedure, the placeholder Z is the character value that should be reporte

If a coder is unsure of which option to select for the substance qualifier utilized during the procedure, Appendix F can be used guide the selection. It is important to note that not all substance qualifier categories are provided by CMS in Appendix F. However, example, the coding scenario indicates that Clolar was introduced percutaneously via the peripheral vein. The coder references Tal 3E0 (Introduction in Physiological Systems and Anatomical Regions) under the peripheral vein, percutaneous approach, anti-neoplast Clolar is not a substance qualifier choice. However, the coder can then locate the substance qualifier categories in Appendix F. T category Clofarabine includes Clolar. Therefore, the coder should select P - Clofarabine for the 7th character.

Important Definitions for the Administration Section

Administration Root Operation	Qualifier	Definition
Transfusion (302)	0 - Autologous	Derived or transferred from the same individual's body*
	1 - Nonautologous	Derived or transferred from another individual's body

*Taken from The Free Dictionary by Farlex at www.thefreedictionary.com

Coding Guideline References

Before reporting Transfusion procedures for embryonic stem cells (6th character A), bone marrow (6th character G), cord blood stem ce (6th character X) or hematopoietic stem cells (6th character Y) users should review coding guideline B3.16.

Before reporting Administration codes for all Biliary and Pancreatic Tract (4th character value of J) procedures with a 6th character val of U (Pancreatic Islet Cells), users should review coding guideline B3.16.

Before reporting Irrigation procedures in this section, users should review coding guideline B6.1c.

dministration Tables 302–3E1

ction 3 **Administration**
dy System 0 **Circulatory**
peration 2 **Transfusion:** Putting in blood or blood products

Body System / Region (4th)	Approach (5th)	Substance (6th)	Qualifier (7th)
3 Peripheral Vein 4 Central Vein	0 Open 3 Percutaneous	A Stem Cells, Embryonic	Z No Qualifier
3 Peripheral Vein 4 Central Vein	0 Open 3 Percutaneous	G Bone Marrow X Stem Cells, Cord Blood Y Stem Cells, Hematopoietic	0 Autologous 2 Allogeneic, Related 3 Allogeneic, Unrelated 4 Allogeneic, Unspecified
3 Peripheral Vein 4 Central Vein	0 Open 3 Percutaneous	H Whole Blood J Serum Albumin K Frozen Plasma L Fresh Plasma M Plasma Cryoprecipitate N Red Blood Cells P Frozen Red Cells Q White Cells R Platelets S Globulin T Fibrinogen V Antihemophilic Factors W Factor IX	0 Autologous 1 Nonautologous
5 Peripheral Artery 6 Central Artery	0 Open 3 Percutaneous	G Bone Marrow H Whole Blood J Serum Albumin K Frozen Plasma L Fresh Plasma M Plasma Cryoprecipitate N Red Blood Cells P Frozen Red Cells Q White Cells R Platelets S Globulin T Fibrinogen V Antihemophilic Factors W Factor IX X Stem Cells, Cord Blood Y Stem Cells, Hematopoietic	0 Autologous 1 Nonautologous
7 Products of Conception, Circulatory	3 Percutaneous 7 Via Natural or Artificial Opening	H Whole Blood J Serum Albumin K Frozen Plasma L Fresh Plasma M Plasma Cryoprecipitate N Red Blood Cells P Frozen Red Cells Q White Cells R Platelets S Globulin T Fibrinogen V Antihemophilic Factors W Factor IX	1 Nonautologous
8 Vein	0 Open 3 Percutaneous	B 4-Factor Prothrombin Complex Concentrate	1 Nonautologous

ection 3 **Administration**
ody System C **Indwelling Device**
peration 1 **Irrigation:** Putting in or on a cleansing substance

Body System / Region (4th)	Approach (5th)	Substance (6th)	Qualifier (7th)
Z None	X External	8 Irrigating Substance	Z No Qualifier

Section 3 **Administration**
Body System E **Physiological Systems and Anatomical Regions**
Operation 0 **Introduction:** Putting in or on a therapeutic, diagnostic, nutritional, physiological, or prophylactic substance except blood or blood products

Body System / Region (4th)	Approach (5th)	Substance (6th)	Qualifier (7th)
0 Skin and Mucous Membranes	**X** External	**0** Antineoplastic	**5** Other Antineoplastic **M** Monoclonal Antibody
0 Skin and Mucous Membranes	**X** External	**2** Anti-infective	**8** Oxazolidinones **9** Other Anti-infective
0 Skin and Mucous Membranes	**X** External	**3** Anti-inflammatory **B** Anesthetic Agent **K** Other Diagnostic Substance **M** Pigment **N** Analgesics, Hypnotics, Sedatives **T** Destructive Agent	**Z** No Qualifier
0 Skin and Mucous Membranes	**X** External	**G** Other Therapeutic Substance	**C** Other Substance
1 Subcutaneous Tissue	**0** Open	**2** Anti-infective	**A** Anti-Infective Envelope
1 Subcutaneous Tissue	**3** Percutaneous	**0** Antineoplastic	**5** Other Antineoplastic **M** Monoclonal Antibody
1 Subcutaneous Tissue	**3** Percutaneous	**2** Anti-infective	**8** Oxazolidinones **9** Other Anti-infective **A** Anti-Infective Envelope
1 Subcutaneous Tissue	**3** Percutaneous	**3** Anti-inflammatory **6** Nutritional Substance **7** Electrolytic and Water Balance Substance **B** Anesthetic Agent **H** Radioactive Substance **K** Other Diagnostic Substance **N** Analgesics, Hypnotics, Sedatives **T** Destructive Agent	**Z** No Qualifier
1 Subcutaneous Tissue	**3** Percutaneous	**4** Serum, Toxoid and Vaccine	**0** Influenza Vaccine **Z** No Qualifier
1 Subcutaneous Tissue	**3** Percutaneous	**G** Other Therapeutic Substance	**C** Other Substance
1 Subcutaneous Tissue	**3** Percutaneous	**V** Hormone	**G** Insulin **J** Other Hormone
2 Muscle	**3** Percutaneous	**0** Antineoplastic	**5** Other Antineoplastic **M** Monoclonal Antibody
2 Muscle	**3** Percutaneous	**2** Anti-infective	**8** Oxazolidinones **9** Other Anti-infective
2 Muscle	**3** Percutaneous	**3** Anti-inflammatory **6** Nutritional Substance **7** Electrolytic and Water Balance Substance **B** Anesthetic Agent **H** Radioactive Substance **K** Other Diagnostic Substance **N** Analgesics, Hypnotics, Sedatives **T** Destructive Agent	**Z** No Qualifier

Continued →

ection 3 **Administration**
ody System E **Physiological Systems and Anatomical Regions**
peration 0 **Introduction:** Putting in or on a therapeutic, diagnostic, nutritional, physiological, or prophylactic substance except blood or blood products

Body System / Region (4th)	Approach (5th)	Substance (6th)	Qualifier (7th)
2 Muscle	**3** Percutaneous	**4** Serum, Toxoid and Vaccine	**0** Influenza Vaccine **Z** No Qualifier
2 Muscle	**3** Percutaneous	**G** Other Therapeutic Substance	**C** Other Substance
3 Peripheral Vein	**0** Open	**0** Antineoplastic	**2** High-dose Interleukin-2 **3** Low-dose Interleukin-2 **5** Other Antineoplastic **M** Monoclonal Antibody **P** Clofarabine
3 Peripheral Vein	**0** Open	**1** Thrombolytic	**6** Recombinant Human-activated Protein C **7** Other Thrombolytic
3 Peripheral Vein	**0** Open	**2** Anti-infective	**8** Oxazolidinones **9** Other Anti-infective
3 Peripheral Vein	**0** Open	**3** Anti-inflammatory **4** Serum, Toxoid and Vaccine **6** Nutritional Substance **7** Electrolytic and Water Balance Substance **F** Intracirculatory Anesthetic **H** Radioactive Substance **K** Other Diagnostic Substance **N** Analgesics, Hypnotics, Sedatives **P** Platelet Inhibitor **R** Antiarrhythmic **T** Destructive Agent **X** Vasopressor	**Z** No Qualifier
3 Peripheral Vein	**0** Open	**G** Other Therapeutic Substance	**C** Other Substance **N** Blood Brain Barrier Disruption
3 Peripheral Vein	**0** Open	**U** Pancreatic Islet Cells	**0** Autologous **1** Nonautologous
3 Peripheral Vein	**0** Open	**V** Hormone	**G** Insulin **H** Human B-type Natriuretic Peptide **J** Other Hormone
3 Peripheral Vein	**0** Open	**W** Immunotherapeutic	**K** Immunostimulator **L** Immunosuppressive
3 Peripheral Vein	**3** Percutaneous	**0** Antineoplastic	**2** High-dose Interleukin-2 **3** Low-dose Interleukin-2 **5** Other Antineoplastic **M** Monoclonal Antibody **P** Clofarabine
3 Peripheral Vein	**3** Percutaneous	**1** Thrombolytic	**6** Recombinant Human-activated Protein C **7** Other Thrombolytic
3 Peripheral Vein	**3** Percutaneous	**2** Anti-infective	**8** Oxazolidinones **9** Other Anti-infective

Continued →

Section 3 **Administration**
Body System E **Physiological Systems and Anatomical Regions**
Operation 0 **Introduction:** Putting in or on a therapeutic, diagnostic, nutritional, physiological, or prophylactic substance except blood or blood products

Body System / Region (4th)	Approach (5th)	Substance (6th)	Qualifier (7th)
3 Peripheral Vein	**3** Percutaneous	**3** Anti-inflammatory **4** Serum, Toxoid and Vaccine **6** Nutritional Substance **7** Electrolytic and Water Balance Substance **F** Intracirculatory Anesthetic **H** Radioactive Substance **K** Other Diagnostic Substance **N** Analgesics, Hypnotics, Sedatives **P** Platelet Inhibitor **R** Antiarrhythmic **T** Destructive Agent **X** Vasopressor	**Z** No Qualifier
3 Peripheral Vein	**3** Percutaneous	**G** Other Therapeutic Substance	**C** Other Substance **N** Blood Brain Barrier Disruption **Q** Glucarpidase
3 Peripheral Vein	**3** Percutaneous	**U** Pancreatic Islet Cells	**0** Autologous **1** Nonautologous
3 Peripheral Vein	**3** Percutaneous	**V** Hormone	**G** Insulin **H** Human B-type Natriuretic Peptide **J** Other Hormone
3 Peripheral Vein	**3** Percutaneous	**W** Immunotherapeutic	**K** Immunostimulator **L** Immunosuppressive
4 Central Vein	**0** Open	**0** Antineoplastic	**2** High-dose Interleukin-2 **3** Low-dose Interleukin-2 **5** Other Antineoplastic **M** Monoclonal Antibody **P** Clofarabine
4 Central Vein	**0** Open	**1** Thrombolytic	**6** Recombinant Human-activated Protein C **7** Other Thrombolytic
4 Central Vein	**0** Open	**2** Anti-infective	**8** Oxazolidinones **9** Other Anti-infective
4 Central Vein	**0** Open	**3** Anti-inflammatory **4** Serum, Toxoid and Vaccine **6** Nutritional Substance **7** Electrolytic and Water Balance Substance **F** Intracirculatory Anesthetic **H** Radioactive Substance **K** Other Diagnostic Substance **N** Analgesics, Hypnotics, Sedatives **P** Platelet Inhibitor **R** Antiarrhythmic **T** Destructive Agent **X** Vasopressor	**Z** No Qualifier
4 Central Vein	**0** Open	**G** Other Therapeutic Substance	**C** Other Substance **N** Blood Brain Barrier Disruption

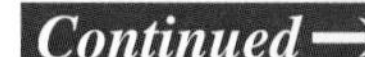
Continued →

ction 3 Administration
dy System E Physiological Systems and Anatomical Regions
eration 0 Introduction: Putting in or on a therapeutic, diagnostic, nutritional, physiological, or prophylactic substance except blood or blood products

Body System / Region (4th)	Approach (5th)	Substance (6th)	Qualifier (7th)
4 Central Vein	0 Open	V Hormone	G Insulin H Human B-type Natriuretic Peptide J Other Hormone
4 Central Vein	0 Open	W Immunotherapeutic	K Immunostimulator L Immunosuppressive
4 Central Vein	3 Percutaneous	0 Antineoplastic	2 High-dose Interleukin-2 3 Low-dose Interleukin-2 5 Other Antineoplastic M Monoclonal Antibody P Clofarabine
4 Central Vein	3 Percutaneous	1 Thrombolytic	6 Recombinant Human-activated Protein C 7 Other Thrombolytic
4 Central Vein	3 Percutaneous	2 Anti-infective	8 Oxazolidinones 9 Other Anti-infective
4 Central Vein	3 Percutaneous	3 Anti-inflammatory 4 Serum, Toxoid and Vaccine 6 Nutritional Substance 7 Electrolytic and Water Balance Substance F Intracirculatory Anesthetic H Radioactive Substance K Other Diagnostic Substance N Analgesics, Hypnotics, Sedatives P Platelet Inhibitor R Antiarrhythmic T Destructive Agent X Vasopressor	Z No Qualifier
4 Central Vein	3 Percutaneous	G Other Therapeutic Substance	C Other Substance N Blood Brain Barrier Disruption Q Glucarpidase
4 Central Vein	3 Percutaneous	V Hormone	G Insulin H Human B-type Natriuretic Peptide J Other Hormone
4 Central Vein	3 Percutaneous	W Immunotherapeutic	K Immunostimulator L Immunosuppressive
5 Peripheral Artery 6 Central Artery	0 Open 3 Percutaneous	0 Antineoplastic	2 High-dose Interleukin-2 3 Low-dose Interleukin-2 5 Other Antineoplastic M Monoclonal Antibody P Clofarabine
5 Peripheral Artery 6 Central Artery	0 Open 3 Percutaneous	1 Thrombolytic	6 Recombinant Human-activated Protein C 7 Other Thrombolytic

Continued →

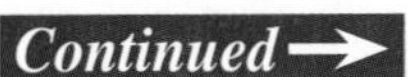

Section 3 **Administration**
Body System E **Physiological Systems and Anatomical Regions**
Operation 0 **Introduction:** Putting in or on a therapeutic, diagnostic, nutritional, physiological, or prophylactic substance except blood or blood products

Body System / Region (4th)	Approach (5th)	Substance (6th)	Qualifier (7th)
5 Peripheral Artery **6** Central Artery	**0** Open **3** Percutaneous	**2** Anti-infective	**8** Oxazolidinones **9** Other Anti-infective
5 Peripheral Artery **6** Central Artery	**0** Open **3** Percutaneous	**3** Anti-inflammatory **4** Serum, Toxoid and Vaccine **6** Nutritional Substance **7** Electrolytic and Water Balance Substance **F** Intracirculatory Anesthetic **H** Radioactive Substance **K** Other Diagnostic Substance **N** Analgesics, Hypnotics, Sedatives **P** Platelet Inhibitor **R** Antiarrhythmic **T** Destructive Agent **X** Vasopressor	**Z** No Qualifier
5 Peripheral Artery **6** Central Artery	**0** Open **3** Percutaneous	**G** Other Therapeutic Substance	**C** Other Substance **N** Blood Brain Barrier Disruption
5 Peripheral Artery **6** Central Artery	**0** Open **3** Percutaneous	**V** Hormone	**G** Insulin **H** Human B-type Natriuretic Peptide **J** Other Hormone
5 Peripheral Artery **6** Central Artery	**0** Open **3** Percutaneous	**W** Immunotherapeutic	**K** Immunostimulator **L** Immunosuppressive
7 Coronary Artery **8** Heart	**0** Open **3** Percutaneous	**1** Thrombolytic	**6** Recombinant Human-activated Protein C **7** Other Thrombolytic
7 Coronary Artery **8** Heart	**0** Open **3** Percutaneous	**G** Other Therapeutic Substance	**C** Other Substance
7 Coronary Artery **8** Heart	**0** Open **3** Percutaneous	**K** Other Diagnostic Substance **P** Platelet Inhibitor	**Z** No Qualifier
7 Coronary Artery **8** Heart	**4** Percutaneous Endoscopic	**G** Other Therapeutic Substance	**C** Other Substance
9 Nose	**3** Percutaneous **7** Via Natural or Artificial Opening **X** External	**0** Antineoplastic	**5** Other Antineoplastic **M** Monoclonal Antibody
9 Nose	**3** Percutaneous **7** Via Natural or Artificial Opening **X** External	**2** Anti-infective	**8** Oxazolidinones **9** Other Anti-infective
9 Nose	**3** Percutaneous **7** Via Natural or Artificial Opening **X** External	**3** Anti-inflammatory **4** Serum, Toxoid and Vaccine **B** Anesthetic Agent **H** Radioactive Substance **K** Other Diagnostic Substance **N** Analgesics, Hypnotics, Sedatives **T** Destructive Agent	**Z** No Qualifier
9 Nose	**3** Percutaneous **7** Via Natural or Artificial Opening **X** External	**G** Other Therapeutic Substance	**C** Other Substance

Continued →

tion 3 **Administration**
ly System E **Physiological Systems and Anatomical Regions**
eration 0 **Introduction:** Putting in or on a therapeutic, diagnostic, nutritional, physiological, or prophylactic substance except blood or blood products

Body System / Region (4th)	Approach (5th)	Substance (6th)	Qualifier (7th)
Bone Marrow	**3** Percutaneous	**0** Antineoplastic	**5** Other Antineoplastic **M** Monoclonal Antibody
Bone Marrow	**3** Percutaneous	**G** Other Therapeutic Substance	**C** Other Substance
Ear	**3** Percutaneous **7** Via Natural or Artificial Opening **X** External	**0** Antineoplastic	**4** Liquid Brachytherapy Radioisotope **5** Other Antineoplastic **M** Monoclonal Antibody
Ear	**3** Percutaneous **7** Via Natural or Artificial Opening **X** External	**2** Anti-infective	**8** Oxazolidinones **9** Other Anti-infective
Ear	**3** Percutaneous **7** Via Natural or Artificial Opening **X** External	**3** Anti-inflammatory **B** Anesthetic Agent **H** Radioactive Substance **K** Other Diagnostic Substance **N** Analgesics, Hypnotics, Sedatives **T** Destructive Agent	**Z** No Qualifier
Ear	**3** Percutaneous **7** Via Natural or Artificial Opening **X** External	**G** Other Therapeutic Substance	**C** Other Substance
Eye	**3** Percutaneous **7** Via Natural or Artificial Opening **X** External	**0** Antineoplastic	**4** Liquid Brachytherapy Radioisotope **5** Other Antineoplastic **M** Monoclonal Antibody
Eye	**3** Percutaneous **7** Via Natural or Artificial Opening **X** External	**2** Anti-infective	**8** Oxazolidinones **9** Other Anti-infective
Eye	**3** Percutaneous **7** Via Natural or Artificial Opening **X** External	**3** Anti-inflammatory **B** Anesthetic Agent **H** Radioactive Substance **K** Other Diagnostic Substance **M** Pigment **N** Analgesics, Hypnotics, Sedatives **T** Destructive Agent	**Z** No Qualifier
Eye	**3** Percutaneous **7** Via Natural or Artificial Opening **X** External	**G** Other Therapeutic Substance	**C** Other Substance
Eye	**3** Percutaneous **7** Via Natural or Artificial Opening **X** External	**S** Gas	**F** Other Gas
Mouth and Pharynx	**3** Percutaneous **7** Via Natural or Artificial Opening **X** External	**0** Antineoplastic	**4** Liquid Brachytherapy Radioisotope **5** Other Antineoplastic **M** Monoclonal Antibody

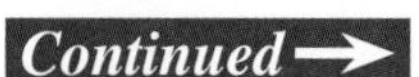

Section 3 **Administration**
Body System E **Physiological Systems and Anatomical Regions**
Operation 0 **Introduction:** Putting in or on a therapeutic, diagnostic, nutritional, physiological, or prophylactic substance except blood or blood products

Body System / Region (4th)	Approach (5th)	Substance (6th)	Qualifier (7th)
D Mouth and Pharynx	**3** Percutaneous **7** Via Natural or Artificial Opening **X** External	**2** Anti-infective	**8** Oxazolidinones **9** Other Anti-infective
D Mouth and Pharynx	**3** Percutaneous **7** Via Natural or Artificial Opening **X** External	**3** Anti-inflammatory **4** Serum, Toxoid and Vaccine **6** Nutritional Substance **7** Electrolytic and Water Balance Substance **B** Anesthetic Agent **H** Radioactive Substance **K** Other Diagnostic Substance **N** Analgesics, Hypnotics, Sedatives **R** Antiarrhythmic **T** Destructive Agent	**Z** No Qualifier
D Mouth and Pharynx	**3** Percutaneous **7** Via Natural or Artificial Opening **X** External	**G** Other Therapeutic Substance	**C** Other Substance
E Products of Conception **G** Upper GI **H** Lower GI **K** Genitourinary Tract **N** Male Reproductive	**3** Percutaneous **7** Via Natural or Artificial Opening **8** Via Natural or Artificial Opening Endoscopic	**0** Antineoplastic	**4** Liquid Brachytherapy Radioisotope **5** Other Antineoplastic **M** Monoclonal Antibody
E Products of Conception **G** Upper GI **H** Lower GI **K** Genitourinary Tract **N** Male Reproductive	**3** Percutaneous **7** Via Natural or Artificial Opening **8** Via Natural or Artificial Opening Endoscopic	**2** Anti-infective	**8** Oxazolidinones **9** Other Anti-infective
E Products of Conception **G** Upper GI **H** Lower GI **K** Genitourinary Tract **N** Male Reproductive	**3** Percutaneous **7** Via Natural or Artificial Opening **8** Via Natural or Artificial Opening Endoscopic	**3** Anti-inflammatory **6** Nutritional Substance **7** Electrolytic and Water Balance Substance **B** Anesthetic Agent **H** Radioactive Substance **K** Other Diagnostic Substance **N** Analgesics, Hypnotics, Sedatives **T** Destructive Agent	**Z** No Qualifier
E Products of Conception **G** Upper GI **H** Lower GI **K** Genitourinary Tract **N** Male Reproductive	**3** Percutaneous **7** Via Natural or Artificial Opening **8** Via Natural or Artificial Opening Endoscopic	**G** Other Therapeutic Substance	**C** Other Substance
E Products of Conception **G** Upper GI **H** Lower GI **K** Genitourinary Tract **N** Male Reproductive	**3** Percutaneous **7** Via Natural or Artificial Opening **8** Via Natural or Artificial Opening Endoscopic	**S** Gas	**F** Other Gas

Continued

ction 3 **Administration**
dy System E **Physiological Systems and Anatomical Regions**
peration 0 **Introduction:** Putting in or on a therapeutic, diagnostic, nutritional, physiological, or prophylactic substance except blood or blood products

Body System / Region (4th)	Approach (5th)	Substance (6th)	Qualifier (7th)
E Products of Conception G Upper GI H Lower GI K Genitourinary Tract N Male Reproductive	4 Percutaneous Endoscopic	G Other Therapeutic Substance	C Other Substance
F Respiratory Tract	3 Percutaneous 7 Via Natural or Artificial Opening 8 Via Natural or Artificial Opening Endoscopic	0 Antineoplastic	4 Liquid Brachytherapy Radioisotope 5 Other Antineoplastic M Monoclonal Antibody
F Respiratory Tract	3 Percutaneous 7 Via Natural or Artificial Opening 8 Via Natural or Artificial Opening Endoscopic	2 Anti-infective	8 Oxazolidinones 9 Other Anti-infective
F Respiratory Tract	3 Percutaneous 7 Via Natural or Artificial Opening 8 Via Natural or Artificial Opening Endoscopic	3 Anti-inflammatory 6 Nutritional Substance 7 Electrolytic and Water Balance Substance B Anesthetic Agent H Radioactive Substance K Other Diagnostic Substance N Analgesics, Hypnotics, Sedatives T Destructive Agent	Z No Qualifier
F Respiratory Tract	3 Percutaneous 7 Via Natural or Artificial Opening 8 Via Natural or Artificial Opening Endoscopic	G Other Therapeutic Substance	C Other Substance
F Respiratory Tract	3 Percutaneous 7 Via Natural or Artificial Opening 8 Via Natural or Artificial Opening Endoscopic	S Gas	D Nitric Oxide F Other Gas
F Respiratory Tract	4 Percutaneous Endoscopic	G Other Therapeutic Substance	C Other Substance
J Biliary and Pancreatic Tract	3 Percutaneous 7 Via Natural or Artificial Opening 8 Via Natural or Artificial Opening Endoscopic	0 Antineoplastic	4 Liquid Brachytherapy Radioisotope 5 Other Antineoplastic M Monoclonal Antibody
J Biliary and Pancreatic Tract	3 Percutaneous 7 Via Natural or Artificial Opening 8 Via Natural or Artificial Opening Endoscopic	2 Anti-infective	8 Oxazolidinones 9 Other Anti-infective

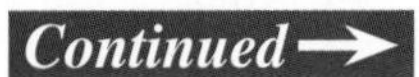
Continued →

Section 3 **Administration**
Body System E **Physiological Systems and Anatomical Regions**
Operation 0 **Introduction:** Putting in or on a therapeutic, diagnostic, nutritional, physiological, or prophylactic substance except blood or blood products

Body System / Region (4th)	Approach (5th)	Substance (6th)	Qualifier (7th)
J Biliary and Pancreatic Tract	**3** Percutaneous **7** Via Natural or Artificial Opening **8** Via Natural or Artificial Opening Endoscopic	**3** Anti-inflammatory **6** Nutritional Substance **7** Electrolytic and Water Balance Substance **B** Anesthetic Agent **H** Radioactive Substance **K** Other Diagnostic Substance **N** Analgesics, Hypnotics, Sedatives **T** Destructive Agent	**Z** No Qualifier
J Biliary and Pancreatic Tract	**3** Percutaneous **7** Via Natural or Artificial Opening **8** Via Natural or Artificial Opening Endoscopic	**G** Other Therapeutic Substance	**C** Other Substance
J Biliary and Pancreatic Tract	**3** Percutaneous **7** Via Natural or Artificial Opening **8** Via Natural or Artificial Opening Endoscopic	**S** Gas	**F** Other Gas
J Biliary and Pancreatic Tract	**3** Percutaneous **7** Via Natural or Artificial Opening **8** Via Natural or Artificial Opening Endoscopic	**U** Pancreatic Islet Cells	**0** Autologous **1** Nonautologous
J Biliary and Pancreatic Tract	**4** Percutaneous Endoscopic	**G** Other Therapeutic Substance	**C** Other Substance
L Pleural Cavity **M** Peritoneal Cavity	**0** Open	**5** Adhesion Barrier	**Z** No Qualifier
L Pleural Cavity **M** Peritoneal Cavity	**3** Percutaneous	**0** Antineoplastic	**4** Liquid Brachytherapy Radioisotope **5** Other Antineoplastic **M** Monoclonal Antibody
L Pleural Cavity **M** Peritoneal Cavity	**3** Percutaneous	**2** Anti-infective	**8** Oxazolidinones **9** Other Anti-infective
L Pleural Cavity **M** Peritoneal Cavity	**3** Percutaneous	**3** Anti-inflammatory **6** Nutritional Substance **7** Electrolytic and Water Balance Substance **B** Anesthetic Agent **H** Radioactive Substance **K** Other Diagnostic Substance **N** Analgesics, Hypnotics, Sedatives **T** Destructive Agent	**Z** No Qualifier
L Pleural Cavity **M** Peritoneal Cavity	**3** Percutaneous	**G** Other Therapeutic Substance	**C** Other Substance
L Pleural Cavity **M** Peritoneal Cavity	**3** Percutaneous	**S** Gas	**F** Other Gas
L Pleural Cavity **M** Peritoneal Cavity	**4** Percutaneous Endoscopic	**5** Adhesion Barrier	**Z** No Qualifier

Continued →

tion 3 **Administration**
dy System E **Physiological Systems and Anatomical Regions**
eration 0 **Introduction:** Putting in or on a therapeutic, diagnostic, nutritional, physiological, or prophylactic substance except blood or blood products

Body System / Region (4th)	Approach (5th)	Substance (6th)	Qualifier (7th)
L Pleural Cavity **M** Peritoneal Cavity	**4** Percutaneous Endoscopic	**G** Other Therapeutic Substance	**C** Other Substance
L Pleural Cavity **M** Peritoneal Cavity	**7** Via Natural or Artificial Opening	**0** Antineoplastic	**4** Liquid Brachytherapy Radioisotope **5** Other Antineoplastic **M** Monoclonal Antibody
L Pleural Cavity **M** Peritoneal Cavity	**7** Via Natural or Artificial Opening	**S** Gas	**F** Other Gas
P Female Reproductive	**0** Open	**5** Adhesion Barrier	**Z** No Qualifier
P Female Reproductive	**3** Percutaneous	**0** Antineoplastic	**4** Liquid Brachytherapy Radioisotope **5** Other Antineoplastic **M** Monoclonal Antibody
P Female Reproductive	**3** Percutaneous	**2** Anti-infective	**8** Oxazolidinones **9** Other Anti-infective
P Female Reproductive	**3** Percutaneous	**3** Anti-inflammatory **5** Adhesion Barrier **6** Nutritional Substance **7** Electrolytic and Water Balance Substance **B** Anesthetic Agent **H** Radioactive Substance **K** Other Diagnostic Substance **L** Sperm **N** Analgesics, Hypnotics, Sedatives **T** Destructive Agent **V** Hormone	**Z** No Qualifier
P Female Reproductive	**3** Percutaneous	**G** Other Therapeutic Substance	**C** Other Substance
P Female Reproductive	**3** Percutaneous	**Q** Fertilized Ovum	**0** Autologous **1** Nonautologous
P Female Reproductive	**3** Percutaneous	**S** Gas	**F** Other Gas
P Female Reproductive	**4** Percutaneous Endoscopic	**5** Adhesion Barrier	**Z** No Qualifier
P Female Reproductive	**4** Percutaneous Endoscopic	**G** Other Therapeutic Substance	**C** Other Substance
P Female Reproductive	**7** Via Natural or Artificial Opening	**0** Antineoplastic	**4** Liquid Brachytherapy Radioisotope **5** Other Antineoplastic **M** Monoclonal Antibody
P Female Reproductive	**7** Via Natural or Artificial Opening	**2** Anti-infective	**8** Oxazolidinones **9** Other Anti-infective
P Female Reproductive	**7** Via Natural or Artificial Opening	**5** Adhesion Barrier **6** Nutritional Substance **7** Electrolytic and Water Balance Substance **B** Anesthetic Agent **H** Radioactive Substance **K** Other Diagnostic Substance **L** Sperm **N** Analgestics, Hypnotics, Sedatives **T** Destructive Agent **V** Hormone	**Z** No Qualifier

Continued →

Section 3 **Administration**
Body System E **Physiological Systems and Anatomical Regions**
Operation 0 **Introduction:** Putting in or on a therapeutic, diagnostic, nutritional, physiological, or prophylactic substance except blood or blood products

3E0 Contin

Body System / Region (4th)	Approach (5th)	Substance (6th)	Qualifier (7th)
P Female Reproductive	**7** Via Natural or Artificial Opening	**G** Other Therapeutic Substance	**C** Other Substance
P Female Reproductive	**7** Via Natural or Artificial Opening	**Q** Fertilized Ovum	**0** Autologous **1** Nonautologous
P Female Reproductive	**7** Via Natural or Artificial Opening	**S** Gas	**F** Other Gas
P Female Reproductive	**8** Via Natural or Artificial Opening Endoscopic	**0** Antineoplastic	**4** Liquid Brachytherapy Radioisotope **5** Other Antineoplastic **M** Monoclonal Antibody
P Female Reproductive	**8** Via Natural or Artificial Opening Endoscopic	**2** Anti-infective	**8** Oxazolidinones **9** Other Anti-infective
P Female Reproductive	**8** Via Natural or Artificial Opening Endoscopic	**3** Anti-inflammatory **6** Nutritional Substance **7** Electrolytic and Water Balance Substance **B** Anesthetic Agent **H** Radioactive Substance **K** Other Diagnostic Substance **N** Analgesics, Hypnotics, Sedatives **T** Destructive Agent	**Z** No Qualifier
P Female Reproductive	**8** Via Natural or Artificial Opening Endoscopic	**G** Other Therapeutic Substance	**C** Other Substance
P Female Reproductive	**8** Via Natural or Artificial Opening Endoscopic	**S** Gas	**F** Other Gas
Q Cranial Cavity and Brain	**0** Open **3** Percutaneous	**0** Antineoplastic	**4** Liquid Brachytherapy Radioisotope **5** Other Antineoplastic **M** Monoclonal Antibody
Q Cranial Cavity and Brain	**0** Open **3** Percutaneous	**2** Anti-infective	**8** Oxazolidinones **9** Other Anti-infective
Q Cranial Cavity and Brain	**0** Open **3** Percutaneous	**3** Anti-inflammatory **6** Nutritional Substitute **7** Electrolytic and Water Balance Substitute **A** Stem Cells, Embryonic **B** Anesthetic Agent **H** Radioactive Substance **K** Other Diagnostic Substance **N** Analgesics, Hypnotics, Sedatives **T** Destructive Agent	**Z** No Qualifier
Q Cranial Cavity and Brain	**0** Open **3** Percutaneous	**E** Stem Cells, Somatic	**0** Autologous **1** Nonautologous
Q Cranial Cavity and Brain	**0** Open **3** Percutaneous	**G** Other Therapeutic Substance	**C** Other Substance
Q Cranial Cavity and Brain	**0** Open **3** Percutaneous	**S** Gas	**F** Other Gas

Continued →

tion	3	Administration
dy System	E	Physiological Systems and Anatomical Regions
eration	0	Introduction: Putting in or on a therapeutic, diagnostic, nutritional, physiological, or prophylactic substance except blood or blood products

Body System / Region (4th)	Approach (5th)	Substance (6th)	Qualifier (7th)
Q Cranial Cavity and Brain	7 Via Natural or Artificial Opening	0 Antineoplastic	4 Liquid Brachytherapy Radioisotope 5 Other Antineoplastic M Monoclonal Antibody
Q Cranial Cavity and Brain	7 Via Natural or Artificial Opening	S Gas	F Other Gas
R Spinal Canal	0 Open	A Stem Cells, Embryonic	Z No Qualifier
R Spinal Canal	0 Open	E Stem Cells, Somatic	0 Autologous 1 Nonautologous
R Spinal Canal	3 Percutaneous	0 Antineoplastic	2 High-dose Interleukin-2 3 Low-dose Interleukin-2 4 Liquid Brachytherapy Radioisotope 5 Other Antineoplastic M Monoclonal Antibody
R Spinal Canal	3 Percutaneous	2 Anti-infective	8 Oxazolidinones 9 Other Anti-infective
R Spinal Canal	3 Percutaneous	3 Anti-inflammatory 6 Nutritional Substance 7 Electrolytic and Water Balance Substance A Stem Cells, Embryonic B Anesthetic Agent H Radioactive Substance K Other Diagnostic Substance N Analgesics, Hypnotics, Sedatives T Destructive Agent	Z No Qualifier
R Spinal Canal	3 Percutaneous	E Stem Cells, Somatic	0 Autologous 1 Nonautologous
R Spinal Canal	3 Percutaneous	G Other Therapeutic Substance	C Other Substance
R Spinal Canal	3 Percutaneous	S Gas	F Other Gas
R Spinal Canal	7 Via Natural or Artificial Opening	S Gas	F Other Gas
S Epidural Space	3 Percutaneous	0 Antineoplastic	2 High-dose Interleukin-2 3 Low-dose Interleukin-2 4 Liquid Brachytherapy Radioisotope 5 Other Antineoplastic M Monoclonal Antibody
S Epidural Space	3 Percutaneous	2 Anti-infective	8 Oxazolidinones 9 Other Anti-infective
S Epidural Space	3 Percutaneous	3 Anti-inflammatory 6 Nutritional Substance 7 Electrolytic and Water Balance Substance B Anesthetic Agent H Radioactive Substance K Other Diagnostic Substance N Analgesics, Hypnotics, Sedatives T Destructive Agent	Z No Qualifier
S Epidural Space	3 Percutaneous	G Other Therapeutic Substance	C Other Substance

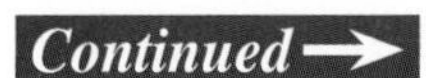

Section 3 **Administration**
Body System E **Physiological Systems and Anatomical Regions**
Operation 0 **Introduction:** Putting in or on a therapeutic, diagnostic, nutritional, physiological, or prophylactic substance except blood or blood products

3E0 Contin

Body System / Region (4th)	Approach (5th)	Substance (6th)	Qualifier (7th)
S Epidural Space	**3** Percutaneous	**S** Gas	**F** Other Gas
S Epidural Space	**7** Via Natural or Artificial Opening	**S** Gas	**F** Other Gas
T Peripheral Nerves and Plexi **X** Cranial Nerves	**3** Percutaneous	**3** Anti-inflammatory **B** Anesthetic Agent **T** Destructive Agent	**Z** No Qualifier
T Peripheral Nerves and Plexi **X** Cranial Nerves	**3** Percutaneous	**G** Other Therapeutic Substance	**C** Other Substance
U Joints	**0** Open	**2** Anti-infective	**8** Oxazolidinones **9** Other Anti-infective
U Joints	**0** Open	**G** Other Therapeutic Substance	**B** Recombinant Bone Morphogenetic Protein
U Joints	**3** Percutaneous	**0** Antineoplastic	**4** Liquid Brachytherapy Radioisotope **5** Other Antineoplastic **M** Monoclonal Antibody
U Joints	**3** Percutaneous	**2** Anti-infective	**8** Oxazolidinones **9** Other Anti-infective
U Joints	**3** Percutaneous	**3** Anti-inflammatory **6** Nutritional Substance **7** Electrolytic and Water Balance Substance **B** Anesthetic Agent **H** Radioactive Substance **K** Other Diagnostic Substance **N** Analgesics, Hypnotics, Sedatives **T** Destructive Agent	**Z** No Qualifier
U Joints	**3** Percutaneous	**G** Other Therapeutic Substance	**B** Recombinant Bone Morphogenetic Protein **C** Other Substance
U Joints	**3** Percutaneous	**S** Gas	**F** Other Gas
U Joints	**4** Percutaneous Endoscopic	**G** Other Therapeutic Substance	**C** Other Substance
V Bones	**0** Open	**G** Other Therapeutic Substance	**B** Recombinant Bone Morphogenetic Protein
V Bones	**3** Percutaneous	**0** Antineoplastic	**5** Other Antineoplastic **M** Monoclonal Antibody
V Bones	**3** Percutaneous	**2** Anti-infective	**8** Oxazolidinones **9** Other Anti-infective
V Bones	**3** Percutaneous	**3** Anti-inflammatory **6** Nutritional Substance **7** Electrolytic and Water Balance Substance **B** Anesthetic Agent **H** Radioactive Substance **K** Other Diagnostic Substance **N** Analgesics, Hypnotics, Sedatives **T** Destructive Agent	**Z** No Qualifier

Continued →

Section	**3**	**Administration**
Body System	**E**	**Physiological Systems and Anatomical Regions**
Operation	**0**	**Introduction:** Putting in or on a therapeutic, diagnostic, nutritional, physiological, or prophylactic substance except blood or blood products

Body System / Region (4th)	Approach (5th)	Substance (6th)	Qualifier (7th)
V Bones	**3** Percutaneous	**G** Other Therapeutic Substance	**B** Recombinant Bone Morphogenetic Protein **C** Other Substance
W Lymphatics	**3** Percutaneous	**0** Antineoplastic	**5** Other Antineoplastic **M** Monoclonal Antibody
W Lymphatics	**3** Percutaneous	**2** Anti-infective	**8** Oxazolidinones **9** Other Anti-infective
W Lymphatics	**3** Percutaneous	**3** Anti-inflammatory **6** Nutritional Substance **7** Electrolytic and Water Balance Substance **B** Anesthetic Agent **H** Radioactive Substance **K** Other Diagnostic Substance **N** Analgesics, Hypnotics, Sedatives **T** Destructive Agent	**Z** No Qualifier
W Lymphatics	**3** Percutaneous	**G** Other Therapeutic Substance	**C** Other Substance
Y Pericardial Cavity	**3** Percutaneous	**0** Antineoplastic	**4** Liquid Brachytherapy Radioisotope **5** Other Antineoplastic **M** Monoclonal Antibody
Y Pericardial Cavity	**3** Percutaneous	**2** Anti-infective	**8** Oxazolidinones **9** Other Anti-infective
Y Pericardial Cavity	**3** Percutaneous	**3** Anti-inflammatory **6** Nutritional Substance **7** Electrolytic and Water Balance Substance **B** Anesthetic Agent **H** Radioactive Substance **K** Other Diagnostic Substance **N** Analgesics, Hypnotics, Sedatives **T** Destructive Agent	**Z** No Qualifier
Y Pericardial Cavity	**3** Percutaneous	**G** Other Therapeutic Substance	**C** Other Substance
Y Pericardial Cavity	**3** Percutaneous	**S** Gas	**F** Other Gas
Y Pericardial Cavity	**4** Percutaneous Endoscopic	**G** Other Therapeutic Substance	**C** Other Substance
Y Pericardial Cavity	**7** Via Natural or Artificial Opening	**0** Antineoplastic	**4** Liquid Brachytherapy Radioisotope **5** Other Antineoplastic **M** Monoclonal Antibody
Y Pericardial Cavity	**7** Via Natural or Artificial Opening	**S** Gas	**F** Other Gas

Section 3 **Administration**
Body System E **Physiological Systems and Anatomical Regions**
Operation 1 **Irrigation:** Putting in or on a cleansing substance

Body System / Region (4th)	Approach (5th)	Substance (6th)	Qualifier (7th)
0 Skin and Mucous Membranes **C** Eye	**3** Percutaneous **X** External	**8** Irrigating Substance	**X** Diagnostic **Z** No Qualifier
9 Nose **B** Ear **F** Respiratory Tract **G** Upper GI **H** Lower GI **J** Biliary and Pancreatic Tract **K** Genitourinary Tract **N** Male Reproductive **P** Female Reproductive	**3** Percutaneous **7** Via Natural or Artificial Opening **8** Via Natural or Artificial Opening Endoscopic	**8** Irrigating Substance	**X** Diagnostic **Z** No Qualifier
L Pleural Cavity **Q** Cranial Cavity and Brain **R** Spinal Canal **S** Epidural Space **U** Joints **Y** Pericardial Cavity	**3** Percutaneous	**8** Irrigating Substance	**X** Diagnostic **Z** No Qualifier
M Peritoneal Cavity	**3** Percutaneous	**8** Irrigating Substance	**X** Diagnostic **Z** No Qualifier
M Peritoneal Cavity	**3** Percutaneous	**9** Dialysate	**Z** No Qualifier

AHA Coding Clinic

3E013GC Introduction of Other Therapeutic Substance into Subcutaneous Tissue, Percutaneous Approach - AHA CC: 2Q, 2014, 10
3E0234Z Introduction of Serum, Toxoid and Vaccine into Muscle, Percutaneous Approach - AHA CC: 4Q, 2014, 16
3E03317 Introduction of Other Thrombolytic into Peripheral Vein, Percutaneous Approach - AHA CC: 4Q, 2013, 124
3E033VJ Introduction of Other Hormone into Peripheral Vein, Percutaneous Approach - AHA CC: 4Q, 2014, 17-18
3E05305 Introduction of Other Antineoplastic into Peripheral Artery, Percutaneous Approach - AHA CC: 1Q, 2015, 38
3E06305 Introduction of Other Antineoplastic into Central Artery, Percutaneous Approach - AHA CC: 3Q, 2014 26-27
3E06317 Introduction of Other Thrombolytic into Central Artery, Percutaneous Approach - AHA CC: 4Q, 2014, 19-20
3E0G76Z Introduction of Nutritional Substance into Upper GI, Via Natural or Artificial Opening - AHA CC: 2Q, 2015, 29
3E0G8GC Introduction of Other Therapeutic Substance into Upper GI, via Natural or Artificial Opening Endoscopic - AHA CC: 3Q, 2015, 24-
3E0G8TZ Introduction of Destructive Agent into Upper GI, Via Natural or Artificial Opening Endoscopic - AHA CC: 1Q, 2013, 27
3E0H3GC Introduction of Other Therapeutic Substance into Lower GI, Percutaneous Approach - AHA CC: 1Q, 2017, 37
3E0L3GC Introduction of Other Therapeutic Substance into Pleural Cavity, Percutaneous Approach - AHA CC: 2Q, 2015, 3 2Q, 2017, 14-15
3E0M3GC Introduction of Other Therapeutic Substance into Peritoneal Cavity, Percutaneous Approach - AHA CC: 4Q, 2014, 38
3E0P7GC Introduction of Other Therapeutic Substance into Female Reproductive, Via Natural or Artificial Opening - AHA CC: 2Q, 2014, 8
3E0Q005 Introduction of Other Antineoplastic into Cranial Cavity and Brain, Open Approach - AHA CC: 4Q, 2016, 114
3E0Q305 Introduction of Other Antineoplastic into Cranial Cavity and Brain, Percutaneous Approach - AHA CC: 4Q, 2014, 34-35
3E0R305 Introduction of Other Antineoplastic into Spinal Canal, Percutaneous Approach - AHA CC: 1Q, 2015, 31
3E0U0GB Introduction of Recombinant Bone Morphogenetic Protein into Joints, Open Approach— AHA CC: 1Q, 2018, 8
3E0V0GB Introduction of Recombinant Bone Morphogenetic Protein into Bones, Open Approach -AHA CC: 3Q, 2016, 29-30

ithin each section of ICD-10-PCS the characters have different meanings. The seven character meanings for the Measurement and onitoring section are illustrated here through the procedure example of *External electrocardiogram (EKG), single reading*.

Section	Body System	Root Operation	Body System	Approach	Function / Device	Qualifier
Measurement and Monitoring	Physiological Systems	Measurement	Cardiac	External	Electrical Activity	None
4	**A**	**0**	**2**	**X**	**4**	**Z**

ction (Character 1)

l Measurement and Monitoring procedure codes have a first character value of 4.

ody System (Character 2)

e alphanumeric character for the body system is placed in the second position. There are two character values applicable for the easurement and Monitoring section. The character value of A is reported for physiological systems. The character value B is reported r physiological devices.

oot Operations (Character 3)

e alphanumeric character value for root operations is placed in the third position. Listed here are the root operations applicable to the easurement and Monitoring section with their associated meaning.

Character Value	Root Operation	Root Operation Definition
0	Measurement	Determining the level of a physiological or physical function at a point in time
1	Monitoring	Determining the level of a physiological or physical function repetitively over a period of time

ody System/Region (Character 4)

r each body system the applicable body part character values will be available for procedure code construction. An example of a body gion for this section is Respiratory.

pproach (Character 5)

he approach is the technique used to reach the procedure site. The following are the approach character values for the Measurement and onitoring section with the associated definitions.

Character Value	Approach	Approach Definition
0	Open	Cutting through the skin or mucous membrane and any other body layers necessary to expose the site of the procedure
3	Percutaneous	Entry, by puncture or minor incision, of instrumentation through the skin or mucous membrane and any other body layers necessary to reach the site of the procedure
4	Percutaneous Endoscopic	Entry, by puncture or minor incision, of instrumentation through the skin or mucous membrane and any other body layers necessary to reach and visualize the site of the procedure
7	Via Natural or Artificial Opening	Entry of instrumentation through a natural or artificial external opening to reach the site of the procedure
8	Via Natural or Artificial Opening Endoscopic	Entry of instrumentation through a natural or artificial external opening to reach and visualize the site of the procedure
X	External	Procedures performed directly on the skin or mucous membrane and procedures performed indirectly by the application of external force through the skin or mucous membrane

Function/Device (Character 6)

In the Measurement and Monitoring section a function or device is always utilized. The function or device is reported in the sixth charac position by the type of function monitored or measured or by the device utilized. The following is a sample list of the functions and devi included in this section:

- Conductivity
- Flow
- Metabolism
- Pressure
- Sound

Qualifier (Character 7)

The qualifier represents an additional attribute for the procedure when applicable. There are several qualifiers included in the Measurem and Monitoring section. For example, measurement procedures in this section include several qualifiers including stress that is repor with the character value of 4. If there is no qualifier for a procedure, the placeholder Z is the character valve that should be reported.

Measurement and Monitoring Section Tables

Measurement and Monitoring Tables 4A0–4B0

Section 4 **Measurement and Monitoring**
Body System A **Physiological Systems**
Operation 0 **Measurement:** Determining the level of a physiological or physical function at a point in time

Body System (4th)	Approach (5th)	Function / Device (6th)	Qualifier (7th)
0 Central Nervous	**0** Open	**2** Conductivity **4** Electrical Activity **B** Pressure	**Z** No Qualifier
0 Central Nervous	**3** Percutaneous **7** Via Natural or Artificial Opening **8** Via Natural or Artificial Opening Endoscopic	**4** Electrical Activity	**Z** No Qualifier
0 Central Nervous	**3** Percutaneous **7** Via Natural or Artificial Opening **8** Via Natural or Artificial Opening Endoscopic	**B** Pressure **K** Temperature **R** Saturation	**D** Intracranial
0 Central Nervous	**X** External	**2** Conductivity **4** Electrical Activity	**Z** No Qualifier
1 Peripheral Nervous	**0** Open **3** Percutaneous **7** Via Natural or Artificial Opening **8** Via Natural or Artificial Opening Endoscopic **X** External	**2** Conductivity	**9** Sensory **B** Motor
1 Peripheral Nervous	**0** Open **3** Percutaneous **7** Via Natural or Artificial Opening **8** Via Natural or Artificial Opening Endoscopic **X** External	**4** Electrical Activity	**Z** No Qualifier
2 Cardiac	**0** Open **3** Percutaneous **7** Via Natural or Artificial Opening **8** Via Natural or Artificial Opening Endoscopic	**4** Electrical Activity **9** Output **C** Rate **F** Rhythm **H** Sound **P** Action Currents	**Z** No Qualifier
2 Cardiac	**0** Open **3** Percutaneous **7** Via Natural or Artificial Opening **8** Via Natural or Artificial Opening Endoscopic	**N** Sampling and Pressure	**6** Right Heart **7** Left Heart **8** Bilateral
2 Cardiac	**X** External	**4** Electrical Activity	**A** Guidance **Z** No Qualifier

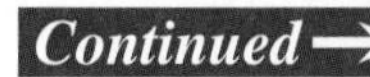

Body System (4th)	Approach (5th)	Function / Device (6th)	Qualifier (7th)
2 Cardiac	X External	9 Output C Rate F Rhythm H Sound P Action Currents	Z No Qualifier
2 Cardiac	X External	M Total Activity	4 Stress
3 Arterial	0 Open 3 Percutaneous	5 Flow J Pulse	1 Peripheral 3 Pulmonary C Coronary
3 Arterial	0 Open 3 Percutaneous	B Pressure	1 Peripheral 3 Pulmonary C Coronary F Other Thoracic
3 Arterial	0 Open 3 Percutaneous	H Sound R Saturation	1 Peripheral
3 Arterial	X External	5 Flow B Pressure H Sound J Pulse R Saturation	1 Peripheral
4 Venous	0 Open 3 Percutaneous	5 Flow B Pressure J Pulse	0 Central 1 Peripheral 2 Portal 3 Pulmonary
4 Venous	0 Open 3 Percutaneous	R Saturation	1 Peripheral
4 Venous	X External	5 Flow B Pressure J Pulse R Saturation	1 Peripheral
5 Circulatory	X External	L Volume	Z No Qualifier
6 Lymphatic	0 Open 3 Percutaneous 7 Via Natural or Artificial Opening 8 Via Natural or Artificial Opening Endoscopic	5 Flow B Pressure	Z No Qualifier
7 Visual	X External	0 Acuity 7 Mobility B Pressure	Z No Qualifier
8 Olfactory	X External	0 Acuity	Z No Qualifier
9 Respiratory	7 Via Natural or Artificial Opening 8 Via Natural or Artificial Opening Endoscopic X External	1 Capacity 5 Flow C Rate D Resistance L Volume M Total Activity	Z No Qualifier
B Gastrointestinal	7 Via Natural or Artificial Opening 8 Via Natural or Artificial Opening Endoscopic	8 Motility B Pressure G Secretion	Z No Qualifier

Continued →

Section 4 **Measurement and Monitoring**
Body System A **Physiological Systems**
Operation 0 **Measurement:** Determining the level of a physiological or physical function at a point in time

Body System (4th)	Approach (5th)	Function / Device (6th)	Qualifier (7th)
C Biliary	**3** Percutaneous **4** Percutaneous Endoscopic **7** Via Natural or Artificial Opening **8** Via Natural or Artificial Opening Endoscopic	**5** Flow **B** Pressure	**Z** No Qualifier
D Urinary	**7** Via Natural or Artificial Opening **8** Via Natural or Artificial Opening Endoscopic	**3** Contractility **5** Flow **B** Pressure **D** Resistance **L** Volume	**Z** No Qualifier
F Musculoskeletal	**3** Percutaneous **X** External	**3** Contractility	**Z** No Qualifier
H Products of Conception, Cardiac	**7** Via Natural or Artificial Opening **8** Via Natural or Artificial Opening Endoscopic **X** External	**4** Electrical Activity **C** Rate **F** Rhythm **H** Sound	**Z** No Qualifier
J Products of Conception, Nervous	**7** Via Natural or Artificial Opening **8** Via Natural or Artificial Opening Endoscopic **X** External	**2** Conductivity **4** Electrical Activity **B** Pressure	**Z** No Qualifier
Z None	**7** Via Natural or Artificial Opening	**6** Metabolism **K** Temperature	**Z** No Qualifier
Z None	**X** External	**6** Metabolism **K** Temperature **Q** Sleep	**Z** No Qualifier

Section 4 **Measurement and Monitoring**
Body System A **Physiological Systems**
Operation 1 **Monitoring:** Determining the level of a physiological or physical function repetitively over a period of time

Body System (4th)	Approach (5th)	Function / Device (6th)	Qualifier (7th)
0 Central Nervous	**0** Open	**2** Conductivity **B** Pressure	**Z** No Qualifier
0 Central Nervous	**0** Open	**4** Electrical Activity	**G** Intraoperative **Z** No Qualifier
0 Central Nervous	**3** Percutaneous **7** Via Natural or Artificial Opening **8** Via Natural or Artificial Opening Endoscopic	**4** Electrical Activity	**G** Intraoperative **Z** No Qualifier
0 Central Nervous	**3** Percutaneous **7** Via Natural or Artificial Opening **8** Via Natural or Artificial Opening Endoscopic	**B** Pressure **K** Temperature **R** Saturation	**D** Intracranial
0 Central Nervous	**X** External	**2** Conductivity	**Z** No Qualifier
0 Central Nervous	**X** External	**4** Electrical Activity	**G** Intraoperative **Z** No Qualifier
1 Peripheral Nervous	**0** Open **3** Percutaneous **7** Via Natural or Artificial Opening **8** Via Natural or Artificial Opening Endoscopic **X** External	**2** Conductivity	**9** Sensory **B** Motor

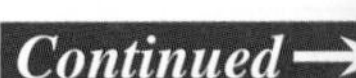
Continued →

Body System (4th)	Approach (5th)	Function / Device (6th)	Qualifier (7th)
1 Peripheral Nervous	0 Open 3 Percutaneous 7 Via Natural or Artificial Opening 8 Via Natural or Artificial Opening Endoscopic X External	4 Electrical Activity	G Intraoperative Z No Qualifier
2 Cardiac	0 Open 3 Percutaneous 7 Via Natural or Artificial Opening 8 Via Natural or Artificial Opening Endoscopic	4 Electrical Activity 9 Output C Rate F Rhythm H Sound	Z No Qualifier
2 Cardiac	X External	4 Electrical Activity	5 Ambulatory Z No Qualifier
2 Cardiac	X External	9 Output C Rate F Rhythm H Sound	Z No Qualifier
2 Cardiac	X External	M Total Activity	4 Stress
2 Cardiac	X External	S Vascular Perfusion	H Indocyanine Green Dye
3 Arterial	0 Open 3 Percutaneous	5 Flow B Pressure J Pulse	1 Peripheral 3 Pulmonary C Coronary
3 Arterial	0 Open 3 Percutaneous	H Sound R Saturation	1 Peripheral
3 Arterial	X External	5 Flow B Pressure H Sound J Pulse R Saturation	1 Peripheral
4 Venous	0 Open 3 Percutaneous	5 Flow B Pressure J Pulse	0 Central 1 Peripheral 2 Portal 3 Pulmonary
4 Venous	0 Open 3 Percutaneous	R Saturation	0 Central 2 Portal 3 Pulmonary
4 Venous	X External	5 Flow B Pressure J Pulse	1 Peripheral
6 Lymphatic	0 Open 3 Percutaneous 7 Via Natural or Artificial Opening 8 Via Natural or Artificial Opening Endoscopic	5 Flow B Pressure	Z No Qualifier
9 Respiratory	7 Via Natural or Artificial Opening X External	1 Capacity 5 Flow C Rate D Resistance L Volume	Z No Qualifier

Continued →

Section 4 **Measurement and Monitoring**
Body System A **Physiological Systems**
Operation 1 **Monitoring:** Determining the level of a physiological or physical function repetitively over a period of time

Body System (4th)	Approach (5th)	Function / Device (6th)	Qualifier (7th)
B Gastrointestinal	**7** Via Natural or Artificial Opening **8** Via Natural or Artificial Opening Endoscopic	**8** Motility **B** Pressure **G** Secretion	**Z** No Qualifier
B Gastrointestinal	**X** External	**S** Vascular Perfusion	**H** Indocyanine Green Dye
D Urinary	**7** Via Natural or Artificial Opening **8** Via Natural or Artificial Opening Endoscopic	**3** Contractility **5** Flow **B** Pressure **D** Resistance **L** Volume	**Z** No Qualifier
G Skin and Breast	**X** External	**S** Vascular Perfusion	**H** Indocyanine Green Dye
H Products of Conception, Cardiac	**7** Via Natural or Artificial Opening **8** Via Natural or Artificial Opening Endoscopic **X** External	**4** Electrical Activity **C** Rate **F** Rhythm **H** Sound	**Z** No Qualifier
J Products of Conception, Nervous	**7** Via Natural or Artificial Opening **8** Via Natural or Artificial Opening Endoscopic **X** External	**2** Conductivity **4** Electrical Activity **B** Pressure	**Z** No Qualifier
Z None	**7** Via Natural or Artificial Opening	**K** Temperature	**Z** No Qualifier
Z None	**X** External	**K** Temperature **Q** Sleep	**Z** No Qualifier

Section 4 **Measurement and Monitoring**
Body System B **Physiological Devices**
Operation 0 **Measurement:** Determining the level of a physiological or physical function at a point in time

Body System (4th)	Approach (5th)	Function / Device (6th)	Qualifier (7th)
0 Central Nervous **1** Peripheral Nervous **F** Musculoskeletal	**X** External	**V** Stimulator	**Z** No Qualifier
2 Cardiac	**X** External	**S** Pacemaker **T** Defibrillator	**Z** No Qualifier
9 Respiratory	**X** External	**S** Pacemaker	**Z** No Qualifier

AHA Coding Clinic

4A023N8 Measurement of Cardiac Sampling and Pressure, Bilateral, Percutaneous Approach—AHA CC: 1Q, 2018, 12-13

4A02X4Z Measurement of Cardiac Electrical Activity, External Approach - AHA CC: 3Q, 2015, 29

4A033BC Measurement of Arterial Pressure, Coronary, Percutaneous Approach - AHA CC: 3Q, 2016, 37

4A103BD Monitoring of Intracranial Pressure, Percutaneous Approach - AHA CC: 2Q, 2016, 29

4A1134G Monitoring of Peripheral Nervous Electrical Activity, Intraoperative, Percutaneous Approach - AHA CC: 4Q, 2014, 28-29

4A11X4G Monitoring of Peripheral Nervous Electrical Activity, Intraoperative, External Approach - AHA CC: 1Q, 2015, 26; 2Q, 2015,

4A1239Z Monitoring of Cardiac Output, Percutaneous Approach - AHA CC: 3Q, 2015, 35

4A133B1 Monitoring of Arterial Pressure, Peripheral, Percutaneous Approach, for Continuous Monitoring of Pressure - AHA CC: 2Q, 2016, 33

4A133B3 Monitoring of Arterial Pressure, Pulmonary, Percutaneous Approach - AHA CC: 3Q, 2015, 35

4A133J1 Monitoring of Arterial Pulse, Peripheral, Percutaneous Approach, for Continuous Monitoring of Pulse - AHA CC: 2Q, 2016,

Extracorporeal or Systemic Assistance and Performance Section (5A0–5A2)

ithin each section of ICD-10-PCS the characters have different meanings. The seven character meanings for the Extracorporeal or stemic Assistance and Performance section are illustrated here through the procedure example of *Hyperbaric oxygenation of wound.*

Section	Body System	Root Operation	Body System	Duration	Function	Qualifier
Extracorporeal or Systemic Assistance and Performance	Physiological Systems	Assistance	Circulatory	Intermittent	Oxygenation	Hyperbaric
5	A	0	5	1	2	1

ction (Character 1)

l Extracorporeal or Systemic Assistance and Performance procedure codes have a first character value of 5.

dy System (Character 2)

e alphanumeric character for the body system is placed in the second position. There is one character value applicable for the tracorporeal or Systemic Assistance and Performance section. The character value of A is reported for physiological systems.

oot Operations (Character 3)

e alphanumeric character value for root operations is placed in the third position. Listed here are the root operations applicable to the tracorporeal or Systemic Assistance and Performance section with their associated meaning.

Character Value	Root Operation	Root Operation Definition
0	Assistance	Taking over a portion of a physiological function by extracorporeal means
1	Performance	Completely taking over a physiological function by extracorporeal means
2	Restoration	Returning, or attempting to return, a physiological function to its original state by extracorporeal means

dy System (Character 4)

r each body system, the applicable body part character values will be available for procedure code construction. An example of a body gion for this section is respiratory.

uration (Character 5)

e duration represents the length of time or frequency for which the assistance or performance is utilized. Some examples of duration Intermittent, Continuous, or Less than 24 consecutive hours.

nction (Character 6)

the Extracorporeal or Systemic Assistance and Performance section a function is always reported. The function is reported in the sixth aracter position. The following is a sample list of the functions utilized in this section:

- Output
- Oxygenation
- Pacing
- Ventilation

ualifier (Character 7)

e qualifier represents an additional attribute for the procedure when applicable. There are several qualifiers included in the Extracorporeal Systemic Assistance and Performance section. For example, assistance procedures in this section include several qualifiers including lloon Pump, which is reported with the character value of 0. If there is no qualifier for a procedure, the placeholder Z is the character lve that should be reported.

Extracorporeal or Systemic Assistance and Performance Section Tables

Extracorporeal or Systemic Assistance and Performance Tables 5A0–5A2

Section 5 **Extracorporeal or Systemic Assistance and Performance**
Body System A **Physiological Systems**
Operation 0 **Assistance:** Taking over a portion of a physiological function by extracorporeal means

Body System (4th)	Duration (5th)	Function (6th)	Qualifier (7th)
2 Cardiac	**1** Intermittent **2** Continuous	**1** Output	**0** Balloon Pump **5** Pulsatile Compression **6** Other Pump **D** Impeller Pump
5 Circulatory	**1** Intermittent **2** Continuous	**2** Oxygenation	**1** Hyperbaric **C** Supersaturated
9 Respiratory	**2** Continuous	**0** Filtration	**Z** No Qualifier
9 Respiratory	**3** Less than 24 Consecutive Hours **4** 24-96 Consecutive Hours **5** Greater than 96 Consecutive Hours	**5** Ventilation	**7** Continuous Positive Airway Pressure **8** Intermittent Positive Airway Pressure **9** Continuous Negative Airway Pressure **B** Intermittent Negative Airway Pressure **Z** No Qualifier

Section 5 **Extracorporeal or Systemic Assistance and Performance**
Body System A **Physiological Systems**
Operation 1 **Performance:** Completely taking over a physiological function by extracorporeal means

Body System (4th)	Duration (5th)	Function (6th)	Qualifier (7th)
2 Cardiac	**0** Single	**1** Output	**2** Manual
2 Cardiac	**1** Intermittent	**3** Pacing	**Z** No Qualifier
2 Cardiac	**2** Continuous	**1** Output **3** Pacing	**Z** No Qualifier
5 Circulatory	**2** Continuous	**2** Oxygenation	**F** Membrane, Central **G** Membrane, Periphera Veno-arterial **H** Membrane, Periphera Veno-venous
9 Respiratory	**0** Single	**5** Ventilation	**4** Nonmechanical
9 Respiratory	**3** Less than 24 Consecutive Hours **4** 24-96 Consecutive Hours **5** Greater than 96 Consecutive Hours	**5** Ventilation	**Z** No Qualifier
C Biliary	**0** Single **6** Multiple	**0** Filtration	**Z** No Qualifier
D Urinary	**7** Intermittent, Less than 6 Hours Per Day **8** Prolonged Intermittent, 6-18 Hours Per Day **9** Continuous, Greater than 18 Hours Per Day	**0** Filtration	**Z** No Qualifier

Section 5 **Extracorporeal or Systemic Assistance and Performance**
Body System A **Physiological Systems**
Operation 2 **Restoration:** Returning, or attempting to return, a physiological function to its original state by extracorporeal means.

Body System (4th)	Duration (5th)	Function (6th)	Qualifier (7th)
2 Cardiac	**0** Single	**4** Rhythm	**Z** No Qualifier

HA Coding Clinic

A02210 Assistance with Cardiac Output using Balloon Pump, Continuous - AHA CC: 3Q, 2013, 18-19; 2Q, 2018, 4-5

A0221D Assistance with Cardiac Output using Impeller Pump, Continuous - AHA CC: 3Q, 2014, 19; 4Q, 2016, 138-139; 1Q, 2017, 11-12; 4Q, 2017, 43-45

A09357 Assistance with Respiratory Ventilation, <24 Hrs, CPAP - AHA CC: 4Q, 2014, 9-10

A09457 Assistance with Respiratory Ventilation, 24-96 Hrs, CPAP - AHA CC: 4Q, 2014, 9-10

A09557 Assistance with Respiratory Ventilation, >96 Hrs, CPAP - AHA CC: 4Q, 2014, 9-10

A1221Z Performance of Cardiac Output, Continuous - AHA CC: 3Q, 2013, 18-19; 1Q, 2014, 10-11; 3Q, 2014, 16-17, 20-21; 4Q, 2015, 22-25; 1Q, 2016, 27-28; 1Q, 2017, 19-20; 3Q, 2017, 7-8

A1223Z Performance of Cardiac Pacing, Continuous - AHA CC: 3Q, 2013, 18-19

A1935Z Respiratory Ventilation, Less than 24 Consecutive Hours - AHA CC: 4Q, 2014, 3-15; 1Q, 2018, 13-14

A1945Z Respiratory Ventilation, 24-96 Consecutive Hours - AHA CC: 4Q, 2014, 3-15

A1955Z Respiratory Ventilation, Greater than 96 Consecutive Hours - AHA CC: 4Q, 2014, 3-15

A1C00Z Performance of Biliary Filtration, Single - AHA CC: 1Q, 2016, 28-29

A1D60Z Performance of Urinary Filtration, Multiple - AHA CC: 1Q, 2016, 29

A1D70Z Performance of Urinary Filtration, Intermittent, Less than 6 Hours Per Day—AHA CC: 4Q, 2017, 72-73

A1D80Z Performance of Urinary Filtration, Prolonged Intermittent, 6-18 hours Per Day—AHA CC: 4Q, 2017, 72

A1D90Z Performance of Urinary Filtration, Continuous, Greater than 18 hours Per Day—AHA CC: 4Q, 2017, 72-73

Extracorporeal or Systemic Therapies Section (6A0–6AB)

Within each section of ICD-10-PCS the characters have different meanings. The seven character meanings for the Extracorporeal Systemic Therapies section are illustrated here through the procedure example of *Ultraviolet light phototherapy, series treatment.*

Section	Body System	Root Operation	Body System	Duration	Qualifier	Qualifier
Extracorporeal or Systemic Therapies	Physiological Systems	UV Light Therapy	Skin	Multiple	None	None
6	A	8	0	1	Z	Z

Section (Character 1)

All Extracorporeal or Systemic Therapies procedure codes have a first character value of 6.

Body System (Character 2)

The alphanumeric character for the body system is placed in the second position. There is one character value applicable for t Extracorporeal or Systemic Therapies section. The character value of A is reported for physiological systems.

Root Operations (Character 3)

The alphanumeric character value for root operations is placed in the third position. Listed below are the root operations applicable to t Extracorporeal or Systemic Therapies section with their associated meaning.

Character Value	Root Operation	Root Operation Definition
0	Atmospheric Control	Extracorporeal control of atmospheric pressure and composition
1	Decompression	Extracorporeal elimination of undissolved gas from body fluids
2	Electromagnetic Therapy	Extracorporeal treatment by electromagnetic rays
3	Hyperthermia	Extracorporeal raising of body temperature
4	Hypothermia	Extracorporeal lowering of body temperature
5	Pheresis	Extracorporeal separation of blood products
6	Phototherapy	Extracorporeal treatment by light rays
7	Ultrasound Therapy	Extracorporeal treatment by ultrasound
8	Ultraviolet Light Therapy	Extracorporeal treatment by ultraviolet light
9	Shock Wave Therapy	Extracorporeal treatment by shock waves
B	Perfusion	Extracorporeal treatment by diffusion of therapeutic fluid

Body System (Character 4)

For each body system the applicable body part character values will be available for procedure code construction. An example of a bo region for this section is Skin.

Duration (Character 5)

The duration represents the number of therapy sessions performed. Single is reported with character value 0; Multiple is reported wi character value 1.

Qualifier (Character 6)

Character 6 is the first of two qualifier characters for the Extracorporeal or Systemic Therapies section. The qualifier represents additional attribute for the procedure when applicable. There are currently no qualifier values for the sixth character position, so t character value of Z is always reported.

Qualifier (Character 7)

Character 7 is the second of two qualifier characters for the Extracorporeal or Systemic Therapies section. The qualifier represents additional attribute for the procedure when applicable. There are some qualifiers included in the Extracorporeal or Systemic Therapi section. For example, pheresis procedures in this section include several qualifiers including Plasma that is reported with the charact value of 3. If there is no qualifier for a procedure, the placeholder Z is the character valve that should be reported.

Extracorporeal or Systemic Therapies Tables 6A0–6AB

Section 6 **Extracorporeal or Systemic Therapies**
Body System A **Physiological Systems**
Operation 0 **Atmospheric Control:** Extracorporeal control of atmospheric pressure and composition

Body System (4th)	Duration (5th)	Qualifier (6th)	Qualifier (7th)
Z None	0 Single 1 Multiple	Z No Qualifier	Z No Qualifier

Section 6 **Extracorporeal or Systemic Therapies**
Body System A **Physiological Systems**
Operation 1 **Decompression:** Extracorporeal elimination of undissolved gas from body fluids

Body System (4th)	Duration (5th)	Qualifier (6th)	Qualifier (7th)
5 Circulatory	0 Single 1 Multiple	Z No Qualifier	Z No Qualifier

Section 6 **Extracorporeal or Systemic Therapies**
Body System A **Physiological Systems**
Operation 2 **Electromagnetic Therapy:** Extracorporeal treatment by electromagnetic rays

Body System (4th)	Duration (5th)	Qualifier (6th)	Qualifier (7th)
1 Urinary 2 Central Nervous	0 Single 1 Multiple	Z No Qualifier	Z No Qualifier

Section 6 **Extracorporeal or Systemic Therapies**
Body System A **Physiological Systems**
Operation 3 **Hyperthermia:** Extracorporeal raising of body temperature

Body System (4th)	Duration (5th)	Qualifier (6th)	Qualifier (7th)
Z None	0 Single 1 Multiple	Z No Qualifier	Z No Qualifier

Section 6 **Extracorporeal or Systemic Therapies**
Body System A **Physiological Systems**
Operation 4 **Hypothermia:** Extracorporeal lowering of body temperature

Body System (4th)	Duration (5th)	Qualifier (6th)	Qualifier (7th)
Z None	0 Single 1 Multiple	Z No Qualifier	Z No Qualifier

Section 6 **Extracorporeal or Systemic Therapies**
Body System A **Physiological Systems**
Operation 5 **Pheresis:** Extracorporeal separation of blood products

Body System (4th)	Duration (5th)	Qualifier (6th)	Qualifier (7th)
5 Circulatory	0 Single 1 Multiple	Z No Qualifier	0 Erythrocytes 1 Leukocytes 2 Platelets 3 Plasma T Stem Cells, Cord Blood V Stem Cells, Hematopoietic

Section 6 **Extracorporeal or Systemic Therapies**
Body System A **Physiological Systems**
Operation 6 **Phototherapy:** Extracorporeal treatment by light rays

Body System (4th)	Duration (5th)	Qualifier (6th)	Qualifier (7th)
0 Skin **5** Circulatory	**0** Single **1** Multiple	**Z** No Qualifier	**Z** No Qualifier

Section 6 **Extracorporeal or Systemic Therapies**
Body System A **Physiological Systems**
Operation 7 **Ultrasound Therapy:** Extracorporeal treatment by ultrasound

Body System (4th)	Duration (5th)	Qualifier (6th)	Qualifier (7th)
5 Circulatory	**0** Single **1** Multiple	**Z** No Qualifier	**4** Head and Neck Vessels **5** Heart **6** Peripheral Vessels **7** Other Vessels **Z** No Qualifier

Section 6 **Extracorporeal or Systemic Therapies**
Body System A **Physiological Systems**
Operation 8 **Ultraviolet Light Therapy:** Extracorporeal treatment by ultraviolet light

Body System (4th)	Duration (5th)	Qualifier (6th)	Qualifier (7th)
0 Skin	**0** Single **1** Multiple	**Z** No Qualifier	**Z** No Qualifier

Section 6 **Extracorporeal or Systemic Therapies**
Body System A **Physiological Systems**
Operation 9 **Shock Wave Therapy:** Extracorporeal treatment by shock waves

Body System (4th)	Duration (5th)	Qualifier (6th)	Qualifier (7th)
3 Musculoskeletal	**0** Single **1** Multiple	**Z** No Qualifier	**Z** No Qualifier

Section 6 **Extracorporeal or Systemic Therapies**
Body System A **Physiological Systems**
Operation B **Perfusion:** Extracorporeal treatment by diffusion of therapeutic fluid

Body System (4th)	Duration (5th)	Qualifier (6th)	Qualifier (7th)
5 Circulatory **B** Respiratory System **F** Hepatobiliary System and Pancreas **T** Urinary System	**0** Single	**B** Donor Organ	**Z** No Qualifier

AHA Coding Clinic

6A750Z7 Ultrasound Therapy of Other Vessels, Single - AHA CC: 4Q, 2014, 19-20

ithin each section of ICD-10-PCS, the characters have different meanings. The seven character meanings for the Osteopathic section are ustrated below through the procedure example of Indirect osteopathic treatment of sacrum.

Section	Body System	Root Operation	Body Region	Approach	Method	Qualifier
Osteopathic	Anatomical Regions	Treatment	Sacrum	External	Indirect	None
7	W	0	4	X	4	Z

ction (Character 1)

l Osteopathic procedure codes have a first character value of 7.

ody System (Character 2)

e alphanumeric character for the body system is placed in the second position. There is one character value applicable for the Osteopathic ction. The character value of W is reported for anatomical regions.

oot Operations (Character 3)

e alphanumeric character value for root operations is placed in the third position. Listed here is the root operation applicable to the steopathic section with its associated meaning.

Character Value	Root Operation	Root Operation Definition
0	Treatment	Manual treatment to eliminate or alleviate somatic dysfunction and related disorders

ody Region (Character 4)

r each body region the applicable body part character values will be available for procedure code construction. An example of a body gion for this section is Head.

pproach (Character 5)

e approach is the technique used to reach the procedure site. The following are the approach character values for the Osteopathic section ith the associated definitions.

Character Value	Approach	Approach Definition
X	External	Procedures performed directly on the skin or mucous membrane and procedures performed indirectly by the application of external force through the skin or mucous membrane

lethod (Character 6)

he method identifies the treatment method used to complete the osteopathic procedure. The available methods are:

- Articulatory-Raising
- Fascial Release
- General Mobilization
- High Velocity-Low Amplitude
- Indirect
- Low Velocity-High Amplitude
- Lymphatic Pump
- Muscle Energy-Isometric
- Muscle Energy-Isotonic
- Other

Qualifier (Character 7)

The qualifier represents an additional attribute for the procedure when applicable. Currently, there are no qualifiers in the Osteopathic section; therefore, the placeholder character value of Z should be reported.

Osteopathic Section Table

Osteopathic Table 7W0

Section 7 **Osteopathic**
Body System W **Anatomical Regions**
Operation 0 **Treatment:** Manual treatment to eliminate or alleviate somatic dysfunction and related disorders

Body Region (4th)	Approach (5th)	Method (6th)	Qualifier (7th)
0 Head **1** Cervical **2** Thoracic **3** Lumbar **4** Sacrum **5** Pelvis **6** Lower Extremities **7** Upper Extremities **8** Rib Cage **9** Abdomen	**X** External	**0** Articulatory-Raising **1** Fascial Release **2** General Mobilization **3** High Velocity-Low Amplitude **4** Indirect **5** Low Velocity-High Amplitude **6** Lymphatic Pump **7** Muscle Energy-Isometric **8** Muscle Energy-Isotonic **9** Other Method	**Z** None

AHA Coding Clinic

No references have been issued for the Osteopathic Section.

Other Procedures Section (8C0–8E0)

ithin each section of ICD-10-PCS the characters have different meanings. The seven character meanings for the Other Procedures section are illus-ated here through the procedure example of Yoga therapy.

Section	Body System	Root Operation	Body Region	Approach	Method	Qualifier
Other Procedures	Physiological Systems and Anatomical Regions	Other Procedures	None	External	Other Method	Yoga Therapy
8	E	0	Z	X	Y	4

ection (Character 1)

ll Other Procedures codes have a first character value of 8.

ody System (Character 2)

he alphanumeric character for the body system is placed in the second position. There are two character values applicable for the Other rocedures section. The character value of C is reported for indwelling device. The character value of E is reported for physiological /stem and anatomical regions.

oot Operations (Character 3)

he alphanumeric character value for root operations is placed in the third position. Listed here is the root operation applicable to the ther Procedures section with its associated meaning.

Character Value	Root Operation	Root Operation Definition
0	Other Procedures	Methodologies which attempt to remediate or cure a disorder or disease

ody Region (Character 4)

or each body region the applicable body part character values will be available for procedure code construction. An example of a body egion for this section is Lower Extremity.

pproach (Character 5)

he approach is the technique used to reach the procedure site. The following are the approach character values for the Other Procedures ection with the associated definitions.

Character Value	Approach	Approach Definition
0	Open	Cutting through the skin or mucous membrane and any other body layers necessary to expose the site of the procedure
3	Percutaneous	Entry, by puncture or minor incision, of instrumentation through the skin or mucous membrane and any other body layers necessary to reach the site of the procedure
4	Percutaneous Endoscopic	Entry, by puncture or minor incision, of instrumentation through the skin or mucous membrane and any other body layers necessary to reach and visualize the site of the procedure
7	Via Natural or Artificial Opening	Entry of instrumentation through a natural or artificial external opening to reach the site of the procedure
8	Via Natural or Artificial Opening Endoscopic	Entry of instrumentation through a natural or artificial external opening to reach and visualize the site of the procedure
X	External	Procedures performed directly on the skin or mucous membrane and procedures performed indirectly by the application of external force through the skin or mucous membrane

Method (Character 6)

The method identifies the treatment method used to complete the other procedure. The available methods are:

- Acupuncture
- Collection
- Computer Assisted Procedure
- Near Infrared Spectroscopy
- Robotic Assisted procedure
- Therapeutic Massage
- Other

Qualifier (Character 7)

The qualifier represents an additional attribute for the procedure when applicable. In the preceding example of Yoga therapy, the qualif of 4 was used to report that the other procedure was Yoga therapy. If there is no qualifier for a procedure, the placeholder Z is the charac valve that should be reported.

Other Procedures Section Tables

Other Procedures Tables 8C0–8E0

Section 8 **Other Procedures**
Body System C **Indwelling Device**
Operation 0 **Other Procedures:** Methodologies which attempt to remediate or cure a disorder or disease

Body Region (4th)	Approach (5th)	Method (6th)	Qualifier (7th)
1 Nervous System	**X** External	**6** Collection	**J** Cerebrospinal Fluid **L** Other Fluid
2 Circulatory System	**X** External	**6** Collection	**K** Blood **L** Other Fluid

Section 8 **Other Procedures**
Body System E **Physiological Systems and Anatomical Regions**
Operation 0 **Other Procedures:** Methodologies which attempt to remediate or cure a disorder or disease

Body Region (4th)	Approach (5th)	Method (6th)	Qualifier (7th)
1 Nervous System **U** Female Reproductive System	**X** External	**Y** Other Method	**7** Examination
2 Circulatory System	**3** Percutaneous	**D** Near Infrared Spectroscopy	**Z** No Qualifier
9 Head and Neck Region **W** Trunk Region	**0** Open **3** Percutaneous **4** Percutaneous Endoscopic **7** Via Natural or Artificial Opening **8** Via Natural or Artificial Opening Endoscopic	**C** Robotic Assisted Procedure	**Z** No Qualifier
9 Head and Neck Region **W** Trunk Region	**X** External	**B** Computer Assisted Procedure	**F** With Fluoroscopy **G** With Computerized Tomography **H** With Magnetic Resonance Imaging **Z** No Qualifier
9 Head and Neck Region **W** Trunk Region	**X** External	**C** Robotic Assisted Procedure	**Z** No Qualifier
9 Head and Neck Region **W** Trunk Region	**X** External	**Y** Other Method	**8** Suture Removal

Continued →

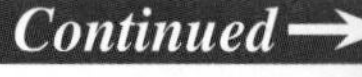

tion 8 **Other Procedures**
ly System E **Physiological Systems and Anatomical Regions**
eration 0 **Other Procedures:** Methodologies which attempt to remediate or cure a disorder or disease

Body Region (4th)	Approach (5th)	Method (6th)	Qualifier (7th)
Integumentary System and Breast	**3** Percutaneous	**0** Acupuncture	**0** Anesthesia **Z** No Qualifier
Integumentary System and Breast	**X** External	**6** Collection	**2** Breast Milk
Integumentary System and Breast	**X** External	**Y** Other Method	**9** Piercing
Musculoskeletal System	**X** External	**1** Therapeutic Massage	**Z** No Qualifier
Musculoskeletal System	**X** External	**Y** Other Method	**7** Examination
Male Reproductive System	**X** External	**1** Therapeutic Massage	**C** Prostate **D** Rectum
Male Reproductive System	**X** External	**6** Collection	**3** Sperm
Upper Extremity Lower Extremity	**0** Open **3** Percutaneous **4** Percutaneous Endoscopic	**C** Robotic Assisted Procedure	**Z** No Qualifier
Upper Extremity Lower Extremity	**X** External	**B** Computer Assisted Procedure	**F** With Fluoroscopy **G** With Computerized Tomography **H** With Magnetic Resonance Imaging **Z** No Qualifier
Upper Extremity Lower Extremity	**X** External	**C** Robotic Assisted Procedure	**Z** No Qualifier
Upper Extremity Lower Extremity	**X** External	**Y** Other Method	**8** Suture Removal
None	**X** External	**Y** Other Method	**1** In Vitro Fertilization **4** Yoga Therapy **5** Meditation **6** Isolation

IA Coding Clinic

0W4CZ Robotic Assisted Procedure of Trunk Region, Percutaneous Endoscopic Approach - AHA CC: 4Q, 2014, 33-34; 1Q, 2015, 33-34

Chiropractic Section (9WB)

Within each section of ICD-10-PCS the characters have different meanings. The seven character meanings for the Chiropractic section illustrated here through the procedure example of Chiropractic treatment of cervical spine, short lever specific contact.

Section	Body System	Root Operation	Body Region	Approach	Method	Qualifier
Chiropractic	Anatomical Regions	Manipulation	Cervical	External	Short Lever Specific Contact	None
9	W	B	1	X	H	Z

Section (Character 1)

All Chiropractic procedure codes have a first character value of 9.

Body System (Character 2)

The alphanumeric character for the body system is placed in the second position. There is one character value applicable for the Chiropra section. The character value of W is reported for anatomical regions.

Root Operations (Character 3)

The alphanumeric character value for root operations is placed in the third position. The following is the root operation applicable to Chiropractic section with its associated meaning.

Character Value	Root Operation	Root Operation Definition
B	Manipulation	Manual procedure that involves a directed thrust to move a joint past the physiological range of motion, without exceeding the anatomical limit

Body Region (Character 4)

For each body region the applicable body part character values will be available for procedure code construction. An example of a bo region for this section is Rib Cage.

Approach (Character 5)

The approach is the technique used to reach the procedure site. The following are the approach character values for the Chiroprac section with the associated definitions.

Character Value	Approach	Approach Definition
X	External	Procedures performed directly on the skin or mucous membrane and procedures performed indirectly by the application of external force through the skin or mucous membrane

Method (Character 6)

The method identifies the treatment method used to complete the chiropractic procedure. The available methods are:

- Non-Manual
- Indirect Visceral
- Extra-Articular
- Direct-Visual
- Long Lever Specific Contact
- Short Lever Specific Contact
- Long and Short Lever Specific Contact
- Mechanically Assisted
- Other

alifier (Character 7)

qualifier represents an additional attribute for the procedure when applicable. Currently, there are no qualifiers in the Chiropractic tion; therefore, the placeholder character value of Z should be reported.

iropractic Section Table

iropractic Table 9WB

tion 9 **Chiropractic**
ly System W **Anatomical Regions**
eration B **Manipulation:** Manual procedure that involves a directed thrust to move a joint past the physiological range of motion, without exceeding the anatomical limit

Body Region (4th)	Approach (5th)	Method (6th)	Qualifier (7th)
Head Cervical Thoracic Lumbar Sacrum Pelvis Lower Extremities Upper Extremities Rib Cage Abdomen	**X** External	**B** Non-Manual **C** Indirect Visceral **D** Extra-Articular **F** Direct Visceral **G** Long Lever Specific Contact **H** Short Lever Specific Contact **J** Long and Short Lever Specific Contact **K** Mechanically Assisted **L** Other Method	**Z** None

IA Coding Clinic

references have been issued for the Chiropractic Section.

Imaging Section (B00–BY4)

Within each section of ICD-10-PCS the characters have different meanings. The seven character meanings for the Imaging section illustrated here through the procedure example of X-ray right clavicle, limited study.

Section	Body System	Root Type	Body Part	Contrast	Qualifier	Qualifie
Imaging	Non-Axial Upper Bones	Plain Radiography	Clavicle, right	None	None	None
B	P	0	4	Z	Z	Z

Section (Character 1)

All Imaging procedure codes have a first character value of B.

Body System (Character 2)

The alphanumeric character for the body system is placed in the second position. The following are the body systems applicable to Imaging section.

Character Value	Character Value Description
0	Central Nervous System
2	Heart
3	Upper Arteries
4	Lower Arteries
5	Veins
7	Lymphatic System
8	Eye
9	Ear, Nose, Mouth and Throat
B	Respiratory System
D	Gastrointestinal System
F	Hepatobiliary System and Pancreas
G	Endocrine System
H	Skin, Subcutaneous Tissue and Breast
L	Connective Tissue
N	Skull and Facial Bones
P	Non-Axial Upper Bones
Q	Non-Axial Lower Bones
R	Axial Skeleton, Except Skull and Facial Bones
T	Urinary System
U	Female Reproductive System
V	Male Reproductive System
W	Anatomical Regions
Y	Fetus and Obstetrical

Root Types (Character 3)

The alphanumeric character value for root types is placed in the third position. Listed here are the root types applicable to the Imag section with their associated meaning.

Character Value	Root Type	Root Type Definition
0	Plain Radiography	Planar display of an image developed from the capture of external ionizing radiatio on photographic or photoconductive plate
1	Fluoroscopy	Single plane or bi-plane real time display of an image developed from the capture o external ionizing radiation on a fluorescent screen. The image may also be stored by either digital or analog means

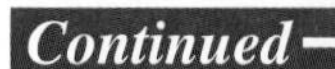

Character Value	Root Type	Root Type Definition
2	Computerized Tomography (CT Scan)	Computer reformatted digital display of multiplanar images developed from the capture of multiple exposures of external ionizing radiation
3	Magnetic Resonance Imaging (MRI)	Computer reformatted digital display of multiplanar images developed from the capture of radiofrequency signals emitted by nuclei in a body site excited within a magnetic field
4	Ultrasonography	Real time display of images of anatomy or flow information developed from the capture of reflected and attenuated high frequency sound waves

ody Part (Character 4)

›r each body part the applicable body part character values will be available for procedure code construction. An example of a body part r this section is Spinal Cord.

ontrast (Character 5)

'hen contrast is utilized during an imaging procedure, the corresponding contrast character value should be reported in the fifth character ›sition. The following are the contrast character values for the Imaging section:

- High Osmolar
- Low Osmolar
- Other Contrast

contrast is not utilized, the placeholder character value of Z should be reported.

ualifier (Character 6)

nis qualifier character specifies when an image taken without contrast is followed by one with contrast. The character value of 0 is ported for Unenhanced and Enhanced.

ualifier (Character 7)

he qualifier represents an additional attribute for the procedure when applicable. For example, ultrasonography procedures in this section clude the qualifier Densitometry that is reported with the character value of 1 for some body parts. If there is no qualifier for a procedure, e placeholder Z is the character valve that should be reported.

maging Section Tables

naging Tables B00–BY4

ection **B** **Imaging**
ody System **0** **Central Nervous System**
ype **0** **Plain Radiography:** Planar display of an image developed from the capture of external ionizing radiation on photographic or photoconductive plate

Body Part (4th)	Contrast (5th)	Qualifier (6th)	Qualifier (7th)
B Spinal Cord	**0** High Osmolar **1** Low Osmolar **Y** Other Contrast **Z** None	**Z** None	**Z** None

ection **B** **Imaging**
ody System **0** **Central Nervous System**
ype **1** **Fluoroscopy:** Single plane or bi-plane real time display of an image developed from the capture of external ionizing radiation on a fluorescent screen. The image may also be stored by either digital or analog means

Body Part (4th)	Contrast (5th)	Qualifier (6th)	Qualifier (7th)
B Spinal Cord	**0** High Osmolar **1** Low Osmolar **Y** Other Contrast **Z** None	**Z** None	**Z** None

Section B **Imaging**
Body System 0 **Central Nervous System**
Type 2 **Computerized Tomography (CT Scan):** Computer reformatted digital display of multiplanar images developed from th capture of multiple exposures of external ionizing radiation

Body Part (4th)	Contrast (5th)	Qualifier (6th)	Qualifier (7th)
0 Brain **7** Cisterna **8** Cerebral Ventricle(s) **9** Sella Turcica/Pituitary Gland **B** Spinal Cord	**0** High Osmolar **1** Low Osmolar **Y** Other Contrast	**0** Unenhanced and Enhanced **Z** None	**Z** None
0 Brain **7** Cisterna **8** Cerebral Ventricle(s) **9** Sella Turcica/Pituitary Gland **B** Spinal Cord	**Z** None	**Z** None	**Z** None

Section B **Imaging**
Body System 0 **Central Nervous System**
Type 3 **Magnetic Resonance Imaging (MRI):** Computer reformatted digital display of multiplanar images developed from the capture of radiofrequency signals emitted by nuclei in a body site excited within magnetic field

Body Part (4th)	Contrast (5th)	Qualifier (6th)	Qualifier (7th)
0 Brain **9** Sella Turcica/Pituitary Gland **B** Spinal Cord **C** Acoustic Nerves	**Y** Other Contrast	**0** Unenhanced and Enhanced **Z** None	**Z** None
0 Brain **9** Sella Turcica/Pituitary Gland **B** Spinal Cord **C** Acoustic Nerves	**Z** None	**Z** None	**Z** None

Section B **Imaging**
Body System 0 **Central Nervous System**
Type 4 **Ultrasonography:** Real time display of images of anatomy or flow information developed from the capture of reflected a attenuated high frequency sound waves

Body Part (4th)	Contrast (5th)	Qualifier (6th)	Qualifier (7th)
0 Brain **B** Spinal Cord	**Z** None	**Z** None	**Z** None

Section B **Imaging**
Body System 2 **Heart**
Type 0 **Plain Radiography:** Planar display of an image developed from the capture of external ionizing radiation on photographi or photoconductive plate

Body Part (4th)	Contrast (5th)	Qualifier (6th)	Qualifier (7th)
0 Coronary Artery, Single **1** Coronary Arteries, Multiple **2** Coronary Artery Bypass Graft, Single **3** Coronary Artery Bypass Grafts, Multiple **4** Heart, Right **5** Heart, Left **6** Heart, Right and Left **7** Internal Mammary Bypass Graft, Right **8** Internal Mammary Bypass Graft, Left **F** Bypass Graft, Other	**0** High Osmolar **1** Low Osmolar **Y** Other Contrast	**Z** None	**Z** None

ection B Imaging
ody System 2 Heart
ype 1 **Fluoroscopy:** Single plane or bi-plane real time display of an image developed from the capture of external ionizing radiation on a fluorescent screen. The image may also be stored by either digital or analog means

Body Part (4th)	Contrast (5th)	Qualifier (6th)	Qualifier (7th)
0 Coronary Artery, Single **1** Coronary Arteries, Multiple **2** Coronary Artery Bypass Graft, Single **3** Coronary Artery Bypass Grafts, Multiple	**0** High Osmolar **1** Low Osmolar **Y** Other Contrast	**1** Laser	**0** Intraoperative
0 Coronary Artery, Single **1** Coronary Arteries, Multiple **2** Coronary Artery Bypass Graft, Single **3** Coronary Artery Bypass Grafts, Multiple	**0** High Osmolar **1** Low Osmolar **Y** Other Contrast	**Z** None	**Z** None
4 Heart, Right **5** Heart, Left **6** Heart, Right and Left **7** Internal Mammary Bypass Graft, Right **8** Internal Mammary Bypass Graft, Left **F** Bypass Graft, Other	**0** High Osmolar **1** Low Osmolar **Y** Other Contrast	**Z** None	**Z** None

ection B Imaging
ody System 2 Heart
ype 2 **Computerized Tomography (CT Scan):** Computer reformatted digital display of multiplanar images developed from the capture of multiple exposures of external ionizing radiation

Body Part (4th)	Contrast (5th)	Qualifier (6th)	Qualifier (7th)
1 Coronary Arteries, Multiple **3** Coronary Artery Bypass Grafts, Multiple **6** Heart, Right and Left	**0** High Osmolar **1** Low Osmolar **Y** Other Contrast	**0** Unenhanced and Enhanced **Z** None	**Z** None
1 Coronary Arteries, Multiple **3** Coronary Artery Bypass Grafts, Multiple **6** Heart, Right and Left	**Z** None	**2** Intravascular Optical Coherence **Z** None	**Z** None

ection B Imaging
ody System 2 Heart
ype 3 **Magnetic Resonance Imaging (MRI):** Computer reformatted digital display of multiplanar images developed from the capture of radiofrequency signals emitted by nuclei in a body site excited within a magnetic field

Body Part (4th)	Contrast (5th)	Qualifier (6th)	Qualifier (7th)
1 Coronary Arteries, Multiple **3** Coronary Artery Bypass Grafts, Multiple **6** Heart, Right and Left	**Y** Other Contrast	**0** Unenhanced and Enhanced **Z** None	**Z** None
1 Coronary Arteries, Multiple **3** Coronary Artery Bypass Grafts, Multiple **6** Heart, Right and Left	**Z** None	**Z** None	**Z** None

Section B **Imaging**
Body System 2 **Heart**
Type 4 **Ultrasonography:** Real time display of images of anatomy or flow information developed from the capture of reflected a[nd] attenuated high frequency sound waves

Body Part (4th)	Contrast (5th)	Qualifier (6th)	Qualifier (7th)
0 Coronary Artery, Single **1** Coronary Arteries, Multiple **4** Heart, Right **5** Heart, Left **6** Heart, Right and Left **B** Heart with Aorta **C** Pericardium **D** Pediatric Heart	**Y** Other Contrast	**Z** None	**Z** None
0 Coronary Artery, Single **1** Coronary Arteries, Multiple **4** Heart, Right **5** Heart, Left **6** Heart, Right and Left **B** Heart with Aorta **C** Pericardium **D** Pediatric Heart	**Z** None	**Z** None	**3** Intravascular **4** Transesophageal **Z** None

Section B **Imaging**
Body System 3 **Upper Arteries**
Type 0 **Plain Radiography:** Planar display of an image developed from the capture of external ionizing radiation on photographi[c] or photoconductive plate

Body Part (4th)	Contrast (5th)	Qualifier (6th)	Qualifier (7th)
0 Thoracic Aorta **1** Brachiocephalic-Subclavian Artery, Right **2** Subclavian Artery, Left **3** Common Carotid Artery, Right **4** Common Carotid Artery, Left **5** Common Carotid Arteries, Bilateral **6** Internal Carotid Artery, Right **7** Internal Carotid Artery, Left **8** Internal Carotid Arteries, Bilateral **9** External Carotid Artery, Right **B** External Carotid Artery, Left **C** External Carotid Arteries, Bilateral **D** Vertebral Artery, Right **F** Vertebral Artery, Left **G** Vertebral Arteries, Bilateral **H** Upper Extremity Arteries, Right **J** Upper Extremity Arteries, Left **K** Upper Extremity Arteries, Bilateral **L** Intercostal and Bronchial Arteries **M** Spinal Arteries **N** Upper Arteries, Other **P** Thoraco-Abdominal Aorta **Q** Cervico-Cerebral Arch **R** Intracranial Arteries **S** Pulmonary Artery, Right **T** Pulmonary Artery, Left	**0** High Osmolar **1** Low Osmolar **Y** Other Contrast **Z** None	**Z** None	**Z** None

ection B Imaging
ody System 4 Lower Arteries
ype 1 **Fluoroscopy:** Single plane or bi-plane real time display of an image developed from the capture of external ionizing radiation on a fluorescent screen. The image may also be stored by either digital or analog means

Body Part (4th)	Contrast (5th)	Qualifier (6th)	Qualifier (7th)
0 Abdominal Aorta **2** Hepatic Artery **3** Splenic Arteries **4** Superior Mesenteric Artery **5** Inferior Mesenteric Artery **6** Renal Artery, Right **7** Renal Artery, Left **8** Renal Arteries, Bilateral **9** Lumbar Arteries **B** Intra-Abdominal Arteries, Other **C** Pelvic Arteries **D** Aorta and Bilateral Lower Extremity Arteries **F** Lower Extremity Arteries, Right **G** Lower Extremity Arteries, Left **J** Lower Arteries, Other	**Z** None	**Z** None	**Z** None

ection B Imaging
ody System 4 Lower Arteries
ype 2 **Computerized Tomography (CT Scan):** Computer reformatted digital display of multiplanar images developed from the capture of multiple exposures of external ionizing radiation

Body Part (4th)	Contrast (5th)	Qualifier (6th)	Qualifier (7th)
0 Abdominal Aorta **1** Celiac Artery **4** Superior Mesenteric Artery **8** Renal Arteries, Bilateral **C** Pelvic Arteries **F** Lower Extremity Arteries, Right **G** Lower Extremity Arteries, Left **H** Lower Extremity Arteries, Bilateral **M** Renal Artery Transplant	**0** High Osmolar **1** Low Osmolar **Y** Other Contrast	**Z** None	**Z** None
0 Abdominal Aorta **1** Celiac Artery **4** Superior Mesenteric Artery **8** Renal Arteries, Bilateral **C** Pelvic Arteries **F** Lower Extremity Arteries, Right **G** Lower Extremity Arteries, Left **H** Lower Extremity Arteries, Bilateral **M** Renal Artery Transplant	**Z** None	**2** Intravascular Optical Coherence **Z** None	**Z** None

ection B Imaging
Body System 4 Lower Arteries
Type 3 **Magnetic Resonance Imaging (MRI):** Computer reformatted digital display of multiplanar images developed from the capture of radiofrequency signals emitted by nuclei in a body site excited within a magnetic field

Body Part (4th)	Contrast (5th)	Qualifier (6th)	Qualifier (7th)
0 Abdominal Aorta **1** Celiac Artery **4** Superior Mesenteric Artery **8** Renal Arteries, Bilateral **C** Pelvic Arteries **F** Lower Extremity Arteries, Right **G** Lower Extremity Arteries, Left **H** Lower Extremity Arteries, Bilateral	**Y** Other Contrast	**0** Unenhanced and Enhanced **Z** None	**Z** None

Continued →

Section B **Imaging**
Body System 4 **Lower Arteries**
Type 3 **Magnetic Resonance Imaging (MRI):** Computer reformatted digital display of multiplanar images developed from the capture of radiofrequency signals emitted by nuclei in a body site excited within a magnetic field

Body Part (4th)	Contrast (5th)	Qualifier (6th)	Qualifier (7th)
0 Abdominal Aorta **1** Celiac Artery **4** Superior Mesenteric Artery **8** Renal Arteries, Bilateral **C** Pelvic Arteries **F** Lower Extremity Arteries, Right **G** Lower Extremity Arteries, Left **H** Lower Extremity Arteries, Bilateral	**Z** None	**Z** None	**Z** None

Section B **Imaging**
Body System 4 **Lower Arteries**
Type 4 **Ultrasonography:** Real time display of images of anatomy or flow information developed from the capture of reflected a attenuated high frequency sound waves

Body Part (4th)	Contrast (5th)	Qualifier (6th)	Qualifier (7th)
0 Abdominal Aorta **4** Superior Mesenteric Artery **5** Inferior Mesenteric Artery **6** Renal Artery, Right **7** Renal Artery, Left **8** Renal Arteries, Bilateral **B** Intra-Abdominal Arteries, Other **F** Lower Extremity Arteries, Right **G** Lower Extremity Arteries, Left **H** Lower Extremity Arteries, Bilateral **K** Celiac and Mesenteric Arteries **L** Femoral Artery **N** Penile Arteries	**Z** None	**Z** None	**3** Intravascular **Z** None

tion	**B**	**Imaging**
dy System	**5**	**Veins**
pe	**0**	**Plain Radiography:** Planar display of an image developed from the capture of external ionizing radiation on photographic or photoconductive plate

Body Part (4th)	Contrast (5th)	Qualifier (6th)	Qualifier (7th)
Epidural Veins Cerebral and Cerebellar Veins Intracranial Sinuses Jugular Veins, Right Jugular Veins, Left Jugular Veins, Bilateral Subclavian Vein, Right Subclavian Vein, Left Superior Vena Cava Inferior Vena Cava Lower Extremity Veins, Right Lower Extremity Veins, Left Lower Extremity Veins, Bilateral Pelvic (Iliac) Veins, Right Pelvic (Iliac) Veins, Left Pelvic (Iliac) Veins, Bilateral Renal Vein, Right Renal Vein, Left Renal Veins, Bilateral Upper Extremity Veins, Right Upper Extremity Veins, Left Upper Extremity Veins, Bilateral Pulmonary Vein, Right Pulmonary Vein, Left Pulmonary Veins, Bilateral Portal and Splanchnic Veins Veins, Other W Dialysis Shunt/Fistula	**0** High Osmolar **1** Low Osmolar **Y** Other Contrast	**Z** None	**Z** None

ction	**B**	**Imaging**
dy System	**5**	**Veins**
pe	**1**	**Fluoroscopy:** Single plane or bi-plane real time display of an image developed from the capture of external ionizing radiation on a fluorescent screen. The image may also be stored by either digital or analog means

Body Part (4th)	Contrast (5th)	Qualifier (6th)	Qualifier (7th)
0 Epidural Veins **1** Cerebral and Cerebellar Veins **2** Intracranial Sinuses **3** Jugular Veins, Right **4** Jugular Veins, Left **5** Jugular Veins, Bilateral **6** Subclavian Vein, Right **7** Subclavian Vein, Left **8** Superior Vena Cava **9** Inferior Vena Cava **B** Lower Extremity Veins, Right **C** Lower Extremity Veins, Left **D** Lower Extremity Veins, Bilateral **F** Pelvic (Iliac) Veins, Right **G** Pelvic (Iliac) Veins, Left **H** Pelvic (Iliac) Veins, Bilateral **J** Renal Vein, Right **K** Renal Vein, Left **L** Renal Veins, Bilateral **M** Upper Extremity Veins, Right **N** Upper Extremity Veins, Left **P** Upper Extremity Veins, Bilateral **Q** Pulmonary Vein, Right **R** Pulmonary Vein, Left **S** Pulmonary Veins, Bilateral **T** Portal and Splanchnic Veins **V** Veins, Other **W** Dialysis Shunt/Fistula	**0** High Osmolar **1** Low Osmolar **Y** Other Contrast **Z** None	**Z** None	**A** Guidance **Z** None

Section B **Imaging**
Body System 5 **Veins**
Type 2 **Computerized Tomography (CT Scan):** Computer reformatted digital display of multiplanar images developed from t capture of multiple exposures of external ionizing radiation

Body Part (4th)	Contrast (5th)	Qualifier (6th)	Qualifier (7th)
2 Intracranial Sinuses **8** Superior Vena Cava **9** Inferior Vena Cava **F** Pelvic (Iliac) Veins, Right **G** Pelvic (Iliac) Veins, Left **H** Pelvic (Iliac) Veins, Bilateral **J** Renal Vein, Right **K** Renal Vein, Left **L** Renal Veins, Bilateral **Q** Pulmonary Vein, Right **R** Pulmonary Vein, Left **S** Pulmonary Veins, Bilateral **T** Portal and Splanchnic Veins	**0** High Osmolar **1** Low Osmolar **Y** Other Contrast	**0** Unenhanced and Enhanced **Z** None	**Z** None
2 Intracranial Sinuses **8** Superior Vena Cava **9** Inferior Vena Cava **F** Pelvic (Iliac) Veins, Right **G** Pelvic (Iliac) Veins, Left **H** Pelvic (Iliac) Veins, Bilateral **J** Renal Vein, Right	**Z** None	**2** Intravascular Optical Coherence **Z** None	**Z** None
K Renal Vein, Left **L** Renal Veins, Bilateral **Q** Pulmonary Vein, Right **R** Pulmonary Vein, Left **S** Pulmonary Veins, Bilateral **T** Portal and Splanchnic Veins			

Section B **Imaging**
Body System 5 **Veins**
Type 3 **Magnetic Resonance Imaging (MRI):** Computer reformatted digital display of multiplanar images developed from the capture of radiofrequency signals emitted by nuclei in a body site excited within magnetic field

Body Part (4th)	Contrast (5th)	Qualifier (6th)	Qualifier (7th)
1 Cerebral and Cerebellar Veins **2** Intracranial Sinuses **5** Jugular Veins, Bilateral **8** Superior Vena Cava **9** Inferior Vena Cava **B** Lower Extremity Veins, Right **C** Lower Extremity Veins, Left **D** Lower Extremity Veins, Bilateral **H** Pelvic (Iliac) Veins, Bilateral **L** Renal Veins, Bilateral **M** Upper Extremity Veins, Right **N** Upper Extremity Veins, Left **P** Upper Extremity Veins, Bilateral **S** Pulmonary Veins, Bilateral **T** Portal and Splanchnic Veins **V** Veins, Other	**Y** Other Contrast	**0** Unenhanced and Enhanced **Z** None	**Z** None

Continued →

Section B **Imaging**
Body System 5 **Veins**
Type 3 **Magnetic Resonance Imaging (MRI):** Computer reformatted digital display of multiplanar images developed from the capture of radiofrequency signals emitted by nuclei in a body site excited within a magnetic field

Body Part (4th)	Contrast (5th)	Qualifier (6th)	Qualifier (7th)
1 Cerebral and Cerebellar Veins 2 Intracranial Sinuses 5 Jugular Veins, Bilateral 8 Superior Vena Cava 9 Inferior Vena Cava B Lower Extremity Veins, Right C Lower Extremity Veins, Left D Lower Extremity Veins, Bilateral H Pelvic (Iliac) Veins, Bilateral L Renal Veins, Bilateral M Upper Extremity Veins, Right N Upper Extremity Veins, Left P Upper Extremity Veins, Bilateral S Pulmonary Veins, Bilateral T Portal and Splanchnic Veins V Veins, Other	Z None	Z None	Z None

Section B **Imaging**
Body System 5 **Veins**
Type 4 **Ultrasonography:** Real time display of images of anatomy or flow information developed from the capture of reflected and attenuated high frequency sound waves

Body Part (4th)	Contrast (5th)	Qualifier (6th)	Qualifier (7th)
3 Jugular Veins, Right 4 Jugular Veins, Left 6 Subclavian Vein, Right 7 Subclavian Vein, Left 8 Superior Vena Cava 9 Inferior Vena Cava B Lower Extremity Veins, Right C Lower Extremity Veins, Left D Lower Extremity Veins, Bilateral J Renal Vein, Right K Renal Vein, Left L Renal Veins, Bilateral M Upper Extremity Veins, Right N Upper Extremity Veins, Left P Upper Extremity Veins, Bilateral T Portal and Splanchnic Veins	Z None	Z None	3 Intravascular A Guidance Z None

Section B **Imaging**
Body System 7 **Lymphatic System**
Type 0 **Plain Radiography:** Planar display of an image developed from the capture of external ionizing radiation on photographic or photoconductive plate

Body Part (4th)	Contrast (5th)	Qualifier (6th)	Qualifier (7th)
0 Abdominal/Retroperitoneal Lymphatics, Unilateral 1 Abdominal/Retroperitoneal Lymphatics, Bilateral 4 Lymphatics, Head and Neck 5 Upper Extremity Lymphatics, Right 6 Upper Extremity Lymphatics, Left 7 Upper Extremity Lymphatics, Bilateral 8 Lower Extremity Lymphatics, Right 9 Lower Extremity Lymphatics, Left B Lower Extremity Lymphatics, Bilateral C Lymphatics, Pelvic	0 High Osmolar 1 Low Osmolar Y Other Contrast	Z None	Z None

Section B **Imaging**
Body System 8 **Eye**
Type 0 **Plain Radiography:** Planar display of an image developed from the capture of external ionizing radiation on photographi or photoconductive plate

Body Part (4th)	Contrast (5th)	Qualifier (6th)	Qualifier (7th)
0 Lacrimal Duct, Right **1** Lacrimal Duct, Left **2** Lacrimal Ducts, Bilateral	**0** High Osmolar **1** Low Osmolar **Y** Other Contrast	**Z** None	**Z** None
3 Optic Foramina, Right **4** Optic Foramina, Left **5** Eye, Right **6** Eye, Left **7** Eyes, Bilateral	**Z** None	**Z** None	**Z** None

Section B **Imaging**
Body System 8 **Eye**
Type 2 **Computerized Tomography (CT Scan):** Computer reformatted digital display of multiplanar images developed from the capture of multiple exposures of external ionizing radiation

Body Part (4th)	Contrast (5th)	Qualifier (6th)	Qualifier (7th)
5 Eye, Right **6** Eye, Left **7** Eyes, Bilateral	**0** High Osmolar **1** Low Osmolar **Y** Other Contrast	**0** Unenhanced and Enhanced **Z** None	**Z** None
5 Eye, Right **6** Eye, Left **7** Eyes, Bilateral	**Z** None	**Z** None	**Z** None

Section B **Imaging**
Body System 8 **Eye**
Type 3 **Magnetic Resonance Imaging (MRI):** Computer reformatted digital display of multiplanar images developed from the capture of radiofrequency signals emitted by nuclei in a body site excited within a magnetic field

Body Part (4th)	Contrast (5th)	Qualifier (6th)	Qualifier (7th)
5 Eye, Right **6** Eye, Left **7** Eyes, Bilateral	**Y** Other Contrast	**0** Unenhanced and Enhanced **Z** None	**Z** None
5 Eye, Right **6** Eye, Left **7** Eyes, Bilateral	**Z** None	**Z** None	**Z** None

Section B **Imaging**
Body System 8 **Eye**
Type 4 **Ultrasonography:** Real time display of images of anatomy or flow information developed from the capture of reflected an attenuated high frequency sound waves

Body Part (4th)	Contrast (5th)	Qualifier (6th)	Qualifier (7th)
5 Eye, Right **6** Eye, Left **7** Eyes, Bilateral	**Z** None	**Z** None	**Z** None

ection B Imaging
ody System 9 Ear, Nose, Mouth and Throat
ype 0 **Plain Radiography:** Planar display of an image developed from the capture of external ionizing radiation on photographic or photoconductive plate

Body Part (4th)	Contrast (5th)	Qualifier (6th)	Qualifier (7th)
2 Paranasal Sinuses **F** Nasopharynx/Oropharynx **H** Mastoids	**Z** None	**Z** None	**Z** None
4 Parotid Gland, Right **5** Parotid Gland, Left **6** Parotid Glands, Bilateral **7** Submandibular Gland, Right **8** Submandibular Gland, Left **9** Submandibular Glands, Bilateral **B** Salivary Gland, Right **C** Salivary Gland, Left **D** Salivary Glands, Bilateral	**0** High Osmolar **1** Low Osmolar **Y** Other Contrast	**Z** None	**Z** None

ection B Imaging
ody System 9 Ear, Nose, Mouth and Throat
ype 1 **Fluoroscopy:** Single plane or bi-plane real time display of an image developed from the capture of external ionizing radiation on a fluorescent screen. The image may also be stored by either digital or analog means

Body Part (4th)	Contrast (5th)	Qualifier (6th)	Qualifier (7th)
G Pharynx and Epiglottis **J** Larynx	**Y** Other Contrast **Z** None	**Z** None	**Z** None

ection B Imaging
ody System 9 Ear, Nose, Mouth and Throat
ype 2 **Computerized Tomography (CT Scan):** Computer reformatted digital display of multiplanar images developed from the capture of multiple exposures of external ionizing radiation

Body Part (4th)	Contrast (5th)	Qualifier (6th)	Qualifier (7th)
0 Ear **2** Paranasal Sinuses **6** Parotid Glands, Bilateral **9** Submandibular Glands, Bilateral **D** Salivary Glands, Bilateral **F** Nasopharynx/Oropharynx **J** Larynx	**0** High Osmolar **1** Low Osmolar **Y** Other Contrast	**0** Unenhanced and Enhanced **Z** None	**Z** None
0 Ear **2** Paranasal Sinuses **6** Parotid Glands, Bilateral **9** Submandibular Glands, Bilateral **D** Salivary Glands, Bilateral **F** Nasopharynx/Oropharynx **J** Larynx	**Z** None	**Z** None	**Z** None

ection B Imaging
ody System 9 Ear, Nose, Mouth and Throat
ype 3 **Magnetic Resonance Imaging (MRI):** Computer reformatted digital display of multiplanar images developed from the capture of radiofrequency signals emitted by nuclei in a body site excited within a magnetic field

Body Part (4th)	Contrast (5th)	Qualifier (6th)	Qualifier (7th)
0 Ear **2** Paranasal Sinuses **6** Parotid Glands, Bilateral **9** Submandibular Glands, Bilateral **D** Salivary Glands, Bilateral **F** Nasopharynx/Oropharynx **J** Larynx	**Y** Other Contrast	**0** Unenhanced and Enhanced **Z** None	**Z** None

Continued →

B93 Continu

Section B **Imaging**
Body System 9 **Ear, Nose, Mouth and Throat**
Type 3 **Magnetic Resonance Imaging (MRI):** Computer reformatted digital display of multiplanar images developed from the capture of radiofrequency signals emitted by nuclei in a body site excited within a magnetic field

Body Part (4th)	Contrast (5th)	Qualifier (6th)	Qualifier (7th)
0 Ear **2** Paranasal Sinuses **6** Parotid Glands, Bilateral **9** Submandibular Glands, Bilateral **D** Salivary Glands, Bilateral **F** Nasopharynx/Oropharynx **J** Larynx	**Z** None	**Z** None	**Z** None

Section B **Imaging**
Body System B **Respiratory System**
Type 0 **Plain Radiography:** Planar display of an image developed from the capture of external ionizing radiation on photographi or photoconductive plate

Body Part (4th)	Contrast (5th)	Qualifier (6th)	Qualifier (7th)
7 Tracheobronchial Tree, Right **8** Tracheobronchial Tree, Left **9** Tracheobronchial Trees, Bilateral	**Y** Other Contrast	**Z** None	**Z** None
D Upper Airways	**Z** None	**Z** None	**Z** None

Section B **Imaging**
Body System B **Respiratory System**
Type 1 **Fluoroscopy:** Single plane or bi-plane real time display of an image developed from the capture of external ionizing radiation on a fluorescent screen. The image may also be stored by either digital or analog means

Body Part (4th)	Contrast (5th)	Qualifier (6th)	Qualifier (7th)
2 Lung, Right **3** Lung, Left **4** Lungs, Bilateral **6** Diaphragm **C** Mediastinum **D** Upper Airways	**Z** None	**Z** None	**Z** None
7 Tracheobronchial Tree, Right **8** Tracheobronchial Tree, Left **9** Tracheobronchial Trees, Bilateral	**Y** Other Contrast	**Z** None	**Z** None

Section B **Imaging**
Body System B **Respiratory System**
Type 2 **Computerized Tomography (CT Scan):** Computer reformatted digital display of multiplanar images developed from the capture of multiple exposures of external ionizing radiation

Body Part (4th)	Contrast (5th)	Qualifier (6th)	Qualifier (7th)
4 Lungs, Bilateral **7** Tracheobronchial Tree, Right **8** Tracheobronchial Tree, Left **9** Tracheobronchial Trees, Bilateral **F** Trachea/Airways	**0** High Osmolar **1** Low Osmolar **Y** Other Contrast	**0** Unenhanced and Enhanced **Z** None	**Z** None
4 Lungs, Bilateral **7** Tracheobronchial Tree, Right **8** Tracheobronchial Tree, Left **9** Tracheobronchial Trees, Bilateral **F** Trachea/Airways	**Z** None	**Z** None	**Z** None

tion	B	**Imaging**
dy System	B	**Respiratory System**
pe	3	**Magnetic Resonance Imaging (MRI):** Computer reformatted digital display of multiplanar images developed from the capture of radiofrequency signals emitted by nuclei in a body site excited within a magnetic field

Body Part (4th)	Contrast (5th)	Qualifier (6th)	Qualifier (7th)
G Lung Apices	**Y** Other Contrast	**0** Unenhanced and Enhanced **Z** None	**Z** None
G Lung Apices	**Z** None	**Z** None	**Z** None

tion	B	**Imaging**
dy System	B	**Respiratory System**
pe	4	**Ultrasonography:** Real time display of images of anatomy or flow information developed from the capture of reflected and attenuated high frequency sound waves

Body Part (4th)	Contrast (5th)	Qualifier (6th)	Qualifier (7th)
B Pleura C Mediastinum	**Z** None	**Z** None	**Z** None

ction	B	**Imaging**
dy System	D	**Gastrointestinal System**
pe	1	**Fluoroscopy:** Single plane or bi-plane real time display of an image developed from the capture of external ionizing radiation on a fluorescent screen. The image may also be stored by either digital or analog means

Body Part (4th)	Contrast (5th)	Qualifier (6th)	Qualifier (7th)
1 Esophagus 2 Stomach 3 Small Bowel 4 Colon 5 Upper GI 6 Upper GI and Small Bowel 9 Duodenum B Mouth/Oropharynx	**Y** Other Contrast **Z** None	**Z** None	**Z** None

ction	B	**Imaging**
dy System	D	**Gastrointestinal System**
pe	2	**Computerized Tomography (CT Scan):** Computer reformatted digital display of multiplanar images developed from the capture of multiple exposures of external ionizing radiation

Body Part (4th)	Contrast (5th)	Qualifier (6th)	Qualifier (7th)
4 Colon	**0** High Osmolar **1** Low Osmolar **Y** Other Contrast	**0** Unenhanced and Enhanced **Z** None	**Z** None
4 Colon	**Z** None	**Z** None	**Z** None

ction	B	**Imaging**
dy System	D	**Gastrointestinal System**
pe	4	**Ultrasonography:** Real time display of images of anatomy or flow information developed from the capture of reflected and attenuated high frequency sound waves

Body Part (4th)	Contrast (5th)	Qualifier (6th)	Qualifier (7th)
1 Esophagus 2 Stomach 7 Gastrointestinal Tract 8 Appendix 9 Duodenum C Rectum	**Z** None	**Z** None	**Z** None

Section **B** **Imaging**
Body System **F** **Hepatobiliary System and Pancreas**
Type **0** **Plain Radiography:** Planar display of an image developed from the capture of external ionizing radiation on photograp
or photoconductive plate

Body Part (4th)	Contrast (5th)	Qualifier (6th)	Qualifier (7th)
0 Bile Ducts **3** Gallbladder and Bile Ducts **C** Hepatobiliary System, All	**0** High Osmolar **1** Low Osmolar **Y** Other Contrast	**Z** None	**Z** None

Section **B** **Imaging**
Body System **F** **Hepatobiliary System and Pancreas**
Type **1** **Fluoroscopy:** Single plane or bi-plane real time display of an image developed from the capture of external ionizing radiation on a fluorescent screen. The image may also be stored by either digital or analog means

Body Part (4th)	Contrast (5th)	Qualifier (6th)	Qualifier (7th)
0 Bile Ducts **1** Biliary and Pancreatic Ducts **2** Gallbladder **3** Gallbladder and Bile Ducts **4** Gallbladder, Bile Ducts and Pancreatic Ducts **8** Pancreatic Ducts	**0** High Osmolar **1** Low Osmolar **Y** Other Contrast	**Z** None	**Z** None

Section **B** **Imaging**
Body System **F** **Hepatobiliary System and Pancreas**
Type **2** **Computerized Tomography (CT Scan):** Computer reformatted digital display of multiplanar images developed from th
capture of multiple exposures of external ionizing radiation

Body Part (4th)	Contrast (5th)	Qualifier (6th)	Qualifier (7th)
5 Liver **6** Liver and Spleen **7** Pancreas **C** Hepatobiliary System, All	**0** High Osmolar **1** Low Osmolar **Y** Other Contrast	**0** Unenhanced and Enhanced **Z** None	**Z** None
5 Liver **6** Liver and Spleen **7** Pancreas **C** Hepatobiliary System, All	**Z** None	**Z** None	**Z** None

Section **B** **Imaging**
Body System **F** **Hepatobiliary System and Pancreas**
Type **3** **Magnetic Resonance Imaging (MRI):** Computer reformatted digital display of multiplanar images developed from the capture of radiofrequency signals emitted by nuclei in a body site excited within magnetic field

Body Part (4th)	Contrast (5th)	Qualifier (6th)	Qualifier (7th)
5 Liver **6** Liver and Spleen **7** Pancreas	**Y** Other Contrast	**0** Unenhanced and Enhanced **Z** None	**Z** None
5 Liver **6** Liver and Spleen **7** Pancreas	**Z** None	**Z** None	**Z** None

ection B Imaging
ody System F Hepatobiliary System and Pancreas
ype 4 **Ultrasonography:** Real time display of images of anatomy or flow information developed from the capture of reflected and attenuated high frequency sound waves

Body Part (4th)	Contrast (5th)	Qualifier (6th)	Qualifier (7th)
0 Bile Ducts **2** Gallbladder **3** Gallbladder and Bile Ducts **5** Liver **6** Liver and Spleen **7** Pancreas **C** Hepatobiliary System, All	**Z** None	**Z** None	**Z** None

ection B Imaging
ody System G Endocrine System
ype 2 **Computerized Tomography (CT Scan):** Computer reformatted digital display of multiplanar images developed from the capture of multiple exposures of external ionizing radiation

Body Part (4th)	Contrast (5th)	Qualifier (6th)	Qualifier (7th)
2 Adrenal Glands, Bilateral **3** Parathyroid Glands **4** Thyroid Gland	**0** High Osmolar **1** Low Osmolar **Y** Other Contrast	**0** Unenhanced and Enhanced **Z** None	**Z** None
2 Adrenal Glands, Bilateral **3** Parathyroid Glands **4** Thyroid Gland	**Z** None	**Z** None	**Z** None

ection B Imaging
ody System G Endocrine System
ype 3 **Magnetic Resonance Imaging (MRI):** Computer reformatted digital display of multiplanar images developed from the capture of radiofrequency signals emitted by nuclei in a body site excited within a magnetic field

Body Part (4th)	Contrast (5th)	Qualifier (6th)	Qualifier (7th)
2 Adrenal Glands, Bilateral **3** Parathyroid Glands **4** Thyroid Gland	**Y** Other Contrast	**0** Unenhanced and Enhanced **Z** None	**Z** None
2 Adrenal Glands, Bilateral **3** Parathyroid Glands **4** Thyroid Gland	**Z** None	**Z** None	**Z** None

ection B Imaging
ody System G Endocrine System
ype 4 **Ultrasonography:** Real time display of images of anatomy or flow information developed from the capture of reflected and attenuated high frequency sound waves

Body Part (4th)	Contrast (5th)	Qualifier (6th)	Qualifier (7th)
0 Adrenal Gland, Right **1** Adrenal Gland, Left **2** Adrenal Glands, Bilateral **3** Parathyroid Glands **4** Thyroid Gland	**Z** None	**Z** None	**Z** None

Section B **Imaging**
Body System H **Skin, Subcutaneous Tissue and Breast**
Type 0 **Plain Radiography:** Planar display of an image developed from the capture of external ionizing radiation on photographi or photoconductive plate

Body Part (4th)	Contrast (5th)	Qualifier (6th)	Qualifier (7th)
0 Breast, Right **1** Breast, Left **2** Breasts, Bilateral	**Z** None	**Z** None	**Z** None
3 Single Mammary Duct, Right **4** Single Mammary Duct, Left **5** Multiple Mammary Ducts, Right **6** Multiple Mammary Ducts, Left	**0** High Osmolar **1** Low Osmolar **Y** Other Contrast **Z** None	**Z** None	**Z** None

Section B **Imaging**
Body System H **Skin, Subcutaneous Tissue and Breast**
Type 3 **Magnetic Resonance Imaging (MRI):** Computer reformatted digital display of multiplanar images developed from the capture of radiofrequency signals emitted by nuclei in a body site excited within a magnetic field

Body Part (4th)	Contrast (5th)	Qualifier (6th)	Qualifier (7th)
0 Breast, Right **1** Breast, Left **2** Breasts, Bilateral **D** Subcutaneous Tissue, Head/Neck **F** Subcutaneous Tissue, Upper Extremity **G** Subcutaneous Tissue, Thorax **H** Subcutaneous Tissue, Abdomen and Pelvis **J** Subcutaneous Tissue, Lower Extremity	**Y** Other Contrast	**0** Unenhanced and Enhanced **Z** None	**Z** None
0 Breast, Right **1** Breast, Left **2** Breasts, Bilateral **D** Subcutaneous Tissue, Head/Neck **F** Subcutaneous Tissue, Upper Extremity **G** Subcutaneous Tissue, Thorax **H** Subcutaneous Tissue, Abdomen and Pelvis **J** Subcutaneous Tissue, Lower Extremity	**Z** None	**Z** None	**Z** None

Section B **Imaging**
Body System H **Skin, Subcutaneous Tissue and Breast**
Type 4 **Ultrasonography:** Real time display of images of anatomy or flow information developed from the capture of reflected a attenuated high frequency sound waves

Body Part (4th)	Contrast (5th)	Qualifier (6th)	Qualifier (7th)
0 Breast, Right **1** Breast, Left **2** Breasts, Bilateral **7** Extremity, Upper **8** Extremity, Lower **9** Abdominal Wall **B** Chest Wall **C** Head and Neck	**Z** None	**Z** None	**Z** None

ction B **Imaging**
dy System L **Connective Tissue**
pe 3 **Magnetic Resonance Imaging (MRI):** Computer reformatted digital display of multiplanar images developed from the capture of radiofrequency signals emitted by nuclei in a body site excited within a magnetic field

Body Part (4th)	Contrast (5th)	Qualifier (6th)	Qualifier (7th)
Connective Tissue, Upper Extremity Connective Tissue, Lower Extremity Tendons, Upper Extremity Tendons, Lower Extremity	Y Other Contrast	0 Unenhanced and Enhanced Z None	Z None
Connective Tissue, Upper Extremity Connective Tissue, Lower Extremity Tendons, Upper Extremity Tendons, Lower Extremity	Z None	Z None	Z None

ction B **Imaging**
dy System L **Connective Tissue**
pe 4 **Ultrasonography:** Real time display of images of anatomy or flow information developed from the capture of reflected and attenuated high frequency sound waves

Body Part (4th)	Contrast (5th)	Qualifier (6th)	Qualifier (7th)
Connective Tissue, Upper Extremity Connective Tissue, Lower Extremity Tendons, Upper Extremity Tendons, Lower Extremity	Z None	Z None	Z None

ction B **Imaging**
dy System N **Skull and Facial Bones**
pe 0 **Plain Radiography:** Planar display of an image developed from the capture of external ionizing radiation on photographic or photoconductive plate

Body Part (4th)	Contrast (5th)	Qualifier (6th)	Qualifier (7th)
0 Skull 1 Orbit, Right 2 Orbit, Left 3 Orbits, Bilateral 4 Nasal Bones 5 Facial Bones 6 Mandible B Zygomatic Arch, Right C Zygomatic Arch, Left D Zygomatic Arches, Bilateral G Tooth, Single H Teeth, Multiple J Teeth, All	Z None	Z None	Z None
7 Temporomandibular Joint, Right 8 Temporomandibular Joint, Left 9 Temporomandibular Joints, Bilateral	0 High Osmolar 1 Low Osmolar Y Other Contrast Z None	Z None	Z None

ction B **Imaging**
dy System N **Skull and Facial Bones**
pe 1 **Fluoroscopy:** Single plane or bi-plane real time display of an image developed from the capture of external ionizing radiation on a fluorescent screen. The image may also be stored by either digital or analog means

Body Part (4th)	Contrast (5th)	Qualifier (6th)	Qualifier (7th)
7 Temporomandibular Joint, Right 8 Temporomandibular Joint, Left 9 Temporomandibular Joints, Bilateral	0 High Osmolar 1 Low Osmolar Y Other Contrast Z None	Z None	Z None

Section B **Imaging**
Body System N **Skull and Facial Bones**
Type 2 **Computerized Tomography (CT Scan):** Computer reformatted digital display of multiplanar images developed from the capture of multiple exposures of external ionizing radiation

Body Part (4th)	Contrast (5th)	Qualifier (6th)	Qualifier (7th)
0 Skull **3** Orbits, Bilateral **5** Facial Bones **6** Mandible **9** Temporomandibular Joints, Bilateral **F** Temporal Bones	**0** High Osmolar **1** Low Osmolar **Y** Other Contrast **Z** None	**Z** None	**Z** None

Section B **Imaging**
Body System N **Skull and Facial Bones**
Type 3 **Magnetic Resonance Imaging (MRI):** Computer reformatted digital display of multiplanar images developed from the capture of radiofrequency signals emitted by nuclei in a body site excited within magnetic field

Body Part (4th)	Contrast (5th)	Qualifier (6th)	Qualifier (7th)
9 Temporomandibular Joints, Bilateral	**Y** Other Contrast **Z** None	**Z** None	**Z** None

Section B **Imaging**
Body System P **Non-Axial Upper Bones**
Type 0 **Plain Radiography:** Planar display of an image developed from the capture of external ionizing radiation on photographic or photoconductive plate

Body Part (4th)	Contrast (5th)	Qualifier (6th)	Qualifier (7th)
0 Sternoclavicular Joint, Right **1** Sternoclavicular Joint, Left **2** Sternoclavicular Joints, Bilateral **3** Acromioclavicular Joints, Bilateral **4** Clavicle, Right **5** Clavicle, Left **6** Scapula, Right **7** Scapula, Left **A** Humerus, Right **B** Humerus, Left **E** Upper Arm, Right **F** Upper Arm, Left **J** Forearm, Right **K** Forearm, Left **N** Hand, Right **P** Hand, Left **R** Finger(s), Right **S** Finger(s), Left **X** Ribs, Right **Y** Ribs, Left	**Z** None	**Z** None	**Z** None
8 Shoulder, Right **9** Shoulder, Left **C** Hand/Finger Joint, Right **D** Hand/Finger Joint, Left **G** Elbow, Right **H** Elbow, Left **L** Wrist, Right **M** Wrist, Left	**0** High Osmolar **1** Low Osmolar **Y** Other Contrast **Z** None	**Z** None	**Z** None

Section **B** **Imaging**
Body System **P** **Non-Axial Upper Bones**
Type **1** **Fluoroscopy:** Single plane or bi-plane real time display of an image developed from the capture of external ionizing radiation on a fluorescent screen. The image may also be stored by either digital or analog means

Body Part (4th)	Contrast (5th)	Qualifier (6th)	Qualifier (7th)
0 Sternoclavicular Joint, Right **1** Sternoclavicular Joint, Left **2** Sternoclavicular Joints, Bilateral **3** Acromioclavicular Joints, Bilateral **4** Clavicle, Right **5** Clavicle, Left **6** Scapula, Right **7** Scapula, Left **A** Humerus, Right **B** Humerus, Left **E** Upper Arm, Right **F** Upper Arm, Left **J** Forearm, Right **K** Forearm, Left **N** Hand, Right **P** Hand, Left **R** Finger(s), Right **S** Finger(s), Left **X** Ribs, Right **Y** Ribs, Left	**Z** None	**Z** None	**Z** None
8 Shoulder, Right **9** Shoulder, Left **L** Wrist, Right **M** Wrist, Left	**0** High Osmolar **1** Low Osmolar **Y** Other Contrast **Z** None	**Z** None	**Z** None
C Hand/Finger Joint, Right **D** Hand/Finger Joint, Left **G** Elbow, Right **H** Elbow, Left	**0** High Osmolar **1** Low Osmolar **Y** Other Contrast	**Z** None	**Z** None

Section **B** **Imaging**
Body System **P** **Non-Axial Upper Bones**
Type **2** **Computerized Tomography (CT Scan):** Computer reformatted digital display of multiplanar images developed from the capture of multiple exposures of external ionizing radiation

Body Part (4th)	Contrast (5th)	Qualifier (6th)	Qualifier (7th)
0 Sternoclavicular Joint, Right **1** Sternoclavicular Joint, Left **W** Thorax	**0** High Osmolar **1** Low Osmolar **Y** Other Contrast	**Z** None	**Z** None

Continued →

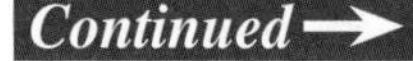

BP2 Continu

Section B **Imaging**
Body System P **Non-Axial Upper Bones**
Type 2 **Computerized Tomography (CT Scan):** Computer reformatted digital display of multiplanar images developed from the capture of multiple exposures of external ionizing radiation

Body Part (4th)	Contrast (5th)	Qualifier (6th)	Qualifier (7th)
2 Sternoclavicular Joints, Bilateral **3** Acromioclavicular Joints, Bilateral **4** Clavicle, Right **5** Clavicle, Left **6** Scapula, Right **7** Scapula, Left **8** Shoulder, Right **9** Shoulder, Left **A** Humerus, Right **B** Humerus, Left **E** Upper Arm, Right **F** Upper Arm, Left **G** Elbow, Right **H** Elbow, Left **J** Forearm, Right **K** Forearm, Left **L** Wrist, Right **M** Wrist, Left **N** Hand, Right **P** Hand, Left **Q** Hands and Wrists, Bilateral **R** Finger(s), Right **S** Finger(s), Left **T** Upper Extremity, Right **U** Upper Extremity, Left **V** Upper Extremities, Bilateral **X** Ribs, Right **Y** Ribs, Left	**0** High Osmolar **1** Low Osmolar **Y** Other Contrast **Z** None	**Z** None	**Z** None
C Hand/Finger Joint, Right **D** Hand/Finger Joint, Left	**Z** None	**Z** None	**Z** None

Section B **Imaging**
Body System P **Non-Axial Upper Bones**
Type 3 **Magnetic Resonance Imaging (MRI):** Computer reformatted digital display of multiplanar images developed from the capture of radiofrequency signals emitted by nuclei in a body site excited within magnetic field

Body Part (4th)	Contrast (5th)	Qualifier (6th)	Qualifier (7th)
8 Shoulder, Right **9** Shoulder, Left **C** Hand/Finger Joint, Right **D** Hand/Finger Joint, Left **E** Upper Arm, Right **F** Upper Arm, Left **G** Elbow, Right **H** Elbow, Left **J** Forearm, Right **K** Forearm, Left **L** Wrist, Right **M** Wrist, Left	**Y** Other Contrast	**0** Unenhanced and Enhanced **Z** None	**Z** None

Continued →

ection B Imaging
ody System P Non-Axial Upper Bones
ype 3 **Magnetic Resonance Imaging (MRI):** Computer reformatted digital display of multiplanar images developed from the capture of radiofrequency signals emitted by nuclei in a body site excited within a magnetic field

Body Part (4th)	Contrast (5th)	Qualifier (6th)	Qualifier (7th)
8 Shoulder, Right **9** Shoulder, Left **C** Hand/Finger Joint, Right **D** Hand/Finger Joint, Left **E** Upper Arm, Right **F** Upper Arm, Left **G** Elbow, Right **H** Elbow, Left **J** Forearm, Right **K** Forearm, Left **L** Wrist, Right **M** Wrist, Left	**Z** None	**Z** None	**Z** None

ection B Imaging
ody System P Non-Axial Upper Bones
ype 4 **Ultrasonography:** Real time display of images of anatomy or flow information developed from the capture of reflected and attenuated high frequency sound waves

Body Part (4th)	Contrast (5th)	Qualifier (6th)	Qualifier (7th)
8 Shoulder, Right **9** Shoulder, Left **G** Elbow, Right **H** Elbow, Left **L** Wrist, Right **M** Wrist, Left **N** Hand, Right **P** Hand, Left	**Z** None	**Z** None	**1** Densitometry **Z** None

ection B Imaging
ody System Q Non-Axial Lower Bones
ype 0 **Plain Radiography:** Planar display of an image developed from the capture of external ionizing radiation on photographic or photoconductive plate

Body Part (4th)	Contrast (5th)	Qualifier (6th)	Qualifier (7th)
0 Hip, Right **1** Hip, Left	**0** High Osmolar **1** Low Osmolar **Y** Other Contrast	**Z** None	**Z** None
0 Hip, Right **1** Hip, Left	**Z** None	**Z** None	**1** Densitometry **Z** None
3 Femur, Right **4** Femur, Left	**Z** None	**Z** None	**1** Densitometry **Z** None
7 Knee, Right **8** Knee, Left **G** Ankle, Right **H** Ankle, Left	**0** High Osmolar **1** Low Osmolar **Y** Other Contrast **Z** None	**Z** None	**Z** None
D Lower Leg, Right **F** Lower Leg, Left **J** Calcaneus, Right **K** Calcaneus, Left **L** Foot, Right **M** Foot, Left **P** Toe(s), Right **Q** Toe(s), Left **V** Patella, Right **W** Patella, Left	**Z** None	**Z** None	**Z** None

Continued →

BQ0 Continued

Section B **Imaging**
Body System Q **Non-Axial Lower Bones**
Type 0 **Plain Radiography:** Planar display of an image developed from the capture of external ionizing radiation on photographic or photoconductive plate

Body Part (4th)	Contrast (5th)	Qualifier (6th)	Qualifier (7th)
X Foot/Toe Joint, Right **Y** Foot/Toe Joint, Left	**0** High Osmolar **1** Low Osmolar **Y** Other Contrast	**Z** None	**Z** None

Section B **Imaging**
Body System Q **Non-Axial Lower Bones**
Type 1 **Fluoroscopy:** Single plane or bi-plane real time display of an image developed from the capture of external ionizing radiation on a fluorescent screen. The image may also be stored by either digital or analog means

Body Part (4th)	Contrast (5th)	Qualifier (6th)	Qualifier (7th)
0 Hip, Right **1** Hip, Left **7** Knee, Right **8** Knee, Left **G** Ankle, Right **H** Ankle, Left **X** Foot/Toe Joint, Right **Y** Foot/Toe Joint, Left	**0** High Osmolar **1** Low Osmolar **Y** Other Contrast **Z** None	**Z** None	**Z** None
3 Femur, Right **4** Femur, Left **D** Lower Leg, Right **F** Lower Leg, Left **J** Calcaneus, Right **K** Calcaneus, Left **L** Foot, Right **M** Foot, Left **P** Toe(s), Right **Q** Toe(s), Left **V** Patella, Right **W** Patella, Left	**Z** None	**Z** None	**Z** None

Section B **Imaging**
Body System Q **Non-Axial Lower Bones**
Type 2 **Computerized Tomography (CT Scan):** Computer reformatted digital display of multiplanar images developed from the capture of multiple exposures of external ionizing radiation

Body Part (4th)	Contrast (5th)	Qualifier (6th)	Qualifier (7th)
0 Hip, Right **1** Hip, Left **3** Femur, Right **4** Femur, Left **7** Knee, Right **8** Knee, Left **D** Lower Leg, Right **F** Lower Leg, Left **G** Ankle, Right **H** Ankle, Left **J** Calcaneus, Right **K** Calcaneus, Left **L** Foot, Right **M** Foot, Left **P** Toe(s), Right **Q** Toe(s), Left **R** Lower Extremity, Right **S** Lower Extremity, Left **V** Patella, Right **W** Patella, Left **X** Foot/Toe Joint, Right **Y** Foot/Toe Joint, Left	**0** High Osmolar **1** Low Osmolar **Y** Other Contrast **Z** None	**Z** None	**Z** None

Continued →

ction B **Imaging**
dy System Q **Non-Axial Lower Bones**
pe 2 **Computerized Tomography (CT Scan):** Computer reformatted digital display of multiplanar images developed from the capture of multiple exposures of external ionizing radiation

Body Part (4th)	Contrast (5th)	Qualifier (6th)	Qualifier (7th)
B Tibia/Fibula, Right **C** Tibia/Fibula, Left	**0** High Osmolar **1** Low Osmolar **Y** Other Contrast	**Z** None	**Z** None

ction B **Imaging**
dy System Q **Non-Axial Lower Bones**
pe 3 **Magnetic Resonance Imaging (MRI):** Computer reformatted digital display of multiplanar images developed from the capture of radiofrequency signals emitted by nuclei in a body site excited within a magnetic field

Body Part (4th)	Contrast (5th)	Qualifier (6th)	Qualifier (7th)
0 Hip, Right **1** Hip, Left **3** Femur, Right **4** Femur, Left **7** Knee, Right **8** Knee, Left **D** Lower Leg, Right **F** Lower Leg, Left **G** Ankle, Right **H** Ankle, Left **J** Calcaneus, Right **K** Calcaneus, Left **L** Foot, Right **M** Foot, Left **P** Toe(s), Right **Q** Toe(s), Left **V** Patella, Right **W** Patella, Left	**Y** Other Contrast	**0** Unenhanced and Enhanced **Z** None	**Z** None
0 Hip, Right **1** Hip, Left **3** Femur, Right **4** Femur, Left **7** Knee, Right **8** Knee, Left **D** Lower Leg, Right **F** Lower Leg, Left **G** Ankle, Right **H** Ankle, Left **J** Calcaneus, Right **K** Calcaneus, Left **L** Foot, Right **M** Foot, Left **P** Toe(s), Right **Q** Toe(s), Left **V** Patella, Right **W** Patella, Left	**Z** None	**Z** None	**Z** None

Section B **Imaging**
Body System Q **Non-Axial Lower Bones**
Type 4 **Ultrasonography:** Real time display of images of anatomy or flow information developed from the capture of reflected attenuated high frequency sound waves

Body Part (4th)	Contrast (5th)	Qualifier (6th)	Qualifier (7th)
0 Hip, Right **1** Hip, Left **2** Hips, Bilateral **7** Knee, Right **8** Knee, Left **9** Knees, Bilateral	**Z** None	**Z** None	**Z** None

Section B **Imaging**
Body System R **Axial Skeleton, Except Skull and Facial Bones**
Type 0 **Plain Radiography:** Planar display of an image developed from the capture of external ionizing radiation on photographic or photoconductive plate

Body Part (4th)	Contrast (5th)	Qualifier (6th)	Qualifier (7th)
0 Cervical Spine **7** Thoracic Spine **9** Lumbar Spine **G** Whole Spine	**Z** None	**Z** None	**1** Densitometry **Z** None
1 Cervical Disc(s) **2** Thoracic Disc(s) **3** Lumbar Disc(s) **4** Cervical Facet Joint(s) **5** Thoracic Facet Joint(s) **6** Lumbar Facet Joint(s) **D** Sacroiliac Joints	**0** High Osmolar **1** Low Osmolar **Y** Other Contrast **Z** None	**Z** None	**Z** None
8 Thoracolumbar Joint **B** Lumbosacral Joint **C** Pelvis **F** Sacrum and Coccyx **H** Sternum	**Z** None	**Z** None	**Z** None

Section B **Imaging**
Body System R **Axial Skeleton, Except Skull and Facial Bones**
Type 1 **Fluoroscopy:** Single plane or bi-plane real time display of an image developed from the capture of external ionizing radiation on a fluorescent screen. The image may also be stored by either digital or analog means

Body Part (4th)	Contrast (5th)	Qualifier (6th)	Qualifier (7th)
0 Cervical Spine **1** Cervical Disc(s) **2** Thoracic Disc(s) **3** Lumbar Disc(s) **4** Cervical Facet Joint(s) **5** Thoracic Facet Joint(s) **6** Lumbar Facet Joint(s) **7** Thoracic Spine **8** Thoracolumbar Joint **9** Lumbar Spine **B** Lumbosacral Joint **C** Pelvis **D** Sacroiliac Joints **F** Sacrum and Coccyx **G** Whole Spine **H** Sternum	**0** High Osmolar **1** Low Osmolar **Y** Other Contrast **Z** None	**Z** None	**Z** None

ction **B** **Imaging**
dy System **R** **Axial Skeleton, Except Skull and Facial Bones**
pe **2** **Computerized Tomography (CT Scan):** Computer reformatted digital display of multiplanar images developed from the capture of multiple exposures of external ionizing radiation

Body Part (4th)	Contrast (5th)	Qualifier (6th)	Qualifier (7th)
0 Cervical Spine 7 Thoracic Spine 9 Lumbar Spine C Pelvis D Sacroiliac Joints F Sacrum and Coccyx	0 High Osmolar 1 Low Osmolar Y Other Contrast Z None	Z None	Z None

ction **B** **Imaging**
ody System **R** **Axial Skeleton, Except Skull and Facial Bones**
ype **3** **Magnetic Resonance Imaging (MRI):** Computer reformatted digital display of multiplanar images developed from the capture of radiofrequency signals emitted by nuclei in a body site excited within a magnetic field

Body Part (4th)	Contrast (5th)	Qualifier (6th)	Qualifier (7th)
0 Cervical Spine 1 Cervical Disc(s) 2 Thoracic Disc(s) 3 Lumbar Disc(s) 7 Thoracic Spine 9 Lumbar Spine C Pelvis F Sacrum and Coccyx	Y Other Contrast	0 Unenhanced and Enhanced Z None	Z None
0 Cervical Spine 1 Cervical Disc(s) 2 Thoracic Disc(s) 3 Lumbar Disc(s) 7 Thoracic Spine 9 Lumbar Spine C Pelvis F Sacrum and Coccyx	Z None	Z None	Z None

ection **B** **Imaging**
ody System **R** **Axial Skeleton, Except Skull and Facial Bones**
ype **4** **Ultrasonography:** Real time display of images of anatomy or flow information developed from the capture of reflected and attenuated high frequency sound waves

Body Part (4th)	Contrast (5th)	Qualifier (6th)	Qualifier (7th)
0 Cervical Spine 7 Thoracic Spine 9 Lumbar Spine F Sacrum and Coccyx	Z None	Z None	Z None

ection **B** **Imaging**
ody System **T** **Urinary System**
ype **0** **Plain Radiography:** Planar display of an image developed from the capture of external ionizing radiation on photographic or photoconductive plate

Body Part (4th)	Contrast (5th)	Qualifier (6th)	Qualifier (7th)
0 Bladder 1 Kidney, Right 2 Kidney, Left 3 Kidneys, Bilateral 4 Kidneys, Ureters and Bladder 5 Urethra 6 Ureter, Right 7 Ureter, Left 8 Ureters, Bilateral B Bladder and Urethra C Ileal Diversion Loop	0 High Osmolar 1 Low Osmolar Y Other Contrast Z None	Z None	Z None

Section B **Imaging**
Body System T **Urinary System**
Type 1 **Fluoroscopy:** Single plane or bi-plane real time display of an image developed from the capture of external ionizing radiation on a fluorescent screen. The image may also be stored by either digital or analog means

Body Part (4th)	Contrast (5th)	Qualifier (6th)	Qualifier (7th)
0 Bladder **1** Kidney, Right **2** Kidney, Left **3** Kidneys, Bilateral **4** Kidneys, Ureters and Bladder **5** Urethra **6** Ureter, Right **7** Ureter, Left **B** Bladder and Urethra **C** Ileal Diversion Loop **D** Kidney, Ureter and Bladder, Right **F** Kidney, Ureter and Bladder, Left **G** Ileal Loop, Ureters and Kidneys	**0** High Osmolar **1** Low Osmolar **Y** Other Contrast **Z** None	**Z** None	**Z** None

Section B **Imaging**
Body System T **Urinary System**
Type 2 **Computerized Tomography (CT Scan):** Computer reformatted digital display of multiplanar images developed from the capture of multiple exposures of external ionizing radiation

Body Part (4th)	Contrast (5th)	Qualifier (6th)	Qualifier (7th)
0 Bladder **1** Kidney, Right **2** Kidney, Left **3** Kidneys, Bilateral **9** Kidney Transplant	**0** High Osmolar **1** Low Osmolar **Y** Other Contrast	**0** Unenhanced and Enhanced **Z** None	**Z** None
0 Bladder **1** Kidney, Right **2** Kidney, Left **3** Kidneys, Bilateral **9** Kidney Transplant	**Z** None	**Z** None	**Z** None

Section B **Imaging**
Body System T **Urinary System**
Type 3 **Magnetic Resonance Imaging (MRI):** Computer reformatted digital display of multiplanar images developed from the capture of radiofrequency signals emitted by nuclei in a body site excited within a magnetic field

Body Part (4th)	Contrast (5th)	Qualifier (6th)	Qualifier (7th)
0 Bladder **1** Kidney, Right **2** Kidney, Left **3** Kidneys, Bilateral **9** Kidney Transplant	**Y** Other Contrast	**0** Unenhanced and Enhanced **Z** None	**Z** None
0 Bladder **1** Kidney, Right **2** Kidney, Left **3** Kidneys, Bilateral **9** Kidney Transplant	**Z** None	**Z** None	**Z** None

ection B Imaging
ody System T Urinary System
ype 4 **Ultrasonography:** Real time display of images of anatomy or flow information developed from the capture of reflected and attenuated high frequency sound waves

Body Part (4th)	Contrast (5th)	Qualifier (6th)	Qualifier (7th)
0 Bladder 1 Kidney, Right 2 Kidney, Left 3 Kidneys, Bilateral 5 Urethra 6 Ureter, Right 7 Ureter, Left 8 Ureters, Bilateral 9 Kidney Transplant J Kidneys and Bladder	Z None	Z None	Z None

ection B Imaging
ody System U Female Reproductive System
ype 0 **Plain Radiography:** Planar display of an image developed from the capture of external ionizing radiation on photographic or photoconductive plate

Body Part (4th)	Contrast (5th)	Qualifier (6th)	Qualifier (7th)
0 Fallopian Tube, Right 1 Fallopian Tube, Left 2 Fallopian Tubes, Bilateral 6 Uterus 8 Uterus and Fallopian Tubes 9 Vagina	0 High Osmolar 1 Low Osmolar Y Other Contrast	Z None	Z None

ection B Imaging
ody System U Female Reproductive System
ype 1 **Fluoroscopy:** Single plane or bi-plane real time display of an image developed from the capture of external ionizing radiation on a fluorescent screen. The image may also be stored by either digital or analog means

Body Part (4th)	Contrast (5th)	Qualifier (6th)	Qualifier (7th)
0 Fallopian Tube, Right 1 Fallopian Tube, Left 2 Fallopian Tubes, Bilateral 6 Uterus 8 Uterus and Fallopian Tubes 9 Vagina	0 High Osmolar 1 Low Osmolar Y Other Contrast Z None	Z None	Z None

ection B Imaging
ody System U Female Reproductive System
ype 3 **Magnetic Resonance Imaging (MRI):** Computer reformatted digital display of multiplanar images developed from the capture of radiofrequency signals emitted by nuclei in a body site excited within a magnetic field

Body Part (4th)	Contrast (5th)	Qualifier (6th)	Qualifier (7th)
3 Ovary, Right 4 Ovary, Left 5 Ovaries, Bilateral 6 Uterus 9 Vagina B Pregnant Uterus C Uterus and Ovaries	Y Other Contrast	0 Unenhanced and Enhanced Z None	Z None
3 Ovary, Right 4 Ovary, Left 5 Ovaries, Bilateral 6 Uterus 9 Vagina B Pregnant Uterus C Uterus and Ovaries	Z None	Z None	Z None

Section B **Imaging**
Body System U **Female Reproductive System**
Type 4 **Ultrasonography:** Real time display of images of anatomy or flow information developed from the capture of reflected and attenuated high frequency sound waves

Body Part (4th)	Contrast (5th)	Qualifier (6th)	Qualifier (7th)
0 Fallopian Tube, Right **1** Fallopian Tube, Left **2** Fallopian Tubes, Bilateral **3** Ovary, Right **4** Ovary, Left **5** Ovaries, Bilateral **6** Uterus **C** Uterus and Ovaries	**Y** Other Contrast **Z** None	**Z** None	**Z** None

Section B **Imaging**
Body System V **Male Reproductive System**
Type 0 **Plain Radiography:** Planar display of an image developed from the capture of external ionizing radiation on photographic or photoconductive plate

Body Part (4th)	Contrast (5th)	Qualifier (6th)	Qualifier (7th)
0 Corpora Cavernosa **1** Epididymis, Right **2** Epididymis, Left **3** Prostate **5** Testicle, Right **6** Testicle, Left **8** Vasa Vasorum	**0** High Osmolar **1** Low Osmolar **Y** Other Contrast	**Z** None	**Z** None

Section B **Imaging**
Body System V **Male Reproductive System**
Type 1 **Fluoroscopy:** Single plane or bi-plane real time display of an image developed from the capture of external ionizing radiation on a fluorescent screen. The image may also be stored by either digital or analog means

Body Part (4th)	Contrast (5th)	Qualifier (6th)	Qualifier (7th)
0 Corpora Cavernosa **8** Vasa Vasorum	**0** High Osmolar **1** Low Osmolar **Y** Other Contrast **Z** None	**Z** None	**Z** None

Section B **Imaging**
Body System V **Male Reproductive System**
Type 2 **Computerized Tomography (CT Scan):** Computer reformatted digital display of multiplanar images developed from the capture of multiple exposures of external ionizing radiation

Body Part (4th)	Contrast (5th)	Qualifier (6th)	Qualifier (7th)
3 Prostate	**0** High Osmolar **1** Low Osmolar **Y** Other Contrast	**0** Unenhanced and Enhanced **Z** None	**Z** None
3 Prostate	**Z** None	**Z** None	**Z** None

tion	**B**	**Imaging**
dy System	**V**	**Male Reproductive System**
pe	**3**	**Magnetic Resonance Imaging (MRI):** Computer reformatted digital display of multiplanar images developed from the capture of radiofrequency signals emitted by nuclei in a body site excited within a magnetic field

Body Part (4th)	Contrast (5th)	Qualifier (6th)	Qualifier (7th)
Corpora Cavernosa Prostate Scrotum Testicle, Right Testicle, Left Testicles, Bilateral	**Y** Other Contrast	**0** Unenhanced and Enhanced **Z** None	**Z** None
Corpora Cavernosa Prostate Scrotum Testicle, Right Testicle, Left Testicles, Bilateral	**Z** None	**Z** None	**Z** None

ction	**B**	**Imaging**
dy System	**V**	**Male Reproductive System**
pe	**4**	**Ultrasonography:** Real time display of images of anatomy or flow information developed from the capture of reflected and attenuated high frequency sound waves

Body Part (4th)	Contrast (5th)	Qualifier (6th)	Qualifier (7th)
4 Scrotum Prostate and Seminal Vesicles **B** Penis	**Z** None	**Z** None	**Z** None

ction	**B**	**Imaging**
dy System	**W**	**Anatomical Regions**
pe	**0**	**Plain Radiography:** Planar display of an image developed from the capture of external ionizing radiation on photographic or photoconductive plate

Body Part (4th)	Contrast (5th)	Qualifier (6th)	Qualifier (7th)
Abdomen Abdomen and Pelvis **3** Chest **B** Long Bones, All **C** Lower Extremity **J** Upper Extremity **K** Whole Body **L** Whole Skeleton **M** Whole Body, Infant	**Z** None	**Z** None	**Z** None

ction	**B**	**Imaging**
dy System	**W**	**Anatomical Regions**
pe	**1**	**Fluoroscopy:** Single plane or bi-plane real time display of an image developed from the capture of external ionizing radiation on a fluorescent screen. The image may also be stored by either digital or analog means

Body Part (4th)	Contrast (5th)	Qualifier (6th)	Qualifier (7th)
1 Abdomen and Pelvis **9** Head and Neck **C** Lower Extremity **J** Upper Extremity	**0** High Osmolar **1** Low Osmolar **Y** Other Contrast **Z** None	**Z** None	**Z** None

Section B **Imaging**
Body System W **Anatomical Regions**
Type 2 **Computerized Tomography (CT Scan):** Computer reformatted digital display of multiplanar images developed from the capture of multiple exposures of external ionizing radiation

Body Part (4th)	Contrast (5th)	Qualifier (6th)	Qualifier (7th)
0 Abdomen **1** Abdomen and Pelvis **4** Chest and Abdomen **5** Chest, Abdomen and Pelvis **8** Head **9** Head and Neck **F** Neck **G** Pelvic Region	**0** High Osmolar **1** Low Osmolar **Y** Other Contrast	**0** Unenhanced and Enhanced **Z** None	**Z** None
0 Abdomen **1** Abdomen and Pelvis **4** Chest and Abdomen **5** Chest, Abdomen and Pelvis **8** Head **9** Head and Neck **F** Neck **G** Pelvic Region	**Z** None	**Z** None	**Z** None

Section B **Imaging**
Body System W **Anatomical Regions**
Type 3 **Magnetic Resonance Imaging (MRI):** Computer reformatted digital display of multiplanar images developed from the capture of radiofrequency signals emitted by nuclei in a body site excited within magnetic field

Body Part (4th)	Contrast (5th)	Qualifier (6th)	Qualifier (7th)
0 Abdomen **8** Head **F** Neck **G** Pelvic Region **H** Retroperitoneum **P** Brachial Plexus	**Y** Other Contrast	**0** Unenhanced and Enhanced **Z** None	**Z** None
0 Abdomen **8** Head **F** Neck **G** Pelvic Region **H** Retroperitoneum **P** Brachial Plexus	**Z** None	**Z** None	**Z** None
3 Chest	**Y** Other Contrast	**0** Unenhanced and Enhanced **Z** None	**Z** None

Section B **Imaging**
Body System W **Anatomical Regions**
Type 4 **Ultrasonography:** Real time display of images of anatomy or flow information developed from the capture of reflected and attenuated high frequency sound waves

Body Part (4th)	Contrast (5th)	Qualifier (6th)	Qualifier (7th)
0 Abdomen **1** Abdomen and Pelvis **F** Neck **G** Pelvic Region	**Z** None	**Z** None	**Z** None

ection **B** **Imaging**
ody System **Y** **Fetus and Obstetrical**
ype **3** **Magnetic Resonance Imaging (MRI):** Computer reformatted digital display of multiplanar images developed from the capture of radiofrequency signals emitted by nuclei in a body site excited within a magnetic field

Body Part (4th)	Contrast (5th)	Qualifier (6th)	Qualifier (7th)
0 Fetal Head **1** Fetal Heart **2** Fetal Thorax **3** Fetal Abdomen **4** Fetal Spine **5** Fetal Extremities **6** Whole Fetus	**Y** Other Contrast	**0** Unenhanced and Enhanced **Z** None	**Z** None
0 Fetal Head **1** Fetal Heart **2** Fetal Thorax **3** Fetal Abdomen **4** Fetal Spine **5** Fetal Extremities **6** Whole Fetus	**Z** None	**Z** None	**Z** None

ection **B** **Imaging**
ody System **Y** **Fetus and Obstetrical**
ype **4** **Ultrasonography:** Real time display of images of anatomy or flow information developed from the capture of reflected and attenuated high frequency sound waves

Body Part (4th)	Contrast (5th)	Qualifier (6th)	Qualifier (7th)
7 Fetal Umbilical Cord **8** Placenta **9** First Trimester, Single Fetus **B** First Trimester, Multiple Gestation **C** Second Trimester, Single Fetus **D** Second Trimester, Multiple Gestation **F** Third Trimester, Single Fetus **G** Third Trimester, Multiple Gestation	**Z** None	**Z** None	**Z** None

HA Coding Clinic

2151ZZ Fluoroscopy of Left Heart using Low Osmolar Contrast—AHA CC: 1Q, 2018, 12-13

518ZZA Fluoroscopy of Superior Vena Cava, Guidance, for Fluoroscopic Guidance used to Place the Renal Dialysis Catheter - AHA CC: 4Q, 2015, 30

Nuclear Medicine Section (C01–CW7)

Within each section of ICD-10-PCS the characters have different meanings. The seven character meanings for the Nuclear Medicine section are illustrated here through the procedure example of *Technetium tomo scan of liver*.

Section	Body System	Root Type	Body Part	Radionuclide	Qualifier	Qualifier
Nuclear Medicine	Hepatobiliary and Pancreas	Tomographic (Tomo)	Liver	Technetium 99m	None	None
C	F	2	5	1	Z	Z

Section (Character 1)

All Nuclear Medicine procedure codes have a first character value of C.

Body System (Character 2)

The alphanumeric character for the body system is placed in the second position. The following are the body systems applicable to the Nuclear Medicine section.

Character Value	Character Value Description
0	Central Nervous System
2	Heart
5	Veins
7	Lymphatic System
8	Eye
9	Ear, Nose, Mouth and Throat
B	Respiratory System
D	Gastrointestinal System
F	Hepatobiliary System and Pancreas
G	Endocrine System
H	Skin, Subcutaneous Tissue and Breast
P	Musculoskeletal
T	Urinary System
V	Male Reproductive System
W	Anatomical Regions

Root Types (Character 3)

The alphanumeric character value for root types is placed in the third position. The following are the root types applicable to the Nuclear Medicine section with their associated meaning.

Character Value	Root Type	Root Type Definition
1	Planar Nuclear Medicine Imaging	Introduction of radioactive materials into the body for single plane display of images developed from the capture of radioactive emissions
2	Tomographic (Tomo) Nuclear Medicine Imaging	Introduction of radioactive materials into the body for three dimensional display of images developed from the capture of radioactive emissions
3	Positron Emission Tomographic (PET) Imaging	Introduction of radioactive materials into the body for three dimensional display of images developed from the simultaneous capture, 180 degrees apart, of radioactive emissions
4	Nonimaging Nuclear Medicine Uptake	Introduction of radioactive materials into the body for measurements of organ function, from the detection of radioactive emissions
5	Nonimaging Nuclear Medicine Probe	Introduction of radioactive materials into the body for the study of distribution and fate of certain substances by the detection of radioactive emissions; or, alternatively, measurement of absorption of radioactive emissions from an external source

Continued→

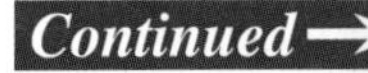

Character Value	Root Type	Root Type Definition
6	Nonimaging Nuclear Medicine Assay	Introduction of radioactive materials into the body for the study of body fluids and blood elements, by the detection of radioactive emissions
7	Systemic Nuclear Medicine Therapy	Introduction of unsealed radioactive materials into the body for treatment

Body Part (Character 4)

For each body part the applicable body part character values will be available for procedure code construction. An example of a body part Cerebrospinal Fluid.

Radionuclide (Character 5)

When radionuclide is utilized during a nuclear medicine procedure, the corresponding radionuclide character value should be reported in the fifth character position. The following are examples of the radionuclide character values available for the Nuclear Medicine section.

- Krypton (Kr-81m)
- Technetium 99m (Tc-99m)
- Xenon 127 (Xe-127)
- Xenon 133 (Xe-133)
- Other Radionuclide

If radionuclide is not utilized, the placeholder character value of Z should be reported.

Qualifier (Character 6)

The qualifier represents an additional attribute for the procedure when applicable. Currently, there are no qualifiers in the Nuclear Medicine section; therefore, the placeholder character value of Z should be reported.

Qualifier (Character 7)

The qualifier represents an additional attribute for the procedure when applicable. Currently, there are no qualifiers in the Nuclear Medicine section; therefore, the placeholder character value of Z should be reported.

Nuclear Medicine Section Tables

Nuclear Medicine Tables C01–CW7

Section **C** **Nuclear Medicine**
Body System **0** **Central Nervous System**
Type **1** **Planar Nuclear Medicine Imaging:** Introduction of radioactive materials into the body for single plane display of images developed from the capture of radioactive emissions

Body Part (4th)	Radionuclide (5th)	Qualifier (6th)	Qualifier (7th)
0 Brain	**1** Technetium 99m (Tc-99m) **Y** Other Radionuclide	**Z** None	**Z** None
5 Cerebrospinal Fluid	**D** Indium 111 (In-111) **Y** Other Radionuclide	**Z** None	**Z** None
Y Central Nervous System	**Y** Other Radionuclide	**Z** None	**Z** None

Section C **Nuclear Medicine**
Body System 0 **Central Nervous System**
Type 2 **Tomographic (Tomo) Nuclear Medicine Imaging:** Introduction of radioactive materials into the body for three dimensional display of images developed from the capture of radioactive emissions

Body Part (4th)	Radionuclide (5th)	Qualifier (6th)	Qualifier (7th)
0 Brain	**1** Technetium 99m (Tc-99m) **F** Iodine 123 (I-123) **S** Thallium 201 (Tl-201) **Y** Other Radionuclide	**Z** None	**Z** None
5 Cerebrospinal Fluid	**D** Indium 111 (In-111) **Y** Other Radionuclide	**Z** None	**Z** None
Y Central Nervous System	**Y** Other Radionuclide	**Z** None	**Z** None

Section C **Nuclear Medicine**
Body System 0 **Central Nervous System**
Type 3 **Positron Emission Tomographic (PET) Imaging:** Introduction of radioactive materials into the body for three dimensional display of images developed from the simultaneous capture, 180 degrees apart, of radioactive emissions

Body Part (4th)	Radionuclide (5th)	Qualifier (6th)	Qualifier (7th)
0 Brain	**B** Carbon 11 (C-11) **K** Fluorine 18 (F-18) **M** Oxygen 15 (O-15) **Y** Other Radionuclide	**Z** None	**Z** None
Y Central Nervous System	**Y** Other Radionuclide	**Z** None	**Z** None

Section C **Nuclear Medicine**
Body System 0 **Central Nervous System**
Type 5 **Nonimaging Nuclear Medicine Probe:** Introduction of radioactive materials into the body for the study of distribution and fate of certain substances by the detection of radioactive emissions; or, alternatively, measurement of absorption of radioactive emissions from an exter source

Body Part (4th)	Radionuclide (5th)	Qualifier (6th)	Qualifier (7th)
0 Brain	**V** Xenon 133 (Xe-133) **Y** Other Radionuclide	**Z** None	**Z** None
Y Central Nervous System	**Y** Other Radionuclide	**Z** None	**Z** None

Section C **Nuclear Medicine**
Body System 2 **Heart**
Type 1 **Planar Nuclear Medicine Imaging:** Introduction of radioactive materials into the body for single plane display of imag developed from the capture of radioactive emissions

Body Part (4th)	Radionuclide (5th)	Qualifier (6th)	Qualifier (7th)
6 Heart, Right and Left	**1** Technetium 99m (Tc-99m) **Y** Other Radionuclide	**Z** None	**Z** None
G Myocardium	**1** Technetium 99m (Tc-99m) **D** Indium 111 (In-111) **S** Thallium 201 (Tl-201) **Y** Other Radionuclide **Z** None	**Z** None	**Z** None
Y Heart	**Y** Other Radionuclide	**Z** None	**Z** None

ction C **Nuclear Medicine**
dy System 2 **Heart**
pe 2 **Tomographic (Tomo) Nuclear Medicine Imaging:** Introduction of radioactive materials into the body for three dimensional display of images developed from the capture of radioactive emissions

Body Part (4th)	Radionuclide (5th)	Qualifier (6th)	Qualifier (7th)
6 Heart, Right and Left	**1** Technetium 99m (Tc-99m) **Y** Other Radionuclide	**Z** None	**Z** None
G Myocardium	**1** Technetium 99m (Tc-99m) **D** Indium 111 (In-111) **K** Fluorine 18 (F-18) **S** Thallium 201 (Tl-201) **Y** Other Radionuclide **Z** None	**Z** None	**Z** None
Y Heart	**Y** Other Radionuclide	**Z** None	**Z** None

ction C **Nuclear Medicine**
dy System 2 **Heart**
pe 3 **Positron Emission Tomographic (PET) Imaging:** Introduction of radioactive materials into the body for three dimensional display of images developed from the simultaneous capture, 180 degrees apart, of radioactive emissions

Body Part (4th)	Radionuclide (5th)	Qualifier (6th)	Qualifier (7th)
G Myocardium	**K** Fluorine 18 (F-18) **M** Oxygen 15 (O-15) **Q** Rubidium 82 (Rb-82) **R** Nitrogen 13 (N-13) **Y** Other Radionuclide	**Z** None	**Z** None
Y Heart	**Y** Other Radionuclide	**Z** None	**Z** None

ction C **Nuclear Medicine**
dy System 2 **Heart**
pe 5 **Nonimaging Nuclear Medicine Probe:** Introduction of radioactive materials into the body for the study of distribution and fate of certain substances by the detection of radioactive emissions; or, alternatively, measurement of absorption of radioactive emissions from an external source

Body Part (4th)	Radionuclide (5th)	Qualifier (6th)	Qualifier (7th)
6 Heart, Right and Left	**1** Technetium 99m (Tc-99m) **Y** Other Radionuclide	**Z** None	**Z** None
Y Heart	**Y** Other Radionuclide	**Z** None	**Z** None

ction C **Nuclear Medicine**
dy System 5 **Veins**
pe 1 **Planar Nuclear Medicine Imaging:** Introduction of radioactive materials into the body for single plane display of images developed from the capture of radioactive emissions

Body Part (4th)	Radionuclide (5th)	Qualifier (6th)	Qualifier (7th)
B Lower Extremity Veins, Right **C** Lower Extremity Veins, Left **D** Lower Extremity Veins, Bilateral **N** Upper Extremity Veins, Right **P** Upper Extremity Veins, Left **Q** Upper Extremity Veins, Bilateral **R** Central Veins	**1** Technetium 99m (Tc-99m) **Y** Other Radionuclide	**Z** None	**Z** None
Y Veins	**Y** Other Radionuclide	**Z** None	**Z** None

Section C **Nuclear Medicine**
Body System 7 **Lymphatic and Hematologic System**
Type 1 **Planar Nuclear Medicine Imaging:** Introduction of radioactive materials into the body for single plane display of images developed from the capture of radioactive emissions

Body Part (4th)	Radionuclide (5th)	Qualifier (6th)	Qualifier (7th)
0 Bone Marrow	**1** Technetium 99m (Tc-99m) **D** Indium 111 (In-111) **Y** Other Radionuclide	**Z** None	**Z** None
2 Spleen **5** Lymphatics, Head and Neck **D** Lymphatics, Pelvic **J** Lymphatics, Head **K** Lymphatics, Neck **L** Lymphatics, Upper Chest **M** Lymphatics, Trunk **N** Lymphatics, Upper Extremity **P** Lymphatics, Lower Extremity	**1** Technetium 99m (Tc-99m) **Y** Other Radionuclide	**Z** None	**Z** None
3 Blood	**D** Indium 111 (In-111) **Y** Other Radionuclide	**Z** None	**Z** None
Y Lymphatic and Hematologic System	**Y** Other Radionuclide	**Z** None	**Z** None

Section C **Nuclear Medicine**
Body System 7 **Lymphatic and Hematologic System**
Type 2 **Tomographic (Tomo) Nuclear Medicine Imaging:** Introduction of radioactive materials into the body for three dimensional display of images developed from the capture of radioactive emissions

Body Part (4th)	Radionuclide (5th)	Qualifier (6th)	Qualifier (7th)
2 Spleen	**1** Technetium 99m (Tc-99m) **Y** Other Radionuclide	**Z** None	**Z** None
Y Lymphatic and Hematologic System	**Y** Other Radionuclide	**Z** None	**Z** None

Section C **Nuclear Medicine**
Body System 7 **Lymphatic and Hematologic System**
Type 5 **Nonimaging Nuclear Medicine Probe:** Introduction of radioactive materials into the body for the study of distribution and fate of certain substances by the detection of radioactive emissions; or, alternatively, measurement of absorption of radioactive emissions from an extern source

Body Part (4th)	Radionuclide (5th)	Qualifier (6th)	Qualifier (7th)
5 Lymphatics, Head and Neck **D** Lymphatics, Pelvic **J** Lymphatics, Head **K** Lymphatics, Neck **L** Lymphatics, Upper Chest **M** Lymphatics, Trunk **N** Lymphatics, Upper Extremity **P** Lymphatics, Lower Extremity	**1** Technetium 99m (Tc-99m) **Y** Other Radionuclide	**Z** None	**Z** None
Y Lymphatic and Hematologic System	**Y** Other Radionuclide	**Z** None	**Z** None

ection C **Nuclear Medicine**
ody System 7 **Lymphatic and Hematologic System**
ype 6 **Nonimaging Nuclear Medicine Assay:** Introduction of radioactive materials into the body for the study of body fluids and blood elements, by the detection of radioactive emissions

Body Part (4th)	Radionuclide (5th)	Qualifier (6th)	Qualifier (7th)
3 Blood	**1** Technetium 99m (Tc-99m) **7** Cobalt 58 (Co-58) **C** Cobalt 57 (Co-57) **D** Indium 111 (In-111) **H** Iodine 125 (I-125) **W** Chromium (Cr-51) **Y** Other Radionuclide	**Z** None	**Z** None
Y Lymphatic and Hematologic System	**Y** Other Radionuclide	**Z** None	**Z** None

ection C **Nuclear Medicine**
ody System 8 **Eye**
ype 1 **Planar Nuclear Medicine Imaging:** Introduction of radioactive materials into the body for single plane display of images developed from the capture of radioactive emissions

Body Part (4th)	Radionuclide (5th)	Qualifier (6th)	Qualifier (7th)
9 Lacrimal Ducts, Bilateral	**1** Technetium 99m (Tc-99m) **Y** Other Radionuclide	**Z** None	**Z** None
Y Eye	**Y** Other Radionuclide	**Z** None	**Z** None

ection C **Nuclear Medicine**
ody System 9 **Ear, Nose, Mouth and Throat**
ype 1 **Planar Nuclear Medicine Imaging:** Introduction of radioactive materials into the body for single plane display of images developed from the capture of radioactive emissions

Body Part (4th)	Radionuclide (5th)	Qualifier (6th)	Qualifier (7th)
B Salivary Glands, Bilateral	**1** Technetium 99m (Tc-99m) **Y** Other Radionuclide	**Z** None	**Z** None
Y Ear, Nose, Mouth and Throat	**Y** Other Radionuclide	**Z** None	**Z** None

ection C **Nuclear Medicine**
ody System B **Respiratory System**
ype 1 **Planar Nuclear Medicine Imaging:** Introduction of radioactive materials into the body for single plane display of images developed from the capture of radioactive emissions

Body Part (4th)	Radionuclide (5th)	Qualifier (6th)	Qualifier (7th)
2 Lungs and Bronchi	**1** Technetium 99m (Tc-99m) **9** Krypton (Kr-81m) **T** Xenon 127 (Xe-127) **V** Xenon 133 (Xe-133) **Y** Other Radionuclide	**Z** None	**Z** None
Y Respiratory System	**Y** Other Radionuclide	**Z** None	**Z** None

Section C **Nuclear Medicine**
Body System B **Respiratory System**
Type 2 **Tomographic (Tomo) Nuclear Medicine Imaging:** Introduction of radioactive materials into the body for three dimensional display of images developed from the capture of radioactive emissions

Body Part (4th)	Radionuclide (5th)	Qualifier (6th)	Qualifier (7th)
2 Lungs and Bronchi	**1** Technetium 99m (Tc-99m) **9** Krypton (Kr-81m) **Y** Other Radionuclide	**Z** None	**Z** None
Y Respiratory System	**Y** Other Radionuclide	**Z** None	**Z** None

Section C **Nuclear Medicine**
Body System B **Respiratory System**
Type 3 **Positron Emission Tomographic (PET) Imaging:** Introduction of radioactive materials into the body for three dimensional display of images developed from the simultaneous capture, 180 degree apart, of radioactive emissions

Body Part (4th)	Radionuclide (5th)	Qualifier (6th)	Qualifier (7th)
2 Lungs and Bronchi	**K** Fluorine 18 (F-18) **Y** Other Radionuclide	**Z** None	**Z** None
Y Respiratory System	**Y** Other Radionuclide	**Z** None	**Z** None

Section C **Nuclear Medicine**
Body System D **Gastrointestinal System**
Type 1 **Planar Nuclear Medicine Imaging:** Introduction of radioactive materials into the body for single plane display of images developed from the capture of radioactive emissions

Body Part (4th)	Radionuclide (5th)	Qualifier (6th)	Qualifier (7th)
5 Upper Gastrointestinal Tract **7** Gastrointestinal Tract	**1** Technetium 99m (Tc-99m) **D** Indium 111 (In-111) **Y** Other Radionuclide	**Z** None	**Z** None
Y Digestive System	**Y** Other Radionuclide	**Z** None	**Z** None

Section C **Nuclear Medicine**
Body System D **Gastrointestinal System**
Type 2 **Tomographic (Tomo) Nuclear Medicine Imaging:** Introduction of radioactive materials into the body for three dimensional display of images developed from the capture of radioactive emissions

Body Part (4th)	Radionuclide (5th)	Qualifier (6th)	Qualifier (7th)
7 Gastrointestinal Tract	**1** Technetium 99m (Tc-99m) **D** Indium 111 (In-111) **Y** Other Radionuclide	**Z** None	**Z** None
Y Digestive System	**Y** Other Radionuclide	**Z** None	**Z** None

Section C **Nuclear Medicine**
Body System F **Hepatobiliary System and Pancreas**
Type 1 **Planar Nuclear Medicine Imaging:** Introduction of radioactive materials into the body for single plane display of images developed from the capture of radioactive emissions

Body Part (4th)	Radionuclide (5th)	Qualifier (6th)	Qualifier (7th)
4 Gallbladder **5** Liver **6** Liver and Spleen **C** Hepatobiliary System, All	**1** Technetium 99m (Tc-99m) **Y** Other Radionuclide	**Z** None	**Z** None
Y Hepatobiliary System and Pancreas	**Y** Other Radionuclide	**Z** None	**Z** None

ction C **Nuclear Medicine**
dy System F **Hepatobiliary System and Pancreas**
pe 2 **Tomographic (Tomo) Nuclear Medicine Imaging:** Introduction of radioactive materials into the body for three dimensional display of images developed from the capture of radioactive emissions

Body Part (4th)	Radionuclide (5th)	Qualifier (6th)	Qualifier (7th)
4 Gallbladder 5 Liver 6 Liver and Spleen	**1** Technetium 99m (Tc-99m) **Y** Other Radionuclide	**Z** None	**Z** None
Y Hepatobiliary System and Pancreas	**Y** Other Radionuclide	**Z** None	**Z** None

ction C **Nuclear Medicine**
dy System G **Endocrine System**
pe 1 **Planar Nuclear Medicine Imaging:** Introduction of radioactive materials into the body for single plane display of images developed from the capture of radioactive emissions

Body Part (4th)	Radionuclide (5th)	Qualifier (6th)	Qualifier (7th)
1 Parathyroid Glands	**1** Technetium 99m (Tc-99m) **S** Thallium 201 (Tl-201) **Y** Other Radionuclide	**Z** None	**Z** None
2 Thyroid Gland	**1** Technetium 99m (Tc-99m) **F** Iodine 123 (I-123) **G** Iodine 131 (I-131) **Y** Other Radionuclide	**Z** None	**Z** None
4 Adrenal Glands, Bilateral	**G** Iodine 131 (I-131) **Y** Other Radionuclide	**Z** None	**Z** None
Y Endocrine System	**Y** Other Radionuclide	**Z** None	**Z** None

ction C **Nuclear Medicine**
dy System G **Endocrine System**
ype 2 **Tomographic (Tomo) Nuclear Medicine Imaging:** Introduction of radioactive materials into the body for three dimensional display of images developed from the capture of radioactive emissions

Body Part (4th)	Radionuclide (5th)	Qualifier (6th)	Qualifier (7th)
1 Parathyroid Glands	**1** Technetium 99m (Tc-99m) **S** Thallium 201 (Tl-201) **Y** Other Radionuclide	**Z** None	**Z** None
Y Endocrine System	**Y** Other Radionuclide	**Z** None	**Z** None

ction C **Nuclear Medicine**
ody System G **Endocrine System**
ype 4 **Nonimaging Nuclear Medicine Uptake:** Introduction of radioactive materials into the body for measurements of organ function, from the detection of radioactive emissions

Body Part (4th)	Radionuclide (5th)	Qualifier (6th)	Qualifier (7th)
2 Thyroid Gland	**1** Technetium 99m (Tc-99m) **F** Iodine 123 (I-123) **G** Iodine 131 (I-131) **Y** Other Radionuclide	**Z** None	**Z** None
Y Endocrine System	**Y** Other Radionuclide	**Z** None	**Z** None

Section C **Nuclear Medicine**
Body System H **Skin, Subcutaneous Tissue and Breast**
Type 1 **Planar Nuclear Medicine Imaging:** Introduction of radioactive materials into the body for single plane display of imag developed from the capture of radioactive emissions

Body Part (4th)	Radionuclide (5th)	Qualifier (6th)	Qualifier (7th)
0 Breast, Right **1** Breast, Left **2** Breasts, Bilateral	**1** Technetium 99m (Tc-99m) **S** Thallium 201 (Tl-201) **Y** Other Radionuclide	**Z** None	**Z** None
Y Skin, Subcutaneous Tissue and Breast	**Y** Other Radionuclide	**Z** None	**Z** None

Section C **Nuclear Medicine**
Body System H **Skin, Subcutaneous Tissue and Breast**
Type 2 **Tomographic (Tomo) Nuclear Medicine Imaging:** Introduction of radioactive materials into the body for three dimensional display of images developed from the capture of radioactive emissions

Body Part (4th)	Radionuclide (5th)	Qualifier (6th)	Qualifier (7th)
0 Breast, Right **1** Breast, Left **2** Breasts, Bilateral	**1** Technetium 99m (Tc-99m) **S** Thallium 201 (Tl-201) **Y** Other Radionuclide	**Z** None	**Z** None
Y Skin, Subcutaneous Tissue and Breast	**Y** Other Radionuclide	**Z** None	**Z** None

Section C **Nuclear Medicine**
Body System P **Musculoskeletal System**
Type 1 **Planar Nuclear Medicine Imaging:** Introduction of radioactive materials into the body for single plane display of imag developed from the capture of radioactive emissions

Body Part (4th)	Radionuclide (5th)	Qualifier (6th)	Qualifier (7th)
1 Skull **4** Thorax **5** Spine **6** Pelvis **7** Spine and Pelvis **8** Upper Extremity, Right **9** Upper Extremity, Left **B** Upper Extremities, Bilateral **C** Lower Extremity, Right **D** Lower Extremity, Left **F** Lower Extremities, Bilateral **Z** Musculoskeletal System, All	**1** Technetium 99m (Tc-99m) **Y** Other Radionuclide	**Z** None	**Z** None
Y Musculoskeletal System, Other	**Y** Other Radionuclide	**Z** None	**Z** None

ection C **Nuclear Medicine**
ody System P **Musculoskeletal System**
ype 2 **Tomographic (Tomo) Nuclear Medicine Imaging:** Introduction of radioactive materials into the body for three dimensional display of images developed from the capture of radioactive emissions

Body Part (4th)	Radionuclide (5th)	Qualifier (6th)	Qualifier (7th)
1 Skull **2** Cervical Spine **3** Skull and Cervical Spine **4** Thorax **6** Pelvis **7** Spine and Pelvis **8** Upper Extremity, Right **9** Upper Extremity, Left **B** Upper Extremities, Bilateral **C** Lower Extremity, Right **D** Lower Extremity, Left **F** Lower Extremities, Bilateral **G** Thoracic Spine **H** Lumbar Spine **J** Thoracolumbar Spine	**1** Technetium 99m (Tc-99m) **Y** Other Radionuclide	**Z** None	**Z** None
Y Musculoskeletal System, Other	**Y** Other Radionuclide	**Z** None	**Z** None

ection C **Nuclear Medicine**
ody System P **Musculoskeletal System**
ype 5 **Nonimaging Nuclear Medicine Probe:** Introduction of radioactive materials into the body for the study of distribution and fate of certain substances by the detection of radioactive emissions; or, alternatively, measurement of absorption of radioactive emissions from an external source

Body Part (4th)	Radionuclide (5th)	Qualifier (6th)	Qualifier (7th)
5 Spine **N** Upper Extremities **P** Lower Extremities	**Z** None	**Z** None	**Z** None
Y Musculoskeletal System, Other	**Y** Other Radionuclide	**Z** None	**Z** None

ection C **Nuclear Medicine**
ody System T **Urinary System**
ype 1 **Planar Nuclear Medicine Imaging:** Introduction of radioactive materials into the body for single plane display of images developed from the capture of radioactive emissions

Body Part (4th)	Radionuclide (5th)	Qualifier (6th)	Qualifier (7th)
3 Kidneys, Ureters and Bladder	**1** Technetium 99m (Tc-99m) **F** Iodine 123 (I-123) **G** Iodine 131 (I-131) **Y** Other Radionuclide	**Z** None	**Z** None
H Bladder and Ureters	**1** Technetium 99m (Tc-99m) **Y** Other Radionuclide	**Z** None	**Z** None
Y Urinary System	**Y** Other Radionuclide	**Z** None	**Z** None

ection C **Nuclear Medicine**
ody System T **Urinary System**
ype 2 **Tomographic (Tomo) Nuclear Medicine Imaging:** Introduction of radioactive materials into the body for three dimensional display of images developed from the capture of radioactive emissions

Body Part (4th)	Radionuclide (5th)	Qualifier (6th)	Qualifier (7th)
3 Kidneys, Ureters and Bladder	**1** Technetium 99m (Tc-99m) **Y** Other Radionuclide	**Z** None	**Z** None
Y Urinary System	**Y** Other Radionuclide	**Z** None	**Z** None

Section C **Nuclear Medicine**
Body System T **Urinary System**
Type 6 **Nonimaging Nuclear Medicine Assay:** Introduction of radioactive materials into the body for the study of body fluids a[nd] blood elements, by the detection of radioactive emissions

Body Part (4th)	Radionuclide (5th)	Qualifier (6th)	Qualifier (7th)
3 Kidneys, Ureters and Bladder	**1** Technetium 99m (Tc-99m) **F** Iodine 123 (I-123) **G** Iodine 131 (I-131) **H** Iodine 125 (I-125) **Y** Other Radionuclide	**Z** None	**Z** None
Y Urinary System	**Y** Other Radionuclide	**Z** None	**Z** None

Section C **Nuclear Medicine**
Body System V **Male Reproductive System**
Type 1 **Planar Nuclear Medicine Imaging:** Introduction of radioactive materials into the body for single plane display of image[s] developed from the capture of radioactive emissions

Body Part (4th)	Radionuclide (5th)	Qualifier (6th)	Qualifier (7th)
9 Testicles, Bilateral	**1** Technetium 99m (Tc-99m) **Y** Other Radionuclide	**Z** None	**Z** None
Y Male Reproductive System	**Y** Other Radionuclide	**Z** None	**Z** None

Section C **Nuclear Medicine**
Body System W **Anatomical Regions**
Type 1 **Planar Nuclear Medicine Imaging:** Introduction of radioactive materials into the body for single plane display of image[s] developed from the capture of radioactive emissions

Body Part (4th)	Radionuclide (5th)	Qualifier (6th)	Qualifier (7th)
0 Abdomen **1** Abdomen and Pelvis **4** Chest and Abdomen **6** Chest and Neck **B** Head and Neck **D** Lower Extremity **J** Pelvic Region **M** Upper Extremity **N** Whole Body	**1** Technetium 99m (Tc-99m) **D** Indium 111 (In-111) **F** Iodine 123 (I-123) **G** Iodine 131 (I-131) **L** Gallium 67 (Ga-67) **S** Thallium 201 (Tl-201) **Y** Other Radionuclide	**Z** None	**Z** None
3 Chest	**1** Technetium 99m (Tc-99m) **D** Indium 111 (In-111) **F** Iodine 123 (I-123) **G** Iodine 131 (I-131) **K** Fluorine 18 (F-18) **L** Gallium 67 (Ga-67) **S** Thallium 201 (Tl-201) **Y** Other Radionuclide	**Z** None	**Z** None
Y Anatomical Regions, Multiple	**Y** Other Radionuclide	**Z** None	**Z** None
Z Anatomical Region, Other	**Z** None	**Z** None	**Z** None

ection C **Nuclear Medicine**
ody System W **Anatomical Regions**
ype 2 **Tomographic (Tomo) Nuclear Medicine Imaging:** Introduction of radioactive materials into the body for three dimensional display of images developed from the capture of radioactive emissions

Body Part (4th)	Radionuclide (5th)	Qualifier (6th)	Qualifier (7th)
0 Abdomen **1** Abdomen and Pelvis **3** Chest **4** Chest and Abdomen **6** Chest and Neck **B** Head and Neck **D** Lower Extremity **J** Pelvic Region **M** Upper Extremity	**1** Technetium 99m (Tc-99m) **D** Indium 111 (In-111) **F** Iodine 123 (I-123) **G** Iodine 131 (I-131) **K** Fluorine 18 (F-18) **L** Gallium 67 (Ga-67) **S** Thallium 201 (Tl-201) **Y** Other Radionuclide	**Z** None	**Z** None
Y Anatomical Regions, Multiple	**Y** Other Radionuclide	**Z** None	**Z** None

ection C **Nuclear Medicine**
ody System W **Anatomical Regions**
ype 3 **Positron Emission Tomographic (PET) Imaging:** Introduction of radioactive materials into the body for three dimensional display of images developed from the simultaneous capture, 180 degrees apart, of radioactive emissions

Body Part (4th)	Radionuclide (5th)	Qualifier (6th)	Qualifier (7th)
N Whole Body	**Y** Other Radionuclide	**Z** None	**Z** None

ection C **Nuclear Medicine**
ody System W **Anatomical Regions**
ype 5 **Nonimaging Nuclear Medicine Probe:** Introduction of radioactive materials into the body for the study of distribution and fate of certain substances by the detection of radioactive emissions; or, alternatively, measurement of absorption of radioactive emissions from an external source

Body Part (4th)	Radionuclide (5th)	Qualifier (6th)	Qualifier (7th)
0 Abdomen **1** Abdomen and Pelvis **3** Chest **4** Chest and Abdomen **6** Chest and Neck **B** Head and Neck **D** Lower Extremity **J** Pelvic Region **M** Upper Extremity	**1** Technetium 99m (Tc-99m) **D** Indium 111 (In-111) **Y** Other Radionuclide	**Z** None	**Z** None

ection C **Nuclear Medicine**
ody System W **Anatomical Regions**
ype 7 **Systemic Nuclear Medicine Therapy:** Introduction of unsealed radioactive materials into the body for treatment

Body Part (4th)	Radionuclide (5th)	Qualifier (6th)	Qualifier (7th)
0 Abdomen **3** Chest	**N** Phosphorus 32 (P-32) **Y** Other Radionuclide	**Z** None	**Z** None
G Thyroid	**G** Iodine 131 (I-131) **Y** Other Radionuclide	**Z** None	**Z** None
N Whole Body	**8** Samarium 153 (Sm-153) **G** Iodine 131 (I-131) **N** Phosphorus 32 (P-32) **P** Strontium 89 (Sr-89) **Y** Other Radionuclide	**Z** None	**Z** None
Y Anatomical Regions, Multiple	**Y** Other Radionuclide	**Z** None	**Z** None

HA Coding Clinic

lo references have been issued for the Nuclear Medicine section.

Radiation Therapy Section (D00–DWY)

Within each section of ICD-10-PCS the characters have different meanings. The seven character meanings for the Radiation Thera section are illustrated here through the procedure example of *HDR brachytherapy of prostate using Palladium 103*.

Section	Body System	Modality	Treatment Site	Modality Qualifier	Isotope	Qualifier
Radiation Therapy	Male Reproductive System	Brachytherapy	Prostate	High Dose Rate (HDR)	Palladium 103	None
D	V	1	0	9	B	Z

Section (Character 1)

All Radiation Therapy procedure codes have a first character value of D.

Body System (Character 2)

The alphanumeric character for the body system is placed in the second position. The following are the body systems applicable to t Radiation Therapy section.

Character Value	Character Value Description
0	Central and Peripheral Nervous System
7	Lymphatic and Hematologic System
8	Eye
9	Ear, Nose, Mouth and Throat
B	Respiratory System
D	Gastrointestinal System
F	Hepatobiliary System and Pancreas
G	Endocrine System
H	Skin
M	Breast
P	Musculoskeletal
T	Urinary System
U	Female Reproductive System
V	Male Reproductive System
W	Anatomical Regions

Modality (Character 3)

The alphanumeric character value for root types is placed in the third position. The following are the root types applicable to the Radiati Therapy section with their associated meaning.

Character Value	Modality	Modality Definition
0	Beam Radiation	The external use of high-energy radiation such as x-rays, photons, electrons, or protons
1	Brachytherapy	The use of radioactive sources placed directly into a tumor bearing area to generate local regions of high intensity radiation
2	Stereotactic Radiosurgery	The use of external radiation sources either from a linear accelerator or a special Cobalt-60 irradiator to deliver many beams of radiation directly to an internal structure in a single fraction
Y	Other Radiation	Other types of radiation therapy such as hyperthermia, contact radiation and plaque radiation. *See Modality qualifier, character 5, for specified types of other radiation.*

Source: CSI Navigator for Radiation Oncology, 2010

Treatment Site (Character 4)

For each treatment site the applicable body part character values will be available for procedure code construction. An example of treatment site for this section is Brain Stem.

odality Qualifier (Character 5)

e modality qualifier further specifies the treatment modality. The following are examples of the modality qualifier values available for Radiation Therapy section:

- Photons >10 MeV
- Neutrons
- Electrons
- High Dose Rate
- Hyperthermia

otope (Character 6)

hen an isotope is utilized during a radiation oncology procedure, the corresponding isotope character value should be reported in the th character position. The following are examples of the isotope character values available for the Radiation Therapy section:

- Iridium 192 (Ir-192)
- Iodine 125 (I-125)
- Californium 252 (Cf-252)

ualifier (Character 7)

e qualifier represents an additional attribute for the procedure when applicable. For example, beam radiation procedures in this section clude the qualifier Intraoperative that is reported with the character value of 0 for some body parts. If there is no qualifier for a procedure, placeholder Z is the character value that should be reported.

adiation Therapy Section Tables

adiation Therapy Tables D00–DWY

ction D **Radiation Therapy**
dy System 0 **Central and Peripheral Nervous System**
odality 0 **Beam Radiation**

Treatment Site (4th)	Modality Qualifier (5th)	Isotope (6th)	Qualifier (7th)
0 Brain **1** Brain Stem **6** Spinal Cord **7** Peripheral Nerve	**0** Photons <1 MeV **1** Photons 1 - 10 MeV **2** Photons >10 MeV **4** Heavy Particles (Protons,Ions) **5** Neutrons **6** Neutron Capture	**Z** None	**Z** None
0 Brain **1** Brain Stem **6** Spinal Cord **7** Peripheral Nerve	**3** Electrons	**Z** None	**0** Intraoperative **Z** None

ction D **Radiation Therapy**
dy System 0 **Central and Peripheral Nervous System**
odality 1 **Brachytherapy**

Treatment Site (4th)	Modality Qualifier (5th)	Isotope (6th)	Qualifier (7th)
0 Brain **1** Brain Stem **6** Spinal Cord **7** Peripheral Nerve	**9** High Dose Rate (HDR) **B** Low Dose Rate (LDR)	**7** Cesium 137 (Cs-137) **8** Iridium 192 (Ir-192) **9** Iodine 125 (I-125) **B** Palladium 103 (Pd-103) **C** Californium 252 (Cf-252) **Y** Other Isotope	**Z** None

Section D **Radiation Therapy**
Body System 0 **Central and Peripheral Nervous System**
Modality 2 **Stereotactic Radiosurgery**

Treatment Site (4th)	Modality Qualifier (5th)	Isotope (6th)	Qualifier (7th)
0 Brain **1** Brain Stem **6** Spinal Cord **7** Peripheral Nerve	**D** Stereotactic Other Photon Radiosurgery **H** Stereotactic Particulate Radiosurgery **J** Stereotactic Gamma Beam Radiosurgery	**Z** None	**Z** None

Section D **Radiation Therapy**
Body System 0 **Central and Peripheral Nervous System**
Modality Y **Other Radiation**

Treatment Site (4th)	Modality Qualifier (5th)	Isotope (6th)	Qualifier (7th)
0 Brain **1** Brain Stem **6** Spinal Cord **7** Peripheral Nerve	**7** Contact Radiation **8** Hyperthermia **F** Plaque Radiation **K** Laser Interstitial Thermal Therapy	**Z** None	**Z** None

Section D **Radiation Therapy**
Body System 7 **Lymphatic and Hematologic System**
Modality 0 **Beam Radiation**

Treatment Site (4th)	Modality Qualifier (5th)	Isotope (6th)	Qualifier (7th)
0 Bone Marrow **1** Thymus **2** Spleen **3** Lymphatics, Neck **4** Lymphatics, Axillary **5** Lymphatics, Thorax **6** Lymphatics, Abdomen **7** Lymphatics, Pelvis **8** Lymphatics, Inguinal	**0** Photons <1 MeV **1** Photons 1 - 10 MeV **2** Photons >10 MeV **4** Heavy Particles (Protons,Ions) **5** Neutrons **6** Neutron Capture	**Z** None	**Z** None
0 Bone Marrow **1** Thymus **2** Spleen **3** Lymphatics, Neck **4** Lymphatics, Axillary **5** Lymphatics, Thorax **6** Lymphatics, Abdomen **7** Lymphatics, Pelvis **8** Lymphatics, Inguinal	**3** Electrons	**Z** None	**0** Intraoperative **Z** None

Section D **Radiation Therapy**
Body System 7 **Lymphatic and Hematologic System**
Modality 1 **Brachytherapy**

Treatment Site (4th)	Modality Qualifier (5th)	Isotope (6th)	Qualifier (7th)
0 Bone Marrow **1** Thymus **2** Spleen **3** Lymphatics, Neck **4** Lymphatics, Axillary **5** Lymphatics, Thorax **6** Lymphatics, Abdomen **7** Lymphatics, Pelvis **8** Lymphatics, Inguinal	**9** High Dose Rate (HDR) **B** Low Dose Rate (LDR)	**7** Cesium 137 (Cs-137) **8** Iridium 192 (Ir-192) **9** Iodine 125 (I-125) **B** Palladium 103 (Pd-103) **C** Californium 252 (Cf-252) **Y** Other Isotope	**Z** None

ection **D** **Radiation Therapy**
ody System **7** **Lymphatic and Hematologic System**
odality **2** **Stereotactic Radiosurgery**

Treatment Site (4th)	Modality Qualifier (5th)	Isotope (6th)	Qualifier (7th)
0 Bone Marrow **1** Thymus **2** Spleen **3** Lymphatics, Neck **4** Lymphatics, Axillary **5** Lymphatics, Thorax **6** Lymphatics, Abdomen **7** Lymphatics, Pelvis **8** Lymphatics, Inguinal	**D** Stereotactic Other Photon Radiosurgery **H** Stereotactic Particulate Radiosurgery **J** Stereotactic Gamma Beam Radiosurgery	**Z** None	**Z** None

ection **D** **Radiation Therapy**
ody System **7** **Lymphatic and Hematologic System**
odality **Y** **Other Radiation**

Treatment Site (4th)	Modality Qualifier (5th)	Isotope (6th)	Qualifier (7th)
0 Bone Marrow **1** Thymus **2** Spleen **3** Lymphatics, Neck **4** Lymphatics, Axillary **5** Lymphatics, Thorax **6** Lymphatics, Abdomen **7** Lymphatics, Pelvis **8** Lymphatics, Inguinal	**8** Hyperthermia **F** Plaque Radiation	**Z** None	**Z** None

ection **D** **Radiation Therapy**
ody System **8** **Eye**
odality **0** **Beam Radiation**

Treatment Site (4th)	Modality Qualifier (5th)	Isotope (6th)	Qualifier (7th)
0 Eye	**0** Photons <1 MeV **1** Photons 1 - 10 MeV **2** Photons >10 MeV **4** Heavy Particles (Protons,Ions) **5** Neutrons **6** Neutron Capture	**Z** None	**Z** None
0 Eye	**3** Electrons	**Z** None	**0** Intraoperative **Z** None

ection **D** **Radiation Therapy**
ody System **8** **Eye**
odality **1** **Brachytherapy**

Treatment Site (4th)	Modality Qualifier (5th)	Isotope (6th)	Qualifier (7th)
0 Eye	**9** High Dose Rate (HDR) **B** Low Dose Rate (LDR)	**7** Cesium 137 (Cs-137) **8** Iridium 192 (Ir-192) **9** Iodine 125 (I-125) **B** Palladium 103 (Pd-103) **C** Californium 252 (Cf-252) **Y** Other Isotope	**Z** None

Section D **Radiation Therapy**
Body System 8 **Eye**
Modality 2 **Stereotactic Radiosurgery**

Treatment Site (4th)	Modality Qualifier (5th)	Isotope (6th)	Qualifier (7th)
0 Eye	**D** Stereotactic Other Photon Radiosurgery **H** Stereotactic Particulate Radiosurgery **J** Stereotactic Gamma Beam Radiosurgery	**Z** None	**Z** None

Section D **Radiation Therapy**
Body System 8 **Eye**
Modality Y **Other Radiation**

Treatment Site (4th)	Modality Qualifier (5th)	Isotope (6th)	Qualifier (7th)
0 Eye	**7** Contact Radiation **8** Hyperthermia **F** Plaque Radiation	**Z** None	**Z** None

Section D **Radiation Therapy**
Body System 9 **Ear, Nose, Mouth and Throat**
Modality 0 **Beam Radiation**

Treatment Site (4th)	Modality Qualifier (5th)	Isotope (6th)	Qualifier (7th)
0 Ear **1** Nose **3** Hypopharynx **4** Mouth **5** Tongue **6** Salivary Glands **7** Sinuses **8** Hard Palate **9** Soft Palate **B** Larynx **D** Nasopharynx **F** Oropharynx	**0** Photons <1 MeV **1** Photons 1 - 10 MeV **2** Photons >10 MeV **4** Heavy Particles (Protons,Ions) **5** Neutrons **6** Neutron Capture	**Z** None	**Z** None
0 Ear **1** Nose **3** Hypopharynx **4** Mouth **5** Tongue **6** Salivary Glands **7** Sinuses **8** Hard Palate **9** Soft Palate **B** Larynx **D** Nasopharynx **F** Oropharynx	**3** Electrons	**Z** None	**0** Intraoperative **Z** None

ction	D	Radiation Therapy
dy System	9	Ear, Nose, Mouth and Throat
odality	1	Brachytherapy

Treatment Site (4th)	Modality Qualifier (5th)	Isotope (6th)	Qualifier (7th)
0 Ear 1 Nose 3 Hypopharynx 4 Mouth 5 Tongue 6 Salivary Glands 7 Sinuses 8 Hard Palate 9 Soft Palate B Larynx D Nasopharynx F Oropharynx	9 High Dose Rate (HDR) B Low Dose Rate (LDR)	7 Cesium 137 (Cs-137) 8 Iridium 192 (Ir-192) 9 Iodine 125 (I-125) B Palladium 103 (Pd-103) C Californium 252 (Cf-252) Y Other Isotope	Z None

ction	D	Radiation Therapy
dy System	9	Ear, Nose, Mouth and Throat
odality	2	Stereotactic Radiosurgery

Treatment Site (4th)	Modality Qualifier (5th)	Isotope (6th)	Qualifier (7th)
0 Ear 1 Nose 4 Mouth 5 Tongue 6 Salivary Glands 7 Sinuses 8 Hard Palate 9 Soft Palate B Larynx C Pharynx D Nasopharynx	D Stereotactic Other Photon Radiosurgery H Stereotactic Particulate Radiosurgery J Stereotactic Gamma Beam Radiosurgery	Z None	Z None

ction	D	Radiation Therapy
dy System	9	Ear, Nose, Mouth and Throat
odality	Y	Other Radiation

Treatment Site (4th)	Modality Qualifier (5th)	Isotope (6th)	Qualifier (7th)
0 Ear 1 Nose 5 Tongue 6 Salivary Glands 7 Sinuses 8 Hard Palate 9 Soft Palate	7 Contact Radiation 8 Hyperthermia F Plaque Radiation	Z None	Z None
3 Hypopharynx F Oropharynx	7 Contact Radiation 8 Hyperthermia	Z None	Z None
4 Mouth B Larynx D Nasopharynx	7 Contact Radiation 8 Hyperthermia C Intraoperative Radiation Therapy (IORT) F Plaque Radiation	Z None	Z None
C Pharynx	C Intraoperative Radiation Therapy (IORT) F Plaque Radiation	Z None	Z None

Section D **Radiation Therapy**
Body System B **Respiratory System**
Modality 0 **Beam Radiation**

Treatment Site (4th)	Modality Qualifier (5th)	Isotope (6th)	Qualifier (7th)
0 Trachea **1** Bronchus **2** Lung **5** Pleura **6** Mediastinum **7** Chest Wall **8** Diaphragm	**0** Photons <1 MeV **1** Photons 1 - 10 MeV **2** Photons >10 MeV **4** Heavy Particles (Protons,Ions) **5** Neutrons **6** Neutron Capture	**Z** None	**Z** None
0 Trachea **1** Bronchus **2** Lung **5** Pleura **6** Mediastinum **7** Chest Wall **8** Diaphragm	**3** Electrons	**Z** None	**0** Intraoperative **Z** None

Section D **Radiation Therapy**
Body System B **Respiratory System**
Modality 1 **Brachytherapy**

Treatment Site (4th)	Modality Qualifier (5th)	Isotope (6th)	Qualifier (7th)
0 Trachea **1** Bronchus **2** Lung **5** Pleura **6** Mediastinum **7** Chest Wall **8** Diaphragm	**9** High Dose Rate (HDR) **B** Low Dose Rate (LDR)	**7** Cesium 137 (Cs-137) **8** Iridium 192 (Ir-192) **9** Iodine 125 (I-125) **B** Palladium 103 (Pd-103) **C** Californium 252 (Cf-252) **Y** Other Isotope	**Z** None

Section D **Radiation Therapy**
Body System B **Respiratory System**
Modality 2 **Stereotactic Radiosurgery**

Treatment Site (4th)	Modality Qualifier (5th)	Isotope (6th)	Qualifier (7th)
0 Trachea **1** Bronchus **2** Lung **5** Pleura **6** Mediastinum **7** Chest Wall **8** Diaphragm	**D** Stereotactic Other Photon Radiosurgery **H** Stereotactic Particulate Radiosurgery **J** Stereotactic Gamma Beam Radiosurgery	**Z** None	**Z** None

Section D **Radiation Therapy**
Body System B **Respiratory System**
Modality Y **Other Radiation**

Treatment Site (4th)	Modality Qualifier (5th)	Isotope (6th)	Qualifier (7th)
0 Trachea **1** Bronchus **2** Lung **5** Pleura **6** Mediastinum **7** Chest Wall **8** Diaphragm	**7** Contact Radiation **8** Hyperthermia **F** Plaque Radiation **K** Laser Interstitial Thermal Therapy	**Z** None	**Z** None

ction D Radiation Therapy
dy System D Gastrointestinal System
odality 0 Beam Radiation

Treatment Site (4th)	Modality Qualifier (5th)	Isotope (6th)	Qualifier (7th)
0 Esophagus 1 Stomach 2 Duodenum 3 Jejunum 4 Ileum 5 Colon 7 Rectum	0 Photons <1 MeV 1 Photons 1 - 10 MeV 2 Photons >10 MeV 4 Heavy Particles (Protons,Ions) 5 Neutrons 6 Neutron Capture	Z None	Z None
0 Esophagus 1 Stomach 2 Duodenum 3 Jejunum 4 Ileum 5 Colon 7 Rectum	3 Electrons	Z None	0 Intraoperative Z None

ction D Radiation Therapy
dy System D Gastrointestinal System
odality 1 Brachytherapy

Treatment Site (4th)	Modality Qualifier (5th)	Isotope (6th)	Qualifier (7th)
0 Esophagus 1 Stomach 2 Duodenum 3 Jejunum 4 Ileum 5 Colon 7 Rectum	9 High Dose Rate (HDR) B Low Dose Rate (LDR)	7 Cesium 137 (Cs-137) 8 Iridium 192 (Ir-192) 9 Iodine 125 (I-125) B Palladium 103 (Pd-103) C Californium 252 (Cf-252) Y Other Isotope	Z None

ction D Radiation Therapy
ody System D Gastrointestinal System
odality 2 Stereotactic Radiosurgery

Treatment Site (4th)	Modality Qualifier (5th)	Isotope (6th)	Qualifier (7th)
0 Esophagus 1 Stomach 2 Duodenum 3 Jejunum 4 Ileum 5 Colon 7 Rectum	D Stereotactic Other Photon Radiosurgery H Stereotactic Particulate Radiosurgery J Stereotactic Gamma Beam Radiosurgery	Z None	Z None

ection D Radiation Therapy
ody System D Gastrointestinal System
odality Y Other Radiation

Treatment Site (4th)	Modality Qualifier (5th)	Isotope (6th)	Qualifier (7th)
0 Esophagus	7 Contact Radiation 8 Hyperthermia F Plaque Radiation K Laser Interstitial Thermal Therapy	Z None	Z None
1 Stomach 2 Duodenum 3 Jejunum 4 Ileum 5 Colon 7 Rectum	7 Contact Radiation 8 Hyperthermia C Intraoperative Radiation Therapy (IORT) F Plaque Radiation K Laser Interstitial Thermal Therapy	Z None	Z None

Continued →

Section D **Radiation Therapy**
Body System D **Gastrointestinal System**
Modality Y **Other Radiation**

Treatment Site (4th)	Modality Qualifier (5th)	Isotope (6th)	Qualifier (7th)
8 Anus	**C** Intraoperative Radiation Therapy (IORT) **F** Plaque Radiation **K** Laser Interstitial Thermal Therapy	**Z** None	**Z** None

Section D **Radiation Therapy**
Body System F **Hepatobiliary System and Pancreas**
Modality 0 **Beam Radiation**

Treatment Site (4th)	Modality Qualifier (5th)	Isotope (6th)	Qualifier (7th)
0 Liver **1** Gallbladder **2** Bile Ducts **3** Pancreas	**0** Photons <1 MeV **1** Photons 1 - 10 MeV **2** Photons >10 MeV **4** Heavy Particles (Protons,Ions) **5** Neutrons **6** Neutron Capture	**Z** None	**Z** None
0 Liver **1** Gallbladder **2** Bile Ducts **3** Pancreas	**3** Electrons	**Z** None	**0** Intraoperative **Z** None

Section D **Radiation Therapy**
Body System F **Hepatobiliary System and Pancreas**
Modality 1 **Brachytherapy**

Treatment Site (4th)	Modality Qualifier (5th)	Isotope (6th)	Qualifier (7th)
0 Liver **1** Gallbladder **2** Bile Ducts **3** Pancreas	**9** High Dose Rate (HDR) **B** Low Dose Rate (LDR)	**7** Cesium 137 (Cs-137) **8** Iridium 192 (Ir-192) **9** Iodine 125 (I-125) **B** Palladium 103 (Pd-103) **C** Californium 252 (Cf-252) **Y** Other Isotope	**Z** None

Section D **Radiation Therapy**
Body System F **Hepatobiliary System and Pancreas**
Modality 2 **Stereotactic Radiosurgery**

Treatment Site (4th)	Modality Qualifier (5th)	Isotope (6th)	Qualifier (7th)
0 Liver **1** Gallbladder **2** Bile Ducts **3** Pancreas	**D** Stereotactic Other Photon Radiosurgery **H** Stereotactic Particulate Radiosurgery **J** Stereotactic Gamma Beam Radiosurgery	**Z** None	**Z** None

Section D **Radiation Therapy**
Body System F **Hepatobiliary System and Pancreas**
Modality Y **Other Radiation**

Treatment Site (4th)	Modality Qualifier (5th)	Isotope (6th)	Qualifier (7th)
0 Liver **1** Gallbladder **2** Bile Ducts **3** Pancreas	**7** Contact Radiation **8** Hyperthermia **C** Intraoperative Radiation Therapy (IORT) **F** Plaque Radiation **K** Laser Interstitial Thermal Therapy	**Z** None	**Z** None

Section	D	Radiation Therapy
Body System	G	Endocrine System
Modality	0	Beam Radiation

Treatment Site (4th)	Modality Qualifier (5th)	Isotope (6th)	Qualifier (7th)
0 Pituitary Gland 1 Pineal Body 2 Adrenal Glands 4 Parathyroid Glands 5 Thyroid	0 Photons <1 MeV 1 Photons 1 - 10 MeV 2 Photons >10 MeV 5 Neutrons 6 Neutron Capture	Z None	Z None
0 Pituitary Gland 1 Pineal Body 2 Adrenal Glands 4 Parathyroid Glands 5 Thyroid	3 Electrons	Z None	0 Intraoperative Z None

Section	D	Radiation Therapy
Body System	G	Endocrine System
Modality	1	Brachytherapy

Treatment Site (4th)	Modality Qualifier (5th)	Isotope (6th)	Qualifier (7th)
0 Pituitary Gland 1 Pineal Body 2 Adrenal Glands 4 Parathyroid Glands 5 Thyroid	9 High Dose Rate (HDR) B Low Dose Rate (LDR)	7 Cesium 137 (Cs-137) 8 Iridium 192 (Ir-192) 9 Iodine 125 (I-125) B Palladium 103 (Pd-103) C Californium 252 (Cf-252) Y Other Isotope	Z None

Section	D	Radiation Therapy
Body System	G	Endocrine System
Modality	2	Stereotactic Radiosurgery

Treatment Site (4th)	Modality Qualifier (5th)	Isotope (6th)	Qualifier (7th)
0 Pituitary Gland 1 Pineal Body 2 Adrenal Glands 4 Parathyroid Glands 5 Thyroid	D Stereotactic Other Photon Radiosurgery H Stereotactic Particulate Radiosurgery J Stereotactic Gamma Beam Radiosurgery	Z None	Z None

Section	D	Radiation Therapy
Body System	G	Endocrine System
Modality	Y	Other Radiation

Treatment Site (4th)	Modality Qualifier (5th)	Isotope (6th)	Qualifier (7th)
0 Pituitary Gland 1 Pineal Body 2 Adrenal Glands 4 Parathyroid Glands 5 Thyroid	7 Contact Radiation 8 Hyperthermia F Plaque Radiation K Laser Interstitial Thermal Therapy	Z None	Z None

Section D **Radiation Therapy**
Body System H **Skin**
Modality 0 **Beam Radiation**

Treatment Site (4th)	Modality Qualifier (5th)	Isotope (6th)	Qualifier (7th)
2 Skin, Face **3** Skin, Neck **4** Skin, Arm **6** Skin, Chest **7** Skin, Back **8** Skin, Abdomen **9** Skin, Buttock **B** Skin, Leg	**0** Photons <1 MeV **1** Photons 1 - 10 MeV **2** Photons >10 MeV **4** Heavy Particles (Protons,Ions) **5** Neutrons **6** Neutron Capture	**Z** None	**Z** None
2 Skin, Face **3** Skin, Neck **4** Skin, Arm **6** Skin, Chest **7** Skin, Back **8** Skin, Abdomen **9** Skin, Buttock **B** Skin, Leg	**3** Electrons	**Z** None	**0** Intraoperative **Z** None

Section D **Radiation Therapy**
Body System H **Skin**
Modality Y **Other Radiation**

Treatment Site (4th)	Modality Qualifier (5th)	Isotope (6th)	Qualifier (7th)
2 Skin, Face **3** Skin, Neck **4** Skin, Arm **6** Skin, Chest **7** Skin, Back **8** Skin, Abdomen **9** Skin, Buttock **B** Skin, Leg	**7** Contact Radiation **8** Hyperthermia **F** Plaque Radiation	**Z** None	**Z** None
5 Skin, Hand **C** Skin, Foot	**F** Plaque Radiation	**Z** None	**Z** None

Section D **Radiation Therapy**
Body System M **Breast**
Modality 0 **Beam Radiation**

Treatment Site (4th)	Modality Qualifier (5th)	Isotope (6th)	Qualifier (7th)
0 Breast, Left **1** Breast, Right	**0** Photons <1 MeV **1** Photons 1 - 10 MeV **2** Photons >10 MeV **4** Heavy Particles (Protons,Ions) **5** Neutrons **6** Neutron Capture	**Z** None	**Z** None
0 Breast, Left **1** Breast, Right	**3** Electrons	**Z** None	**0** Intraoperative **Z** None

Section D **Radiation Therapy**
Body System M **Breast**
Modality 1 **Brachytherapy**

Treatment Site (4th)	Modality Qualifier (5th)	Isotope (6th)	Qualifier (7th)
0 Breast, Left **1** Breast, Right	**9** High Dose Rate (HDR) **B** Low Dose Rate (LDR)	**7** Cesium 137 (Cs-137) **8** Iridium 192 (Ir-192) **9** Iodine 125 (I-125) **B** Palladium 103 (Pd-103) **C** Californium 252 (Cf-252) **Y** Other Isotope	**Z** None

ection D **Radiation Therapy**
ody System M **Breast**
odality 2 **Stereotactic Radiosurgery**

Treatment Site (4th)	Modality Qualifier (5th)	Isotope (6th)	Qualifier (7th)
0 Breast, Left **1** Breast, Right	**D** Stereotactic Other Photon Radiosurgery **H** Stereotactic Particulate Radiosurgery **J** Stereotactic Gamma Beam Radiosurgery	**Z** None	**Z** None

ection D **Radiation Therapy**
ody System M **Breast**
odality Y **Other Radiation**

Treatment Site (4th)	Modality Qualifier (5th)	Isotope (6th)	Qualifier (7th)
0 Breast, Left **1** Breast, Right	**7** Contact Radiation **8** Hyperthermia **F** Plaque Radiation **K** Laser Interstitial Thermal Therapy	**Z** None	**Z** None

ection D **Radiation Therapy**
ody System P **Musculoskeletal System**
odality 0 **Beam Radiation**

Treatment Site (4th)	Modality Qualifier (5th)	Isotope (6th)	Qualifier (7th)
0 Skull **2** Maxilla **3** Mandible **4** Sternum **5** Rib(s) **6** Humerus **7** Radius/Ulna **8** Pelvic Bones **9** Femur **B** Tibia/Fibula **C** Other Bone	**0** Photons <1 MeV **1** Photons 1 - 10 MeV **2** Photons >10 MeV **4** Heavy Particles (Protons,Ions) **5** Neutrons **6** Neutron Capture	**Z** None	**Z** None
0 Skull **2** Maxilla **3** Mandible **4** Sternum **5** Rib(s) **6** Humerus **7** Radius/Ulna **8** Pelvic Bones **9** Femur **B** Tibia/Fibula **C** Other Bone	**3** Electrons	**Z** None	**0** Intraoperative **Z** None

ection D **Radiation Therapy**
ody System P **Musculoskeletal System**
odality Y **Other Radiation**

Treatment Site (4th)	Modality Qualifier (5th)	Isotope (6th)	Qualifier (7th)
0 Skull **2** Maxilla **3** Mandible **4** Sternum **5** Rib(s) **6** Humerus **7** Radius/Ulna **8** Pelvic Bones **9** Femur **B** Tibia/Fibula **C** Other Bone	**7** Contact Radiation **8** Hyperthermia **F** Plaque Radiation	**Z** None	**Z** None

Section D **Radiation Therapy**
Body System T **Urinary System**
Modality 0 **Beam Radiation**

Treatment Site (4th)	Modality Qualifier (5th)	Isotope (6th)	Qualifier (7th)
0 Kidney **1** Ureter **2** Bladder **3** Urethra	**0** Photons <1 MeV **1** Photons 1 - 10 MeV **2** Photons >10 MeV **4** Heavy Particles (Protons,Ions) **5** Neutrons **6** Neutron Capture	**Z** None	**Z** None
0 Kidney **1** Ureter **2** Bladder **3** Urethra	**3** Electrons	**Z** None	**0** Intraoperative **Z** None

Section D **Radiation Therapy**
Body System T **Urinary System**
Modality 1 **Brachytherapy**

Treatment Site (4th)	Modality Qualifier (5th)	Isotope (6th)	Qualifier (7th)
0 Kidney **1** Ureter **2** Bladder **3** Urethra	**9** High Dose Rate (HDR) **B** Low Dose Rate (LDR)	**7** Cesium 137 (Cs-137) **8** Iridium 192 (Ir-192) **9** Iodine 125 (I-125) **B** Palladium 103 (Pd-103) **C** Californium 252 (Cf-252) **Y** Other Isotope	**Z** None

Section D **Radiation Therapy**
Body System T **Urinary System**
Modality 2 **Stereotactic Radiosurgery**

Treatment Site (4th)	Modality Qualifier (5th)	Isotope (6th)	Qualifier (7th)
0 Kidney **1** Ureter **2** Bladder **3** Urethra	**D** Stereotactic Other Photon Radiosurgery **H** Stereotactic Particulate Radiosurgery **J** Stereotactic Gamma Beam Radiosurgery	**Z** None	**Z** None

Section D **Radiation Therapy**
Body System T **Urinary System**
Modality Y **Other Radiation**

Treatment Site (4th)	Modality Qualifier (5th)	Isotope (6th)	Qualifier (7th)
0 Kidney **1** Ureter **2** Bladder **3** Urethra	**7** Contact Radiation **8** Hyperthermia **C** Intraoperative Radiation Therapy (IORT) **F** Plaque Radiation	**Z** None	**Z** None

Section D **Radiation Therapy**
Body System U **Female Reproductive System**
Modality 0 **Beam Radiation**

Treatment Site (4th)	Modality Qualifier (5th)	Isotope (6th)	Qualifier (7th)
0 Ovary **1** Cervix **2** Uterus	**0** Photons <1 MeV **1** Photons 1 - 10 MeV **2** Photons >10 MeV **4** Heavy Particles (Protons,Ions) **5** Neutrons **6** Neutron Capture	**Z** None	**Z** None

Continued →

ection D Radiation Therapy
ody System U Female Reproductive System
odality 0 Beam Radiation

Treatment Site (4th)	Modality Qualifier (5th)	Isotope (6th)	Qualifier (7th)
0 Ovary **1** Cervix **2** Uterus	**3** Electrons	**Z** None	**0** Intraoperative **Z** None

ection D Radiation Therapy
ody System U Female Reproductive System
odality 1 Brachytherapy

Treatment Site (4th)	Modality Qualifier (5th)	Isotope (6th)	Qualifier (7th)
0 Ovary **1** Cervix **2** Uterus	**9** High Dose Rate (HDR) **B** Low Dose Rate (LDR)	**7** Cesium 137 (Cs-137) **8** Iridium 192 (Ir-192) **9** Iodine 125 (I-125) **B** Palladium 103 (Pd-103) **C** Californium 252 (Cf-252) **Y** Other Isotope	**Z** None

ection D Radiation Therapy
ody System U Female Reproductive System
odality 2 Stereotactic Radiosurgery

Treatment Site (4th)	Modality Qualifier (5th)	Isotope (6th)	Qualifier (7th)
0 Ovary **1** Cervix **2** Uterus	**D** Stereotactic Other Photon Radiosurgery **H** Stereotactic Particulate Radiosurgery **J** Stereotactic Gamma Beam Radiosurgery	**Z** None	**Z** None

ection D Radiation Therapy
ody System U Female Reproductive System
odality Y Other Radiation

Treatment Site (4th)	Modality Qualifier (5th)	Isotope (6th)	Qualifier (7th)
0 Ovary **1** Cervix **2** Uterus	**7** Contact Radiation **8** Hyperthermia **C** Intraoperative Radiation Therapy (IORT) **F** Plaque Radiation	**Z** None	**Z** None

ection D Radiation Therapy
ody System V Male Reproductive System
odality 0 Beam Radiation

Treatment Site (4th)	Modality Qualifier (5th)	Isotope (6th)	Qualifier (7th)
0 Prostate **1** Testis	**0** Photons <1 MeV **1** Photons 1 - 10 MeV **2** Photons >10 MeV **4** Heavy Particles (Protons,Ions) **5** Neutrons **6** Neutron Capture	**Z** None	**Z** None
0 Prostate **1** Testis	**3** Electrons	**Z** None	**0** Intraoperative **Z** None

Section D **Radiation Therapy**
Body System V **Male Reproductive System**
Modality 1 **Brachytherapy**

Treatment Site (4th)	Modality Qualifier (5th)	Isotope (6th)	Qualifier (7th)
0 Prostate **1** Testis	**9** High Dose Rate (HDR) **B** Low Dose Rate (LDR)	**7** Cesium 137 (Cs-137) **8** Iridium 192 (Ir-192) **9** Iodine 125 (I-125) **B** Palladium 103 (Pd-103) **C** Californium 252 (Cf-252) **Y** Other Isotope	**Z** None

Section D **Radiation Therapy**
Body System V **Male Reproductive System**
Modality 2 **Stereotactic Radiosurgery**

Treatment Site (4th)	Modality Qualifier (5th)	Isotope (6th)	Qualifier (7th)
0 Prostate **1** Testis	**D** Stereotactic Other Photon Radiosurgery **H** Stereotactic Particulate Radiosurgery **J** Stereotactic Gamma Beam Radiosurgery	**Z** None	**Z** None

Section D **Radiation Therapy**
Body System V **Male Reproductive System**
Modality Y **Other Radiation**

Treatment Site (4th)	Modality Qualifier (5th)	Isotope (6th)	Qualifier (7th)
0 Prostate	**7** Contact Radiation **8** Hyperthermia **C** Intraoperative Radiation Therapy (IORT) **F** Plaque Radiation **K** Laser Interstitial Thermal Therapy	**Z** None	**Z** None
1 Testis	**7** Contact Radiation **8** Hyperthermia **F** Plaque Radiation	**Z** None	**Z** None

Section D **Radiation Therapy**
Body System W **Anatomical Regions**
Modality 0 **Beam Radiation**

Treatment Site (4th)	Modality Qualifier (5th)	Isotope (6th)	Qualifier (7th)
1 Head and Neck **2** Chest **3** Abdomen **4** Hemibody **5** Whole Body **6** Pelvic Region	**0** Photons <1 MeV **1** Photons 1 - 10 MeV **2** Photons >10 MeV **4** Heavy Particles (Protons,Ions) **5** Neutrons **6** Neutron Capture	**Z** None	**Z** None
1 Head and Neck **2** Chest **3** Abdomen **4** Hemibody **5** Whole Body **6** Pelvic Region	**3** Electrons	**Z** None	**0** Intraoperative **Z** None

Section D **Radiation Therapy**
Body System W **Anatomical Regions**
Modality 1 **Brachytherapy**

Treatment Site (4th)	Modality Qualifier (5th)	Isotope (6th)	Qualifier (7th)
1 Head and Neck **2** Chest **3** Abdomen **6** Pelvic Region	**9** High Dose Rate (HDR) **B** Low Dose Rate (LDR)	**7** Cesium 137 (Cs-137) **8** Iridium 192 (Ir-192) **9** Iodine 125 (I-125) **B** Palladium 103 (Pd-103) **C** Californium 252 (Cf-252) **Y** Other Isotope	**Z** None

Section D **Radiation Therapy**
Body System W **Anatomical Regions**
Modality 2 **Stereotactic Radiosurgery**

Treatment Site (4th)	Modality Qualifier (5th)	Isotope (6th)	Qualifier (7th)
1 Head and Neck **2** Chest **3** Abdomen **6** Pelvic Region	**D** Stereotactic Other Photon Radiosurgery **H** Stereotactic Particulate Radiosurgery **J** Stereotactic Gamma Beam Radiosurgery	**Z** None	**Z** None

Section D **Radiation Therapy**
Body System W **Anatomical Regions**
Modality Y **Other Radiation**

Treatment Site (4th)	Modality Qualifier (5th)	Isotope (6th)	Qualifier (7th)
1 Head and Neck **2** Chest **3** Abdomen **4** Hemibody **6** Pelvic Region	**7** Contact Radiation **8** Hyperthermia **F** Plaque Radiation	**Z** None	**Z** None
5 Whole Body	**7** Contact Radiation **8** Hyperthermia **F** Plaque Radiation	**Z** None	**Z** None
5 Whole Body	**G** Isotope Administration	**D** Iodine 131 (I-131) **F** Phosphorus 32 (P-32) **G** Strontium 89 (Sr-89) **H** Strontium 90 (Sr-90) **Y** Other Isotope	**Z** None

AHA Coding Clinic

DU11B7Z Low Dose Rate (LDR) Brachytherapy of Cervix using Cesium 137 (Cs-137)—AHA CC: 4Q, 2017, 104

Physical Rehabilitation and Diagnostic Audiology Section (F00–F15)

Within each section of ICD-10-PCS the characters have different meanings. The seven character meanings for the Physical Rehabilitati and Diagnostic Audiology section are illustrated below through the procedure example of *Individual fitting of moveable brace, right kne*

Section	Section Qualifier	Root Type	Body System/ Region	Type Qualifier	Equipment	Qualifier
Physical Rehabilitation and Diagnostic Audiology	Rehabilitation	Device Fitting	None	Dynamic Orthosis	Orthosis	None
F	0	D	Z	6	E	Z

Section (Character 1)

All Physical Rehabilitation and Diagnostic Audiology procedure codes have a first character value of F.

Section Qualifier (Character 2)

The alphanumeric character in the second character position identifies if the procedure is a physical rehabilitation procedure or a diagnost audiology procedure. Physical rehabilitation is reported with character value 0, and diagnostic audiology is reported with character value

Root Type (Character 3)

The alphanumeric character value for root types is placed in the third position. The following are the root types applicable to the Physic Rehabilitation and Diagnostic Audiology section with their associated meaning.

Character Value	Root Type	Root Type Definition
0	Speech Assessment	Measurement of speech and related functions
1	Motor and/or Nerve Function Assessment	Measurement of motor, nerve, and related functions
2	Activities of Daily Living Assessment	Measurement of functional level for activities of daily living
3	Hearing Assessment	Measurement of hearing and related functions
4	Hearing Aid Assessment	Measurement of the appropriateness and/or effectiveness of a hearing device
5	Vestibular Assessment	Measurement of the vestibular system and related functions
6	Speech Treatment	Application of techniques to improve, augment, or compensate for speech and related functional impairment
7	Motor Treatment	Exercise or activities to increase or facilitate motor function
8	Activities of Daily Living Treatment	Exercise or activities to facilitate functional competence for activities of daily living
9	Hearing Treatment	Application of techniques to improve, augment, or compensate for hearing and related functional impairment
B	Cochlear Implant Treatment	Application of techniques to improve the communication abilities of individuals with cochlear implant
C	Vestibular Treatment	Application of techniques to improve, augment, or compensate for vestibular and related functional impairment
D	Device Fitting	Fitting of a device designed to facilitate or support achievement of a higher level of function
F	Caregiver Training	Training in activities to support patient's optimal level of function

Body System/Region (Character 4)

For each body system/region the applicable body part character values will be available for procedure code construction. An example (a body region for this section is Musculoskeletal System—Lower Back/Lower Extremity.

Type Qualifier (Character 5)

Type qualifier further specifies the root type procedure. For example, the type qualifier of Gait Training/Functional Ambulation is use with Motor Treatment (character value 7) when applicable.

quipment (Character 6)

equipment is utilized during the procedure character six is used to report the type. Some examples of equipment are

- Aerobic Endurance and Conditioning
- Electrotherapeutic
- Mechanical
- Orthosis
- Prosthesis

If equipment is not utilized, the placeholder character value of Z should be reported.

ualifier (Character 7)

e qualifier represents an additional attribute for the procedure when applicable. Currently, there are no qualifiers in the Physical habilitation and Diagnostic Audiology section; therefore, the placeholder character value of Z should be reported.

hysical Rehabilitation and Diagnostic Audiology Section Tables

ysical Rehabilitation and Diagnostic Audiology Tables F00–F15

ction F **Physical Rehabilitation and Diagnostic Audiology**
ction Qualifier 0 **Rehabilitation**
pe 0 **Speech Assessment:** Measurement of speech and related functions

Body System / Region (4th)	Type Qualifier (5th)	Equipment (6th)	Qualifier (7th)
3 Neurological System - Whole Body	G Communicative/Cognitive Integration Skills	K Audiovisual M Augmentative / Alternative Communication P Computer Y Other Equipment Z None	Z None
Z None	0 Filtered Speech 3 Staggered Spondaic Word Q Performance Intensity Phonetically Balanced Speech Discrimination R Brief Tone Stimuli S Distorted Speech T Dichotic Stimuli V Temporal Ordering of Stimuli W Masking Patterns	1 Audiometer 2 Sound Field / Booth K Audiovisual Z None	Z None
Z None	1 Speech Threshold 2 Speech/Word Recognition	1 Audiometer 2 Sound Field / Booth 9 Cochlear Implant K Audiovisual Z None	Z None
Z None	4 Sensorineural Acuity Level	1 Audiometer 2 Sound Field / Booth Z None	Z None
Z None	5 Synthetic Sentence Identification	1 Audiometer 2 Sound Field / Booth 9 Cochlear Implant K Audiovisual	Z None
Z None	6 Speech and/or Language Screening 7 Nonspoken Language 8 Receptive/Expressive Language C Aphasia G Communicative/Cognitive Integration Skills L Augmentative/Alternative Communication System	K Audiovisual M Augmentative / Alternative Communication P Computer Y Other Equipment Z None	Z None

Continued →

Section F **Physical Rehabilitation and Diagnostic Audiology**
Section Qualifier 0 **Rehabilitation**
Type 0 **Speech Assessment:** Measurement of speech and related functions

F00 Contin

Body System / Region (4th)	Type Qualifier (5th)	Equipment (6th)	Qualifier (7th)
Z None	**9** Articulation/Phonology	**K** Audiovisual **P** Computer **Q** Speech Analysis **Y** Other Equipment **Z** None	**Z** None
Z None	**B** Motor Speech	**K** Audiovisual **N** Biosensory Feedback **P** Computer **Q** Speech Analysis **T** Aerodynamic Function **Y** Other Equipment **Z** None	**Z** None
Z None	**D** Fluency	**K** Audiovisual **N** Biosensory Feedback **P** Computer **Q** Speech Analysis **S** Voice Analysis **T** Aerodynamic Function **Y** Other Equipment **Z** None	**Z** None
Z None	**F** Voice	**K** Audiovisual **N** Biosensory Feedback **P** Computer **S** Voice Analysis **T** Aerodynamic Function **Y** Other Equipment **Z** None	**Z** None
Z None	**H** Bedside Swallowing and Oral Function **P** Oral Peripheral Mechanism	**Y** Other Equipment **Z** None	**Z** None
Z None	**J** Instrumental Swallowing and Oral Function	**T** Aerodynamic Function **W** Swallowing **Y** Other Equipment	**Z** None
Z None	**K** Orofacial Myofunctional	**K** Audiovisual **P** Computer **Y** Other Equipment **Z** None	**Z** None
Z None	**M** Voice Prosthetic	**K** Audiovisual **P** Computer **S** Voice Analysis **V** Speech Prosthesis **Y** Other Equipment **Z** None	**Z** None
Z None	**N** Non-invasive Instrumental Status	**N** Biosensory Feedback **P** Computer **Q** Speech Analysis **S** Voice Analysis **T** Aerodynamic Function **Y** Other Equipment	**Z** None
Z None	**X** Other Specified Central Auditory Processing	**Z** None	**Z** None

ction F Physical Rehabilitation and Diagnostic Audiology
ction Qualifier 0 Rehabilitation
ype 1 **Motor and/or Nerve Function Assessment:** Measurement of motor, nerve, and related functions

Body System / Region (4th)	Type Qualifier (5th)	Equipment (6th)	Qualifier (7th)
0 Neurological System - Head and Neck 1 Neurological System - Upper Back / Upper Extremity 2 Neurological System - Lower Back / Lower Extremity 3 Neurological System - Whole Body	0 Muscle Performance	E Orthosis F Assistive, Adaptive, Supportive or Protective U Prosthesis Y Other Equipment Z None	Z None
0 Neurological System - Head and Neck 1 Neurological System - Upper Back / Upper Extremity 2 Neurological System - Lower Back / Lower Extremity 3 Neurological System - Whole Body	1 Integumentary Integrity 3 Coordination/Dexterity 4 Motor Function G Reflex Integrity	Z None	Z None
0 Neurological System - Head and Neck 1 Neurological System - Upper Back / Upper Extremity 2 Neurological System - Lower Back / Lower Extremity 3 Neurological System - Whole Body	5 Range of Motion and Joint Integrity 6 Sensory Awareness/ Processing/Integrity	Y Other Equipment Z None	Z None
D Integumentary System - Head and Neck F Integumentary System - Upper Back / Upper Extremity G Integumentary System - Lower Back / Lower Extremity H Integumentary System - Whole Body J Musculoskeletal System - Head and Neck K Musculoskeletal System - Upper Back / Upper Extremity L Musculoskeletal System - Lower Back / Lower Extremity M Musculoskeletal System - Whole Body	0 Muscle Performance	E Orthosis F Assistive, Adaptive, Supportive or Protective U Prosthesis Y Other Equipment Z None	Z None
D Integumentary System - Head and Neck F Integumentary System - Upper Back / Upper Extremity G Integumentary System - Lower Back / Lower Extremity H Integumentary System - Whole Body J Musculoskeletal System - Head and Neck K Musculoskeletal System - Upper Back / Upper Extremity L Musculoskeletal System - Lower Back / Lower Extremity M Musculoskeletal System - Whole Body	1 Integumentary Integrity	Z None	Z None
D Integumentary System - Head and Neck F Integumentary System - Upper Back / Upper Extremity G Integumentary System - Lower Back / Lower Extremity H Integumentary System - Whole Body J Musculoskeletal System - Head and Neck K Musculoskeletal System - Upper Back / Upper Extremity L Musculoskeletal System - Lower Back / Lower Extremity M Musculoskeletal System - Whole Body	5 Range of Motion and Joint Integrity 6 Sensory Awareness/ Processing/Integrity	Y Other Equipment Z None	Z None

Continued →

Section F **Physical Rehabilitation and Diagnostic Audiology**
Section Qualifier 0 **Rehabilitation**
Type 1 **Motor and/or Nerve Function Assessment:** Measurement of motor, nerve, and related functions

Body System / Region (4th)	Type Qualifier (5th)	Equipment (6th)	Qualifier (7th)
N Genitourinary System	**0** Muscle Performance	**E** Orthosis **F** Assistive, Adaptive, Supportive or Protective **U** Prosthesis **Y** Other Equipment **Z** None	**Z** None
Z None	**2** Visual Motor Integration	**K** Audiovisual **M** Augmentative / Alternative Communication **N** Biosensory Feedback **P** Computer **Q** Speech Analysis **S** Voice Analysis **Y** Other Equipment **Z** None	**Z** None
Z None	**7** Facial Nerve Function	**7** Electrophysiologic	**Z** None
Z None	**9** Somatosensory Evoked Potentials	**J** Somatosensory	**Z** None
Z None	**B** Bed Mobility **C** Transfer **F** Wheelchair Mobility	**E** Orthosis **F** Assistive, Adaptive, Supportive or Protective **U** Prosthesis **Z** None	**Z** None
Z None	**D** Gait and/or Balance	**E** Orthosis **F** Assistive, Adaptive, Supportive or Protective **U** Prosthesis **Y** Other Equipment **Z** None	**Z** None

Section F **Physical Rehabilitation and Diagnostic Audiology**
Section Qualifier 0 **Rehabilitation**
Type 2 **Activities of Daily Living Assessment:** Measurement of functional level for activities of daily living

Body System / Region (4th)	Type Qualifier (5th)	Equipment (6th)	Qualifier (7th)
0 Neurological System - Head and Neck	**9** Cranial Nerve Integrity **D** Neuromotor Development	**Y** Other Equipment **Z** None	**Z** None
1 Neurological System - Upper Back / Upper Extremity **2** Neurological System - Lower Back / Lower Extremity **3** Neurological System - Whole Body	**D** Neuromotor Development	**Y** Other Equipment **Z** None	**Z** None
4 Circulatory System - Head and Neck **5** Circulatory System - Upper Back / Upper Extremity **6** Circulatory System - Lower Back / Lower Extremity **8** Respiratory System - Head and Neck **9** Respiratory System - Upper Back / Upper Extremity **B** Respiratory System - Lower Back / Lower Extremity	**G** Ventilation, Respiration and Circulation	**C** Mechanical **G** Aerobic Endurance and Conditioning **Y** Other Equipment **Z** None	**Z** None

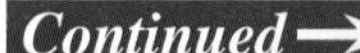
Continued

ction **F** **Physical Rehabilitation and Diagnostic Audiology**
ction Qualifier **0** **Rehabilitation**
pe **2** **Activities of Daily Living Assessment:** Measurement of functional level for activities of daily living

Body System / Region (4th)	Type Qualifier (5th)	Equipment (6th)	Qualifier (7th)
7 Circulatory System - Whole Body C Respiratory System - Whole Body	**7** Aerobic Capacity and Endurance	**E** Orthosis **G** Aerobic Endurance and Conditioning **U** Prosthesis **Y** Other Equipment **Z** None	**Z** None
7 Circulatory System - Whole Body C Respiratory System - Whole Body	**G** Ventilation, Respiration and Circulation	**C** Mechanical **G** Aerobic Endurance and Conditioning **Y** Other Equipment **Z** None	**Z** None
Z None	**0** Bathing/Showering **1** Dressing **3** Grooming/Personal Hygiene **4** Home Management	**E** Orthosis **F** Assistive, Adaptive, Supportive or Protective **U** Prosthesis **Z** None	**Z** None
Z None	**2** Feeding/Eating **8** Anthropometric Characteristics **F** Pain	**Y** Other Equipment **Z** None	**Z** None
Z None	**5** Perceptual Processing	**K** Audiovisual **M** Augmentative / Alternative Communication **N** Biosensory Feedback **P** Computer **Q** Speech Analysis **S** Voice Analysis **Y** Other Equipment **Z** None	**Z** None
Z None	**6** Psychosocial Skills	**Z** None	**Z** None
Z None	**B** Environmental, Home and Work Barriers **C** Ergonomics and Body Mechanics	**E** Orthosis **F** Assistive, Adaptive, Supportive or Protective **U** Prosthesis **Y** Other Equipment **Z** None	**Z** None
Z None	**H** Vocational Activities and Functional Community or Work Reintegration Skills	**E** Orthosis **F** Assistive, Adaptive, Supportive or Protective **G** Aerobic Endurance and Conditioning **U** Prosthesis **Y** Other Equipment **Z** None	**Z** None

ction **F** **Physical Rehabilitation and Diagnostic Audiology**
ction Qualifier **0** **Rehabilitation**
ype **6** **Speech Treatment:** Application of techniques to improve, augment, or compensate for speech and related functional impairment

Body System / Region (4th)	Type Qualifier (5th)	Equipment (6th)	Qualifier (7th)
3 Neurological System - Whole Body	**6** Communicative/Cognitive Integration Skills	**K** Audiovisual **M** Augmentative / Alternative Communication **P** Computer **Y** Other Equipment **Z** None	**Z** None

Continued →

Section F **Physical Rehabilitation and Diagnostic Audiology**
Section Qualifier 0 **Rehabilitation**
Type 6 **Speech Treatment:** Application of techniques to improve, augment, or compensate for speech and related functional impairment

F06 Continu

Body System / Region (4th)	Type Qualifier (5th)	Equipment (6th)	Qualifier (7th)
Z None	**0** Nonspoken Language **3** Aphasia **6** Communicative/Cognitive Integration Skills	**K** Audiovisual **M** Augmentative / Alternative Communication **P** Computer **Y** Other Equipment **Z** None	**Z** None
Z None	**1** Speech-Language Pathology and Related Disorders Counseling **2** Speech-Language Pathology and Related Disorders Prevention	**K** Audiovisual **Z** None	**Z** None
Z None	**4** Articulation/Phonology	**K** Audiovisual **P** Computer **Q** Speech Analysis **T** Aerodynamic Function **Y** Other Equipment **Z** None	**Z** None
Z None	**5** Aural Rehabilitation	**K** Audiovisual **L** Assistive Listening **M** Augmentative / Alternative Communication **N** Biosensory Feedback **P** Computer **Q** Speech Analysis **S** Voice Analysis **Y** Other Equipment **Z** None	**Z** None
Z None	**7** Fluency	**4** Electroacoustic Immitance / Acoustic Reflex **K** Audiovisual **N** Biosensory Feedback **Q** Speech Analysis **S** Voice Analysis **T** Aerodynamic Function **Y** Other Equipment **Z** None	**Z** None
Z None	**8** Motor Speech	**K** Audiovisual **N** Biosensory Feedback **P** Computer **Q** Speech Analysis **S** Voice Analysis **T** Aerodynamic Function **Y** Other Equipment **Z** None	**Z** None
Z None	**9** Orofacial Myofunctional	**K** Audiovisual **P** Computer **Y** Other Equipment **Z** None	**Z** None
Z None	**B** Receptive/Expressive Language	**K** Audiovisual **L** Assistive Listening **M** Augmentative / Alternative Communication **P** Computer **Y** Other Equipment **Z** None	**Z** None

Continued →

ction F Physical Rehabilitation and Diagnostic Audiology
ction Qualifier 0 Rehabilitation
ype 6 Speech Treatment: Application of techniques to improve, augment, or compensate for speech and related functional impairment

Body System / Region (4th)	Type Qualifier (5th)	Equipment (6th)	Qualifier (7th)
Z None	C Voice	K Audiovisual N Biosensory Feedback P Computer S Voice Analysis T Aerodynamic Function V Speech Prosthesis Y Other Equipment Z None	Z None
Z None	D Swallowing Dysfunction	M Augmentative / Alternative Communication T Aerodynamic Function V Speech Prosthesis Y Other Equipment Z None	Z None

ction F Physical Rehabilitation and Diagnostic Audiology
ction Qualifier 0 Rehabilitation
ype 7 Motor Treatment: Exercise or activities to increase or facilitate motor function

Body System / Region (4th)	Type Qualifier (5th)	Equipment (6th)	Qualifier (7th)
0 Neurological System - Head and Neck 1 Neurological System - Upper Back / Upper Extremity 2 Neurological System - Lower Back / Lower Extremity 3 Neurological System - Whole Body D Integumentary System - Head and Neck F Integumentary System - Upper Back / Upper Extremity G Integumentary System - Lower Back / Lower Extremity H Integumentary System - Whole Body J Musculoskeletal System - Head and Neck K Musculoskeletal System - Upper Back / Upper Extremity L Musculoskeletal System - Lower Back / Lower Extremity M Musculoskeletal System - Whole Body	0 Range of Motion and Joint Mobility 1 Muscle Performance 2 Coordination/Dexterity 3 Motor Function	E Orthosis F Assistive, Adaptive, Supportive or Protective U Prosthesis Y Other Equipment Z None	Z None
0 Neurological System - Head and Neck 1 Neurological System - Upper Back / Upper Extremity 2 Neurological System - Lower Back / Lower Extremity 3 Neurological System - Whole Body D Integumentary System - Head and Neck F Integumentary System - Upper Back / Upper Extremity G Integumentary System - Lower Back / Lower Extremity H Integumentary System - Whole Body J Musculoskeletal System - Head and Neck K Musculoskeletal System - Upper Back / Upper Extremity L Musculoskeletal System - Lower Back / Lower Extremity M Musculoskeletal System - Whole Body	6 Therapeutic Exercise	B Physical Agents C Mechanical D Electrotherapeutic E Orthosis F Assistive, Adaptive, Supportive or Protective G Aerobic Endurance and Conditioning H Mechanical or Electromechanical U Prosthesis Y Other Equipment Z None	Z None

Continued →

Section F **Physical Rehabilitation and Diagnostic Audiology**
Section Qualifier 0 **Rehabilitation**
Type 7 **Motor Treatment:** Exercise or activities to increase or facilitate motor function

F07 Continu

Body System / Region (4th)	Type Qualifier (5th)	Equipment (6th)	Qualifier (7th)
0 Neurological System - Head and Neck **1** Neurological System - Upper Back / Upper Extremity **2** Neurological System - Lower Back / Lower Extremity **3** Neurological System - Whole Body **D** Integumentary System - Head and Neck **F** Integumentary System - Upper Back / Upper Extremity **G** Integumentary System - Lower Back / Lower Extremity **H** Integumentary System - Whole Body **J** Musculoskeletal System - Head and Neck **K** Musculoskeletal System - Upper Back / Upper Extremity **L** Musculoskeletal System - Lower Back / Lower Extremity **M** Musculoskeletal System - Whole Body	**7** Manual Therapy Techniques	**Z** None	**Z** None
4 Circulatory System - Head and Neck **5** Circulatory System - Upper Back / Upper Extremity **6** Circulatory System - Lower Back / Lower Extremity **7** Circulatory System - Whole Body **8** Respiratory System - Head and Neck **9** Respiratory System - Upper Back / Upper Extremity **B** Respiratory System - Lower Back / Lower Extremity **C** Respiratory System - Whole Body	**6** Therapeutic Exercise	**B** Physical Agents **C** Mechanical **D** Electrotherapeutic **E** Orthosis **F** Assistive, Adaptive, Supportive or Protective **G** Aerobic Endurance and Conditioning **H** Mechanical or Electromechanical **U** Prosthesis **Y** Other Equipment **Z** None	**Z** None
N Genitourinary System	**1** Muscle Performance	**E** Orthosis **F** Assistive, Adaptive, Supportive or Protective **U** Prosthesis **Y** Other Equipment **Z** None	**Z** None
N Genitourinary System	**6** Therapeutic Exercise	**B** Physical Agents **C** Mechanical **D** Electrotherapeutic **E** Orthosis **F** Assistive, Adaptive, Supportive or Protective **G** Aerobic Endurance and Conditioning **H** Mechanical or Electromechanical **U** Prosthesis **Y** Other Equipment **Z** None	**Z** None
Z None	**4** Wheelchair Mobility	**D** Electrotherapeutic **E** Orthosis **F** Assistive, Adaptive, Supportive or Protective **U** Prosthesis **Y** Other Equipment **Z** None	**Z** None
Z None	**5** Bed Mobility	**C** Mechanical **E** Orthosis **F** Assistive, Adaptive, Supportive or Protective **U** Prosthesis **Y** Other Equipment **Z** None	**Z** None

Continued →

Section	F	**Physical Rehabilitation and Diagnostic Audiology**
Section Qualifier	0	**Rehabilitation**
Type	7	**Motor Treatment:** Exercise or activities to increase or facilitate motor function

Body System / Region (4th)	Type Qualifier (5th)	Equipment (6th)	Qualifier (7th)
Z None	**8** Transfer Training	**C** Mechanical **D** Electrotherapeutic **E** Orthosis **F** Assistive, Adaptive, Supportive or Protective **U** Prosthesis **Y** Other Equipment **Z** None	**Z** None
Z None	**9** Gait Training/Functional Ambulation	**C** Mechanical **D** Electrotherapeutic **E** Orthosis **F** Assistive, Adaptive, Supportive or Protective **G** Aerobic Endurance and Conditioning **U** Prosthesis **Y** Other Equipment **Z** None	**Z** None

Section	F	**Physical Rehabilitation and Diagnostic Audiology**
Section Qualifier	0	**Rehabilitation**
Type	8	**Activities of Daily Living Treatment:** Exercise or activities to facilitate functional competence for activities of daily living

Body System / Region (4th)	Type Qualifier (5th)	Equipment (6th)	Qualifier (7th)
D Integumentary System - Head and Neck **F** Integumentary System - Upper Back / Upper Extremity **G** Integumentary System - Lower Back / Lower Extremity **H** Integumentary System - Whole Body **J** Musculoskeletal System - Head and Neck **K** Musculoskeletal System - Upper Back / Upper Extremity **L** Musculoskeletal System - Lower Back / Lower Extremity **M** Musculoskeletal System - Whole Body	**5** Wound Management	**B** Physical Agents **C** Mechanical **D** Electrotherapeutic **E** Orthosis **F** Assistive, Adaptive, Supportive or Protective **U** Prosthesis **Y** Other Equipment **Z** None	**Z** None
Z None	**0** Bathing/Showering Techniques **1** Dressing Techniques **2** Grooming/Personal Hygiene	**E** Orthosis **F** Assistive, Adaptive, Supportive or Protective **U** Prosthesis **Y** Other Equipment **Z** None	**Z** None
Z None	**3** Feeding/Eating	**C** Mechanical **D** Electrotherapeutic **E** Orthosis **F** Assistive, Adaptive, Supportive or Protective **U** Prosthesis **Y** Other Equipment **Z** None	**Z** None
Z None	**4** Home Management	**D** Electrotherapeutic **E** Orthosis **F** Assistive, Adaptive, Supportive or Protective **U** Prosthesis **Y** Other Equipment **Z** None	**Z** None

Continued →

F08 Continu

Section F **Physical Rehabilitation and Diagnostic Audiology**
Section Qualifier 0 **Rehabilitation**
Type 8 **Activities of Daily Living Treatment:** Exercise or activities to facilitate functional competence for activities of daily livi

Body System / Region (4th)	Type Qualifier (5th)	Equipment (6th)	Qualifier (7th)
Z None	**6** Psychosocial Skills	**Z** None	**Z** None
Z None	**7** Vocational Activities and Functional Community or Work Reintegration Skills	**B** Physical Agents **C** Mechanical **D** Electrotherapeutic **E** Orthosis **F** Assistive, Adaptive, Supportive or Protective **G** Aerobic Endurance and Conditioning **U** Prosthesis **Y** Other Equipment **Z** None	**Z** None

Section F **Physical Rehabilitation and Diagnostic Audiology**
Section Qualifier 0 **Rehabilitation**
Type 9 **Hearing Treatment:** Application of techniques to improve, augment, or compensate for hearing and related functional impairme

Body System / Region (4th)	Type Qualifier (5th)	Equipment (6th)	Qualifier (7th)
Z None	**0** Hearing and Related Disorders Counseling **1** Hearing and Related Disorders Prevention	**K** Audiovisual **Z** None	**Z** None
Z None	**2** Auditory Processing	**K** Audiovisual **L** Assistive Listening **P** Computer **Y** Other Equipment **Z** None	**Z** None
Z None	**3** Cerumen Management	**X** Cerumen Management **Z** None	**Z** None

Section F **Physical Rehabilitation and Diagnostic Audiology**
Section Qualifier 0 **Rehabilitation**
Type B **Cochlear Implant Treatment:** Application of techniques to improve the communication abilities of individuals with cochlear implant

Body System / Region (4th)	Type Qualifier (5th)	Equipment (6th)	Qualifier (7th)
Z None	**0** Cochlear Implant Rehabilitation	**1** Audiometer **2** Sound Field / Booth **9** Cochlear Implant **K** Audiovisual **P** Computer **Y** Other Equipment	**Z** None

Section F **Physical Rehabilitation and Diagnostic Audiology**
Section Qualifier 0 **Rehabilitation**
Type C **Vestibular Treatment:** Application of techniques to improve, augment, or compensate for vestibular and related functiona impairment

Body System / Region (4th)	Type Qualifier (5th)	Equipment (6th)	Qualifier (7th)
3 Neurological System - Whole Body **H** Integumentary System - Whole Body **M** Musculoskeletal System - Whole Body	**3** Postural Control	**E** Orthosis **F** Assistive, Adaptive, Supportive or Protective **U** Prosthesis **Y** Other Equipment **Z** None	**Z** None

Continued →

ction F **Physical Rehabilitation and Diagnostic Audiology**
ction Qualifier 0 **Rehabilitation**
ype C **Vestibular Treatment:** Application of techniques to improve, augment, or compensate for vestibular and related functional impairment

Body System / Region (4th)	Type Qualifier (5th)	Equipment (6th)	Qualifier (7th)
Z None	**0** Vestibular	**8** Vestibular / Balance **Z** None	**Z** None
Z None	**1** Perceptual Processing **2** Visual Motor Integration	**K** Audiovisual **L** Assistive Listening **N** Biosensory Feedback **P** Computer **Q** Speech Analysis **S** Voice Analysis **T** Aerodynamic Function **Y** Other Equipment **Z** None	**Z** None

ction F **Physical Rehabilitation and Diagnostic Audiology**
ction Qualifier 0 **Rehabilitation**
ype D **Device Fitting:** Fitting of a device designed to facilitate or support achievement of a higher level of function

Body System / Region (4th)	Type Qualifier (5th)	Equipment (6th)	Qualifier (7th)
Z None	**0** Tinnitus Masker	**5** Hearing Aid Selection / Fitting / Test **Z** None	**Z** None
Z None	**1** Monaural Hearing Aid **2** Binaural Hearing Aid **5** Assistive Listening Device	**1** Audiometer **2** Sound Field / Booth **5** Hearing Aid Selection / Fitting / Test **K** Audiovisual **L** Assistive Listening **Z** None	**Z** None
Z None	**3** Augmentative/Alternative Communication System	**M** Augmentative / Alternative Communication	**Z** None
Z None	**4** Voice Prosthetic	**S** Voice Analysis **V** Speech Prosthesis	**Z** None
Z None	**6** Dynamic Orthosis **7** Static Orthosis **8** Prosthesis **9** Assistive, Adaptive, Supportive or Protective Devices	**E** Orthosis **F** Assistive, Adaptive, Supportive or Protective **U** Prosthesis **Z** None	**Z** None

Section F **Physical Rehabilitation and Diagnostic Audiology**
Section Qualifier 0 **Rehabilitation**
Type F **Caregiver Training:** Training in activities to support patient's optimal level of function

Body System / Region (4th)	Type Qualifier (5th)	Equipment (6th)	Qualifier (7th)
Z None	**0** Bathing/Showering Technique **1** Dressing **2** Feeding and Eating **3** Grooming/Personal Hygiene **4** Bed Mobility **5** Transfer **6** Wheelchair Mobility **7** Therapeutic Exercise **8** Airway Clearance Techniques **9** Wound Management **B** Vocational Activities and Functional Community or Work Reintegration Skills **C** Gait Training/Functional Ambulation **D** Application, Proper Use and Care of Devices **F** Application, Proper Use and Care of Orthoses **G** Application, Proper Use and Care of Prosthesis **H** Home Management	**E** Orthosis **F** Assistive, Adaptive, Supportive or Protective **U** Prosthesis **Z** None	**Z** None
Z None	**J** Communication Skills	**K** Audiovisual **L** Assistive Listening **M** Augmentative / Alternative Communication **P** Computer **Z** None	**Z** None

Section F **Physical Rehabilitation and Diagnostic Audiology**
Section Qualifier 1 **Diagnostic Audiology**
Type 3 **Hearing Assessment:** Measurement of hearing and related functions

Body System / Region (4th)	Type Qualifier (5th)	Equipment (6th)	Qualifier (7th)
Z None	**0** Hearing Screening	**0** Occupational Hearing **1** Audiometer **2** Sound Field / Booth **3** Tympanometer **8** Vestibular / Balance **9** Cochlear Implant **Z** None	**Z** None
Z None	**1** Pure Tone Audiometry, Air **2** Pure Tone Audiometry, Air and Bone	**0** Occupational Hearing **1** Audiometer **2** Sound Field / Booth **Z** None	**Z** None
Z None	**3** Bekesy Audiometry **6** Visual Reinforcement Audiometry **9** Short Increment Sensitivity Index **B** Stenger **C** Pure Tone Stenger	**1** Audiometer **2** Sound Field / Booth **Z** None	**Z** None
Z None	**4** Conditioned Play Audiometry **5** Select Picture Audiometry	**1** Audiometer **2** Sound Field / Booth **K** Audiovisual **Z** None	**Z** None
Z None	**7** Alternate Binaural or Monaural Loudness Balance	**1** Audiometer **K** Audiovisual **Z** None	**Z** None

Continued →

ection F Physical Rehabilitation and Diagnostic Audiology
ection Qualifier 1 Diagnostic Audiology
ype 3 **Hearing Assessment:** Measurement of hearing and related functions

Body System / Region (4th)	Type Qualifier (5th)	Equipment (6th)	Qualifier (7th)
Z None	**8** Tone Decay **D** Tympanometry **F** Eustachian Tube Function **G** Acoustic Reflex Patterns **H** Acoustic Reflex Threshold **J** Acoustic Reflex Decay	**3** Tympanometer **4** Electroacoustic Immitance / Acoustic Reflex **Z** None	**Z** None
Z None	**K** Electrocochleography **L** Auditory Evoked Potentials	**7** Electrophysiologic **Z** None	**Z** None
Z None	**M** Evoked Otoacoustic Emissions, Screening **N** Evoked Otoacoustic Emissions, Diagnostic	**6** Otoacoustic Emission (OAE) **Z** None	**Z** None
Z None	**P** Aural Rehabilitation Status	**1** Audiometer **2** Sound Field / Booth **4** Electroacoustic Immitance / Acoustic Reflex **9** Cochlear Implant **K** Audiovisual **L** Assistive Listening **P** Computer **Z** None	**Z** None
Z None	**Q** Auditory Processing	**K** Audiovisual **P** Computer **Y** Other Equipment **Z** None	**Z** None

ection F Physical Rehabilitation and Diagnostic Audiology
ection Qualifier 1 Diagnostic Audiology
ype 4 **Hearing Aid Assessment:** Measurement of the appropriateness and/or effectiveness of a hearing device

Body System / Region (4th)	Type Qualifier (5th)	Equipment (6th)	Qualifier (7th)
Z None	**0** Cochlear Implant	**1** Audiometer **2** Sound Field / Booth **3** Tympanometer **4** Electroacoustic Immitance / Acoustic Reflex **5** Hearing Aid Selection / Fitting / Test **7** Electrophysiologic **9** Cochlear Implant **K** Audiovisual **L** Assistive Listening **P** Computer **Y** Other Equipment **Z** None	**Z** None
Z None	**1** Ear Canal Probe Microphone **6** Binaural Electroacoustic Hearing Aid Check **8** Monaural Electroacoustic Hearing Aid Check	**5** Hearing Aid Selection / Fitting / Test **Z** None	**Z** None

Continued →

F14 Continued

Section F **Physical Rehabilitation and Diagnostic Audiology**
Section Qualifier 1 **Diagnostic Audiology**
Type 4 **Hearing Aid Assessment:** Measurement of the appropriateness and/or effectiveness of a hearing device

Body System / Region (4th)	Type Qualifier (5th)	Equipment (6th)	Qualifier (7th)
Z None	**2** Monaural Hearing Aid **3** Binaural Hearing Aid	**1** Audiometer **2** Sound Field / Booth **3** Tympanometer **4** Electroacoustic Immitance / Acoustic Reflex **5** Hearing Aid Selection / Fitting / Test **K** Audiovisual **L** Assistive Listening **P** Computer **Z** None	**Z** None
Z None	**4** Assistive Listening System/ Device Selection	**1** Audiometer **2** Sound Field / Booth **3** Tympanometer **4** Electroacoustic Immitance / Acoustic Reflex **K** Audiovisual **L** Assistive Listening **Z** None	**Z** None
Z None	**5** Sensory Aids	**1** Audiometer **2** Sound Field / Booth **3** Tympanometer **4** Electroacoustic Immitance / Acoustic Reflex **5** Hearing Aid Selection / Fitting / Test **K** Audiovisual **L** Assistive Listening **Z** None	**Z** None
Z None	**7** Ear Protector Attentuation	**0** Occupational Hearing **Z** None	**Z** None

Section F **Physical Rehabilitation and Diagnostic Audiology**
Section Qualifier 1 **Diagnostic Audiology**
Type 5 **Vestibular Assessment:** Measurement of the vestibular system and related functions

Body System / Region (4th)	Type Qualifier (5th)	Equipment (6th)	Qualifier (7th)
Z None	**0** Bithermal, Binaural Caloric Irrigation **1** Bithermal, Monaural Caloric Irrigation **2** Unithermal Binaural Screen **3** Oscillating Tracking **4** Sinusoidal Vertical Axis Rotational **5** Dix-Hallpike Dynamic **6** Computerized Dynamic Posturography	**8** Vestibular / Balance **Z** None	**Z** None
Z None	**7** Tinnitus Masker	**5** Hearing Aid Selection / Fitting / Test **Z** None	**Z** None

AHA Coding Clinic

No references have been issued for the Physical Rehabilitation and Diagnostic Audiology section.

Mental Health Section (GZ1–GZJ)

Within each section of ICD-10-PCS the characters have different meanings. The seven character meanings for the Mental Health section are illustrated here through the procedure example of *Crisis intervention*.

Section	Body System	Root Type	Qualifier	Qualifier	Qualifier	Qualifier
Mental Health	None	Crisis Intervention	None	None	None	None
G	Z	2	Z	Z	Z	Z

Section (Character 1)

All Mental Health procedure codes have a first character value of G.

Body System (Character 2)

The body system is not specified for mental health; therefore, the placeholder character value of Z is reported in the second character position.

Root Type (Character 3)

The alphanumeric character value for root types is placed in the third position. Listed below are the root types applicable to the Mental Health section with their associated meaning.

Character Value	Root Type	Root Type Definition
1	Psychological Tests	The administration and interpretation of standardized psychological tests and measurement instruments for the assessment of psychological function
2	Crisis Intervention	Treatment of a traumatized, acutely disturbed or distressed individual for the purpose of short-term stabilization
3	Medication Management	Monitoring and adjusting the use of medications for the treatment of a mental health disorder
5	Individual Psychotherapy	Treatment of an individual with a mental health disorder by behavioral, cognitive, psychoanalytic, psychodynamic or psychophysiological means to improve functioning or well-being
6	Counseling	The application of psychological methods to treat an individual with normal developmental issues and psychological problems in order to increase function, improve well-being, alleviate distress, maladjustment or resolve crises
7	Family Psychotherapy	Treatment that includes one or more family members of an individual with a mental health disorder by behavioral, cognitive, psychoanalytic, psychodynamic or psychophysiological means to improve functioning or well-being
B	Electroconvulsive Therapy	The application of controlled electrical voltages to treat a mental health disorder
C	Biofeedback	Provision of information from the monitoring and regulating of physiological processes in conjunction with cognitive-behavioral techniques to improve patient functioning or well-being
F	Hypnosis	Induction of a state of heightened suggestibility by auditory, visual and tactile techniques to elicit an emotional or behavioral response
G	Narcosynthesis	Administration of intravenous barbiturates in order to release suppressed or repressed thoughts
H	Group Psychotherapy	Treatment of two or more individuals with a mental health disorder by behavioral, cognitive, psychoanalytic, psychodynamic or psychophysiological means to improve functioning or well-being
J	Light Therapy	Application of specialized light treatments to improve functioning or well-being

Qualifier (Character 4)

This qualifier further specifies the root type procedure. For example, the qualifier of Development further specifies the type of Psychological Tests.

Qualifier (Character 5)

The qualifier represents an additional attribute for the procedure when applicable. Currently, there are no qualifiers in the Mental Health section; therefore, the placeholder character value of Z should be reported.

Qualifier (Character 6)

The qualifier represents an additional attribute for the procedure when applicable. Currently, there are no qualifiers in the Mental Healt section; therefore, the placeholder character value of Z should be reported.

Qualifier (Character 7)

The qualifier represents an additional attribute for the procedure when applicable. Currently, there are no qualifiers in the Mental Healt section; therefore, the placeholder character value of Z should be reported.

Mental Health Tables

Mental Health Tables GZ1–GZJ

Section G **Mental Health**
Body System Z **None**
Type 1 **Psychological Tests:** The administration and interpretation of standardized psychological tests and measurement instruments for the assessment of psychological function

Qualifier (4th)	Qualifier (5th)	Qualifier (6th)	Qualifier (7th)
0 Developmental **1** Personality and Behavioral **2** Intellectual and Psychoeducational **3** Neuropsychological **4** Neurobehavioral and Cognitive Status	**Z** None	**Z** None	**Z** None

Section G **Mental Health**
Body System Z **None**
Type 2 **Crisis Intervention:** Treatment of a traumatized, acutely disturbed or distressed individual for the purpose of short-term stabilization

Qualifier (4th)	Qualifier (5th)	Qualifier (6th)	Qualifier (7th)
Z None	**Z** None	**Z** None	**Z** None

Section G **Mental Health**
Body System Z **None**
Type 3 **Medication Management:** Monitoring and adjusting the use of medications for the treatment of a mental health disorder

Qualifier (4th)	Qualifier (5th)	Qualifier (6th)	Qualifier (7th)
Z None	**Z** None	**Z** None	**Z** None

Section G **Mental Health**
Body System Z **None**
Type 5 **Individual Psychotherapy:** Treatment of an individual with a mental health disorder by behavioral, cognitive, psychoanalytic, psychodynamic or psychophysiological means to improve functioning or well-being

Qualifier (4th)	Qualifier (5th)	Qualifier (6th)	Qualifier (7th)
0 Interactive **1** Behavioral **2** Cognitive **3** Interpersonal **4** Psychoanalysis **5** Psychodynamic **6** Supportive **8** Cognitive-Behavioral **9** Psychophysiological	**Z** None	**Z** None	**Z** None

ction G Mental Health
ody System Z None
pe 6 **Counseling:** The application of psychological methods to treat an individual with normal developmental issues and psychological problems in order to increase function, improve well-being, alleviate distress, maladjustment or resolve crises

Qualifier (4th)	Qualifier (5th)	Qualifier (6th)	Qualifier (7th)
0 Educational 1 Vocational 3 Other Counseling	Z None	Z None	Z None

ction G Mental Health
ody System Z None
pe 7 **Family Psychotherapy:** Treatment that includes one or more family members of an individual with a mental health disorder by behavioral, cognitive, psychoanalytic, psychodynamic or psychophysiological means to improve functioning or well-being

Qualifier (4th)	Qualifier (5th)	Qualifier (6th)	Qualifier (7th)
2 Other Family Psychotherapy	Z None	Z None	Z None

ction G Mental Health
ody System Z None
pe B **Electroconvulsive Therapy:** The application of controlled electrical voltages to treat a mental health disorder

Qualifier (4th)	Qualifier (5th)	Qualifier (6th)	Qualifier (7th)
0 Unilateral-Single Seizure 1 Unilateral-Multiple Seizure 2 Bilateral-Single Seizure 3 Bilateral-Multiple Seizure 4 Other Electroconvulsive Therapy	Z None	Z None	Z None

ction G Mental Health
ody System Z None
ype C **Biofeedback:** Provision of information from the monitoring and regulating of physiological processes in conjunction with cognitive-behavioral techniques to improve patient functioning or well-being

Qualifier (4th)	Qualifier (5th)	Qualifier (6th)	Qualifier (7th)
9 Other Biofeedback	Z None	Z None	Z None

ction G Mental Health
ody System Z None
ype F **Hypnosis:** Induction of a state of heightened suggestibility by auditory, visual and tactile techniques to elicit an emotional or behavioral response

Qualifier (4th)	Qualifier (5th)	Qualifier (6th)	Qualifier (7th)
Z None	Z None	Z None	Z None

ection G Mental Health
ody System Z None
ype G **Narcosynthesis:** Administration of intravenous barbiturates in order to release suppressed or repressed thoughts

Qualifier (4th)	Qualifier (5th)	Qualifier (6th)	Qualifier (7th)
Z None	Z None	Z None	Z None

Section G **Mental Health**
Body System Z **None**
Type H **Group Psychotherapy:** Treatment of two or more individuals with a mental health disorder by behavioral, cognitive, psychoanalytic, psychodynamic or psychophysiological means to improve functioning or well-being

Qualifier (4th)	Qualifier (5th)	Qualifier (6th)	Qualifier (7th)
Z None	Z None	Z None	Z None

Section G **Mental Health**
Body System Z **None**
Type J **Light Therapy:** Application of specialized light treatments to improve functioning or well-being

Qualifier (4th)	Qualifier (5th)	Qualifier (6th)	Qualifier (7th)
Z None	Z None	Z None	Z None

AHA Coding Clinic

No references have been issued for the Mental Health section.

Substance Abuse Treatment Section (HZ2–HZ9)

ʼithin each section of ICD-10-PCS the characters have different meanings. The seven character meanings for the Substance Abuse ·eatment section are illustrated below through the procedure example of *Substance abuse family counseling*.

Section	Body System	Root Type	Qualifier	Qualifier	Qualifier	Qualifier
Substance Abuse	None	Family Counseling	Other Family Counseling	None	None	None
H	Z	6	3	Z	Z	Z

ection (Character 1)

ll Substance Abuse Treatment procedure codes have a first character value of H.

ody System (Character 2)

he body system is not specified for substance abuse treatment; therefore, the placeholder character value of Z is reported in the second aracter position.

oot Type (Character 3)

he alphanumeric character value for root types is placed in the third position. The following are the root types applicable to the Substance buse Treatment section with their associated meaning.

Character Value	Root Type	Root Type Definition
2	Detoxification Services	Detoxification from alcohol and/or drugs
3	Individual Counseling	The application of psychological methods to treat an individual with addictive behavior
4	Group Counseling	The application of psychological methods to treat two or more individuals with addictive behavior
5	Individual Psychotherapy	Treatment of an individual with addictive behavior by behavioral, cognitive, psychoanalytic, psychodynamic or psychophysiological means
6	Family Counseling	The application of psychological methods that includes one or more family members to treat an individual with addictive behavior
8	Medication Management	Monitoring and adjusting the use of replacement medications for the treatment of addiction
9	Pharmacotherapy	The use of replacement medications for the treatment of addiction

ualifier (Character 4)

his qualifier further specifies the root type procedure. For example, the qualifier of Cognitive further specifies the type of Individual ounseling.

ualifier (Character 5)

he qualifier represents an additional attribute for the procedure when applicable. Currently, there are no qualifiers in the Substance Abuse reatment section; therefore, the placeholder character value of Z should be reported.

ualifier (Character 6)

he qualifier represents an additional attribute for the procedure when applicable. Currently, there are no qualifiers in the Substance Abuse reatment section; therefore, the placeholder character value of Z should be reported.

ualifier (Character 7)

he qualifier represents an additional attribute for the procedure when applicable. Currently, there are no qualifiers in the Substance Abuse reatment section; therefore, the placeholder character value of Z should be reported.

Substance Abuse Treatment Section Tables

Substance Abuse Treatment Tables HZ2–HZ9

Section H **Substance Abuse Treatment**
Body System Z **None**
Type 2 **Detoxification Services:** Detoxification from alcohol and/or drugs

Qualifier (4th)	Qualifier (5th)	Qualifier (6th)	Qualifier (7th)
Z None	**Z** None	**Z** None	**Z** None

Section H **Substance Abuse Treatment**
Body System Z **None**
Type 3 **Individual Counseling:** The application of psychological methods to treat an individual with addictive behavior

Qualifier (4th)	Qualifier (5th)	Qualifier (6th)	Qualifier (7th)
0 Cognitive **1** Behavioral **2** Cognitive-Behavioral **3** 12-Step **4** Interpersonal **5** Vocational **6** Psychoeducation **7** Motivational Enhancement **8** Confrontational **9** Continuing Care **B** Spiritual **C** Pre/Post-Test Infectious Disease	**Z** None	**Z** None	**Z** None

Section H **Substance Abuse Treatment**
Body System Z **None**
Type 4 **Group Counseling:** The application of psychological methods to treat two or more individuals with addictive behavior

Qualifier (4th)	Qualifier (5th)	Qualifier (6th)	Qualifier (7th)
0 Cognitive **1** Behavioral **2** Cognitive-Behavioral **3** 12-Step **4** Interpersonal **5** Vocational **6** Psychoeducation **7** Motivational Enhancement **8** Confrontational **9** Continuing Care **B** Spiritual **C** Pre/Post-Test Infectious Disease	**Z** None	**Z** None	**Z** None

ction H **Substance Abuse Treatment**
dy System Z **None**
pe 5 **Individual Psychotherapy:** Treatment of an individual with addictive behavior by behavioral, cognitive, psychoanalytic, psychodynamic or psychophysiological means

Qualifier (4th)	Qualifier (5th)	Qualifier (6th)	Qualifier (7th)
0 Cognitive 1 Behavioral 2 Cognitive-Behavioral 3 12-Step 4 Interpersonal 5 Interactive 6 Psychoeducation 7 Motivational Enhancement 8 Confrontational 9 Supportive B Psychoanalysis C Psychodynamic D Psychophysiological	**Z** None	**Z** None	**Z** None

ction H **Substance Abuse Treatment**
dy System Z **None**
pe 6 **Family Counseling:** The application of psychological methods that includes one or more family members to treat an individual with addictive behavior

Qualifier (4th)	Qualifier (5th)	Qualifier (6th)	Qualifier (7th)
3 Other Family Counseling	**Z** None	**Z** None	**Z** None

ction H **Substance Abuse Treatment**
dy System Z **None**
pe 8 **Medication Management:** Monitoring and adjusting the use of replacement medications for the treatment of addiction

Qualifier (4th)	Qualifier (5th)	Qualifier (6th)	Qualifier (7th)
0 Nicotine Replacement 1 Methadone Maintenance 2 Levo-alpha-acetyl-methadol (LAAM) 3 Antabuse 4 Naltrexone 5 Naloxone 6 Clonidine 7 Bupropion 8 Psychiatric Medication 9 Other Replacement Medication	**Z** None	**Z** None	**Z** None

ction H **Substance Abuse Treatment**
dy System Z **None**
pe 9 **Pharmacotherapy:** The use of replacement medications for the treatment of addiction

Qualifier (4th)	Qualifier (5th)	Qualifier (6th)	Qualifier (7th)
0 Nicotine Replacement 1 Methadone Maintenance 2 Levo-alpha-acetyl-methadol (LAAM) 3 Antabuse 4 Naltrexone 5 Naloxone 6 Clonidine 7 Bupropion 8 Psychiatric Medication 9 Other Replacement Medication	**Z** None	**Z** None	**Z** None

HA Coding Clinic

o references have been issued for the Substance Abuse Treatment section.

New Technology (X2A–XY0)

Within each section of ICD-10-PCS the characters have different meanings. The seven character meanings for the New Technolo section are illustrated below through the procedure example of *Introduction of ceftazidime-avibactam anti-infective into peripheral ve percutaneous approach.*

Section	Body System	Root Operation	Body Part	Approach	Device / Substance / Technology	Qualifier
New Technology	Anatomical Regions	Introduction	Peripheral Vein	Percutaneous	Ceftazidime-Avibactam Anti-infective	New Technolog Group 1
X	W	0	3	3	2	1

Section (Character 1)

All New Technology procedure codes have a first character value of X.

Body System (Character 2)

For each body system the applicable body part character values will be available for procedure code construction.

Root Operations (Character 3)

The alphanumeric character value for root operations is placed in the third position. Listed below are the root operations applicable to New Technology section with their associated meaning.

Character Value	Root Operation	Root Operation Definition
A	Assistance	Taking over a portion of a physiological function by extracorporeal means
C	Extirpation	Taking or cutting out solid matter from a body part
G	Fusion	Joining together portions of an articular body part rendering the articular body part immobile
R	Replacement	Putting in or on biological or synthetic material that physically takes the place and/or function of all o a portion of a body part
S	Reposition	Moving to its normal location, or other suitable location, all or a portion of a body part
0	Introduction	Putting in or on a therapeutic, diagnostic, nutritional, physiological, or prophylactic substance except blood or blood products
2	Monitoring	Determining the level of a physiological or physical function repetitively
5	Destruction	Physical eradication of all or a portion of a body part by the direct use of energy, force, or a destructive agent

Body Part (Character 4)

For each body system the applicable body part character values will be available for procedure code construction.

Approach (Character 5)

The approach is the technique used to reach the procedure site. Listed below are the approach character values for the New Technolo section with the associated definitions.

Character Value	Approach	Approach Definition
0	Open	Cutting through the skin or mucous membrane and any other body layers necessary to expose the site of the procedure
3	Percutaneous	Entry, by puncture or minor incision, of instrumentation through the skin or mucous membran and any other body layers necessary to reach the site of the procedure
4	Percutaneous Endoscopic	Entry, by puncture or minor incision, of instrumentation through the skin or mucous membran and any other body layers necessary to reach and visualize the site of the procedure
8	Via Natural or Artificial Opening Endoscopic	Entry of instrumentation through a natural or artificial external opening to reach and visualize the site of the procedure
X	External	Procedures performed directly on the skin or mucous membrane and procedures performed indirectly by the application of external force through the skin or mucous membrane

)evice/Substance/Technology (Character 6)

'he New Technology section created a place within ICD-10-PCS to include procedure codes for new services that utilize a specific ew device, substance, or technology. Procedures in this section may be part of the Inpatient Prospective Payment System (IPPS) new echnology add-on payment mechanism. Depending on the procedure performed there is either a device, substance, or new technology tilized.

)ualifier (Character 7)

'he qualifier represents the category year in which the new device, substance, or technology was added to the coding system. In federal iscal year 2016 (October 1, 2015) the first group of device, substance, and technology was added and therefore are labeled as New 'echnology Group 1.

New Technology Section Guidelines (section X)

). New Technology Section

;eneral Guidelines

)1. Section X codes are standalone codes. They are not supplemental codes. Section X codes fully represent the specific procedure escribed in the code title, and do not require any additional codes from other sections of ICD-10-PCS. When section X contains a code tle which describes a specific new technology procedure, only that X code is reported for the procedure. There is no need to report a roader, non-specific code in another section of ICD-10-PCS.

:xample: XW04321 Introduction of Ceftazidime-Avibactam Anti-infective into Central Vein, Percutaneous Approach, New Technology ;roup 1 can be coded to indicate that Ceftazidime-Avibactam Anti-infective was administered via a central vein. A separate code from able 3E0 in the Administration section of ICD-10-PCS is not coded in addition to this code.

New Technology Section Tables

New Technology Tables X2A–XY0

ection X **New Technology**
ody System 2 **Cardiovascular System**
peration A **Assistance:** Taking over a portion of a physiological function by extracorporeal means

Body Part (4th)	Approach (5th)	Device/Substance/Technology (6th)	Qualifier (7th)
5 Innominate Artery and Left Common Carotid Artery	3 Percutaneous	1 Cerebral Embolic Filtration, Dual Filter	2 New Technology Group 2

ection X **New Technology**
ody System 2 **Cardiovascular System**
peration C **Extirpation:** Taking or cutting out solid matter from a body part

Body Part (4th)	Approach (5th)	Device/Substance/Technology (6th)	Qualifier (7th)
0 Coronary Artery, One Artery 1 Coronary Artery, Two Arteries 2 Coronary Artery, Three Arteries 3 Coronary Artery, Four or More Arteries	3 Percutaneous	6 Orbital Atherectomy Technology	1 New Technology Group 1

ection X **New Technology**
ody System 2 **Cardiovascular System**
peration R **Replacement:** Putting in or on biological or synthetic material that physically takes the place and/or function of all or a portion of a body part

Body Part (4th)	Approach (5th)	Device/Substance/Technology (6th)	Qualifier (7th)
F Aortic Valve	0 Open 3 Percutaneous 4 Percutaneous Endoscopic	3 Zooplastic Tissue, Rapid Deployment Technique	2 New Technology Group 2

Section X **New Technology**
Body System H **Skin, Subcutaneous Tissue, Fascia and Breast**
Operation R **Replacement:** Putting in or on biological or synthetic material that physically takes the place and/or function of all or a portion of a body part

Body Part (4th)	Approach (5th)	Device/Substance/Technology (6th)	Qualifier (7th)
P Skin	**X** External	**L** Skin Substitute, Porcine Liver Derived	**2** New Technology Group 2

Section X **New Technology**
Body System K **Muscles, Tendons, Bursae and Ligaments**
Operation 0 **Introduction:** Putting in or on a therapeutic, diagnostic, nutritional, physiological, or prophylactic substance except blood or blood products

Body Part (4th)	Approach (5th)	Device/Substance/Technology (6th)	Qualifier (7th)
2 Muscle	**3** Percutaneous	**0** Concentrated Bone Marrow Aspirate	**3** New Technology Group 3

Section X **New Technology**
Body System N **Bones**
Operation S **Reposition:** Moving to its normal location, or other suitable location, all or a portion of a body part

Body Part (4th)	Approach (5th)	Device/Substance/Technology (6th)	Qualifier (7th)
0 Lumbar Vertebra **3** Cervical Vertebra **4** Thoracic Vertebra	**0** Open **3** Percutaneous	**3** Magnetically Controlled Growth Rod(s)	**2** New Technology Group 2

Section X **New Technology**
Body System R **Joints**
Operation 2 **Monitoring:** Determining the level of a physiological or physical function repetitively over a period of time

Body Part (4th)	Approach (5th)	Device/Substance/Technology (6th)	Qualifier (7th)
G Knee Joint, Right **H** Knee Joint, Left	**0** Open	**2** Intraoperative Knee Replacement Sensor	**1** New Technology Group 1

Section X **New Technology**
Body System R **Joints**
Operation G **Fusion:** Joining together portions of an articular body part rendering the articular body part immobile

Body Part (4th)	Approach (5th)	Device/Substance/Technology (6th)	Qualifier (7th)
0 Occipital-cervical Joint	**0** Open	**9** Interbody Fusion Device, Nanotextured Surface	**2** New Technology Group 2
0 Occipital-cervical Joint	**0** Open	**F** Interbody Fusion Device, Radiolucent Porous	**3** New Technology Group 3
1 Cervical Vertebral Joint	**0** Open	**9** Interbody Fusion Device, Nanotextured Surface	**2** New Technology Group 2
1 Cervical Vertebral Joint	**0** Open	**F** Interbody Fusion Device, Radiolucent Porous	**3** New Technology Group 3
2 Cervical Vertebral Joints, 2 or More	**0** Open	**9** Interbody Fusion Device, Nanotextured Surface	**2** New Technology Group 2
2 Cervical Vertebral Joints, 2 or More	**0** Open	**F** Interbody Fusion Device, Radiolucent Porous	**3** New Technology Group 3
4 Cervicothoracic Vertebral Joint	**0** Open	**9** Interbody Fusion Device, Nanotextured Surface	**2** New Technology Group 2

Continued →

ection X New Technology
ody System R Joints
peration G **Fusion:** Joining together portions of an articular body part rendering the articular body part immobile

Body Part (4th)	Approach (5th)	Device/Substance/Technology (6th)	Qualifier (7th)
4 Cervicothoracic Vertebral Joint	0 Open	F Interbody Fusion Device, Radiolucent Porous	3 New Technology Group 3
6 Thoracic Vertebral Joint	0 Open	9 Interbody Fusion Device, Nanotextured Surface	2 New Technology Group 2
6 Thoracic Vertebral Joint	0 Open	F Interbody Fusion Device, Radiolucent Porous	3 New Technology Group 3
7 Thoracic Vertebral Joints, 2 to 7	0 Open	9 Interbody Fusion Device, Nanotextured Surface	2 New Technology Group 2
7 Thoracic Vertebral Joints. 2 to 7	0 Open	F Interbody Fusion Device, Radiolucent Porous	3 New Technology Group 3
8 Thoracic Vertebral Joints, 8 or More	0 Open	9 Interbody Fusion Device, Nanotextured Surface	2 New Technology Group 2
8 Thoracic Vertebral Joints, 8 or More	0 Open	F Interbody Fusion Device, Radiolucent Porous	3 New Technology Group 3
A Thoracolumbar Vertebral Joint	0 Open	9 Interbody Fusion Device, Nanotextured Surface	2 New Technology Group 2
A Thoracolumbar Vertebral Joint	0 Open	F Interbody Fusion Device, Radiolucent Porous	3 New Technology Group 3
B Lumbar Vertebral Joint	0 Open	9 Interbody Fusion Device, Nanotextured Surface	2 New Technology Group 2
B Lumbar Vertebral Joint	0 Open	F Interbody Fusion Device, Radiolucent Porous	3 New Technology Group 3
C Lumbar Vertebral Joints, 2 or More	0 Open	9 Interbody Fusion Device, Nanotextured Surface	2 New Technology Group 2
C Lumbar Vertebral Joints, 2 or More	0 Open	F Interbody Fusion Device, Radiolucent Porous	3 New Technology Group 3
D Lumbosacral Vertebral Joint	0 Open	9 Interbody Fusion Device, Nanotextured Surface	2 New Technology Group 2
D Lumbosacral Vertebral Joint	0 Open	F Interbody Fusion Device, Radiolucent Porous	3 New Technology Group 3

ection X New Technology
ody System V Male Reproductive System
peration 5 **Destruction:** Physical eradication of all or a portion of a body part by the direct use of energy, force, or a destructive agent

Body Part (4th)	Approach (5th)	Device/Substance/Technology (6th)	Qualifier (7th)
0 Prostate	8 Via Natural or Artificial Opening Endoscopic	A Robotic Waterjet Ablation	4 New Technology Group 4

Section X **New Technology**
Body System W **Anatomical Regions**
Operation 0 **Introduction:** Putting in or on a therapeutic, diagnostic, nutritional, physiological, or prophylactic substance except bloo or blood products

Body Part (4th)	Approach (5th)	Device/Substance/Technology (6th)	Qualifier (7th)
3 Peripheral Vein	**3** Percutaneous	**2** Ceftazidime-Avibactam Anti-infective **3** Idarucizumab, Dabigatran Reversal Agent **4** Isavuconazole Anti-infective **5** Blinatumomab Antineoplastic Immunotherapy	**1** New Technology Group
3 Peripheral Vein	**3** Percutaneous	**7** Andexanet Alfa, Factor Xa Inhibitor Reversal Agent **9** Defibrotide Sodium Anticoagulant	**2** New Technology Group
3 Peripheral Vein	**3** Percutaneous	**A** Bezlotoxumab Monoclonal **B** Cytarabine and Daunorubicin Liposome Antineoplastic **C** Engineered Autologous Chimeric Antigen Receptor T-cell Immunotherapy **F** Other New Technology Therapeutic Substance	**3** New Technology Group
3 Peripheral Vein	**3** Percutaneous	**G** Plazomicin Anti-infective **H** Synthetic Human Angiotensin II	**4** New Technology Group
4 Central Vein	**3** Percutaneous	**2** Ceftazidime-Avibactam Anti-infective **3** Idarucizumab, Dabigatran Reversal Agent **4** Isavuconazole Anti-infective **5** Blinatumomab Antineoplastic Immunotherapy	**1** New Technology Group
4 Central Vein	**3** Percutaneous	**7** Andexanet Alfa, Factor Xa Inhibitor Reversal Agent **9** Defibrotide Sodium Anticoagulant	**2** New Technology Group
4 Central Vein	**3** Percutaneous	**A** Bezlotoxumab Monoclonal **B** Cytarabine and Daunorubicin Liposome Antineoplastic **C** Engineered Autologous Chimeric Antigen Receptor T-cell Immunotherapy **F** Other New Technology Therapeutic Substance	**3** New Technology Group
4 Central Vein	**3** Percutaneous	**G** Plazomicin Anti-infective **H** Synthetic Human Angiotensin II	**4** New Technology Group
D Mouth and Pharynx	**X** External	**8** Uridine Triacetate	**2** New Technology Group

Section X **New Technology**
Body System Y **Extracorporeal**
Operation 0 **Introduction: Putting in or on a therapeutic, diagnostic, nutritional, physiological, or prophylactic substance excep blood or blood products**

Body Part (4th)	Approach (5th)	Device/Substance/Technology (6th)	Qualifier (7th)
V Vein Graft	**X** External	**8** Endothelial Damage Inhibitor	**3** New Technology Group

AHA Coding Clinic

X2C0361 Extirpation of Matter from Coronary Artery, One Site Using Orbital Atherectomy Technology, Percutaneous Approach, New Technology Group 1 - AHA CC: 4Q, 2015, 13-14

XNS0032 Reposition of Lumbar Vertebra using Magnetically Controlled Growth Rod(s), Open Approach, New Technology Group 2— AHA CC: 4Q, 2017, 75

RGB0F3 Fusion of Lumbar Vertebral Joint using Radiolucent Porous Interbody Fusion Device, Open Approach, New Technology Group 3— AHA CC: 4Q, 2017, 76-77

RGD0F3 Fusion of Lumbosacral Joint using Radiolucent Porous Interbody Fusion Device, Open Approach, New Technology Group 3— AHA CC: 4Q, 2017, 76-77

W04331 Introduction of Idarucizumab, Dabigatran Reversal Agent into Central Vein, Percutaneous Approach, New Technology Group 1 - AHA CC: 4Q, 2015, 13

W04351 Introduction of Blinatumomab Antineoplastic into Central Vein, Percutaneous Approach, New Technology Group 1 - AHA CC: 4Q, 2015, 14-15

Appendix A: Root Operations Definitions

Section 0 - Medical and Surgical — Character 3 - Root Operation	
Alteration (0)	**Definition:** Modifying the anatomic structure of a body part without affecting the function of the body part **Explanation:** Principal purpose is to improve appearance **Includes/Examples:** Face lift, breast augmentation
Bypass (1)	**Definition:** Altering the route of passage of the contents of a tubular body part **Explanation:** Rerouting contents of a body part to a downstream area of the normal route, to a similar route and body part, or to an abnormal route and dissimilar body part. Includes one or more anastomoses, with or without the use of a device **Includes/Examples:** Coronary artery bypass, colostomy formation
Change (2)	**Definition:** Taking out or off a device from a body part and putting back an identical or similar device in or on the same body part without cutting or puncturing the skin or a mucous membrane **Explanation:** All CHANGE procedures are coded using the approach EXTERNAL **Includes/Examples:** Urinary catheter change, gastrostomy tube change
Control (3)	**Definition:** Stopping, or attempting to stop, postprocedural or other acute bleeding **Explanation:** The site of the bleeding is coded as an anatomical region and not to a specific body part **Includes/Examples:** Control of post-prostatectomy hemorrhage, control of intracranial subdural hemorrhage, control of bleeding duodenal ulcer, control of retroperitoneal hemorrhage
Creation (4)	**Definition:** Putting in or on biological or synthetic material to form a new body part that to the extent possible replicates the anatomic structure or function of an absent body part **Explanation:** Used for gender reassignment surgery and corrective procedures in individuals with congenital anomalies **Includes/Examples:** Creation of vagina in a male, creation of right and left atrioventricular valve from common atrioventricular valve
Destruction (5)	**Definition:** Physical eradication of all or a portion of a body part by the direct use of energy, force, or a destructive agent **Explanation:** None of the body part is physically taken out **Includes/Examples:** Fulguration of rectal polyp, cautery of skin lesion
Detachment (6)	**Definition:** Cutting off all or a portion of the upper or lower extremities **Explanation:** The body part value is the site of the detachment, with a qualifier if applicable to further specify the level where the extremity was detached **Includes/Examples:** Below knee amputation, disarticulation of shoulder
Dilation (7)	**Definition:** Expanding an orifice or the lumen of a tubular body part **Explanation:** The orifice can be a natural orifice or an artificially created orifice. Accomplished by stretching a tubular body part using intraluminal pressure or by cutting part of the orifice or wall of the tubular body part **Includes/Examples:** Percutaneous transluminal angioplasty, internal urethrotomy
Division (8)	**Definition:** Cutting into a body part, without draining fluids and/or gases from the body part, in order to separate or transect a body part **Explanation:** All or a portion of the body part is separated into two or more portions **Includes/Examples:** Spinal cordotomy, osteotomy
Drainage (9)	**Definition:** Taking or letting out fluids and/or gases from a body part **Explanation:** The qualifier DIAGNOSTIC is used to identify drainage procedures that are biopsies **Includes/Examples:** Thoracentesis, incision and drainage
Excision (B)	**Definition:** Cutting out or off, without replacement, a portion of a body part **Explanation:** The qualifier DIAGNOSTIC is used to identify excision procedures that are biopsies **Includes/Examples:** Partial nephrectomy, liver biopsy
Extirpation (C)	**Definition:** Taking or cutting out solid matter from a body part **Explanation:** The solid matter may be an abnormal byproduct of a biological function or a foreign body; it may be imbedded in a body part or in the lumen of a tubular body part. The solid matter may or may not have been previously broken into pieces **Includes/Examples:** Thrombectomy, choledocholithotomy
Extraction (D)	**Definition:** Pulling or stripping out or off all or a portion of a body part by the use of force **Explanation:** The qualifier DIAGNOSTIC is used to identify extraction procedures that are biopsies **Includes/Examples:** Dilation and curettage, vein stripping
Fragmentation (F)	**Definition:** Breaking solid matter in a body part into pieces **Explanation:** Physical force (e.g., manual, ultrasonic) applied directly or indirectly is used to break the solid matter into pieces. The solid matter may be an abnormal byproduct of a biological function or a foreign body. The pieces of solid matter are not taken out **Includes/Examples:** Extracorporeal shockwave lithotripsy, transurethral lithotripsy
Fusion (G)	**Definition:** Joining together portions of an articular body part rendering the articular body part immobile **Explanation:** The body part is joined together by fixation device, bone graft, or other means **Includes/Examples:** Spinal fusion, ankle arthrodesis
Insertion (H)	**Definition:** Putting in a nonbiological appliance that monitors, assists, performs, or prevents a physiological function but does not physically take the place of a body part **Includes/Examples:** Insertion of radioactive implant, insertion of central venous catheter

Continued →

Section 0 - Medical and Surgical — Character 3 - Root Operation

Inspection (J)	**Definition:** Visually and/or manually exploring a body part **Explanation:** Visual exploration may be performed with or without optical instrumentation. Manual exploration may be performed directly or through intervening body layers **Includes/Examples:** Diagnostic arthroscopy, exploratory laparotomy
Map (K)	**Definition:** Locating the route of passage of electrical impulses and/or locating functional areas in a body part **Explanation:** Applicable only to the cardiac conduction mechanism and the central nervous system **Includes/Examples:** Cardiac mapping, cortical mapping
Occlusion (L)	**Definition:** Completely closing an orifice or the lumen of a tubular body part **Explanation:** The orifice can be a natural orifice or an artificially created orifice **Includes/Examples:** Fallopian tube ligation, ligation of inferior vena cava
Reattachment (M)	**Definition:** Putting back in or on all or a portion of a separated body part to its normal location or other suitable location **Explanation:** Vascular circulation and nervous pathways may or may not be reestablished **Includes/Examples:** Reattachment of hand, reattachment of avulsed kidney
Release (N)	**Definition:** Freeing a body part from an abnormal physical constraint by cutting or by the use of force **Explanation:** Some of the restraining tissue may be taken out but none of the body part is taken out **Includes/Examples:** Adhesiolysis, carpal tunnel release
Removal (P)	**Definition:** Taking out or off a device from a body part **Explanation:** If a device is taken out and a similar device put in without cutting or puncturing the skin or mucous membrane, the procedure is coded to the root operation CHANGE. Otherwise, the procedure for taking out a device is coded to the root operation REMOVAL **Includes/Examples:** Drainage tube removal, cardiac pacemaker removal
Repair (Q)	**Definition:** Restoring, to the extent possible, a body part to its normal anatomic structure and function **Explanation:** Used only when the method to accomplish the repair is not one of the other root operations **Includes/Examples:** Colostomy takedown, suture of laceration
Replacement (R)	**Definition:** Putting in or on biological or synthetic material that physically takes the place and/or function of all or a portion of a body part **Explanation:** The body part may have been taken out or replaced, or may be taken out, physically eradicated, or rendered nonfunctional during the Replacement procedure. A Removal procedure is coded for taking out the device used in a previous replacement procedure **Includes/Examples:** Total hip replacement, bone graft, free skin graft
Reposition (S)	**Definition:** Moving to its normal location, or other suitable location, all or a portion of a body part **Explanation:** The body part is moved to a new location from an abnormal location, or from a normal location where it is not functioning correctly. The body part may or may not be cut out or off to be moved to the new location **Includes/Examples:** Reposition of undescended testicle, fracture reduction
Resection (T)	**Definition:** Cutting out or off, without replacement, all of a body part **Includes/Examples:** Total nephrectomy, total lobectomy of lung
Restriction (V)	**Definition:** Partially closing an orifice or the lumen of a tubular body part **Explanation:** The orifice can be a natural orifice or an artificially created orifice **Includes/Examples:** Esophagogastric fundoplication, cervical cerclage
Revision (W)	**Definition:** Correcting, to the extent possible, a portion of a malfunctioning device or the position of a displaced device **Explanation:** Revision can include correcting a malfunctioning or displaced device by taking out or putting in components of the device such as a screw or pin **Includes/Examples:** Adjustment of position of pacemaker lead, recementing of hip prosthesis
Supplement (U)	**Definition:** Putting in or on biological or synthetic material that physically reinforces and/or augments the function of a portion of a body part **Explanation:** The biological material is non-living, or is living and from the same individual. The body part may have been previously replaced, and the Supplement procedure is performed to physically reinforce and/or augment the function of the replaced body part **Includes/Examples:** Herniorrhaphy using mesh, free nerve graft, mitral valve ring annuloplasty, put a new acetabular liner in a previous hip replacement
Transfer (X)	**Definition:** Moving, without taking out, all or a portion of a body part to another location to take over the function of all or a portion of a body part **Explanation:** The body part transferred remains connected to its vascular and nervous supply **Includes/Examples:** Tendon transfer, skin pedicle flap transfer
Transplantation (Y)	**Definition:** Putting in or on all or a portion of a living body part taken from another individual or animal to physically take the place and/or function of all or a portion of a similar body part **Explanation:** The native body part may or may not be taken out, and the transplanted body part may take over all or a portion of its function **Includes/Examples:** Kidney transplant, heart transplant

Section 1 - Obstetrics — Character 3 - Root Operations Unique to Obstetrics

Abortion (A)	**Definition:** Artificially terminating a pregnancy **Explanation:** Subdivided according to whether an additional device such as a laminaria or abortifacient is used, or whether the abortion was performed by mechanical means **Includes/Example:** Transvaginal abortion using vacuum aspiration technique

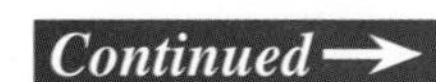
Continued →

Section 1 - Obstetrics — Character 3 - Root Operations Unique to Obstetrics	
Delivery (E)	**Definition:** Assisting the passage of the products of conception from the genital canal **Explanation:** Applies only to manually-assisted, vaginal delivery **Includes/Example:** Manually-assisted delivery

Section 2 - Placement — Character 3 - Root Operation	
Change (0)	**Definition:** Taking out or off a device from a body part and putting back an identical or similar device in or on the same body part without cutting or puncturing the skin or a mucous membrane **Includes/Example:** Change of vaginal packing
Compression (1)	**Definition:** Putting pressure on a body region **Includes/Example:** Placement of pressure dressing on abdominal wall
Dressing (2)	**Definition:** Putting material on a body region for protection **Includes/Example:** Application of sterile dressing to head wound
Immobilization (3)	**Definition:** Limiting or preventing motion of a body region **Includes/Example:** Placement of splint on left finger
Packing (4)	**Definition:** Putting material in a body region or orifice **Includes/Example:** Placement of nasal packing
Removal (5)	**Definition:** Taking out or off a device from a body part **Includes/Example:** Removal of cast from right lower leg
Traction (6)	**Definition:** Exerting a pulling force on a body region in a distal direction **Includes/Example:** Lumbar traction using motorized split-traction table

Section 3 - Administration — Character 3 - Root Operation	
Introduction (0)	**Definition:** Putting in or on a therapeutic, diagnostic, nutritional, physiological, or prophylactic substance except blood or blood products **Includes/Example:** Nerve block injection to median nerve
Irrigation (1)	**Definition:** Putting in or on a cleansing substance **Includes/Example:** Flushing of eye
Transfusion (2)	**Definition:** Putting in blood or blood products **Includes/Example:** Transfusion of cell saver red cells into central venous line

Section 4 - Measurement and Monitoring — Character 3 - Root Operation	
Measurement (0)	**Definition:** Determining the level of a physiological or physical function at a point in time **Includes/Example:** External electrocardiogram (EKG), single reading
Monitoring (1)	**Definition:** Determining the level of a physiological or physical function repetitively over a period of time **Includes/Example:** Urinary pressure monitoring

Section 5 - Extracorporeal Assistance and Performance — Character 3 - Root Operation	
Assistance (0)	**Definition:** Taking over a portion of a physiological function by extracorporeal means **Includes/Example:** Hyperbaric oxygenation of wound
Performance (1)	**Definition:** Completely taking over a physiological function by extracorporeal means **Includes/Example:** Cardiopulmonary bypass in conjunction with CABG
Restoration (2)	**Definition:** Returning, or attempting to return, a physiological function to its original state by extracorporeal means. **Includes/Example:** Attempted cardiac defibrillation, unsuccessful

Section 6 - Extracorporeal Therapies — Character 3 - Root Operation	
Atmospheric Control (0)	**Definition:** Extracorporeal control of atmospheric pressure and composition **Includes/Example:** Atmospheric control, single treatment
Decompression (1)	**Definition:** Extracorporeal elimination of undissolved gas from body fluids **Includes/Example:** Hyperbaric decompression treatment, single
Electromagnetic Therapy (2)	**Definition:** Extracorporeal treatment by electromagnetic rays **Includes/Example:** Electromagnetic therapy, central nervous, multiple treatments
Hyperthermia (3)	**Definition:** Extracorporeal raising of body temperature **Includes/Example:** Hyperthermia, single treatment

Continued →

Section 6 - Extracorporeal Therapies — Character 3 - Root Operation	
Hypothermia (4)	**Definition:** Extracorporeal lowering of body temperature **Includes/Example:** Whole body hypothermia treatment for temperature imbalances, series treatment
Perfusion (B)	**Definition:** Extracorporeal treatment by diffusion of therapeutic fluid
Pheresis (5)	**Definition:** Extracorporeal separation of blood products **Includes/Example:** Therapeutic leukopheresis, single treatment
Phototherapy (6)	**Definition:** Extracorporeal treatment by light rays **Includes/Example:** Phototherapy of circulatory system, series treatment
Shock Wave Therapy (7)	**Definition:** Extracorporeal treatment by shock waves **Includes/Example:** Shock wave therapy, musculoskeletal, single treatment
Ultrasound Therapy (8)	**Definition:** Extracorporeal treatment by ultrasound **Includes/Example:** Ultrasound therapy of the heart, single treatment
Ultraviolet Light Therapy (9)	**Definition:** Extracorporeal treatment by ultraviolet light **Includes/Example:** Ultraviolet light phototherapy, series treatment

Section 7 - Osteopathic — Character 3 - Root Operation	
Treatment (0)	**Definition:** Manual treatment to eliminate or alleviate somatic dysfunction and related disorders **Includes/Example:** Fascial release of abdomen, osteopathic treatment

Section 8 - Other Procedures — Character 3 - Root Operation	
Other Procedures (0)	**Definition:** Methodologies which attempt to remediate or cure a disorder or disease **Includes/Example:** Acupuncture

Section 9 - Chiropractic — Character 3 - Root Operation	
Manipulation (B)	**Definition:** Manual procedure that involves a directed thrust to move a joint past the physiological range of motion, without exceeding the anatomical limit **Includes/Example:** Chiropractic treatment of cervical spine, short lever specific contact

Section X - New Technology — Character 3 - Root Operation	
Assistance (A)	**Definition:** Taking over a portion of a physiological function by extracorporeal means
Destruction (5)	**Definition:** Physical eradication of all or a portion of a body part by the direct use of energy, force, or a destructive agent **Explanation:** None of the body part is physically taken out **Includes/Examples:** Fulguration of rectal polyp, cautery of skin lesion
Extirpation (C)	**Definition:** Taking or cutting out solid matter from a body part **Explanation:** The solid matter may be an abnormal by product of a biological function or a foreign body; it may be imbedded in a body part or in the lumen of a tubular body part. The solid matter may or may not have been previously broken into pieces **Includes/Example:** Thrombectomy, choledocholithotomy
Fusion (G)	**Definition:** Joining together portions of an articular body part rendering the articular body part immobile **Explanation:** The body part is joined together by fixation device, bone graft, or other means **Includes/Examples:** Spinal fusion, ankle arthrodesis
Introduction (0)	**Definition:** Putting in or on a therapeutic, diagnostic, nutritional, physiological, or prophylactic substance except blood or blood products
Monitoring (2)	**Definition:** Determining the level of a physiological or physical function repetitively over a period of time
Replacement (R)	**Definition:** Putting in or on biological or synthetic material that physically takes the place and/or function of all or a portion of a body part **Explanation:** The body part may have been taken out or replaced, or may be taken out, physically eradicated, or rendered nonfunctional during the Replacement procedure. A Removal procedure is coded for taking out the device used in a previous replacement procedure. **Includes/Examples:** Total hip replacement, bone graft, free skin graft
Reposition (S)	**Definition:** Moving to its normal location, or other suitable location, all or a portion of a body part **Explanation:** The body part is moved to a new location from an abnormal location, or from a normal location where it is not functioning correctly. The body part may or may not be cut out or off to be moved to the new location. **Includes/Examples:** Reposition of undescended testicle, fracture reduction

Appendix B: Type and Qualifier Definitions

Section B - Imaging — Character 3 - Root Type	
Computerized Tomography (CT Scan) (2)	**Definition:** Computer reformatted digital display of multiplanar images developed from the capture of multiple exposures of external ionizing radiation
Fluoroscopy (1)	**Definition:** Single plane or bi-plane real time display of an image developed from the capture of external ionizing radiation on a fluorescent screen. The image may also be stored by either digital or analog means
Magnetic Resonance Imaging (MRI) (3)	**Definition:** Computer reformatted digital display of multiplanar images developed from the capture of radiofrequency signals emitted by nuclei in a body site excited within a magnetic field
Plain Radiography (0)	**Definition:** Planar display of an image developed from the capture of external ionizing radiation on photographic or photoconductive plate
Ultrasonography (4)	**Definition:** Real time display of images of anatomy or flow information developed from the capture of reflected and attenuated high frequency sound waves

Section C - Nuclear Medicine — Character 3 - Root Type	
Nonimaging Nuclear Medicine Assay (6)	**Definition:** Introduction of radioactive materials into the body for the study of body fluids and blood elements, by the detection of radioactive emissions
Nonimaging Nuclear Medicine Probe (5)	**Definition:** Introduction of radioactive materials into the body for the study of distribution and fate of certain substances by the detection of radioactive emissions; or, alternatively, measurement of absorption of radioactive emissions from an external source
Nonimaging Nuclear Medicine Uptake (4)	**Definition:** Introduction of radioactive materials into the body for measurements of organ function, from the detection of radioactive emissions
Planar Nuclear Medicine Imaging (1)	**Definition:** Introduction of radioactive materials into the body for single plane display of images developed from the capture of radioactive emissions
Positron Emission Tomographic (PET) Imaging (3)	**Definition:** Introduction of radioactive materials into the body for three dimensional display of images developed from the simultaneous capture, 180 degrees apart, of radioactive emissions
Systemic Nuclear Medicine Therapy (7)	**Definition:** Introduction of unsealed radioactive materials into the body for treatment
Tomographic (Tomo) Nuclear Medicine Imaging (2)	**Definition:** Introduction of radioactive materials into the body for three dimensional display of images developed from the capture of radioactive emissions

Section F - Physical Rehabilitation and Diagnostic Audiology — Character 3 - Root Type	
Activities of Daily Living Assessment	**Definition:** Measurement of functional level for activities of daily living
Activities of Daily Living Treatment	**Definition:** Exercise or activities to facilitate functional competence for activities of daily living
Caregiver Training	**Definition:** Training in activities to support patient's optimal level of function
Cochlear Implant Treatment	**Definition:** Application of techniques to improve the communication abilities of individuals with cochlear implant
Device Fitting	**Definition:** Fitting of a device designed to facilitate or support achievement of a higher level of function
Hearing Aid Assessment	**Definition:** Measurement of the appropriateness and/or effectiveness of a hearing device
Hearing Assessment	**Definition:** Measurement of hearing and related functions
Hearing Treatment	**Definition:** Application of techniques to improve, augment, or compensate for hearing and related functional impairment
Motor and/or Nerve Function Assessment	**Definition:** Measurement of motor, nerve, and related functions
Motor Treatment	**Definition:** Exercise or activities to increase or facilitate motor function
Speech Assessment	**Definition:** Measurement of speech and related functions
Speech Treatment	**Definition:** Application of techniques to improve, augment, or compensate for speech and related functional impairment
Vestibular Assessment	**Definition:** Measurement of the vestibular system and related functions
Vestibular Treatment	**Definition:** Application of techniques to improve, augment, or compensate for vestibular and related functional impairment

Section F - Physical Rehabilitation and Diagnostic Audiology — Character 5 - Type Qualifier

Acoustic Reflex Decay	**Definition:** Measures reduction in size/strength of acoustic reflex over time **Includes/Examples:** Includes site of lesion test
Acoustic Reflex Patterns	**Definition:** Defines site of lesion based upon presence/absence of acoustic reflexes with ipsilateral vs. contralateral stimulation
Acoustic Reflex Threshold	**Definition:** Determines minimal intensity that acoustic reflex occurs with ipsilateral and/or contralateral stimulation
Aerobic Capacity and Endurance	**Definition:** Measures autonomic responses to positional changes; perceived exertion, dyspnea or angina during activity; performance during exercise protocols; standard vital signs; and blood gas analysis or oxygen consumption
Alternate Binaural or Monaural Loudness Balance	**Definition:** Determines auditory stimulus parameter that yields the same objective sensation **Includes/Examples:** Sound intensities that yield same loudness perception
Anthropometric Characteristics	**Definition:** Measures edema, body fat composition, height, weight, length and girth
Aphasia (Assessment)	**Definition:** Measures expressive and receptive speech and language function including reading and writing
Aphasia (Treatment)	**Definition:** Applying techniques to improve, augment, or compensate for receptive/expressive language impairments
Articulation/Phonology (Assessment)	**Definition:** Measures speech production
Articulation/Phonology (Treatment)	**Definition:** Applying techniques to correct, improve, or compensate for speech productive impairment
Assistive Listening Device	**Definition:** Assists in use of effective and appropriate assistive listening device/system
Assistive Listening System/Device Selection	**Definition:** Measures the effectiveness and appropriateness of assistive listening systems/devices
Assistive, Adaptive, Supportive or Protective Devices	**Explanation:** Devices to facilitate or support achievement of a higher level of function in wheelchair mobility; bed mobility; transfer or ambulation ability; bath and showering ability; dressing; grooming; personal hygiene; play or leisure
Auditory Evoked Potentials	**Definition:** Measures electric responses produced by the VIIIth cranial nerve and brainstem following auditory stimulation
Auditory Processing (Assessment)	**Definition:** Evaluates ability to receive and process auditory information and comprehension of spoken language
Auditory Processing (Treatment)	**Definition:** Applying techniques to improve the receiving and processing of auditory information and comprehension of spoken language
Augmentative/Alternative Communication System (Assessment)	**Definition:** Determines the appropriateness of aids, techniques, symbols, and/or strategies to augment or replace speech and enhance communication **Includes/Examples:** Includes the use of telephones, writing equipment, emergency equipment, and TDD
Augmentative/Alternative Communication System (Treatment)	**Includes/Examples:** Includes augmentative communication devices and aids
Aural Rehabilitation	**Definition:** Applying techniques to improve the communication abilities associated with hearing loss
Aural Rehabilitation Status	**Definition:** Measures impact of a hearing loss including evaluation of receptive and expressive communication skills
Bathing/Showering	**Includes/Examples:** Includes obtaining and using supplies; soaping, rinsing, and drying body parts; maintaining bathing position; and transferring to and from bathing positions
Bathing/Showering Techniques	**Definition:** Activities to facilitate obtaining and using supplies, soaping, rinsing and drying body parts, maintaining bathing position, and transferring to and from bathing positions
Bed Mobility (Assessment)	**Definition:** Transitional movement within bed
Bed Mobility (Treatment)	**Definition:** Exercise or activities to facilitate transitional movements within bed
Bedside Swallowing and Oral Function	**Includes/Examples:** Bedside swallowing includes assessment of sucking, masticating, coughing, and swallowing. Oral function includes assessment of musculature for controlled movements, structures and functions to determine coordination and phonation
Bekesy Audiometry	**Definition:** Uses an instrument that provides a choice of discrete or continuously varying pure tones; choice of pulsed or continuous signal
Binaural Electroacoustic Hearing Aid Check	**Definition:** Determines mechanical and electroacoustic function of bilateral hearing aids using hearing aid test box
Binaural Hearing Aid (Assessment)	**Definition:** Measures the candidacy, effectiveness, and appropriateness of a hearing aids **Explanation:** Measures bilateral fit

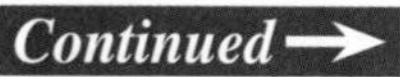
Continued →

Section F - Physical Rehabilitation and Diagnostic Audiology — Character 5 - Type Qualifier	
Binaural Hearing Aid (Treatment)	**Explanation:** Assists in achieving maximum understanding and performance
Bithermal, Binaural Caloric Irrigation	**Definition:** Measures the rhythmic eye movements stimulated by changing the temperature of the vestibular system
Bithermal, Monaural Caloric Irrigation	**Definition:** Measures the rhythmic eye movements stimulated by changing the temperature of the vestibular system in one ear
Brief Tone Stimuli	**Definition:** Measures specific central auditory process
Cerumen Management	**Definition:** Includes examination of external auditory canal and tympanic membrane and removal of cerumen from external ear canal
Cochlear Implant	**Definition:** Measures candidacy for cochlear implant
Cochlear Implant Rehabilitation	**Definition:** Applying techniques to improve the communication abilities of individuals with cochlear implant; includes programming the device, providing patients/families with information
Communicative/Cognitive Integration Skills (Assessment)	**Definition:** Measures ability to use higher cortical functions **Includes/Examples:** Includes orientation, recognition, attention span, initiation and termination of activity, memory, sequencing, categorizing, concept formation, spatial operations, judgment, problem solving, generalization and pragmatic communication
Communicative/Cognitive Integration Skills (Treatment)	**Definition:** Activities to facilitate the use of higher cortical functions **Includes/Examples:** Includes level of arousal, orientation, recognition, attention span, initiation and termination of activity, memory sequencing, judgment and problem solving, learning and generalization, and pragmatic communication
Computerized Dynamic Posturography	**Definition:** Measures the status of the peripheral and central vestibular system and the sensory/motor component of balance; evaluates the efficacy of vestibular rehabilitation
Conditioned Play Audiometry	**Definition:** Behavioral measures using nonspeech and speech stimuli to obtain frequency-specific and ear-specific information on auditory status from the patient **Explanation:** Obtains speech reception threshold by having patient point to pictures of spondaic words
Coordination/Dexterity (Assessment)	**Definition:** Measures large and small muscle groups for controlled goal-directed movements **Explanation:** Dexterity includes object manipulation
Coordination/Dexterity (Treatment)	**Definition:** Exercise or activities to facilitate gross coordination and fine coordination
Cranial Nerve Integrity	**Definition:** Measures cranial nerve sensory and motor functions, including tastes, smell and facial expression
Dichotic Stimuli	**Definition:** Measures specific central auditory process
Distorted Speech	**Definition:** Measures specific central auditory process
Dix-Hallpike Dynamic	**Definition:** Measures nystagmus following Dix-Hallpike maneuver
Dressing	**Includes/Examples:** Includes selecting clothing and accessories, obtaining clothing from storage, dressing, fastening and adjusting clothing and shoes, and applying and removing personal devices, prosthesis or orthosis
Dressing Techniques	**Definition:** Activities to facilitate selecting clothing and accessories, dressing and undressing, adjusting clothing and shoes, applying and removing devices, prostheses or orthoses
Dynamic Orthosis	**Includes/Examples:** Includes customized and prefabricated splints, inhibitory casts, spinal and other braces, and protective devices; allows motion through transfer of movement from other body parts or by use of outside forces
Ear Canal Probe Microphone	**Definition:** Real ear measures
Ear Protector Attentuation	**Definition:** Measures ear protector fit and effectiveness
Electrocochleography	**Definition:** Measures the VIIIth cranial nerve action potential
Environmental, Home and Work Barriers	**Definition:** Measures current and potential barriers to optimal function, including safety hazards, access problems and home or office design
Ergonomics and Body Mechanics	**Definition:** Ergonomic measurement of job tasks, work hardening or work conditioning needs; functional capacity; and body mechanics
Eustachian Tube Function	**Definition:** Measures eustachian tube function and patency of eustachian tube
Evoked Otoacoustic Emissions, Diagnostic	**Definition:** Measures auditory evoked potentials in a diagnostic format
Evoked Otoacoustic Emissions, Screening	**Definition:** Measures auditory evoked potentials in a screening format
Facial Nerve Function	**Definition:** Measures electrical activity of the VIIth cranial nerve (facial nerve)
Feeding/Eating (Assessment)	**Includes/Examples:** Includes setting up food, selecting and using utensils and tableware, bringing food or drink to mouth, cleaning face, hands, and clothing, and management of alternative methods of nourishment

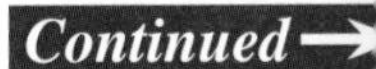

Section F - Physical Rehabilitation and Diagnostic Audiology — Character 5 - Type Qualifier

Feeding/Eating (Treatment)	**Definition:** Exercise or activities to facilitate setting up food, selecting and using utensils and tableware, bringing food or drink to mouth, cleaning face, hands, and clothing, and management of alternative methods of nourishment
Filtered Speech	**Definition:** Uses high or low pass filtered speech stimuli to assess central auditory processing disorders, site of lesion testing
Fluency (Assessment)	**Definition:** Measures speech fluency or stuttering
Fluency (Treatment)	**Definition:** Applying techniques to improve and augment fluent speech
Gait and/or Balance	**Definition:** Measures biomechanical, arthrokinematic and other spatial and temporal characteristics of gait and balance
Gait Training/Functional Ambulation	**Definition:** Exercise or activities to facilitate ambulation on a variety of surfaces and in a variety of environments
Grooming/Personal Hygiene (Assessment)	**Includes/Examples:** Includes ability to obtain and use supplies in a sequential fashion, general grooming, oral hygiene, toilet hygiene, personal care devices, including care for artificial airways
Grooming/Personal Hygiene (Treatment)	**Definition:** Activities to facilitate obtaining and using supplies in a sequential fashion: general grooming, oral hygiene, toilet hygiene, cleaning body, and personal care devices, including artificial airways
Hearing and Related Disorders Counseling	**Definition:** Provides patients/families/caregivers with information, support, referrals to facilitate recovery from a communication disorder **Includes/Examples:** Includes strategies for psychosocial adjustment to hearing loss for clients and families/caregivers
Hearing and Related Disorders Prevention	**Definition:** Provides patients/families/caregivers with information and support to prevent communication disorders
Hearing Screening	**Definition:** Pass/refer measures designed to identify need for further audiologic assessment
Home Management (Assessment)	**Definition:** Obtaining and maintaining personal and household possessions and environment **Includes/Examples:** Includes clothing care, cleaning, meal preparation and cleanup, shopping, money management, household maintenance, safety procedures, and childcare/parenting
Home Management (Treatment)	**Definition:** Activities to facilitate obtaining and maintaining personal household possessions and environment **Includes/Examples:** Includes clothing care, cleaning, meal preparation and clean-up, shopping, money management, household maintenance, safety procedures, childcare/parenting
Instrumental Swallowing and Oral Function	**Definition:** Measures swallowing function using instrumental diagnostic procedures **Explanation:** Methods include videofluoroscopy, ultrasound, manometry, endoscopy
Integumentary Integrity	**Includes/Examples:** Includes burns, skin conditions, ecchymosis, bleeding, blisters, scar tissue, wounds and other traumas, tissue mobility, turgor and texture
Manual Therapy Techniques	**Definition:** Techniques in which the therapist uses his/her hands to administer skilled movements **Includes/Examples:** Includes connective tissue massage, joint mobilization and manipulation, manual lymph drainage, manual traction, soft tissue mobilization and manipulation
Masking Patterns	**Definition:** Measures central auditory processing status
Monaural Electroacoustic Hearing Aid Check	**Definition:** Determines mechanical and electroacoustic function of one hearing aid using hearing aid test box
Monaural Hearing Aid (Assessment)	**Definition:** Measures the candidacy, effectiveness, and appropriateness of a hearing aid **Explanation:** Measures unilateral fit
Monaural Hearing Aid (Treatment)	**Explanation:** Assists in achieving maximum understanding and performance
Motor Function (Assessment)	**Definition:** Measures the body's functional and versatile movement patterns **Includes/Examples:** Includes motor assessment scales, analysis of head, trunk and limb movement, and assessment of motor learning
Motor Function (Treatment)	**Definition:** Exercise or activities to facilitate crossing midline, laterality, bilateral integration, praxis, neuromuscular relaxation, inhibition, facilitation, motor function and motor learning
Motor Speech (Assessment)	**Definition:** Measures neurological motor aspects of speech production
Motor Speech (Treatment)	**Definition:** Applying techniques to improve and augment the impaired neurological motor aspects of speech production
Muscle Performance (Assessment)	**Definition:** Measures muscle strength, power and endurance using manual testing, dynamometry or computer-assisted electromechanical muscle test; functional muscle strength, power and endurance; muscle pain, tone, or soreness; or pelvic-floor musculature **Explanation:** Muscle endurance refers to the ability to contract a muscle repeatedly over time

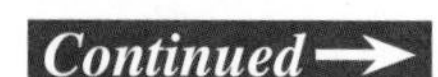

Continued →

Section F - Physical Rehabilitation and Diagnostic Audiology — Character 5 - Type Qualifier	
Muscle Performance (Treatment)	**Definition:** Exercise or activities to increase the capacity of a muscle to do work in terms of strength, power, and/or endurance **Explanation:** Muscle strength is the force exerted to overcome resistance in one maximal effort. Muscle power is work produced per unit of time, or the product of strength and speed. Muscle endurance is the ability to contract a muscle repeatedly over time
Neuromotor Development	**Definition:** Measures motor development, righting and equilibrium reactions, and reflex and equilibrium reactions
Non-invasive Instrumental Status	**Definition:** Instrumental measures of oral, nasal, vocal, and velopharyngeal functions as they pertain to speech production
Nonspoken Language (Assessment)	**Definition:** Measures nonspoken language (print, sign, symbols) for communication
Nonspoken Language (Treatment)	**Definition:** Applying techniques that improve, augment, or compensate spoken communication
Oral Peripheral Mechanism	**Definition:** Structural measures of face, jaw, lips, tongue, teeth, hard and soft palate, pharynx as related to speech production
Orofacial Myofunctional (Assessment)	**Definition:** Measures orofacial myofunctional patterns for speech and related functions
Orofacial Myofunctional (Treatment)	**Definition:** Applying techniques to improve, alter, or augment impaired orofacial myofunctional patterns and related speech production errors
Oscillating Tracking	**Definition:** Measures ability to visually track
Pain	**Definition:** Measures muscle soreness, pain and soreness with joint movement, and pain perception **Includes/Examples:** Includes questionnaires, graphs, symptom magnification scales or visual analog scales
Perceptual Processing (Assessment)	**Definition:** Measures stereognosis, kinesthesia, body schema, right-left discrimination, form constancy position in space, visual closure, figure-ground, depth perception, spatial relations and topographical orientation
Perceptual Processing (Treatment)	**Definition:** Exercise and activities to facilitate perceptual processing **Explanation:** Includes stereognosis, kinesthesia, body schema, right-left discrimination, form constancy, position in space, visual closure, figure-ground, depth perception, spatial relations, and topographical orientation **Includes/Examples:** Includes stereognosis, kinesthesia, body schema, right-left discrimination, form constancy, position in space, visual closure, figure-ground, depth perception, spatial relations, and topographical orientation
Performance Intensity Phonetically Balanced Speech Discrimination	**Definition:** Measures word recognition over varying intensity levels
Postural Control	**Definition:** Exercise or activities to increase postural alignment and control
Prosthesis	**Definition:** Artificial substitutes for missing body parts that augment performance or function **Includes/Examples:** Limb prosthesis, ocular prosthesis
Psychosocial Skills (Assessment)	**Definition:** The ability to interact in society and to process emotions **Includes/Examples:** Includes psychological (values, interests, self-concept); social (role performance, social conduct, interpersonal skills, self expression); self-management (coping skills, time management self-control)
Psychosocial Skills (Treatment)	**Definition:** The ability to interact in society and to process emotions **Includes/Examples:** Includes psychological (values, interests, self-concept); social (role performance, social conduct, interpersonal skills, self expression); self-management (coping skills, time management self-control)
Pure Tone Audiometry, Air	**Definition:** Air-conduction pure tone threshold measures with appropriate masking
Pure Tone Audiometry, Air and Bone	**Definition:** Air-conduction and bone-conduction pure tone threshold measures with appropriate masking
Pure Tone Stenger	**Definition:** Measures unilateral nonorganic hearing loss based on simultaneous presentation of pure tones of differing volume
Range of Motion and Joint Integrity	**Definition:** Measures quantity, quality, grade, and classification of joint movement and/or mobility **Explanation:** Range of Motion is the space, distance or angle through which movement occurs at a joint or series of joints. Joint integrity is the conformance of joints to expected anatomic, biomechanical and kinematic norms
Range of Motion and Joint Mobility	**Definition:** Exercise or activities to increase muscle length and joint mobility
Receptive/Expressive Language (Assessment)	**Definition:** Measures receptive and expressive language
Receptive/Expressive Language (Treatment)	**Definition:** Applying techniques to improve and augment receptive/expressive language

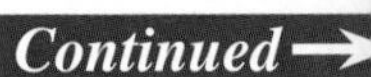

Section F - Physical Rehabilitation and Diagnostic Audiology — Character 5 - Type Qualifier

Reflex Integrity	**Definition:** Measures the presence, absence, or exaggeration of developmentally appropriate, pathologic or normal reflexes
Select Picture Audiometry	**Definition:** Establishes hearing threshold levels for speech using pictures
Sensorineural Acuity Level	**Definition:** Measures sensorineural acuity masking presented via bone conduction
Sensory Aids	**Definition:** Determines the appropriateness of a sensory prosthetic device, other than a hearing aid or assistive listening system/device
Sensory Awareness/Processing/Integrity	**Includes/Examples:** Includes light touch, pressure, temperature, pain, sharp/dull, proprioception, vestibular, visual, auditory, gustatory, and olfactory
Short Increment Sensitivity Index	**Definition:** Measures the ear's ability to detect small intensity changes; site of lesion test requiring a behavioral response
Sinusoidal Vertical Axis Rotational	**Definition:** Measures nystagmus following rotation
Somatosensory Evoked Potentials	**Definition:** Measures neural activity from sites throughout the body
Speech and/or Language Screening	**Definition:** Identifies need for further speech and/or language evaluation
Speech Threshold	**Definition:** Measures minimal intensity needed to repeat spondaic words
Speech-Language Pathology and Related Disorders Counseling	**Definition:** Provides patients/families with information, support, referrals to facilitate recovery from a communication disorder
Speech-Language Pathology and Related Disorders Prevention	**Definition:** Applying techniques to avoid or minimize onset and/or development of a communication disorder
Speech/Word Recognition	**Definition:** Measures ability to repeat/identify single syllable words; scores given as a percentage; includes word recognition/speech discrimination
Staggered Spondaic Word	**Definition:** Measures central auditory processing site of lesion based upon dichotic presentation of spondaic words
Static Orthosis	**Includes/Examples:** Includes customized and prefabricated splints, inhibitory casts, spinal and other braces, and protective devices; has no moving parts, maintains joint(s) in desired position
Stenger	**Definition:** Measures unilateral nonorganic hearing loss based on simultaneous presentation of signals of differing volume
Swallowing Dysfunction	**Definition:** Activities to improve swallowing function in coordination with respiratory function **Includes/Examples:** Includes function and coordination of sucking, mastication, coughing, swallowing
Synthetic Sentence Identification	**Definition:** Measures central auditory dysfunction using identification of third order approximations of sentences and competing messages
Temporal Ordering of Stimuli	**Definition:** Measures specific central auditory process
Therapeutic Exercise	**Definition:** Exercise or activities to facilitate sensory awareness, sensory processing, sensory integration, balance training, conditioning, reconditioning **Includes/Examples:** Includes developmental activities, breathing exercises, aerobic endurance activities, aquatic exercises, stretching and ventilatory muscle training
Tinnitus Masker (Assessment)	**Definition:** Determines candidacy for tinnitus masker
Tinnitus Masker (Treatment)	**Explanation:** Used to verify physical fit, acoustic appropriateness, and benefit; assists in achieving maximum benefit
Tone Decay	**Definition:** Measures decrease in hearing sensitivity to a tone; site of lesion test requiring a behavioral response
Transfer	**Definition:** Transitional movement from one surface to another
Transfer Training	**Definition:** Exercise or activities to facilitate movement from one surface to another
Tympanometry	**Definition:** Measures the integrity of the middle ear; measures ease at which sound flows through the tympanic membrane while air pressure against the membrane is varied
Unithermal Binaural Screen	**Definition:** Measures the rhythmic eye movements stimulated by changing the temperature of the vestibular system in both ears using warm water, screening format
Ventilation, Respiration and Circulation	**Definition:** Measures ventilatory muscle strength, power and endurance, pulmonary function and ventilatory mechanics **Includes/Examples:** Includes ability to clear airway, activities that aggravate or relieve edema, pain, dyspnea or other symptoms, chest wall mobility, cardiopulmonary response to performance of ADL and IAD, cough and sputum, standard vital signs
Vestibular	**Definition:** Applying techniques to compensate for balance disorders; includes habituation, exercise therapy, and balance retraining

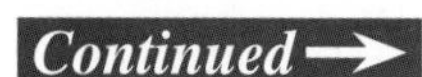
Continued →

Section F - Physical Rehabilitation and Diagnostic Audiology — Character 5 - Type Qualifier

Visual Motor Integration (Assessment)	**Definition:** Coordinating the interaction of information from the eyes with body movement during activit
Visual Motor Integration (Treatment)	**Definition:** Exercise or activities to facilitate coordinating the interaction of information from eyes wit body movement during activity
Visual Reinforcement Audiometry	**Definition:** Behavioral measures using nonspeech and speech stimuli to obtain frequency/ear-specific information on auditory status **Includes/Examples:** Includes a conditioned response of looking toward a visual reinforcer (e.g., lights animated toy) every time auditory stimuli are heard
Vocational Activities and Functional Community or Work Reintegration Skills (Assessment)	**Definition:** Measures environmental, home, work (job/school/play) barriers that keep patients from functioning optimally in their environment **Includes/Examples:** Includes assessment of vocational skill and interests, environment of work (job/school/play), injury potential and injury prevention or reduction, ergonomic stressors, transportation skills, and ability to access and use community resources
Vocational Activities and Functional Community or Work Reintegration Skills (Treatment)	**Definition:** Activities to facilitate vocational exploration, body mechanics training, job acquisition, anc environmental or work (job/school/play) task adaptation **Includes/Examples:** Includes injury prevention and reduction, ergonomic stressor reduction, job coaching and simulation, work hardening and conditioning, driving training, transportation skills, and use of community resources
Voice (Assessment)	**Definition:** Measures vocal structure, function and production
Voice (Treatment)	**Definition:** Applying techniques to improve voice and vocal function
Voice Prosthetic (Assessment)	**Definition:** Determines the appropriateness of voice prosthetic/adaptive device to enhance or facilitate communication
Voice Prosthetic (Treatment)	**Includes/Examples:** Includes electrolarynx, and other assistive, adaptive, supportive devices
Wheelchair Mobility (Assessment)	**Definition:** Measures fit and functional abilities within wheelchair in a variety of environments
Wheelchair Mobility (Treatment)	**Definition:** Management, maintenance and controlled operation of a wheelchair, scooter or other device, in and on a variety of surfaces and environments
Wound Management	**Includes/Examples:** Includes non-selective and selective debridement (enzymes, autolysis, sharp debridement), dressings (wound coverings, hydrogel, vacuum-assisted closure), topical agents, etc.

Section G - Mental Health — Character 3 - Root Type

Biofeedback	**Definition:** Provision of information from the monitoring and regulating of physiological processes in conjunction with cognitive-behavioral techniques to improve patient functioning or well-being **Includes/Examples:** Includes EEG, blood pressure, skin temperature or peripheral blood flow, ECG, electrooculogram, EMG, respirometry or capnometry, GSR/EDR, perineometry to monitor/regulate bowel/bladder activity, electrogastrogram to monitor/regulate gastric motility
Counseling	**Definition:** The application of psychological methods to treat an individual with normal developmental issues and psychological problems in order to increase function, improve well-being, alleviate distress, maladjustment or resolve crises
Crisis Intervention	**Definition:** Treatment of a traumatized, acutely disturbed or distressed individual for the purpose of short-term stabilization **Includes/Examples:** Includes defusing, debriefing, counseling, psychotherapy and/or coordination of care with other providers or agencies
Electroconvulsive Therapy	**Definition:** The application of controlled electrical voltages to treat a mental health disorder **Includes/Examples:** Includes appropriate sedation and other preparation of the individual
Family Psychotherapy	**Definition:** Treatment that includes one or more family members of an individual with a mental health disorder by behavioral, cognitive, psychoanalytic, psychodynamic or psychophysiological means to improv functioning or well-being **Explanation:** Remediation of emotional or behavioral problems presented by one or more family members in cases where psychotherapy with more than one family member is indicated
Group Psychotherapy	**Definition:** Treatment of two or more individuals with a mental health disorder by behavioral, cognitive, psychoanalytic, psychodynamic or psychophysiological means to improve functioning or well-being
Hypnosis	**Definition:** Induction of a state of heightened suggestibility by auditory, visual and tactile techniques to elicit an emotional or behavioral response
Individual Psychotherapy	**Definition:** Treatment of an individual with a mental health disorder by behavioral, cognitive, psychoanalytic, psychodynamic or psychophysiological means to improve functioning or well-being
Light Therapy	**Definition:** Application of specialized light treatments to improve functioning or well-being

Continued →

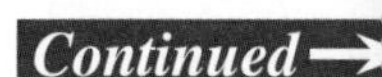

Section G - Mental Health — Character 3 - Root Type	
Medication Management	**Definition:** Monitoring and adjusting the use of medications for the treatment of a mental health disorder
Narcosynthesis	**Definition:** Administration of intravenous barbiturates in order to release suppressed or repressed thoughts
Psychological Tests	**Definition:** The administration and interpretation of standardized psychological tests and measurement instruments for the assessment of psychological function

Section G - Mental Health — Character 4 - Type Qualifier	
Behavioral	**Definition:** Primarily to modify behavior **Includes/Examples:** Includes modeling and role playing, positive reinforcement of target behaviors, response cost, and training of self-management skills
Cognitive	**Definition:** Primarily to correct cognitive distortions and errors
Cognitive-Behavioral	**Definition:** Combining cognitive and behavioral treatment strategies to improve functioning **Explanation:** Maladaptive responses are examined to determine how cognitions relate to behavior patterns in response to an event. Uses learning principles and information-processing models
Developmental	**Definition:** Age-normed developmental status of cognitive, social and adaptive behavior skills
Intellectual and Psychoeducational	**Definition:** Intellectual abilities, academic achievement and learning capabilities (including behaviors and emotional factors affecting learning)
Interactive	**Definition:** Uses primarily physical aids and other forms of non-oral interaction with a patient who is physically, psychologically or developmentally unable to use ordinary language for communication **Includes/Examples:** Includes the use of toys in symbolic play
Interpersonal	**Definition:** Helps an individual make changes in interpersonal behaviors to reduce psychological dysfunction **Includes/Examples:** Includes exploratory techniques, encouragement of affective expression, clarification of patient statements, analysis of communication patterns, use of therapy relationship and behavior change techniques
Neurobehavioral and Cognitive Status	**Definition:** Includes neurobehavioral status exam, interview(s), and observation for the clinical assessment of thinking, reasoning and judgment, acquired knowledge, attention, memory, visual spatial abilities, language functions, and planning
Neuropsychological	**Definition:** Thinking, reasoning and judgment, acquired knowledge, attention, memory, visual spatial abilities, language functions, planning
Personality and Behavioral	**Definition:** Mood, emotion, behavior, social functioning, psychopathological conditions, personality traits and characteristics
Psychoanalysis	**Definition:** Methods of obtaining a detailed account of past and present mental and emotional experiences to determine the source and eliminate or diminish the undesirable effects of unconscious conflicts **Explanation:** Accomplished by making the individual aware of their existence, origin, and inappropriate expression in emotions and behavior
Psychodynamic	**Definition:** Exploration of past and present emotional experiences to understand motives and drives using insight-oriented techniques to reduce the undesirable effects of internal conflicts on emotions and behavior **Explanation:** Techniques include empathetic listening, clarifying self-defeating behavior patterns, and exploring adaptive alternatives
Psychophysiological	**Definition:** Monitoring and alteration of physiological processes to help the individual associate physiological reactions combined with cognitive and behavioral strategies to gain improved control of these processes to help the individual cope more effectively
Supportive	**Definition:** Formation of therapeutic relationship primarily for providing emotional support to prevent further deterioration in functioning during periods of particular stress **Explanation:** Often used in conjunction with other therapeutic approaches
Vocational	**Definition:** Exploration of vocational interests, aptitudes and required adaptive behavior skills to develop and carry out a plan for achieving a successful vocational placement **Includes/Examples:** Includes enhancing work related adjustment and/or pursuing viable options in training education or preparation

Section H - Substance Abuse Treatment — Character 3 - Root Type	
Detoxification Services	**Definition:** Detoxification from alcohol and/or drugs **Explanation:** Not a treatment modality, but helps the patient stabilize physically and psychologically until the body becomes free of drugs and the effects of alcohol
Family Counseling	**Definition:** The application of psychological methods that includes one or more family members to treat an individual with addictive behavior **Explanation:** Provides support and education for family members of addicted individuals. Family member participation is seen as a critical area of substance abuse treatment

Continued →

Section H - Substance Abuse Treatment — Character 3 - Root Type	
Group Counseling	**Definition:** The application of psychological methods to treat two or more individuals with addictive behavi **Explanation:** Provides structured group counseling sessions and healing power through the connection wi others
Individual Counseling	**Definition:** The application of psychological methods to treat an individual with addictive behavior **Explanation:** Comprised of several different techniques, which apply various strategies to address drug addiction
Individual Psychotherapy	**Definition:** Treatment of an individual with addictive behavior by behavioral, cognitive, psychoanalytic, psychodynamic or psychophysiological means
Medication Management	**Definition:** Monitoring and adjusting the use of replacement medications for the treatment of addiction
Pharmacotherapy	**Definition:** The use of replacement medications for the treatment of addiction

Appendix C: Approach Definitions

Section 0 - Medical and Surgical — Character 5 - Approach	
External (X)	**Definition:** Procedures performed directly on the skin or mucous membrane and procedures performed indirectly by the application of external force through the skin or mucous membrane
Open (0)	**Definition:** Cutting through the skin or mucous membrane and any other body layers necessary to expose the site of the procedure
Percutaneous (3)	**Definition:** Entry, by puncture or minor incision, of instrumentation through the skin or mucous membrane and any other body layers necessary to reach the site of the procedure
Percutaneous Endoscopic (4)	**Definition:** Entry, by puncture or minor incision, of instrumentation through the skin or mucous membrane and any other body layers necessary to reach and visualize the site of the procedure
Via Natural or Artificial Opening (7)	**Definition:** Entry of instrumentation through a natural or artificial external opening to reach the site of the procedure
Via Natural or Artificial Opening Endoscopic (8)	**Definition:** Entry of instrumentation through a natural or artificial external opening to reach and visualize the site of the procedure
Via Natural or Artificial Opening With Percutaneous Endoscopic Assistance (F)	**Definition:** Entry of instrumentation through a natural or artificial external opening and entry, by puncture or minor incision, of instrumentation through the skin or mucous membrane and any other body layers necessary to aid in the performance of the procedure

Section 1 - Obstetrics — Character 5 - Approach	
External (X)	**Definition:** Procedures performed directly on the skin or mucous membrane and procedures performed indirectly by the application of external force through the skin or mucous membrane
Open (0)	**Definition:** Cutting through the skin or mucous membrane and any other body layers necessary to expose the site of the procedure
Percutaneous (3)	**Definition:** Entry, by puncture or minor incision, of instrumentation through the skin or mucous membrane and any other body layers necessary to reach the site of the procedure
Percutaneous Endoscopic (4)	**Definition:** Entry, by puncture or minor incision, of instrumentation through the skin or mucous membrane and any other body layers necessary to reach and visualize the site of the procedure
Via Natural or Artificial Opening (7)	**Definition:** Entry of instrumentation through a natural or artificial external opening to reach the site of the procedur
Via Natural or Artificial Opening Endoscopic (8)	**Definition:** Entry of instrumentation through a natural or artificial external opening to reach and visualize the site of the procedure

Section 2 - Placement — Character 5 - Approach	
External (X)	**Definition:** Procedures performed directly on the skin or mucous membrane and procedures performed indirectly by the application of external force through the skin or mucous membrane

Section 3 - Administration — Character 5 - Approach	
External (X)	**Definition:** Procedures performed directly on the skin or mucous membrane and procedures performed indirectly by the application of external force through the skin or mucous membrane
Open (0)	**Definition:** Cutting through the skin or mucous membrane and any other body layers necessary to expose the site of the procedure

Continued →

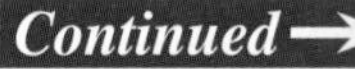

Section 3 - Administration — Character 5 - Approach	
Percutaneous (3)	**Definition:** Entry, by puncture or minor incision, of instrumentation through the skin or mucous membrane and any other body layers necessary to reach the site of the procedure
Percutaneous Endoscopic (4)	**Definition:** Entry, by puncture or minor incision, of instrumentation through the skin or mucous membrane and any other body layers necessary to reach and visualize the site of the procedure
Via Natural or Artificial Opening (7)	**Definition:** Entry of instrumentation through a natural or artificial external opening to reach the site of the procedure
Via Natural or Artificial Opening Endoscopic (8)	**Definition:** Entry of instrumentation through a natural or artificial external opening to reach and visualize the site of the procedure

Section 4 - Measurement and Monitoring — Character 5 - Approach	
External (X)	**Definition:** Procedures performed directly on the skin or mucous membrane and procedures performed indirectly by the application of external force through the skin or mucous membrane
Open (0)	**Definition:** Cutting through the skin or mucous membrane and any other body layers necessary to expose the site of the procedure
Percutaneous (3)	**Definition:** Entry, by puncture or minor incision, of instrumentation through the skin or mucous membrane and any other body layers necessary to reach the site of the procedure
Percutaneous Endoscopic (4)	**Definition:** Entry, by puncture or minor incision, of instrumentation through the skin or mucous membrane and any other body layers necessary to reach and visualize the site of the procedure
Via Natural or Artificial Opening (7)	**Definition:** Entry of instrumentation through a natural or artificial external opening to reach the site of the procedure
Via Natural or Artificial Opening Endoscopic (8)	**Definition:** Entry of instrumentation through a natural or artificial external opening to reach and visualize the site of the procedure

Section 7 - Osteopathic — Character 5 - Approach	
External (X)	**Definition:** Procedures performed directly on the skin or mucous membrane and procedures performed indirectly by the application of external force through the skin or mucous membrane

Section 8 - Other Procedures — Character 5 - Approach	
External (X)	**Definition:** Procedures performed directly on the skin or mucous membrane and procedures performed indirectly by the application of external force through the skin or mucous membrane
Open (0)	**Definition:** Cutting through the skin or mucous membrane and any other body layers necessary to expose the site of the procedure
Percutaneous (3)	**Definition:** Entry, by puncture or minor incision, of instrumentation through the skin or mucous membrane and any other body layers necessary to reach the site of the procedure
Percutaneous Endoscopic (4)	**Definition:** Entry, by puncture or minor incision, of instrumentation through the skin or mucous membrane and any other body layers necessary to reach and visualize the site of the procedure
Via Natural or Artificial Opening (7)	**Definition:** Entry of instrumentation through a natural or artificial external opening to reach the site of the procedure
Via Natural or Artificial Opening Endoscopic (8)	**Definition:** Entry of instrumentation through a natural or artificial external opening to reach and visualize the site of the procedure

Section 9 - Chiropractic — Character 5 - Approach	
External (X)	**Definition:** Procedures performed directly on the skin or mucous membrane and procedures performed indirectly by the application of external force through the skin or mucous membrane

Section X - New Technology — Character 5 - Approach	
External (X)	**Definition:** Procedures performed directly on the skin or mucous membrane and procedures performed indirectly by the application of external force through the skin or mucous membrane
Open (0)	**Definition:** Cutting through the skin or mucous membrane and any other body layers necessary to expose the site of the procedure
Percutaneous (3)	**Definition:** Entry, by puncture or minor incision, of instrumentation through the skin or mucous membrane and any other body layers necessary to reach the site of the procedure
Percutaneous Endoscopic (4)	**Definition:** Entry, by puncture or minor incision, of instrumentation through the skin or mucous membrane and any other body layers necessary to reach and visualize the site of the procedure
Via Natural or Artificial Opening Endoscopic (8)	**Definition:** Entry of instrumentation through a natural or artificial external opening to reach and visualize the site of the procedure

Appendix D: Medical and Surgical Body Parts

Appendices D–F are structured to assist coders with confirming character selections within the Tables. For example, if the coder is considering the body part of Abdomen Muscle, appendix D can be referenced to identify all of the muscles that are included in the body part Abdomen Muscle (see row 2 in the table below). After reviewing the information, the coder can determine if the body part under consideration is correct or if another body part should be reviewed. The same process can be followed for devices which are included in appendix E and substances which are included in appendix F.

Section 0 - Medical and Surgical — Character 4 - Body Part	
1st Toe, Left **1st** Toe, Right	**Includes:** Hallux
Abdomen Muscle, Left **Abdomen** Muscle, Right	**Includes:** External oblique muscle Internal oblique muscle Pyramidalis muscle Rectus abdominis muscle Transversus abdominis muscle
Abdominal Aorta	**Includes:** Inferior phrenic artery Lumbar artery Median sacral artery Middle suprarenal artery Ovarian artery Testicular artery
Abdominal Sympathetic Nerve	**Includes:** **Abdominal** aortic plexus Auerbach's (myenteric) plexus Celiac (solar) plexus Celiac ganglion Gastric plexus Hepatic plexus Inferior hypogastric plexus Inferior mesenteric ganglion Inferior mesenteric plexus Meissner's (submucous) plexus Myenteric (Auerbach's) plexus Pancreatic plexus Pelvic splanchnic nerve Renal plexus Solar (celiac) plexus Splenic plexus Submucous (Meissner's) plexus Superior hypogastric plexus Superior mesenteric ganglion Superior mesenteric plexus Suprarenal plexus
Abducens Nerve	**Includes:** Sixth cranial nerve
Accessory Nerve	**Includes:** Eleventh cranial nerve
Acoustic Nerve	**Includes:** Cochlear nerve Eighth cranial nerve Scarpa's (vestibular) ganglion Spiral ganglion Vestibular (Scarpa's) ganglion Vestibular nerve Vestibulocochlear nerve
Adenoids	**Includes:** Pharyngeal tonsil

Section 0 - Medical and Surgical — Character 4 - Body Part	
Adrenal Gland **Adrenal** Gland, Left **Adrenal** Gland, Right **Adrenal** Glands, Bilateral	**Includes:** Suprarenal gland
Ampulla of Vater	**Includes:** Duodenal ampulla Hepatopancreatic ampulla
Anal Sphincter	**Includes:** External anal sphincter Internal anal sphincter
Ankle Bursa and Ligament, Left **Ankle** Bursa and Ligament, Right	**Includes:** Calcaneofibular ligament Deltoid ligament Ligament of the lateral malleolus Talofibular ligament
Ankle Joint, Left **Ankle** Joint, Right	**Includes:** Inferior tibiofibular joint Talocrural joint
Anterior Chamber, Left **Anterior** Chamber, Right	**Includes:** Aqueous humour
Anterior Tibial Artery, Left **Anterior** Tibial Artery, Right	**Includes:** Anterior lateral malleolar artery Anterior medial malleolar artery Anterior tibial recurrent artery Dorsalis pedis artery Posterior tibial recurrent artery
Anus	**Includes:** Anal orifice
Aortic Valve	**Includes:** Aortic annulus
Appendix	**Includes:** Vermiform appendix
Atrial Septum	**Includes:** Interatrial septum
Atrium, Left	**Includes:** Atrium pulmonale Left auricular appendix
Atrium, Right	**Includes:** Atrium dextrum cordis Right auricular appendix Sinus venosus
Auditory Ossicle, Left **Auditory** Ossicle, Right	**Includes:** Incus Malleus Stapes

Continued →

Section 0 - Medical and Surgical — Character 4 - Body Part	
Axillary Artery, Left **Axillary** Artery, Right	**Includes:** Anterior circumflex humeral artery Lateral thoracic artery Posterior circumflex humeral artery Subscapular artery Superior thoracic artery Thoracoacromial artery
Azygos Vein	**Includes:** Right ascending lumbar vein Right subcostal vein
Basal Ganglia	**Includes:** Basal nuclei Claustrum Corpus striatum Globus pallidus Substantia nigra Subthalamic nucleus
Basilic Vein, Left **Basilic** Vein, Right	**Includes:** Median antebrachial vein Median cubital vein
Bladder	**Includes:** Trigone of bladder
Brachial Artery, Left **Brachial** Artery, Right	**Includes:** Inferior ulnar collateral artery Profunda brachii Superior ulnar collateral artery
Brachial Plexus	**Includes:** Axillary nerve Dorsal scapular nerve First intercostal nerve Long thoracic nerve Musculocutaneous nerve Subclavius nerve Suprascapular nerve
Brachial Vein, Left **Brachial** Vein, Right	**Includes:** Radial vein Ulnar vein
Brain	**Includes:** Cerebrum Corpus callosum Encephalon
Breast, Bilateral **Breast,** Left **Breast,** Right	**Includes:** Mammary duct Mammary gland
Buccal Mucosa	**Includes:** Buccal gland Molar gland Palatine gland
Carotid Bodies, Bilateral **Carotid** Body, Left **Carotid** Body, Right	**Includes:** Carotid glomus
Carpal Joint, Left **Carpal** Joint, Right	**Includes:** Intercarpal joint Midcarpal joint

Section 0 - Medical and Surgical — Character 4 - Body Part	
Carpal, Left **Carpal,** Right	**Includes:** Capitate bone Hamate bone Lunate bone Pisiform bone Scaphoid bone Trapezium bone Trapezoid bone Triquetral bone
Celiac Artery	**Includes:** Celiac trunk
Cephalic Vein, Left **Cephalic** Vein, Right	**Includes:** Accessory cephalic vein
Cerebellum	**Includes:** Culmen
Cerebral Hemisphere	**Includes:** Frontal lobe Occipital lobe Parietal lobe Temporal lobe
Cerebral Meninges	**Includes:** Arachnoid mater, intracranial Leptomeninges, intracranial Pia mater, intracranial
Cerebral Ventricle	**Includes:** Aqueduct of Sylvius Cerebral aqueduct (Sylvius) Choroid plexus Ependyma Foramen of Monro (intraventricular) Fourth ventricle Interventricular foramen (Monro) Left lateral ventricle Right lateral ventricle Third ventricle
Cervical Nerve	**Includes:** Greater occipital nerve Spinal nerve, cervical Suboccipital nerve Third occipital nerve
Cervical Plexus	**Includes:** Ansa cervicalis Cutaneous (transverse) cervical nerve Great auricular nerve Lesser occipital nerve Supraclavicular nerve Transverse (cutaneous) cervical nerve
Cervical Vertebra	**Includes:** Dens Odontoid process Spinous process Transverse foramen Transverse process Vertebral arch Vertebral body Vertebral foramen Vertebral lamina Vertebral pedicle

Continued →

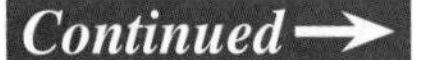

Section 0 - Medical and Surgical — Character 4 - Body Part	
Cervical Vertebral Joint	**Includes:** Atlantoaxial joint Cervical facet joint
Cervical Vertebral Joints, 2 or more	**Includes:** Cervical facet joint
Cervicothoracic Vertebral Joint	**Includes:** Cervicothoracic facet joint
Cisterna Chyli	**Includes:** Intestinal lymphatic trunk Lumbar lymphatic trunk
Coccygeal Glomus	**Includes:** Coccygeal body
Colic Vein	**Includes:** Ileocolic vein Left colic vein Middle colic vein Right colic vein
Conduction Mechanism	**Includes:** Atrioventricular node Bundle of His Bundle of Kent Sinoatrial node
Conjunctiva, Left **Conjunctiva,** Right	**Includes:** Plica semilunaris
Dura Mater	**Includes:** Diaphragma sellae Dura mater, intracranial Falx cerebri Tentorium cerebelli
Elbow Bursa and Ligament, Left **Elbow** Bursa and Ligament, Right	**Includes:** Annular ligament Olecranon bursa Radial collateral ligament Ulnar collateral ligament
Elbow Joint, Left **Elbow** Joint, Right	**Includes:** Distal humerus, involving joint Humeroradial joint Humeroulnar joint Proximal radioulnar joint
Epidural Space, Intracranial	**Includes:** Extradural space, intracranial
Epiglottis	**Includes:** Glossoepiglottic fold
Esophagogastric Junction	**Includes:** Cardia Cardioesophageal junction Gastroesophageal (GE) junction
Esophagus, Lower	**Includes:** Abdominal esophagus
Esophagus, Middle	**Includes:** Thoracic esophagus
Esophagus, Upper	**Includes:** Cervical esophagus
Ethmoid Bone, Left **Ethmoid** Bone, Right	**Includes:** Cribriform plate
Ethmoid Sinus, Left **Ethmoid** Sinus, Right	**Includes:** Ethmoidal air cell

Section 0 - Medical and Surgical — Character 4 - Body Part	
Eustachian Tube, Left **Eustachian** Tube, Right	**Includes:** Auditory tube Pharyngotympanic tube
External Auditory Canal, Left **External** Auditory Canal, Right	**Includes:** External auditory meatus
External Carotid Artery, Left **External** Carotid Artery, Right	**Includes:** Ascending pharyngeal artery Internal maxillary artery Lingual artery Maxillary artery Occipital artery Posterior auricular artery Superior thyroid artery
External Ear, Bilateral **External** Ear, Left **External** Ear, Right	**Includes:** Antihelix Antitragus Auricle Earlobe Helix Pinna Tragus
External Iliac Artery, Left **External** Iliac Artery, Right	**Includes:** Deep circumflex iliac artery Inferior epigastric artery
External Jugular Vein, Left **External** Jugular Vein, Right	**Includes:** Posterior auricular vein
Extraocular Muscle, Left **Extraocular** Muscle, Right	**Includes:** Inferior oblique muscle Inferior rectus muscle Lateral rectus muscle Medial rectus muscle Superior oblique muscle Superior rectus muscle
Eye, Left **Eye,** Right	**Includes:** Ciliary body Posterior chamber
Face Artery	**Includes:** Angular artery Ascending palatine artery External maxillary artery Facial artery Inferior labial artery Submental artery Superior labial artery
Face Vein, Left **Face** Vein, Right	**Includes:** Angular vein Anterior facial vein Common facial vein Deep facial vein Frontal vein Posterior facial (retromandibular) vein Supraorbital vein
Facial Muscle	**Includes:** Buccinator muscle Corrugator supercilii muscle Depressor anguli oris muscle Depressor labii inferioris muscle

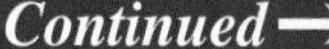
Continued

Section 0 - Medical and Surgical — Character 4 - Body Part	
	Depressor septi nasi muscle Depressor supercilii muscle Levator anguli oris muscle Levator labii superioris alaeque nasi Levator labii superioris alaeque nasi Levator labii superioris alaeque nasi Levator labii superioris muscle Mentalis muscle Nasalis muscle Occipitofrontalis muscle Orbicularis oris muscle Procerus muscle Risorius muscle Zygomaticus muscle
Facial Nerve	**Includes:** Chorda tympani Geniculate ganglion Greater superficial petrosal nerve Nerve to the stapedius Parotid plexus Posterior auricular nerve Seventh cranial nerve Submandibular ganglion
Fallopian Tube, Left **Fallopian** Tube, Right	**Includes:** Oviduct Salpinx Uterine tube
Femoral Artery, Left **Femoral** Artery, Right	**Includes:** Circumflex iliac artery Deep femoral artery Descending genicular artery External pudendal artery Superficial epigastric artery
Femoral Nerve	**Includes:** Anterior crural nerve Saphenous nerve
Femoral Shaft, Left **Femoral** Shaft, Right	**Includes:** Body of femur
Femoral Vein, Left **Femoral** Vein, Right	**Includes:** Deep femoral (profunda femoris) vein Popliteal vein Profunda femoris (deep femoral) vein
Fibula, Left **Fibula,** Right	**Includes:** Body of fibula Head of fibula Lateral malleolus
Finger Nail	**Includes:** Nail bed Nail plate
Finger Phalangeal Joint, Left **Finger** Phalangeal Joint, Right	**Includes:** Interphalangeal (IP) joint
Foot Artery, Left **Foot** Artery, Right	**Includes:** Arcuate artery Dorsal metatarsal artery Lateral plantar artery Lateral tarsal artery Medial plantar artery

Section 0 - Medical and Surgical — Character 4 - Body Part	
Foot Bursa and Ligament, Left **Foot** Bursa and Ligament, Right	**Includes:** Calcaneocuboid ligament Cuneonavicular ligament Intercuneiform ligament Interphalangeal ligament Metatarsal ligament Metatarsophalangeal ligament Subtalar ligament Talocalcaneal ligament Talocalcaneonavicular ligament Tarsometatarsal ligament
Foot Muscle, Left **Foot** Muscle, Right	**Includes:** Abductor hallucis muscle Adductor hallucis muscle Extensor digitorum brevis muscle Extensor hallucis brevis muscle Flexor digitorum brevis muscle Flexor hallucis brevis muscle Quadratus plantae muscle
Foot Vein, Left **Foot** Vein, Right	**Includes:** Common digital vein Dorsal metatarsal vein Dorsal venous arch Plantar digital vein Plantar metatarsal vein Plantar venous arch
Frontal Bone	**Includes:** Zygomatic process of frontal bone
Gastric Artery	**Includes:** Left gastric artery Right gastric artery
Glenoid Cavity, Left **Glenoid** Cavity, Right	**Includes:** Glenoid fossa (of scapula)
Glomus Jugulare	**Includes:** Jugular body
Glossopharyngeal Nerve	**Includes:** Carotid sinus nerve Ninth cranial nerve Tympanic nerve
Hand Artery, Left **Hand** Artery, Right	**Includes:** Deep palmar arch Princeps pollicis artery Radialis indicis Superficial palmar arch
Hand Bursa and Ligament, Left **Hand** Bursa and Ligament, Right	**Includes:** Carpometacarpal ligament Intercarpal ligament Interphalangeal ligament Lunotriquetral ligament Metacarpal ligament Metacarpophalangeal ligament Pisohamate ligament Pisometacarpal ligament Scapholunate ligament Scaphotrapezium ligament
Hand Muscle, Left **Hand** Muscle, Right	**Includes:** Hypothenar muscle Palmar interosseous muscle Thenar muscle

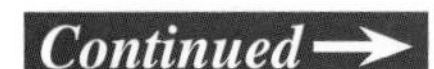

Section 0 - Medical and Surgical — Character 4 - Body Part	
Hand Vein, Left **Hand** Vein, Right	**Includes:** Dorsal metacarpal vein Palmar (volar) digital vein Palmar (volar) metacarpal vein Superficial palmar venous arch Volar (palmar) digital vein Volar (palmar) metacarpal vein
Head and Neck Bursa and Ligament	**Includes:** Alar ligament of axis Cervical interspinous ligament Cervical intertransverse ligament Cervical ligamentum flavum Interspinous ligament cervical Intertransverse ligament, cervical Lateral temporomandibular ligament Ligamentum flavum, cervical Sphenomandibular ligament Stylomandibular ligament Transverse ligament of atlas
Head and Neck Sympathetic Nerve	**Includes:** Cavernous plexus Cervical ganglion Ciliary ganglion Internal carotid plexus Otic ganglion Pterygopalatine (sphenopalatine) ganglion Sphenopalatine (pterygopalatine) ganglion Stellate ganglion Submandibular ganglion Submaxillary ganglion
Head Muscle	**Includes:** Auricularis muscle Masseter muscle Pterygoid muscle Splenius capitis muscle Temporalis muscle Temporoparietalis muscle
Heart, Left	**Includes:** Left coronary sulcus Obtuse margin
Heart, Right	**Includes:** Right coronary sulcus
Hemiazygos Vein	**Includes:** Left ascending lumbar vein Left subcostal vein
Hepatic Artery	**Includes:** Common hepatic artery Gastroduodenal artery Hepatic artery proper
Hip Bursa and Ligament, Left **Hip** Bursa and Ligament, Right	**Includes:** Iliofemoral ligament Ischiofemoral ligament Pubofemoral ligament Transverse acetabular ligament Trochanteric bursa
Hip Joint, Left **Hip** Joint, Right	**Includes:** Acetabulofemoral joint

Section 0 - Medical and Surgical — Character 4 - Body Part	
Hip Muscle, Left **Hip** Muscle, Right	**Includes:** Gemellus muscle Gluteus maximus muscle Gluteus medius muscle Gluteus minimus muscle Iliacus muscle Obturator muscle Piriformis muscle Psoas muscle Quadratus femoris muscle Tensor fasciae latae muscle
Humeral Head, Left **Humeral** Head, Right	**Includes:** Greater tuberosity Lesser tuberosity Neck of humerus (anatomical) (surgical)
Humeral Shaft, Left **Humeral** Shaft, Right	**Includes:** Distal humerus Humerus, distal Lateral epicondyle of humerus Medial epicondyle of humerus
Hypogastric Vein, Left **Hypogastric** Vein, Right	**Includes:** Gluteal vein Internal iliac vein Internal pudendal vein Lateral sacral vein Middle hemorrhoidal vein Obturator vein Uterine vein Vaginal vein Vesical vein
Hypoglossal Nerve	**Includes:** Twelfth cranial nerve
Hypothalamus	**Includes:** Mammillary body
Inferior Mesenteric Artery	**Includes:** Sigmoid artery Superior rectal artery
Inferior Mesenteric Vein	**Includes:** Sigmoid vein Superior rectal vein
Inferior Vena Cava	**Includes:** Postcava Right inferior phrenic vein Right ovarian vein Right second lumbar vein Right suprarenal vein Right testicular vein
Inguinal Region, Bilateral **Inguinal** Region, Left **Inguinal** Region, Right	**Includes:** Inguinal canal Inguinal triangle
Inner Ear, Left **Inner** Ear, Right	**Includes:** Bony labyrinth Bony vestibule Cochlea Round window Semicircular canal

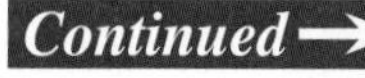

Section 0 - Medical and Surgical — Character 4 - Body Part	
Innominate Artery	**Includes:** Brachiocephalic artery Brachiocephalic trunk
Innominate Vein, Left **Innominate** Vein, Right	**Includes:** Brachiocephalic vein Inferior thyroid vein
Internal Carotid Artery, Left **Internal** Carotid Artery, Right	**Includes:** Caroticotympanic artery Carotid sinus
Internal Iliac Artery, Left **Internal** Iliac Artery, Right	**Includes:** Deferential artery Hypogastric artery Iliolumbar artery Inferior gluteal artery Inferior vesical artery Internal pudendal artery Lateral sacral artery Middle rectal artery Obturator artery Superior gluteal artery Umbilical artery Uterine artery Vaginal artery
Internal Mammary Artery, Left **Internal** Mammary Artery, Right	**Includes:** Anterior intercostal artery Internal thoracic artery Musculophrenic artery Pericardiophrenic artery Superior epigastric artery
Intracranial Artery	**Includes:** Anterior cerebral artery Anterior choroidal artery Anterior communicating artery Basilar artery Circle of Willis Internal carotid artery, intracranial portion Middle cerebral artery Ophthalmic artery Posterior cerebral artery Posterior communicating artery Posterior inferior cerebellar artery (PICA)
Intracranial Vein	**Includes:** Anterior cerebral vein Basal (internal) cerebral vein Dural venous sinus Great cerebral vein Inferior cerebellar vein Inferior cerebral vein Internal (basal) cerebral vein Middle cerebral vein Ophthalmic vein Superior cerebellar vein Superior cerebral vein
Jejunum	**Includes:** Duodenojejunal flexure

Section 0 - Medical and Surgical — Character 4 - Body Part	
Kidney	**Includes:** Renal calyx Renal capsule Renal cortex Renal segment
Kidney Pelvis, Left **Kidney** Pelvis, Right	**Includes:** Ureteropelvic junction (UPJ)
Kidney, Left **Kidney,** Right **Kidneys,** Bilateral	**Includes:** Renal calyx Renal capsule Renal cortex Renal segment
Knee Bursa and Ligament, Left **Knee** Bursa and Ligament, Right	**Includes:** Anterior cruciate ligament (ACL) Lateral collateral ligament (LCL) Ligament of head of fibula Medial collateral ligament (MCL) Patellar ligament Popliteal ligament Posterior cruciate ligament (PCL) Prepatellar bursa
Knee Joint, Femoral Surface, Left **Knee** Joint, Femoral Surface, Right	**Includes:** Femoropatellar joint Patellofemoral joint
Knee Joint, Left **Knee** Joint, Right	**Includes:** Femoropatellar joint Femorotibial joint Lateral meniscus Medial meniscus Patellofemoral joint Tibiofemoral joint
Knee Joint, Tibial Surface, Left **Knee** Joint, Tibial Surface, Right	**Includes:** Femorotibial joint Tibiofemoral joint
Knee Tendon, Left **Knee** Tendon, Right	**Includes:** Patellar tendon
Lacrimal Duct, Left **Lacrimal** Duct, Right	**Includes:** Lacrimal canaliculus Lacrimal punctum Lacrimal sac Nasolacrimal duct
Larynx	**Includes:** Aryepiglottic fold Arytenoid cartilage Corniculate cartilage Cuneiform cartilage False vocal cord Glottis Rima glottidis Thyroid cartilage Ventricular fold
Lens, Left **Lens,** Right	**Includes:** Zonule of Zinn
Liver	**Includes:** Quadrate lobe

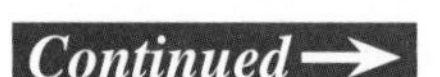

Section 0 - Medical and Surgical — Character 4 - Body Part	
Lower Arm and Wrist Muscle, Left **Lower** Arm and Wrist Muscle, Right	**Includes:** Anatomical snuffbox Brachioradialis muscle Extensor carpi radialis muscle Extensor carpi ulnaris muscle Flexor carpi radialis muscle Flexor carpi ulnaris muscle Flexor pollicis longus muscle Palmaris longus muscle Pronator quadratus muscle Pronator teres muscle
Lower Artery	Umbilical artery
Lower Eyelid, Left **Lower** Eyelid, Right	**Includes:** Inferior tarsal plate Medial canthus
Lower Femur, Left **Lower** Femur, Right	**Includes:** Lateral condyle of femur Lateral epicondyle of femur Medial condyle of femur Medial epicondyle of femur
Lower Leg Muscle, Left **Lower** Leg Muscle, Right	**Includes:** Extensor digitorum longus muscle Extensor hallucis longus muscle Fibularis brevis muscle Fibularis longus muscle Flexor digitorum longus muscle Flexor hallucis longus muscle Gastrocnemius muscle Peroneus brevis muscle Peroneus longus muscle Popliteus muscle Soleus muscle Tibialis anterior muscle Tibialis posterior muscle
Lower Leg Tendon, Left **Lower** Leg Tendon, Right	**Includes:** Achilles tendon
Lower Lip	**Includes:** Frenulum labii inferioris Labial gland Vermilion border
Lower Spine Bursa and Ligament	Iliolumbar ligament Interspinous ligament, lumbar Intertransverse ligament, lumbar Ligamentum flavum, lumbar Sacrococcygeal ligament Sacroiliac ligament Sacrospinous ligament Sacrotuberous ligament Supraspinous ligament
Lumbar Nerve	**Includes:** Lumbosacral trunk Spinal nerve, lumbar Superior clunic (cluneal) nerve
Lumbar Plexus	**Includes:** Accessory obturator nerve Genitofemoral nerve Iliohypogastric nerve Ilioinguinal nerve Lateral femoral cutaneous nerve Obturator nerve Superior gluteal nerve

Section 0 - Medical and Surgical — Character 4 - Body Part	
Lumbar Spinal Cord	**Includes:** Cauda equina Conus medullaris
Lumbar Sympathetic Nerve	**Includes:** Lumbar ganglion Lumbar splanchnic nerve
Lumbar Vertebra	**Includes:** Spinous process Transverse process Vertebral arch Vertebral body Vertebral foramen Vertebral lamina Vertebral pedicle
Lumbar Vertebral Joint	**Includes:** Lumbar facet joint
Lumbosacral Joint	**Includes:** Lumbosacral facet joint
Lymphatic, Aortic	**Includes:** Celiac lymph node Gastric lymph node Hepatic lymph node Lumbar lymph node Pancreaticosplenic lymph node Paraaortic lymph node Retroperitoneal lymph node
Lymphatic, Head	**Includes:** Buccinator lymph node Infraauricular lymph node Infraparotid lymph node Parotid lymph node Preauricular lymph node Submandibular lymph node Submaxillary lymph node Submental lymph node Subparotid lymph node Suprahyoid lymph node
Lymphatic, Left Axillary	**Includes:** Anterior (pectoral) lymph node Apical (subclavicular) lymph node Brachial (lateral) lymph node Central axillary lymph node Lateral (brachial) lymph node Pectoral (anterior) lymph node Posterior (subscapular) lymph node Subclavicular (apical) lymph node Subscapular (posterior) lymph node
Lymphatic, Left Lower Extremity	**Includes:** Femoral lymph node Popliteal lymph node
Lymphatic, Left Neck	**Includes:** Cervical lymph node Jugular lymph node Mastoid (postauricular) lymph node Occipital lymph node Postauricular (mastoid) lymph node Retropharyngeal lymph node Supraclavicular (Virchow's) lymph node Virchow's (supraclavicular) lymph node

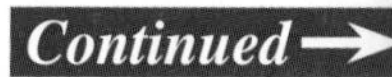
Continued →

Section 0 - Medical and Surgical — Character 4 - Body Part	
Lymphatic, Left Upper Extremity	**Includes:** Cubital lymph node Deltopectoral (infraclavicular) lymph node Epitrochlear lymph node Infraclavicular (deltopectoral) lymph node Supratrochlear lymph node
Lymphatic, Mesenteric	**Includes:** Inferior mesenteric lymph node Pararectal lymph node Superior mesenteric lymph node
Lymphatic, Pelvis	**Includes:** Common iliac (subaortic) lymph node Gluteal lymph node Iliac lymph node Inferior epigastric lymph node Obturator lymph node Sacral lymph node Subaortic (common iliac) lymph node Suprainguinal lymph node
Lymphatic, Right Axillary	**Includes:** Anterior (pectoral) lymph node Apical (subclavicular) lymph node Brachial (lateral) lymph node Central axillary lymph node Lateral (brachial) lymph node Pectoral (anterior) lymph node Posterior (subscapular) lymph node Subclavicular (apical) lymph node Subscapular (posterior) lymph node
Lymphatic, Right Lower Extremity	**Includes:** Femoral lymph node Popliteal lymph node
Lymphatic, Right Neck	**Includes:** Cervical lymph node Jugular lymph node Mastoid (postauricular) lymph node Occipital lymph node Postauricular (mastoid) lymph node Retropharyngeal lymph node Right jugular trunk Right lymphatic duct Right subclavian trunk Supraclavicular (Virchow's) lymph node Virchow's (supraclavicular) lymph node
Lymphatic, Right Upper Extremity	**Includes:** Cubital lymph node Deltopectoral (infraclavicular) lymph node Epitrochlear lymph node Infraclavicular (deltopectoral) lymph node Supratrochlear lymph node
Lymphatic, Thorax	**Includes:** Intercostal lymph node Mediastinal lymph node Parasternal lymph node Paratracheal lymph node Tracheobronchial lymph node

Section 0 - Medical and Surgical — Character 4 - Body Part	
Main Bronchus, Right	**Includes:** Bronchus Intermedius Intermediate bronchus
Mandible, Left **Mandible,** Right	**Includes:** Alveolar process of mandible Condyloid process Mandibular notch Mental foramen
Mastoid Sinus, Left **Mastoid** Sinus, Right	**Includes:** Mastoid air cells
Maxilla	**Includes:** Alveolar process of maxilla
Maxillary Sinus, Left **Maxillary** Sinus, Right	**Includes:** Antrum of Highmore
Median Nerve	**Includes:** Anterior interosseous nerve Palmar cutaneous nerve
Mediastinum	Mediastinal cavity Mediastinal space
Medulla Oblongata	**Includes:** Myelencephalon
Mesentery	**Includes:** Mesoappendix Mesocolon
Metatarsal-Phalangeal Joint, Left **Metatarsal-Phalangeal** Joint, Right	**Includes:** Metatarsophalangeal (MTP) joint
Middle Ear, Left **Middle** Ear, Right	**Includes:** Oval window Tympanic cavity
Minor Salivary Gland	**Includes:** Anterior lingual gland
Mitral Valve	**Includes:** Bicuspid valve Left atrioventricular valve Mitral annulus
Nasal Bone	**Includes:** Vomer of nasal septum
Nasal Mucosa and Soft Tissue	Columella External naris Greater alar cartilage Internal naris Lateral nasal cartilage Lesser alar cartilage Nasal cavity Nostril
Nasal Septum	**Includes:** Quadrangular cartilage Septal cartilage Vomer bone
Nasal Turbinate	**Includes:** Inferior turbinate Middle turbinate Nasal concha Superior turbinate

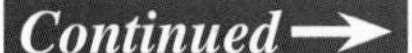
Continued →

Section 0 - Medical and Surgical — Character 4 - Body Part	
Nasopharynx	**Includes:** Choana Fossa of Rosenmuller Pharyngeal recess Rhinopharynx
Neck Muscle, Left **Neck** Muscle, Right	**Includes:** Anterior vertebral muscle Arytenoid muscle Cricothyroid muscle Infrahyoid muscle Levator scapulae muscle Platysma muscle Scalene muscle Splenius cervicis muscle Sternocleidomastoid muscle Suprahyoid muscle Thyroarytenoid muscle
Nipple, Left **Nipple,** Right	**Includes:** Areola
Occipital Bone	**Includes:** Foramen magnum
Oculomotor Nerve	**Includes:** Third cranial nerve
Olfactory Nerve	**Includes:** First cranial nerve Olfactory bulb
Omentum	Gastrocolic ligament Gastrocolic omentum Gastrohepatic omentum Gastrophrenic ligament Gastrosplenic ligament Greater Omentum Hepatogastric liagment Lesser Omentum
Optic Nerve	**Includes:** Optic chiasma Second cranial nerve
Orbit, Left **Orbit,** Right	**Includes:** Bony orbit Orbital portion of ethmoid bone Orbital portion of frontal bone Orbital portion of lacrimal bone Orbital portion of maxilla Orbital portion of palatine bone Orbital portion of sphenoid bone Orbital portion of zygomatic bone
Pancreatic Duct	**Includes:** Duct of Wirsung
Pancreatic Duct, Accessory	**Includes:** Duct of Santorini
Parotid Duct, Left **Parotid** Duct, Right	**Includes:** Stensen's duct
Pelvic Bone, Left **Pelvic** Bone, Right	**Includes:** Iliac crest Ilium Ischium Pubis
Pelvic Cavity	**Includes:** Retropubic space

Section 0 - Medical and Surgical — Character 4 - Body Part	
Penis	**Includes:** Corpus cavernosum Corpus spongiosum
Perineum Muscle	**Includes:** Bulbospongiosus muscle Cremaster muscle Deep transverse perineal muscle Ischiocavernosus muscle Levator ani muscle Superficial transverse perineal muscle
Peritoneum	**Includes:** Epiploic foramen
Peroneal Artery, Left **Peroneal** Artery, Right	**Includes:** Fibular artery
Peroneal Nerve	**Includes:** Common fibular nerve Common peroneal nerve External popliteal nerve Lateral sural cutaneous nerve
Pharynx	**Includes:** Base of Tongue Hypopharynx Laryngopharynx Lignual tonsil Oropharynx Piriform recess (sinus) Tongue, base of
Phrenic Nerve	**Includes:** Accessory phrenic nerve
Pituitary Gland	**Includes:** Adenohypophysis Hypophysis Neurohypophysis
Pons	**Includes:** Apneustic center Basis pontis Locus ceruleus Pneumotaxic center Pontine tegmentum Superior olivary nucleus
Popliteal Artery, Left **Popliteal** Artery, Right	**Includes:** Inferior genicular artery Middle genicular artery Superior genicular artery Sural artery
Portal Vein	**Includes:** Hepatic portal vein
Prepuce	**Includes:** Foreskin Glans penis
Pudendal Nerve	**Includes:** Posterior labial nerve Posterior scrotal nerve
Pulmonary Artery, Left	**Includes:** Arterial canal (duct) Botallo's duct Pulmoaortic canal
Pulmonary Valve	**Includes:** Pulmonary annulus Pulmonic valve

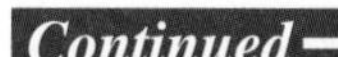

Section 0 - Medical and Surgical — Character 4 - Body Part	
Pulmonary Vein, Left	**Includes:** Left inferior pulmonary vein Left superior pulmonary vein
Pulmonary Vein, Right	**Includes:** Right inferior pulmonary vein Right superior pulmonary vein
Radial Artery, Left **Radial** Artery, Right	**Includes:** Radial recurrent artery
Radial Nerve	**Includes:** Dorsal digital nerve Musculospiral nerve Palmar cutaneous nerve Posterior interosseous nerve
Radius, Left **Radius,** Right	**Includes:** Ulnar notch
Rectum	**Includes:** Anorectal junction
Renal Artery, Left **Renal** Artery, Right	**Includes:** Inferior suprarenal artery Renal segmental artery
Renal Vein, Left	**Includes:** Left inferior phrenic vein Left ovarian vein Left second lumbar vein Left suprarenal vein Left testicular vein
Retina, Left **Retina,** Right	**Includes:** Fovea Macula Optic disc
Retroperitoneum	**Includes:** Retroperitoneal cavity Retroperitoneal space
Rib(s) Bursa and Ligament	Costotransverse ligament
Sacral Nerve	**Includes:** Spinal nerve, sacral
Sacral Plexus	**Includes:** Inferior gluteal nerve Posterior femoral cutaneous nerve Pudendal nerve
Sacral Sympathetic Nerve	**Includes:** Ganglion impar (ganglion of Walther) Pelvic splanchnic nerve Sacral ganglion Sacral splanchnic nerve
Sacrococcygeal Joint	**Includes:** Sacrococcygeal symphysis
Saphenous Vein, Left **Saphenous** Vein, Right	External pudendal vein Great(er) saphenous vein Lesser saphenous vein Small saphenous vein Superficial circumflex iliac vein Superficial epigastric vein
Scapula, Left **Scapula,** Right	**Includes:** Acromion (process) Coracoid process
Sciatic Nerve	**Includes:** Ischiatic nerve

Section 0 - Medical and Surgical — Character 4 - Body Part	
Shoulder Bursa and Ligament, Left **Shoulder** Bursa and Ligament, Right	**Includes:** Acromioclavicular ligament Coracoacromial ligament Coracoclavicular ligament Coracohumeral ligament
	Costoclavicular ligament Glenohumeral ligament Interclavicular ligament Sternoclavicular ligament Subacromial bursa Transverse humeral ligament Transverse scapular ligament
Shoulder Joint, Left **Shoulder** Joint, Right	**Includes:** Glenohumeral joint Glenoid ligament (labrum)
Shoulder Muscle, Left **Shoulder** Muscle, Right	**Includes:** Deltoid muscle Infraspinatus muscle Subscapularis muscle Supraspinatus muscle Teres major muscle Teres minor muscle
Sigmoid Colon	**Includes:** Rectosigmoid junction Sigmoid flexure
Skin	**Includes:** Dermis Epidermis Sebaceous gland Sweat gland
Sphenoid Bone	**Includes:** Greater wing Lesser wing Optic foramen Pterygoid process Sella turcica
Spinal Canal	**Includes:** Epidural space, spinal Extradural space, spinal Subarachnoid space, spinal Subdural space, spinal Vertebral canal
Spinal Meninges	**Includes:** Arachnoid mater, spinal Denticulate (dentate) ligament Dura mater, spinal Filum terminale Leptomeninges, spinal Pia mater, spinal
Spleen	**Includes:** Accessory spleen
Splenic Artery	**Includes:** Left gastroepiploic artery Pancreatic artery Short gastric artery
Splenic Vein	**Includes:** Left gastroepiploic vein Pancreatic vein

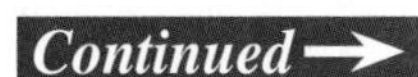
Continued →

Section 0 - Medical and Surgical — Character 4 - Body Part	
Sternum	**Includes:** Manubrium Suprasternal notch Xiphoid process
Sternum Bursa and Ligament	Costotransverse ligament Costoxiphoid ligament Sternocostal ligament
Stomach, Pylorus	**Includes:** Pyloric antrum Pyloric canal Pyloric sphincter
Subclavian Artery, Left **Subclavian** Artery, Right	**Includes:** Costocervical trunk Dorsal scapular artery Internal thoracic artery
Subcutaneous Tissue and Fascia, Chest	**Includes:** Pectoral fascia
Subcutaneous Tissue and Fascia, Face	**Includes:** Masseteric fascia Orbital fascia
Subcutaneous Tissue and Fascia, Left Foot	**Includes:** Plantar fascia (aponeurosis)
Subcutaneous Tissue and Fascia, Left Hand	**Includes:** Palmar fascia (aponeurosis)
Subcutaneous Tissue and Fascia, Left Lower Arm	**Includes:** Antebrachial fascia Bicipital aponeurosis
Subcutaneous Tissue and Fascia, Left Neck	Deep cervical fascia Pretracheal fascia Prevertebral fascia
Subcutaneous Tissue and Fascia, Left Upper Arm	**Includes:** Axillary fascia Deltoid fascia Infraspinatus fascia Subscapular aponeurosis Supraspinatus fascia
Subcutaneous Tissue and Fascia, Left Upper Leg	**Includes:** Crural fascia Fascia lata Iliac fascia Iliotibial tract (band)
Subcutaneous Tissue and Fascia, Right Foot	**Includes:** Plantar fascia (aponeurosis)
Subcutaneous Tissue and Fascia, Right Hand	**Includes:** Palmar fascia (aponeurosis)
Subcutaneous Tissue and Fascia, Right Lower Arm	**Includes:** Antebrachial fascia Bicipital aponeurosis
Subcutaneous Tissue and Fascia, Right Neck	Deep cervical fascia Pretracheal fascia Prevertebral fascia
Subcutaneous Tissue and Fascia, Right Upper Arm	**Includes:** Axillary fascia Deltoid fascia Infraspinatus fascia Subscapular aponeurosis Supraspinatus fascia

Section 0 - Medical and Surgical — Character 4 - Body Part	
Subcutaneous Tissue and Fascia, Right Upper Leg	**Includes:** Crural fascia Fascia lata Iliac fascia Iliotibial tract (band)
Subcutaneous Tissue and Fascia, Scalp	**Includes:** Galea aponeurotica
Subcutaneous Tissue and Fascia, Trunk	**Includes:** External oblique aponeurosis Transversalis fascia
Submaxillary Gland, Left **Submaxillary** Gland, Right	**Includes:** Submandibular gland
Superior Mesenteric Artery	**Includes:** Ileal artery Ileocolic artery Inferior pancreaticoduodenal artery Jejunal artery
Superior Mesenteric Vein	**Includes:** Right gastroepiploic vein
Superior Vena Cava	**Includes:** Precava
Tarsal Joint, Left **Tarsal** Joint, Right	**Includes:** Calcaneocuboid joint Cuboideonavicular joint Cuneonavicular joint Intercuneiform joint Subtalar (talocalcaneal) joint Talocalcaneal (subtalar) joint Talocalcaneonavicular joint
Tarsal, Left **Tarsal,** Right	**Includes:** Calcaneus Cuboid bone Intermediate cuneiform bone Lateral cuneiform bone Medial cuneiform bone Navicular bone Talus bone
Temporal Artery, Left **Temporal** Artery, Right	**Includes:** Middle temporal artery Superficial temporal artery Transverse facial artery
Temporal Bone, Left **Temporal** Bone, Right	**Includes:** Mastoid process Petrous part of temoporal bone Tympanic part of temoporal bone Zygomatic process of temporal bone
Thalamus	**Includes:** Epithalamus Geniculate nucleus Metathalamus Pulvinar
Thoracic Aorta Ascending/ Arch	**Includes:** Aortic arch Ascending aorta

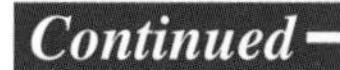

Section 0 - Medical and Surgical — Character 4 - Body Part	
Thoracic Duct	**Includes:** Left jugular trunk Left subclavian trunk
Thoracic Nerve	**Includes:** Intercostal nerve Intercostobrachial nerve Spinal nerve, thoracic Subcostal nerve
Thoracic Sympathetic Nerve	**Includes:** Cardiac plexus Esophageal plexus Greater splanchnic nerve Inferior cardiac nerve Least splanchnic nerve Lesser splanchnic nerve Middle cardiac nerve Pulmonary plexus Superior cardiac nerve Thoracic aortic plexus Thoracic ganglion
Thoracic Vertebra	**Includes:** Spinous process Transverse process Vertebral arch Vertebral body Vertebral foramen Vertebral lamina Vertebral pedicle
Thoracic Vertebral Joint	**Includes:** Costotransverse joint Costovertebral joint Thoracic facet joint
Thoracolumbar Vertebral Joint	**Includes:** Thoracolumbar facet joint
Thorax Muscle, Left **Thorax** Muscle, Right	**Includes:** Intercostal muscle Levatores costarum muscle Pectoralis major muscle Pectoralis minor muscle Serratus anterior muscle Subclavius muscle Subcostal muscle Transverse thoracis muscle
Thymus	**Includes:** Thymus gland
Thyroid Artery, Left **Thyroid** Artery, Right	**Includes:** Cricothyroid artery Hyoid artery Sternocleidomastoid artery Superior laryngeal artery Superior thyroid artery Thyrocervical trunk
Tibia, Left **Tibia,** Right	**Includes:** Lateral condyle of tibia Medial condyle of tibia Medial malleolus
Tibial Nerve	**Includes:** Lateral plantar nerve Medial plantar nerve Medial popliteal nerve Medial sural cutaneous nerve

Section 0 - Medical and Surgical — Character 4 - Body Part	
Toe Nail	**Includes:** Nail bed Nail plate
Toe Phalangeal Joint, Left **Toe** Phalangeal Joint, Right	**Includes:** Interphalangeal (IP) joint
Tongue	**Includes:** Frenulum linguae
Tongue, Palate, Pharynx Muscle	**Includes:** Chondroglossus muscle Genioglossus muscle Hyoglossus muscle Inferior longitudinal muscle Levator veli palatini muscle Palatoglossal muscle Palatopharyngeal muscle Pharyngeal constrictor muscle Salpingopharyngeus muscle Styloglossus muscle Stylopharyngeus muscle Superior longitudinal muscle Tensor veli palatini muscle
Tonsils	**Includes:** Palatine tonsil
Trachea	**Includes:** Cricoid cartilage
Transverse Colon	**Includes:** Hepatic flexure Splenic flexure
Tricuspid Valve	**Includes:** Right atrioventricular valve Tricuspid annulus
Trigeminal Nerve	**Includes:** Fifth cranial nerve Gasserian ganglion Mandibular nerve Maxillary nerve Ophthalmic nerve Trifacial nerve
Trochlear Nerve	**Includes:** Fourth cranial nerve
Trunk Muscle, Left **Trunk** Muscle, Right	**Includes:** Coccygeus muscle Erector spinae muscle Interspinalis muscle Intertransversarius muscle Latissimus dorsi muscle Quadratus lumborum muscle Rhomboid major muscle Rhomboid minor muscle Serratus posterior muscle Transversospinalis muscle Trapezius muscle
Tympanic Membrane, Left **Tympanic** Membrane, Right	**Includes:** Pars flaccida
Ulna, Left **Ulna,** Right	**Includes:** Olecranon process Radial notch

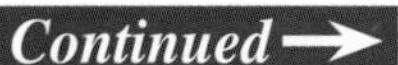

Section 0 - Medical and Surgical — Character 4 - Body Part	
Ulnar Artery, Left **Ulnar** Artery, Right	**Includes:** Anterior ulnar recurrent artery Common interosseous artery Posterior ulnar recurrent artery
Ulnar Nerve	**Includes:** Cubital nerve
Upper Arm Muscle, Left **Upper** Arm Muscle, Right	**Includes:** Biceps brachii muscle Brachialis muscle Coracobrachialis muscle Triceps brachii muscle
Upper Artery	**Includes:** Aortic intercostal artery Bronchial artery Esophageal artery Subcostal artery
Upper Eyelid, Left **Upper** Eyelid, Right	**Includes:** Lateral canthus Levator palpebrae superioris muscle Orbicularis oculi muscle Superior tarsal plate
Upper Femur, Left **Upper** Femur, Right	**Includes:** Femoral head Greater trochanter Lesser trochanter Neck of femur
Upper Leg Muscle, Left **Upper** Leg Muscle, Right	**Includes:** Adductor brevis muscle Adductor longus muscle Adductor magnus muscle Biceps femoris muscle Gracilis muscle Pectineus muscle Quadriceps (femoris) Rectus femoris muscle Sartorius muscle Semimembranosus muscle Semitendinosus muscle Vastus intermedius muscle Vastus lateralis muscle Vastus medialis muscle
Upper Lip	**Includes:** Frenulum labii superioris Labial gland Vermilion border
Upper Spine Bursa and Ligament	Interspinous ligament, thoracic Intertransverse ligament, thoracic Ligamentum flavum, thoracic Supraspinous ligament
Ureter **Ureter,** Left **Ureter,** Right **Ureters,** Bilateral	**Includes:** Ureteral orifice Ureterovesical orifice
Urethra	**Includes:** Bulbourethral (Cowper's) gland Cowper's (bulbourethral) gland External urethral sphincter Internal urethral sphincter Membranous urethra Penile urethra Prostatic urethra

Section 0 - Medical and Surgical — Character 4 - Body Part	
Uterine Supporting Structure	**Includes:** Broad ligament Infundibulopelvic ligament Ovarian ligament Round ligament of uterus
Uterus	**Includes:** Fundus uteri Myometrium Perimetrium Uterine cornu
Uvula	**Includes:** Palatine uvula
Vagus Nerve	**Includes:** Anterior vagal trunk Pharyngeal plexus Pneumogastric nerve Posterior vagal trunk Pulmonary plexus Recurrent laryngeal nerve Superior laryngeal nerve Tenth cranial nerve
Vas Deferens **Vas** Deferens, Bilateral **Vas** Deferens, Left **Vas** Deferens, Right	**Includes:** Ductus deferens Ejaculatory duct
Ventricle, Right	**Includes:** Conus arteriosus
Ventricular Septum	**Includes:** Interventricular septum
Vertebral Artery, Left **Vertebral** Artery, Right	**Includes:** Anterior spinal artery Posterior spinal artery
Vertebral Vein, Left **Vertebral** Vein, Right	**Includes:** Deep cervical vein Suboccipital venous plexus
Vestibular Gland	**Includes:** Bartholin's (greater vestibular) gland Greater vestibular (Bartholin's) gland Paraurethral (Skene's) gland Skene's (paraurethral) gland
Vitreous, Left **Vitreous,** Right	**Includes:** Vitreous body
Vocal Cord, Left **Vocal** Cord, Right	**Includes:** Vocal fold
Vulva	**Includes:** Labia majora Labia minora
Wrist Bursa and Ligament, Left **Wrist** Bursa and Ligament, Right	**Includes:** Palmar ulnocarpal ligament Radial collateral carpal ligament Radiocarpal ligament Radioulnar ligament Ulnar collateral carpal ligament
Wrist Joint, Left **Wrist** Joint, Right	**Includes:** Distal radioulnar joint Radiocarpal joint

Appendix E: Medical and Surgical Device Table (Device Key) and Device Aggregation Table

Section 0 - Medical and Surgical — Character 6 - Device	
Articulating Spacer in Lower Joints	**Includes:** Articulating Spacer (Antibiotic) Spacer, Articulating (Antibiotic)
Artificial Sphincter in Gastrointestinal System	**Includes:** Artificial anal sphincter (AAS) Artificial bowel sphincter (neosphincter)
Artificial Sphincter in Urinary System	**Includes:** AMS 800® Urinary Control System Artificial urinary sphincter (AUS)
Autologous Arterial Tissue in Heart and Great Vessels	**Includes:** Autologous artery graft
Autologous Arterial Tissue in Lower Arteries	**Includes:** Autologous artery graft
Autologous Arterial Tissue in Lower Veins	**Includes:** Autologous artery graft
Autologous Arterial Tissue in Upper Arteries	**Includes:** Autologous artery graft
Autologous Arterial Tissue in Upper Veins	**Includes:** Autologous artery graft
Autologous Tissue Substitute	**Includes:** Autograft Cultured epidermal cell autograft Epicel® cultured epidermal autograft
Autologous Venous Tissue in Heart and Great Vessels	**Includes:** Autologous vein graft
Autologous Venous Tissue in Lower Arteries	**Includes:** Autologous vein graft
Autologous Venous Tissue in Lower Veins	**Includes:** Autologous vein graft
Autologous Venous Tissue in Upper Arteries	**Includes:** Autologous vein graft
Autologous Venous Tissue in Upper Veins	**Includes:** Autologous vein graft
Bone Growth Stimulator in Head and Facial Bones	**Includes:** Electrical bone growth stimulator (EBGS) Ultrasonic osteogenic stimulator Ultrasound bone healing system
Bone Growth Stimulator in Lower Bones	**Includes:** Electrical bone growth stimulator (EBGS) Ultrasonic osteogenic stimulator Ultrasound bone healing system
Bone Growth Stimulator in Upper Bones	**Includes:** Electrical bone growth stimulator (EBGS) Ultrasonic osteogenic stimulator Ultrasound bone healing system
Cardiac Lead in Heart and Great Vessels	**Includes:** Cardiac contractility modulation lead
Cardiac Lead, Defibrillator for Insertion in Heart and Great Vessels	**Includes:** ACUITY™ Steerable Lead Attain Ability® lead Attain StarFix® (OTW) lead Cardiac resynchronization therapy (CRT) lead Corox (OTW) Bipolar Lead Durata® Defibrillation Lead ENDOTAK RELIANCE® (G) Defibrillation Lead
Cardiac Lead, Pacemaker for Insertion in Heart and Great Vessels	**Includes:** ACUITY™ Steerable Lead Attain Ability® lead Attain StarFix® (OTW) lead Cardiac resynchronization therapy (CRT) lead Corox (OTW) Bipolar Lead
Cardiac Resynchronization Defibrillator Pulse Generator for Insertion in Subcutaneous Tissue and Fascia	**Includes:** COGNIS® CRT-D Concerto II CRT-D Consulta CRT-D CONTAK RENEWAL® 3 RF (HE) CRT-D LIVIAN™ CRT-D Maximo II DR CRT-D Ovatio™ CRT-D Protecta XT CRT-D Viva (XT)(S)
Cardiac Resynchronization Pacemaker Pulse Generator for Insertion in Subcutaneous Tissue and Fascia	**Includes:** Consulta CRT-P Stratos LV Synchra CRT-P
Contraceptive Device in Female Reproductive System	**Includes:** Intrauterine device (IUD)
Contraceptive Device in Subcutaneous Tissue and Fascia	**Includes:** Subdermal progesterone implant
Contractility Modulation Device for Insertion in Subcutaneous Tissue and Fascia	**Includes:** Optimizer™ III implantable pulse generator
Defibrillator Generator for Insertion in Subcutaneous Tissue and Fascia	**Includes:** Evera (XT)(S)(DR/VR) Implantable cardioverter-defibrillator (ICD) Maximo II DR (VR) Protecta XT DR (XT VR) Secura (DR) (VR) Virtuoso (II) (DR) (VR)
Diaphragmatic Pacemaker Lead in Respiratory System	**Includes:** Phrenic nerve stimulator lead
Drainage Device	**Includes:** Cystostomy tube Foley catheter Percutaneous nephrostomy catheter Thoracostomy tube

Continued →

Section 0 - Medical and Surgical — Character 6 - Device	
External Fixation Device in Head and Facial Bones	**Includes:** External fixator
External Fixation Device in Lower Bones	**Includes:** External fixator
External Fixation Device in Lower Joints	**Includes:** External fixator
External Fixation Device in Upper Bones	**Includes:** External fixator
External Fixation Device in Upper Joints	**Includes:** External fixator
External Fixation Device, Hybrid for Insertion in Upper Bones	**Includes:** Delta frame external fixator Sheffield hybrid external fixator
External Fixation Device, Hybrid for Insertion in Lower Bones	**Includes:** Delta frame external fixator Sheffield hybrid external fixator
External Fixation Device, Hybrid for Reposition in Upper Bones	**Includes:** Delta frame external fixator Sheffield hybrid external fixator
External Fixation Device, Hybrid for Reposition in Lower Bones	**Includes:** Delta frame external fixator Sheffield hybrid external fixator
External Fixation Device, Limb Lengthening for Insertion in Upper Bones	**Includes:** Ilizarov-Vecklich device
External Fixation Device, Limb Lengthening for Insertion in Lower Bones	**Includes:** Ilizarov-Vecklich device
External Fixation Device, Monoplanar for Insertion in Upper Bones	**Includes:** Uniplanar external fixator
External Fixation Device, Monoplanar for Insertion in Lower Bones	**Includes:** Uniplanar external fixator
External Fixation Device, Monoplanar for Reposition in Upper Bones	**Includes:** Uniplanar external fixator
External Fixation Device, Monoplanar for Reposition in Lower Bones	**Includes:** Uniplanar external fixator
External Fixation Device, Ring for Insertion in Upper Bones	**Includes:** Ilizarov external fixator Sheffield ring external fixator
External Fixation Device, Ring for Insertion in Lower Bones	**Includes:** Ilizarov external fixator Sheffield ring external fixator
External Fixation Device, Ring for Reposition in Upper Bones	**Includes:** Ilizarov external fixator Sheffield ring external fixator
External Fixation Device, Ring for Reposition in Lower Bones	**Includes:** Ilizarov external fixator Sheffield ring external fixator

Section 0 - Medical and Surgical — Character 6 - Device	
Extraluminal Device	**Includes:** AtriClip LAA Exclusion System LAP-BAND® adjustable gastric banding system REALIZE® Adjustable Gastric Band
Feeding Device in Gastrointestinal System	**Includes:** Percutaneous endoscopic gastrojejunostomy (PEG/J) tube Percutaneous endoscopic gastrostomy (PEG) tube
Hearing Device in Ear, Nose, Sinus	**Includes:** Esteem® implantable hearing system
Hearing Device in Head and Facial Bones	**Includes:** Bone anchored hearing device
Hearing Device, Bone Conduction for Insertion in Ear, Nose, Sinus	**Includes:** Bone anchored hearing device
Hearing Device, Multiple Channel Cochlear Prosthesis for Insertion in Ear, Nose, Sinus	**Includes:** Cochlear implant (CI), multiple channel (electrode)
Hearing Device, Single Channel Cochlear Prosthesis for Insertion in Ear, Nose, Sinus	**Includes:** Cochlear implant (CI), single channel (electrode)
Implantable Heart Assist System in Heart and Great Vessels	**Includes:** Berlin Heart Ventricular Assist Device DeBakey Left Ventricular Assist Device DuraHeart Left Ventricular Assist System HeartMate II® Left Ventricular Assist Device (LVAD) HeartMate 3® LVAS HeartMate XVE® Left Ventricular Assist Device (LVAD) MicroMed HeartAssist Novacor Left Ventricular Assist Device Thoratec IVAD (Implantable Ventricular Assist Device)
Infusion Device	**Includes:** Ascenda Intrathecal Catheter InDura, intrathecal catheter (1P) (spinal) Non-tunneled central venous catheter Peripherally inserted central catheter (PICC) Tunneled spinal (intrathecal) catheter
Infusion Device, Pump in Subcutaneous Tissue and Fascia	**Includes:** Implantable drug infusion pump (anti-spasmodic)(chemotherapy)(pain) Injection reservoir, pump Pump reservoir Subcutaneous injection reservoir, pump SynchroMed pump
Interbody Fusion Device in Lower Joints	**Includes:** Axial Lumbar Interbody Fusion System AxiaLIF® System CoRoent® XL Direct Lateral Interbody Fusion (DLIF) device EXtreme Lateral Interbody Fusion (XLIF) device Interbody fusion (spine) cage XLIF® System

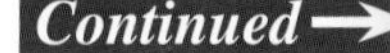
Continued →

Section 0 - Medical and Surgical — Character 6 - Device	
Interbody Fusion Device in Upper Joints	**Includes:** BAK/C® Interbody Cervical Fusion System Interbody fusion (spine) cage
Internal Fixation Device in Head and Facial Bones	**Includes:** Bone screw (interlocking)(lag)(pedicle) (recessed) Kirschner wire (K-wire) Neutralization plate
Internal Fixation Device in Lower Bones	**Includes:** Bone screw (interlocking)(lag)(pedicle) (recessed) Clamp and rod internal fixation system (CRIF) Kirschner wire (K-wire) Neutralization plate
Internal Fixation Device in Lower Joints	**Includes:** Fusion screw (compression)(lag) (locking) Joint fixation plate Kirschner wire (K-wire)
Internal Fixation Device in Upper Bones	**Includes:** Bone screw (interlocking)(lag)(pedicle) (recessed) Clamp and rod internal fixation system (CRIF) Kirschner wire (K-wire) Neutralization plate
Internal Fixation Device in Upper Joints	**Includes:** Fusion screw (compression)(lag) (locking) Joint fixation plate Kirschner wire (K-wire)
Internal Fixation Device, Intramedullary in Lower Bones	**Includes:** Intramedullary (IM) rod (nail) Intramedullary skeletal kinetic distractor (ISKD) Kuntscher nail
Internal Fixation Device, Intramedullary in Upper Bones	**Includes:** Intramedullary (IM) rod (nail) Intramedullary skeletal kinetic distractor (ISKD) Kuntscher nail
Internal Fixation Device, Rigid Plate for Insertion in Upper Bones	**Includes:** Titanium Sternal Fixation System (TSFS)
Internal Fixation Device, Rigid Plate for Reposition in Upper Bones	**Includes:** Titanium Sternal Fixation System (TSFS)

Section 0 - Medical and Surgical — Character 6 - Device	
Intraluminal Device	**Includes:** Absolute Pro Vascular (OTW) Self-Expanding Stent System Acculink (RX) Carotid Stent System AFX® Endovascular AAA System AneuRx® AAA Advantage® Assurant (Cobalt) stent Carotid WALLSTENT® Monorail® Endoprosthesis CoAxia NeuroFlo catheter Colonic Z-Stent® Complete (SE) stent Cook Zenith AAA Endovascular Graft Driver stent (RX) (OTW) E-Luminexx™ (Biliary)(Vascular) Stent Embolization coil(s) Endologix AFX® Endovascular AAA System Endurant® II AAA stent graft system Endurant® Endovascular Stent Graft EXCLUDER® AAA Endoprosthesis Express® (LD) Premounted Stent System Express® Biliary SD Monorail® Premounted Stent System Express® SD Renal Monorail® Premounted Stent System FLAIR® Endovascular Stent Graft Formula™ Balloon-Expandable Renal Stent System GORE EXCLUDER® AAA Endoprosthesis GORE TAG® Thoracic Endoprosthesis Herculink (RX) Elite Renal Stent System LifeStent® (Flexstar)(XL) Vascular Stent System Medtronic Endurant® II AAA stent graft system Micro-Driver stent (RX) (OTW) MULTI-LINK (VISION)(MINI-VISION) (ULTRA) Coronary Stent System Omnilink Elite Vascular Balloon Expandable Stent System Pipeline™ Embolization device (PED) Protégé® RX Carotid Stent System Stent, intraluminal (cardiovascular) (gastrointestinal)(hepatobiliary) (urinary) Talent® Converter Talent® Occluder Talent® Stent Graft (abdominal)(thoracic) Therapeutic occlusion coil(s) Ultraflex™ Precision Colonic Stent System Valiant Thoracic Stent Graft WALLSTENT® Endoprosthesis Xact Carotid Stent System Zenith AAA Endovascular Graft Zenith Flex® AAA Endovascular Graft Zenith® Renu™ AAA Ancillary Graft Zenith TX2® TAA Endovascular Graft
Intraluminal Device, Airway in Ear, Nose, Sinus	**Includes:** Nasopharyngeal airway (NPA)

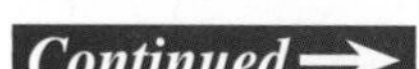

Section 0 - Medical and Surgical — Character 6 - Device	
Intraluminal Device, Airway in Gastrointestinal System	**Includes:** Esophageal obturator airway (EOA)
Intraluminal Device, Airway in Mouth and Throat	**Includes:** Guedel airway Oropharyngeal airway (OPA)
Intraluminal Device, Bioactive in Upper Arteries	**Includes:** Bioactive embolization coil(s) Micrus CERECYTE microcoil
Intraluminal Device, Branched or Fenestrated, One or Two Arteries for Restriction in Lower Arteries	**Includes:** Cook Zenith AAA Endovascular Graft EXCLUDER® AAA Endoprosthesis EXCLUDER® IBE Endoprosthesis GORE EXCLUDER® AAA Endoprosthesis GORE EXCLUDER® IBE Endoprosthesis Zenith AAA Endovascular Graft
Intraluminal Device, Branched or Fenestrated, Three or More Arteries for Restriction in Lower Arteries	**Includes:** Cook Zenith AAA Endovascular Graft EXCLUDER® AAA Endoprosthesis GORE EXCLUDER® AAA Endoprosthesis Zenith AAA Endovascular Graft
Intraluminal Device, Drug-eluting in Heart and Great Vessels	**Includes:** CYPHER® Stent Endeavor® (III)(IV) (Sprint) Zotarolimus-eluting Coronary Stent System Everolimus-eluting coronary stent Paclitaxel-eluting coronary stent Sirolimus-eluting coronary stent TAXUS® Liberté® Paclitaxel-eluting Coronary Stent System XIENCE Everolimus Eluting Coronary Stent System Zotarolimus-eluting coronary stent
Intraluminal Device, Drug-eluting in Lower Arteries	**Includes:** Paclitaxel-eluting peripheral stent Zilver® PTX® (paclitaxel) Drug-Eluting Peripheral Stent
Intraluminal Device, Drug-eluting in Upper Arteries	**Includes:** Paclitaxel-eluting peripheral stent Zilver® PTX® (paclitaxel) Drug-Eluting Peripheral Stent
Intraluminal Device, Endobronchial Valve in Respiratory System	**Includes:** Spiration IBV™ Valve System
Intraluminal Device, Pessary in Female Reproductive System	**Includes:** Pessary ring Vaginal pessary
Intraluminal Device, Endotracheal Airway in Respiratory System	**Includes:** Endotracheal tube (cuffed)(double-lumen)
Liner in Lower Joints	**Includes:** Acetabular cup Hip (joint) liner Joint liner (insert) Knee (implant) insert Tibial insert

Section 0 - Medical and Surgical — Character 6 - Device	
Monitoring Device	**Includes:** Blood glucose monitoring system Cardiac event recorder Continuous Glucose Monitoring (CGM) device Implantable glucose monitoring device Loop recorder, implantable Reveal (DX)(XT)
Monitoring Device, Hemodynamic for Insertion in Subcutaneous Tissue and Fascia	**Includes:** Implantable hemodynamic monitor (IHM Implantable hemodynamic monitoring system (IHMS)
Monitoring Device, Pressure Sensor for Insertion in Heart and Great Vessels	**Includes:** CardioMEMS® pressure sensor EndoSure® sensor
Neurostimulator Lead in Central Nervous System and Cranial Nerves	**Includes:** Cortical strip neurostimulator lead DBS lead Deep brain neurostimulator lead RNS System lead Spinal cord neurostimulator lead
Neurostimulator Lead in Peripheral Nervous System	**Includes:** InterStim® Therapy lead
Neurostimulator Generator in Head and Facial Bones	**Includes:** RNS system neurostimulator generator
Nonautologous Tissue Substitute	**Includes:** Acellular Hydrated Dermis Bone bank bone graft Cook Biodesign® Fistula Plug(s) Cook Biodesign® Hernia Graft(s) Cook Biodesign® Layered Graft(s) Cook Zenapro™ Layered Grafts(s) Tissue bank graft
Pacemaker, Dual Chamber for Insertion in Subcutaneous Tissue and Fascia	**Includes:** Advisa (MRI) EnRhythm Kappa Revo MRI™ SureScan® pacemaker Two lead pacemaker Versa
Pacemaker, Single Chamber for Insertion in Subcutaneous Tissue and Fascia	**Includes:** Single lead pacemaker (atrium)(ventricle)
Pacemaker, Single Chamber Rate Responsive for Insertion in Subcutaneous Tissue and Fascia	**Includes:** Single lead rate responsive pacemaker (atrium)(ventricle)
Radioactive Element	**Includes:** Brachytherapy seeds
Radioactive Element, Cesium-131 Collagen Implant for Insertion in Central Nervous System and Cranial Nerves	Cesium-131 Collagen Implant GammaTile™
Resurfacing Device in Lower Joints	**Includes:** CONSERVE® PLUS Total Resurfacing Hip System Cormet Hip Resurfacing System

Continued →

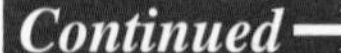

Section 0 - Medical and Surgical — Character 6 - Device	
Short-term External Heart Assist System in Heart and Great Vessels	Biventricular external heart assist system BVS 5000 Ventricular Assist Device Centrimag® Blood Pump Impella® heart pump TandemHeart® System Thoratec Paracorporeal Ventricular Assist Device
Spacer in Lower Joints	**Includes:** Joint spacer (antibiotic) Spacer, Static (Antibiotic) Static Spacer (Antibiotic)
Spacer in Upper Joints	**Includes:** Joint spacer (antibiotic)
Spinal Stabilization Device, Facet Replacement for Insertion in Upper Joints	**Includes:** Facet replacement spinal stabilization device
Spinal Stabilization Device, Facet Replacement for Insertion in Lower Joints	**Includes:** Facet replacement spinal stabilization device
Spinal Stabilization Device, Interspinous Process for Insertion in Upper Joints	**Includes:** Interspinous process spinal stabilization device X-STOP® Spacer
Spinal Stabilization Device, Interspinous Process for Insertion in Lower Joints	**Includes:** Interspinous process spinal stabilization device X-STOP® Spacer
Spinal Stabilization Device, Pedicle-Based for Insertion in Upper Joints	**Includes:** Dynesys® Dynamic Stabilization System Pedicle-based dynamic stabilization device
Spinal Stabilization Device, Pedicle-Based for Insertion in Lower Joints	**Includes:** Dynesys® Dynamic Stabilization System Pedicle-based dynamic stabilization device
Stimulator Generator in Subcutaneous Tissue and Fascia	**Includes:** Baroreflex Activation Therapy® (BAT®) Diaphragmatic pacemaker generator Mark IV Breathing Pacemaker System Phrenic nerve stimulator generator Rheos® System device
Stimulator Generator, Multiple Array for Insertion in Subcutaneous Tissue and Fascia	**Includes:** Activa PC neurostimulator Enterra gastric neurostimulator Neurostimulator generator, multiple channel PrimeAdvanced neurostimulator (SureScan)(MRI Safe)
Stimulator Generator, Multiple Array Rechargeable for Insertion in Subcutaneous Tissue and Fascia	**Includes:** Activa RC neurostimulator Neurostimulator generator, multiple channel rechargeable RestoreAdvanced neurostimulator (SureScan)(MRI Safe) RestoreSensor neurostimulator (SureScan)(MRI Safe) RestoreUltra neurostimulator (SureScan) (MRI Safe)
Stimulator Generator, Single Array for Insertion in Subcutaneous Tissue and Fascia	**Includes:** Activa SC neurostimulator InterStim® Therapy neurostimulator Itrel (3)(4) neurostimulator Neurostimulator generator, single channel

Section 0 - Medical and Surgical — Character 6 - Device	
Stimulator Generator, Single Array Rechargeable for Insertion in Subcutaneous Tissue and Fascia	**Includes:** Neurostimulator generator, single channel rechargeable
Stimulator Lead in Gastrointestinal System	**Includes:** Gastric electrical stimulation (GES) lead Gastric pacemaker lead
Stimulator Lead in Muscles	**Includes:** Electrical muscle stimulation (EMS) lead Electronic muscle stimulator lead Neuromuscular electrical stimulation (NEMS) lead
Stimulator Lead in Upper Arteries	**Includes:** Baroreflex Activation Therapy® (BAT®) Carotid (artery) sinus (baroreceptor) lead Rheos® System lead
Stimulator Lead in Urinary System	**Includes:** Sacral nerve modulation (SNM) lead Sacral neuromodulation lead Urinary incontinence stimulator lead
Synthetic Substitute	**Includes:** AbioCor® Total Replacement Heart AMPLATZER® Muscular VSD Occluder Annuloplasty ring Bard® Composix® (E/X)(LP) mesh Bard® Composix® Kugel® patch Bard® Dulex™ mesh Bard® Ventralex™ hernia patch BRYAN® Cervical Disc System Ex-PRESS™ mini glaucoma shunt Flexible Composite Mesh GORE® DUALMESH® Holter valve ventricular shunt MitraClip valve repair system Nitinol framed polymer mesh Open Pivot Aortic Valve Graft (AVG) Open Pivot (mechanical) valve Partially absorbable mesh PHYSIOMESH™ Flexible Composite Mesh Polymethylmethacrylate (PMMA) Polypropylene mesh PRESTIGE® Cervical Disc PROCEED™ Ventral Patch Prodisc-C Prodisc-L PROLENE Polypropylene Hernia System (PHS) Rebound HRD® (Hernia Repair Device) SynCardia Total Artificial Heart Total artificial (replacement) heart ULTRAPRO Hernia System (UHS) ULTRAPRO Partially Absorbable Lightweight Mesh ULTRAPRO Plug Ventrio™ Hernia Patch Zimmer® NexGen® LPS Mobile Bearing Knee Zimmer® NexGen® LPS-Flex Mobile Knee
Synthetic Substitute, Ceramic for Replacement in Lower Joints	**Includes:** Ceramic on ceramic bearing surface Novation® Ceramic AHS® (Articulation Hip System)

Continued →

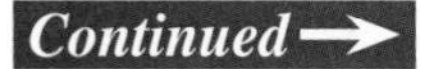

Section 0 - Medical and Surgical — Character 6 - Device	
Synthetic Substitute, Intraocular Telescope for Replacement in Eye	**Includes:** Implantable Miniature Telescope™ (IMT)
Synthetic Substitute, Metal for Replacement in Lower Joints	**Includes:** Cobalt/chromium head and socket Metal on metal bearing surface
Synthetic Substitute, Metal on Polyethylene for Replacement in Lower Joints	**Includes:** Cobalt/chromium head and polyethylene socket
Synthetic Substitute, Oxidized Zirconium on Polyethylene for Replacement in Lower Joints	OXINIUM
Synthetic Substitute, Polyethylene for Replacement in Lower Joints	**Includes:** Polyethylene socket
Synthetic Substitute, Reverse Ball and Socket for Replacement in Upper Joints	**Includes:** Delta III Reverse shoulder prosthesis Reverse® Shoulder Prosthesis
Tissue Expander in Skin and Breast	**Includes:** Tissue expander (inflatable)(injectable)
Tissue Expander in Subcutaneous Tissue and Fascia	**Includes:** Tissue expander (inflatable)(injectable)
Tracheostomy Device in Respiratory System	**Includes:** Tracheostomy tube

Section 0 - Medical and Surgical — Character 6 - Device	
Vascular Access Device, Totally Implantable in Subcutaneous Tissue and Fascia	**Includes:** Implanted (venous)(access) port Injection reservoir, port Subcutaneous injection reservoir, port
Vascular Access Device, Tunneled in Subcutaneous Tissue and Fascia	Tunneled central venous catheter Vectra® Vascular Access Graft
Zooplastic Tissue in Heart and Great Vessels	**Includes:** 3f (Aortic) Bioprosthesis valve Bovine pericardial valve Bovine pericardium graft Contegra Pulmonary Valved Conduit CoreValve transcatheter aortic valve Epic™ Stented Tissue Valve (aortic) Freestyle (Stentless) Aortic Root Bioprosthesis Hancock Bioprosthesis (aortic) (mitral) valve Hancock Bioprosthetic Valved Conduit Melody® transcatheter pulmonary valve Mitroflow® Aortic Pericardial Heart Valve Mosaic Bioprosthesis (aortic) (mitral) valve Porcine (bioprosthetic) valve SAPIEN transcatheter aortic valve SJM Biocor® Stented Valve System Stented tissue valve Trifecta™ Valve (aortic) Xenograft

Device Aggregation Table

Specific Device	for Operation	in Body System	General Device
Autologous Arterial Tissue	All applicable	Heart and Great Vessels Lower Arteries Lower Veins Upper Arteries Upper Veins	**7** Autologous Tissue Substitute
Autologous Venous Tissue	All applicable	Heart and Great Vessels Lower Arteries Lower Veins Upper Arteries Upper Veins	**7** Autologous Tissue Substitute
Cardiac Lead, Defibrillator	Insertion	Heart and Great Vessels	**M** Cardiac Lead
Cardiac Lead, Pacemaker	Insertion	Heart and Great Vessels	**M** Cardiac Lead
Cardiac Resynchronization Defibrillator Pulse Generator	Insertion	Subcutaneous Tissue and Fascia	**P** Cardiac Rhythm Related Device
Cardiac Resynchronization Pacemaker Pulse Generator	Insertion	Subcutaneous Tissue and Fascia	**P** Cardiac Rhythm Related Device
Contractility Modulation Device	Insertion	Subcutaneous Tissue and Fascia	**P** Cardiac Rhythm Related Device
Defibrillator Generator	Insertion	Subcutaneous Tissue and Fascia	**P** Cardiac Rhythm Related Device
Epiretinal Visual Prosthesis	All applicable	Eye	**J** Synthetic Substitute
External Fixation Device, Hybrid	Insertion	Lower Bones Upper Bones	**5** External Fixation Device
External Fixation Device, Hybrid	Reposition	Lower Bones Upper Bones	**5** External Fixation Device
External Fixation Device, Limb Lengthening	Insertion	Lower Bones Upper Bones	**5** External Fixation Device
External Fixation Device, Monoplanar	Insertion	Lower Bones Upper Bones	**5** External Fixation Device
External Fixation Device, Monoplanar	Reposition	Lower Bones Upper Bones	**5** External Fixation Device
External Fixation Device, Ring	Insertion	Lower Bones Upper Bones	**5** External Fixation Device
External Fixation Device, Ring	Reposition	Lower Bones Upper Bones	**5** External Fixation Device
Hearing Device, Bone Conduction	Insertion	Ear, Nose, Sinus	**S** Hearing Device
Hearing Device, Multiple Channel Cochlear Prosthesis	Insertion	Ear, Nose, Sinus	**S** Hearing Device
Hearing Device, Single Channel Cochlear Prosthesis	Insertion	Ear, Nose, Sinus	**S** Hearing Device
Internal Fixation Device, Intramedullary	All applicable	Lower Bones Upper Bones	**4** Internal Fixation Device
Internal Fixation Device, Rigid Plate	Insertion	Upper Bones	**4** Internal Fixation Device
Internal Fixation Device, Rigid Plate	Reposition	Upper Bones	**4** Internal Fixation Device
Intraluminal Device, Airway	All applicable	Ear, Nose, Sinus Gastrointestinal System Mouth and Throat	**D** Intraluminal Device

Specific Device	for Operation	in Body System	General Device
Intraluminal Device, Bioactive	All applicable	Upper Arteries	**D** Intraluminal Device
Intraluminal Device, Branched or Fenestrated, One or Two Arteries	Restriction	Heart and Great Vessels Lower Arteries	**D** Intraluminal Device
Intraluminal Device, Branched or Fenestrated, Three or More Arteries	Restriction	Heart and Great Vessels Lower Arteries	**D** Intraluminal Device
Intraluminal Device, Drug-eluting	All applicable	Heart and Great Vessels Lower Arteries Upper Arteries	**D** Intraluminal Device
Intraluminal Device, Drug-eluting, Four or More	All applicable	Heart and Great Vessels Lower Arteries Upper Arteries	**D** Intraluminal Device
Intraluminal Device, Drug-eluting, Three	All applicable	Heart and Great Vessels Lower Arteries Upper Arteries	**D** Intraluminal Device
Intraluminal Device, Drug-eluting, Two	All applicable	Heart and Great Vessels Lower Arteries Upper Arteries	**D** Intraluminal Device
Intraluminal Device, Endobronchial Valve	All applicable	Respiratory System	**D** Intraluminal Device
Intraluminal Device, Endotracheal Airway	All applicable	Respiratory System	**D** Intraluminal Device
Intraluminal Device, Four or More	All applicable	Heart and Great Vessels Lower Arteries Upper Arteries	**D** Intraluminal Device
Intraluminal Device, Pessary	All applicable	Female Reproductive System	**D** Intraluminal Device
Intraluminal Device, Radioactive	All applicable	Heart and Great Vessels	**D** Intraluminal Device
Intraluminal Device, Three	All applicable	Heart and Great Vessels Lower Arteries Upper Arteries	**D** Intraluminal Device
Intraluminal Device, Two	All applicable	Heart and Great Vessels Lower Arteries Upper Arteries	**D** Intraluminal Device
Monitoring Device, Hemodynamic	Insertion	Subcutaneous Tissue and Fascia	**2** Monitoring Device
Monitoring Device, Pressure Sensor	Insertion	Heart and Great Vessels	**2** Monitoring Device
Pacemaker, Dual Chamber	Insertion	Subcutaneous Tissue and Fascia	**P** Cardiac Rhythm Related Device
Pacemaker, Single Chamber	Insertion	Subcutaneous Tissue and Fascia	**P** Cardiac Rhythm Related Device
Pacemaker, Single Chamber Rate Responsive	Insertion	Subcutaneous Tissue and Fascia	**P** Cardiac Rhythm Related Device
Spinal Stabilization Device, Facet Replacement	Insertion	Lower Joints Upper Joints	**4** Internal Fixation Device
Spinal Stabilization Device, Interspinous Process	Insertion	Lower Joints Upper Joints	**4** Internal Fixation Device
Spinal Stabilization Device, Pedicle-Based	Insertion	Lower Joints Upper Joints	**4** Internal Fixation Device

pecific Device	for Operation	in Body System	General Device
timulator Generator, Multiple Array	Insertion	Subcutaneous Tissue and Fascia	**M** Stimulator Generator
timulator Generator, Iultiple Array Rechargeable	Insertion	Subcutaneous Tissue and Fascia	**M** Stimulator Generator
timulator Generator, ingle Array	Insertion	Subcutaneous Tissue and Fascia	**M** Stimulator Generator
timulator Generator, Single Array echargeable	Insertion	Subcutaneous Tissue and Fascia	**M** Stimulator Generator
ynthetic Substitute, Ceramic	Replacement	Lower Joints	**J** Synthetic Substitute
ynthetic Substitute, Ceramic n Polyethylene	Replacement	Lower Joints	**J** Synthetic Substitute
ynthetic Substitute, ntraocular Telescope	Replacement	Eye	**J** Synthetic Substitute
ynthetic Substitute, Metal	Replacement	Lower Joints	**J** Synthetic Substitute
ynthetic Substitute, Ietal on Polyethylene	Replacement	Lower Joints	**J** Synthetic Substitute
ynthetic Substitute, Oxidized Zirconium on olyethylene	Replacement	Lower Joints	**J** Synthetic Substitute
ynthetic Substitute, Polyethylene	Replacement	Lower Joints	**J** Synthetic Substitute
ynthetic Substitute, Reverse Ball nd Socket	Replacement	Upper Joints	**J** Synthetic Substitute

Appendix F: Substance Qualifier Table (Key)

Section 3 – Administration Character 6 – Substance	
4-Factor Prothrombin Complex Concentrate	**Includes:** Kcentra
Adhesion Barrier	**Includes:** Seprafilm
Anti-Infective Envelope	**Includes:** AIGISRx Antibacterial Envelope Antimicrobial envelope
Clofarabine	**Includes:** Clolar
Glucarpidase	**Includes:** Voraxaze
Human B-type Natriuretic Peptide	**Includes:** Nesiritide
Other Thrombolytic	**Includes:** Tissue Plasinogen Activator (tPA)(r-tPA)
Oxazolidinones	**Includes:** Zyvox
Recombinant Bone Morphogenetic Protein	**Includes:** Bone morphogenetic protein 2 (BMP 2) rhBMP-2

Section X - New Technology - Character 6 - Device/ Substance/Technology	
Andexanet Alfa, Factor Xa Inhibitor Reversal Agent	Factor Xa Inhibitor Reversal Agent, Andexanet Alfa
Bezlotoxumab Monoclonal Antibody	ZINPLAVA™
Concentrated Bone Marrow Aspirate	CBMA (Concentrated Bone Marrow Aspirate)
Cytarabine and Daunorubicin Liposome Antineoplastic	VYXEOS™
Defibrotide Sodium Anticoagulant	Defitelio
Endothelial Damage Inhibitor	DuraGraft® Endothelial Damage Inhibitor
Engineered Autologous Chimeric Antigent Receptor T-cell Immunotherapy	Axicabtagene Ciloeucel KYMRIAH Tisagenlecleucel
Interbody Fusion Device, Nanotextured Surface in New Technology	nanoLOCK™ interbody fusion device
Interbody Fusion Device, Radiolucent Porous in New Technology	COALESCE® radiolucent interbody fusion device COHERE® radiolucent interbody fusion device
Magnetically Controlled Growth Rod(s) in New Technology	MAGEC® Spinal Bracing and Distraction System Spinal growth rods, magnetically controlled
Other New Technology Therapeutic Substance	STELARA® Ustekinumab
Skin Substitute, Porcine Liver Derived in New Technology	MIRODERM™ Biologic Wound Matrix
Synthetic Human Angiotensin II	Angiotensin II GIAPREZA™ Human angiotensin II, synthetic
Uridine Triacetate	Vistogard®
Zooplastic Tissue, Rapid Deployment Technique in New Technology	**Includes:** EDWARDS INTUITY Elite valve system INTUITY elite valve system, EDWARDS Perceval sutureless valve Sutureless valve, Perceval

Appendix G: New ICD-10-PCS Codes FY2019

pendix G is provided online in a format suitable for spreadsheet and/or database use. Go to http://ahimapress.org/casto6709, click the "Online Resources" link, and er case sensitive password AHIMA7Cf3m2018 to download files.

Appendix H: Deleted ICD-10-PCS Codes FY2019

Appendix H is provided online in a format suitable for spreadsheet and/or database use. Go to http://ahimapress.org/casto6709, click the "Online Resources" link, and enter case sensitive password AHIMA7Cf3m2018 to download files.